Practical Pain Management

THIRD EDITION

Practical Pain Management

THIRD EDITION

C. David Tollison, Ph.D.

Carolinas Center for Advanced Management of Pain
Greenville, South Carolina

John R. Satterthwaite, M.D.

Carolinas Center for Advanced Management of Pain
Greenville, South Carolina

Joseph W. Tollison, M.D.

Professor Emeritus
Medical College of Georgia
Augusta, Georgia

◆ LIPPINCOTT WILLIAMS & WILKINS
A **Wolters Kluwer** Company

Philadelphia · Baltimore · New York · London
Buenos Aires · Hong Kong · Sydney · Tokyo

Acquisitions Editor: R. Craig Percy
Developmental Editor: Selina M. Bush
Supervising Editor: Mary Ann McLaughlin
Production Editor: Diane Ratto/Michael Bass & Associates
Manufacturing Manager: Ben Rivera
Cover Designer: David Levy
Compositor: Michael Bass & Associates
Printer: Maple Press

© 2002 by LIPPINCOTT WILLIAMS & WILKINS
530 Walnut Street
Philadelphia, PA 19106 USA
LWW.com

Printed in the USA

Library of Congress Cataloging-in-Publication Data
  Practical Pain Management / [edited by] C. David Tollison, John R. Satterthwaite, Joseph W. Tollison.—3rd ed.
     p. ; cm.
  Rev. ed. of: Handbook of pain management. c1994. 2nd ed.
  Includes bibliographical references and index.
  ISBN 0-7817-3160-7
  1. Intractable pain—Handbooks, manuals, etc. 2. Pain—Handbooks, manuals, etc. 3. Analgesia—Handbooks, manuals, etc. I. Tollison, C. David 1949– II. Satterthwaite, John R. III. Tollison, Joseph W. IV. Handbook of pain management.
  [DNLM: 1. Pain—therapy. WL 704 C641 2001]
RB127.H353 2001
616'.0472—dc21   2001050203
                                                              CIP

Care has been taken to confirm the accuracy of the information presented and to describe generally accepted practices. However, the authors, editors, and publisher are not responsible for errors or omissions or for any consequences from application of the information in this book and make no warranty, expressed or implied, with respect to the currency, completeness, or accuracy of the contents of the publication. Application of this information in a particular situation remains the professional responsibility of the practitioner.

The authors, editors, and publisher have exerted every effort to ensure that drug selection and dosage set forth in this text are in accordance with current recommendations and practice at the time of publication. However, in view of ongoing research, changes in government regulations, and the constant flow of information relating to drug therapy and drug reactions, the reader is urged to check the package insert for each drug for any change in indications and dosage and for added warnings and precautions. This is particularly important when the recommended agent is a new or infrequently employed drug.

Some drugs and medical devices presented in this publication have Food and Drug Administration (FDA) clearance for limited use in restricted research settings. It is the responsibility of health care providers to ascertain the FDA status of each drug or device planned for use in their clinical practice.

10 9 8 7 6 5 4 3 2 1

To my wife, Linda Surett Tollison, and children, Courtney Louise Tollison and C. David Tollison, Jr.

To my wife, Sharon Roe Satterthwaite, and children, Michael Joseph, Jennifer Satterthwaite Revels and Joel Walter Satterthwaite.

In memory of my wife, Betty Browning Tollison, and in honor of our children, J. Wade, Stephanie Tollison and Julie Elisabeth Tollison.

Contents

Section IV   Pharmacologic Intervention

Section V   The Treatment of Selected Pain Disorders

Section VIII   Selected Topics

Contributing Authors

Tim A. Ahles, PhD *Professor, Department of Psychiatry, Dartmouth Medical School, Lebanon, NH (Chapter 42)*

Gerald M. Aronoff, MD *Assistant Clinical Professor, Department of Psychiatry, Tufts Medical School, Boston, MA; Medical Director, Carolina Pain Associates, Presbyterian Orthopedic Hospital, Charlotte, NC (Chapter 19)*

John Aryanpur, MD *Northcoast Neurosurgical Association, Arcata, CA (Chapter 26)*

David B. Boyd, MD *Adjunct Professor, Department of Medicine, University of Western Ontario, London, Ontario, Canada; General Internist, Department of Medicine, London Health Sciences Centre, Victoria Campus, London, Ontario, Canada (Chapter 4)*

Kim J. Burchiel, MD *Professor and Chairman, Neurological Surgery, Oregon Health Sciences University, Portland, OR (Chapter 25)*

Jeffrey A. Burgess, MD, DDS *Department of Neurological Surgery, Oregon Health Sciences University, Portland, OR (Chapter 25)*

Roger W. Catlin, MD *Medical Director, Chattanooga Center for Pain Medicine, Chattanooga, TN (Chapter 8)*

Stanley L. Chapman, PhD *Associate Professor, Department of Anesthesiology, Emory University School of Medicine, Center for Pain Medicine, Atlanta, GA (Chapter 52)*

Paola M. Conte, PhD *Pediatric Psychologist, The David Center for Children's Pain and Palliative Care, Hackensack University Medical Center, Hackensack, NJ (Chapter 50)*

Sarah E. DeRossett, MD, PhD *Assistant Professor and Program Director, Department of Neurology, Emory University School of Medicine, Atlanta, GA (Chapter 30)*

Satvinder S. Dhesi, MD *Assistant Professor, Department of Anesthesia and Critical Care, The University of Chicago, Chicago, IL (Chapter 2)*

Daniel M. Doleys, PhD *Director, Pain and Rehabilitation Institute, Birmingham, AL (Chapter 3)*

Thomas B. Ducker, MD *Clinical Professor of Neurosurgery, The Johns Hopkins Hospital, Baltimore, MD (Chapter 26)*

Will T. Dunn, Jr., JD *Attorney at Law, Greenville, SC (Chapter 43)*

Tony Y. Eng, MD *Assistant Professor, Department of Radiation Oncology, University of Texas Health Science Center at San Antonio, San Antonio, TX; Staff, Department of Radiation Oncology, Cancer Therapy and Research Center, San Antonio, TX (Chapter 41)*

Perry G. Fine, MD *Professor, Department of Anesthesiology, University of Utah, Salt Lake City, UT; Associate Medical Director, Pain Management Center, University of Utah, Salt Lake City, UT (Chapter 23)*

Gerald M. Finkel *Attorney at Law, Columbia, SC (Chapter 45)*

xi

David A. Fishbain, MD, FAPA *Professor of Psychiatry and Adjunct Professor, Department of Neurological Surgery and Anesthesiology, University of Miami School of Medicine, Miami Beach, FL; University of Miami Comprehensive Pain Center, Miami Beach, FL (Chapters 22 and 39)*

Richard H. Fitzgerald, Jr., MD *Director, Radiation Oncology Department, Roper Hospital, Charleston, SC (Chapter 41)*

Rollin M. Gallagher, MD, MPH *Professor of Psychiatry, Anesthesiology and Public Health, Director of Pain Medicine, MCP Hahnemann University, Philadelphia, PA; Director, Pain Medicine and Rehabilitation Center, Graduate Hospital—Teuet, Philadelphia, PA (Chapter 19)*

R. Michael Gallagher, DO *Professor, Department of Family Medicine, University of Medicine and Dentistry of New Jersey, School of Osteopathic Medicine, Stratford, NJ; Director, University Headache Center, University of Medicine and Dentistry of New Jersey, School of Osteopathic Medicine, Moorestown, NJ (Chapter 20)*

Martin Grabois, MD *Professor and Chairman, Department of Physical Medicine and Rehabilitation, Baylor College of Medicine, Houston, TX; Chief, Physical Medicine and Rehabilitation, The Methodist Hospital, Houston, TX (Chapter 47)*

Carmen R. Green, MD *Assistant Professor, Department of Anesthesiology, University of Michigan Medical Center, Ann Arbor, MI; Director, Acute Pain Service, University of Michigan Medical Center, Ann Arbor, MI (Chapter 21)*

John C. Haasis, MD *Carolinas Center for Advanced Management of Pain, Spartanburg, SC (Chapter 15)*

James L. Hall, PhD *Professor Emeritus, Department of Anatomy and Neurobiology, University of Cincinatti, Cincinatti, OH (Chapter 1)*

Steven L. Halpern, MD *Assistant Professor, Department of Pediatrics, University of Medicine and Dentistry of New Jersey, Hackensack, NJ; Associate Director, The David Center for Children's Pain and Palliative Care, Hackensack University Medical Center, Hackensack, NJ (Chapter 50)*

Leslie J. Heinberg, PhD *Assistant Professor, Department of Psychiatry & Behavioral Sciences, The Johns Hopkins University School of Medicine, Baltimore, MD (Chapter 17)*

Donald W. Hinnant, PhD *Behavioral Associates (private practice), Charleston, SC (Chapters 7 and 48)*

Allen H. Hord, MD *Associate Professor, Department of Anesthesiology, Emory University School of Medicine, Atlanta, GA (Chapter 33)*

Fred M. Howard, MD, MS *Professor, Obstetrics and Gynecology, University of Rochester School of Medicine and Dentistry, Rochester, NY; Division Director, Gynecologic Specialties, Strong Memorial Hospital, Rochester, NY (Chapter 31)*

Frank P. K. Hsu, MD, PhD *Resident, Department of Neurological Surgery, Oregon Health Sciences University, Portland, OR (Chapter 25)*

Robert W. Hurley, PhD *Postdoctoral Fellow, Committee on Neurobiology, Department of Anesthesia and Critical Care, University of Chicago, Chicago, IL (Chapter 2)*

Zvi H. Israel, MBBS *Department of Neurological Surgery, Oregon Health Sciences University, Portland, OR (Chapter 25)*

Kenneth C. Jackson, II, Pharm D *Assistant Professor of Pharmacy Practice, Department of Pharmacy Practice, Texas Tech University Health Sciences Center, School of Pharmacy, Lubbock, TX; Clinical Pharmacy Specialist, International Pain Institute, Texas Tech Medical Center, Lubbock, TX (Chapter 16)*

Erin M. Joyner *Attorney at Law, Columbia, SC (Chapter 45)*

Kenneth Kemp, MD *Assistant Professor, Department of Physical Medicine and Rehabilitation, Baylor College of Medicine, Houston, TX (Chapter 47)*

Robert L. Knobler, MD, PhD   *Professor, Department of Neurology, Thomas Jefferson University, Philadelphia, PA; Director, The K.I.N.D. Clinic, Knobler Institute of Neurological Disease, PC, Fort Washington, PA (Chapter 38)*

Angela J. Koestler, PhD   *Director, Behavioral Health Services, Mississippi Methodist Rehabilitation Center, Jackson, MS (Chapter 3)*

Phillip LaTourette, MD   *Carolinas Center for Advanced Management of Pain, Spartanburg, SC (Chapter 5)*

Victor C. Lee, MD   *Medical Director, Pain Management, Augusta Medical Center, Fisherville, VA (Chapter 51)*

Arthur G. Lipman, Pharm D   *Professor, College of Pharmacy, University of Utah, Salt Lake City, UT; Director of Clinical Pharmacology, Pain Management Center, University Health Science Center, Salt Lake City, UT (Chapter 16)*

Brenda C. McClain, MD, DABPM   *Associate Professor, Department of Anesthesiology, Yale University, New Haven, CT; Director of Pediatric Pain Management, Department of Anesthesiology, Yale-New Haven Children's Hospital, New Haven, CT (Chapter 21)*

John A. McCulloch, MD, FRCSC   *Medical Director, Institute for Spinal Microsurgery, Presbyterian/St. Luke's Medical Center, Denver Orthopedic Clinic, Denver, CO (Chapter 27)*

Ralph C. McCullough, II   *Attorney at Law, Columbia, SC (Chapter 45)*

Y. Eugene Mironer, MD   *Medical Director, Carolinas Center for Advanced Management of Pain, Spartanburg, SC (Chapters 11 and 12)*

Richard K. Osenbach, MD   *Assistant Professor, Department of Neurological Surgery, Medical University of South Carolina, Charleston, SC (Chapter 13)*

Marco Pappagallo, MD   *Associate Professor of Clinical Neurology; Department of Neurology, NYU, New York, NY; Director, Comprehensive Pain Treatment Center, Department of Neurosciences, Hospital for Joint Diseases–Orthopedic Institute, New York, NY (Chapter 29)*

Tom Parrott, MD   *Assistant Professor, Community and Family Medicine, Dartmouth Medical School, Hanover, NH; Active Clinical Staff, Family and Community Medicine, Dartmouth Hitchcock Medical Center, Lebanon, NH (Chapter 49)*

Jashvant G. Patel, MD, MBBS, MS   *Fellow in Pain Medicine, MCP Hahnemann School of Medicine, Philadelphia, PA (Chapter 19)*

Richard B. Patt, MD   *President and Chief Medical Officer, The Patt Center for Cancer Pain and Wellness, Houston, TX; Inpatient Medical Director, The Hospice at the Texas Medical Center, Houston, TX (Chapter 40)*

Jacqueline H. Peat, DIP COT   *Clinical Specialist Occupational Therapist, Human Focus Return to Work, Lancastrian Office Centre, Manchester, UK (Chapter 10)*

Marzban Rad, BA   *Psychiatry and Behavorial Sciences, The Johns Hopkins University School of Medicine, Baltimore, MD (Chapter 17)*

P. Prithvi Raj, MD   *Professor, Department of Anesthesiology/Pain Medicine, Texas Tech University, Lubbock, TX; Co-director of Pain Services, Anesthesiology/Pain Medicine, Texas Tech University Health Sciences Center, Lubbock, TX (Chapter 35)*

Albert L. Ray, MD   *Medical Director, Miami Pain and Integrative Medicine Center, Miami, FL (Chapter 14)*

Marcel Reischer, MD   *Assistant Professor, Division of Rehabilitation Medicine, University of Maryland School of Medicine, Baltimore, MD; Chief, Division of Rehabilitation Medicine, Franklin Square Hospital, Baltimore, MD (Chapter 6)*

Hubert L. Rosomoff, MD, DMedSc *Professor and Chairman Emeritus, Neurological Surgery, Anesthesiology, Orthopedics and Rehabilitation, University of Miami School of Medicine, Miami, FL; Medical Director, Comprehensive Pain and Rehabilitation Center, South Shore Hospital, Miami, FL (Chapter 53)*

Renee Steele Rosomoff, BSN, MBA, CRC, CDMS, CRRN *Adjunct Associate Professor, Neurological Surgery, Anesthesiology, University of Miami, Miami, FL; Program Director, Comprehensive Pain and Rehabilitation Center, South Shore Hospital, Miami Beach, FL (Chapter 53)*

Richard A. Schmidt, MD *Private Practice, Blessing Hospital, Quincy, IL (Chapter 32)*

Janette L. Seville, PhD *Assistant Professor, Department of Psychiatry, Dartmouth Medical School, Lebanon, NH (Chapter 42)*

Lynn Shook, Esquire, PC *Attorney, Greenville, SC (Chapter 44)*

Maureen J. Simmonds, PT, PhD *Associate Professor, School of Physical Therapy, Texas Woman's University, Houston, TX (Chapter 10)*

Robert W. Simms, MD *Associate Professor of Medicine, Clinical Director, Rheumatology Section, Boston University School of Medicine, Boston, MA (Chapter 37)*

Derek Snook, MD *Resident Orthopedics, Department of Orthopedic Surgery, Akron General Medical Center, Akron, OH (Chapter 27)*

Glen D. Solomon, MD *Associate Professor, Department of Medicine, The Ohio State University, Columbus, OH; Consultant, Departments of Neurology and General Internal Medicine, Cleveland Clinic Foundation, Cleveland, OH (Chapter 18)*

Judson Jeffrey Somerville, MD *Director, The Pain Management Clinic of Loredo, Loredo, TX (Chapter 28)*

Henry A. Spindler, MD *Assistant Professor, Division of Rehabilitation Medicine, University of Maryland School of Medicine, Baltimore, MD; Division of Rehabilitation Medicine, Franklin Square Hospital, Baltimore, MD (Chapter 6)*

Charles R. Thomas, Jr., MD *Associate Professor & Vice-Chairman, Department of Radiation Oncology, Adjunct Associate Professor, Division of Medical Oncology, Department of Medicine, University of Texas Health Sciences Center at San Antonio, San Antonio, TX; Member, San Antonio Cancer Institute, Cancer Therapy and Cancer Center, San Antonio, TX (Chapter 41)*

C. David Tollison, PhD *Carolinas Center for Advanced Management of Pain, Greenville and Spartanburg, SC (Chapter 48)*

Roger B. Traycoff *Division of Rheumatology, Southern Illinois University School of Medicine, Springfield, IL (Chapter 36)*

John J. Triano, DC, PhD *Adjunct Faculty, Joint Biomedical Engineering Program, University of Texas Southwestern Medical Center and University of Texas at Arlington, Dallas, TX; Co-Director, Conservative Medicine, Director, Chiropractic Division, Chiropractic Division, Texas Back Institute, Plano, TX (Chapter 9)*

David M. Vaughn *Managing Partner, Vaughn, Dupree & Miller, Baton Rouge, LA (Chapter 46)*

Gary A. Walco, PhD *Associate Professor, Department of Pediatrics, University of Medicine and Dentistry of New Jersey, New Jersey Medical School, Newark, NJ; Director, The David Center for Children's Pain and Palliative Care, Hackensack University Medical Center, Hackensack, NJ (Chapter 50)*

Katherine A. Waldman, OTR, MBA *Pain Consortium of Greater Kansas City, Leawood, KS (Chapter 54)*

Steven D. Waldman, MD, JD *Clinical Professor, Department of Anesthesiology, University of Missouri-Kansas City, Kansas City, MO; Director, Pain Consortium of Greater Kansas City, Leawood, KS (Chapter 54)*

Linda H. Wang, MD, PhD   *Assistant Professor, Department of Anesthesiology, Emory University Hospital, Atlanta, GA (Chapter 33)*

Bradley K. Weiner, MD   *Assistant Professor, Department of Orthopedics, Northeastern Ohio Universities, College of Medicine, Rootstown, OH; Attending Orthopedic Spine Surgeon, Department of Orthopaedics, Summa Health Systems, St. Thomas Hospital, Akron, OH (Chapter 27)*

Steve D. Wheeler, MD   *Director and Co-Founder, Ryan Wheeler Headache Treatment Center, Miami, FL (Chapter 24)*

Peter G. Wilson, MD   *Associate Professor, Department of Psychiatry, Cornell University Medical College, New York, NY; Associate Attending, Department of Psychiatry, New York Presbyterian Hospital, New York, NY (Chapter 34)*

Lisa M. Yacono Freeman, PhD   *Post-Doctoral Fellow, Department of Psychiatry and Behavioral Sciences, The Johns Hopkins University School of Medicine, Baltimore, MD (Chapter 17)*

Albert Zbik, PsyD   *Clinical Psychologist, Neuro Psychologist, Miami Pain and Integrative Medicine Center, Miami, FL (Chapter 14)*

Dirk Zerman, MD   *Private Practice, Blessing Hospital, Quincy, IL (Chapter 32)*

Preface

It has been said that the only thing constant in life is change. Certainly this well summarizes the continually evolving discipline of pain medicine.

The first edition of this book was published in 1989. At the time, the book was credited with representing state-of-the-art knowledge of clinical pain practice. However, the discipline of clinical pain practice rapidly changed. Consequently, the second edition of the text was published in 1994. In only five relatively short years between the first and second editions, the discipline of pain practice had changed so markedly that the second edition's table of contents outlines 15 chapter changes from the original text. And the continued growth and evolution of our discipline shows no signs of slowing. This third edition is marked by an additional 20 new chapters and major revision of 29 chapters.

Today, the discipline of pain medicine involves more health practitioners of various disciplines than at any time before. The diagnosis and treatment of pain is growing as a clinical discipline and becoming more sophisticated as a science. Truly we have come a long way from our early helpless days of informing patients that pain was something they would need to "learn to live with." Research into the causes and mechanisms of pain has flourished, technical expertise into altering the neural transmission of pain has progressed, and our collective thinking regarding the role and utilization of narcotic and other pharmacologic interventions has changed. Yet, we have not lost sight of the basic fact that pain, ultimately, is a perception and is influenced by numerous psychologic, sociologic, and related factors. The third edition of this book marks these major changes with new chapters on neurostimulation techniques, neuroaxial pharmacology, issues and controversies in opioid analgesia, advancements in psychological diagnosis and psychopharmacology, and other contemporary issues. In addition, the third edition explores the new challenges to pain practice with chapters on reimbursement facilitation and surviving and thriving within our era of managed care.

Much has changed in the practice of pain diagnosis and treatment and much has changed in the third edition of this text. However, what has not changed in the challenge that faces every pain practitioner is staying abreast of new clinical developments that improve the lives of our patients. The objectives in developing the third edition were to assess the current state of clinical pain practice, predict and provide applied information on future trends, collect the considerable expertise of a multidisciplinary and heralded faculty of authors, and to orchestrate that expertise into a comprehensive clinical resource for the diagnosis and treatment of pain. We expect that the reader will find the third edition of this book to have a particularly strong, applied clinical practice orientation.

One of the joys of editing a major clinical text with multiple editions is the opportunity to interact with clinicians from across the world and, in so doing, to solicit recommendations for future text editions. We are grateful to the countless number of colleagues who have offered valuable criticism of the first two editions of this book, and who have made recommendations on this third edition. The many changes and advancements that are obvious in this third edition reflect, in large part, their collective recommendations.

The editors wish to express our gratitude to Craig Percy, Executive Editor, and to Selina Bush, Associate Development Editor, Lippincott Williams & Wilkins. Craig Percy quarterbacked the idea of a third edition and championed the effort through to completion. Selina Bush demonstrated uncommon organizational skills and considerable patience. Both have been a true pleasure to work with and we are in their debt.

Particular appreciation is extended to the chapter authors. The editors of this text also occasionally serve as chapter authors, not only for our own books but for texts edited by other professionals. When the telephone rings with an invitation to author a book chapter, the feeling generated usually involves a strange combination of honor and dread. Writing a chapter for a major text while maintaining a busy clinical practice and countless additional responsibilities is not an easy chore. The authors whose work is presented in this third edition have honored each of us by sharing their considerable knowledge and expertise. As editors of the third edition and on behalf of all health professionals who shall benefit from this book, we extend to each author our sincere appreciation.

C. David Tollison, Ph.D.
John R. Satterthwaite, M.D.
Joseph W. Tollison, M.D.

SECTION I

Foundations

CHAPTER 1

Anatomy of Pain

James L. Hall

The desired objective of this chapter is to acquaint the reader with the principal central and peripheral anatomic structures involved in the perception of painful stimuli. The mechanism of pain is perhaps one of the more complex topics in medicine. In many areas, complete anatomic and physiologic explanations are not yet known or are inadequate.

This, then, is an attempt by an anatomist to set forth the anatomic substrates that will be more exhaustively dealt with in subsequent sections of this book. It is instructive to note that the word *pain* is derived from a Greek word meaning "penalty." We can easily imagine a penalty in the form of pain being visited upon some poor mortal for his effronteries to the gods of Mt. Olympus.

PERIPHERAL STRUCTURES

Receptors

We are now aware that most receptors on the peripheral endings of afferent nerves respond to a variety of stimuli. However, their shape, location, and field of reception indicate that they are able to perceive one type of stimulus more efficiently than many other types. The specific receptor type that is incriminated in the reception of the pain stimulus is said to be an unencapsulated nerve ending. Although this receptor, in many examples, has a thin myelin covering, it is usually referred to as an unmyelinated or "naked" nerve ending.

The pain receptor is a primitive, unorganized nerve ending and often has a weedlike appearance. It has many branches and often overlaps the territory of other nerve endings from cord segments above and below it. Here, it is important to realize that the strength of the stimulus is a critical factor in the production of pain in this and other types of receptors. When a certain threshold of intensity of the stimulus is surpassed, any stimulus can be inter-

preted as painful to most receptors. This specific threshold, referred to as a noxious stimulus, is one that will elicit tissue damage. At that point, the receptor is referred to as nociceptive. Pressure, for example, if increased, can become painful, and an encapsulated pacinian corpuscle, which is admirably modified by its onionlike capsule to have a large receptive field for pressure, can at a specific threshold level become a nociceptive receptor and generate an impulse of pain along its afferent nerve.

Afferent Pain Fibers

All nerve fibers are classified as to their age and conduction rate. They are called A, B, and C fibers, with A fibers being the largest in diameter and the most rapidly conducting fibers. B fibers are intermediate-sized fibers and have a somewhat slower conducting rate. C fibers are the smallest in caliber and the slowest conducting. There are apparently two types of pain-conducting fiber: an A-delta fiber, which is the most rapid of the pain-conducting fibers but the slowest of the alpha-conducting fibers, and C fibers, which are the slowest conducting fibers.

The pain conducted by the A-delta fibers is a quick, "bright" pain. It is often described as sharp, shooting, or even intense. C fiber pain, on the other hand, is described as steady, slow, and constant.

Somatic Pain Classification

Since the days of Henry Head in 1920, two other types of classifications of somatic pain have been used. Head proposed using the terms *epicritic* and *protopathic* to describe somatic pain. Head suggested that epicritic pain could be discriminated and localized; thus, such pain must usually come from the skin or more superficial areas. Protopathic pain, conversely, can only be discriminated in a generalized way and cannot always be localized.

Spinal or Dorsal Root Ganglia

Dorsal root ganglia are found on the dorsal or posterior root of all spinal nerves. These are the sensory roots conducting the central process of the spinal ganglion cell into the central nervous system. The spinal or segmental nerve conducts epicritic pain from a specific area of the skin called the *dermatome*.

There may be some individual variation in size and contours of the dermatome, but dermatomic areas are always segmental and have distinct boundaries. A given spinal ganglion supplies a specific dermatome in a one-to-one relationship, but there may be overlap between the sensory roots. A ganglion may carry some information from the dermatome above and below it; this is usually true in the conduction of pain. Thus, when a specific ganglion is destroyed, there may be only a slight loss of pain from the dermatome it supplies.

Protopathic or deep somatic and visceral pain are less rigidly related to the nerve roots. This is at least in part due to the migration of structures during embryonic development (e.g., the diaphragm, supplied by C-3–C-5 via the phrenic nerve). The segmental division of deep pain is called a *sclerotome*. Because the pain fibers from a sclerotome enter the cord through several posterior roots, a more generalized or nonlocalizing pattern results.

Visceral pain is conducted by the peripheral process of the dorsal root ganglia traveling with the autonomic fibers that supply the target tissue. If they are bound in the same sheath as the sympathetic fibers, they may travel some distance from their origin in the spinal ganglia via the white ramus of the sympathetic chain and the very long preganglionic fibers before they reach the specific viscera they supply.

An example of this arrangement is the afferent fibers from spinal ganglia T-5–T-10 that travel with the greater splanchnic nerve to reach the celiac ganglia in the abdomen. The afferent fibers pass through the celiac ganglia without synapsing and supply the derivatives of embryonic foregut. It is useful to conceptualize the sympathetic innervation of viscera to be somewhat like a cascade or waterfall, with the viscera in the cavities being supplied by sympathetic fibers that originate at higher levels. The afferent fibers to these same viscera accompany the sympathetic fibers. Thoracic fibers cascade down into abdominal viscera, and fibers from lumbar sympathetic ganglia, called lumbar splanchnics, cascade down into pelvic viscera via the hypogastric fibers.

Although this concept also holds for afferents conducted in the parasympathetic vagus nerve, which is also supplying afferent innervation to some structures in the thorax and abdomen from its cranial origin via its two sensory ganglia, it is not entirely true for parasympathetic supply to the embryonic hindgut and pelvic splanchnic nerves. These arise from sacral segments S-2–S-4 and travel superiorly to supply the embryonic hindgut through the inferior mesenteric plexus. Nevertheless, the axiom that the efferent sympathetic response is regional or widespread and the parasympathetic response is usually local or confined has some validity when applied to afferent impulses as well. Cranial sympathetics, of course, arise at lower levels in the cord and ascend via the anterior and posterior cerebral circulation to higher levels. Thoracic sympathetics, usually above T-5 or T-6, supply thoracic viscera at those levels even though to do so they may ascend in the chain some distance, as in the case of the cardioaccelerator nerves.

The relationship between pain-conducting afferent fibers and sympathetic efferent fibers is thought to be involved in the condition known as *causalgia*. The patient complains of a persistent and burning pain, usually following the course of the nerve fibers in the region. It is thought that the integrity of the afferent pain fibers has been compromised so that the neurotransmitter of the afferent fibers (in this case, acetylcholine) is noxious to the sympathetic fiber, thus producing the burning sensation. The condition is usually relieved by a sympathectomy.

Receptors of pain are sparse in the viscera, and this generally contributes to a poorly localized sensation from most of the viscera. There are two notable exceptions to this rule: Distention of the gut and pain from the heart can readily be localized by the physician. However, the sensory innervation of the heart is now known to be much more elegant than was previously thought.

Referred Pain

Referred pain is a troublesome topic in the interpretation and diagnosis of pain. In essence, it means that the originating pain from one region of the body is referred to another region of the body that is not receiving the noxious stimulus directly. A classic example is that of pain from the gallbladder being referred to the tip of the right shoulder, because the C-3–C-5 nerve roots are distributed to both the diaphragm and the shoulder area. Anatomically, the usual reason given for referred pain is that the pain-conducting fibers are distributed to different localities by portions of the same spinal nerves. These pain fibers then converge on the same neurons in the dorsal gray horn of the spinal cord. There, based on the patient's past experience and the breakdown of the integrity of the neuronal pool, a message is sent to the cortex that the pain is coming from point "A," which the cortex is preferentially structured to handle with ease, when the pain is really coming from point "B," which it is not so well equipped to handle. The referred pain is finally localized correctly when somatic pain receptors are involved. Pain from the appendix, for example, may initially be perceived as originating from the umbilicus because the T-10 nerve supplies both structures. Eventually, when the pain involves the peritoneum or the anterior abdominal wall, which are more densely supplied with afferent receptors, the pain will be correctly perceived as coming from the appendix.

SPINAL CORD

Pain fibers enter the spinal cord in the medial portion of the dorsal roots of spinal nerves. They enter in the dorsolateral funiculus, just dorsal to the dorsal gray horn. Here they usually give off collaterals that descend in the dorsolateral funiculus or the tract of Lissauer for one or two cord segments. The main group of fibers, however, ascend in the tract of Lissauer for about two cord segments before entering the dorsal gray horn to synapse. They do so on cells lying in Rexed's laminae II, III, IV, and V on a group of small neurons called the nucleus proprius. The ascent in the cord prior to synapsing is the anatomic reason given as to why patients perceive somatic pain at a higher level than the origin of the spinal nerve that is involved.

The axons of the cells in the nucleus proprius, following the law of neurobiotaxis, leave diagonally opposite the point of the incoming stimulus and travel across the midline of the cord in the ventral gray and white commissurae just below the central canal of the spinal cord.

As these fibers cross just below the central canal they are vulnerable to a condition in which the central canal enlarges or cavitates, known as *syringomyelia*. This would cause a loss of pain and temperature in the patient two cord segments below the cord segment in which the cavitation occurs. Typically this occurs in the cervical cord, and the deficit is a bilateral loss of pain and temperature in the upper extremities; usually other sensory modalities are spared.

The fibers then pass to the ventral lateral portion of the contralateral lateral funiculus, where they form two separate tracks or pathways to the thalamus. These are the classic ventral and lateral spinothalamic pathways. In the current literature, these are also referred to as the paleo- and neospinothalamic tracts. The two tracts are joined, and some think that the fibers are mixed in each tract. The neospinothalamic or lateral tract is the more rapidly conducting tract that produces so-called bright, quick pain and the paleospinothalamic or ventral tract elicits dull, aching pain. The ventral tract is sometimes thought to be clinically unimportant, but is now receiving more attention.

The spinothalamic tracts are the principal pain-conducting pathways in the cord, but not the only ones. A phylogenetically older tract that conducts visceral pain may be found closely applied to the gray matter of the cord in all funiculi. This is the fasciculus proprius, and its axons travel up or down one cord segment, then synapse in the dorsal gray horn to again travel up one more segment. The reticulospinal tract may also conduct pain impulses, again usually from the viscera, and its axons travel up or down the cord a few segments to eventually reach the thalamus and even the cerebral cortex itself. The fasciculus proprius system ends at the medulla, and the impulses conducted by it are conducted rostrally by the reticular formation.

Pain of visceral origin, therefore, can be conducted rostrally in one of three alternative pathways. This is given as the anatomic explanation as to why visceral pain may persist after a surgical procedure to cut the lateral spinothalamic tract, as in a cordotomy.

It should be noted that within the spinal cord the lateral spinothalamic tract is topographically laminated. As the axons from the nucleus proprius in the sacral segments cross the midline and ascend, they take a dorsolateral position in the newly formed tract. Fibers from higher cord segments, as they assume their positions, become more medially placed. The final configuration of the tract would then have sacral segments represented more laterally and cervical segments more ventromedially. A space-occupying extramedulary neoplasm that compresses the ventrolateral spinal cord at any level therefore might compromise the conduction of pain and temperature from the sacral and lumbar regions of the body.

BRAINSTEM PAIN SYSTEMS

An exhaustive treatment of brainstem form systems is not within the intended scope of this chapter. Principal mechanisms and systems are presented with a view to elucidating a very voluminous and complex topic.

Spinothalamic Pathways in the Brainstem

We have seen that there are two spinothalamic tracts, a ventral or paleospinothalamic and a more significant lateral or neospinothalamic tract. Both conduct pain, although of different types, in the spinal cord. These two tracts diverge in the medulla, then come in close proximity in the lateral pons and are eventually associated with the medial lemniscus in either the rostral pons or the caudal mesencephalon. En route to this association, both tracts are greatly diminished in size, with the ventral spinothalamic tract probably very modest in the mesencephalon.

The impulse from both tracts ends in the ventrobasal nuclear complex of the thalamus, with most fibers terminating in the ventral posterior lateral nucleus. Many studies have shown that the paleospinothalamic tract is polysynaptic and gives off many collaterals to reticular nuclei in the medulla, chiefly to the nucleus gigantoreticularis and the lateral reticular nucleus. These in turn project to the centromedian nucleus of the thalamus.

There are also many pain-conducting fibers of the reticular formation of both spinal and brainstem origin projecting to the intralaminar nuclei of the thalamus. The reticular formation of the brainstem is a monitoring or modulating mechanism. All modalities pass through its network and are in some way affected by it. It is thought that, by its projections to the thalamus and the cortex directly, the reticular formation contributes to a better total image of the body and its parts. Certainly, it accentuates or inhibits certain stimuli to produce a focus of attention or awareness of some impulses that are filtered through its all-encompassing network. Some specific reticular mechanisms, such as the nucleus of the median raphe in the pons, play down on other structures, such as the neurons in laminae II, III, IV, and V of the dorsal gray horn of the cord, to inhibit the transmission of pain. Other reticular nuclei around the periaqueductal gray of the midbrain do the same to the neo- and paleospinothalamic tracts as they pass through the midbrain.

A noteworthy relationship between the spinothalamic tracts and the spinal or descending nucleus of the trigeminal complex is found in the caudal medulla. The spinal nucleus of the trigeminal complex is a pain-conducting nucleus from the ipsilateral face. Its presence usually produces a small, but grossly visible, lateral bulge in the medulla called the tuberculum cinereum. Just ventral to the tuberculum cinereum is another smaller bulge or protuberance, called Monakow's area, that indicates the location of the spinothalamic tracts. At this level, in the medulla the spinothalamic tracts are conducting pain from the contralateral body, because all of the fibers originating from the dorsal gray horn have crossed the midline of the cord and are ascending contralaterally. Both of these areas are supplied by small branches of the posterior inferior cerebellar artery. Both structures are vulnerable to a deficit in the blood supply from the same artery. When this occurs (as the well-known lateral medullary syndrome), the patient complains of a loss of pain and temperature sensation from the ipsilateral face and the contralateral body. Other complaints, such as difficulty swallowing or loss of taste on the ipsilateral side of the tongue, may also be present if the lesioned area is more extensive and involves the nucleus ambiguous and the nucleus of the solitary tract. This is a classic neuroanatomic deficit and is also known as Weber's syndrome.

Trigeminal System

Perhaps the most significant neuroanatomic structure involved in pain in the brainstem is the trigeminal system. The trigeminal nuclear complex has components in the midbrain, pons, and medulla, and even extends down into the upper cervical segments of the spinal cord. There are three sensory nuclei and one motor nucleus. The sensory nuclei are a mesencephalic nucleus lying along the cerebral aqueduct that is functionally associated with proprioception; the chief or principal sensory nucleus in the pons, which receives impulses of touch and pressure, but also some impulses of pain; and a long, attenuated spinal or descending nucleus that descends to the upper cervical segments as far as C-4 to blend with the substantia gelatinosa

of the cervical cord. The spinal nucleus is the nucleus usually associated with pain conduction. The motor nucleus also lies in the pons, and through reflex connections with the spinal nucleus can produce activity of the muscles of mastication (e.g., clenching of the jaw or chattering of the teeth) in response to noxious stimuli to the face.

The sensory nuclei receive their input from the pseudounipolar neurons of the trigeminal gasserian ganglion lying in Meckel's cavity in the middle cranial fossa. The peripheral processes of the ganglion are distributed via the ophthalmic maxillary and mandibular divisions of the trigeminal nerve to those regions of the face anterior to the ears. All three divisions conduct pain from their area of distribution. An irritative lesion of one of these divisions may produce a severe episodic pain in the patient, a condition called *trigeminal neuralgia*. The mandibular division is very commonly affected; the patient would complain of severe pain from the region of the lower lip and jaw. The pain is so severe and debilitating that some patients have contemplated suicide to escape its ravages.

The descending fibers of the pseudounipolar cells in the ganglion descend along the lateral aspect of the spinal nucleus through the pons and the medulla. They enter the spinal nucleus as they descend to synapses on the secondary cells of the nucleus. They, too, descend as far caudally as the C-4 segment of the spinal cord.

The spinal nucleus has been described as having a rostral portion called the *nucleus oralis,* a caudal portion called the caudalis or subcaudalis, and an intermediate portion called the interpolaris. The nucleus appears to be laminated or organized in both a rostral-to-caudal and a dorsal-to-ventral fashion. The *nucleus oralis* portion would be comprised mainly of secondary neurons receiving pain impulses from the mandibular division of the nerve, whereas the subcaudalis would be receiving much of its input from the ophthalmic division. Hence, the lamination represents an innervated face. Lesions involving the upper cervical cord may sometimes cause either production of pain or loss of pain in the ophthalmic region of the face along with other manifestations of spinal cord involvement.

The secondary fibers then sweep caudally from their origin from the neurons in the elongated spinal nucleus and cross the midline. As they cross the midline in the pons and medulla, they are called the ventral central trigeminal tract and are anatomically and physiologically separate from the fibers originating from the principal sensory nucleus conducting primarily impulses of touch and pressure, some of which also cross the midline to ascend to the thalamus as the dorsal central trigeminal tract. The remainder of the fibers originating from the principal sensory nucleus do cross the midline and ascend ipsilaterally. Hence, touch and pressure impulses are found bilaterally represented above the location of the principal sensory nucleus, whereas pain-conducting fibers are found contralaterally only. Touch and pressure perception may often be perceived in a patient with a brainstem lesion because of its bilateral representation, while the pain-conducting pathway may be compromised.

As both pathways ascend to the thalamus, they are called the trigeminal thalamic pathways. They will come to be so close to the medial lemniscus in the caudal midbrain that they cannot be anatomically distinguished from it. However, physiologically they maintain their integrity and can be identified. The medial lemniscus is located on the lateral aspect of the midbrain above the level of the inferior colliculus, which is the auditory relay nucleus; above this level, the trigeminal thalamic or lemniscal fibers are vulnerable to compromise. They may be severed or compressed by the sharp and firm edge of the dura mater as it forms the incisura to allow the brainstem to pass through. The extensions of the tentorium cerebelli rostrally to the clinoid processes forming the incisura pass alongside the lateral surface of the midbrain to form a formidable presence if there should be any sudden movement of the midbrain such as might occur in some types of trauma. A meningioma at this point could slowly compress the laterally placed medial lemniscus, with the trigeminal fibers at first producing pain through irritation, and eventually causing a contralateral loss of pain in the face as the compression slowly destroyed integrity of the axons to conduct the impulses. The deficit produced by the destruction of the medial lemniscus would be loss of conscious proprioception: position sense, two-point discrimination, and vibratory sense.

The secondary pain and touch axons of the trigeminal thalamic pathway terminate in the posterior ventral medial nucleus of the thalamus. This conforms to a phylogenetic pattern: The older structures in the central nervous system have a more favored position, that is, they are more medially placed. Most neurologic structures concerned with the head and neck are phylogenetically older and more medially placed than others that have to do mainly with other body parts.

THALAMUS

The two groups of thalamic nuclei that are of interest to us are in the posterior basal complex: the posterior ventral lateral and the posterior ventral medial nuclei. They are mainly concerned with the perception and integration of the pain impulse from the body and from the face, respectively. Other thalamic nuclei may be involved after the impulses reach these primary targets, but which nuclei and to what degree are not clear at the present time. Pain is perceived on a conscious level at the thalamus. However, it is not recognized there as completely as it is in the cortex. Thalamic pain perception is a low-level type of appreciation. The thalamus tends to synchronize all incoming stimuli and place them in a particular order for transmission to the cerebral cortex. Otherwise, much of what we perceive would produce neurologic chaos.

The frailties of the thalamus are well documented. The *thalamic syndrome* can produce amplification of various stimuli so that many normally innocuous stimuli, such as putting a spoon to the lips, can be interpreted as a very painful experience. Patients may go to great lengths to prevent exposure to these stimuli and to protect themselves from the very real pain produced by ordinary events. The thalamic syndrome is thought to be elicited by an altered blood supply to the nuclei involved. The blood supply is primarily from the thalamostriate branch of the posterior cerebral artery. It is presumed to be diminished but not completely absent, thus causing an improper functioning of the nuclei.

Reticular nuclei are found in the external and internal medullary lamina of the thalamus. These nuclei project to the various thalamic nuclei and modulate their activity. The reticular nuclei apparently can either excite or inhibit the thalamic nuclei and the various impulses that are received by them. The reticular formation also modulates the impulses conducted through it by the specific pain-conducting tracts in the brainstem, that is, the spinothalamic and trigeminothalamic tracts. The attention of the thalamus can thereby be focused on a specific stimulus or the stimulus could be significantly downgraded both at the brainstem and the thalamic level.

The reticular nuclei also receive input from the corticothalamic fibers arising from the cortex. These fibers are found in the anterior limb of the internal capsule. The thalamic nuclei also receive input from this feedback loop. The cortex then monitors, through this feedback loop, much of the information that comes to it both at the reticular and the thalamic level. The thalamocortical loop could play a major role in the patient's ability to tolerate pain at various thresholds.

INTERNAL CAPSULE

The pain impulse, along with other general sensory impulses, is projected to the cerebral cortex through the posterior limb of the internal capsule. At this point, the exquisite orderliness of neurologic organization observed at the brainstem level breaks down. There is little or no organization to the arrangement of the general sensory-conducting fibers in the posterior limb of the internal capsule. The fibers are found alongside the lateral border of the thalamus in the posterior limb. The pain-conducting fibers are spread diffusely in this area. Lesions of the posterior limb of the internal capsule can produce either a diffuse loss of pain or general sensations in the case of irritative lesions such as edema or blood from hemorrhage eliciting the production of pain.

In either instance, the deficit may be puzzling to the diagnostician. The irritated fibers may represent conduction from a knee, a shoulder, a hand, or other widely separated parts of the body. The fact that the patient does have these very unusual deficits may be useful in localizing the lesion to the internal capsule.

It should also be recalled that portions of the optic radiations and the auditory radiations pass through the posterior limb as well as the corticobulbar and cortiocospinal portions of the voluntary motor system. The motor deficits, especially supranuclear facial paralysis, need no elaboration here. However, the possible involvement of the optic radiations, producing visual field deficits, or the auditory radiations, producing hearing deficits or hallucinations, might be useful to keep in mind when presented with patients who have seemingly nonlocalizable signs.

CEREBRAL CORTEX

The general sensory impulses, including pain, project through the internal capsule and the corona radiata to the postcentral gyrus and posterior paracentral lobule of the cerebral cortex. Other areas of the cerebral cortex have also been incriminated in the pain pathway. The centromedian nucleus is thought to project some pain conducted by the reticular formation to the frontal lobe. Pain is also projected to the parietal operculum just posterior to the postcentral gyrus. It would appear that many cortical areas, not just the primary sensory strip, can be involved in pain. In this respect, pain is unique as a general sensory sensation.

Visceral pain is projected to the insular cortex, which is hidden deep in the lateral fissure. The insular cortex, or island of Reil, is known to be associated with the autonomic nervous system and may produce autonomic responses such as nausea and vomiting when stimulated.

The model of the homunculus, or "little man," is laid out on the postcentral gyrus in an inverted fashion. The head, at the base of the gyrus, and the body parts are represented disproportionately as one moves superiorly along the gyrus to the superior longitudinal fissure. For example, the lower extremity below the knee is represented on the medial surface in the posterior part of the paracentral gyrus. The main portion of the lateral convexity of the hemisphere is supplied by the middle cerebral artery and its branches; this would include most of the postcentral gyrus. The superior aspect of the gyrus, however, is supplied by the anterior cerebral artery, as is the postcentral gyrus.

The pariental operculum and the insular cortex as well as the lateral aspect of the frontal lobe are also supplied by branches of the middle cerebral artery. The anterior and middle cerebral arteries are portions of the anterior cerebral circulation and are direct terminal branches of the internal carotid artery. It is worthy of note that cortical areas incriminated in the analytic recognition of pain are supplied by two different branches of the internal carotid, whereas some of the thalamic nuclei involved with rela-

tively crude but conscious recognition of pain are supplied by branches of the posterior cerebral artery.

The thalamic relay nuclei, involved in the projection of pain, project to very specific areas of the cortex on a point-to-point basis. If the nuclei are destroyed, there is degeneration of cortical neurons in the specific area to which that nucleus projects its axons.

The pain fibers from the thalamus project to the fourth layer of cortical cells of the postcentral gyrus, the posterior paracentral lobule, and the parietal operculum. Here the impulse is conducted first to the more superficial layers of the cortex for further integration. In a sensory cortex, the layers above the fourth layer or granule layer are perhaps more significant in processing the information that comes to that area of the cortex. Because they are superficial, they are more vulnerable to some types of injuries and difficulties within the cranial cavity than the deeper layers (e.g., layers five and six in a mammalian neocortex).

The impulse for pain and other general sensations is then conducted to the superior parietal lobule on the ipsilateral side for integration. This is interpreted to mean the critical recognition of the stimulus, and the specific body part from which that stimulus has been perceived in the other areas of the cortex may be relevant to its significance to a given individual based on his or her past experiences. Interpretation of the stimulus or impulse above and beyond recognition is a function of the parietal lobe. Various forms of aphasia are examples of this type of activity. The primary cortical receptor area is intact, as are the secondary and perhaps tertiary areas. The stimulus is perceived correctly, but when conducted to the parietal lobe, as in the case of pain, its true meaning or significance may not be interpreted correctly.

Impulses are then conducted from the parietal lobe via association bundles in the white matter to other areas of the cortex and specifically to the frontal lobe for further cortical activity and perhaps decision making. The long association bundles of the cerebral hemisphere are very important in the production of unified activity within the nervous system. The long association bundles involved in transmission, in this case, would be the superior frontooccipital bundle and the superior longitudinal fasciculus. Lesions of these structures would not alter the perception of the pain or its meaning but would have an effect on the patient's response to it or his or her attitude toward the pain.

These same association bundles could also send collaterals to the medial portions of the limbic system and evoke an emotional or autonomic response to somatic pain.

DESCENDING PATHWAYS

The periaqueductal gray of the midbrain appears to have an ameliorative effect on pain. When stimulated, these neurons have an analgesic effect on ascending pain pathways.

CONCLUSIONS

The elementary basis of neurologic structures involved in the conduction, recognition, and integration of pain have been identified. The role of each of the anatomic entities involved in the process is difficult to understand because there is a duality or overlap of activities that makes clarification elusive.

There are two pathways for conduction of somatic and visceral pain in the spinal cord, the paleo- and neo-spinothalamic tracts. A third, the fasciculus proprius, conducts visceral pain. A fourth system, the reticular formation, can conduct either type of pain impulse rostrally or caudally. There are several brainstem structures involved: tracts (both ascending and descending), and cranial nerve nuclei and their secondary nuclear axons. All of these have differing arterial supplies that can, when compromised, involve one structure and spare another, and can either produce pain or cause (or "reduce pain") loss of pain. These entities pass through the reticular formation, which monitors all impulses passing through to all-encompassing networks. This, in turn, can excite or inhibit the production of pain.

Two nuclei are primarily involved at the thalamic level, but other nuclei participate. Their role is uncertain; however, they project to areas other than the postcentral gyrus and the paracentral lobule, the classic cortical centers for recognition of pain. In the cortex itself, there are many areas involved in pain perception and their roles differ from recognition to integration to attitudes and response. Even in the white matter, two or more association bundles may be involved in even the most straightforward pathway.

An anatomic description of the structures involved in the pain pathway presents a picture that is very different from most other sensory pathways. The structures involved have evolved and been modified and enhanced over a very long time and probably are still being modified to deal with a specific type of stimulus that is disturbing to the usual functions of the brain. Yet as we learn more about the structures and their connections, their role may become clearer, and more enlightened diagnoses and treatments should be forthcoming.

There cannot be many more causes in medicine more worthy of the attention and efforts of all physicians and scientists than the reflex of pain. The author hopes he has made a contribution to that cause.

SUGGESTED READING

Adams RD, Victor M. *Principles of neurology.* New York: McGraw-Hill, 1977:1041.

Bond MR. *Pain: its nature and treatment.* New York: Churchill Livingstone, 1979:185.

Gilman S, Newman SW. *Manter and Gatz's essentials of clinical neuroanatomy and neurophysiology,* 7th ed. Philadelphia: FA Davis, 1987:256.

Hall JL. Peripheral pain pathways. In: Lee JF, ed. *Pain management.* Baltimore: Williams & Wilkins, 1977:1–11.

Holden AV, Winlow N, eds. *The neurobiology of pain.* Manchester, England: Manchester University Press, 1983:414.

Kandel ER, Schwartz JH. *Principles of neural sciences.* New York: Elsevier, 1985:979.

Keller JT. The anatomy of central pain pathways. In: Lee JF, ed. *Pain management.* Baltimore: Williams & Wilkins, 1977:12–24.

Pawl RP. *Chronic pain primer.* Chicago: Year Book, 1979:106.

CHAPTER **2**

The Neurobiology of Pain

Satvinder S. Dhesi and Robert W. Hurley

We live in an exciting era of medicine. With the imminent decoding of the human genome (1,2), much promise lies along the molecular avenues through which science is taking us. We have entered a second millenium in which many previously unanswered questions about pain medicine are gradually becoming elucidated via these scientific avenues.

The purpose of this chapter is to provide a comprehensive, yet brief, review of the neurobiological and neuroanatomical mechanisms of pain with a strong emphasis on their application to the clinical care of patients. We intend to provide the pain clinician with the fundamental scientific principles on which the practice of pain medicine is based. More importantly, we intend to relate this information in a meaningful way to guide therapeutic options focusing on pharmacological measures. In the process of explaining practical therapies, we will address relevant pain taxonomy and drug pharmacology where appropriate. Certainly, some redundancy will be evident in sections of the chapter. However, this is necessary in order to both parallel the repetitive nature of our nervous system and provide a reinforcing tool for the clinician to learn as much as possible efficiently.

From an organization standpoint, we will follow an anatomical model in which we will start at the periphery—at the level of stimuli and receptor—and then progress centrally toward the spinal cord. We will explore the synaptic interactions at the spinal cord level in substantial detail with relevance to therapies that affect this dynamic processing system. We will investigate the major brainstem structures involved in pain processing and modulation. In doing so, we will explain how the brain's central medullary descending system plays a role in the inhibition of noxious peripheral stimuli. We will also explain how the physician can pharmacologically manipulate this complex circuitry and augment its endogenous analgesic capacities. Throughout the chapter, we intend to provide therapeutic options at their respective neuroanatomical sites of action. Wher-

ever we do so, we will attempt to provide the commonly accepted rationale behind these respective treatments.

We would like to emphasize that the therapeutic approaches we suggest in this chapter are the result of a combination of elements. These include personal experience and guidelines attained from practice. A strong emphasis is placed on appropriate patient selection and care deemed to be reasonable and logical, factoring in both time and resource costs to the health care "system." Wherever possible, reliance will be on evidence-based medicine and, above all, adherence to the strictest ethical care of the patient and professional standards. Our goal from the outset is to attempt to present approaches that focus on the best possible outcome based on science as we understand it.

ACUTE VERSUS CHRONIC PAIN

While the focus of this textbook is the treatment of chronic painful conditions, we feel it is important to mention that a substantial portion of the available therapies also applies to injuries of an acute nature. Furthermore, acute and chronic pain states are not necessarily dichotomous, but may coexist or represent a continuum of pain states. Acute pain generally refers to that which is of shorter duration or is temporary. Examples include postoperative surgical pain after an appendectomy or bone pain from a nondisplaced fracture of the fibula. In either case, an immediate onset of pain after the initial injury is expected. The causative agent, more often than not, is known or understood. Pain sensation is usually limited to the area of trauma or damage or that area which immediately surrounds it. Perhaps, most importantly, the painful sensations associated with such an injury are expected to resolve on their own over time when adequate wound healing has occurred. In contrast, chronic pain persists beyond either the course of an acute injury or illness, or its expected time for healing and repair. Examples include persistent radicular spinal pain after surgical laminectomy or discectomy, or "phantom" limb pain after amputation of a lower limb for irreversible ischemia. Chronic pain is believed to be associated with a pathologic process that results in aberrant signaling from a previously injured location or site of trauma. Chronic pain may persist or recur for months to years.

PRIMARY AFFERENTS AND PERIPHERAL STIMULATION

A variety of mechanical, thermal, or chemical stimuli can result in the sensation of pain. Information about these painful or noxious stimuli is carried to higher brain centers by receptors and neurons that are distinct from those that carry innocuous somatic sensory information. The mammalian somatosensory system is subserved by four groups of afferent fibers differentiated by their anatomy, rate of transmission, and sensory modality transduced (Table 2-1). Stimulus intensity within each group is frequently encoded as afferent fiber firing rate or frequency; "frequency encoding" (3–5).

The first group, the heavily myelinated large-diameter *Aα fibers*, have specialized terminals incorporated within muscle spindles, Golgi tendon organs, and joints that transduce proprioceptive information. The second group, the heavily myelinated large-diameter *Aβ fibers*, have specialized encapsulated nerve endings, including the Meissner, Pacinian, and Ruffini corpuscles and the Merkel disk, that transduce innocuous or low-threshold mechanical stimulation. Aβ fibers do not ordinarily participate in signaling pain sensations to the central nervous system (CNS). However, the activation of Aβ, and possibly Aα, fibers has been invoked as part of the mechanism for the production of pain relief by *transcutaneous electrical nerve stimulation* (TENS) (6), which may implicate their role in pain signal processing. Furthermore, it is becoming increasingly apparent that in chronic pathologic pain states, these fibers may indeed participate in pain signaling by adopting a "phenotype" similar to that of a C fiber (7). This attribute is important since its consideration is at least indirectly involved in therapeutic management of injuries involving the peripheral skin tissues and the extremities. The final two groups have greater relevance for this chapter and represent the specialized sensory neurons that respond to actual or potential tissue damage, the *nociceptors*.

The third group, the lightly myelinated medium-diameter *Aδ fibers*, has free nerve endings that transduce noxious or high-threshold thermal, mechanical, and chemical stimulation. The final group, the unmyelinated small-diameter *C fibers*, also has free nerve endings that transduce noxious thermal, mechanical, and chemical signals. Again, like their larger myelinated counterparts, stimulus intensity is frequently encoded as afferent fiber firing rate or frequency; "frequency encoding" (3–5). For instance, for a given thermal stimulus, a higher firing frequency can be observed following a 55°C than a 47°C exposure. The nociceptive primary afferents, the Aδ and C fibers, represent the principal target of pharmacological manipulation by the physician treating pain. Although we have focused on the transmission of nociceptive information by the Aδ and C fibers, the reader should be aware of a subset of the Aδ and C fibers that are thermoreceptors that transduce *innocuous* cold and warm information, respectively (8). Unlike receptors in the first two groups, Aδ and C fibers respond to stimulation of their receptive fields in a characteristic manner with slow adaptation and residual firing following the withdrawal of the stimulus. Although these two fiber groups respond similarly to stimulation, they mediate different aspects of pain sensation (9). The rapidly conducting Aδ fibers mediate the "first" pain, or epicritic pain, which is well localized and is characterized as sharp or prickling. The slowly conducting C fibers mediate the "second" pain, or protopathic pain, which temporally

TABLE 2-1. *Primary afferent fibers and their function*

Modality	Receptor	Fiber type	Conduction velocity and diameter	Rate of adaptation	Function
Proprioceptive	Golgi and Ruffini endings, muscle spindle afferents	Aα	70–120 m/s 15–20 microns	Slow and rapid	Muscle tension, length, and velocity
Mechanosensitive	Meissner, Ruffini, Pacinian corpuscles and Merkel disk	Aβ	40–70 m/s 5–15 microns	Rapid (slow–Merkel)	Touch, flutter, motion, pressure, and vibration
Thermoreceptive	Free nerve endings	Aδ	10–35 m/s 1–5 microns	Slow	Innocuous cold
	Free nerve endings	C	0.5–1 m/s < 1 micron	Slow	Innocuous warmth
Nociceptive	Free nerve endings	Aδ	10–35 m/s 1–5 microns	Slow	Sharp pain
	Free nerve endings	C	0.5–1 m/s < 1 micron	Slow	Burning pain

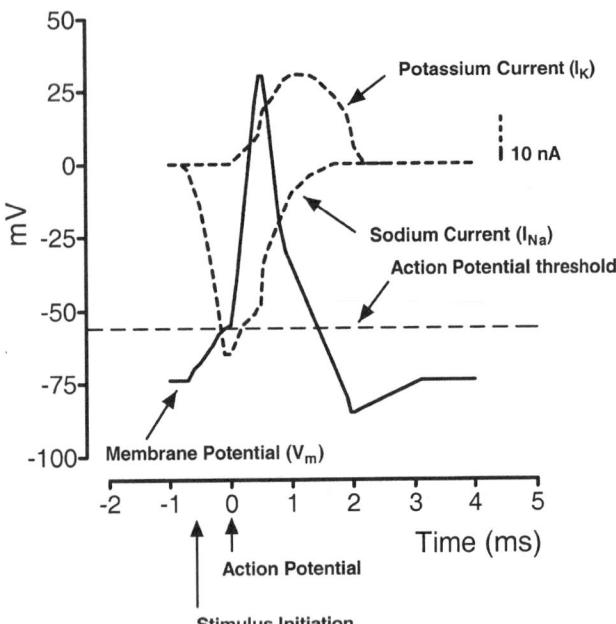

FIG. 2-1. The nerve action potential and associated ion currents. Membrane potential (V_m) of the nerve in millivolts (blue, solid line). The action potential (AP) is produced with sufficient depolarization to cross the AP threshold (horizontal dashed line). Depolarization is achieved by a rapid increase in the influx of sodium ions through voltage-gated sodium channels depicted as an increase (downward deflection) in sodium current (I_{Na}) in nanoamperes (red dashed line). Repolarization and hyperpolarization result from the slow and delayed increase in the outward potassium current (I_K) through voltage-gated potassium channels.

follows the epicritic pain, is poorly localized or diffuse, and is characterized as burning or dull (10).

The majority of Aδ and C nociceptors are polymodal and therefore are responsible for the transduction of noxious stimuli of different modalities into the action potential (Fig. 2-1). The noxious thermal threshold for humans

is approximately 45°C to 47°C, and the subject's ratings of the painful stimulus increase linearly with increasing temperature (11). These data correlate well with the responsiveness of C fibers in monkeys to the same temperature stimuli (11).

Chemical mediators of pain are numerous. These mediators come from sources intrinsic to the neuron, including various neurotransmitters such as *serotonin* and *substance P*, and extrinsic to the nervous system, including substances from inflammatory/immune cells and red blood cells such as *prostaglandins, kinins, cytokines, chemokines,* and *ATP* that are released following injury to the tissue (Table 2-2).

Although mechanical transduction has been less well studied than either thermal or chemical transduction of nociceptive signals, there is some evidence of a mechanically activated molecule, *degenerins*, in the nematode *Caenorhabditis elegans* as well as in human homologues. This compound may have a role in the transduction of mechanical stimuli in humans (12–14). It is unknown whether these molecules are involved in the transduction of noxious or nonnoxious mechanical stimuli in primary afferents. Therefore, the therapeutic benefit we may garner by antagonism of this class of molecule remains an open question. More recently, a mechanosensitive stretch-inactivated channel has been localized to small-diameter sensory neurons (15). This channel is inactivated by cell shrinkage and may therefore have a role in signaling hypertonic stimuli exposure following injury to the organism.

Although the sensory modalities (chemical, thermal, and mechanical) may appear quite disparate at first glance, the recent animal literature has begun to focus on their similarities. The recent cloning and characterization of the rat (16) and human (17) "capsaicin" receptor, vanilloid receptor subtype 1 (VR1), which not only responds to capsaicin and other vanilloid compounds, but also is activated by acid and heat, provides an excellent example of the integration of multiple sensory modalities within a single neuron. More recent studies have localized the VR1 receptor

TABLE 2-2. *Chemical mediators of pain and associated receptors*

Intrinsic to nervous system	Primary afferent receptor	Extrinsic to nervous system	Extrinsic source
Substance P	Neurokinin$_{1-3}$	Leukotriene B$_4$	Neutrophils
ATP	P2X$_3$	Interleukin 1α, 1β	Leukocytes
Glutamate	NMDA, AMPA	Serotonin	Mast cells, activated platelets
Serotonin	5-HT$_{1A, 3, 7}$	Histamine	Mast cells
Norepinephrine	Alpha$_1$	Tumor necrosis factor α (TNF α)	Macrophages
		Bradykinin	Plasma
		Hydrogen ions	
		Prostaglandins (incl. PGE$_2$)	Synthesized *de novo* from cell membrane
		Chemokines (RANTES, gp120, SDC)	Infection

protein to small- and medium-diameter unmyelinated (C fiber) and myelinated (Aδ fiber) primary afferent neurons (18,19). Furthermore, the authors demonstrate that heat directly opens and activates the VR1 channel in a temperature-dependent manner and, more importantly, an acidic environment can lower the activation threshold of the channel to the same heat stimuli. Although the integrative function of the VR1 receptor is certainly important in acute pain conditions, a more interesting and theoretically possible avenue to target for therapeutic intervention is its role in inflammatory pain conditions where the tissue surrounding the primary afferent may be of a lower (acidic) pH (20). Mice lacking the VR1 receptor are deficient in their response to thermal, but not to mechanical or other noxious stimuli (21). This deficiency, in an appropriate response to noxious thermal stimuli, is especially prominent in mice suffering from inflammatory pain. These data suggest that the capsaicin receptor (VR1) may play a role in the integration of noxious chemical and thermal stimuli, while having relatively little to do with mechanical transduction. Further, mice lacking this receptor appeared otherwise normal, which bodes well for the possibility of drug development targeting the antagonism of the VR1 receptor.

ALLODYNIA AND HYPERALGESIA

Pain sensation is unique among the somatosensory modalities in that it does not rapidly adapt to prolonged stimulation as do the other sensory modalities, such as fine touch. In fact, continued stimulation may produce greater noxious sensation or reduce the stimulus threshold or intensity that is necessary for the appreciation of the sensation as noxious (Fig. 2-2). For instance, previously innocuous thermal or mechanical stimulation may be perceived as painful following a prior noxious stimulus. This is termed *allodynia*. An example of allodynia that commonly occurs is increased sensitivity to thermal or mechanical stimuli in an area of sunburned skin. The warm water of a shower or the light touch of a towel produces a painful sensation that may persist for a few minutes following the stimulation. Although painful stimuli are transmitted to the spinal cord via Aδ and C fibers (Table 2-1), the presence of allodynia is thought to be mediated by the activation of large-diameter Aβ fibers through what has been termed a "phenotypic" switch (7, 22). Prior to this peripheral injury, the Aβ fibers, unlike the C fibers, do *not* express substance P. However, following injury, these fibers are able to express this neuropeptide (Table 2-2) (23). These data therefore implicate Aβ fibers in the transmission of *noxious* peripheral stimulation and provide further support for the involvement of somatic Aβ fibers in at least some forms of allodynic pain states. Furthermore, the blockade of Aβ fibers results in a reduction in light touch-evoked allodynia (24). This phenotypic switch of Aβ fibers may represent another avenue for therapeutic intervention. However, the difficulty will be

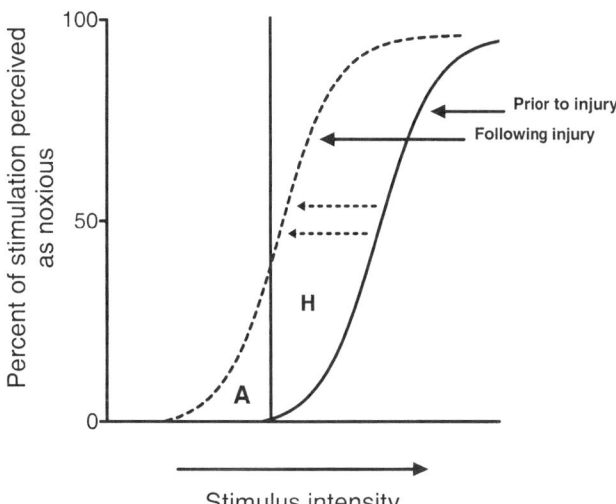

FIG. 2-2. Allodynia and hyperalgesia. A stimulus-response curve of a person prior to an injury is depicted as a positive sigmoidal relationship (solid line). As the stimulus intensity increases so does the percentage of stimuli that are perceived as painful. The vertical solid line represents the division of between noxious (to the right) and nonnoxious stimuli (to the left) in an uninjured person. Following injury, the stimulus-response relationship (dashed line) shifts to the left. This shift to the left results in an increased percentage of stimuli perceived as painful. Previously nonnoxious stimuli are perceived as painful (this is termed allodynia [A]), and previously noxious stimuli are perceived as more noxious (termed hyperalgesia [H]).

in differentiating between those Aβ fibers involved in noxious versus nonnoxious sensory information.

Another example of an altered pain state that may follow an acute injury is that of *hyperalgesia*, in which previously noxious stimuli are perceived as more painful. The sensation of increased intensity of noxious stimulation at the site of the injury is the result of the sensitization of the peripheral nociceptors. This sensitization is the result of the release of chemical mediators such as bradykinin, histamine, serotonin, and prostaglandins stimulated by the injury acting on the peripheral nociceptor. As discussed earlier, an acidic environment, similar to one found following an injury, decreases the temperature required to activate the capsaicin receptor (VR1). This is one additional mechanism by which a hyperalgesic state may develop.

THERAPEUTIC INTERVENTIONS AT PERIPHERAL SITES OF INJURY

Now that we have discussed some of the neurophysiology and neuroanatomy at the peripheral level, it is appropriate to mention some of the commonly available therapies that can have a significant effect in palliation of pain at this site. We mentioned previously that an area of injury can be painful both at the site of injury and in the area surrounding the trauma. This leads us into our first preventive measure option for the periphery, *avoidance*. If a behavior optimizes our physical well-being by eliminating a potential for injury or further trauma, then it is an adaptive. Although this seems intuitively obvious, we frequently encounter clinical scenarios in which our patients repeatedly expose themselves to an injurious element. A classic example is a patient who has both radiologically and clinically confirmed signs of lumbar disc herniation, and yet continues to perform work-related activities that involve lumbar spinal flexion and heavy lifting that result in exacerbation of his or her pain. Our role is to advise the patient to modify his or her environment so that injured tissue is protected from further destruction or injury. Increasingly, evidence is showing that a multidisciplinary approach to treating pain patients, including a strong psychological foundation, is best at controlling a patient's pain and his or her responses to it (25).

Our next level of therapeutic intervention is *physical barriers*. These can be effective because they may decrease or eliminate the possibility of further tissue damage or pain receptor activation. Barriers may include splints, dressings, and bandages. Any injury that breaches the skin must be appropriately managed from a healing and functional standpoint, as well as from the analgesic perspective. Extreme caution must be taken to decrease the possible atrophy or dysfunction of an affected limb. It is therefore appropriate to consult specialists for surgical wound management as well as physical medical practitioners, especially if splint placement is being considered or such care is necessary. Physical therapy can also be instrumental in maintaining limb function, range of motion, and strength. If a patient suffers from lumbar facet arthropathy pain, lumbar-stretching exercises performed twice daily may aid in strengthening the anterior muscle groups of the lumbar spine. This can decrease the "load" placed on the posterior bony elements of the spine, and thus contribute to reducing the pain related to facet opposition and loading. In addition, routine home exercise may improve overall functioning capacity (26). Another simple alternative or adjunct, often overlooked by the clinician, are the *topical agents*. Topical agents can be a source of significant intervention at the cutaneous level, especially in painful conditions with a substantial *neuropathic* pain component. Although one may argue that all pain is invariably neuropathic in nature, here we refer to that pain that is substantially propagated by the aberrant processing, signaling, or reconfiguration of neurons from their normal disease-free state, as discussed above. The topical agent delivery site should also be as proximate as possible to the site of injury, allowing for good penetration into the damaged tissue and the nociceptors supplying the area.

Topical compounds may include a variety of mixtures including local anesthetics. The rationale here is clearly related to their ability to be absorbed through the skin, and then cause a conduction blockade of the peripheral afferent pain nerve fibers. Local anesthetic ability to provide nerve conduction block is well documented (27). Once taken into the cutaneous tissue, they penetrate the perineurium and then the nerve fiber itself. The propagation of nerve impulses in the form of an action potential to carry sensory or motor information requires ionic flux through specific channels in the nerve membrane. As illustrated in Figure 2-1, the generation of an action potential is dependent on the electrical potential of the membrane. After sufficient membrane depolarization, the membrane crosses the electrical threshold and an action potential is produced. The inward current of sodium ions through the voltage-gated ion channels predominantly determines the action potential. Local anesthetic agents reversibly bind to these channels and block the conductance of sodium ions through the channels, thereby inhibiting nerve conduction (28). Sodium channels are complex, three-dimensional structures that are integral membrane proteins in the lipid bilayer of cells. Local anesthetics can access the sodium channel from either the plasma or the cytoplasmic side of the channel protein and bind within the pore of the channel (28). The binding of sodium channels by local anesthetics is state dependent; in other words, they can bind to the channel when it is open, allowing sodium ion conductance, closed (inactivated), or in a resting state. Specifically, a conformational or allosteric model, in which the receptor has the highest affinity when the channel is open or closed, can explain the state-dependent binding while also explaining why weakest binding occurs in the resting state (29). The delivery route of any topical agent occurs via the skin; therefore, the pharmacological properties of these drugs are determined by their speed of onset and systemic washout. The lipid solubility of the compound determines its ability to traverse the skin and penetrate the perineurium of the nerve tissue. Determinants of lipid solubility of a drug include the charge (ionization) of the compound, hydrophobicity, pK_a, local tissue pH, and its molecular structure and size.

Commercially prepared standard mixtures are available, but it may be necessary to have solutions custom prepared by specialist pharmacies to meet specific patient needs. Custom preparations include, for example, varying percent combinations of two or more local anesthetics in a cream base, or varying concentrations of capsaicin cream (discussed below). We prefer a combination of a relatively rapid onset agent, such as *lidocaine*, combined with a longer acting agent, such as *bupivacaine*. Exact concentrations of various agents are not as important as appropriate clinical application, with a keen eye on possible toxicity from systemic absorption. Toxicity to these drugs includes minor and often subtle signs of confusion, circumoral numbness, glossal paresthesia, tinnitus, dizziness, and blurred vision. Much more serious symptoms may include cardiac arrhythmias, apnea, and circulatory collapse.

Also included in this class of topically applied drugs are various preparations of compounds based on *non-*

steroidal antiinflammatory drugs (NSAIDs). These drugs can be especially effective for painful conditions involving a substantial inflammatory component such as osteoarthritis or burn injuries. Injurious mechanical, chemical, thermal, and other types of tissue damage stimuli result in the liberation of arachidonic acid (AA) by the activation of cellular phospholipase A_2 (PLA_2) (Fig. 2-3). The AA metabolites—the eicosanoids (thromboxanes, prostaglandins, and leukotrienes)—are all involved in the development of inflammation. The thromboxanes and prostaglandins are produced through the action of the *cyclooxygenase* enzymes, *COX-I* and *COX-II*, which represent the molecular target of NSAIDs. The leukotrienes, which are involved in neutrophil chemotaxis, leukocyte aggregation and adhesion, as well as vasoconstriction and vascular permeability, are not inhibited by NSAIDs. NSAIDs can be categorized into two broad subtypes: nonselective and selective agents. Nonselective NSAID agents inhibit both the constitutive (COX-I) and inducible (COX-II) form of

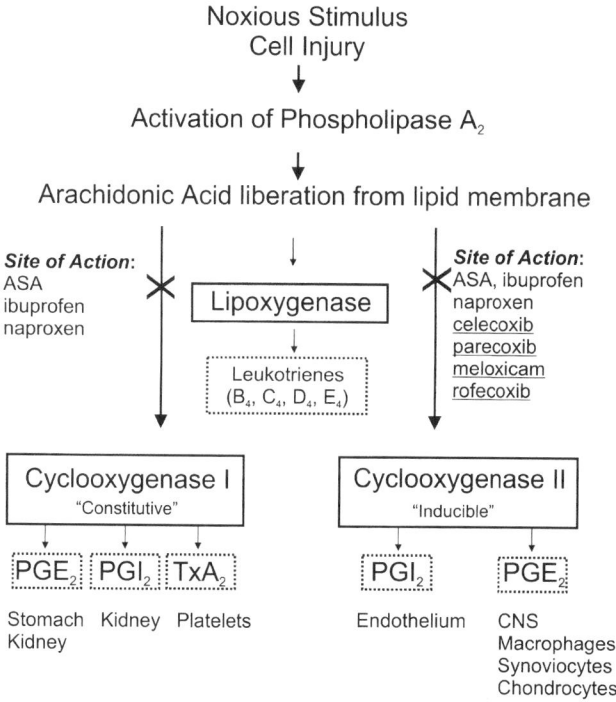

FIG. 2-3. The cyclooxygenase I and II pathways. The site of action of the nonselective cyclooxygenase (COX) inhibitors—including aspirin, naproxen, and ibuprofen—are depicted inhibiting both the predominantly constitutive COX-I and the inducible COX-II enzymes resulting in effects impacting numerous tissue and organ systems. Celecoxib, parecoxib, rofecoxib, and meloxicam have greater selectivity for the inducible form of COX, COX-II, and therefore have an effect on a more select group of tissues. Parecoxib is an intravenous formulation; celecoxib, meloxicam, and rofecoxib exist as oral formulations at this time. Neither group of drugs reduces the production of the third major category of the arachidonic acid metabolism, the leukotrienes. Abbreviations: CNS, central nervous system; ASA, acetylsalicylic acid.

the cyclooxygenase enzyme. As a result, they not only produce analgesia mediated through COX-II mechanisms involving inflammatory pain mediators, but also may cause undesirable systemic effects secondary to their inhibition of COX-I. COX-I is involved with the production of platelet-aggregating factors and protective prostaglandins in the gastrointestinal tract. Lack of these protective compounds and platelet-aggregating factors in patients may result in an increased risk of gastrointestinal ulceration and bleeding. In the kidney, the "traditional" nonselective NSAID agents have long been known to potentially cause nephrotoxicity. Although the newer COX-II specific inhibitors have far greater selectivity, they are not immune from potentially contributing to nephrotoxicity since the COX-II enzyme is constitutively expressed in the renal tissues (30). In platelets, nonselective NSAID agents inhibit COX-I production of end products involved with platelet functioning. As a result, an iatrogenic coagulopathy may result from platelet inhibition. COX-II is not thought to be present in any significant quantities, if any, in platelets (31). As a result, platelet function inhibition does not appear to occur with these COX-II selective agents (32). Again, prudence must be used to avoid these potentially harmful effects from the nonselective NSAID compounds. COX-II agents are approximately two orders of magnitude more selective for cyclooxygenase-II than cyclooxygenase-I (33). As a result of their specificity, they are able to aid in analgesia without many of the untoward systemic side effects associated with their nonselective counterparts. Currently, there are no commercially available topical COX-II selective agents, but they are under development.

Common nonselective agents that are available in a topical cream include, but are not limited to, acetylsalicylic acid and ibuprofen. Again, these agents should be applied as close as possible to the target area, with cautions to avoid open tissue. They are useful in conditions where cutaneous or superficial muscle inflammation and pain exist. An example would be biceps tendinitis after overexertion. Undesirable effects from systemic absorption, again, need to be avoided. Undesirable systemic side effects resemble those of systemically administered NSAID agents, which we mentioned earlier. There is a significant body of literature well known to the medical community substantiating the risks, incidence, and mortality related to episodes of severe/massive gastrointestinal bleeding caused by long-term NSAID use.

Another interesting compound, which has been clinically shown to have analgesic activity in the periphery, is *capsaicin*. Capsaicin is thought to work by the VR1 receptor, as discussed above. It is absorbed through the skin and depletes the peripheral terminal substance P (34). Capsaicin is also a neurotoxin selective for C fiber afferents (35) and epidermal nerve fibers (36). The analgesic effect of capsaicin cream may result from a combination of these actions on nociceptive afferents. It is available in several concentrations of a topical cream up to about 10%, which can be readily applied to affected extremities or areas. However, extreme caution must be exercised with this compound. Unless the area of application is either anesthetized or in some fashion rendered senseless by injury or disease, capsaicin application will result in a very painful burning sensation that can last for hours. Application must be kept in place for approximately 30 minutes to allow the compound to be absorbed and reach its target receptor. The effects of analgesia can be observed for up to 2 weeks, a time frame more consistent with its neurotoxic effects. To achieve a more prolonged effect, some practitioners perform a series of applications in patients who show a good response to the treatments.

Another frequently used class of topical agents is the *corticosteroids* (CS). Hydrocortisone cream in assorted concentrations is the most frequently used agent. Similar to NSAID, CS works by modulating the inflammatory mediator pathways, although these agents affect this system more globally. They not only affect the cyclooxygenase pathways, but also inhibit the lipoxygenase and peroxidase pathways, and thus their respective resultant inflammatory/algogenic mediator end products. End products of the lipoxygenase and peroxidase pathways include 12-hydroperoxyeicosatetraenoic acid and leukotrienes B4, C4, and D4 (Fig. 2-3) (37). Care must be exercised to not overutilize these agents due to their potential for systemic absorption and adrenal suppression. In addition, these agents are known to be catabolic to tissues and can lead to breach in skin integrity, myopathy, and cartilage and ligament damage.

Nonpharmacological interventions in the periphery are also available and can range from completely noninvasive to more aggressive and invasive interventions reserved for refractory patients. *Massage therapy,* one nonpharmacological therapy that is often overlooked, can be a powerful adjunct for certain pain states evolving from musculoskeletal origin. Massage is known to locally deform muscle myofibrils, stretching them beyond their normal fiber length and therefore providing intense stimulation to the spinal cord via Aα fibers. As mentioned above, stimulation of this fiber type can be involved in "closing the gate" on painful transmission via the C and Aδ fibers. Further, when massage therapy is done consistently, it can improve a patient's flexibility and limb range of motion (ROM). In addition, the positive sensations of massage seldom, if ever, result in worsening a patient's mood since most people feel that these manipulations actually feel very good. Other forms of cutaneous stimulation include *transcutaneous electrical nerve stimulation* (TENS) and *interferential* (IF) therapy. TENS and IF therapy are delivered by means of an electrical device that is capable of providing a variable voltage, pulse width, and amperage from a pulse generator to a semiviscous contact pad gel. The pads are attached on or near the painful areas. Extreme caution must be used when placing the stimulation pads near the head. The pads should never be placed on the scalp due to

the possibility of seizure propagation. TENS is less penetrating than IF therapy and does not activate myofibril contraction. The underlying mechanism of action in TENS is thought to be related to the gate control theory of pain first proposed by Melzak and Wall (38). As discussed above, this theory is based on the notion that the activation of large-diameter, nonnoxious fibers results in the inhibition of the transmission of small-diameter, noxious fiber signals to the dorsal horn of the spinal cord, and therefore a decrease in the perception of pain. IF therapy, on the other hand, directly causes myofibril contraction and even muscle spasm. Patients describe the sensation as "electrical hands" pinching and pulling their tissues. IF is used to purposefully cause the rapid, cyclical contraction and relaxation of muscle groups that are in constant spasm or are persistently sore. Although there is no well-defined neurophysiology to explain its mechanism, there is some clinical evidence that suggests IF is an effective adjunctive tool to improve pain of myalgic origin and to improve function (39). Again, electrical parameters can be adjusted to patient comfort level and desired effect.

We have already discussed the mechanism of action of local anesthetics and their use as topical agents. However, in clinical practice, their most common use is in the form of injectable solutions for peripheral tissue infiltration or neural blockade. Here, we bypass the need for topical application and cutaneous absorption, and instead, deliver the drugs directly, close to their sites of action. Just as with the topical creams, solutions of injectable local anesthetics can be adjusted according to the specific goal. We frequently like to use a combination of a more rapid onset agent with a longer acting drug. This allows the patients to better tolerate the injection itself, provides them with some relatively immediate relief, and provides them with a more sustained analgesia for a longer time. One-percent lidocaine mixed with equal volumes of 0.5% bupivacaine is a mixture that we frequently employ. Depending on individual circumstances, we can also modify solutions with bicarbonate to alter the local tissue pH to provide a more favorable balance between the ionized and nonionized neutral species of the compound. This alters the rate of blockade onset, and therefore, onset of pain relief. This more rapid onset occurs because the increased availability of the nonionized form of the drug translates to an increased amount of "active" compound that can then readily enter and occupy its respective sodium channels to block them. This is important if the practitioner needs to have diagnostic information available as soon as possible before proceeding with further management. In addition, epinephrine can also be added to mixtures to prolong the effects of local anesthetics secondary to the production of local vasoconstriction, thereby slowing the rate of washout and redistribution away from the nerve fibers. Epinephrine is also useful to rule out intravascular injection. Systemic delivery of significant doses of epinephrine must be carefully avoided to prevent potentially harmful side effects that include extreme anxiety, paroxysmal tachycardia, hypertension, and even myocardial ischemia and stroke.

Another group of drugs that are frequently injected into peripheral tissues are the corticosteroids (CS). The mechanism of action is identical to those of their topical counterparts. Arthritis of the major joints, tendinitis, and severe myofascial spasm are all conditions that may be responsive to local corticosteroid injections. One agent we frequently use is methylprednisolone. We typically dilute 20 to 40 mg in 10cc of a local anesthetic mixture. The major advantage of adding steroids to the mixture is having an agent with potent antiinflammatory activity present in an affected area for extended periods. These steroid formulations are typically carried in a preservative suspension, which allows their slow release over time. Again, care must be taken to not overutilize these agents as to avoid tissue breakdown and the previously discussed systemic side effects.

NEUROBIOLOGY OF THE SPINAL CORD AND SUPRASPINAL STRUCTURES

We have previously discussed the various types of peripheral stimulation, their respective receptors, and the transduction of these stimuli via the different types of afferent fibers. We will now shift our focus to the level of the spinal cord and the synapse of the primary afferent "pain" fibers onto their respective secondary projection neurons and interneurons. We will also begin our discussion of some of the properties and functional roles of the intrinsic descending pain inhibition systems.

Aδ and C fiber neurons synapse primarily within *laminae I, II, and V* of the dorsal horn of the spinal cord (Fig. 2-4). These primary afferents release neurotransmitters and neuropeptides (Fig. 2-5), which activate the second-order projection neurons of the spinal cord. Nociceptive transmission through the spinal cord may be modulated by an endogenous descending pain inhibitory system and may be influenced by exogenously administered medications (Figs. 2-6, 2-7). Here, we will expand our discussion of this modulating system and include the fundamentals of its contributions to analgesia and our ability to manipulate this system.

The primary components of this descending pain inhibition system—though certainly not all-inclusive—are the "triad" of the *periaqueductal gray* (PAG), the *rostral ventromedial medulla* (RVM), and the *dorsal lateral pontine tegmentum* (DLPT), which includes the *locus coeruleus* (LC) and the *A7* nuclei (40,41). The PAG is an important site for the production of antinociception following electrical or chemical activation, or the injection of opioid receptor agonists in animals (42,43). The endogenous opioid, [Met⁵] enkephalin, is present within this nucleus (44) and opioid receptors of each subtype are present in this region (45). The PAG provides dense projections to the

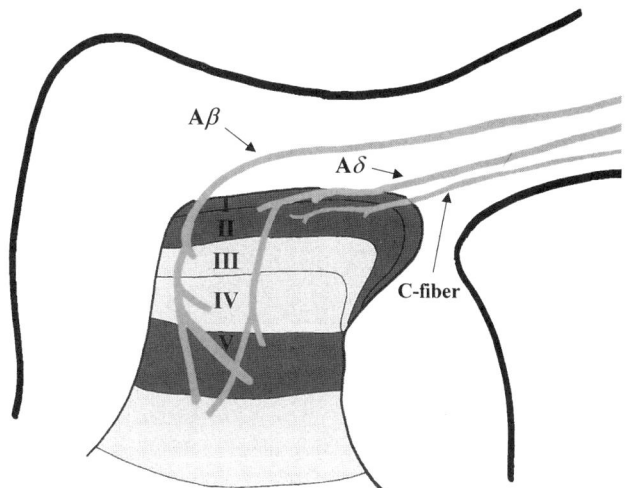

FIG. 2-4. The spinal cord terminations of primary afferent fibers. The three types of sensory primary afferent synapse upon distinct areas of the spinal cord dorsal horn; the afferents associated with the transmission of pain—the Aδ and C fibers—primarily synapse in laminae I, II, and V and the afferents primarily involved in transmission of nonnoxious information—the Aβ fibers—synapse in laminae III, IV, V, and VI. (Adapted from Benzon. *Essentials of pain medicine and regional anesthesia.* New York: Churchill Livingstone, 1999, with permission.)

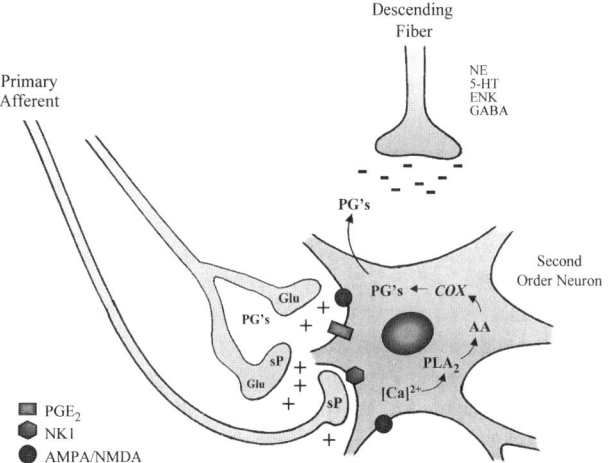

FIG. 2-5. Neurotransmitters involved with the transmission of noxious information. Primary afferents release multiple neurotransmitters, including substance P and glutamate, resulting in the activation of the spinal cord second-order neuron and the transmission of the noxious information to higher brain structures. Activation of the spinal cord neuron may also result in the production of prostaglandins (PG), including prostaglandin E₂, which sensitizes the second-order neuron to further noxious stimulation. The processes of the spinal cord neuron may be modulated by higher brain structures via descending fibers that release numerous neurotransmitters, including norepinephrine (NE), serotonin (5-HT), enkephalin (ENK), or γ-aminobutyric acid (GABA). These substances can act to limit the activation of the spinal cord neuron and thereby reduce the transmission of noxious information from the periphery. (Adapted from Wall and Melzack. *Textbook of pain,* 4th ed. London: Churchill Livingstone, 1999, with permission.)

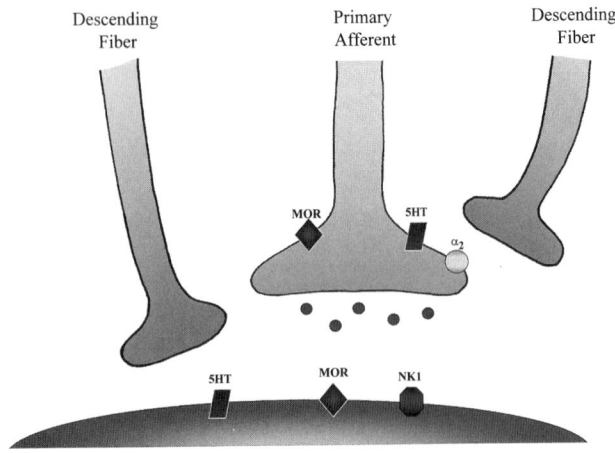

Descending Fiber   Primary Afferent   Descending Fiber

MOR   5HT   α₂

5HT   MOR   NK1

Second Order Neuron

FIG. 2-6. Higher brain structure influence on the transmission of noxious information from the periphery. Descending fibers from higher brain structures can modulate both the primary afferent and the second-order spinal cord neuron. Inhibition of the primary afferent reduces the amount of transmitter released, whereas inhibition of the second-order neuron can function independent of the release of neurotransmitter. (Adapted from Wall and Melzack. *Textbook of pain*, 4th ed. London: Churchill Livingstone, 1999, with permission.)

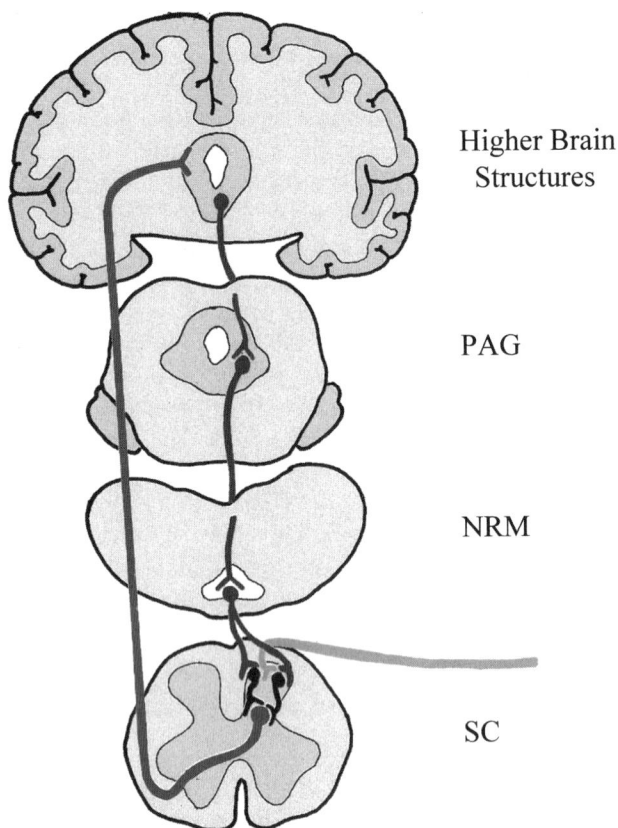

Higher Brain Structures

PAG

NRM

SC

FIG. 2-7. Ascending and descending pain pathways. The primary afferents, C and Aδ fibers (yellow), synapse onto spinal cord interneurons (black) and/or second-order neurons (green). The second-order neurons (wide-dynamic range or nociceptive specific) then cross the midline and ascend to terminate in higher brain structures, including the thalamus. The descending pain control system may begin in the frontal cortices and hypothalamus. These neurons (red) then project to the periaqueductal gray (PAG), which projects to the nucleus raphe magnus (NRM) and on to the spinal cord dorsal horn. Pharmacological therapies, including the use of *mu* opioid receptor agonists, have an impact at each of these sites, resulting in the activation of descending pain inhibitory fibers. (Adapted from Wall and Melzack. *Textbook of pain*, 4th ed. London: Churchill Livingstone, 1999, with permission.)

RVM (46) and the brainstem noradrenergic nuclei LC and A7 (47). Although each of these regions has direct projections to the spinal cord, it has been proposed that their projections to the RVM, and to the NRM (see below) in particular, are important components in the modulation of nociception by these regions. For example, chemical or electrical inactivation of the RVM results in the attenuation of the antinociceptive effects produced by the activation of these midbrain structures (48). The RVM consists of the *nucleus raphe magnus* (NRM), the nucleus reticularis gigantocellularis pars alpha (NGCpα), and the nucleus reticularis gigantocellularis pars lateralis (40). It is a functionally heterogeneous region that has been reported to modulate cardiovascular activity and thermoregulation. However, it is the role of the NRM and NGCpα in the modulation of nociceptive transmission that has made this region the subject of considerable interest and investigation to pain researchers. Although the RVM can function as a relay nucleus in the production of antinociception by more rostral midbrain structures (PAG), it also has a primary role in the suppression of nociceptive transmission at the level of the spinal cord. The suppression of nociceptive reflex behavior is thought to be mediated by the axons of RVM neurons that descend within the dorsolateral funiculus and terminate bilaterally in laminae I, II, V, VI, and VII of the spinal cord (Fig. 2-7). Anatomical studies have shown these axons terminate coincident with spinothalamic tract cells and interneurons of the dorsal horn that are related to nociceptive transmission (49,50) (Fig. 2-7). Consistent with the anatomical terminations of

the RVM axons, physiological studies have shown that stimulation of the RVM results in the inhibition of a population of nociceptive-specific neurons within the dorsal horn, as well as selective inhibition of the nociceptive responses of wide-dynamic range (WDR) neurons (51, 52). Additionally, the primary source of serotonergic projections to the dorsal horn of the spinal cord is the NRM (49, 50). However, spinally projecting neurons of the RVM also possess numerous transmitters other than serotonin. These neurotransmitters include enkephalin, GABA, glutamate, and substance P (53–55) (Figs. 2-5, 2-6). The DLPT contains all of the noradrenergic neurons that project to the RVM and the spinal cord (56,57). In animal models, electrical stimulation of the DLPT sites produces analgesia (41,58) and the analgesia produced by the activation of these nuclei is mediated by the α_2 adrenergic receptor (58,59). The physician, then, in order to alleviate or reduce a patient's pain, can pharmacologically manipulate each of these neurotransmitters to play a role in the modulation of nociceptive transmission at the level of the spinal cord.

INTERVENTIONS TO MODULATE NOCICEPTIVE TRANSMISSION

Now that we have discussed some of the neurophysiology and neuroanatomy at the spinal cord synaptic level, as well as higher brainstem influences on the spinal cord, it is appropriate to discuss how some of the commonly available therapies manipulate or accentuate this physiology and anatomy. First, we will discuss an assortment of systemic pharmacological agents. These include the "traditionally" labeled *antidepressants* as well as other agents we will discuss later.

Although there are numerous compounds within the antidepressant family, we will limit our discussion to several of the more common ones that are representative of this class. A given agent may alter either the 5-HT or the NE pathways. There are also those that may alter both systems. Of the assorted pathologic pain states, these antidepressant agents are most effective against neuropathic pain states. However, these agents can also be used to manage myofascial pain, and data from animal studies suggest that these agents may even produce acute analgesic effects (60). Some of the most commonly used agents are the *tricyclic-antidepressants* (TCA), which include amitriptyline, nortriptyline, and desipramine. All of these are "mixed" agents in the sense that they increase available serotonin and norepinephrine, but individual agents may preferentially affect one monoamine pathway more than another (61). Amitriptyline is predominantly serotonergic, while the remaining two agents are primarily noradrenergic agents (61–63). It is thought that the effects of TCA on the monoamine systems produce pain relief through an accentuation of the descending pain inhibition system.

Administration of these agents to patients, as with any medication, needs to be accompanied by appropriate vigilance for their respective side effects. The most common clinical side effects reported by patients receiving these medications include xerostomia, urinary retention or urinary hesitancy, changes in libido, and sexual dysfunction. Other side effects may portend more ominous consequences, including cardiac rhythm disturbances. It is therefore important, prior to initiating this therapy, to carefully evaluate patients for any significant cardiac disease history, focusing on the potential for cardiac arrhythmias. Although cognitive impairment and the sensation of excessive fatigue or daytime somnolence are also commonly reported, this can be a significant benefit to the chronically sleep-deprived patient with a history of insomnia. Chronic pain

patients often have a history of significant comorbid reactive or primary depression. Patients who have these conditions may also benefit from the addition of these agents.

Older patients can be particularly sensitive to the sedative effects of these drugs. Therefore, when prescribing to this group, additional prudence should be exercised. Although amitriptyline is the more investigated drug in this group, and perhaps one of the more effective, it unfortunately is also associated with the least desirable side effect profile. Nortriptyline is "intermediate" in this regard, with desipramine usually being the most well-tolerated agent in terms of side effects. These agents also may have significant interactions with other concomitantly administered systemic drugs. Therefore, it is necessary to periodically determine the patient's blood levels to verify therapeutic effect. Also, if given with drugs of similar activity, it is important to observe for additive or synergistic toxicity.

The dosing of these agents also requires some careful titration. In general, we do not immediately start with the target dosages. In most cases, the target dose is 150 mg at bedtime. This is usually achieved by gradually increasing the dose of an agent by 10 to 25 mg every 5 to 14 days or so. As a general rule, the drug should be increased to the goal dose as limited by patient tolerance or when desired efficacy is achieved. If a patient complains of excessive daytime sleepiness or grogginess, one measure to combat this problem is to have the patient take the medication earlier in the evening before sleeping, allowing the symptoms to coincide with the patient's normal sleep cycle.

A second class of drugs, which we categorize as part of the systemic group, is the *anticonvulsants*. While we have several drugs available in this group, we will limit our discussion to one of the most frequently prescribed agents, *gabapentin*. Like antidepressants, anticonvulsants can be particularly effective in treating pain of neuropathic origin. Pain stemming from neuropathies and neurodegenerative disease states, such as diabetic neuropathy and even herpes zoster, can be especially responsive to therapy with this group of agents, gabapentin in particular (64,65). The mechanism by which gabapentin exerts its analgesic effect is somewhat controversial. Although it was originally designed as a structural analog of the inhibitory neurotransmitter γ-aminobutyric acid (GABA) (66), it is inactive at the $GABA_A$ and $GABA_B$ receptors (67) and, in contrast with the mechanism of action of other anticonvulsants (68,69), gabapentin inhibits neither the metabolism nor the uptake of GABA (70,71). However, it has been suggested that gabapentin may produce its effects by the disinhibition of glutamic acid decarboxylase (GAD), which may result in an increase in the synthesis or release of GABA (72) leading to the production of antinociception. Recently, it has been observed that gabapentin binds to the $\alpha_2\delta$ subunit of high-intensity, voltage-activated calcium channels (73) and that these calcium channels are involved in the development of the enhanced pain state after the induction of inflammation (74,75). Therefore, an alternate or possible complementary explanation for the antihyperalgesic effects produced by this compound is the result of its action at this calcium channel subunit. Similar to findings with calcium channel antagonists, gabapentin is ineffective in altering baseline nociceptive thresholds in animal models of acute pain (76,77). However, several studies using animal models of persistent nociception report that both compounds can relieve hyperalgesia and allodynia of inflammatory (77) and neuropathic origin (76,78).

Just as with the antidepressants, gabapentin must be slowly titrated to the point of reaching the desired effect, maximal dose, or patient intolerability. Side effects of this drug include cognitive impairment, which typically manifests as inability to "focus" or short-term memory impairment; significant degrees of sedation or even unresponsiveness; and edema of the upper and lower extremities. Again, elderly patients are usually far more sensitive to the sedative and cognitive effects, and therefore require more vigilance. Dosing is started at or close to the lowest doses so that patients are not overcome by side effects due to acute loading of the drug. Older patients are started on even lower doses than their younger adult counterparts. Doses are typically started at 100 to 300 mg per day. These are gradually increased by a total dose of 100 to 300 mg per day, and each total dose increase is usually done no less than 5 to 7 days apart. The end point of dosing is the maximal dose of 3600 mg per day (although some clinicians have reported higher doses), or the highest tolerated dose.

NSAIDs represent another class of systemically administered analgesics. As discussed above, nonselective NSAID agents inhibit both of the cyclooxygenase enzymes. In general, when agents are equally efficacious, we prefer to use those with the most favorable side effect profile. It has been shown that the COX-II selective inhibitors (Fig. 2-3) are equally as effective as their "traditional" NSAID counterparts (79,80). Given the recent availability of COX-II selective inhibitors, and the less desirable side effect profile of traditional NSAID drugs, we will focus on only the COX-II selective agents.

Clinically then, we have a more desirable alternative. The currently available oral COX-II selective agents include celecoxib, meloxicam, and rofecoxib. Celecoxib can be dosed, at the low end, 100 mg per day orally, or up to 200 mg twice per day orally. Common side effects may include gastrointestinal discomfort, peripheral extremity edema, and rashes. In addition, a less common but potentially more severe reaction can be allergic in nature. It is related to the sulfonamide side group present in celecoxib (81). Thus, caution and careful vigilance must be observed in prescribing this drug to patients with a history of allergic reactions to sulfa-containing drugs. Meloxicam is dosed at 7.5 mg per day orally. Rofecoxib can be dosed in a range of 12.5 mg per day to 25 mg per day. It can also be used in acute settings in doses up to 50 mg per day for up to

5 days. Both meloxicam and rofecoxib have a side effects profile similar to that of celecoxib, mentioned above.

A parenteral COX-II selective inhibitor, parecoxib, which appears to be as effective as its oral predecessors, and perhaps even as effective as morphine in some settings, is anticipated to reach market in the spring of 2001 (82, 83). This agent is currently under efficacy and safety study trials in healthy adult volunteers in 4 doses of up to 50 mg twice per day for up to 9 days (82).

One additional topic we would like to address is the issue of concomitant use of these COX-II selective agents and the use of aspirin. A frequent misconception among physicians, and other clinical care team staff, is that these two agents cannot be used in combination because of their theoretic redundant effects with regard to antiplatelet activity. As we have previously mentioned, cyclooxygenase II is not present in human platelets (31,32). Therefore, these agents are likely to have no antiplatelet effect, although this is still under extensive investigation. The removal of aspirin therapy and the use of COX-II therapy as a substitute may place patients with a history of coronary artery or cerebrovascular disease at unnecessary risk for an adverse effect. If these patients have a medical indication for such antiplatelet therapy, they should continue that therapy, regardless of whether they are receiving concomitant COX-II inhibitor therapy. Of course, care must always be tailored to individual patients, and medical management may dictate exceptions to this practice.

While on the topic of antiinflammatory agents, we would like to briefly mention the role of *corticosteriods* (CS) in systemic therapy. We have already explained some of the mechanisms by which these compounds affect pain signal processing and their effects on the inflammatory pathway. Their activity at the spinal cord and CNS levels, when given systemically, is the same as their peripheral counterparts. Typical CS agents, which are employed for their systemic effects, include dexamethasone and prednisone. CS agents have long been known to be potent antiinflammatory agents. However, recent clinical work strongly suggests that they may one day also play an important role in the treatment of chronic neuropathic pain states, such as that of postherpetic neuralgia (PHN), when administered through an intrathecal route (84). Thus, the future may hold additional promise for specific application of these agents to a variety of other pain disorders.

Opioids have been investigated for a sufficiently long period such that a fair amount of information is available about them. This knowledge includes mechanisms of action, sites of activity, and receptor biology. The existence of multiple types of opioid receptors was originally proposed by Martin and colleagues (85). Subsequent studies using both *in vitro* and *in vivo* pharmacological methods, employing alkaloid-derived as well as synthetic compounds, provided support for the existence of *mu, delta,* and *kappa* opioid receptors (86,87). These data were provided by radioligand binding (88, 89), *in vitro* bioassays (86), and pharmacological cross-tolerance (90) studies. These studies also provided evidence for the existence of multiple subtypes of each receptor including mu_1, mu_2, $delta_1$, $delta_2$, and $kappa_{1-3}$ (91–94). In addition, there is evidence for additional opioid receptor classes. More recently, molecular cloning techniques have identified three gene families that encode for these receptors (95–97). Also, an "orphan" opioid receptor (ORL1), which shares substantial sequence homology but does not bind prototypic opioid receptor agonists with high affinity, has also been identified (98). All of these receptors belong to the GTP-binding protein superfamily of metabotropic receptors (99). Agonist binding to an opioid receptor results in activation of inwardly rectifying K^+ channels (100), the inhibition of the N-type (101) and L-type (102) calcium channels, and/or the inhibition of adenyl cyclase activity (95,97), all processes by which neuronal excitability can be suppressed (103).

Numerous endogenous opioid peptides have been isolated and determined to have high affinity for one or more of the identified opioid receptors (Table 2-3) (104–106). Enkephalin, dynorphin, and beta-endorphin are derived from three precursor proteins: proenkephalin, prodynorphin, and proopiomelanocortin, respectively. The precursor molecule for the most recently isolated peptides, endomorphin-1 and -2, has not yet been isolated. However, the small size of these peptides, four amino acids, would lead one to predict that they are the cleavage products of a much larger precursor peptide or protein (106).

Although multiple opioid receptors and their respective endogenous agonists have been identified and isolated, we will focus predominantly on the *mu* opioid receptor-related activities of the clinically available medications. *Mu* opioid receptors are present throughout the central nervous system (CNS) (45). One of the most important locations is in the periaqueductal gray (PAG) tissue of the brain, which encompasses the cerebral aqueduct. This area

of the brain has an abundance of *mu* opioid receptors present (45). The PAG is one of the primary components of the descending pain inhibition system to which we alluded earlier. When opioid compounds are able to penetrate into the CNS, they can bind and "activate" *mu* opioid receptors. Activation of these receptors results in "activation" via disinhibition of the PAG with resultant increased "activation" of the RVM, as well as direct action within the RVM and spinal cord to produce analgesia. Neurons of the RVM project down to the spinal cord level and have an inhibitory influence on spinal cord pain transmission at the level of the dorsal gray horn. This provides a basic understanding of one of the many opioid-mediated circuits involved in the descending control of nociceptive transmission.

Before any patient is placed on opioid medications, the clinician must first assess the appropriateness of a specific therapy for that individual. Narcotics are not innocuous medications and are associated with a significant pattern of misuse, addiction, and physical dependence, especially the shorter-acting agents (107). Therefore, it is imperative to be extremely judicious prior to committing an individual to these agents. In the event a clinician feels unable to render such a judgment, consulting with a specially trained individual, such as a pain psychologist, is recommended. Since the entire discussion of opioid use in chronic "nonmalignant" pain is an ongoing controversy with regard to efficacy and outcome, we will defer this portion of the treatment protocol to the individual practitioner and his or her experience. The aim here is not to avoid the use of such agents, but to minimize the risks of inappropriate and ineffective use, to maximize efficacy, and to guard patient safety. We have enclosed an opioid conversion table (Table 2-4) which includes some of the more commonly used agents, with their relative potencies compared to morphine sulfate (MSO_4) and their approximate range of duration in hours.

Once the decision has been made to use opioid therapy, we must proceed to find a regimen that maximizes analgesic efficacy while minimizing side effects. There are numerous opioid agonists from which the clinician can choose (Table 2-4). Rather than individually covering each, we will use morphine sulfate (MSO_4) as our prototype.

TABLE 2-3. *Endogenous opioid peptides*

Endogenous opioid peptide	Amino acid sequence	Receptor
[Leu^5]enkephalin	Tyr-Gly-Gly-Phe-Leu	$\delta > \mu$
[Met^5]enkephalin	Tyr-Gly-Gly-Phe-Met	$\delta > \mu$
Endomorphin-1	Tyr-Pro-Trp-Phe-NH$_2$	μ
Endomorphin-2	Tyr-Pro-Phe-Phe-NH$_2$	μ
β-endorphin	Tyr-Gly-Gly-Phe-Met-Thr-Ser-Glu-Lys-Ser-Gln-Thr-Pro-Leu-Val-Thr-Leu-Phe-Lys-Asn-Ile-Ile-Lys-Asn-Tyr-Lys-Lys-Gly-Glu	μ, ε
Dynorphin A (1–17)	Tyr-Gly-Gly-Phe-Leu-Arg-Arg-Ile-Arg-Pro-Lys-Leu-Lys-Trp-Asp-Asn-Gln	κ
Dynorphin A (1–13)	Tyr-Gly-Gly-Phe-Leu-Arg-Arg-Ile-Arg-Pro-Lys-Leu-Lys	κ

TABLE 2-4. *Commonly used* mu *opioid receptor agonists*

Agent	Duration of effect (hr)	Route	Morphine equivalent dosage
Fentanyl	0.5–1	IV/TD	~100×
Codeine	2–4	PO	~1/3×
Hydrocodone	2–4	PO	~3–8×
Hydromorphone	2–4	IV/PO	~3–7× / ~3-8×
Meperidine	2–4	IV/PO	~1/8× / 1/5×
Oxycodone	3–5	PO	~1–2×
Methadone	8–12	IV/PO	~1–3× / 3×

Abbrev.: IV, Intravenous; PO, Oral administration; TD, Transdermal

Some agents are available in a form that may be administered orally, intravenously, intramuscular, or by another parenteral route. Parenteral dosing includes epidural or intrathecal administration of an agent. This "central" administration is usually reserved for patients in whom conventional routes are either not possible, or in whom these drugs have limited use secondary to their respective systemic side effects. Central administration has the advantage of directly administering these agents to their major sites of action. As a result, we are able to produce analgesia with only a fraction of the oral or intravenous doses. This generally maintains efficacy while minimizing systemic side effects. Once we have selected an appropriate patient, our first objective will then be to find (a) route(s) of administration that is acceptable for the patient. Since we have several routes of administration available to us, we can usually tailor an opioid regimen even in patients where other classes of drugs are impossible to administer.

Another common phenomenon we often need to overcome in the clinical setting is the problem of varying plasma levels of an opioid analgesic. This is seen with patients who are taking relatively short-acting agents, and who therefore require more frequent dosing as the drug's effect wears off toward the end of its analgesic halflife. This not only is inconvenient for the patient because of the need to repeatedly self-administer doses, but risks reinforcing behavior that may later become problematic in terms of dependence and misuse (107). One of the methods we use to minimize or eliminate the risk of this problem is to use agents that are "long acting." This is thought to maintain a more consistent and sustained plasma level of the drug. In addition, this practice can eliminate or minimize the need for shorter-acting "break through" opioids. To illustrate this point, let us use a clinical case example.

> A 66-year-old male has metastatic prostate cancer to the spine. He is admitted for spinal pain, with the goal of discharge home in a few days. Let us assume he has no allergies, and that he has no problems with oral intake. He has never been on any opioids, but at home was taking maximal doses of acetaminophen and NSAIDs. Let us say we started him on a long-acting morphine preparation 15 mg orally every 8 hours. In addition, we allow him to take 15 mg of a rapid-acting MSO_4 preparation orally every 6 hours as needed. After 48 hours, we note that he is comfortable if he takes both the long-acting agent and three additional doses per day of the short-acting morphine. We would then increase his long-acting agent to 30 mg every 8 hours, and still allow him the short-acting opioid as needed.

The agent we choose to use is not as important as individualizing the therapy to a particular patient. Our next, and perhaps greatest, concern involving the use of opioids is the risk of side effects.

The most frequently reported side effects include constipation, pruritus, nausea, and urinary retention. Common side effects that are more ominous include confusion, sedation, unresponsiveness, and respiratory depression.

Although all of these can be quite common, they tend to be very patient specific and thus should be individually addressed. The side effect that is perhaps the most consistently resistant to therapy is often opioid-induced constipation. Patients who experience this side effect may even need to be referred to a gastroenterologist who can aid in its management if conventional approaches fail. Symptomatic management can usually be used to successfully treat the other common side effects. In the event that a patient continues to experience an unacceptable degree of side effects, consideration should be given to trying an alternate compound, or even the possibility of intrathecal opioids, if appropriate for the particular patient. Some of the more common side effects may be attributable to the different opioid receptor subtypes. *Mu* opioid receptors may be involved in respiratory depression, muscle rigidity, and physical dependence; *kappa* receptors may play a role in sedation; and *delta* receptors may be involved with epileptogenic phenomena (108). Other side effects mentioned above can be attributable to the anticholinergic effects of opioid compounds. Now that we have completed a brief review of the rationale behind opioid use, we will begin our discussion of the last class of pharmacological compounds we will cover, the *alpha*-2 agonists.

Alpha-adrenergic receptors are widely distributed in a ubiquitous fashion throughout the body tissues. *Alpha*-1 receptors play an essential role in the regulation of systemic vascular resistance (SVR). Their presence on vascular tissue allows them to participate in blood pressure and blood flow regulation. Their *alpha*-2 counterparts are present throughout a variety of peripheral and central nervous system structures. The *alpha*-2 spinal cord receptor sites may be active in pain-signaling processes. There is also a substantial distribution of these receptors on primary afferent pain fibers, and their location here is thought to contribute to analgesic activity.

It is thought that agonist binding to these *alpha*-2 receptors results in activation of a G-protein-modulated second messenger system. However, depending on the particular *alpha* subunit—2a, 2b, or 2c—different physiologic consequences may occur, and responses can be either inhibitory or excitatory (109). For example, The *alpha*-2b "adrenoceptor" produces hemodynamic responses to the *alpha*-2 agonists, while the *alpha*-2a receptor is responsible for the anesthetic response (109). Thus, both neuronal activation and inactivation can occur and, depending on the system, may or may not produce analgesia. In other words, in an inhibitory system, neuronal inactivation would result in a net activation, and in an excitatory system, neuronal inactivation would result in net inhibition.

There is one agent, clonidine, that is routinely used for its analgesic properties. In particular, due to its effect on pain transmission through the spinal cord, it makes a useful adjunct in treating neuropathic pain. Clonidine may be administered by several different routes: orally, transdermally, epidurally, and intrathecally. Any dosing schedule is very carefully titrated because of the risks of hemodynamic consequences (orthostatic hypotension). Oral dosing is started at 0.1 mg twice per day up to 1–2 mg per day. Cutaneous patches are typically started at 0.1 mg/day/week and titrated up accordingly. Central delivery of these agents starts at approximately 10 mcg per day in trathecally and usually requires close monitoring for the first 24 to 48 hours to observe for hemodynamic disturbances and excessive sedation. Side effects to be expected can include sedation, bradycardia, and hypotension. Avoiding abrupt cessation of the drug should prevent rebound hypertension.

Another agent, dexmedetomidine, has only recently been approved by the FDA (December 1999) for clinical use as an intravenous preparation. Although it is currently being used for sedation and hemodynamic control, dexmedetomidine appears to have substantial application for analgesia given its selectivity for the *alpha*-2 receptor, approximately (1000 × alpha-2:alpha-1) (109). Again, any time a drug is as effective as another, or even more so, while having a more desirable side effect profile, then it would be preferable over the other. In other words, since dexmedetomidine is so much more *alpha*-2 selective, we would anticipate not only increased analgesic potency and efficacy, but also fewer non-*alpha*-2-related side effects.

CONCLUSIONS

We hope that after review of this chapter, the reader will come away with a sound understanding of the most commonly used analgesic agents and the basic science and clinical rationale behind their use. Although it is impossible to provide a complete review of all available therapies, our goal was to focus on the most practical and rational. In addition, we hope we have provided the reader with an understanding of some of the neurophysiology, neurochemistry, and neuroanatomy behind the efficacy of some of the pharmacological therapies used by the pain clinician.

It is clear from the rapidly expanding volume of material addressing pain medicine and pain research that we are in a germinal phase of our specialty. Although scientists and clinicians have been investigating and treating pain for over two decades, long before its popular acceptance, we still feel that we are at only the foothills of what will be a very exciting future for our discipline. We find it exhilarating that we may play even a small role in the expansion of the body of knowledge that will hopefully one day become a solid foundation for future pain clinicians and investigators.

ACKNOWLEDGMENT

U.S. Public Health Service Grant / NIH DA05784 to RWH supported this work.

REFERENCES

1. Altshuler D, Pollara VJ, Cowles CR, et al. An SNP map of the human genome generated by reduced representation shotgun sequencing. *Nature* 2000;407(6803):513–516.
2. Dunham I, Shimizu N, Roe BA, et al. The DNA sequence of human chromosome 22. *Nature* 1999;402(6761):489–495.
3. Tillman DB, Treede RD, Meyer RA, Campbell JN. Response of C fibre nociceptors in the anaesthetized monkey to heat stimuli: correlation with pain threshold in humans. *J Physiol (Lond,* 1995;485(pt 3): 767–774.
4. Bromm B, Treede RD. Nerve fibre discharges, cerebral potentials and sensations induced by CO2 laser stimulation. *Hum Neurobiol* 1984; 3(1)33–40.
5. LaMotte RH, Campbell JN. Comparison of responses of warm and nociceptive C-fiber afferents in monkey with human judgments of thermal pain. *J Neurophysiol* 1978;41(2):509–528.
6. Melzack R. Prolonged relief of pain by brief, intense transcutaneous somatic stimulation. *Pain* 1975;1(4):357–373.
7. Neumann S, Doubell TP, Leslie T, Woolf CJ. Inflammatory pain hypersensitivity mediated by phenotypic switch in myelinated primary sensory neurons. *Nature* 1996;384(6607):360–364.
8. Darian-Smith I. Thermal sensibility. In: Darian-Smith I, Brookhart JM, Mouncastle VB, eds. Handbook of physiology. Bethesda, MD: *American Physiological Society*, 1984:879–914.
9. Torebjork HE, Hallin RG. Perceptual changes accompanying controlled preferential blocking of A and C fibre responses in intact human skin nerves. *Exp Brain Res* 1973; 16(3):321–332.
10. Fields HL, ed. Pain syndromes in neurology. London: Butterworths, 1990.
11. Meyer RA, Campbell JN. Myelinated nociceptive afferents account for the hyperalgesia that follows a burn to the hand. *Science* 1981; 213(4515):1527–1529.
12. Garcia-Anoveros J, Derler B, Neville-Golden J, et al. BNaC1 and BNaC2 constitute a new family of human neuronal sodium channels related to degenerins and epithelial sodium channels. *Proc Natl Acad Sci USA* 1997;94(4):1459–1464.
13. Garcia-Anoveros J, Corey DP. The molecules of mechanosensation. *Annu Rev Neurosci* 1997;20:567–594.
14. Mano I, Driscoll M. DEG/ENaC channels: a touchy superfamily that watches its salt. *Bioessays* 1999;21(7):568–578.
15. Schumacher MA, Jong BE, Frey SL, et al. The stretch-inactivated channel, a vanilloid receptor variant, is expressed in small-diameter sensory neurons in the rat. *Neurosci Lett* 2000;287(3):215–218.
16. Caterina MJ, Schumacher MA, Tominaga M, et al. The capsaicin receptor: a heat-activated ion channel in the pain pathway. *Nature* 1997;389(6653): 816–824.
17. Hayes P, Meadows HJ, Gunthorpe MJ, et al. Cloning and functional expression of a human orthologue of rat vanilloid receptor-1. *Pain* 2000;88(2):205–215.
18. Helliwell RJ, McLatchie LM, Clarke M, et al. Capsaicin sensitivity is associated with the expression of the vanilloid (capsaicin) receptor (VR1) mRNA in adult rat sensory ganglia. *Neurosci Lett* 1998;250(3): 177–180.
19. Tominaga M, Caterina MJ, Malmberg AB, et al. The cloned capsaicin receptor integrates multiple pain-producing stimuli. *Neuron* 1998; 21(3):531–543.
20. Jacobus WE, Taylor GJ, Hollis DP, Nunnally RL. Phosphorus nuclear magnetic resonance of perfused working rat hearts. *Nature* 1977; 265(5596):756–758.
21. Caterina MJ, Leffler A, Malmberg AB, et al. Impaired nociception and pain sensation in mice lacking the capsaicin receptor. *Science* 2000; 288(5464):306–313.
22. Ma QP, Woolf CJ. Progressive tactile hypersensitivity: an inflammation-induced incremental increase in the excitability of the spinal cord. *Pain* 1996;67(1):97–106.
23. Basbaum AI. Spinal mechanisms of acute and persistent pain. *Reg Anesth Pain Med* 1999;24(1):59–67.
24. Torebjork HE, Lundberg LE, LaMotte RH. Central changes in processing of mechanoreceptive input in capsaicin-induced secondary hyperalgesia in humans. J *Physiol (Lond)* 1992;448:765–780.
25. Park TL. Effectiveness of a multidisciplinary program for the young and old with chronic pain. In: *American pain society*. 2000. Atlanta, 93.

26. Papaioannou A, Parkinson W, McCartney N, et al. Effects of home exercise on functional status of older women with back pain associated with osteoporosis related vertebral fractures. In: *American pain society*. 2000. Atlanta, 169.
27. Eappen S, Datta S. Pharmacology of Local Anesthetics. *Semin Anesth, Periop Med Pain* 1998;17(1):10–17.
28. Ragsdale DS, McPhee JC, Scheuer T, Catterall WA. Molecular determinants of state-dependent block of Na+ channels by local anesthetics. *Science* 1994;265(5179):1724–1728.
29. Butterworth JFT, Strichartz GR. Molecular mechanisms of local anesthesia: a review. *Anesthesiology* 1990;72(4):711–734.
30. Payne R. Limitations of NSAIDs for pain management: toxicity or lack of efficacy. *J Pain* 2000;1(3) (Suppl 1):14–18.
31. Patrignani P. Nonsteroidal anti-inflammatory drugs, COX-2 and colorectal cancer. *Toxicol Lett* 2000;112–113:493–498.
32. Leese PT, Hubbard RC, Karim A, et al. Effects of celecoxib, a novel cyclooxygenase-2 inhibitor, on platelet function in healthy adults: a randomized, controlled trial. *J Clin Pharmacol* 2000;40(2):124–132.
33. Marnett LJ, Kalgutkar AS. Cyclooxygenase 2 inhibitors: discovery, selectivity and the future. *Trends Pharmacol Sci* 1999;20(11):465–469.
34. Zhao ZQ, Yand HQ, Zhang KM, Zhuang XX. Release and depletion of substance P by capsaicin in substantia gelatinosa studied with the antibody microprobe technique and immunohistochemistry. *Neuropeptides* 1992;23(3):161–167.
35. Lynn B. Capsaicin: actions on nociceptive C-fibres and therapeutic potential. *Pain* 1990;41(1):61–69.
36. Simone DA, Khalili N, Brederson J-D, et al. Sensory functions of epidermal nerve fibers in humans. In: Devor M, Rowbotham MC, Wiesenfeld-Hallin Z, eds. *Proceedings of the 9th world congress on pain*. Seattle: IASP Press, 2000:207–213.
37. Wong H. Nonsteroidal anti-inflammatory drugs. In: Benson HT, ed. *Essentials of pain medicine and regional anesthesia*. New York: Churchill Livingston, 1999:74–77.
38. Melzack R, Wall PD. Pain mechanisms: a new theory. *Science* 1965;150(699): 971–979.
39. Werners R, Pynsent PB, Bulstrode CJ. Randomized trial comparing interferential therapy with motorized lumbar traction and massage in the management of low back pain in a primary care setting. *Spine* 1999;24(15):1579–1584.
40. Basbaum AI, Fields HL. Endogenous pain control systems: brainstem spinal pathways and endorphin circuitry. *Annu Rev Neurosci* 1984;7:309–338.
41. Proudfit HK. In: Fields HL, Besson J-M, eds., *Progress in brain research*. Elsevier: New York, 1988:357–370.
42. Yeung JC, Yaksh TL, Rudy TA. Concurrent mapping of brain sites for sensitivity to the direct application of morphine and focal electrical stimulation in the production of antinociception in the rat. *Pain* 1977;4(1):23–40.
43. Reynolds DV. Surgery in the rat during electrical analgesia induced by focal brain stimulation. *Science* 1969;164(878):444–445.
44. Beitz AJ. The nuclei of origin of brain stem enkephalin and substance P projections to the rodent nucleus raphe magnus. *Neuroscience* 1982;7(11):2753–2768.
45. Mansour A, Fox CA, Akil H, Watson SJ. Opioid-receptor mRNA expression in the rat CNS: anatomical and functional implications. *Trends Neurosci* 1995;18(1):22–29.
46. Beitz AJ, Mullett MA, Weiner LL. The periaqueductal gray projections to the rat spinal trigeminal, raphe magnus, gigantocellular pars alpha and paragigantocellular nuclei arise from separate neurons. *Brain Res* 1983;288(1–2):307–314.
47. Bajic D, Proudfit HK. Projections of neurons in the periaqueductal gray to pontine and medullary catecholamine cell groups involved in the modulation of nociception. *J Comp Neurol* 1999;405(3):359–379.
48. Gebhart GF. Recent developments in the neurochemical bases of pain and analgesia. *NIDA Res Monogr* 1983;45:19–35.
49. Skagerberg G, Bjorklund A. Topographic principles in the spinal projections of serotonergic and non-serotonergic brainstem neurons in the rat. *Neuroscience* 1985;15(2):445–480.
50. Basbaum AI, Clanton CH, Fields HL. Three bulbospinal pathways from the rostral medulla of the cat: an autoradiographic study of pain modulating systems. *J. Comp Neurol* 1978;178(2):209–224.
51. Light AR, Casale EJ, Menetrey DM. The effects of focal stimulation in nucleus raphe magnus and periaqueductal gray on intracellularly

52. recorded neurons in spinal laminae I and II. *J. Neurophysiol* 1986; 56(3):555–571.
52. Duggan AW, Griersmith BT. Inhibition of the spinal transmission of nociceptive information by supraspinal stimulation in the cat. *Pain* 1979;6(2):149–161.
53. Antal M, Petko M, Polgar E, et al. Direct evidence of an extensive GABAergic innervation of the spinal dorsal horn by fibres descending from the rostral ventromedial medulla. *Neuroscience* 1996;73:509–518.
54. Bowker RM, Abbott LC, Dilts RP. Peptidergic neurons in the nucleus raphe magnus and the nucleus gigantocellularis: their distributions, interrelationships, and projections to the spinal cord. *Prog. Brain Res* 1988;77:95–127.
55. Menetrey D, Basbaum AI. The distribution of substance P-, enkephalin- and dynorphin- immunoreactive neurons in the medulla of the rat and their contribution to bulbospinal pathways. *Neuroscience* 1987;23(1):173–187.
56. Kwiat GC, Basbaum AI. The origin of brainstem noradrenergic and serotonergic projections to the spinal cord dorsal horn in the rat. *Somatosens Mot Res* 1992;9(2):157–173.
57. Clark FM, Proudfit, HK. The projection of noradrenergic neurons in the A7 catecholamine cell group to the spinal cord in the rat demonstrated by anterograde tracing combined with immunocytochemistry. *Brain Res* 1991;547(2):279–288.
58. Yeomans DC, Clark FM, Paice JA, et al. Antinociception induced by electrical stimulation of spinally projecting noradrenergic neurons in the A7 catecholamine cell group of the rat. *Pain* 1992;48(3): 449–461.
59. Yeomans DC, Proudfit HK. Antinociception induced by microinjection of substance P into the A7 catecholamine cell group in the rat. *Neuroscience* 1992;9(3):681–691.
60. Abdi S, Lee DH, Chung JM. The anti-allodynic effects of amitriptyline, gabapentin, and lidocaine in a rat model of neuropathic pain. *Anesth Analg* 1998;87(6):1360–1366.
61. Sanchez C, Hyttel J. Comparison of the effects of antidepressants and their metabolites on reuptake of biogenic amines and on receptor binding. *Cell Mol Neurobiol* 1999;19(4):467–489.
62. Di Matteo V, Di Mascio M, Di Giovanni G, Esposito E. Acute administration of amitriptyline and mianserin increases dopamine release in the rat nucleus accumbens: possible involvement of serotonin2C receptors. *Psychopharmacology (Berl)* 2000;150(1):45–51.
63. Yau JL, Olsson T, Noble J, Seckl JR. Serotonin receptor subtype gene expression in the hippocampus of aged rats following chronic amitriptyline treatment. *Brain Res Mol Brain Res* 1999;70(2):282–287.
64. Rowbotham M, Harden N, Stacey B, et al. Gabapentin for the treatment of postherpetic neuralgia: a randomized controlled trial. *JAMA* 1998;280(21):1837–1842.
65. Backonja M, Beydoun A, Edwards KR, et al. Gabapentin for the symptomatic treatment of painful neuropathy in patients with diabetes mellitus: a randomized controlled trial. *JAMA* 1998;280(21):1831–1836.
66. Satzinger G. Antiepileptics from gamma-aminobutyric acid. *Arzneimittelforschung* 1994;44(3):261–266.
67. Suman-Chauhan N, Webdale L, Hill DR, Woodruff GN. Characterisation of [3H]gabapentin binding to a novel site in rat brain: homogenate binding studies. *Eur J Pharmacol* 1993;244(3):293–301.
68. Suzdak PD, Jansen JA. A review of the preclinical pharmacology of tiagabine: a potent and selective anticonvulsant GABA uptake inhibitor. *Epilepsia* 1995;36(6):612–626.
69. Tunnicliff G. Molecular basis of buspirone's anxiolytic action. *Pharmacol Toxicol* 1991;69(3):149–156.
70. Goldlust A, Su TZ, Welty DF, et al. Effects of anticonvulsant drug gabapentin on the enzymes in metabolic pathways of glutamate and GABA. *Epilepsy Res* 1995;22(1):1–11.
71. Su TZ, Lunney E, Campbell G, Oxender DL. Transport of gabapentin, a gamma-amino acid drug, by system l alpha-amino acid transporters: a comparative study in astrocytes, synaptosomes, and CHO cells. *J Neurochem* 1995;64(5):2125–2131.
72. Taylor CP, Gee NS, Su TZ, et al. A summary of mechanistic hypotheses of gabapentin pharmacology. *Epilepsy Res* 1998;29(3):233–249.
73. Gee NS, Brown JP, Dissanayake VU, et al. The novel anticonvulsant drug, gabapentin (Neurontin), binds to the alpha2delta subunit of a calcium channel. *J Biol Chem* 1996;271(10):5768–5776.
74. Neugebauer V, Vanegas H, Nebe J, et al. Effects of N- and L-type calcium channel antagonists on the responses of nociceptive spinal cord

neurons to mechanical stimulation of the normal and the inflamed knee joint. *J Neurophysiol* 1996;76(6):3740–3749.

75. Nebe J, Vanegas H, Schaible HG. Spinal application of omega-cono-toxin GVIA, an N-type calcium channel antagonist, attenuates enhancement of dorsal spinal neuronal responses caused by intra-articular injection of mustard oil in the rat. *Exp Brain Res* 1998;120(1):61–69.

76. Hunter JC, Gogas KR, Hedley LR, et al. The effect of novel antiepileptic drugs in rat experimental models of acute and chronic pain. *Eur J Pharmacol* 1997;324(2–3):153–160.

77. Jun JH, Yaksh TL. The effect of intrathecal gabapentin and 3-isobutyl gamma-aminobutyric acid on the hyperalgesia observed after thermal injury in the rat. *Anesth Analg* 1998;86(2):348–354.

78. Field MJ, McCleary S, Hughes J, Singh L. Gabapentin and pregabalin, but not morphine and amitriptyline, block both static and dynamic components of mechanical allodynia induced by streptozocin in the rat. *Pain* 1999;80(1–2):391–398.

79. Lefkowith J, Albrecht L, Wendt H, et al. Celecoxib is as effective as diclofenac for the treatment of acute pain of OA flare. In: *American pain society*. 2000. Atlanta, 97.

80. Morrison BW, Christensen S, Yuan W, et al. Analgesic efficacy of the cyclooxygenase-2-specific inhibitor rofecoxib in post-dental surgery pain: a randomized, controlled trial. *Clin Ther* 1999;21(6):943–953.

81. Hawkey CJ. COX-2 inhibitors. *Lancet* 1999;353(9149):307–314.

82. Hubbard R, Laurent A, Kuss M, et al. A pharmacokinetic study of analgesic doses of parecoxib, a new COX-2 specific inhibitor, in heathy subjects. In: *American pain society*. 2000. Atlanta,110.

83. Langeland F, Brown J, Waller P, et al. A comparative analgesic efficacy study of parecoxib, a new COX-2 specific inhibitor, in post-gynecologic surgery patients. In: *American pain society*. 2000. Atlanta, 180.

84. Kotani N, Kushikata T, Hashimoto H, et al. Intrathecal Methylprednisolone for Intractable Postherpetic Neuralgia. *N Engl J Med* 2000; 343(21):1514–1519.

85. Martin WR, Eades CG, Thompson JA, et al. The effects of morphine- and nalorphine-like drugs in the nondependent and morphine-dependent chronic spinal dog. *J Pharmacol. Exp Ther* 1976;197(3):517–532.

86. Lord JA, Waterfield AA, Hughes J, Kosterlitz HW. Endogenous opioid peptides: multiple agonists and receptors. *Nature* 1977;267(5611): 495–499.

87. Martin WR, Eades CG, Thompson WO. Morphine physical dependence in the dog. *J Pharmacol Exp Ther* 1974;189(3):759–771.

88. Change KJ, Cooper BR, Hazum E, Cuatrecasas P. Multiple opiate receptors: different regional distribution in the brain and differential binding of opiates and opioid peptides. *Mol. Pharmacol* 1979;16(1):91–104.

89. Chang KJ, Cuatrecasas P. Multiple opiate receptors. Enkephalins and morphine bind to receptors of different specificity. *J Biol Chem* 1979; 254(8):2610–2618.

90. Schulz R, Wuster M, Krenss H, Herz A. Selective development of tolerance without dependence in multiple opiate receptors of mouse vas deferens. *Nature* 1980;285(5762):242–243.

91. Zaki PA, Bilsky EJ, Vanderah TW, et al. Opioid receptor types and subtypes: the δ opioid receptor as a model. *Ann Rev Pharmacol Toxicol* 1996;36:379–401.

92. Paul D, Bodnar RJ, Gistrak MA, Pasternak GW. Different mu receptor subtypes mediate spinal and supraspinal analgesia in mice. *Eur J Pharmacol* 1989;168(3):307–314.

93. Gintzler AR, Pasternak GW. Multiple mu receptors: evidence for mu2 sites in the guinea pig ileum. *Neurosci Lett* 1983;39(1): 51–56.

94. Pasternak GW. Pharmacological mechanisms of opioid analgesics. *Clin Neuropharmacol* 1993;16(1):1–18.

95. Chen Y, Mestek A, Liu J, Hurley JA, Yu L. Molecular cloning and functional expression of a mu-opioid receptor from rat brain. *Mol Pharmacol* 1993;44(1):8–12.

96. Chen Y, Mestek A, Liu J, Yu L. Molecular cloning of a rat kappa opioid receptor reveals sequence similarities to the mu and delta opioid receptors. *Biochem J* 1993;295(pt 3):625–628.

97. Kieffer BL, Befort K, Gaveriaux-Ruff C, Hirth CG. The delta-opioid receptor: isolation of a cDNA by expression cloning and pharmacological characterization. *Proc Natl Acad Sci U S A* 1992;89 (24):12048–12052.

98. Mollereau C, Parmentier M, Mailleux P, et al. ORL1, a novel member of the opioid receptor family. Cloning, functional expression and localization. *FEBS Lett* 1994;341(1):33–38.

99. Standifer KM, Pasternak GW. G proteins and opioid receptor-mediated signalling. *Cell Signal* 1997;9(3-4):237–248.

100. Henry DJ, Grandy DK, Lester HA, et al. Kappa-opioid receptors couple to inwardly rectifying potassium channels when coexpressed by Xenopus oocytes. *Mol Pharmacol* 1995;47(3):551–557.

101. Tallent M, Dichter MA, Bell GI, Reisine T. The cloned kappa opioid receptor couples to an N-type calcium current in undifferentiated PC-12 cells. *Neuroscience* 1994;63(4):1033–1040.

102. Piros ET, Prather PL, Law PY, et al. Voltage-dependent inhibition of Ca2+ channels in GH3 cells by cloned mu- and delta-opioid receptors. *Mol Pharmacol* 1996;50(4):947–956.

103. North RA. Opioid actions on membrane ion channels. In: Herz A, ed. *Handbook of experimental pharmacology*. Berlin: Springer-Verlag, 1993:773–797.

104. Corbett AD, Gillan MGC, Kosterlitz HW, et al. Selectivities of opioid peptide analogues as agonists and antagonists at the δ-receptor. *Br J Pharmacol* 1984;83:271–279.

105. Hughes J, Smith TW, Kosterlitz HW, et al. Identification of two related pentapeptides from the brain with potent opiate agonist activity. *Nature* 1975;258(5536):577–580.

106. Zadina JE, Hackler L, GE L-J, Kastin AJ. A potent and selective endogenous agonist for the μ-opiate receptor. *Nature* 1997;386: 499–502.

107. Mironer Y, Brown C, Satterthwaite J, et al. Relative misuse potential of different opioids: A large pain clinic experience. In: *American pain society*. 2000. Atlanta, 128.

108. Pasternak GW. Multiple morphine and enkephalin receptors and the relief of pain. *Jama* 1988;259(9):1362–1367.

109. Kamibayashi T, Maze M. Clinical uses of alpha2-adrenergic agonists. *Anesthesiology* 2000;93(5):1345–1349.

CHAPTER 3

The Psychology of Pain

Angela J. Koestler and Daniel M. Doleys

A 35-year-old electrician sustained a work-related injury to his lower back and subsequently underwent a laminectomy. His pain intensity level decreased significantly following surgery, but began to worsen 3 months later. Six months postsurgery he described a pain level of 8 on a 0-to 10-point scale. Following further medical evaluation by four physicians, he was diagnosed with "failed back" and was referred to a multidisciplinary pain center 2 years after his initial injury. He presented with intense pain that ranged from a 7 to a 10. Although no history of depression was reported, the patient presented with vegetative symptoms of depression and admitted to suicidal ideation. He stated, "I've never had any depression. I've always worked and I've never been sick." He was selling his home as he was 2 months behind on the payments and was concerned that he may lose his truck. Although his wife was employed, she was making minimum wage, and they had three children below the age of 12. The patient frequently commented, "nothing helps my pain. My life is ruined. I can't work. I can't help around the house. I can't play with my kids. They'd be better off without me." His wife was quite angry that "no one" would help her husband and "fix the problem." She was also angry with the insurance company and stated, "Our check is always late and sometimes they don't send it." Shortly after the patient was injured, he was fired from his job. The patient had retained an attorney and was planning to file for temporary disability.

A forklift operator injured his lower back at work and after 2 months of conservative treatment underwent a laminectomy. His pain intensity level decreased significantly following surgery, but would fluctuate in intensity and worsen at times in the evening. After participating in a physical therapy program, he returned to his job approximately 6 months after his initial injury. The patient stated, "My employer is very supportive and is willing to work with the temporary restrictions given me by the physician until I'm up to full steam. My pain interferes with my job

sometimes, but my job helps me keep my mind off my pain. Work isn't as easy as it was before, but it's all going to be okay."

A middle-aged woman developed mild to moderate abdominal pain with nausea that persisted for several days. She attributed her pain to a virus. Although her symptoms were uncomfortable, she continued in her normal activities and felt her problem would eventually subside.

A 58-year-old female developed mild to moderate abdominal pain with nausea that persisted for several days. She became extremely focused on her pain and quite anxious. With a history of ovarian cancer in her family, she was quite fearful that something could be terribly wrong with her. She saw her physician who told her she had a virus. Although he reassured her that it was unlikely her symptoms represented anything to be concerned about since several patients had recently presented with similar symptoms, she continued to be preoccupied with her pain and felt she should see a specialist.

Johnny was a top-notch soccer player and was on a select team. They were in the play-offs for the district championship. In the final game his team was tied 2 to 2 with only minutes left in the game. While attempting to make a goal, he was fouled by another player who tripped him and fell on top of him. Johnny played hard for the remaining time and scored the final point for his team's victory. While celebrating with his team at dinner, he rose from his chair and found that his leg was very stiff and that it was quite painful to walk. After medical evaluation several days later, he was scheduled for anterior cruciate ligament (ACL) reconstruction and was also treated for a sprained wrist. He asked the physician how long his recovery period would be as practice for the next soccer season was scheduled to begin in 3 months.

Mr. Smith was painting the eaves of his home when he slipped and fell off of a ladder. He twisted his knee and felt immediate, unbearable pain. After sitting on the ground for several minutes rubbing his knee, he called to his wife to help him. His wife drove him to the emergency room of the local hospital where after evaluation he was told that he probably needed surgery for an ACL tear. Mr. Smith asked if they could give him crutches and wrap his knee in a supportive bandage as he was afraid he might fall. He also stated that his pain was unbearable and he needed medication.

People respond differently to pain, despite similarities in the characteristics and course of the pain or in the medical interventions rendered. Throughout history a variety of reasons have been attributed to the occurrence and persistence of pain. It has been viewed as a form of possession or spiritual punishment, as well as the result of character deficiencies and emotional illness. Thirty years ago this chapter, "The Psychology of Pain," would not have appeared in the foundations section of a text on pain. If included, the chapter, or more likely a section, would have reviewed psychopathological states related to the production or continuation of physical symptoms and complaints without known organic cause.

Previously, the biomedical model and specificity theory were of primary influence on approaches to pain treatment and research. Both theoretical models developed from Descartes's conceptualization of the mind and body as separate entities. According to these models, physical complaints and symptoms are viewed as either somatogenic (originating from the body) or psychogenic (originating from the mind). A patient's symptoms are assumed to be directly related to a specific disease state that can be confirmed by medical evaluation. The physician's role is therefore to determine the source of the complaint, diagnose, and implement medical intervention directed toward correcting the pathology, thereby eliminating the patient's symptoms.

Specificity theory and earlier pain models support a view that the level of pain an individual experiences varies in accordance with the degree of actual tissue damage. Pain receptors in body tissue project by pain fibers and a pain pathway to a pain center in the brain. The analogy of a telephone system has been used to suggest that if the wire transmitting the message is cut, the transmission is interrupted and stopped. This implies that a painful condition should be eliminated through appropriate medical treatment or surgical intervention. For instance, if someone were complaining of back pain thought to be generated from a herniated disk, repair or removal of that disk should eliminate the pain. Or, in the case of nerve pain, the pain should be eliminated if the nerve were severed or ablated. Again, the presentation of symptoms should be in direct correlation to the injury or amount of tissue damage sustained. Previously, if pain persisted after medical intervention, the patient was thought to be exaggerating or malingering and was assigned a psychiatric label, such as hysteria. Although a paradigm shift is underway, these positions continue to receive some support today.

Beginning with the observations of several physicians, particularly during and after World War II, of individuals whose injuries could not explain the amount of or lack of pain they experienced, traditional pain theories and disease models began to fall under greater scrutiny and the role of psychological variables began to be seen as possibly instrumental to the understanding of pain. As in the examples of Johnny and Mr. Smith, individuals vary in their responses to injury and pain. Tissue damage is not always a predictor of when and how an individual will experience pain. Cognitive variables, such as attention and meaning, appear to affect individual responses. Additionally, psychosocial and environmental influences, such as relationships with employers, spouses, insurance companies, attorneys, and health care providers, may influence treatment outcome and return to work in work-related injuries. Why did treatment outcome differ for the two workers who sustained similar work injuries and received similar treatment?

The introduction and subsequent modifications of the gate control theory of pain (1–6) have underscored the complexity of pain and expanded pain from an entirely sensory phenomenon to a multidimensional one. The gate control theory has generated interest in rethinking the physiological mechanisms of pain to include psychological processes. Today, pain is seen as an ongoing chain of events that can be modified by ascending and descending activity in the central nervous system. Psychological processes are considered an integral part of pain perception and not merely a reaction to pain. With imaging technology, areas of the brain are being investigated that may play a crucial role in identifying the reciprocal and interactive nature of psychological variables in the perception of pain. This chapter will review theoretical models related to understanding the psychology of pain and psychological factors that have been found to influence pain and suffering.

THEORIES OF PAIN

Gate Control Theory

There are, in fact, many types of theories (7). Some provide a generalized explanatory principle, whereas others refer to a group of logically organized laws, and yet others merely summarize statements that give order to a cluster of empirically developed laws. Our own "theory" of pain, regardless of how well formalized, will influence our approach to patients (8). Those without, or who claim to be "eclectic," may have both feet firmly planted in mid-air. Scientific advancement in a specific area may, at least in part, be judged by the longevity of any particular theory. One would expect the theories and concepts to evolve coincident with cumulative observations and advancing technology. This is no less true in the study of pain (9).

Descartes (10) is credited with one of the earliest formulations of the theory of pain. His specificity theory encouraged the notion that injury activates very specific pain receptors or fibers, which in turn project unencumbered impulses to pain centers in the brain. This theory remained relatively unchallenged until the middle 1900s. Central summation, reverberatory circuits, and pattern theory emerged as possible alternatives (6). These, however, gave way to what has become one of the most widely known and heuristic theories, the *gate control theory* (1). In general, the gate control theory hypothesized that pain was initiated by nerve impulses from afferent fibers in the periphery to spinal cord transmission cells modulated by a spinal gating mechanism in the dorsal horn of the spinal cord. This gating mechanism was in turn influenced by large- and small-diameter fibers. Large fibers tended to inhibit transmission (close the gate) while small-fiber activity facilitated transmission (open the gate). Furthermore, it was recognized that nerve impulses descending from the brain could also influence this mechanism. It was noted that certain fibers could activate cognitive processes, which in turn could modulate the activity of the spinal gating mechanism. When the output of the transmission cell exceeded a critical value, the system was put into motion. The acknowledgment of this type of modulatory system gave credibility to the influences of psychological factors. This was a clear departure from previous thinking. Shortly after, Melzack and Casey (2) advanced the notion of three specialized systems in the brain involved in the processing of nociceptive stimulation, which included the sensory-discriminative, motivational-affective, and cognitive-evaluative systems. The experience of pain, while remaining basically subjective, was catapulted from the arena of unimpaired sensory transmission to a complex interaction between peripheral and central nervous system mechanisms. Suddenly, there was a framework for understanding the commonly observed variation in individual responses to comparable pain-inducing injuries.

The gate control theory emphasized the dynamic relationship among sensory input, affect, cognitions, and observable behavior. No longer was pain a static reflexive response. The implications for developing a broader range of therapeutic interventions were obvious. Expectations, learning, and past experiences began to take on importance heretofore unimagined.

The gate control theory, however, was not without its critics (11,12). The theory has undergone critical analysis and modification as a result of new scientific data. It is highly unlikely that Melzack and Wall expected it to remain unchanged. Indeed, this is highlighted by Melzack's own recent formulation in which he postulates the existence of a neuromatrix, defined as a network of neurons consisting of loops between the thalamus and cortex, and cortex and limbic system. Repeated processing and synthesis of nerve impulses results in the development of a characteristic pattern labeled by Melzack as a *neurosignature* (6). It is the activation of these neurosignatures that may account for certain types of pain experiences.

Biopsychosocial Model

The gate control theory of pain helped to provide a framework within which to understand the complex and dynamic relationship between nerve impulses created by the activation of peripheral nociceptors (i.e., nociception) and the experience of pain. The awareness of the role of psychological processes encouraged the development of a biopsychosocial perspective of pain (13). Heretofore, the medical model emphasized the relationship between anatomic and physiologic abnormalities in the experience of pain. It restricted the view of pain therapies to the arena of medical interventions, including surgical and pharmacological. There is somewhat of a reawakening of this view. However unintended, the current jargon that encourages the identification of a "pain generator" through provocative testing (e.g., discography) or disruptive procedures (e.g., selective nerve root blocks) can, in the absence of equal emphasis on psychological and social contributions, return us to a Descartian approach wherein the disruption of impulses seems to be the most if not only logical approach to "pain management." The biopsychosocial perspective reminds us that pain, whether acute or chronic, caused by cancer or nonmalignant factors, is always a product of the societal attitude and guidelines regarding pain and disability (14). Societies with governmental agencies and laws designed to support the disabled or impaired individual, such as workers' compensation and Social Security disability, may experience a higher percentage of pain and disability in response to similar injuries compared to societies with no such programs. Some patients develop an attitude of entitlement in these circumstances. This possibility itself creates another maladaptive reaction. That is, claims adjusters and others involved in the adjudication of such programs are susceptible to overgeneralization, assuming that any and all patients eligible for support, such as workers' compensation, are motivated only by financial gain and in fact have no medical basis for their complaints and disability.

We hope that this brief discussion not only highlights but justifies the importance of applying the biopsychosocial model in the assessment and treatment of the patient with pain. Furthermore, the existence of a particular factor does not automatically imply its relevance. The relative contribution of biological, psychological, and sociological factors may be ever changing. However elusive the goal may be, we must continue to understand patients with pain in this context.

PSYCHOLOGICAL THEORY

Learning/Conditioning

The manner in which organisms come to know what they know and behave as they do is the proper subject matter of psychology, more specifically learning theory. Early explanations, such as those of Darwin and Freud, seemed either unsatisfactory or lacking in scientific foundation. The early 1900s witnessed an unprecedented interest in the scientific analysis of human behavior. Scientifically rigorous experiments under controlled laboratory conditions involving both human and animal subjects began to discover predictable and lawful patterns. As these observations were formalized, they gave way to theories of learning and principles of conditioning.

In general, there are three conditioning paradigms: instrumental, operant, and classical conditioning. Many of the early experiments conducted by researchers such as Thorndike, Hall, Spence, and Watson required the organism to engage in some response that was instrumental in achieving or producing an outcome, thus the term *instrumental conditioning* (15). Negotiating mazes of different complexity, discrimination tasks, and serial learning were commonly relied upon experimental strategies. Skinner (16) became interested in developing a field of study examining behavior in an ongoing fashion rather than through discreet trials. He wished to observe the effects of various contingencies on behavior and outcomes. He referred to these behaviors as *operants,* indicating the importance of how the organism operates in the environment. This approach formed the basis for operant conditioning, which became characterized by the specification of presenting contingencies in a structured fashion in an effort to define relationships between these contingencies and behavior. Both instrumental and operant conditioning differed from classical conditioning. The classical conditioning paradigm examined the apparent inextricable and reflexive relationship between physiological responses and their eliciting stimuli. The parameters governing this apparent reflexive relationship became the subject of study.

Operant Conditioning

There are several basic principles/procedures in operant conditioning (16–18). The principle of reinforcement states that whenever a behavior is followed by desirable consequences, it is likely to be strengthened or increased in frequency. Therefore, the occurrence of pain behaviors such as grimacing, posturing, guarding, or verbal utterances, is likely to occur with more regularity even in the absence of identifiable physical pathology if followed by reinforcing consequences such as attention, massage, and medication. The manner in which these consequences are programmed constitutes *schedules of reinforcement* (19). Schedules of reinforcement may be based on the number or frequency of a response (i.e., ratio schedules of reinforcement) or on the first response occurring after a specific time (i.e., interval schedules of reinforcement). In some instances, the number of responses or time interval required is *fixed* and in others may be unpredictable or *variable*. Skinner and others (16,18,19) have repeatedly demonstrated the influence of these schedules of reinforcement on behavior. The strongest and most robust behavior is generated by provid-

ing immediate and frequent reinforcement initially, and then gradually "thinning" the schedule of reinforcement. These behaviors are most resistant to extinction, or the removal of reinforcement. The pattern created is reminiscent of addictive behavior seen in gamblers wherein the payoff, although inevitable, is highly unpredictable.

Another principle of operant conditioning is negative reinforcement. This principle describes the strengthening of behavior, such as rest or inactivity, by virtue of being associated with avoidance or withdrawal of negative, aversive, or punitive consequences. In the clinical setting, a patient may continue to experience or report pain if it results in the avoidance of unpleasant work (20). Fordyce and colleagues (21) noted that patients scoring high on scale 3 of the Minnesota Multiphasic Personality Inventory, the hysteria scale, were more likely to perceive life circumstances as undesirable and tended to demonstrate higher complaints of pain and disability. Perhaps, what is viewed as a "hysterical personality" may in fact be a pattern of behavior that was strongly reinforced by the immediate removal of undesirable tasks in response to even minimal objection.

Punishment is another well-recognized principle. It states that any behavior followed by negative or aversive consequences will diminish in strength or frequency. To the extent that patients perceive or experience the loss or reduction of income, absenteeism from work, or negative comments from co-workers as negative, one would predict a lower rate of pain behavior. This is often seen in sporting events where athletes are admonished by their fellow players and sometimes coaches if they complain of pain and do not practice or play because of it. It is important to remember that the presentation of an aversive event, that is, punishment, may result in a variety of emotional responses. This is easily observed when animals are exposed to a painfully, though not necessarily damaging, brief electric shock. We do not ordinarily think of human behavior in these terms. Nonetheless, a negative reaction to a patient's complaint of pain, such as questioning the authenticity of their pain, may result in a variety of emotional responses, including depression or aggression.

The withdrawal of positive reinforcement is referred to as extinction. This has been viewed as one mechanism of treating pain behavior. Behavioral research has identified what is referred to as an *extinction burst* characterized by an increase in the targeted behavior and perhaps accompanying emotional behavior when extinction is introduced (18). This may help to explain why patients in our experience appear, at least initially, to complain more and evidence greater distress when introduced to a therapeutic environment wherein the customary rewards (e.g., spousal attention, avoidance of activity, uncontrolled consumption of medications) are no longer present.

Another important and relevant concept is that of *stimulus control*. Simply stated, this principle notes the relationship between certain antecedent conditions and the presence of specific responses. For example, behaviors such as complaining, rubbing, or grimacing may become associated with certain external or internal events, settings, or circumstances. Research has documented differential frequency and probabilities of these pain behaviors in the presence of an attentive versus inattentive spouse (22,23). The differential application of reinforcement across different situations (e.g., physician's office, workplace, social settings, and home) may help to explain the frequently observed inconsistencies in patients' pain behaviors. These inconsistencies are often interpreted as evidence of malingering or symptom magnification when, in fact, they may present direct evidence of the role of conditioning and be unrelated to any deliberate attempt at dissimulation or misrepresentation.

Fordyce was one of the first to elaborate the potential role of conditioning theory and principles, and in particular operant conditioning, to the problem of chronic pain (24). For example, Fordyce noted that patients were more likely to exercise to a specific number of repetitions or duration. If patients were responding only to the experience of pain or some internal sensation, the termination point of exercise would be expected to be randomly distributed. Expanding on this observation, Doleys and colleagues (25) demonstrated the benefit of utilizing a quota system, that is, preexercise goals, in rehabilitation. Despite the fact that various pain behaviors could be shown to be related to environmental versus internal circumstances, such behavior continues to be used to justify invasive procedures such as surgery. There is no reason to believe that verbal behavior cannot be brought under the control of external versus internal (physiological) stimuli. In this case, a patient's description of pain as having burning, shooting, electrical qualities thought to correlate with neuropathic or nerve-related pain may be a product of the situation (i.e., physical examination and prior consequences). To assume that such statements are somewhat different from other behavior and reflect a one-to-one correspondence to physiological events may be an error. In the same fashion that morphological findings do not necessarily correlate with the experience of pain (26), so it is that pain behaviors do not always correlate with subjective pain ratings (27).

In summarizing learning or conditioning factors as they relate to pain, Fordyce has identified four key principles. First, in the operant-respondent distinction, respondents have their specific stimuli and occur automatically when the stimulus is adequate. Respondents can, therefore, be said to be controlled by antecedent stimuli. Operants, in contrast, are responsible to the influence of the consequences that systematically follow their occurrence. Second, conditioning effects are temporary in that they can be made stronger or weaker by virtue of arranging the stimuli and consequences. Third, conditioning effects are generally related to specific stimulus conditions under which they arise. And, fourth, stimuli that are present when positive or negative consequences are applied may acquire pos-

itive or negative properties of their own. This phenomenon, referred to as *conditioned* or secondary reinforcement or punishment, has been well studied (28–29). Although there may be controversy over the meaning and emphasis on overt behaviors in the analysis of pain and pain management (30,31), the validity and reproducibility of these principles and their effects are undeniable.

The above represents only a subset of operant conditioning principles. In effect, there are no less than 16 operant conditioning procedures (32). Many of these procedures have not been systematically applied to the study of pain and pain behavior. Their presence, however, must be acknowledged when performing a *functional analysis*. A functional analysis is a systematic analysis of the relationship among behaviors (overt or covert), their controlling antecedents (discriminative stimuli), and consequences (over or covert) (33). These principles have been demonstrated to be effective at modifying not only observable overt behavior, but also covert or cognitive behavior and psychological activity. As can be imagined, a true functional analysis of pain behavior is much more complicated than merely hypothesizing the reinforcing aspects of attention or financial gain (17,24,27,34,35). The potential relevance of operant conditioning procedures and principles is only now beginning to be realized. A good deal of evidence, for example, supports the notion of conditioned nociception (36).

Classical Conditioning

Classical conditioning represents a quite different paradigm in learning theory. Perhaps the most recognizable example is that of Pavlov (37) in which the presentation of food to a dog resulted in the reflexive response of salivation. By associating a bell with the food, the bell eventually came to elicit salivation in the absence of food. In this experiment, the food represented the unconditioned stimulus (UCS), so defined because it automatically elicits a predictable response, unconditioned response (UCR). The bell or conditioned stimulus (CS), which previously had no effect on salivation, through repeated association or pairing with food eventually comes to acquire the property of being able to elicit all or some of the same degree of salivation, conditioned response (CR), as previously provoked only by the food.

There are a variety of variations on this typical paradigm. For example, forward conditioning is defined by the conditioned stimulus (CS) always preceding the unconditioned stimulus (UCS). In backward conditioning, the UCS precedes the CS. This latter method has proven much less effective in producing a conditioned response. A second subtype is defined by the duration of the CS. In delayed conditioning, the CS comes on prior to the UCS and continues until the UCS is present. By contrast, in trace conditioning, the CS is presented only momentarily and terminated prior to the onset of the UCS. These various methodologies and manner in which they compare and contrast with instrumental and operant conditioning have been the subject of systematic investigation for decades (38).

Such principles have formed the foundation for certain behavioral therapy techniques such as systematic desensitization. For example, patients experiencing the unfortunate consequence of nausea secondary to chemotherapy often experience a similar response even upon approaching the facility wherein chemotherapy is given. Once chemotherapy has been concluded, it may take repeated trips to this same facility before this conditioned nausea is extinguished. Similarly, it is not improbable that the stimuli associated with acute pain states, including emergency rooms, doctors' offices, hospital beds, and the like, may come to elicit the experience of pain even in the presence of resolving pathology. *Preemptive analgesia*, administration of anesthetics and analgesics preoperatively, in part is an attempt to control and suppress the experience of postoperative pain so as to minimize the development of these types of associations.

The classical conditioning paradigm has been repeatedly applied in pharmacological studies. Various conditioned stimuli, including tactile and visual, when paired with morphine may eventually come to elicit a similar analgesic response (39–40). In some cases, the presentation of a CS in association with the morphine has actually resulted in a state of hyperalgesia or enhanced pain (41). Valone and colleagues (42) provided an illustration of conditioned analgesia in rats. In this experiment, banana extract odor served as the CS and was associated with the presentation of morphine (US). The hot-plate test was used in which analgesia was defined as the latency between the presentation of aversive heat to the rat's paw and the paw-lick response. After only four CS–UCS pairings, the banana extract odor (CS) resulted in a delayed latency, characteristic of the morphine injection and considered to be evidence of analgesia. Such experiments are common and have formed the basis for explaining certain outcomes in pharmacotherapy (43). Classical conditioning paradigms have been used as a framework to understand the often-observed placebo response (44–45). This explanation has not been without its critics (46). In some instances, however, it has been incorporated into the broader theory, such as the psychological behaviorism explanation of the placebo effect (47).

A wide variety of responses are susceptible to conditioning. There is evidence of alteration in neurochemical activity, such as the release of cholecystokinin (CCK) that is frequently associated with the development of tolerance and/or hyperalgesia (48). Further evidence of the impact of classical conditioning was recently presented in an article demonstrating the activation of "addiction centers" of the brain as measured by functional MRI (fMRI) when cocaine addicts were merely exposed to videotaped representations of cocaine paraphernalia compared to neutral videotapes (49).

Most often it is the combination of operant and classical conditioning that has drawn attention. The importance of learning theory and its principles is dramatically stated by Birbaumer and Flor (36) as they note ". . . these learning induced alterations have not only been demonstrated for behavioral expressions of pain, but also for accompanying physiological and neurochemical changes and the central mechanism of these learned changes in pain sensitivity . . ." (p. 442). Generalization of learned pain sensitivity, hyperalgesia, hypoalgesia, and central reorganization have been demonstrated via the application of these conditioning principles.

Social Learning Theory

The social learning approach assumes that human behavior is developed and maintained by three separate but interactive systems (50). These systems include response patterns regulated through pained experience (i.e., classical conditioning); the influence of external reinforcement (i.e., operant conditioning); and regulatory influences brought about by cognitive remediational processes. The latter is deemed to be the most important. In this context, environmental events acquire their importance largely through cognitive processes. These processes determine which events will be attended to, how they will be perceived, and the effect they will have on future action. Classical conditioning does not occur automatically but is attributed to self-activated, learned expectations. Likewise, reinforcement is viewed not as an event that automatically strengthens behavior but as a source of information and incentives used by the organism to regulate its own behavior.

Some of the more common principles of social learning theory include modeling and vicarious learning. Learning, in this case, occurs predominantly through observation. Individuals observing the presence of pain or suffering behavior in response to a procedure they are yet to be exposed to may report and/or experience a greater intensity of pain than would be the case if observing a more stoic model.

In this model of behavior, cognitive processes and environmental factors are interactive. The individual is neither driven by irresistible internal forces nor a mere passive reactor to environmental events. Cognitive processes assume a central role in explaining learning experiences and their lasting effects.

Some of the key concepts in the social learning model are self-efficacy and expectancy. Briefly, self-efficacy relates to the individual's belief in his or her ability to respond in a beneficial and adaptive fashion to a given situation or set of circumstances (51). Expectancy or expectations may be related to and include such phenomenon as beliefs, anticipations, and appraisals. Expectancy theory has formed the cornerstone of one approach to the placebo effect (52,53). The assessment and modification of these beliefs, expectations, appraisals, and attributions have occupied center stage in cognitive behavioral therapy (54).

Self-expectancies and anticipatory concern (e.g., fear as to the consequences of engaging in certain activities) were examined in a series of studies by Dolce and Doleys. Self-expectancies were found to be a better predictor of cold pain tolerance in college students than subjective pain ratings (55). The use of preset exercise quotas in the treatment of chronic pain patients was shown to be associated with an increase in positive self-expectancies and a decrease in the level of anticipatory concern (56). Finally, self-efficacy and anticipatory concern ratings were found to be positively correlated with medication use, exercise levels, and work status 6 to 12 months posttreatment. However, these variables did not account for a significant amount of the variance in a regression model (57).

To some degree, when we expound the effectiveness of a given pain management procedure, invite the patient to discuss this with someone who has undergone a successful outcome to a procedure, and identify all of the existing characteristics that are associated with positive outcomes, we are employing aspects of a social learning model. One should not find it surprising for a patient to mimic the pain behaviors of some other patient, deriving what the first patient would consider to be reinforcing consequences in response to the pain behaviors. This scenario is played out in pain clinic waiting rooms as patients discuss their various problems and witness the manner in which treatment may be differentially applied.

Summary

Learning and conditioning theories and principles have their foundation in and are considered part of the basic science of psychology. These principles have formed the basis for the development of a broad variety of therapeutic approaches applicable in the treatment of medical disorders (58). Systematic application of learning theory and principles has shown them to be effective in altering observable behavior and biochemical and physiological activity. To conceptualize these principles as applicable and of interest only in mutually observable behavior, such as groaning, posturing, and guarding, in the chronic pain patient is to impose unnecessary restrictions on their general applicability. This type of restrictive application is tantamount to saying that certain mathematical manipulations, such as addition and subtraction, only apply to a subset of physical objects when in fact such maneuvers have all but universal utility.

PSYCHOLOGICAL FACTORS

Affective Processes

According to the International Association for the Study of Pain, pain is "an unpleasant sensory and emotional experience associated with actual or potential tissue damage" (59). It is considered a subjective, perceptual experience characterized by sensory and affective qualities. That is, pain is experienced not only on a physical level (intensity, duration, location, and quality), but also with emotional feelings such as fear, despair, frustration, anger, anxiety, and depression.

The central and interactive roles of the sensory and affective dimensions of pain are widely supported (60). However, there continues to be some controversy regarding the separability of these two components and whether they can be measured independently (61). By definition, the physical sensation of pain evokes unpleasant emotion that in turn has an impact on sensory perception (62,63). Although there is interdependence, the separability of these dimensions has received support from studies using multivariate statistical analyses, signal detection, and paired scaling (60). For instance, factor analytic studies of the McGill Pain Questionnaire (MPQ) descriptors provided evidence of independent measurability, suggesting a *pure* affective factor (64–66).

The affective dimension of pain is considered the end product of multiple contributing processes, including the pain sensation itself, arousal, autonomic and somatomotor activation, and cognitive appraisal, which is considered most critical (67,68). Several authors have proposed conceptual models that differentiate stages of pain affect in relation to the temporal progression of the pain experience (66–69). These models address questions about the relationship and interaction of affective and sensory variables.

Price (66,67) proposed that two quite different affective stages of pain exist. The first stage is related to the immediate appraisal and emotional reaction to the sensory feature of pain and the second stage is related to the longer term implications of having pain. Gracely (69) suggested three types of pain affect, which include feelings associated with the immediate pain sensation, feelings associated with the way in which pain experiences are cognitively integrated into an individual's life, and the adverse effects of chronic or severe pain on psychological health. Terms associated with immediate pain affect include unpleasantness, discomfort, aversive, and motivational. Uncertainty, fear, and dread are used to describe the second type of pain affect. The third affective stage in Gracely's model is characterized by depression, anhedonia, irritability, and paranoia.

Gatchel presented a broad conceptual model of three stages that may be involved in the transition from acute low back pain into chronic low back pain disability and accompanying psychosocial distress (68). Like Price and Gracely, Gatchel's model provides a description of pain affect following a continuum from initial noxious stimulation to more chronic pain states. Furthermore, all three models underscore the importance of cognitive variables in different stages of pain affect. Price suggested that cognitive factors affect both the immediate affective response to noxious stimuli and affective responses associated with later stages of the pain experience. Both Gracely and

Gatchel separate Price's second affective stage into two components that reflect subacute and chronic pain stages. Regardless of the model used to describe various phases or stages of pain affect, it appears that the identification of associated specific reactions and emotions are important to the development and application of appropriate treatment interventions and to the prevention of more chronic pain states.

Greater specificity and clarification are needed with regard to the terminology and definitions used in the literature and in future studies on pain affect. Gracely (69) suggested that the term *affective* is somewhat confusing as it has several different usages and all are applied at different times to describe pain experience. Within psychology and psychiatry *affective* is used to denote affective disorder or observable behavior as related to mood. *Affective* is also used to describe the "emotional component" of pain in immediate, acute, and chronic pain phases, but does not implicitly signify psychopathology or emotional disturbance. Gracely's point is important, particularly in view of the confusion that could arise among researchers, health care providers, and third-party entities. Additional clarification is also important with the use of other terms such as *emotional disturbance*.

As previously indicated, the affective dimension of pain includes many different emotions that primarily have an unpleasant and negative valence. Anxiety, depression, anger, fear, frustration, and other emotions have been investigated, but anxiety and depression have received the greatest amount of attention (70–80).

In definition, anxiety is a feeling of apprehension or fear occurring in conjunction with patterns of heightened autonomic arousal. It is associated both with increased pain perception, threat of bodily harm, increased risk to physical health, and the prolongation of the pain experience. Additionally, anxiety affects physiology and can increase the risk of other medical complications (81). For instance, cortically mediated increases in blood viscosity and clotting time, fibrinolysis, and platelet aggregation can lead to increased risk of thromboembolism. Anxiety can cause increases in the neuroendocrine secretion of catecholamines and cortisol, resulting in significant increases in cardiac output, abnormally high sympathetic tone, shock, excessive vasoconstriction, intestinal ischemia, and hypoxic tissue damage. Moreover, anxiety can lower the pain threshold, causing the patient to interpret any sensation as pain.

Anxiety has been studied more frequently in acute pain and injury and as it relates to fear/avoidance. Wall (5) proposed three stages of response following an acute injury that include the immediate, secondary, and tertiary stages. Individuals may report the absence of pain immediately after injury, which may represent an adaptive survival mechanism. The absence of pain in the immediate response stage may permit the individual to fight, escape, or seek help. The secondary response is marked by tissue damage, pain, and anxiety. It is during this phase that the individual can mentally process the events leading up to the injury and seek coping responses to aid in recovery. In the tertiary stage, the individual may experience limited activity, excessive sleep, poor appetite, and diminished attention span, which may serve a protective function of limiting mobility and preparing the body for recovery. This model suggests that anxiety plays a significant role in acute pain states, particularly in the secondary stage. Additionally, cognitive appraisal is involved in this stage and may serve to mediate anxiety.

Many individuals with pain experience symptoms of depression. As reported, authors suggest that the occurrence and severity of affective factors in pain patients are related to the severity or temporal progression of the pain condition (66–69). Whereas anxiety has been studied more frequently in patients with acute pain, more studies have investigated depression in chronic pain states. Investigators have shown that the incidence of depression is common among chronic pain patients (82–84). Depression has also been associated with specific pain conditions, including chronic abdominal pain (85), rheumatoid arthritis (86), and other musculoskeletal conditions (75).

The incidence of depression in chronic pain patients is reported to range from 10% to 100% (87) with most studies reporting prevalence rates between 30% and 60% (88). These variations appear related to the type of pain condition investigated, diagnostic criteria, assessment tools, and the population sample studied (75). Since chronic pain imposes significant limitations on patients' lives, it is puzzling why all patients do not experience depression. Several studies addressed this question and determined that patients who felt that they could continue to function despite their pain, and maintain some control over their pain and their lives, did not become depressed (89–90). Their appraisal of the pain and its impact was instrumental in mediating the pain–depression relationship.

Although the association between pain and depression is well established, the nature of the relationship remains unclear. Some researchers have inferred that depression precedes pain or that pain is an alternate expression of a depressive disturbance (75). Others have attempted to explain the relationship between pain and depression by suggesting a pain-prone disorder (71), somatization (91), psychogenic pain (92–94), masked depression (95), psychosomatic illness (96), and chronic pain syndrome (97).

A more widely held view of the pain–depression relationship is that the two are interrelated and interact on multiple levels. For instance, neurotransmitters involved in depression have also been implicated in the modulation of pain. This suggests that the transmission of pain signals may be altered by depressive disturbance, while nociceptive input may induce or exacerbate a depressed state (98). From a behavioral perspective, it has been suggested that depression occurs secondary to impaired social role performance and activity levels as a form of learned helplessness

(24,89). Furthermore, patients with somatosensory amplification have been found to have a greater propensity to experience and report depressive symptoms and pain. Somatosensory amplification is proposed to have both a trait component similar to neuroticism and a state component in which amplification covaries with psychological distress (99).

Currently, there is inadequate evidence to substantiate that depression precedes and generates pain. In most cases depression appears to be patients' reaction to pain and its consequences (72,100). Fields proposed a systems perspective, suggesting that pain and depression have reciprocal psychological effects. Pain may precipitate worry and pessimism, while depression impairs patients' ability to cope with pain. The combined action of chronic pain and depression contribute to increased deterioration and, ultimately, to decreased function and disability (101). In a review of epidemiological studies of the pain–depression relationship, VonKorff and Simon (73) concluded that pain and psychological illness have reciprocal psychological and behavioral effects on illness expression and adaptation, and pain has specific effects on emotional state and behavioral function.

Personality Factors

Many studies have suggested that personality disturbances precipitate and perpetuate pain (71,102–107), and others have shown that chronic pain patients exhibit a wide range of personality problems (108–111). Attempts have been made to identify personality factors associated with specific pain problems or to chronic pain in general (e.g., RA personality, pain-prone personality) (71).

In two studies (112,113) the relationship of extroversion and neuroticism on chronic pain was examined. In both cases, results showed that neither of these personality traits affects sensory mechanisms of nociceptive processes, but tend to exert their influence on later stages of the pain experience. These traits were shown to influence the ways in which people cognitively process the meanings and implications of pain on their lives. Although the studies demonstrated an association between these two personality factors and suffering, a causal relationship was not identified.

Gamsa (72) investigated the relationship between psychological factors and pain to assess the contribution of emotional disturbance to the perpetuation of pain. Overall, pain was related to more current depression and less current life satisfaction, but was not associated with personal history. Results of this study suggest that emotional disturbance in pain patients is more likely to be a consequence than a cause of chronic pain. Efforts to identify specific personality disturbances related to various pain problems have received little empirical support (72,100). For example, many studies suggesting that an underlying personality disturbance precedes pain have used inade-

quate conceptualizations and have other methodological problems (e.g., no controls, inappropriate assessment tools). Furthermore, Turk (13) has suggested that based on prior experiences, people develop unique ways of appraising information and coping with stress that influence their perceptions and responses to pain and suffering.

Cognitive Processes

Cognitive processes include beliefs and assumptions that influence the way an individual perceives and reacts to the world. They play a major role in the perception of pain by influencing mood and behavior. In turn, they directly affect people's response to pain from initial onset through acute and chronic pain stages. For instance, when individuals have pain, they actively respond by evaluating their condition and seeking an explanation of what is causing their discomfort. They then interpret and assign meaning to their pain. This interpretation is influenced by the socioenvironmental and interpersonal context in which the pain occurs, prior learning history, and the potential impact pain may have on their lives.

People respond differently to pain. Two individuals who sustain the same type of injury and receive similar interventions may have different treatment outcomes. One individual may view pain as disabling, whereas the other continues to function in spite of his or her pain and returns to a productive lifestyle. Several studies have shown that many individuals with chronic pain continue to function satisfactorily in daily activities (25,114) Furthermore, many people in the general population experience pain, but continue to work and rarely seek medical treatment (115). Variations in individuals' response to pain may be a function of cognitive factors that can serve to either promote adaptive functioning despite the presence of pain or lead to increased dysfunction and disability. A great deal of research has focused on identifying cognitive factors that contribute to pain and disability (e.g., 57, 116–120). These studies offer strong support that patients' cognitions (beliefs, attitudes, expectations) affect reports of pain, activity level, coping, and treatment outcome.

Cognitive theories relevant to pain and pain control have been reviewed by several authors (121,122). Included are theories developed by Ellis (123), Beck (124), Beck et al. (125,126), Roskies and Lazarus (127), Folkman (128), Folkman et al. (129), Lazarus and Folkman (130), Michenbaum (131,132), and Bandura (50,133,134). Overall, belief systems are thought to affect the appraisal of pain that in turn affects mood, behavior, and coping.

Beliefs

Beliefs are uniquely formed cognitive schemes that are shaped by sociocultural experiences and learning history. They form a person's perception of his or her relationship to the environment. Beliefs influence appraisal by determining what is factual about an event and by shaping an understanding of its meaning. As previously mentioned, beliefs, appraisals, and expectancies about the consequences of an event and the ability to cope with it may influence mood (123,135) and coping efforts (130,136). Negative thoughts that emphasize the catastrophic consequences of events and one's inability to control those consequences can lead to depression. Research has shown that the interpretation of pain as ongoing tissue damage, rather than the result of a stable condition, tends to increase suffering and dysfunction (137). Additionally, if patients are uncertain of what is wrong with them, they tend to negatively evaluate their own abilities to manage or decrease their pain (138).

The relationship between perceived pain control and pain has been supported by several studies. In a review of the literature, Jensen and colleagues (119) found that patients who endorse an internal locus of control and believe that they have control over pain appear to function better than those who do not. There is evidence that the specific expectation of uncontrollable pain stimulation may cause the following nociceptive input to be perceived as more intense (139,140). Turk (140) has suggested that patients who associate activity with pain may anticipate increased levels of pain when they begin an activity, and they may actually perceive higher levels of pain or avoid activity all together. Flor and Turk (117) examined the relationship between general and situation-specific pain-related cognitions, including convictions of personal control in patients with chronic low back pain and rheumatoid arthritis. They found that the general and situation-specific convictions of uncontrollability and helplessness were more highly related to pain and disability than disease-related variables for both samples.

Self-efficacy and Outcome Expectancies

Many studies have supported a relationship between self-efficacy and pain. Bandura (50) differentiated between an efficacy expectation and outcome expectancy. An outcome expectancy is defined as a person's estimate that a given behavior will lead to certain outcomes. An efficacy expectation is the conviction that one can successfully execute a behavior required to produce an outcome. This differentiation is important because individuals can come to believe that a particular action will produce certain outcomes, but question whether they can perform those activities.

According to Bandura (141), self-efficacy beliefs can bring relief from pain in three ways. First, those who believe they can relieve their pain are more likely to search for skills and information that will enable them to manage their pain and persist in those activities. Second, feelings of self-efficacy reduce expectations of distress along with anxiety and physical tension, which has positive effects on the relief of pain. Last, those with strong self-efficacy beliefs

tend to view unpleasant sensations as more benign and fear them less, which may lessen their pain levels.

Self-efficacy beliefs have been associated with less depression, stress, pain, and disability (120,142–144). In a longitudinal study, Keefe and Williams (144) found that high levels of coping efficacy were related to decreases in pain and negative mood among 53 rheumatoid arthritis patients. Kores and colleagues (120) asked two groups of chronic pain patients to rate their perceived ability to engage in five activities (walking, lifting, coping with pain, work and family, or avocational activities) during treatment in a multidisciplinary pain treatment program. In the first group, those with higher self-efficacy ratings displayed longer concurrent sitting and standing times than those with lower self-efficacy scores. These patients also rated themselves as having improved more in their ability to work, participate in social activities, and use fewer medications 3 to 11 months following treatment. In the second group of patients studied, measures of self-efficacy were associated with lower rates of observed pain behavior at 2- to 14-month follow-up.

With regard to outcome expectancies, social learning theory (50) has suggested that behaviors thought to have beneficial outcomes are more likely to occur than those thought to result in negative outcomes. Council and colleagues (116) found support for the hypothesis that self-efficacy expectancies mediate the relationship between outcome expectancies and functioning. For instance, patients' beliefs about the outcome of an activity on pain may influence their beliefs about their ability to engage in that activity, which then influences the actual initiation of a behavior.

Coping

Individuals who experience pain develop adaptive and maladaptive ways of coping with their pain and the effects it has on their lives. Coping is thought to affect pain perception, the ability to manage pain and pain tolerance, and activity level (122). In the literature on pain and coping, pain is defined as a source of stress, whereas coping is defined as purposeful overt (e.g., rest, activity, taking medication) and covert (e.g., self-statements, seeking information, problem solving) efforts to manage it (13,130).

Active or passive coping strategies may be employed by patients who have pain (145). Active pain coping is considered adaptive and requires the patient to assume self-management responsibilities. In contrast, passive coping is considered maladaptive and involves withdrawal from activities and dependency on others for pain relief. Studies have found active coping to be related to lower levels of pain severity, depression, and functional disability, whereas passive coping has been associated positively with greater pain and depression (74,145,146). Additionally, a review of the literature (54) demonstrated that if individuals are instructed in the use of adaptive coping strategies, pain intensity ratings decrease and pain tolerance increases.

Cognitive Errors

The assumption underlying the cognitive-behavioral therapies of Beck, Ellis, Goldfried, Meichenbaum, and Novaco suggests that how we act and feel depends on the way we think, specifically how we appraise the significance of encounters for our well-being (130). Cognitive errors are defined as negatively distorted beliefs about oneself or one's situation (123). Such errors have been shown to influence the severity and maintenance of depression (123,124, 147) These cognitive distortions include selective abstraction, in which the person ignores contradictory evidence and forms a conclusion about an event on the basis of an isolated negative detail; overgeneralization, whereby a general, negative conclusion is drawn from a single event and applied in an unjustified way to dissimilar situations; catastrophizing, in which the significance of a negative event is overestimated or magnified; and personalization, in which personal responsibility is inappropriately taken for a negative event.

The role of cognitive errors in the adjustment to chronic pain has been strongly supported by a number of studies. The Pain Anxiety Symptoms Scale (PASS) was developed to measure cognitive, physiologic, and motoric aspects of fear of pain (148). Correlations were found with measures of anxiety, cognitive errors, depression, and disability. A second study with chronic low back pain patients found a significant overlap between the Coping Strategies Questionnaire (CSQ) (149) factor catastrophizing and anxiety symptoms (150). Keefe and colleagues (151) examined the relationship between catastrophizing and adjustment in a longitudinal study and found that pain-related catastrophizing was associated positively with pain intensity, physical disability, and depression. Other studies have also supported a relationship between cognitive distortions and pain severity (117, 152), as well as depression (152–155).

Jensen and colleagues (119) summarized a review of the literature on cognitive errors by stating that more sophisticated longitudinal, path analytic, and mediational analyses suggest a strong relationship between negative thoughts and adjustment. The authors suggested that cognitive errors can predict long-term adjustment to chronic pain, mediate part of the relationship between disease severity and adjustment, and make a unique contribution (over and above other cognitive factors) to the prediction of adjustment.

CONCLUSIONS

We began this chapter with case examples that highlight the role of psychological, social, and environmental processes in the pain experience. Both the electrician and forklift operator sustained similar injuries and received similar treatments, but their treatment outcomes were not the same. In the case of abdominal pain, one patient viewed her pain as an interference, while the other inter-preted her pain as a symptom of a life-threatening disease. And with similar injuries, Johnny and Mr. Smith responded quite differently to their pain. Without question, individuals respond differently to pain and treatment interventions. As clearly stated elsewhere, we must work toward developing specific treatments for specific pain disorders tailored for specific patient populations. Furthermore, within specific patient populations, treatment must be individualized. Our approach to treatment must incorporate an understanding of the patient's cognitive and behavioral responses to pain and the sociocultural and environmental context within which it occurs.

Our understanding of the mechanisms of pain is incomplete, but our approaches to improving that understanding and ultimately finding ways of effectively alleviating human pain and suffering have greatly improved over the last few decades. It is in the coming together of thinking and research across multiple disciplines that we will unravel the complexities pain. In our respective disciplines, we must mete out the specifics of certain phenomenon, but not minimize or ignore outside factors that may play crucial roles in our outcomes. Both from a clinical and scientific position, we must not be so rigid in our haste to find answers or be influenced by sociocultural and economic forces that we relegate possible explanations as secondary or unimportant. Communication and cooperation among the many disciplines involved in research and treatment efforts are vital in successfully meeting the challenges that lay before us.

REFERENCES

1. Melzack R, Wall P. Pain mechanisms: a new theory. *Science* 1965;50: 971–979.
2. Melzack R, Casey KL. Sensory, motivational and central control determinants of pain: a new conceptual model. In: Kenshalo D, ed. *The skin senses*. Springfield: Charles C Thomas, 1968:423–439.
3. Wall PD. The gate control theory of pain mechanism: a re-examination and restatement. *Brain* 1978;101:1–18.
4. Melzack R, Dennis SG: Neurophysiological foundations of pain. In: Sternbach RA, ed. *The Psychology of Pain*. New York: Raven, 1978: 1–24.
5. Wall PD. On the relation of injury to pain: the John Bonica lecture. *Pain* 1979;6: 253–264.
6. Melzack R. Gate control theory: on the evolution of pain concepts. *Pain Forum* 1999;5: 128–138.
7. Marx MH. The general nature of theory construction. In: Marx MH, ed *Theories in Contemporary Psychology*. New York: McMillan, 1963:4-45.
8. Shapiro GS. Implications of our definition of pain. *Pain Forum* 1999; 8:100–102.
9. Doleys DM. Pain: An evolving concept. *Southern Pain Society Newsletter* 2000(Winter);5–7.
10. Descartes R. *L'Homme*. Paris, 1664.
11. Nathan PW. The gate control theory of pain: a critical review. *Brain* 1976;99:123–158.
12. Schmidt RF. The gate control theory of pain: an unlikely hypothesis. In: Jansen R, Keidel WD, Harz A, Streichele C, Payne JT, Burt RB, eds. *Pain: basic principles of pharmacological therapy*. Stuttgart: Theime, 1972:57–71.
13. Turk DC. Biopsychosocial perspective on chronic pain. In: Gatchel RJ, Turk DC, eds. *Psychological approaches to pain management: a practitioner's handbook*. New York: Guilford Press, 1996:33–52.

14. Gallagher RM, Williams RA, Skelly J, et al. Worker's compensation and return to work in low back pain. *Pain* 1995;61:299–306.
15. Marx MH, ed. *Learning Theories.* New York: McMillan, 1970.
16. Skinner BF. *Science and Human Behavior.* New York: Free Press/McMillan, 1953.
17. Skinner BF. The operant side of behavioral therapy. *J Behav Ther Experi Psychia* 1998;18:171–179.
18. Honig WK, ed. *Operant Behavior: Areas of Research and Application.* New York: Appleton-Century-Crofts, 1966.
19. Ferster CB, Skinner BF. *Schedules of Reinforcement.* New York: Appleton-Century-Crofts, 1957.
20. Waddell G, Newton M, Henderson I, et al. A fear-avoidance beliefs questionnaire (FABQ) and the role of fear-avoidance in chronic low back pain and disability. *Pain* 1993;52:157–168.
21. Fordyce WE, Bogis S, Battie M, Fisher L. MMPI scale 3 as a predictor of back injury report: what does it tell us? *Clin J Pain* 1992;8:222–230.
22. Block AR. An investigation of the response of the spouse to chronic pain behavior. *Psychosom Med* 1981;43:415–419.
23. Gil KM, Keefe FJ, Chrisson JE, Van-Dalfsen PJ. Social support and pain behavior. *Pain* 1987;29:209–212.
24. Fordyce WE. *Behavioral Methods for Chronic Pain and Illness.* St. Louis: Mosby, 1976.
25. Doleys DM, Crocker MF, Patton D. Response of patients with chronic pain to exercise quotas. *Phys Ther* 1982;62:1111–1115.
26. Carragee EJ, Kimm DH. A perspective analysis of magnetic resonance imaging findings in patients with sciatica and lumbar disc herniation: correlation of outcomes with disc fragments and canal morphology. *Spine* 1997;22:1650–1660.
27. Linton SJ. The relationship between activity and chronic pain. *Pain* 1985;21:289–294.
28. Hendry DP, ed. *Conditioned reinforcement.* Homewood, Ill: Dorsey Press, 1969.
29. Wike EL, ed. *Secondary reinforcement: selected experiments.* New York: Harper and Row, 1966.
30. Merskey H. Limitations on pain behavior. *Am Pain Soc J* 1992;1:101–104.
31. Turk DC, Flor H. Pain greater than pain behaviors: the utility and limitations of the pain behavior construct. *Pain* 1987;31:277–295.
32. Woods PJ. A taxonomy of instrumental conditioning. *Am Psychol* 1974;29:584–597.
33. Sanders SH. Operant conditioning with chronic pain: back to basics. In: Gatchel RJ, Turk DC, eds. *Psychological approaches to pain management: a practitioner's handbook.* New York: Guilford Press, 1996:112–130.
34. Doleys DM, Doherty D. Psychological and behavioral assessment. In: Raj PP, ed. *Practical management of pain.* St. Louis: Mosby, 2000: 408–426.
35. Tryon WW. Observing contingencies: taxonomy and methods. *Clin Psychol Rev* 1966;16:215–230.
36. Birbaumer N, Flor H. A leg to stand on: learning creates pain. *Behav Brain Sci* 1997;20:441–442.
37. Pavlov IP. *Conditioned reflexes.* London: Oxford University Press, 1927.
38. Kimble GA. *Hilgard and Marquis' conditioning and learning.* New York: Appleton-Century-Crofts, 1961.
39. Rossi NA, Reid LD: Affective states associated with morphine injections. *Phys Psychol* 1976;4:269–274.
40. Spear LP, Horowitz GP, Lipovsky J. Altered behavioral responsivity to morphine during peri adolescent behavior in rats. *Behav and Brain Res* 1982;4:279–288.
41. Frank MD, Hinson RE, Siegel S. Conditioned hyperalgesia is elicited by environmental signals of morphine. *Behavior and Natural Biology* 1981;32:148–157.
42. Valone JM, Randall CK, Kramer PJ, Bardo MT. Olfactory cues and morphine induced conditioned analgesia in rats. *Pharmacol Biochem and Behav* 1998;60:115–118.
43. Ader A. The role of conditioning in pharmacotherapy. In: Harrington A, ed. *The placebo effect.* Cambridge: Harvard University Press, 1997:139–163.
44. Suchman AL, Ader AA. Classical conditioning in the placebo effect in crossover studies. *Clin Pharmacol Ther* 1992;(Oct):372–377.
45. Montgomery GH, Kirsch I. Classical conditioning in the placebo effect. *Pain* 1997;71:107–113.
46. Brewer WF. There is no convincing evidence for operant classical conditioning in adult humans. In: Weiner WB, Polermo DS, eds. *Cognition and the symbolic process.* New York:Wiley, 1974:1–42.
47. Staats PS, Doleys D, Hekmat H, Staats AW. The powerful placebo: friend or foe. In: Warfield C, Rice A, McGrath P, Justins D, eds. *Clinical pain management.* London: Arnold. (in press.)
48. Wiertelak EP, Mayer SF, Watkins LR. Cholecystokinine antialgesia: safety cues abolish morphine analgesia. *Science* 1992;256:830–833.
49. Childress AR, Mozley PD, McElgin W, et al. Limbic activation during cue-induced cocaine craving. *Am J Psychia* 1999;157:11–18.
50. Bandura A. *Social learning theory.* New Jersey: Prentice-Hall, 1977.
51. Bandura A. Self-efficacy: toward a unifying theory of behavior change. *Psychol Rev* 1977;84:191–215.
52. Kirsch I. Response expectancy as a determinate of experience and behavior. *Am Psychol* 1985;40:1189–1202.
53. Kirsch I. *Changing expectations: a key in effective psychotherapy.* Pacific Grove, Calif.: Brooks/Cole, 1999.
54. Fernandez E, Turk DC. The utility of cognitive coping strategies for altering pain perception: a meta-analysis. *Pain* 1989;38:123–135.
55. Dolce JJ, Doleys DM, Raczynski JM, et al. The role of self-efficacy expectancies in the prediction of pain tolerance. *Pain* 1986;27: 261–266.
56. Dolce JJ, Crocker MF, Moletteire M, Doleys DM. Exercise quotas, anticipatory concern and self-efficacy expectancies in chronic pain: a preliminary report. *Pain* 1986;24:365–372.
57. Dolce JJ, Crocker MF, Doleys DM. Prediction of outcome among chronic pain patients. *Behav Res Ther* 1986;24:313–319.
58. Doleys DM, Meredith RL, Ciminero A. *Behavioral medicine: assessment and treatment strategies.* New York: Plenum, 1982.
59. Merskey H, Bogduk N. *Classification of chronic pain.* Seattle: IASP Press, 1994.
60. Fernandez E, Turk DC. Sensory and affective components of pain. *Psychol Bull* 1992;112(2):205–217.
61. Merskey H, Spear FG. The concept of pain. *J Psychosom Res* 1967; 11:59–67.
62. Craig KD. Emotional aspects of pain. In: Wall PD, Melzack R, eds. *Textbook of pain.* London: Churchill Livingston, 1984:153–161.
63. Gross RT, Collins FL. On the relationship between anxiety and pain: a methodological confounding. *Clin Psychol Rev* 1981;1:375–387.
64. Leavitt F, Garron DC, Whisler WW, Skeinkop MB. Affective and sensory dimensions of back pain. *Pain* 1978;4:273–281.
65. Reading, AE. The internal structure of the McGill Pain Questionnaire in dysmennorhoea patients. *Pain* 1979;7:353–358.
66. Price DD, Harkins, SW. The affective-motivational dimension of pain. *APS J* 1992;1(4):229–239.
67. Price DD. *Psychological mechanisms of pain and analgesia.* Seattle: IASP Press, 1999.
68. Gatchel RJ. Psychological disorders and chronic pain: cause-and-effect relationships. In: Gatchel RJ, Turk DC, eds. *Psychological approaches to pain management: a practitioner's guide.* New York: Guilford Press, 1996.
69. Gracely RH. Affective dimensions of pain. *APS J* 1992;1(4):243–247.
70. Ales TA, Yunus MB, Masi AT. Is chronic pain a variant of depressive disease? The case of primary fibromyalgia syndrome. *Pain* 1987;29: 105–111.
71. Blumer D, Heilbronn M. Chronic pain as a variant of depressive disease: the pain prone disorder. *J Nerv Ment Dis* 1982;170(7):381–406.
72. Gamsa A. Is emotional disturbance a precipitator or a consequence of chronic pain. *Pain.* 42: 183-195, 1990.
73. Vonkorff M, Simon G: The relationship between pain and depression. *Br J Psychia* 1996;168 (30):101–108.
74. Brown GK, Nicassio PM, Wallston KA. Pain coping strategies and depression in rheumatoid arthritis. *J Consult Clin Psychol* 1989;57(5): 652–657.
75. Magni G, Caldieron C, Rigatti-Luchini S, Merskey H. Chronic musculoskeletal pain and depressive symptoms in the general population. An analysis of the 1st national health and nutrition examination survey data. *Pain* 1990;43:299–307.
76. Flor H, Birbammer N, Turk DC. The psychobiology of chronic pain. *Adv Behav Res Ther* 1990;12:47–84.
77. Lentham J, Slade PO, Troup JPG, Bentley G. Outline of fear-avoidance model of exaggerated pain perception. *Behav Res Ther* 1983;21:401–408.
78. Phillips HC. Avoidance behavior and its role in sustaining chronic pain. *Behav Res Ther* 1987;25:273–279.
79. Asmundson GJG, Kuperos JL, Norton GR. Do patients with chronic pain selectively attend to pain-related information?: preliminary evidence for the mediating role of fear. *Pain* 1997;72:27–32.

80. Chapman CR, Turner JA. Psychologic and psychosocial aspects of acute pain. In: Bonica JJ, ed. *The management of pain*. Philadelphia: Lea & Febiger, 1990:122–132.
81. Bonica JJ. General considerations of acute pain. In: Bonica JJ, ed. *The management of pain*. Philadelphia: Lea & Febiger, 1990: 159–179.
82. Pilowsky I, Chapman CR, Bonica JJ. Pain, depression, and illness behavior in a pain clinic population. *Pain* 1977;4:183–192.
83. Benjamin S, Barnes D, Berger S, Clarke I, Jeacock J. The relationship of chronic pain, mental illness and organic disorders. *Pain* 1988;32:185–195.
84. Tyrer SP, Capon M, Peterson DM, Charlton JE, Thompson JW. The detection of psychiatric illness and psychological handicaps in a British pain clinic population. *Pain* 1989;36:63–74.
85. Magni G, Rossi MR, Rigatti-Luchini S, Merskey H. Chronic abdominal pain and depression. Hispanic Health and Nutrition Examination Survey. *Pain* 1992;49:77–85.
86. Anderson L, Bradley LA, Young LD, McDaniel LK, Wise WM. Rheumatoid arthritis: review of psychological factors related to etiology, effects, and treatment. *Psychol Bull* 1985;98:358–387.
87. Romano JM, Turner JA. Chronic pain and depression: does the evidence support a relationship. *Psychol Bull* 1985;97:18–34.
88. Magni G. On the relationship between chronic pain and depression when there is no organic lesion. *Pain* 1987;31:1–21.
89. Rudy TE, Kerns RJ, Turk DC. Chronic pain and depression: toward a cognitive behavioral mediation model. *Pain* 1988;35: 179–183.
90. Turk DC, Okifuji A, Scharff L. Chronic pain and depression: role of perceived impact and perceived control in different age cohorts. *Pain* 1995;61:93–102.
91. Kellner R. Functional somatic symptoms and hypochondriasis. *Arch Gen Psychia* 1985;42:821–833.
92. Drossman DA. Patients with psychogenic abdominal pain: six years' observation in the medical setting. *Am J Psychia* 1982;139: 1549–1557.
93. Feinmann C. Psychogenic facial pain: presentation and treatment. *J Psychosom Res* 1983;27:403–410.
94. Haber J, Kuczmierczy KA, Adams H. Tension headaches: muscle overactivity or psychogenic pain. *Headache* 1985;25:23–29.
95. Lesse S. The masked depression syndrome—results of a seventeen year clinical study. *Am J Psychother* 1983;37:456–475.
96. Webb JW. Chronic pain: psychosomatic illness review. *Psychosom* 1983;24:1053–1063.
97. Addison R. Chronic pain syndrome. *Am J Med* 1984;77:54–58.
98. Fields H. Depression and pain: a neurobiological model. *Neuropsychiatry, Neuropsychology, Behavior Neurology* 1991;4:83–92.
99. Fordyce WE. *Behavioral methods in chronic pain and illness*. St. Louis: Mosby, 1976.
48. Barksy A. Amplification, somatization, somatoform disorders. *Psychosom* 1992;33:24–34.
100. Turk DC, Salovey P. Chronic pain as a variant of depressive disease: a critical reappraisal. *J Nerv Ment Dis* 1984;172:398–404.
101. Fields H. *Pain*. New York: McGraw Hill, 1987.
102. Blazer D. Narcissism and the development of chronic pain. *Int J Psychiatr Med* 1980–81;10:69–77.
103. Catchlove RF, Cohen KR, Braha R, Demers-Desrosiers L. Incidence and implications of alexythymia on chronic pain patients. *J Nerv Ment Dis* 1985;173:246–248.
104. Freeman, CW, Calsyn DA, Louks J. The use of the MMPI with low back pain patients. *J Clin Psychol* 1976;32:294–298.
105. Gentry WD, Shows WD, Thomas M. Chronic low back pain: a psychological profile. *Psychosom* 1974;15:174–177.
106. Hudson JI, Hudson MS, Pliner LF, Goldenberg DL, Pope HG. Fibromyalgia and major affective disorder: a controlled phenomenology and family history study. *Am J Psychia* 1985;142:441–446.
107. Violon A, Giurgea D. Familial models for chronic pain. *Pain* 1984; 18:199–203.
108. Bond MR, Pearson IB. Psychological aspects of pain in women with advanced cancer of the cervix. *J. Psychosom Res* 1969;13:13–39.
109. Merskey H. Pain and personality. In: RA Sternback, ed. *The psychology of pain*. New York: Raven Press, 1978:111–127.
110. Payne TC, Leavitt FG, Katz RS, Golden HE, Glickman PB, Vanderplate C. Fibrositis and psychological disturbance. *Arthr Rheum* 1982;25:213–217.

111. Pilowsky I, Spence ND. Is illness behaviour related to chronicity in patients with intractable pain? *Pain* 1976;2:61–71.
112. Harkins SW, Price DD, Braith J. Effects of extraversion and neuroticism on experimental pain, clinical pain, and illness behavior. *Pain* 1989;36:209–218.
113. Wade JB, Dougherty LM, Hart RP, Rafii A, Price DD. A canonical correlation analysis of the influence of neuroticism and extraversion on chronic pain, suffering, and pain behavior. *Pain* 1992;51: 67–73.
114. Fordyce WE, Brockway, JA, Bergman JA, Spengler D. Acute back pain: a control-group comparison of behavioral versus traditional management methods. *J Behav Med* 1986;9:127–140.
115. Taylor H, Curran NM. *The Nuprin pain report*. New York: Louis Harris, 1985.
116. Council JR, Ahern DK, Follick MJ, Kline CL. Expectancies and functional impairment in chronic low back pain. *Pain* 1988;33: 323–331.
117. Flor H, Turk DC. Chronic back pain and rheumatoid arthritis: predicting pain and disability from cognitive variables. *J Behav Med* 1988;11:251–265.
118. Gil KM, Williams DA, Keefe FJ, Beckham JC. The relationship of negative thoughts to pain and psychological distress. *Behav Ther* 1990;21:349–352.
119. Jensen MP, Turner JA, Romano JM, Karoly, P. Coping with chronic pain: a critical review of the literature. *Pain* 1991;47:249–283.
120. Kores, RC, Murphy, WD, Rosenthal TL, Elias, DB, North WC. Predicting outcome of chronic pain treatment via a modified self-efficacy scale. *Behav Res Ther* 1990;28:165–169.
121. Weisenberg M. Cognitive aspects of pain. In Wall PD, Melzack R, eds. *Textbook of pain*. London: Churchill Livingston, 1989:231–241.
122. Turk DC, Meichenbaum D, Genest M. *Pain and behavioral medicine: a cognitive-behavioral perspective*. New York: Guilford Press, 1983.
123. Ellis A. *Reason and emotion in psychotherapy*. New York: Lyle Stuart, 1962.
124. Beck AT. *Cognitive therapy and the emotional disorders*. New York: International Universities Press, 1976.
125. Beck AT, Rush AJ, Shaw BF, Emery G. *Cognitive therapy of depression*. New York: Guilford Press, 1979.
126. Beck A, Emery G, Greenberg RI. *Anxiety disorders and phobia*. New York: Basic Books, 1985.
127. Roskies E, Lazarus RS. Coping theory and the teaching of coping skills. In: Davidson PO, Davidson SM, eds. *Behavioral medicine: changing health lifestyles*. New York: Brunner/Mazel, 1980.
128. Folkman S. Personal control and stress and coping processes: a theoretical analysis. *J Pers Soc Psychol* 1984;46:839–852.
129. Folkman S, Lazarus RS, Dunkel-Schemer C, DeLongis A, Gruen RJ. Dynamics of a stressful encounter: cognitive appraisal, coping and encounter outcomes. *J Pers Soc Psychol* 1986;50:992–1003.
130. Lazarus R S, Folkman S. *Stress, appraisal, and coping*. New York: Springer, 1984.
131. Meichenbaum D. *Cognitive behavior modification*. New York: Plenum Press, 1977.
132. Meichenbaum D. *Stress inoculation training*. New York: Pergamon Press, 1985.
133. Bandura A. Self-efficacy mechanism in human agency. *Am Psychol* 1982;37:122–147.
134. Bandura A. Recycling misconceptions of perceived self-efficacy. *Cogn Ther Res* 1984;8:231–255.
135. Seligman MEP. *Helplessness*. San Francisco: WH Freeman, 1975.
136. Bandura, A. *Social foundations of thought and action: a social cognitive theory*. Englewood Cliffs, NJ: Prentice-Hall, 1986.
137. Spiegel D, Bloom JR. Pain in metastatic breast cancer. *Cancer* 1983; 52:341–345.
138. Williams DA, Keefe FJ. Pain beliefs and the use of cognitive-behavioral coping strategies. *Pain* 1991;46:185–190.
139. Leventhal H, Everhart D. Emotion, pain, and physical illness. In Izard CE, ed. *Emotions in personality and psychopathology*. New York: Plenum Press, 1979.
140. Turk SM. Controllability and human stress: method, evidence, and theory. *Behav Res Ther* 17:287–304, 1981.
141. Bandura A. Self-efficacy mechanisms in physiological activation and health promoting behavior. In: Madden J, ed. *Neurobiology of learning, emotion and affect*. New York: Raven Press, 1991:229–269.

142. Lackner JM, Carosella AM, Feurerstein M. Pain expectancies, pain and functional self-efficacy expectancies as determinants of disability in patients with chronic low back disorders. *J Consult Clin Psychol* 1996;64:212–220.

143. Buckelew SP, Murray SE, Hewett JE, Johnson J, Huyser B. Self-efficacy, pain and physical activity among fibromyalgia subjects. *Arthri Care Res* 1995;8:43–50.

144. Keefe FJ, Williams DA. Pain behavior assessment. In: Turk DC, Melzack R, eds. *Handbook of pain assessment.* New York: Guilford Press, 1992:277–292.

145. Brown, GK, Nicassio PM. The development of a questionnaire for the assessment of active and passive coping strategies in chronic pain patients. *Pain* 1987;31:53–65.

146. Tota-Faucette ME, Gil KM, Williams FJ, Goli V. Predictors of response to pain management treatment: the role of family environment and changes in cognitive processes. *Clin J Pain* 1993;9:115–123.

147. Beck AT. *Depression: causes and treatment.* Philadelphia: University of Pennsylvania Press, 1967.

148. McCracken LM, Zayfert C, Gross RT. The Pain Anxiety Symptoms Scale: development and validation of a scale to measure fear of pain. *Pain* 1992;50:67–73.

149. Rosenstiel AK, Keefe FJ. The use of coping strategies in chronic low back pain patients: relationship to patient characteristics and current adjustment. *Pain* 1983;17:33–44.

150. McCracken LM, Gross RT, Sorg PJ, Edmands TA. Prediction of pain in patients with chronic low back pain: effects of inaccurate prediction and pain-related anxiety. *Behav Res Ther* 1993;31:647–652.

151. Keefe FJ, Brown GK, Wallston KA, Caldwell DS. Coping with rheumatoid arthritis pain: catastrophizing as a maladaptive strategy. *Pain* 1989;37:51–56.

152. Keefe FJ, Williams DA. A comparison of coping strategies in chronic pain patients in different age groups. *J Gerontol* 1990;45:161–165.

153. Lefebvre, MF. Cognitive distortion and cognitive errors in depressed psychiatric and low back pain patients. *J Consult Clin Psychol* 1981;49:517–525.

154. Smith TW, Aberger EW, Follick MJ, Ahern BK. Cognitive distortion and psychological distress in chronic low back pain. *J Consult Clin Psychol* 1986;54:573–575.

155. Smith TW, Peck JR, Ward JR. Helplessness and depression in rheumatoid arthritis. *Health Psychol* 1990;9:377–389.

CHAPTER 4

Taxonomy and Classification of Pain

David B. Boyd

There are two primary concerns regarding pain taxonomy. One is the intellectual exercise of trying to precisely sort out and classify a common complaint. The other is the more political exercise of trying to get everyone to agree on and use one major organizational model.

This chapter will attempt to examine different approaches to classifying pain and will then conclude by reinforcing the use of Classification of Chronic Pain—Descriptions of Chronic Pain Syndromes and Definitions of Pain Terms (1).

As a complaint, pain is of interest to all of us as individuals and to most of us as students, therapists, practitioners, etc. Each clinical discipline carries its own body of knowledge, language, attitudes, and approach to problem solving. Trying to get different disciplines to relate to each other is challenging but not impossible. Most of us dealing with chronic pain would agree that a multidisciplinary approach to understanding and treating pain is essential if a complete picture is to be obtained. Much as the three blind men examining the elephant, looking at pain is like inspecting different facets of a finely cut diamond; each viewpoint is valid but different.

Philosophically, if happiness is the greatest good, pain is the worst evil. No medical problem causes poorer quality of life than chronic pain. Pain is something everyone knows about, and many feel they are pain experts. "Pain is what hurts" or defined with Harold Merskey's linguistic finesse: "Pain is an unpleasant sensory and emotional experience associated with actual or potential tissue damage, or described in terms of such damage" (2).

Pain is a thought, a feeling, a behavior. We all know what it is, but it is hard to measure. There are potentially many ways to try to measure it, both qualitatively and quantitatively. "This is the worst pain I have ever had—worse than my worst headache, toothache, or bellyache." Visual analogue scales may come closest: "0 out of 10 is no pain, 10 out of 10 is the worst, most excruciating pain possible."

Any approach to classification will have its advocates and its critics. Some are "lumpers" (wanting a few large, rather mixed groups), whereas others are "splitters" (in the extreme, individualizing groups to just one). Pain is vague and intrinsically difficult to measure and categorize.

Do we approach classification by location of pain, character of pain, etiology, pathophysiology, or response to treatment? The approach to, for example, low back pain will be somewhat different for the physiotherapist, the chiropractor, the rheumatologist, the anesthesiologist, the neurosurgeon, the orthopedic surgeon, or the psychologist (to name just a few potential caregivers). Often we can only speculate about the aspects of pain. All clinical medicine is confronted with attempts at classification. Perhaps artificially we dichotomize: pain is acute or chronic, benign or malignant, mild or severe, treatable or intractable. One-dimensional models are common in medicine, such as the classification by pathophysiology and system in Figure 4-1; the two-dimensional model often used as a grid in psychiatry is shown in Figure 4-2.

Pain is classified as chronic if it lasts longer than 6 months and is generally regarded as permanent (or at least likely to be so) if it lasts longer than 2 years. Chronic pain may be divided into malignant and nonmalignant (nonmalignant is probably a better term than benign since any pain is hardly benign to the patient). There has been considerable recent interest into classifying chronic pain as neuropathic pain and nonneuropathic pain. One can think of pain as organic-structural, organic-physiological, or psychiatric in origin. Perhaps as neurochemistry improves, pain will be classified by the type of opioid receptor involved.

The International Association for Study of Pain (IASP) pain classification uses a five-axis model similar to *DSM-IV* (Fig. 4-3) (1).

There is a numerical code, starting with the hundreds digit (Fig. 4-4) for pain site. Then a tens digits (Fig. 4-5) is used for the system involved. Next a units digits (Fig. 4-6) is

Congenital

Acquired
   Infectious (viral, bacterial, fungal, or protozoal)
   Toxic—endocrine-metabolic
   Allergic/autoimmune
   Traumatic
   Collagen vascular
   Vascular
   Neoplastic
   Hematologic
   Neurologic
   Psychiatric
   Degenerative
   Iatrogenic
   Other
      sarcoid
      amyloid

FIG. 4-1. Sample list classification often used in internal medicine—an example of a one-dimensional system.

	Biologic	Psychologic	Sociocultural
Predisposing			
Precipitating			
Perpetuating			

FIG. 4-2. Sample grid classification often used in psychiatry—an example of a two-dimensional system.

Axis I: Region

Axis II: System

Axis III: Temporal characteristics of pain: pattern of occurrence

Axis IV: Patient's statement of intensity: time since onset of pain

Axis V: Etiology

FIG. 4-3. Overview of the IASP five-axis pain taxonomy.

Head, face, and mouth	000
Cervical region	100
Upper shoulder and upper limbs	200
Thoracic region	300
Abdominal region	400
Lower back, lumbar spine, sacrum, and coccyx	500
Lower limbs	600
Pelvic region	700
Anal, perineal, and genital region	800
More than three major sites	900

FIG. 4-4. Axis I: Region. Record main site first; record two important regions separately. If there is more than one site of pain, separate coding will be necessary. (From Merskey H, Bogduk N. *Classification of chronic pain,* 2nd ed. Seattle: IASP, 1994 with permission.)

Nervous system (central, peripheral and autonomic) and special senses; physical disturbance or dysfunction	00
Nervous system (psychological and social)	10
Respiratory and cardiovascular systems	20
Musculoskeletal system and connective tissue	30
Cutaneous and subcutaneous and associated glands (breast, apocrine, etc.)	40
Gastrointestinal system	50
Genito-urinary system	60
Other organs or viscera (e.g., thyroid, lymphatic, hemopoietic)	70
More than one system	80

FIG. 4-5. Axis II: System. The system coded is that in which abnormal functioning produces the pain (e.g., claudication = vascular). Similarly, the nervous system is to be coded only when a pathologic disturbance in it produces pain. Thus pain from a pancreatic carcinoma = gastrointestinal; pain from a metastatic deposit affecting bones = musculoskeletal. (From Merskey H, Bogduk N. *Classification of chronic pain*—2nd ed. Seattle: IASP, 1994 with permission.)

Not recorded, not applicable, or not known	0
Single episode, limited duration (e.g., ruptured aneurysm, sprained ankle)	1
Continuous or nearly continuous, nonfluctuating (e.g., low back pain, some cases)	2
Continuous or nearly continuous, fluctuating severity (e.g., ruptured intervertebral disc)	3
Recurring, irregularly (e.g., headache, mixed type)	4
Recurring, regularly (e.g., premenstrual pain)	5
Paroxysmal (e.g., tic douloureux)	6
Sustained with superimposed paroxysms	7
Other combinations	8
None of the above	9

FIG. 4-6. Axis III: Temporal characteristics of pain, pattern of occurrence. (From Merskey H, Bogduk N. *Classification of chronic pain*, 2nd ed. Seattle: IASP, 1994 with permission.)

Not recorded, not applicable, or not known		.0
Mild—	1 month or less	.1
	1 month to 6 months	.2
	more than 6 months	.3
Medium—	1 month or less	.4
	1 month to 6 months	.5
	more than 6 months	.6
Severe—	1 month or less	.7
	1 month to 6 months	.8
	more than 6 months	.9

FIG. 4-7. Axis IV: Patient's statement of intensity, time since onset of pain. (From Merskey H, Bogduk N. *Classification of chronic pain*, 2nd ed. Seattle: IASP, 1994 with permission.)

used for the temporal characteristics of the pain. Following that is a tenths digit (Fig. 4-7) used for duration and intensity. And finally, a hundreds digits (Fig. 4-8) is used for etiology.

Any patient's pain can be described by all five of these axes in sequence—for example, a low back pain (Axis I),

Genetic or congenital disorders (e.g., congenital dislocation)	.00
Trauma, operation, burns	.01
Infective, parasitic	.02
Inflammatory (no known infective agent), immune reactions	.03
Neoplasm	.04
Toxic, metabolic (e.g., alcoholic neuropathy, anoxia, vascular, nutritional, endocrine), radiation	.05
Degenerative, mechanical	.06
Dysfunctional (including psychophysiologic)	.07
Unknown or other	.08
Psychological origin (e.g., conversion hysteria, depressive hallucination)	.09
(Note: No physical cause should be held to be present nor any pathophysiological mechanism.)	

FIG. 4-8. Axis V: Etiology. (From Merskey H, Bogduk N. *Classification of chronic pain*, 2nd ed. Seattle: IASP, 1994 with permission.)

of neurologic origin (Axis II, occurring continuously and severely (Axis III) for 6 months (Axis IV) from degenerative disk disease (Axis V).

Table 4-1 overviews pain syndromes commonly seen clinically and discussed in greater detail in the *IASP Taxonomy and Descriptions of Pain Syndromes* (1).

The ideal classification system would have a specific location for each pain syndrome with no chance of omission or overlap. Clinical medicine rarely lends itself to such precise dissection. Nonetheless, by continual reexamination by various groups, even pain gradually becomes more understandable. The IASP pain classification proposed above has several noteworthy advantages. First of all, it was developed by a multidisciplinary association. Second, this association is widely based in terms of both geography and expertise. Third, it publishes a respected and well-circulated journal and has already published a proposed pain taxonomy. The five axes follow criteria that are currently used in pain problems, and so should be easy to adopt by most clinicians. This classification will be modified as knowledge expands but offers a firm starting point.

There has been recent debate about pain in the uncommunicative patient and in animals, but these are specific corollary activities.

Attempt to familiarize yourself to the IASP classification and use it!

TABLE 4-1. *Syndromes by group according to IASP taxonomy*

I.	Relatively Generalized Syndromes
II.	Neuralgias of the Head and Face
III.	Craniofacial Pain of Musculoskeletal Origin
IV.	Lesions of the Ear, Nose, and Oral Cavity
V.	Primary Headache Syndromes
VI.	Pain of Psychological Origin in the Head and Face
VII.	Suboccipital and Cervical Musculoskeletal Disorders
VIII.	Visceral Pain in the Neck
IX.	Pain of Neurologic Origin in Neck, Shoulder, and Upper Extremity
X.	Lesions of the Brachial Plexus
XI.	Pain in the Shoulder, Arm, and Hand
XII.	Vascular Disease of the Limbs
XIII.	Collagen Disease of the Limbs
XIV.	Vasodilating Functional Disease of the Limbs
XV.	Arterial Insufficiencies in the Limbs
XVI.	Pain in the Limbs of Psychological Origin
XVII.	Chest Pain
XVIII.	Chest Pain of Psychological Origin
XIX.	Chest Pain: Referred from Abdomen or Gastrointestinal Tract
XX.	Abdominal Pain of Neurologic Origin
XXI.	Abdominal Pain of Visceral Origin
XXII.	Abdominal Pain Syndromes of Generalized Diseases
XXIII.	Abdominal Pain of Psychological Origin
XXIV.	Disease of Uterus, Ovaries, and Adnexa
XXV.	Pain in the Rectum, Perineum, and External Genitalia
XXVI.	Backache and Pain of Neurologic Origin in Trunk and Back
XXVII.	Back Pain of Musculoskeletal Origin
XXVIII.	Back Pain of Visceral Origin
XXIX.	Low Back Pain of Psychological Origin
XXX.	Local Syndromes in the Leg or Foot—Pain of Neurologic Origin
XXXI.	Pain Syndromes of Hip and Thigh of Musculoskeletal Origin
XXXII.	Musculoskeletal Syndromes of the Leg

(From Merskey H, Bogduk N. *Classification of chronic pain*, 2nd ed. Seattle: IASP, 1994, with permission.)

REFERENCES

1. Merskey H, Bogduk N. *Classification of chronic pain*, 2nd ed. Seattle: IASP, 1994:6–36.
2. Merskey H. Classification of chronic pain, descriptions of chronic pain syndromes and definitions of pain terms. *PAIN* 1986;(Suppl 3): S10–S24.

SECTION II

Diagnostics

CHAPTER **5**

Focused Evaluation of the Pain Patient

Phillip LaTourette

Evaluation of the pain patient with a headache, neck pain, or low back pain need not be complicated, abstract, or only for the specialist. Pain, especially spinal pain, is not the "black box" it was just a few years ago. The fact that the psychological, social, and financial factors are strong influences on a patient's perception of pain does not mean one should abandon hope of defining a patient's pain generator. Only after the pain generator has been defined can a physician lead the patient through the appropriate education and timely, cost-efficient treatment of that pain condition. Furthermore, the specific diagnosis of the pain condition gives medical and legal credence to the ongoing use of specific treatment modalities.

A targeted history and physical examination should not be limited in scope or time, nor should it be dominated by the physician. Listening is the most important aspect of beginning a targeted history and physical examination. Listening should be an active process of interpretation and guidance of the patient as the patient presents the problem from his or her unique perspective. Listening generates trust in a caring atmosphere, which is crucial for patient education; compliance with medications, activity levels, exercise; and generation of appropriate expectation of therapy. The history and physical examination is a much less costly approach to the diagnosis of the pain generator than most imaging studies or neurodiagnostic studies. Furthermore, imaging studies without a sound history and physical examination may be very misleading and may identify pathology that may, in fact, have nothing to do with the generation of pain. For example, a magnetic resonance imaging (MRI) of an elderly male may reveal multiple pain generators, including multilevel lumbar degenerative disc disease, herniated nucleus pulposus at L-5 segments, and spinal stenosis at L-4 segments. Without the history of neurogenic claudication, initiation of therapy or surgery for treatment of the wrong generator, let's

say the herniated disc at L-5, may create misery for the patient; a proper history and physical exam may save him from undue risk and expense.

SETTING

The physical office surroundings are very important to the evaluation of the pain patient. A warm, quiet atmosphere will help relax an anxious patient. The relaxed patient is better able to recall events, understand and relate to the physician, and probably give a more reliable exam than a patient who is apprehensive. A quiet, comfortable atmosphere also promotes a more intimate relationship between physician and patient, as well as promotes the art of listening. Often pain patients are dissatisfied with their previous care, not necessarily with previous diagnostic or therapeutic interventions, but with the amount and quality of time they spend with their physicians and with the explanations of their diagnosis and treatment. Recent studies have shown that the patient's overall office experience, including interactions with the physician, staff, and billing department, all have a significant impact on the patient's perceived quality of care and satisfaction of treatment.

TAKING THE HISTORY

Chief Complaint and Associated Symptoms

This is the initial information collected from the patient. This may include a complaint of pain or possibly weakness or numbness, or a diagnosis given to the patient by another physician (degenerative disc disease). This helps focus the exam on the specific body region and gives an idea of the degree of insight the patient has on his or her condition. Patients often present to a pain management physician for reasons other than pain itself. They may wish to medically document a condition or injury that occurred at work or in a motor vehicle accident, for example. Occasionally, the fear of cancer or recurrence of treated cancer brings patients to the office. Many patients also present for psychological reasons. Some patients may not require much in the way of new or different treatment options, only needing assurance that their pain is not secondary to some malignancy or life-threatening disease. Many of my patients are not necessarily seeking new or different treatment options. Their present medications manage their pain well, but the referring physician may be leaving the area, retiring, or feeling uncomfortable about prescribing narcotics for a long period. (We try to make sure, by calling the referring physician, that there are no issues of abuse or diversion of drugs.) To have a targeted history and physical, the physician must begin with a clear idea of the patient's motives for coming to seek medical attention.

Duration of Symptoms

The duration of pain may be the most important aspect of a targeted history to determine whether the patient needs urgent care versus routine evaluation and treatment. The patient presenting with any type of pain that is rapidly worsening or changing in character or location should receive a higher level of urgency of care than a patient with a stable pattern of pain for 20 years. In fact, one challenging aspect of pain management is to care for patients with chronic low back pain or headaches who are seen on a regular basis over an extended period and be able to identify significant changes in their pain patterns so that their low back pain, secondary to degenerative disc disease, can be differentiated from an expanding abdominal aortic aneurysm, or their chronic tension headache is not confused with a subarachnoid hemorrhage. One must take into account patients' personality. Are they anxious, histrionic, stoic? Certainly the addition of objective neurological findings on physical examination should have significant weight in determining the urgency of evaluation and treatment.

Location of Pain

Is the pain localized to a specific region or is there a referred pain pattern? Do the projected pain and neurological changes of nerve root injury neatly fit into a dermatomal, myotomal, or sclerotomal distribution, or is this a peripheral nerve injury? Is this more of a vague upper abdominal pain, with shoulder pain, indicating referred diaphragmatic irritation? The use of a pain diagram in which the patient can draw the areas of pain on a picture of the human body can be most helpful with the localization of the pain generator. Initially, I used the pain diagram to help differentiate organic verses nonorganic causes of pain; however, as I have learned more about pain generators and their referral patterns, especially referred pain from facet joints, shoulder, hip and knee joints, and myofascial pain, the pain diagram has become more and more useful to me to locate the pain generator itself.

Quality/Pain Descriptors

The McGill Pain Questionnaire short form is an excellent format to differentiate the emotional component of pain from the sensory component of pain. However, to some extent, the emotional aspect of pain may change in importance over time. How long the patient has suffered pain, and the amount of disability, social, and financial hardship the pain has caused, has significant effect on the ratio of emotional to sensory component of pain. The patient's description of pain is another key aspect in orienting and focusing the physician on the cause and location of the pain generator. Descriptors such as pins and needles, tingling, electric, numbing, cramping at night, or burning are often indicators of neurological processes or nerve damage. Throbbing and pounding often refer to vascular processes. Sharp, stabbing pain that occurs with every movement and deep breaths may indicate musculoskeletal problems, especially those of muscle spasm. Describing pain as aching in nature appears to be quite nonspecific. However, the location of pain can focus the exam as to the anatomic location of the pain generator. The description of how the pain evolves through the patient's daily activities may give more insight as to the diagnosis of the pain generator. For instance, aching and stiffness on the day after activity may indicate tendonitis, bursitis, or overuse of muscles. Aching pain and stiffness in the morning, which improves as the day progresses, is often observed in patients with inflammatory joint disease, such as rheumatoid arthritis. The duration of gelling (the reports of stiffness) often helps give an idea of activity of the inflammation and response to treatment. Increased aching with activity is more indicative of degenerative disorders of the joints or spine. Abdominal pain secondary to obstructional bowel, ureter, or biliary tree problems, coming in rhythmic waves resulting in colic, is unique to the pathology associated with obstruction of a hollow viscus.

Mechanism of Injury

It is critical in motor vehicle accidents to identify speed and direction of impact, type of vehicles involved, and whether safety belts were in use or air bags deployed. Further information as to whether the patient required an ambulance or hospitalization and if there were associated injuries help provide an estimate of the severity of the impact. Work-related injuries must be clearly defined as to the time and place of the injury and the routine duties of the worker. Does the worker have a position that calls for highly repetitive motions or can a history be extracted from the patient detailing the lifting injury, including the size and weight of the object and the body position of the patient during the motion used to lift the object? Understanding injuries caused by a fall certainly requires information as to the height of the fall, how the patient landed, and the surface the patient struck. One should not forget to ask the patient why he or she fell. Was it loss of consciousness secondary to dysrhythmia or seizure, or did he or she simply trip on an electrical cord?

Provocative/Exacerbating Factors

Information from this aspect of the history is useful in developing and understanding the patient's disability and also helps gauge the success of the treatment regimen. Pertinent questions about activities are important. Can the patient walk through the entire mall, get groceries, sleep in his or her own bed instead of a recliner, work an 8-hour day, or sleep more comfortably with treatment? Factors that exacerbate pain may be mechanical, such as walking, bending, lifting, and sports, or psychological, including social stressors, financial problems, anxiety, and depression. Obviously, if many of the factors the patient cites are psychological in nature, counseling may be quite beneficial in helping the patient manage pain.

Palliative Factors

Determining what, if anything, has relieved pain in the past may be very helpful in diagnosing the patient's pain generator. Response to opiates verses nonsteroidals verses anticonvulsants can give a hint as to what is the most important component of the patient's pain. Response to physical therapy, aquatic verses land therapy, facet injections, epidural steroid injections, and chiropractic care all give clues as to what may be causing the patient's pain. Did the surgery on a herniated disc help relieve the patient's pain for 4 to 6 months, only to have the pain return now in a more constant nature in the same distribution, indicating possible epidural fibrosis or scar tissue formation after surgery? Sometimes determining what has been tried and what has not helped the patient can be equally as important. Did surgery on the back help the patient at all? Perhaps the microdiscectomy on the herniated disc at L-5 was an asymptomatic generator and the real pain generator was a discogenic pain caused by an annular tear at L-4. Were facet injections or epidural steroid injections administered properly? Review of the patient's chart and fluoroscopic records may be quite revealing in that the injections may never have reached their intended targets.

Review of Systems

The review of systems allows the patient to bring to light complaints that may involve systems seemingly unrelated to the pain generator. Often patients may be completely unaware of an association with their medical problems that may be causing the pain, but may give the alert physician clues as to the multiple system effect some pain generators bring to bear on the body. Certainly, many pain patients will not associate a facial rash or hair loss with joint pain caused by lupus erythematosus, for instance.

Past Medical History

The past medical history provides the pain practitioner with an appraisal of the patient's health status. The treatment for these medical problems also gives an understanding of what the patient has availed himself or herself to and the extent of the patient's understanding of the health care system and medicine in general. In this section it is essential to include past surgical history. A critical aspect to the past medical history is also determining whether the patient is currently or has previously been treated for mental health problems. It is important to understand why they required psychiatric treatment, who their health care provider is, and whether they have required impatient treatment in the past and what prompted the need for inpatient treatment. It is also appropriate to question the patient about previous or ongoing alcohol and substance abuse. According to David (1), it is essential to obtain an accurate history of injury and illness, especially when worker's compensation or personal injury is involved, to give the patient an extra opportunity to admit to old symptoms in the same body region as a recent compensable injury that is supposedly the sole cause of current suffering.

Medication History

A very important component of the history and physical examination is medication history. Which medications relieve pain, how long do they relieve pain, and what side effects do they cause? Are these side effects tolerable or intolerable? Does the patient take his or her medications in prescribed patterns or use his or her own system? Does the patient mix medication with alcohol or illicit drugs? Often I use this time to understand how and why the patient uses pain medications and the patient's understanding of the risk and side effects of medications. It is also important to document where they get their medications: physician offices, emergency rooms, friends/relatives. Is there a history of substance abuse: alcohol, drugs, tobacco?

Allergy

Much insight can be gained about patient preferences when questioned about allergies or adverse side effects caused by medications. Certainly, agents that cause life-threatening cardiovascular or respiratory effects must be identified and avoided at all cost. In contrast, dyspepsia after one administration of a nonsteroidal is quite different from EGD proven gastritis, ulcer, or documented GI bleeding.

Family History

Focus should be made on family members with chronic pain. Are they disabled? How do they manage their pain and social problems? Ascertaining the mental health of family members is another critical factor in obtaining an informative family history.

Social History

In my experience, the key aspect in determining the success in rehabilitation of a patient is the patient's support systems. Does the patient have parents, brothers, sisters, spouse, and friends on whom he or she can depend; conversely, does the patient have children or a debilitated spouse or parents who depend on him or her? Is the patient isolated? What favorite activities does the patient avoid because of this disability or fear of inducing pain? Are the patient's financial problems causing severe stress? The patient's criminal history and history of motor vehicle accidents can be potentially revealing.

Occupational History

Education and vocational history give insight about a patient's intelligence, upbringing, and ability to understand medical explanation. Further questioning needs to be made as to the patient's vocational status. Is he or she on disability and for how long? What caused the patient's disability? Is it the same problem he or she is being evaluated for or something else? Is the patient on medical leave or have work restrictions? What are the activities the patient is normally expected to perform on the job?

Physical Examination

The physical examination begins the moment I lay eyes on a patient. It may not end until I watch the patient walk out to his or her car in the parking lot. The evaluation of gait is very important. Is it smooth, balanced, coordinated? Is it antalgic, does it favor the appropriate leg, or injured body part, and is it consistent? Is this more of a neurological process causing a broad-based ataxic gait? Does the patient use assistance to walk or hold on to the walls to maintain balance?

The vital signs are just that. Many medications we prescribe alter blood pressure and/or heart rate including nonsteroidals, antidepressants, steroids, calcium channel blockers, and beta blockers for headaches. It is imperative that we follow these vital signs for side effects and, in the meantime, we may uncover hypertension or poorly controlled hypertensive patients. The pain patient expects a complete evaluation. There is much research indicating patients with chronic pain have altered immune status and overall depressed states of health. These patients require a high index of suspicion for many medical problems (2).

PAIN BEHAVIOR

Much has been written about pain behavior and what it reflects in terms of the patient's actual pain experience (3). Accuracy and credibility of these scoring systems are questionable. My normal limits for pain behaviors are quite wide. A 2-minute, five-step, sight-unseen evaluation of a pain patient to evaluate them for organic versus nonorganic pain, malingering or drug-seeking behavior are of little value. Rather, multiple visits over time, constancy of behavior, drug-use pattern, response to medications and therapy—including injections, education, social stressors, surgery, and appropriateness of expectations of therapy—give far more insight than a single simple test or snap-shot evaluation of a patient. Anxiety, depression, and previous unpleasant interaction with health care professionals can influence behavior significantly. Many patients are simply unsure as to how to behave in front of health care professionals to convey to them that they are indeed having significant pain. Obviously suicidal, homicidal, erotic desire, delusional, or hallucinatory behavior need to be addressed immediately. Inappropriate expectations also need to be addressed early (e.g., expecting one pill, one injection, or one operation to cure or fix the patient).

Examination of the head, in a headache patient, requires closer scrutiny than the average examination. Palpation of the head can be extremely important. Finding a Tinel sign over the greater occipital nerve or exquisite tenderness over the temporomandibular joint can be extremely helpful in making a diagnosis. Obviously, a careful cranial nerve evaluation is essential to the evaluation of the patient with headache or facial pain. Checking the patient's teeth for excessive wear caused by bruxism or malocclusion is extremely important in patients with jaw pain. Palpation of the sinuses and vision check can be extremely helpful.

The importance of a good examination of the neck certainly can't be overemphasized. The musculoskeletal exam is much more extensive for pain management physicians than the usual examination. The patient with neck pain deserves a careful range-of-motion examination. I believe it is not just the range of motion that is important, but also the direction that elicits the most pain. The patient with decreased flexion and increased pain may have an underlying herniated disc or myofascial problems. Patients with decreased extension may be suffering from facet joint arthropathy, posterior herniated disc, or possibly ligamentous instability. Significant pain with rotation may be associated with spondylosis, herniated disc, or myofascial pain. Range of motion also gives some appraisal of the patient's response to treatment. Careful palpation, mindful of underlying anatomy, can give some significant clues as to where the generator lies. Certainly, midline tenderness may indicate true spinal pathology. Tenderness over structures lateral to the spine may be more specific for musculoskeletal problems involving the facet joints or musculature.

Evaluation of patients with thoracic or chest pain requires palpation of the midline thoracic spine, costovertebral and costochondral joints, and the ribs themselves. Careful examination of previous incisions may elicit paresthesia. Also, careful evaluation of the chest wall for changes in sensation and rocking the chest wall for possible instability are keys to the evaluation of the patient with chest pain.

The patient with abdominal pain also deserves more than just the standard abdominal evaluation for bowel sounds and hepatosplenomegaly. Careful palpation of incisions for neuromas and stitch abscesses and asking the patient to perform an abdominal crunch may elicit increased pain and help determine whether a patient has *abdominal wall* pathology. Palpation during the crunch may help localize the lesion. Again, a thorough search for changes in sensation needs to be performed to evaluate for a low thoracic or upper lumbar radiculopathy versus a peripheral nerve injury, such as ilioinguinal nerve or genitofemoral nerve damage.

Examination of the patient with back pain is similar to that of a musculoskeletal exam for neck pain. The patient should be inspected carefully for kyphosis, lordosis, scoliosis, and poor posture. Palpation of the patient's back, always keeping in mind the patient's anatomy, gives further insight as to which structures are generating pain. Systematic palpation of the patient's midline spine, facet joints, paraspinal musculature, sciatic notches, and sacroiliac joints are a must to help elucidate the patient's pain. Again, range of motion, in association with what position elicits the most pain, can be very revealing as to the cause of pain. Decreased flexion, with increased pain in the low back, often indicates herniated disc or myofascial dysfunctional pain syndrome of the paraspinal musculature, multifidus muscles, or rotatorebrevis muscles. Pain and reduced extension, or difficulty arising from a flexed position, often indicate a facet joint problem or possibly posterior herniation of a lumbar disc. Pain elicited ipsilateral to the direction of lateral bending often indicates facet joint arthropathy. Pain contralateral to the direction of bending often indicates facet joint myofascial pain. Patients who have pain and reduced range of motion in all directions often suffer from degenerative disc disease.

The neurologic exam is not necessarily different from a general medical examination, except it is probably more intensive with the purpose of defining the level of neurological insult. Careful testing using light touch, cold and pinprick, comparing the contralateral limb and different dermatomes on the same limb are extremely important to the pain management physician. It is also very important to measure the circumference of the limbs involved to document atrophy. Finally, because of ongoing spinal pathology and the interventions of the pain management specialist including spinal injections, spinal cord stimulators, and intrathecal pumps, it is extremely important to evaluate for long tract signs, including clonus and/or

Babinski's signs. Documentation of clonus or up-going toes in patients complaining of new back pain, new extremity weakness, or incontinence of bowel or bladder after a new injury or a spinal procedure necessitates immediate spinal imaging and neurosurgical evaluation.

Probably the most unusual aspect to the neurological evaluation is the evaluation of the autonomic system. Changes in autonomic outflow may cause significant temperature changes of the skin. The patient may also have unusual sensory symptoms to light touch, including hyperesthesia, which describes the stinging sensation when the skin is just lightly touched over the involved area. The patient may also complain of allodynia, which is an abnormal painful sensation to a stimulus such as light touch, which would not be expected to cause pain. Often when the allodynia or hyperesthesia is in a nondermatonal pattern, it is associated with complex regional pain syndrome, sympathetically maintained pain, whereas allodynia or hyperesthesia in a more dermatonal peripheral nerve distribution indicates neuralgia or neuropathy.

DIAGNOSTIC WORKUP

Most patients come into a pain management specialist having had recent imaging studies. Much can be learned from personal review of the imaging studies and explaining to the patient what is found on these studies. Presently, most authorities agree that MRIs are probably more useful in patients with true radicular qualities to their pain, whereas standard x-rays of the spine are more cost effective and, generally, just as informative for patients who have axial-type pain. I am certainly more likely to order an MRI, or possibly a bone scan, in patients with a history of cancer, such as breast or lung cancer, which often metastasizes to the bone. It is often very useful to consider flexion/extension films of the neck or lumbar spine, as it is important to keep in mind the MRI is only a static image. It often misses important instability. If the patient has had previous spinal surgery, it is important to obtain MRI imaging with contrast, which will help delineate whether the patient's pain is from scar tissue from previous surgery or a recurrent disc problem. Bone scans seem to be most helpful in identifying inflammation and infection or in dating occult fractures that may not be picked up on routine x-rays or MRIs. I restrict the use of electromyography (EMGs) mainly for medical-legal documentation of radiculopathy or peripheral neuropathies. Usually if the patient's symptoms on physical examination respond to spinal injections, that can serve as adequate documentation of a radiculopathy.

In terms of laboratory assessment of patients, I think that it is most important to find what studies they have had prior to coming to be seen by the pain management physician. Certainly the type of patients we see with hypertension and diabetes deserve electrolyte and renal function checks two to three times per year during treatment with nonsteroidal antiinflammatory medications or while they are on Neurontin, which is excreted renally. Certainly liver function tests are important while patients are taking nonsteroidal antiinflammatories and anticonvulsants. Occasionally, thyroid function tests are very important in patients who have not been completely evaluated for the cause of depression or neuropathy. Finally, the patient with possible connective tissue disease or lupus-type illnesses deserves a CBC because they may have thrombocytopenia, anemia, or depressed white cell counts. Evaluation of their antinucleic acid antibody (ANA) status, sedimentation rate, rheumatoid factor, and, if it is an acute flare of lupus, complement levels may be in order. More specific DNA and anti-body testing should be relegated to the rheumatologist. Occasionally human lymphocytic antigen (HLA) profiles can be useful in the diagnosis of Reiter's syndrome for patients who are expected to have ankylosing spondylitis.

REFERENCES

1. Longmire DR. Evaluation of the pain patient. In: Raj P, ed. *Pain medicine, a comprehensive review*, 1996.
2. Donoboc CD. Evaluation of the patient in pain. In: Waldman S, Winnie A, eds. *Interventional pain management*.
3. Bowen J, Loeser J. Evaluation of the patient with pain. In: *The management of pain*.

CHAPTER 6

Medical Electrodiagnostics

Henry A. Spindler and Marcel Reischer

Patients are referred for electrodiagnostic evaluation of a variety of complaints, including pain, weakness, sensory complaints, gait disturbances, headache, and bowel and bladder dysfunction (1). These electrical studies are frequently of great help in diagnosing acute and chronic pain involving the neck, back, and extremities. The most useful tests are electromyography (EMG) and nerve conduction studies (NCS), including H reflex and F wave measurement. Somatosensory evoked potentials may also sometimes be helpful in evaluating patients with pain syndromes. Older methods of electrodiagnosis (reaction of degeneration, chronaxy, rheobase, galvanic-tetanus ratio, strength-duration curves) are rarely, if ever, used for the evaluation of pain in a modern electrodiagnostic laboratory. However, they are certainly of historical interest, and nerve excitability studies continue to be used for evaluation of Bell's palsy (2,3).

The primary function of an electrodiagnostic evaluation using electromyography and nerve conduction studies is to evaluate the functional integrity of the motor unit. The term *motor unit* was first used by Liddell and Sherrington in 1925 to describe the functional unit of the peripheral nervous system (4). The motor unit is defined as an anterior horn cell, its axon, and all of the muscle fibers innervated by that axon. Electrodiagnostic studies attempt to localize sites of pathology within the motor unit (e.g., root, plexus, peripheral nerve, etc.) to diagnose the presence of a lesion causing the clinical pain syndrome.

In this chapter we will explore the basic physiology and techniques of electrodiagnostic medicine, the expected findings in specific disorders, and the clinical usefulness of these studies.

ELECTROMYOGRAPHY

Electromyography is the technique of recording voltage changes within a muscle. Resting mammalian muscle fibers have a transmembrane potential of 70 to 90 millivolts in the resting state. The inside of the cell is negative with respect to the outside. This resting potential arises because the membrane is impermeable to the large organic anions within the cell and because of the active transport mechanism that maintains the internal sodium (Na+) concentration at a low level. When a nerve impulse reaches the neuromuscular junction, acetylcholine is released across the enAd plate zone. This initiates an action potential, or reversal of polarity across the muscle membrane, which rapidly spreads over the length of the muscle fiber initiating contraction. The amplitude of this voltage change may be 100 mV or more when measured with an intracellular electrode.

Intracellular muscle potential recording is technically difficult and unsuited to the clinical situation. Extracellular electromyographic recordings are performed clinically with a needle electrode. Adrian and Bronk in 1929 introduced the concentric needle electrode (5). This electrode consists of a hypodermic needle serving as the cannula with a wire located centrally in the needle but completely insulated from it. Voltage is recorded as the potential difference between the exposed tip of the central wire and the cannula. Since the recording is made extracellularly at a distance from the muscle fiber, the voltage changes recorded are much smaller and range from 500 µv to 5 mV. Also, with standard recording electrodes, the recording surface at the tip is quite large with respect to the muscle fiber, and potentials from several muscle fibers are recorded simultaneously. Specialized electrodes with very small recording areas have been developed for recording single muscle fiber potentials. Single fiber recordings, however, are quite specialized studies and are not used routinely in the electrodiagnostic examination.

Today, the most commonly used needle electrode is of the monopolar type. This is a small-diameter wire electrode that is coated with insulating Teflon except at the tip where recording is done. Potential measurements are made between the exposed tip of the needle within the muscle compared to a surface electrode taped to the skin. This electrode arrangement has largely replaced the concentric electrode in most clinical conditions due to the much greater patient comfort.

Electrical activity measured within the muscle is fed into a suitable amplifier and then displayed on an oscilloscope. The activity is also monitored through a loudspeaker, since the various potential changes encountered have characteristic sounds. Electromyographic activity is measured during needle insertion, during complete rest of the muscle without needle movement, and during various grades of active muscle contraction.

Insertional Activity

The electrical response seen when a needle electrode is inserted into resting muscle is termed the *insertional activity*. This appears as a burst of spike potentials, which continues for 100 to 300 millisecond (ms) after needle motion has ceased. This electrical activity is produced by mechanical damage or deformation of the muscle membrane by the advancing needle. While the evaluation of insertional activity may appear simple, it is actually a quite difficult procedure. With careful analysis, a great deal of information may be gained by an experienced electromyographer.

The duration of insertional activity may be normal, increased, or decreased. The exact duration of normal insertional activity cannot be given since it depends on many factors, including the velocity of needle insertion and the degree of tissue deformation that occurs. Each electromyographer must therefore to some degree determine "normal" insertional activity with his or her equipment and technique. Increase in the duration of insertional activity may be the first or only sign of neuromuscular disease. Decrease in the duration of insertional activity is also significant. It most commonly indicates a loss of muscle tissue and is usually a late finding in neuromuscular disease.

The character of the electrical discharges seen with needle insertion must also be examined. Occasional positive sharp waves may be seen during insertional activity as the first sign of denervation.

Since abnormal insertional activity may not be uniform throughout the muscle, at least 10 to 20 needle insertions must be performed at various sites within the muscle. Electromyographers must be aware of the *end plate noise*, which is the normal electrical activity seen in the end plate zone of the muscle, and not report this as abnormal insertional activity.

RESTING MUSCLE

With the needle electrode at rest in relaxed muscle, there is normally no electrical activity seen. Resting activity is observed during pauses between needle insertions. During this procedure, the electromyographer is searching for the presence of abnormal spontaneous activity at rest, but may also encounter normal spontaneous activity, which must be recognized as such.

Normal Spontaneous Activity

Normal spontaneous activity can be recorded if the needle electrode is near the motor end plate region (6). Two types of end plate noise are commonly seen. The first appears as a widening of the baseline, but at closer inspection is a series of 8 to 10 µv negative potentials that exhibit a characteristic "seashell" sound over the loudspeaker. This electrical activity corresponds to the miniature end plate potentials caused by acetylcholine release. Occasionally, large spike potentials may be seen superimposed on the end plate noise. These are most likely due to the needle electrode provoking enough acetylcholine release to depolarize the entire muscle membrane, resulting in the recording of a propagated single muscle fiber nerve action potential.

Abnormal Spontaneous Activity

Fibrillation Potentials

Fibrillation potentials are the electrical activity recorded from the spontaneous depolarization of single muscle fibers. They are usually bi- or triphasic potentials, 50 to 500 uv in amplitude, with a duration of less than 1.5 ms. The initial deflection is positive when recording away from the end plate zone. Each muscle fiber depolarizes at a regular rate varying from 1 to 30 per second, but in some cases the firing may be irregular (7). However, since in most cases, multiple fibrillations are seen simultaneously, an irregular-appearing pattern appears on the oscilloscope with a characteristic crackling, "rain on a tin roof" sound from the loudspeaker. Fibrillations have been most commonly associated with lower motor neuron disease such as anterior horn cell pathology, radiculopathies, and neuropathies. In these disorders muscle fiber has lost continuity with its motor nerve fiber allowing spontaneous depolarization. However, it is now known that fibrillations can occur in the presence of myopathies, especially polymyositis, where splitting of the muscle fiber occurs. Fibrillations may also be seen in electrolyte disorders as hypokalemia or hyperkalemia. Fibrillations have also been reported in spinal cord injury and stroke, but this finding is still controversial (8,9).

Positive Sharp Waves

Positive sharp waves are seen in the same conditions and have the same significance as fibrillation potentials. They are biphasic potentials with an initial sharp positive phase of from 50 µv to 1 mV followed by a low amplitude, long duration negative phase commonly exceeding 10 ms before returning to baseline. Positive waves fire regularly, commonly at a rate of 2 to 10 per second. Positive waves are felt to arise from spontaneously depolarizing single muscle fibers that have been damaged by needle insertion.

Fasciculation Potentials

Fasciculation potentials are the electrical activity recorded from the spontaneous firing of a motor unit. When these occur near the surface of the muscle, a visible twitch can be seen. The neural discharge initiating the fasciculation is most commonly in the distal axon, but it may be anywhere within the motor unit (10). Thus, while they are usually associated with motor neuron disease, fasciculations may be present in radiculopathies or peripheral neuropathies. They may be occasionally seen in otherwise normal muscle, especially with fatigue. Fasciculations are not seen in primary muscle disorders.

Complex Repetitive Discharges

Complex repetitive discharges (previously called bizarre high-frequency discharges) can be seen in many forms of lower motor neuron disorders or myopathies. These are trains of potentials that begin and end abruptly. Their amplitude may range from 50 µv to several mV. The individual potentials may assume many forms and may be 50 to 100 ms in duration. They may fire at rates ranging from 5 to 100 cycles per second. These discharges most likely arise within a group of denervated muscle fibers where one muscle fiber acts as a pacemaker with spread of depolarization to the neighboring denervated muscle fibers (11). Myotonic discharges are felt to be a distinct repetitive discharge due to muscle membrane instability as seen in disorders such as myotonic dystrophy and myotonia congenita. These discharges wax and wane in frequency and amplitude, whereas complex repetitive discharges display constant rate and amplitude. Myotonic discharges also differ in that the trains of potentials slowly decrease in frequency until they stop, instead of suddenly ceasing.

VOLUNTARY MUSCLE CONTRACTION

After the muscle being examined has been studied at rest, the patient is asked to produce a minimal contraction with the needle electrode in place. The number of motor unit potentials seen is proportional to the strength of contraction; and therefore to examine individual motor unit potentials, the contraction must be kept minimal. The normal motor unit potential usually contains up to four phases. A potential with five or more phases is termed *polyphasic*. A small proportion of normal motor units may be polyphasic (5 to 15%). An increase in the percentage of polyphasic motor unit potentials is considered abnormal. This may occur with either neuropathic disease or myopathy. In neuropathy, impaired conduction in the terminal nerve fibers of the motor unit will result in asynchrony of firing and an increase in the number of phases seen on electromyography (12). In primary muscle disorders, loss of muscle fibers contributing to the motor unit potential may result in an increased number of phases.

The amplitude of the normal motor unit action potential ranges from 500 µv to 5 mV. This amplitude will vary with the density of the muscle fibers in the region of the tip of the electrode as well as with the synchrony of firing of the individual muscle fibers in the unit. In lower motor neuron disorders, reinnervation frequently leads to an increase in fiber density, resulting in increased motor unit potential amplitudes. In myopathy, loss of muscle fibers from the unit will result in decreased amplitude. Normal motor unit potential duration ranges from 5 to 12 ms as defined from the first deviation from the baseline to the final return to baseline. In neuropathy, with slowing in terminal nerve fiber conduction, there will be an increase in the duration of the potential. In myopathy, the common finding is a decrease in potential duration.

As the strength of voluntary contraction increases, the number of motor units firing increases proportionally. The first recruited motor unit potentials fire at a rate of approximately five per second. As the strength of contraction increases, the initial unit begins firing at a higher rate, and simultaneously other motor units are recruited. In neuropathic disease, when fewer motor units are available for recruitment, the first unit will be seen firing at a higher-than-normal rate before the second unit appears. In myopathy, where the strength produced by each motor unit is reduced, the second motor unit will be recruited much earlier. With maximal voluntary contraction in normal muscle, the oscilloscope will be obscured by electrical activity, and individual motor units cannot be seen (complete interference pattern). In neuropathic disorders, at maximal contraction there may not be a complete obliteration of the baseline with electrical activity (incomplete interference pattern); or in severe cases, individual motor units may still be discernible (single unit interference pattern). In myopathies, as previously discussed, there is decreased strength produced by contraction by each motor unit. Therefore, for a contraction of fixed strength, more motor units will need to be recruited than in normal muscle. This causes a complete interference pattern with less-than-maximal effort.

Although evaluation of the interference pattern is important, it must be interpreted with caution, because lack of patient cooperation from anxiety or pain may influence the results.

NERVE CONDUCTION STUDIES

Nerve conduction studies are safe, reliable, and reproducible in assessing peripheral nerve function. They are used to determine the presence and type of neuropathy, to localize lesions, and to determine their severity. The nerve is stimulated electrically, and various parameters are measured to determine the nerve's ability to carry the impulse. Stimulation may be done either with needle or surface electrodes. In most laboratories, surface stimulation is the method of choice. However, with deeply placed nerves, as the sciatic in the gluteal region, near nerve needle stimulation is easier and more comfortable for the patient. At rest the nerve is charged with a 90 mV transmembrane potential, positive externally. When the negatively applied stimulus exceeds threshold, an action potential is generated. This potential is then self-propagated proximally and distally.

Motor conduction studies are performed by stimulating the nerve and recording the evoked response from a distal muscle. The time from stimulation to the onset of the evoked response is termed *the latency*. Conduction velocity from the distal stimulation site to the muscle cannot be determined because of the presence of the neuromuscular junction. However, if the nerve is stimulated at two points, the velocity between these points is easily determined by subtracting the distal from the proximal latency and dividing this into the distance between the stimulus sites. Conduction velocities can thus be determined over multiple segments of the nerve to localize a lesion.

Sensory conduction studies are performed by placing recording electrodes directly over the sensory nerve being examined. The nerve may be stimulated either proximally (antidromic conduction) or distally (orthodromic conduction) to these electrodes, and the time is measured from the onset of the stimulus to the onset of the action potential that is being recorded. Dividing this time into the distance between the recording and stimulating electrodes yields the sensory conduction velocity. The sensory nerve action potential is usually bi- or triphasic. Latency measurements are frequently made to both the onset and the peak of the first negative phase. As in motor studies, the amplitude of the evoked response is recorded.

Decrease in nerve conduction velocity is most commonly associated with disorders of the myelin. However, this may also occur with diseases affecting the large, rapidly conducting axons. Axonal disorders more commonly cause a decrease in the amplitude of the evoked motor and sensory responses since fewer fibers are available to contribute to the response.

Sensory nerves commonly studied include the median, ulnar, radial, medial and lateral antebrachial cutaneous, lateral femoral cutaneous, sural, superficial peroneal, and tibial. Motor studies may be done on the median, ulnar, radial, tibial, peroneal, and sciatic nerves. Motor latency studies may be done on the femoral, axillary, suprascapular, accessory, and facial nerves.

Proximal Conduction Studies

The conduction studies discussed thus far allow evaluation of peripheral nerve function in the extremities.

Nerve root stimulation, H reflex, and F wave measurements allow examination of proximal segments at the root and plexus level.

Nerve Root Stimulation

Nerve root stimulation may be performed in either the cervical or lumbar region. In the cervical region, the C-8 nerve root is the most frequently studied; but C-6 and C-7 may also be evaluated. In the lumbar region, L-4, L-5, or S-1 may be examined. A stimulating needle cathode is placed into the paraspinal musculature at the proper level. The anode is placed on the skin. A recording of the evoked response from an appropriate muscle in the limb is made in the normal manner. Side-to-side latency comparisons are made to determine abnormality (13).

H Reflex

The H reflex, first discovered by Hoffman in 1918, was later named and further investigated by Magladery and associates in the 1950s (14). Since then hundreds of articles have been published on the further investigation and use of this reflex. Most investigators feel that this is the electrical counterpart of the muscle stretch reflex, but it differs in several ways. In infancy, an H reflex can be obtained from most nerves, but after age 2, it can easily be found only in the tibial nerve. In spinal shock, when reflexes may be absent, the H reflex may still be present.

The tibial H reflex is normally obtained by stimulating the tibial nerve at the knee with recording from the gastrocnemius or soleus muscles. It is felt that the impulse is carried proximally by the Ia fibers to the spinal cord. There they synapse with the alpha motor neurons and the impulse is conducted back to the muscle, resulting in a muscle twitch. The latency measurement between the stimulus and twitch is therefore a measure of the integrity of both the S-1 motor and sensory roots. This study is most commonly used for evaluating S-1 radiculopathies. However, it has also been described as useful in diagnosing C-6–C-7 lesions by stimulating the median nerve with recording from the flexor carpi radialis and L-3–L-4 by stimulating the femoral nerve and recording from the vastus medialis.

F Wave

The F wave was first described by Magladery and McDougal (14). When any motor nerve is stimulated with recording from a distal muscle, a late response may be seen following the initial muscle response. The amplitude and latency of this late response is quite variable, and it may not be present with each stimulation. In contrast, the H reflex is identical with each stimulus. It is believed that the F wave results from antidromic conduction of the stimulus in the alpha motor neurons to the spinal cord. There they cause firing of the anterior horn cells. These impulses are then carried orthodromically by the alpha motor neurons causing discharge of the muscle fibers that they innervate. The same alpha motor neurons may not fire with each stimulus, thus resulting in a variable response. Since only alpha motor neurons are involved, the F wave is a measurement of motor function only. F waves are commonly studied in the median, ulnar, peroneal, and tibial nerves. They are most valuable in examining proximal nerve function in neuropathy, but they may also be abnormal in radiculopathy. If distal conduction studies are normal but the F wave latency is prolonged, a proximal lesion may exist. This is commonly helpful in evaluating proximal neuropathies such as Guillain-Barré syndrome.

Somatosensory Evoked Potentials

Somatosensory evoked potentials (SEP) may be obtained by stimulating a peripheral nerve, usually the median or ulnar at the wrist or tibial or peroneal at the ankle, and recording wave forms from proximal areas of the extremity, plexus, spine or contralateral scalp. It is felt that these potentials are carried by sensory fibers in the peripheral nerves and in the dorsal column-lemniscal system centrally. They can therefore be theoretically used to measure function distally or proximally in the peripheral nervous system or in the spinal cord or brain. They are most commonly used for aid in diagnosing multiple sclerosis (15) along with auditory and visual evoked potentials. They also have proved very useful in monitoring spinal cord function during spinal surgery.

Somatosensory evoked potentials continue to undergo evaluation as to their clinical usefulness in diagnosing plexus and root lesions, especially when only sensory fibers are involved. Limited success has been achieved thus far, and the clinical usefulness of these studies in radiculopathy is very controversial. Studies in several centers are presently underway to evaluate dermatomal cutaneous stimulation to better localize lesions to a single root, especially in patients with multilevel pathology as in spinal stenosis, but these studies are still in an experimental stage. At this point, few electromyographers would be willing to diagnose a radiculopathy based on somatosensory abnormalities alone.

Magnetic Stimulation

Magnetic stimulation studies of the peripheral and central nervous system, while still investigational, deserve mention. Magnetic coils have been developed that induce current flow in tissue with essentially no patient discomfort. Deeply seated structures such as the brachial plexus can be stimulated with ease. The major problem with this technique is the inability to determine the exact point of nerve stimulation since a broad area of current flow is induced. Therefore conduction velocities cannot be accurately calculated and the value of this procedure will be limited in peripheral nerve studies until more focused stimulators can be developed.

Transcranial stimulation of the motor cortex with magnetic coils has also been accomplished. Recording motor evoked responses from appropriate contralateral muscles should allow another method of evaluating central and peripheral pathways complementary to somatosensory studies.

ELECTRODIAGNOSTIC FINDINGS IN SPECIFIC DISORDERS

Electrodiagnostic studies were originally developed for evaluation and localization of peripheral nerve injuries. While this continues to be an important use of these studies, they are more frequently used to diagnose radiculopathies, entrapment syndromes, peripheral neuropathies, and myopathies in patients with acute and chronic pain, paresthesias, and weakness.

Radiculopathies

Neck and low back pain are the most common forms of musculoskeletal disability. Cervical and lumbar radiculopathies may cause acute and chronic back pain, headaches, extremity pain, numbness, paresthesias, and weakness. Thoracic radiculopathies, while less common, may cause noncardiac chest pain and abdominal pain.

Electrodiagnostic studies have proven very useful in diagnosing radiculopathy. While myelography, computerized axial tomography, and magnetic resonance imaging (MRI) all examine the anatomy of the spine, spinal cord, and roots, electrical testing is the only widely accepted method of assessing the physiologic function of the nerve roots. Since 15 to 20% of asymptomatic patients will show evidence of disc herniation on MRI, electrodiagnostic studies are necessary to document which of these are causing significant neural compromise. Although radiculopathy is usually due to a compressive lesion, such as a herniated disc, it may also be due to a noncompressive lesion as in diabetic radiculopathy. It has been found that electrodiagnostic studies and myelography are equal in their sensitivity and accuracy in diagnosing compressive root lesions (16). Comparisons with computerized tomography have shown electrical studies to be the more accurate study in localizing a radiculopathy (17). Most studies have shown that both anatomical and electrical studies have approximately a 75 to 80% accuracy; but when a combination of the two types of study are performed, a much higher degree of accuracy will be obtained. Therefore, when evaluating the patient with chronic pain, both imaging and physiological studies should be employed.

In evaluating for a possible radiculopathy, the examiner performs electromyography on multiple muscles innervated by each of the roots supplying the extremity involved. While this will evaluate function in the anterior primary ramus, the corresponding paraspinal musculature must also be examined to evaluate the posterior primary ramus. If root compression is causing damage to motor fibers within the root, EMG abnormalities will be seen in the muscles supplied by that root, allowing the level of the lesion to be localized. In some cases, EMG abnormalities will be seen only in the paraspinal musculature. This localizes the lesion to the root level, but the exact root involved cannot be determined since there is a large overlap in innervation of the paraspinal musculature. In an acute nerve root lesion, EMG abnormalities in the paraspinal musculature will not occur until approximately 7 to 10 days after onset. In the extremity musculature, abnormalities such as fibrillations and positive waves may not occur for 3 to 4 weeks. However, if weakness is present, a decrease in motor unit recruitment may be seen in a myotomal pattern during this early phase. Medicolegally, it may be worthwhile performing electromyography during the first week after injury to determine whether abnormalities are present from a preexisting lesion. This is especially true in the chronic pain patient who may have had multiple previous injuries or surgery. If no fibrillations are found on this initial examination, but are then present 3 weeks later, they can be ascribed to the present illness.

Since most peripheral nerves contain fibers from multiple nerve roots, standard peripheral nerve conduction studies are usually normal. However, they may be abnormal if multiple roots are involved with loss of a large number of nerve fibers. H reflex, F wave, and somatosensory studies in the affected nerve root distribution may be abnormal and aid in the diagnosis.

Cervical Radiculopathy

The C-7 nerve root is probably the most commonly involved in cervical radiculopathy, followed by C-6, C-8, and C-5 (18). With C-5 radiculopathies, pain is usually felt radiating into the shoulder. Weakness may be seen in the deltoid and possibly the biceps. The biceps jerk may be depressed. Sensory complaints are uncommon, but there may be some dysesthesias over the lateral aspect of the forearm. EMG abnormalities may be seen in the rhomboids, supraspinatus, infraspinatus, deltoid, and possibly the biceps. C-6 radiculopathies give a similar pain pattern, but paresthesias are frequently complained of in the thumb. EMG abnormalities are commonly seen in the biceps, pronator teres, and extensor carpi radialis, but may also be seen in the deltoid and supraspinatus. C-7 radiculopathy frequently presents with pain radiating into the triceps, forearm, and hand. Paresthesias are commonly present in the index and long fingers. Weakness may be prominent in the triceps with an absent triceps jerk. EMG abnormalities are likely to be found in the triceps, pronator teres, flexor carpi radialis, and extensor digitorum communis. A prolonged median H reflex latency to the flexor carpi radialis may be seen with C-6–C-7 lesions. With both C-6 and C-7 lesions, median, radial and musculocutaneous sensory conduction, and median and radial motor conduction studies should be normal to rule out carpal tunnel syndrome or other nerve entrapment. With C-8 radiculopathy, the patient frequently presents with pain and paresthesias radiating down the ulnar aspect of the arm into the fourth and fifth digits. The triceps tendon jerk may be absent. EMG abnormalities may be seen in the extensor digitorum communis, extensor and flexor carpi ulnaris, and in all the intrinsic hand musculature. Median and ulnar F wave latencies may be prolonged to the thenar and hypothenar musculature, respectively, but these must be interpreted with caution since thoracic outlet syndrome may also cause F wave abnormalities in the C-8 distribution. Ulnar motor and sensory conduction studies should be normal to exclude ulnar entrapment mimicking a C-8 lesion. Since C-8 radiculopathies are uncommon, one must be sure to evaluate the patient for possible lower brachial plexopathy as seen with a Pancoast tumor.

Although fibrillations and positive waves are the hallmark of an acute radiculopathy, increased insertional activity and an increased number of polyphasic motor unit potentials may be the only abnormality seen. With chronic radiculopathies, these are commonly the only abnormalities present (19).

Lumbosacral Radiculopathies

Electrodiagnostic studies are of great use in the evaluation of low back and leg pain. They can differentiate radiculopathy from the many other causes of back and leg pain such as vascular lesions, mechanical or muscular low back pain, arthritis of the spine and hip, or disc disease without nerve root compression.

In L-4 radiculopathy, the patient commonly experiences pain in the hip radiating into the groin, anterior thigh, and knee. Sensory complaints are not common, but paresthesias may be experienced over the medial aspect of the knee. The patient may complain that bearing weight on the knee causes buckling. Interestingly, the patient with primary hip pathology will have many of these same complaints. On physical examination, the knee jerk may be decreased and weakness may be appreciated in the quadriceps. Electromyography may show abnormalities in the quadriceps and femoral adductors. The femoral H reflex latency to the vastus medialis may be prolonged. Femoral motor conduction should be normal to differentiate this from a femoral neuropathy.

With L-5 radiculopathies, the patient will commonly complain of pain radiating from the back to the lateral hip and thigh and anterior tibial region. Paresthesias may be felt over the dorsum of the foot, and weakness may be noted in the ankle. On physical examination, weakness in the ankle and toe dorsiflexors may be appreciated. There may also be weakness of hip abduction. The medial hamstring reflex may be reduced. Electrically, EMG abnormalities will be seen in the ankle and toe dorsiflexors, flexor digitorum longus, medial hamstrings, tensor fascia latae, and hip abductors. The peroneal F wave latency recorded from the extensor digitorum brevis may be prolonged on the affected side. Differentiation from peroneal neuropathy is made by normal peroneal conduction and by EMG abnormalities in the proximal L-5 innervated musculature at the hip.

In S-1 radiculopathy, the patient experiences pain radiating to the hip, posterior thigh, and calf. There may be complaints of paresthesias over the lateral aspect of the foot. Weakness is uncommon, but there may be some difficulty with toe standing on the affected side. Electrical abnormalities are most commonly found in the gastrocnemius and soleus. They may also be found in the lateral hamstrings and gluteus maximus as well as the intrinsic foot musculature. However, findings localized to the foot musculature must be interpreted with caution, since the extensor digitorum brevis is subject to much trauma, and tarsal tunnel syndrome may cause abnormality in the tibial innervated foot musculature. The tibial H reflex latency will commonly be prolonged or absent with stimulation of the tibial nerve at the knee recording from the gastrocnemius or soleus. Normal tibial motor conduction will indicate that this tibial H reflex abnormality is due to a proximal lesion. Normal sural sensory conduction will confirm that the sensory abnormalities on the lateral aspect of the foot are due to a proximal lesion.

In all patients who have undergone spinal surgery, electromyographic abnormalities found in the paraspinal musculature must be interpreted with caution. Electrical abnormalities may persist in these muscles for years after surgery. Some researchers feel that performing the EMG needle examination at 3 cm from the scar at a 3- to 5-cm depth will avoid abnormalities due to the trauma of surgery. However, in most circumstances it is safest to avoid examination of these muscles once surgery has been performed. In the distribution of the anterior primary ramus, EMG abnormalities tend to subside faster than clinical abnormalities (20). However, with severe root lesions, EMG abnormalities may persist as long as 3 to 4 years after surgery. Therefore, in examining a patient with recurrent back or leg pain, it is very helpful to have a preoperative examination for comparison of the distribution of the abnormalities.

In some patients with radicular symptoms, EMG abnormalities may only be seen in the paraspinals. This indicates there is root level pathology, but most electromyographers agree that in the absence of extremity muscle findings, the root involved cannot be accurately identified since the paraspinals have broadly overlapping innervation.

Thoracic Radiculopathies

Thoracic radiculopathies are much less common than cervical or lumbosacral radiculopathies. They may be the cause of chest or abdominal pain, which usually begins in the spine and radiates anteriorly, or spinal pain may be the only symptom. Compressive root lesions can occur with a herniated disc or tumor, but the lesion may also be on the basis of herpes zoster or diabetes. In patients with abdominal pain, but an otherwise normal examination, a radiculopathy must be considered, especially in diabetics. The classical findings in diabetic thoracic radiculopathy include mild peripheral nerve conduction abnormalities with fibrillation in the thoracic paraspinal musculature on the symptomatic side (21).

Entrapment Syndromes

Peripheral nerve entrapment syndromes are a frequent cause of extremity paresthesias, pain, and weakness (22). Median nerve entrapment at the wrist—carpal tunnel syndrome—is the most commonly encountered nerve entrapment syndrome, but many others have also been described. Both the median and ulnar nerves may be entrapped at the wrist and elbow. The radial nerve may be entrapped at the elbow, and its superficial sensory branch may be entrapped in the forearm. The sensory division of the musculocutaneous nerve may be entrapped at the elbow. The femoral, lateral femoral cutaneous, and tibial nerves may be entrapped in the lower extremities.

The classic electrodiagnostic finding in an entrapment syndrome is segmental slowing of conduction across the area of entrapment due to focal demyelination as in carpal tunnel syndrome. Conduction in segments proximal and distal to the lesion are frequently normal; but with a severe nerve compression, conduction in the distal segment may also be affected. Sensory conduction is commonly affected before motor conduction. Electromyographic abnormalities may be found in the muscle supplied by the entrapped nerve, but this is usually a late finding when demyelination is the primary pathology. In recent years it has come to be realized that the basic pathology in some nerve entrapments is axonal loss in which amplitude decrease is the first change seen. This makes diagnosis much more difficult since there is a wide range of normal amplitude in any conduction study. Most cases of tarsal tunnel syndrome, pronator syndrome, and radial entrapment are axonal lesions. Occasionally ulnar entrapment, and more rarely carpal tunnel syndrome, may be axonal. This would help explain why a few patients with classical symptoms and physical exam have normal nerve conduction studies.

Median Nerve

Median nerve entrapment at the wrist (carpal tunnel syndrome) must be differentiated from entrapment at the elbow. Patients with carpal tunnel syndrome usually present with paresthesias in the hand. This should be confined to the thumb, index, long finger, and radial half of the ring finger. However, many patients have difficulty localizing their symptoms and complain of generalized numbness in the entire hand. While this should alert the examiner to consider other lesions, carpal tunnel syndrome is frequently the only problem found. There may be pain in the hand and wrist with radiation up the arm to the shoulder. Occasionally, shoulder pain may be prominent, and it may be confused with cervical radiculopathy. In a small group of patients, shoulder pain will be the only symptom. There are frequent complaints of weakness in the hand and dropping of small objects. Patients commonly complain that their symptoms awaken them at night or are most severe on arising in the morning. The symptoms may be brought on by use of the hand as in knitting, driving, or with any repetitive activity. Complaints are often bilateral with the dominant hand more involved. Carpal tunnel syndrome may be associated with trauma, arthritis and connective tissue disease, or hypothyroidism, but it is frequently idiopathic.

Hundreds of articles have been written on the electrodiagnostic evaluation of carpal tunnel syndrome. Many methods exist for evaluating median conduction across the wrist, and each laboratory will have its preferred procedure. Since carpal tunnel syndrome is often bilateral and associated with other entrapment neuropathies, median, ulnar, and radial sensory studies as well as median and ulnar motor conduction studies should be performed in both hands. Slowing of median sensory and motor conduction across the wrist with normal conduction proximal and distal to the transverse carpal ligament is the classical finding in carpal tunnel syndrome. Sensory conduction will be abnormal before motor in the vast majority of patients. Frequently, in early cases, the absolute values of median conduction may be within the normal range, but comparison to the asymptomatic hand or to radial or ulnar conduction in the same hand may yield evidence of relative slowing of median conduction, which may be diagnostic (23). Again, it cannot be emphasized too strongly that when assessing a patient for possible carpal tunnel syndrome, conduction studies should not be limited to the median nerve. In addition to finding other entrapments, it is not at all unusual for the electromyographer to discover an unsuspected peripheral polyneuropathy.

Electromyography must always be performed along with nerve conduction studies for a complete evaluation. EMG may sometimes show denervation of the thenar musculature in carpal tunnel syndrome, but usually only in severe cases. In addition to the hand musculature, the entire extremity should be examined to rule out the presence of a radiculopathy simulating carpal tunnel syndrome or coexisting with it. Persistent symptoms after carpal tunnel release may be due to a root lesion that was not recognized.

In very early or mild carpal tunnel syndrome, all electrical studies may be normal in a small percentage of patients. This occurs because significant demyelination or axonal damage may not have taken place. Detailed cutaneous sensory testing, when combined with the electrical studies, may improve the diagnostic yield (24), but there still may be the exceptional case with no abnormal findings. In this event, the exam should be repeated at a later date to differentiate psychogenic symptoms from neuropathology.

Median nerve entrapments in the proximal forearm are rare, but they may be confused with carpal tunnel syndrome. At the elbow, the median nerve may be entrapped within the pronator teres (pronator syndrome) or, very rarely, by the ligament of Struthers at the level of the medial epicondyle. Patients with these proximal entrapments may have very similar symptoms to carpal tunnel syndrome, but pain in the forearm is more prominent. These patients frequently perform work that requires repetitive pronation of the forearm, but other cases have been related to fractures, dislocations, and trauma to the elbow. Electrodiagnosticly, median conduction slowing may be seen across the elbow or in the forearm. In the pronator syndrome, EMG abnormalities may be seen in the forearm musculature distal to the innervation of the pronator teres. More proximal entrapment at the ligament of Struthers would be necessary for EMG abnormalities to be seen in the pronator teres. In both these elbow entrapments, EMG abnormalities have been reported to be of more diagnostic significance than nerve conduction studies (25).

The anterior interosseus nerve is a motor branch of the median nerve that arises below the pronator teres. The nerve may be entrapped at this point or, more commonly, may be involved in trauma. Clinically, weakness is found in the pronator quadratus, flexor pollicis longus, and flexor digitorum profundus to digits II and III. Electromyographic abnormalities will be seen in these muscles, while the remainder of the median musculature will be normal. Standard median motor and sensory conduction studies will be normal because they bypass the anterior interosseus nerve. Stimulation of the median nerve at the elbow and recording from the flexor pollicis longus may occasionally reveal a prolonged latency, but this is not frequent (26).

Ulnar Nerve Entrapments

Entrapment of the ulnar nerve at the elbow is the second most common entrapment neuropathy. However, the ulnar nerve may also be entrapped at the wrist and in the palm. While not truly an entrapment neuropathy, thoracic outlet syndrome commonly causes symptoms primarily in the ulnar distribution.

Ulnar neuropathy at the elbow may be the result of a long-standing deformity of the elbow (tardy ulnar palsy) or entrapment of the nerve under the aponeurosis connecting the two heads of the flexor carpi ulnaris (cubital tunnel syndrome) (27). Patients commonly complain of pain in the elbow with numbness and paresthesias in the fourth and fifth digits as well as weakness in the hands. These symptoms are often bilateral. Nerve conduction studies will classically show slowing of ulnar motor and/or sensory conduction velocity across the elbow as compared to the proximal and distal segments or as compared to the opposite ulnar nerve. This slowing should be at least 10 meters per second (28). There will usually be a decrease in the amplitude of the ulnar sensory nerve action potential recorded from the fifth digit when stimulating at the wrist. Severe ulnar neuropathies may have slowing in the distal segments as well as across the elbow due to wallerian degeneration. EMG abnormalities in advanced cases will be seen in the ulnar portion of the flexor digitorum profundus and the ulnar innervated intrinsic hand musculature. The flexor carpi ulnaris will be spared since this muscle is innervated by a branch of the ulnar nerve arising above the elbow.

The ulnar nerve may also be compressed at the wrist in the Guyon canal. The sensory complaints and weakness in the hand are similar to lesions at the elbow, but discomfort proximal to the wrist is unusual. Electrical studies will show slowing of ulnar motor and sensory conduction across the wrist, and there may be EMG changes in the ulnar innervated intrinsic hand musculature. Proximal ulnar conduction studies should be normal.

The deep motor branch of the ulnar nerve may also be traumatized or compressed by a ganglion distal to the Guyon canal. In this case ulnar motor distal latency from the wrist to the abductor digiti quinti may be normal, whereas conduction to the first dorsal interosseus may be prolonged. Sensory conduction to the fifth digit may be normal or abnormal depending on the site of the lesion.

Thoracic outlet syndrome is defined as compression of the neurovascular bundle in the thoracic outlet, which results in pain, dysesthesias, and occasionally weakness in the arm. In most cases, this is a vascular syndrome, but in a small percentage, neurological symptoms may be prominent. When this occurs, paresthesias are most prominent in the ulnar distribution and weakness may be seen in the hand. Because this syndrome is most often primarily vascular, electrodiagnostic studies are frequently normal. When there is neurologic involvement, slowing of ulnar conduction through the thoracic outlet may occur. However, the best method to detect this is controversial. It has been proposed that stimulation of the ulnar nerve in the supraclavicular fossa and in the axilla will allow for measurement of ulnar motor conduction velocity through the thoracic outlet (29). However, other authors have found this unreliable because stimulation at the supraclavicular fossa may be distal to the actual area of compression (30). Nerve root stimulation may be a better method of demonstrating slowing of conduction through the thoracic outlet. Well-documented electrical abnormalities found in patients with clear-cut neurogenic thoracic outlet syndrome include reduced ulnar sensory and perhaps motor evoked amplitudes, decreased motor evoked amplitude from the abductor pollicis brevis, and denervation of the median and ulnar innervated intrinsic hand musculature in the presence of normal median and ulnar motor conduction velocities and latencies (31). The ulnar F wave

latency may also be prolonged on the affected side as compared to the normal side (32). These are essentially the findings expected in a lower brachial plexus lesion. Thoracic outlet syndrome has classically been felt to be rare, but in recent years this syndrome appears to be invoked in patients involved in minor trauma, especially when litigation is involved. They usually have vague, poorly documented neck and extremity pain as well as paresthesias. Objective studies are usually normal. Many of these patients are subjected to first rib resection, when conservative treatment until the litigation is resolved would appear to be more appropriate.

Since the ulnar nerve may be injured or entrapped at many points along its course, patients with symptoms in an ulnar distribution should receive segmental conduction studies throughout the course of the nerve to best localize the lesion. Also, studies should be done in both arms since these syndromes are frequently bilateral. Electromyography should also be performed on the extremities and cervical paraspinals to rule out a C-8 cervical radiculopathy, which may give a clinical picture identical to an ulnar neuropathy.

Radial Nerve

While not a true entrapment neuropathy, the radial nerve is most commonly injured in the spiral groove. Prolonged pressure in this area results in the classic "Saturday night palsy." Triceps strength and the reflex will be normal, while the brachioradialis and all distal radial innervated muscles will be weak. There may be sensory loss over the radial aspect of the dorsum of the hand. Radial motor conduction studies may show slowing across the spiral groove, and radial sensory conduction may also be abnormal. EMG abnormalities will be found from the brachioradialis distally in the radial distribution.

True entrapments of the radial nerve occur in the region of the elbow. Compression of the recurrent branch of the radial nerve at the elbow gives rise to local pain and is felt to be one of the causes of tennis elbow. This is a rather small branch, and it cannot be tested electrically.

The posterior interosseus syndrome is entrapment of the terminal motor branch of the radial nerve as it passes through the arcade of Froshe between the two heads of the supinator. A lesion at this level will cause weakness of the extensor carpi ulnaris and finger extensors, but the extensor carpi radialis will be spared. Since the superficial radial sensory nerve has already exited the main trunk at this level, there should be no sensory complaints. Motor nerve conduction studies may show slowing in the distal portion with normal proximal conduction. Electromyography will show abnormalities distal to the innervation of the extensor carpi radialis longus and brevis.

Compression of the radial nerve at the wrist (cheiralgia paresthetica) by a wrist band is well documented, and radial sensory conduction studies are useful in demonstrating this lesion (33). Recently, an entrapment of the radial sensory nerve in the forearm has been described (34). These patients usually present with pain or burning over the dorsoradial aspect of the forearm and wrist. The etiology is felt to be local trauma, twisting injuries, or repetitive pronation-supination movements at work. On physical examination, there is usually a positive Tinel's sign over the radial sensory nerve in the distal forearm. There is often a positive Finklestein test, which may lead to a misdiagnosis of de Quervain syndrome. Sensation may be impaired in the radial distribution of the hand, but strength should be normal. Hyperpronation of the forearm may reproduce the symptoms. It is felt that the superficial radial sensory nerve is compressed between the tendons of the extensor carpi radialis longus and brachioradialis when the wrist is pronated. Radial sensory conduction studies may be abnormal with slowing of radial sensory conduction in the forearm, but with normal conduction from the wrist to the thumb. Comparison to musculocutaneous sensory conduction is often helpful, since they have a similar course. Decrease in the amplitude of the radial sensory nerve action potential may be the only abnormality found. Radial motor conduction studies should be normal, and no EMG abnormalities should be seen.

Suprascapular Nerve

The suprascapular nerve is composed of nerve fibers from the C-5 and C-6 roots. This nerve leaves the upper trunk of the brachial plexus and passes under the trapezius muscle, eventually passing through the suprascapular foramen to innervate the supra- and infraspinatus muscles. The nerve may be entrapped in this foramen under the transverse scapular ligament, or it may be subjected to a stretch injury at this site. Entrapment of this nerve will result in shoulder pain, which may be misdiagnosed as bursitis or cervical radiculopathy. Nerve conduction studies may show prolongation of the suprascapular nerve latency from Erb's point to the supra- or infraspinatus. Electromyography will show abnormalities confined to the supra- and infraspinatus with no other C-5 and C-6 innervated muscles involved.

Musculocutaneous Nerve

The musculocutaneous nerve is occasionally injured with local trauma, but can also be damaged by heavy exercise. Rarely, the musculocutaneous nerve may be entrapped by the coracobrachialis. Weakness will be seen in the biceps with sensory loss over the lateral aspect of the forearm. The biceps stretch reflex should be absent. This diagnosis may be confirmed by musculocutaneous motor conduction with stimulation in the axilla and at Erb's

point. Sensory conduction may also be abnormal. Electromyographic abnormalities will be seen in the biceps, brachialis, and coracobrachialis muscles.

An uncommon lesion of the musculocutaneous nerve at the elbow involves only the sensory division, the lateral antebrachial cutaneous nerve. These patients experience pain in the region of the biceps tendon insertion with paresthesias over the radial aspect of the forearm. The biceps tendon jerk and strength will be normal. There is frequently tenderness over the tendon of insertion of the biceps with clinical sensory loss in the distribution of the sensory branch. Musculocutaneous sensory conduction will be abnormal while motor conduction is within normal limits (35,36). No EMG abnormalities will be present.

Lateral Femoral Cutaneous Nerve

The lateral femoral cutaneous nerve arises from the L-2 and L-3 nerve roots. It emerges through the inguinal ligament near the anterior superior iliac spine to innervate the skin over the lateral thigh from the hip to the knee. Compression of this nerve in the inguinal ligament results in burning pain and paresthesias over the lateral thigh (meralgia paresthetica). Objective sensory loss can usually be demonstrated in this area. Since the nerve is purely sensory, there will be no weakness. Nerve conduction studies may show abnormalities in this nerve (37). Comparison should always be made between the symptomatic and asymptomatic legs, since conduction in this nerve is frequently difficult to obtain in obese patients. Electromyography must be performed to rule out a lumbar radiculopathy.

Femoral Nerve

The femoral nerve may be compressed within the pelvis by tumor, psoas abscess, retroperitoneal lymphadenopathy, or hemorrhage into iliacus or psoas muscles. The nerve may also be entrapped at the level of the inguinal ligament. These patients complain of pain, paresthesias, and weakness in the groin and anterior thigh. Femoral motor conduction studies may show abnormal distal latencies, and slowing may be able to be demonstrated across the inguinal ligament (38). Abnormalities on electromyography will be confined to the femoral distribution. Commonly, L3-4 radiculopathies or plexopathies, especially in diabetics, can mimic femoral neuropathy; and electromyography of the entire extremity with emphasis on the quadriceps, femoral adductors, and lumbar paraspinals should make this differentiation.

Obturator Nerve

The obturator nerve is most commonly injured during labor, but may also be injured with pelvic fractures and pelvic surgery. Obturator hernias may entrap the nerve in the obturator canal. Patients complain of pain in the groin radiating along the medial aspect of the thigh. There may be dysesthesias in the medial aspect of the upper thigh. Reproducible obturator conduction studies have not been reported. However, electromyographic examination will show abnormalities confined to the femoral adductors.

Peroneal Nerve

The peroneal nerve is commonly injured at the level of the fibular head where it is very superficial. The nerve may also be compressed at the level of the biceps femoris tendon after prolonged squatting. Pain and numbness may be experienced in the anterior aspect of the leg and foot. Weakness of the ankle and toe dorsiflexors is prominent. Peroneal motor conduction studies may show segmental slowing across the fibular head. With more severe lesions, distal peroneal motor conduction will also be abnormal. Superficial peroneal sensory conduction may also be affected. EMG abnormalities should be confined to the peroneal innervated musculature. Since this may easily be confused with an L-5 radiculopathy, the entire extremity must be examined. Electromyography should always be performed on the short head of the biceps femoris, since this is innervated by a branch from the common peroneal nerve. Involvement of this muscle suggests a lesion proximal to the fibular head.

The deep peroneal nerve is commonly traumatized at the ankle. Many patients may have a prolonged distal peroneal motor latency with no symptoms whatsoever. Fibrillations may be found in the extensor digitorum brevis in approximately 25% of otherwise normal patients, and in older patients the muscle may be completely atrophied. The deep peroneal nerve has been reported to be involved in an entrapment neuropathy at the ankle (39), and this was termed the *anterior tarsal tunnel syndrome*. Patients complain of pain on the dorsum of the foot with numbness between the first and second toes. Since, as previously mentioned, many "normal" individuals have electrical abnormalities in this segment, this diagnosis must only be made when the clinical picture is compatible.

Tibial Nerve

The tibial nerve may be entrapped in the tarsal tunnel, which lies posterior to the medial malleolus and is covered by the laciniate ligament. This entrapment is termed the *tarsal tunnel syndrome* (40). This may be idiopathic or follow fractures of the ankle. The patient will frequently complain of pain in the ankle, heel, and foot with paresthesias on the sole of the foot and toes. A positive Tinel's sign may be present over the tarsal tunnel. Classically, it was felt that motor or sensory tibial distal latencies should be abnormal in either the medial or lateral plantar division. This

assumed the lesion was demyelinating as in carpal tunnel syndrome. However, this is not analogous to carpal tunnel syndrome, and very frequently latencies and velocities are normal, even when comparing to the asymptomatic side.

In 1994 we performed a literature review on the history of electrodiagnosis in tarsal tunnel syndrome (41). It quickly became evident that the few early studies reporting latency abnormalities were based on very few cases, and that axonal changes actually seemed more prominent than demyelination.

Unfortunately, in the 1960s, it became dogma that latency prolongation was necessary to diagnose tarsal tunnel syndrome. Because this is so rarely seen, even today some electromyographers believe tarsal tunnel syndrome is very rare or nonexistent.

In our experience, motor and sensory amplitude changes will be seen much more commonly than latency prolongation. In a series of 104 patients with classic tarsal tunnel syndrome seen in our lab, 95% had evidence of an axonal lesion, whereas only 4.8% had evidence only of demyelination. An additional 24% had evidence of both an axonal and myelin lesion. Electromyography of the abductor hallucis and abductor digiti minimi may also help establish this diagnosis. Fibrillations confined to these muscles on the involved side with normal extensor digitorum brevis examination (peroneal innervated) and a normal examination of the opposite foot suggest tarsal tunnel syndrome. Positive waves alone are not enough to establish this diagnosis since these are frequently seen in otherwise normal patients (42).

In all patients being evaluated for possible tarsal tunnel syndrome, an electromyographic exam should be performed on the entire extremity and lumbar paraspinals to rule out a radiculopathy, which may give a similar clinical picture.

Peripheral Polyneuropathy

Peripheral polyneuropathy may be a cause of severe acute or chronic pain, especially in diabetics. However, it may also be a prominent cause of pain with alcoholic neuropathy, vasculitis, or nutritional neuropathies. The clinical and electrical findings may be diffuse and symmetric or more localized. In mononeuritis multiplex, one nerve may be severely abnormal with other nearby nerves relatively spared. If the basic pathology is axonal loss, the EMG will show abnormalities, and nerve conduction studies will show decreased amplitude of the evoked responses. If the myelin sheath is primarily affected, nerve conduction slowing will be the most prominent finding. Commonly, both types of pathology are seen together. Occasionally, small, fiber-type neuropathies are seen in which no electrical abnormalities can be demonstrated. This occurs because nerve conduction studies primarily measure conduction in the large myelinated fibers. In addition to the naturally occurring neuropathies, iatrogenic peripheral neuropathies or plexopathies may be due to chemotherapy or radiation.

Myopathies

Myopathies are generally not considered when evaluating a patient with chronic pain. However, dermatomyositis and polymyositis may result in chronic pain and weakness. Electromyographic examination would demonstrate fibrillations, positive waves, and repetitive discharges at rest. Motor unit action potentials tend to be polyphasic with decreased amplitude and duration. Proximal muscles are involved more than distal, and the paraspinal musculature is also involved. Myopathy may also be associated with other connective tissue diseases such as scleroderma or rheumatoid arthritis. It may also be secondary to chronic steroid treatment.

CLINICAL APPLICATIONS

At this point we would like to discuss the use of the electrodiagnostic exam in a variety of clinical situations where the test will be helpful and what the referring clinician may expect to learn from the study. For a detailed discussion of typical findings in each disorder, the reader is referred to the previous section.

Neck Pain or Headache Without Radicular Symptoms

Many patients in this category are referred for electrical studies, usually to investigate possible radiculopathy, but the yield of positive findings is quite low. EMG findings may rarely be present in the cervical paraspinals suggesting root level pathology, but nothing more specific is usually learned. Only rarely will a radiculopathy be documented. Screening nerve conduction studies will usually be done on the symptomatic side, but any incidental abnormalities will usually be unrelated to the primary complaint.

Back Pain Without Radicular Symptoms

Electrodiagnostic evaluation of this group may be more rewarding. EMG abnormalities in the paraspinals indicating radiculopathy are more common than in the cervical area and can confirm that there is local pathology causing the patient's symptoms, even if imaging studies are not diagnostic. Without radicular symptoms there will commonly be a lack of extremity muscle abnormalities, making identification of the root involved very difficult. However, this is not absolute, especially if radicular pain was present and has cleared. Some electromyographers believe a technique called *paraspinal mapping* may be of help in these cases, but this is not widely accepted. Again, standard screening nerve conduction studies will usually be performed, but only infrequently will be helpful. How-

ever, H reflex and F wave abnormalities may help identify the abnormal root.

Neck or Low Back Pain with Radicular Symptoms

This group of patients is ideal for electrodiagnostic evaluation. When extremity pain, numbness, paresthesias, or especially weakness is associated with axial pain, much useful information can be gained. It is very common to be able to localize a radiculopathy to a single root. This is extremely helpful when MRI or other imaging studies have shown multilevel pathology or are equivocal. Patients with diabetes may be found to have a radiculoneuropathy with electrical studies when imaging is normal. Also, since up to 20% of asymptomatic people may have disc herniation causing no problems, it is incumbent on the clinician to establish that any MRI abnormality is the actual cause of the patient's symptoms. If an imaging abnormality does not correlate exactly with the patient's physical findings, EMG may be very helpful in resolving the conflict. We have seen a patient with arm pain and weakness with a large C6-7 disc herniation who did not improve postoperatively. No preop electrical study was done. The exam in our lab after surgery showed a C-8 plexus lesion, and the patient was found to have a Pancoast tumor. While many neurosurgeons will operate based on clinical and imaging findings, reserving electrical studies for difficult cases, others insist on them in most cases.

As seen above, in addition to being able to confirm a radiculopathy in this group, EMG and NCS will be able to evaluate for plexopathy or nerve entrapment as the cause of, or as a contributing factor to, the symptoms. It is not at all uncommon to see patients with both carpal tunnel syndrome and C6-7 radiculopathy. If this is known preoperatively, the patient can be forewarned that all symptoms may not clear postdiscectomy, and a second surgery may be needed. Therefore, although EMG is the most likely electrical study to identify a radiculopathy, nerve conduction studies are needed for a complete evaluation, and the referring physician should never accept a study without them.

Shoulder Pain

Electrodiagnostic studies can be very helpful in evaluating the patient with shoulder pain. This is especially true when the patient has been felt to have a localized tendinitis or arthritis but has not responded to standard treatment. C5 radiculopathy, suprascapular nerve entrapment, serratus anterior palsy, accessory nerve injury, or even more commonly carpal tunnel syndrome (CTS) may cause this complaint. It is well known that a small number of CTS patients may present with shoulder pain as their main or only complaint.

Thoracic outlet syndrome (TOS), a frequently controversial diagnosis, may be divided into three subtypes: true neurogenic, vascular, and controversial. Patients with the neurogenic form initially have shoulder and arm pain and paresthesias, and later weakness, primarily in a C-8, ulnar distribution. EMG and NCS will show evidence of a lower brachial plexus lesion (low amplitude ulnar sensory response, low amplitude median and possibly ulnar motor response, and EMG abnormalities in a C8 distribution). In addition, they will frequently show loss of the radial pulse with hyperabduction of the arm at the shoulder and hyperemia on return of the arm to the side. Patients with the vascular type have none of the electrical abnormalities but do have the same vascular changes, which can be documented by Doppler studies. Severe vascular cases have been reported with ischemia and emboli requiring immediate surgical intervention, but these are very rare. In the author's opinion, these two forms may represent the progression of the disorder from a mild vascular to the worsened neurogenic form. The controversial form is just that. Patients with minor trauma complain of vague discomfort and paresthesias, which are poorly localized. Litigation or emotional problems are commonly present. All studies are usually normal and conservative treatment is not helpful. Unfortunately, many of these patients are subjected to thoracic outlet decompression, and it is not unusual to see this done after they have already had median, ulnar, and even radial nerve releases without improvement.

Elbow Pain

Ulnar nerve entrapment at the elbow can easily be documented in most cases and is a frequent cause of medial elbow pain. Both EMG and NCS are needed to do this adequately.

Entrapment of the recurrent branch of the radial nerve at the elbow has been postulated as a cause of lateral elbow pain as differentiated from tennis elbow or tendinitis, but electrical studies have not been able to clearly document this. It is possible that this is an axonal lesion and therefore difficult to document, but electrical studies will probably not be helpful if the referring physician is considering this diagnosis. Radial nerve injury or entrapment in the spiral grove is easily diagnosed electrically, but is rarely a cause of pain. Entrapment of the posterior interosseus nerve, a branch of the radial, will cause weakness in the finger extensors but infrequent pain.

The sensory branch of the musculocutaneous nerve may be entrapped at the elbow, causing paresthesias in the lateral forearm and occasionally pain.

The pronator syndrome, or entrapment of the median nerve at the elbow, causes symptoms very similar to carpal tunnel syndrome, although pain in the flexor muscle mass is more common. Since this is probably an axonal lesion, EMG and NCS will have difficulty, and in most cases, be unable to document this. Therefore, this is usually a diag-

nosis of exclusion with the electromyographer ruling out carpal tunnel syndrome, radiculopathy, etc.

Wrist and Hand Pain

Obviously, wrist and hand pain have a broad range of etiologies. While arthritis and tendinitis are probably more common, neurogenic causes should always be considered since they are very frequent and treatment is rewarding. Both EMG and NCS must be performed to adequately explore the possibilities.

Carpal tunnel syndrome, ulnar nerve entrapment at Guyon's canal, or a lesion of the deep branch of the ulnar nerve in the palm are the most commonly recognized entrapments causing hand pain. Of course, entrapments at the elbow and possible radiculopathy or plexopathy must also be investigated. A less commonly recognized entrapment is that of the radial sensory nerve at the wrist, which can mimic de Quervain's syndrome and may explain cases of failed tendon release (43).

Carpal tunnel syndrome, or median nerve entrapment at the wrist, is the most common and easily diagnosed. Unfortunately, this frequently leads to an incomplete electrical exam being performed. It is not at all uncommon to see patients with hand paresthesias have only median distal latencies and perhaps an ulnar performed. If the patient appears to have carpal tunnel syndrome, the study is terminated. While this abbreviated form of exam is being encouraged by the insurance industry as well as Medicare, it is not in the patient's best interest, and it should not be accepted by the referring physician. Patients commonly have more than one nerve entrapment, may have a concomitant radiculopathy or plexopathy; or they may actually have a polyneuropathy that only at first glance appears to be an entrapment. It is well known that patients frequently, for unknown reasons, are unable to localize hand paresthesias to the correct dermatome corresponding to the nerve entrapped. Carpal tunnel patients may state the entire hand is involved, rather than just the median distribution, and some will actually localize their complaints entirely to the ulnar distribution. Therefore limiting the exam to the area of the symptoms is never justified.

Hip Pain

Very commonly hip pain may be secondary to a lumbar radiculopathy. Even though the patient may have evidence of local arthritis or tendinitis, if they do not respond to conservative treatment, EMG and NCS may be helpful. Pain radiating from the hip to the groin and thigh may be caused by an L-4 radiculopathy due to disc herniation, but clinically be indistinguishable from osteoarthritis of the hip. A femoral neuropathy, plexopathy, or diabetic amyotrophy may give the same clinical picture but be fairly easily diagnosed electrically. Commonly these patients will have sensory or motor complaints in addition to the pain, but this is not always seen.

Irritation of the sciatic nerve as it passes under the piriformis muscle has been advocated as a cause of posterior hip and buttock pain (piriformis syndrome), but if this truly exists, it has not been clearly demonstrated electrically.

Knee Pain

The same conditions mentioned causing hip pain must also be considered here. In addition, entrapment of the peroneal nerve at the fibular head may cause knee pain, but more commonly causes numbness and weakness. Irritation of the tibial nerve in the popliteal fossa due to a Baker's cyst is occasionally questioned as a cause of pain, but is extremely uncommon.

Calf Pain

Neurologically, lumbar radiculopathy should be considered, even if the symptoms do not seem typical. Patients will usually have more proximal leg or back pain, but not always. Neurogenic pain may also mimic vascular compromise. We are frequently referred patients who seem to have classic intermittent claudication but have had normal vascular studies. If there is electrical evidence of multiple radiculopathies by EMG, dermatomal somatosensory evoked potentials (SEP), or F or H reflex abnormalities, spinal stenosis can be inferred as the cause of the pain (neurogenic claudication).

Ankle and Foot Pain

Radiculopathy, polyneuropathy, or nerve entrapment may cause pain in this area; and therefore a very complete electrical study must be performed to delineate this. The most common nerve entrapment at the ankle is tarsal tunnel syndrome (TTS), or entrapment of the tibial nerve. The peroneal nerve may also be entrapped (anterior tarsal tunnel syndrome), but this is an uncommon cause of pain.

As mentioned earlier in this chapter, TTS is more difficult to document than CTS since it is an axonal lesion rather than a demyelinating one. In younger, basically healthy individuals, the diagnosis is more easily achieved than in the elderly who may already have an underlying age-related mild axonal neuropathy. This is especially true in diabetic patients with neuropathy since the findings in TTS may be easily masked by the neuropathy. Elderly diabetic patients with leg and foot pain are especially challenging to diagnose completely and precisely and frequently require an extensive examination.

THE ELECTRODIAGNOSTIC EXAMINATION

Most patients approach the electrodiagnostic examination with some degree of fear and anxiety, because many have some fear of needle puncture and/or electrical stimuli. Frequently, patients have been subjected to "horror stories" involving electrodiagnostic studies by their acquaintances. This may have been either in jest or in an attempt to gain sympathy. Since patient cooperation is important to a successful examination, the electromyographer must be able to allay the patient's fears. While some complaints of discomfort are to be expected, most patients will agree that their fears were unwarranted and that many other medical diagnostic and therapeutic procedures are much more uncomfortable.

Timing is very important when ordering and interpreting electrodiagnostic studies. After a nerve is severed, conduction velocity in the distal segment will remain normal for 7 to 10 days. However, during that time the amplitude of the evoked response will begin to decline. EMG will not show fibrillations for 3 to 4 weeks postinjury. With radiculopathy, the paraspinal EMG may begin to show abnormalities 7 to 10 days after onset, but the extremity musculature will probably be normal until 4 to 6 weeks later. Most electromyographers will usually prefer to postpone electrical studies until the full development of electrical abnormalities can be expected. However, if a patient presents with both an old and an acute injury, it may be advisable to perform an immediate exam and another in 4 weeks to differentiate the age of the findings.

An electrodiagnostic examination, unlike other studies such as electrocardiography or electroencephalography, cannot be performed in a preset, routine manner. Each examination must be individualized according to the clinical picture. To properly plan the study, a complete history and physical examination must be done by the physician performing the study. The structure of the examination may be changed several times during the procedure as new information is gained. A patient may initially be felt to have an entrapment neuropathy, but further examination may reveal the presence of a polyneuropathy, radiculopathy, etc. Screening nerve conduction studies are performed on the symptomatic extremity as the first step in most examinations. If abnormalities are found, the opposite extremity is also studied. Should abnormal findings again be present, the other limbs may be examined. Electromyography is then conducted on the symptomatic extremity and corresponding paraspinal musculature. Again, other areas will need to be studied if the first limb is abnormal. The results of the examination must then be interpreted in the light of the history and clinical findings.

Ideally, the clinical neurophysiologist performing the electrodiagnostic study will have met the minimal training criteria established by the American Association of Electromyography and Electrodiagnosis (43). These criteria recognize that the electrodiagnostic examination is essentially a neuromuscular disease consultation utilizing electrophysiological methods. The examiner must, therefore, have special expertise in diagnosis of neuromuscular disease. Completion of an approved residency in neurology or physical medicine and rehabilitation is recommended. This training should include adequate instruction in anatomy and physiology of muscle and nerve, electrophysiology, and clinical aspects of neuromuscular disease as they pertain to electrodiagnostic studies. A minimum of 6 months supervised training with performance of at least 200 examinations is recommended. In spite of these recommendations, one can find electrodiagnostic studies being performed by physicians with little or no formal training. In some states, these studies may legally be performed by technicians. It therefore behooves the physician requesting the electrodiagnostic examination to know the qualifications of the examiner. If an experienced clinical neurophysiologist is to perform the examination, it is best to allow him or her to plan and carry out the examination as appropriate to the clinical picture. In this chapter we have specifically not mentioned normal values for most studies, because each clinical neurophysiologist will have established these for his or her own laboratory and will be able to advise the referring physician as to the outcome of the examination. If the electrodiagnostic study is to be performed by a technician, a detailed outline of the examination requested should be given to the technician. All of the diagnostic possibilities should be outlined, and the specific nerves and muscles to be examined must be listed. If a detailed outline is not provided for the technician, an incomplete examination may well be done. This is illustrated by the following case reports.

Case 1

A 54-year-old female received electrodiagnostic studies because of a one-month history of numbness in the right thumb and index finger. She also complained of pain in the hand and shoulder, but no neck pain. Right median sensory conduction to the index finger could not be obtained, while ulnar sensory conduction and median motor conduction were normal. Electromyography of the thenar musculature was also normal. This was the full extent of the examination, and on the basis of these findings the diagnosis of carpal tunnel syndrome was made.

On admission to the hospital for surgery, a new exam was requested. In addition to the studies outlined above, radial and musculocutaneous conduction were measured, and EMG was performed on the entire extremity and cervical paraspinal musculature. Both median and musculocutaneous sensory conduction were absent while all other conduction studies were normal. EMG showed the presence of fibrillations and positive waves in the right biceps, brachialis, and pronator teres with sparing of the paraspinals. These findings indicated that the lesion was in the lateral cord of the brachial plexus, rather than at the wrist. Further workup revealed a metastatic breast carcinoma to the plexus.

This case points out that the study should not be cut short as soon as one abnormality is found or the clinical impression is "confirmed." Multiple lesions may be missed or an incorrect diagnosis made.

Case 2

A 62-year-old female patient was referred to a technician for nerve conduction studies because of weakness. She had fallen on several occasions and fractured her right hip. Extensive motor and sensory conduction studies were done on the upper and lower extremities with no abnormalities found. This was reported as a "Normal Study." This patient was later seen in another laboratory where the normal conduction studies were confirmed. However, electromyography was also done and showed the presence of diffuse fibrillations and fasciculations, which led to the diagnosis of amyotrophic lateral sclerosis.

This case illustrates the need to know your examiner. The initial referring physician assumed his patient would be seen by a physician-clinical neurophysiologist and used the term "Nerve Conduction Study" in a generic sense. Unfortunately the technician took him literally, and hence the inadequate study and delay in diagnosis.

In summary, routine performance of only brief, limited electrical studies is analogous to ordering a limb x-ray and examining only the bones while ignoring the soft-tissue structures. Since so much information is to be gained, especially in the evaluation of the patient with chronic pain, the full potential of the electrodiagnostic examination should be utilized.

REFERENCES

1. Johnson EW. Use of the electrodiagnostic examination in a university hospital. *Arch Phys Med Rahabil* 1965;46:573.
2. Rogoff J. Traditional electrodiagnosis. In: Johnson EW, ed. *Practical Electromyography*. Baltimore: Williams & Wilkins, 1980:326.
3. Licht S. History. In: Johnson EW, ed. *Practical Electromyography*. Baltimore: Williams & Wilkins, 1980:403.
4. Liddell E, Sherrington C. Recruitment and some other features of reflex inhibition. *Proc Roy Soc London (Biol)* 1925;97:488–518.
5. Adrian E, Bronk D. The discharge of impulses in motor nerve fibers. Part II. The frequency of discharge in reflex and voluntary conduction. *J Physiol (London)* 1929;67:119–151.
6. Brown W, Varkey G. The origin of spontaneous electrical activity at the endplate zone. *Ann Neurol* 1981;10:557–570.
7. Buchthal F, Rosenfalk P. Spontaneous electrical activity of human muscle. *Electroenceph Clin Neurophysiol* 1966;20:321–326.
8. Johnson EW, Denny ST, Kelley JP. Sequence of electromyographic abnormalities in stroke syndrome. *Arch Phys Med Rehabil* 1975;56:468.
9. Chokroverty S, Medina T. Electrophysiological study of hemiplegia. *Arch Neurol* 1978;35:360.
10. Wettstein A. The origin of fasciculations in motor neuron disease. *Ann Neurol* 1979;5:295.
11. Stalberg E, Trontel JV. *Single fiber electromyography*. Old Woking, Surrey U.K: Mirvalle Press Limited, 1979.
12. Borenstein S, Desmedt J. Range variations in motor unit potentials during reinnervation after traumatic nerve lesions in humans. *Ann Neurol* 1980;8:460.
13. MacLean I. Nerve root stimulation to evaluate conduction across the brachial and lumbosacral plexuses. *Third Annual Continuing Educa-*

tion Course, American Association of Electromyography and Electrodiagnosis. Sept. 25, 1980, Philadelphia.

14. Magladery JW, McDougal DB. Electrophysiological studies of nerve and reflex activity in normal man: I. Identification of certain reflexes in electromyogram and conduction velocity of peripheral nerve fibers. *Bull Johns Hopkins Hospital* 1950;86:265.
15. Namerow HS. Somatosensory evoked responses in multiple sclerosis patients with varying sensory loss. *Neurology* 1968;18:1197.
16. Knutson B. Comparative values of electromyographic, myelographic and clinical-neurological examinations of lumbar root compression syndromes. *Acta Orthop Scand Suppl* 1961;49:1.
17. Khatri B, Baruah J, McQuillen P. Correlation of Electromyography with computed tomography in evaluation of lower back pain. *Arch Neurol* 1984;41:594.
18. Marinacci A. *Applied electromyography.* Philadelphia: Lea & Febiger, 1968.
19. Waylonis G. Electromyographic findings in chronic cervical radicular syndrome. *Arch Phys Med Rehabil* 1968;49:407.
20. Johnson E, Burkhart J, Earl W. Electromyography in postlaminectomy patients. *Arch Phys Med Rehabil* 1972;53:407.
21. Langstreth G, Newcomer A. Abdominal pain caused by diabetic radiculopathy. *Ann Intern Med* 1977;86:166.
22. Kopell HP, Thompson WA. *Peripheral entrapment neuropathies.* Baltimore: Williams & Wilkins, 1963.
23. Felsenthal G. Median and ulnar distal motor and sensory latencies in the same normal subject. *Arch Phys Med Rehabil* 1977;58:297.
24. Spindler H, Dellon AL. Nerve conduction studies and sensibility testing in carpal tunnel syndrome. *J Hand Surg* 1982;7:260.
25. Hartz CR. The pronator teres syndrome: compressive neurology of the median nerve. *J Bone Joint Surg* 1981;63A:885.
26. Nakano KK. Anterior interosseous nerve syndrome. *Arch Neorol* 1977;34:477.
27. Feindel W, Stratford J. The role of the cubital tunnel in tardy ulnar palsy. *Canad J Surg* 1958;1:287.
28. Eisen A. Early diagnosis of ulnar nerve palsy. An electrophysiological study. *Neurology* 1974;24:256.
29. Caldwell JW, Crane CR, Krasen EM. Nerve conduction studies: an aid in the diagnosis of thoracic outlet syndrome. *South Med J* 1971;64:210.
30. Daube JR. Nerve conduction studies in the thoracic outlet syndrome. *Neurology* 1975;25:347.
31. Gilliat RW. Peripheral nerve conduction in patients with a cervical rib or band. *J Neurol Neurosurg Psychiat* 1970;33:615.
32. Dorfman LJ. F-wave latency in the cervical rib-and-band syndrome. Letter to the Editor. *Muscle and Nerve* 1979;2:158.
33. Dorfman LJ, Jayaram AR. Handcuff neuropathy. *JAMA* 1978;239:957.
34. Dellon AL, MacKinnon SE. Radial sensory nerve entrapment. *Arch Neurol* 1986;43:833.
35. Spindler HA, Felsenthal G. Sensory conduction in the musculocutaneous nerve. *Arch Phys Med Rehabil* 1978;59:70.
36. Felsenthal G, Mondell DL. Forearm pain secondary to compression syndrome of lateral cutaneous nerve of the forearm. *Arch Phys Med Rehabil* 1984;65:139.
37. Butler ET, Johnson EW, Kaye ZA. Normal conduction velocity in the lateral femoral cutaneous nerve. *Arch Phys Med Rehabil* 1974;55:31.
38. Johnson EW, Wood P, Pomeus J. Femoral nerve conduction studies. *Arch Phys Med Rehabil* 1968;49:528.
39. Krause KH, Witt T, Ross A. The anterior tarsal tunnel syndrome. *J Neurol* 1977;217:67.
40. Delisa JA, Saeed MA. AAEE case report #8: The tarsal tunnel syndrome. *Muscle Nerve* 1983;6:664.
41. Spindler HA, Reischer MA, Felsenthal G. Electrodiagnostic assessment in suspected tarsal tunnel syndrome. *Phys Med Rehabil Clin North Am* 1994;5,3:595–612.
42. Gatens PF, Saeed MA. Electromyographic findings in the intrinsic muscles of normal feet. *Arch Phys Med Rehabil* 1982;63:317.
43. Guidelines in electrodiagnostic medicine, Rochester, Minn.: American Association of Electromyography and Electrodiagnosis, 1984.

CHAPTER **7**

Psychological Evaluation and Assessment of Pain

Donald W. Hinnant

This chapter provides a framework for the evaluation of patients who have pain and describes psychological instruments that are helpful in pain evaluation. The recognition of emotional variables, especially the negative ones, in the etiology, maintenance, and exacerbation of pain has promoted the psychology of pain as a science and has generated much research. Evaluation of pain is facilitated by a combination of measures. The psychological evaluation should be comprised of a variety of behavioral, observational, and psychometric techniques. Health care professionals are aware that a fairly minor injury or painful disorder may initiate a series of events with negative consequences that result in biological, psychological, and social disruption of the individual's life. Early recognition of this series of events and changes by the medical professional may help avoid intractable physical and psychological complications. The foundation for pain assessment provided by researchers Melzack and Wall has provided a better understanding of the multidimensional aspects of pain, including the motivational-affective, sensory-discriminative, and cognitive-evaluative processes inherent in pain (1). Their theory demonstrated the highly complex nature of pain perception and pain responses. The involvement of multiple pathways and the effects of interacting systems on nociceptive impulses and higher cortical processes are known to modify perception and emotional reaction to pain. The gate control theory placed an emphasis on central neuromechanisms and helped to focus attention on the brain as an active system that filters, selects, and modulates pain input. Recently, Melzack proposed a more complex neuronetwork referred to as the *body-self neuromatrix* (2). The system accepts stimulus inputs to produce the output pattern that evokes pain. Melzack's neuromatrix theory certainly does not simplify our evaluation and understanding of pain, but does help to explain the highly complicated interactive systems, including both sensory input and output, that influence the cognitive interpretation of pain. This system, in conjunction with phasic and tonic cognitive and emotional inputs from other areas of the brain, activates an intrinsic neuroinhibitory modulation system in the brain. In addition, the neuromatrix system highlights the importance of stress regulation of systems, including endocrine, autonomic, immune, and opioid systems (Fig 7-1).

From a psychological perspective, the neurosignature pattern is modulated by sensory inputs and cognitive events, such as psychological stress. The theory continues to emphasize multidimensional factors involved in pain, including genetic and neurohormonal mechanisms. Melzack has recommended that interdisciplinary pain clinics should expand to "include specialists in endocrinology and immunology" (2).

PSYCHOLOGICAL REFERRAL PROCESS

A psychological evaluation is frequently requested when an individual's pain symptoms or complaints are considered to be in excess of physical findings and explanation based on diagnostic procedures. Physicians who have attempted various forms of treatment and obtained numerous diagnostic tests may become challenged and perhaps frustrated. They may begin to question whether the patient's pain is real or psychological. This frustration is easily conveyed to the patient in pain. Issues of trust may develop at this stage, adding to the psychological components of the patient's pain syndrome. From the patient's perspective, suggestions that the pain should have been alleviated or controlled are often interpreted as an accusation that the patient may have other causes for continued

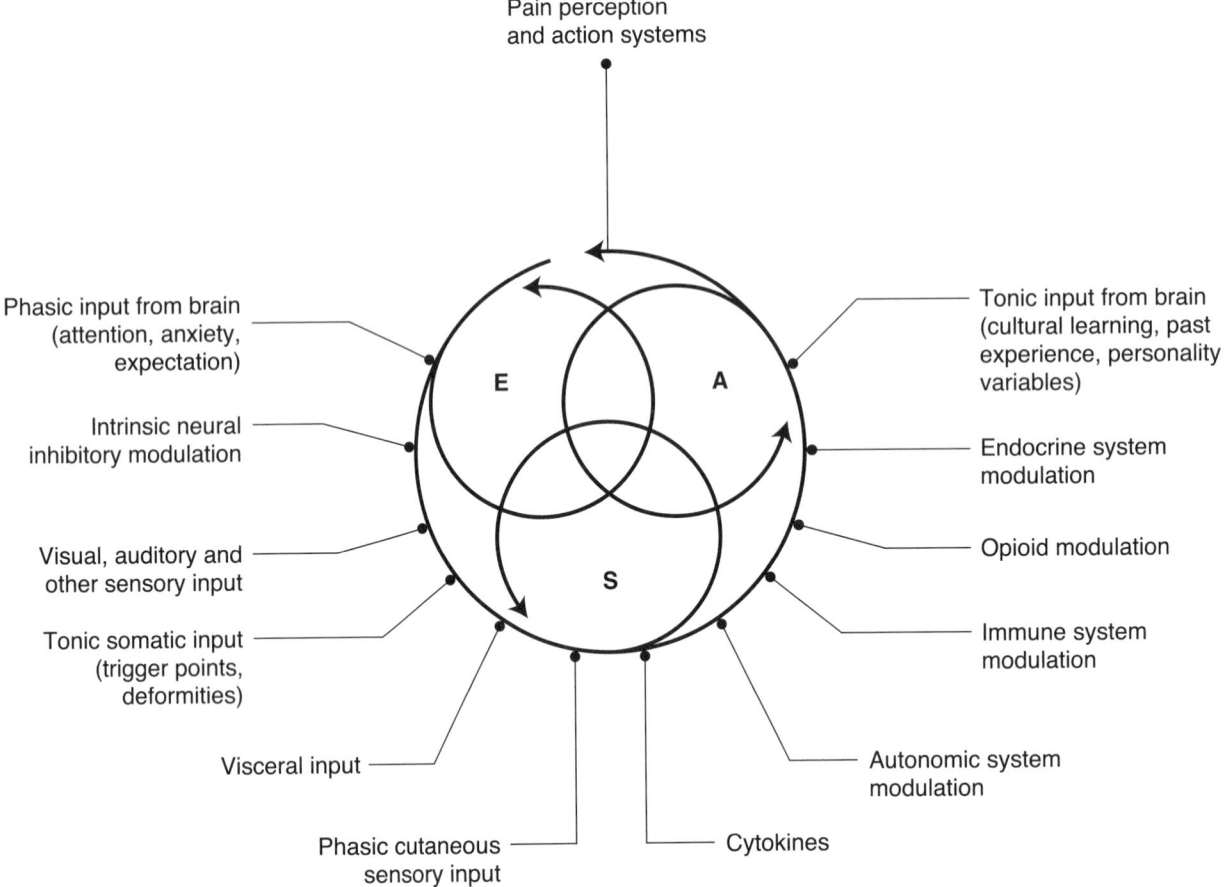

FIG. 7-1. The body-self neuromatrix. The body-self neuromatrix, which comprises a widely distributed neural network that includes somatosensory, limbic, and thalamocortical components, is schematically depicted as a circle containing smaller parallel networks that contribute to the sensory-discriminative (S), affective-motivational (A), and evaluative-cognitive (E) dimensions of pain experience. The synaptic architecture of the neuromatrix is determined by genetic and sensory influences. The "neurosignature" output of the neuromatrix—patterns of nerve impulses of varying temporal and spacial dimensions—is produced by neural programs genetically built into the neuromatrix and determines the particular qualities and other properties of the pain experience and behavior. Multiple inputs that act on the neuromatrix programs and contribute to the output neurosignature include (1) sensory inputs from somatic receptors (phasic cutaneous, visceral and tonic somatic inputs); (2) visual and other sensory inputs that influence the cognitive interpretation of the situation; (3) phasic and tonic cognitive and emotional inputs from other areas of the brain; (4) intrinsic neural inhibitary modulation inherent in all brain function; and (5) the activity of the body's stress-regulation systems, including cytokines as well as the endocrine, autonomic, immune, and opioid systems.

pain complaints. Although poor coping skills and mood disorders clearly have an impact on a patient's experience of pain, the clinician should be aware that chronic pain is, in fact, similar to other chronic medical disorders that have comparable psychological estimates of comorbidity. Physical and psychological signs and symptoms are not mutually exclusive, and clinicians should avoid the use of such diagnostic labels as hypochondriacal, hysterical, and functional. The psychiatric diagnosis of psychogenic pain is relatively rare in the general population, and the *DSM-IV* (3) diagnosis of "pain disorder" awaits further clarification because the majority of individuals who are given this somatoform diagnosis often meet the criteria for other psychiatric diagnoses. The pain disorder diagnosis is vague and omits important factors, such as pain duration, intensity, and level of impairment. When the clinician is making a determination about referring a patient for psychological evaluation or intervention, it is best to consider the symptoms and quality-of-life issues that may have potential for improvement. We know that chronic pain patients may improve in their functional capacity without directly reducing the pain intensity. Pain assessment is complex, and attempts to categorize the pain as functional versus organic are meaningless and may lead to confusion, possible inappropriate treatment, or lack of appropriate treatment.

IMPORTANCE OF TIMING

When should referral for psychological evaluation be made? Often psychological referral is delayed until traditional treatment methods have been exhausted. The consequences of delayed medical treatment and, just as importantly, delayed psychological intervention are well known. Delays in psychological referral often lead to factors that increase the risk for long-term disability and associated personal and financial costs. An acute pain condition may become chronic under certain psychological and environmental conditions. Physicians and insurance carriers, including managed care programs, must be responsible for early recognition and response to these factors. Cost containment efforts made by insurance adjusters who deny psychological referral or involvement in treating painful conditions may lead to exorbitant costs common to chronic pain syndromes. Delayed referrals also lead to a strong sense of entitlement carried by many individuals who feel that they have not been treated fairly. When this occurs, it is often difficult to obtain improvement with any form of treatment, and the condition may enter into the realm of the medical-legal system, which is seen frequently in workers' compensation cases.

The medical practitioner should explain to the patient in pain that stress, emotional reactions, and pain assessment require a multidisciplinary approach. A psychological evaluation may provide information regarding reactions to pain, such as work problems, family stress, depression, and other psychological disorders. Often, behavioral problems such as smoking, obesity, and insomnia are associated with the pain and can be managed through behavior modification, counseling, biofeedback, and hypnosis, which are valid adjunctive treatments available for the patient (See Appendix A).

Referral Guidelines for Psychological Evaluation (4)

1. Emphasize the multidimensional nature of pain and need for multidisciplinary treatment.
2. Present the referral as a positive move to obtain additional opinions for optimal improvement. Recognize the fact that pain causes life disruption and stress and that the referral is being made out of genuine concern for the patient.
3. Explain that the psychological evaluation may provide helpful information about the patient's response to medications and potential benefit from alternative forms of treatment.
4. Ensure that office personnel and medical staff maintain the same positive attitude and behavior regarding referral for psychological evaluation.
5. Emphasize to the patient that the referral does not imply that his or her pain is considered "psychological" or that he or she is being transferred or abandoned.

THE PSYCHOLOGICAL EVALUATION

The Psychological Interview

The evaluation should begin with a review of medical records and history taking with an emphasis on the physical aspects of the patient's problem. It is important to alleviate any fear the patient may have about being referred to a mental health practitioner. Pain patients may present with the expectations that their physician believes that they have "psychological" pain; they are not believed or possibly faking; or their physician believes that they must "learn to live with the pain." Specific interview topics should include descriptions of the patient's pain experience outlining pain intensity, quality of the pain, and pain pattern. Environmental situations and conditions that increase and decrease the pain should be elicited. Prior treatment experience and response to interventions need to be addressed, and the practitioner should keep in mind that patients often report that "nothing has helped" due to their discouragement. It is helpful to remind them that single modality treatments may have had some effect on their pain, but one function of the psychological evaluation is to consider a combination of treatments that may be effective. Careful review of medications, side effects, potential for substance abuse, problems with sleep, and sexual functioning should be obtained. Information about the family background and parents or siblings who may have chronic pain is needed. The individual's education, work history, and job satisfaction are critical in the assessment. Issues related to workers' compensation and how the patient perceives that he or she has been treated by both the insurance carrier and former employer is important. The patient's potential for returning to a job on which he or she was injured must be carefully assessed due to the high percentage of return to work failures that are seen in this population of pain patients. Often, work-related injuries become very complicated and the injured worker may not return to his or her prior occupation because of psychosocial problems, as opposed to clearly defined physical impairments.

As a general outline for the interview, particular strengths and weaknesses should be assessed. Potential negative aspects of coping may include

1. a tendency toward catastrophization of symptoms and pain;
2. poor coping based on prior medical problems or surgery;
3. a weak support system, including family, employer, marital difficulties, etc.;
4. a tendency toward "blaming" or "entitlement";
5. a history of physical and/or emotional abuse;
6. substance abuse history;
7. psychiatric disorder.

Positive coping responses include

1. willingness to appreciate, or interest in understanding, multidisciplinary treatment of pain;

2. compliance with treatment;
3. willingness to accept responsibility;
4. active involvement in treatment;
5. interest in cooperative development of a treatment plan, with realistic expectations.

Measurement of Pain Sensation, Location, and Intensity

Four primary methods of measurement of pain include visual analog scales, verbal rating scales, pain drawings, and numerical rating scales. The strengths of these scales and their proper use by pain clinicians are due to their simplicity. They also are brief to administer and scoring is usually simple and straightforward. Various techniques may be adapted for use with children and the elderly. Many clinicians use a pain diary for ongoing assessment, which describes daily activity level, changes in pain and other symptoms, and often, exercise, medication usage, and other self-management techniques.

Limitations with these single-dimension instruments such as the visual analog scale, numerical pain scales, and verbal scales are due to the potential influences of the emotional state of the patient, and simplified pain rating scales may hide complex idiosyncratic meanings. The multidimensional nature of pain defies accurate assessment of intensity based on a single verbal or numerical rating. The pain practitioner may often find that these scales are obviously invalid due to tendencies toward embellishment, such as rating the pain as an 11 on a 0 to 10 point scale! Attempts to sample a patient's pain experience by the use of a single-dimension tool eliminates the social components of the pain, and in essence, we are attempting to have patients place a number or use a verbal description of a very complex symptom in simple terminology. Self-reporting of pain is influenced by many factors, including confusion, cultural factors, and treatment expectations.

Pain Drawings

Pain drawings require individuals to identify symptoms related to their pain by marking specific locations or characteristics on human figures, which may present various perspectives of the body or views and regions of the body. Use of these drawings has been controversial. Unusual pain drawings may actually be more of an expression of psychological problems or pain embellishment than actual pain location or description. Ransford et al. (5) developed a point scoring system for unusual pain patterns in an effort to classify patients as having abnormal symptoms. It is difficult to diagnose accurately those patients who have obvious psychological problems and physical pathology. Ohnmeiss (6) et al performed an interesting study using pain location and drawings as they correlate to specific lumbar disc abnormalities. In their study, drawings were completed unassisted, and those that reflected psychologi-

cal problems were analyzed separately. Drawings were collected from a sample of patients considered surgical candidates who were undergoing computed tomograpic/discography (Fig. 7-2).

Obviously pain drawings should be used in conjunction with multiple assessment techniques. When properly used, they may provide helpful information. The author recommends the pain drawing as a guide to assist in a discussion of pain symptoms and specific characteristics of pain intensity and quality. Drawings may be used as a component of a daily pain diary that is helpful in ongoing assessment.

Personality Tests and Questionnaires

The Minnesota Multiphasic Personality Inventory (MMPI, MMPI-2)

The Minnesota Multiphasic Personality Inventory (MMPI) has a long history of use with chronic pain patients. The MMPI was revised in 1989 and is now referred to as the MMPI-2 (7), which provides the benefit of a more current normative sample and modernization of language and wording. The test is quite long (60 to 90 minutes, 567 true/false items), yet it remains the most widely used and researched test of adult psychopathology. Although the MMPI has been used to describe "functional" as compared to "organic" patients, a more sound practice has been used to identify specific forms of psychological distress, such as depression, and those symptoms that may be particularly responsive to psychologic intervention. Fordyce (8) originated MMPI interpretations based on the degree to which pain patients were found to have pain rewarded by their symptoms. Specific scales on the MMPI have been reported to correlate with treatment outcome, particularly scales 1 and 3 representing hypochondriasis and hysteria. In the conversion V profile, the individual may have responded in a manner suggesting multiple physical symptoms with reduced levels of reported emotional distress. There is much support in the literature for poor treatment outcome among groups of patients with elevated scores on scales Hs and Hy, and these individuals may be oversensitive to pain or report high levels of pain and somatic symptoms because of environmental reinforcement of these symptoms. Individuals with elevations on scale 2 for depression are suggestive of a low threshold for pain and, based on cognitive theory, focus on negative perceptions and events. These individuals report decreased motivation, low energy, and poor self-esteem. Elevations on the depression scale are frequently encountered in the chronic pain population. Many individuals who have chronic pain may have premorbid problems with depression (7,10).

In several studies, cluster analysis statistical techniques have identified four MMPI-2 profiles that suggest various responses to treatment and patterns of coping. Outcome

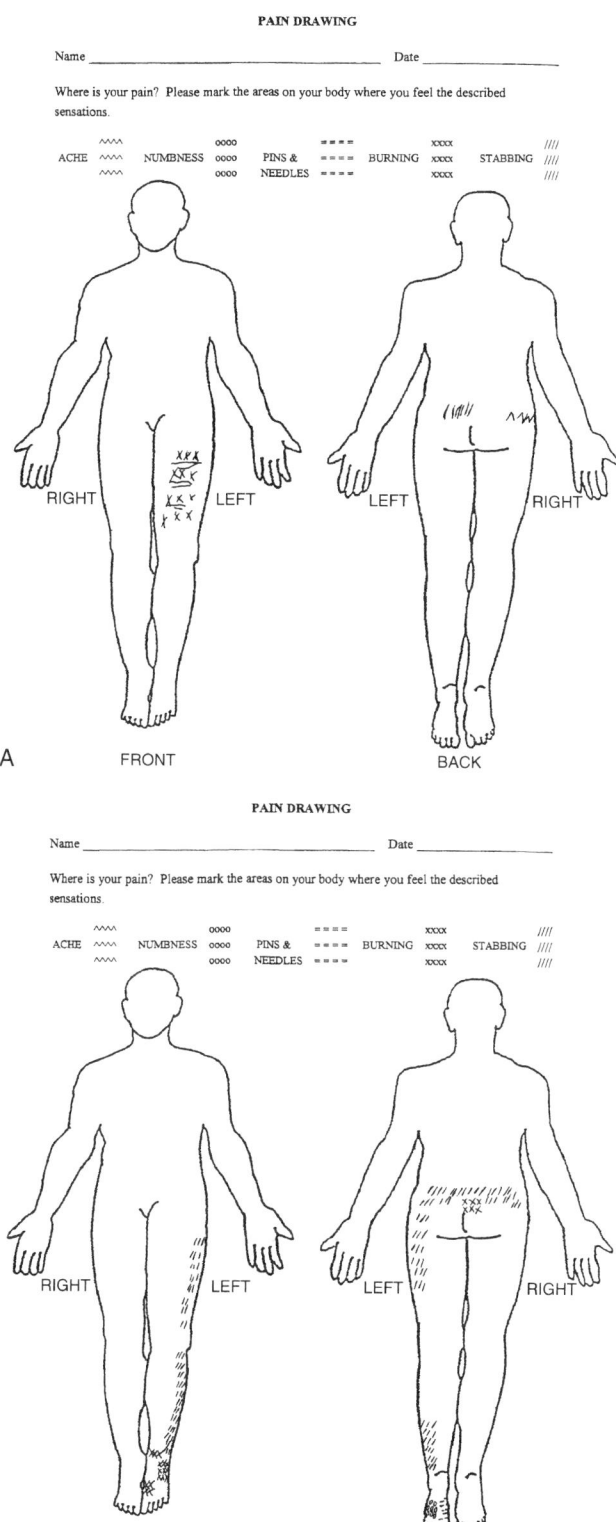

FIG. 7-2. Pain drawings and computed tomographic.disco-graphic images from patients with symptomatic disc disruption at the L3-4 (**A, B**) levels.

studies for low back surgery suggest that the MMPI scale elevations on hypochondriasis, hysteria, and depression are most predictive of outcome. A study by Riley et al. (11) demonstrated that cluster analysis of MMPI-2 profiles are predictive of a number of surgical outcome measures. Patients with a normal profile (scores below T-score of 70) and patients identified by elevations on the three scales considered the "neurotic triad" (Hs, D, and Hy) reported greater satisfaction with postsurgical improvement following lumbar fusion. Patients who had primary elevations on schizophrenia (Sc), psychasthenia (Pt), and depression (D) scales were referred to as the depressed-pathological subgroup with a reported poor outcome. The reader is referred to the works of Riley et al. for detailed comparisons of these profile subgroups.

The MMPI should be used as one component of a psychological assessment for pain. This test is intimidating to some individuals because of its length and the psychiatric nature of many questions. New scales have been developed for the MMPI-2 and an expanded version of an interpretative report is provided by National Computer Systems (12) for use in various settings, including chronic pain and general medical. The tests should be used only by clinicians who are trained specifically in its use and with experience in the area of pain.

The McGill Pain Questionnaire

The McGill Pain Questionnaire (MPQ) was developed by Melzack (13) to provide detailed information about the intensity and quality of pain. Three classes of adjectives used to describe pain include sensory adjectives that focus on temporal, spatial, thermal, and other sensory qualities. Affective adjectives refer to the emotional (fear, tension, anxiety) and autonomic properties of the experience. Evaluative words allow the patient to report the subjective intensity of their total pain experience. Patients are asked to locate their pain on a human pain drawing, and an added component includes questions regarding pain experience, location, and medication. The questionnaire utilizes a pain intensity index, which is a visual rating scale based on a number value of 0 to 5. Although the construct validity, reliability, and other factors of the McGill Pain Questionnaire have been criticized, the questionnaire is widely applicable and has been used in laboratory research. The questionnaire has been used to evaluate particular pain syndromes that could be differentiated among groups of patients with various disorders, including neuralgia, arthritis, reflex sympathetic dystrophy, and radiculopathy (14).

Battery for Health Improvement

The Battery for Health Improvement (BHI) (15) is a self-report inventory designed to identify multiple factors that may interfere with a patient's recovery from physical injury.

The test has been found to be valid and reliable and provides comprehensive assessment. Both psychological and psychosocial factors are included that are known impediments to recovery. The impact of physical, environmental, and psychological factors is included in the report, which identifies patient's symptoms, satisfaction with treatment, and readiness for vocational training. Clinical scales include symptom dependency, chronic maladjustment, family dysfunction, job satisfaction, doctor satisfaction, muscular bracing, somatic complaints, pain complaints, and perseverance. The computerized report compares a patient to normative samples from the community, as well as a sample of physical rehabilitation patients. An interesting study using the BHI focused on violent ideation and hostility found among workers' compensation and personal injury patients (16). Higher rates of hostility were observed in workers' compensation patients. Although a psychological test may not be necessary to detect hostility or frustration exhibited by patients in pain, these are issues that must be considered in the assessment.

Millon Behavioral Medicine Diagnostic

The Millon Behavioral Medicine Diagnostic (MBMD) (17) is a recently developed test that provides information on the patient's coping style and, in addition, provides scales regarding stress moderators, treatment prognostics, psychiatric information, negative health habits, and a management guide. The interpretative report is designed to provide information that may be helpful for improving treatment outcomes by identifying personal and social assets that may facilitate adjustment to physical limitations and/or lifestyle changes. The test was developed on a sample of cancer, diabetic, organ transplant, cardiac, and HIV/AIDS patients. The test is unique with its one-page health care provider summary that is designed for physicians and other health care providers to use much as they would a lab report. The advantage of the MBMD is information provided on a patient's coping style with suggestions regarding prognostics and behavioral factors that influence recovery and predictions tailored for the health care provider. This information should also be useful for objective information to provide to insurance carriers for treatment authorization and demonstration of treatment effectiveness (Fig. 7-3).

Pain Patient Profile

The Pain Patient Profile (P-3) (18) was designed as a cost-efficient screening tool to identify psychological factors that may be impeding the pain patient's recovery from chronic disorders, primarily psychological factors such as depression, anxiety, and somatization. These three psychological disorders are very common with chronic pain patients. The test is designed to screen individuals who

may have symptoms that warrant further psychological and behavioral assessment. The P-3 is designed for use by a broad range of health care professionals. The test has been used as a screening instrument for "readiness" for surgery, and the interpretive report is designed for repeated assessment over time, demonstrating treatment effectiveness. A unique characteristic of the P-3 is the interpretative report that compares the subject to a normative sample of patients used in the test development that were in treatment for persistent pain. The individual's scores are compared to a large community sample of "normal patients." This comparison allows the health care provider to evaluate the patient relative to other pain patients.

The P-3 has been used in clinical research with neurosurgery patients. In a pilot study based on 119 individuals tested as part of their intake during their initial visit with a neurosurgeon, multivariant analysis was predictive of insurance status (workers' compensation or "other insurance"), gender, and smoker/nonsmoker. In the study, symptoms of depression and somatization were statistically significant predictors of medical and psychological factors that are known to impact treatment outcome. At 6-month follow-up, the P-3 scale elevations declined following various types of intervention. The somatization scale was most predictive of outcome and demonstrated that behavioral interventions, medication, epidurals, and surgery were correlated with improvement. Physical therapy, bed rest, and time were not correlated significantly with treatment success. Current research is being conducted using the test as a screening instrument and predictor of long-term treatment success with spinal cord stimulation and implantable pump system (19) (Fig. 7-4).

Presurgical Psychological Evaluation and Screening

Waddell (20) presented evidence that the correlation between impairment and pain, impairment and disability, and pain and disability were relatively weak, providing the implication that disability is related more to nonphysical factors than to physical pathology with chronic back pain. Waddell's research on nonorganic signs has been popularized and is often integrated into the evaluation of spine pain patients by physicians, especially spine surgeons. Nonorganic or "atypical" pain has been associated with poor outcome following surgery. Behavioral factors such as frequency of medical utilization, obesity, and smoking have been found to increase risk for failed back surgery. In addition, behavioral factors, such as poor overall physical fitness and prior psychological treatment, are found to increase risk for chronicity and/or failed surgical intervention in spine patients. A history of physical, sexual, and emotional abuse negatively influence the treatment of spine pain. Schofferman et al. (21) reported that childhood psychological trauma was found to be associated with unsuccessful surgical outcome in 85% of their patients evaluated. The patients in this study had a history of

MBMD™
Samual J. Sample (ID 9099)

Race: White
Medical Problem(s): Heart Disease, Other
CODE:-**BB*//-**7*//ABE**C*DF+//-**-*HIG+//

Valid Profile

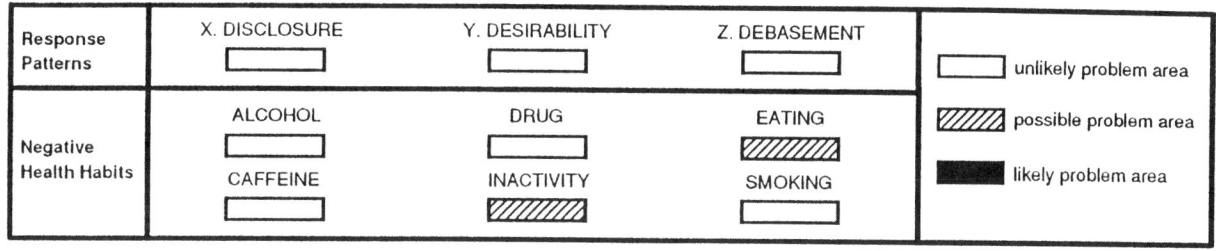

		SCORE		PROFILE OF PREVALENCE SCORES			CLINICAL SCALES
		RAW	PS	0 35 75 85 100+			
Psychiatric Indications	AA	3	45				ANXIETY-TENSION
	BB	12	83				DEPRESSION
	CC	4	44				COGNITIVE DYSFUNCTION
	DD	6	55				EMOTIONAL LABILITY
	EE	4	30				GUARDEDNESS
Coping Styles	1	4	50				INTROVERSIVE
	2A	1	40				INHIBITED
	2B	0	5				DEJECTED
	3	8	60				COOPERATIVE
	4	15	70				SOCIABLE
	5	11	56				CONFIDENT
	6A	4	30				NONCONFORMING
	6B	5	25				FORCEFUL
	7	25	80				RESPECTFUL
	8A	10	67				OPPOSITIONAL
	8B	3	55				DENIGRATED
Stress Moderators	A	27	95				ILLNESS APPREHENSION
	B	22	90				FUNCTIONAL DEFICITS
	C	15	75				PAIN SENSITIVITY
	D	0	5				SOCIAL ISOLATION
	E	20	86				FUTURE PESSIMISM
	F	0	5				SPIRITUAL ABSENCE
Treatment Prognostics	G	2	15				INTERVENTIONAL FRAGILITY
	H	0	5				MEDICATION ABUSE
	I	0	5				INFORMATION DISCOMFORT
	J	7	70				UTILIZATION EXCESS
	K	3	40				PROBLEMATIC COMPLIANCE
Management Guide	L	6	77				ADJUSTMENT DIFFICULTIES
	M	5	69				PSYCH REFERRAL

◄━━━━━━ *Increasingly Problematic* ━━━━━━►

FIG. 7-3. Millon Behavioral Medicine Diagnostic (MBMD)

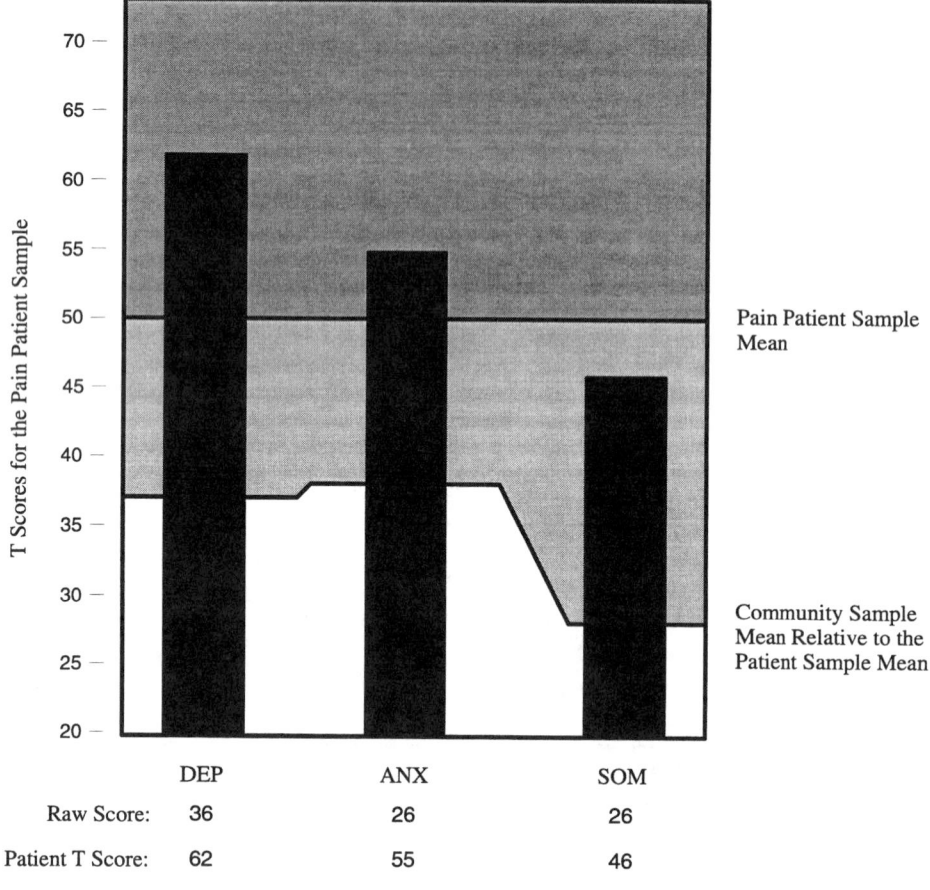

Pain Patient Profile

The Individual Compared to the Patient Sample

	DEP	ANX	SOM
Raw Score:	36	26	26
Patient T Score:	62	55	46

A   Validity Index (raw):   6

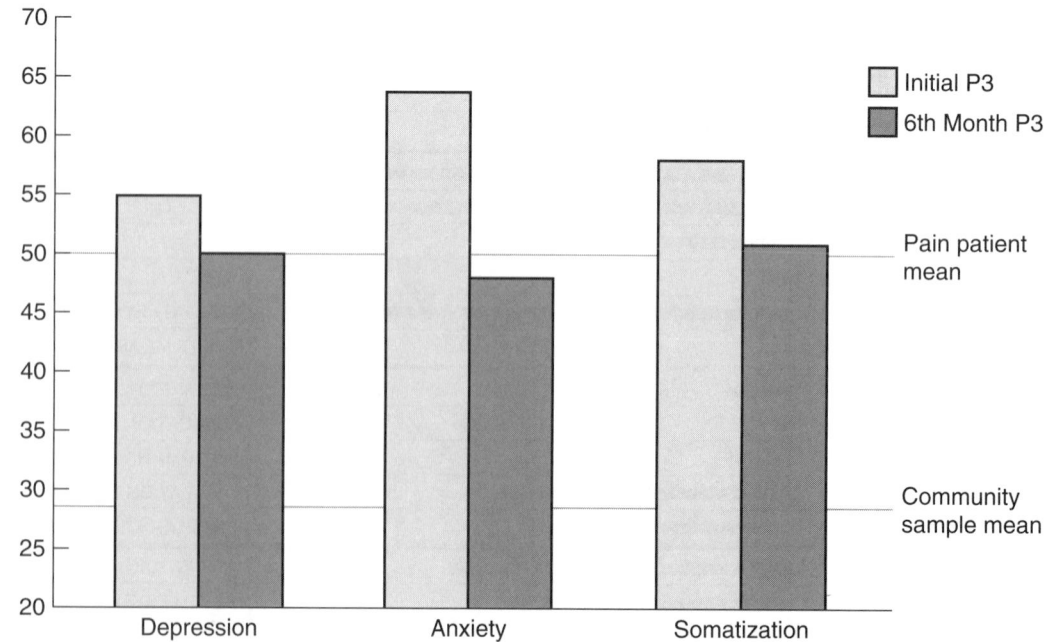

FIG. 7-4. **A.** Pain patient profile **B.** P3: Pre-post treatment results

trauma, including emotional, sexual, physical, parental substance abuse, and abandonment.

Obviously from a presurgical viewpoint, psychological factors are important for evaluation. Premorbid psychological disorders increase the risk of development of chronic pain and failed treatment outcome. The reader is encouraged to review the excellent text by Block (22) on presurgical psychological evaluation of chronic pain syndrome. His work has provided a systematic protocol for psychological screening prior to surgery that is detailed, yet readily accessible to psychologists and other health practitioners. The presurgical psychological scale developed by Block integrates well-investigated factors that place patients at risk for poor outcome with chronic pain syndromes (Fig. 7-5).

Certainly, all surgical candidates for treatment of painful disorders do not require a full psychological evaluation. Specific pain syndromes do warrant at least a psychological screening prior to surgical intervention, such as chronic syndromes that may require neurostimulation implants or implantable infusion devices and pumps, and with individuals undergoing complicated repeated surgical procedures. *Psychological Assessment and Intervention in Implantable Pain Therapies* edited by Doleys and Olsen (23) is highly recommended. This publication, sponsored by Medtronic, Inc., is an insightful and useful guide for the clinician, with specific recommendations regarding patient selection, interviewing, and assessment techniques with an emphasis on multidisciplinary treatment for chronic pain syndromes.

Name: _____ Oswestry _____ Date _____
Med DX: _____ Onset _____ ID _____
MD: _____ Surg. Type _____ Psych _____

Medical	Risk	Interview	Risk	Testing	Risk
Chronicity		**Litig./SSDI**		**MMPI (T>70)**	
6-12 mos	med	present	high	(max. 4 points)	
> 12 mos	high	**Work Comp**			
Prev. Spine Surg.		working	med	*Hs*	high
One	med	non working	high	*D* (pre-inj.)	high
Two +	high	**Job Disatis**		*D* (reactive)	med
Destructiveness		moderate	med	*Hy*	high
Min-Mod	med	extreme	high	*Pd*	high
Highly	high	**Heavy Job**		*Pt*	med
Salvage	high	>50 lb lift	high		
Non organic		**Sub. Abuse**		**CSQ**	
Present	high	pre injury	med	(max. 2 points)	
Non spine Med		current	high		
moderate	med	**Family Rein.**		low self-rel	high
multiple	high	moderate	med	low cont.	high
Smoking		extreme	high		
< 1 pack/day	med	**Mar. Disatis.**			
> 1 pack/day	high	present	med		
Obesity		**Abuse**		**Test Total**	____
>50% over	med	pre injury	med		
		current	high	**Psych total**	
Med Total	____	**Pre injury Psy**		(Int. + Test)	____
Threshold	= 8 ± 2	outpatient	med	Threshold =	10 ± 3
		inpatient	high		
MED RISK = ____		**INTER TOT.** ____		**PSYCH RISK** = ____	

PROGNOSIS

GOOD
FAIR
POOR

MED TREATMENT RECOMMENDATIONS

Clear for surgery, no psych necessary
Clear for surgery, post-op psych
Hold, pending psych intervention
Do not operate, conservative care only
Do not operate, recommend discharge

FIG. 7-5. Presurgical psychological scale.

It is often helpful for the evaluating psychologist to maintain follow-up visits following surgical procedures to assist in the patient's recovery. Adjustment issues such as vocational and other social/lifestyle changes may benefit from counseling and support.

Assessment of Malingering

According to the *Diagnostic and Statistical Manual* (3), malingering should be strongly suspected if any of the following features are present:

1. Medical/legal context of presentation (e.g., the individual is referred by an attorney to the clinician for examination).
2. Marked discrepancy between the person's claim, stress, or disability and the objective findings.
3. Lack of cooperation during the diagnostic evaluation and non-compliance with the prescribed treatment regimen.
4. The presence of antisocial personality disorder. (p. 683)

Malingering is not a mental disorder; it is differentiated from the *DSM-IV* listings of factitious disorders by the intentional production of symptoms in order to gain obvious external incentives. No single test is a true indicator of malingering. Certain psychological tests, such as the MMPI-2, have validity scales that demonstrate tendencies toward exaggeration or denial ("faking bad," "faking good"). Neuropsychologists have traditionally used simple tests for detecting malingering, which indicate the subject's motivation to complete a simple task, and often their results are compared to individuals who have severe or well-known organic cognitive pathology. The Validity Indicator Profile (24) was designed to provide empirical support based on the test subject's performance on test responses that measure malingering and other response styles. The Validity Indicator Profile (VIP) consists of verbal and nonverbal subtests and is helpful due to categorization of response styles, including compliance, carelessness, irrelevance, and malingering.

The detection of malingering cannot be determined by any specific psychological instruments or battery of tests. History, behavioral observations, and other obvious factors need to be included with the assessment for malingering or for detection of a factitious disorder. Pain is a very common sensory disturbance presented by patients who have a conversion disorder. Traditionally, conversion disorder suggests a physical disturbance; however, the symptoms are considered an expression of underlying psychological conflict, or need. A conversion disorder is not diagnosed typically when conversion symptoms are limited to pain. Traditional conversion symptoms are more often those that suggest neurologic disease, such as seizures, paralysis, coordination disturbance, dyskinesia, akinesia, blindness, and paresthesia. The onset of symptoms usually occurs when there is extreme psychological stress.

Untreated conversion reactions may produce serious complications, such as contractures or disuse atrophy. The conversion reaction is usually characterized by nonverbal communication and symbolic representation reflecting the patient's knowledge of the body and systems. This diagnosis is not confirmed by exclusion or personality traits, but when the physician demonstrates clinically that the symptoms do not conform to known anatomic and physiologic patterns. Psychogenic sensory deficits are diagnosed by their variability, sharp midline transition, and unusual dermatomal distribution. Motor deficits are typically diagnosed by their nonanatomic distribution, as well as variability and reserve strength. Some authors believe that conversion reactions have changed over the years to conform to our present litigious society, and it is not as common to see the traditional conversion reactions, such as paralysis, blindness, deafness, and convulsions, as once before (25). Emphasis should be placed on the fact that a broad range of neurological disorders may be misdiagnosed as a conversion disorder. Conversion disorder may be diagnosed in the presence of a known neurologic or medical disorder if the symptoms are not completely explained by the nature of the disorder or severity of the medical condition.

The diagnostic criteria for conversion disorder are (3)

E. One or more symptoms or deficits affecting voluntary motor or sensory function that suggest a neurological or other medical condition.
F. Psychological factors are judged to be associated with symptoms of deficits because the initiation or exacerbation of the symptom or deficit is preceded by conflicts or other stressors.
G. The symptom or deficit is not intentionally produced or feigned (as in factitious disorder or malingering).
H. The symptom or deficit cannot, after appropriate investigation, be fully explained by general medical condition or by the direct effects of a substance, or as a culturally sanctioned behavior experience.
I. The symptom or deficit causes clinically significant distress or impairment in social, occupational, or other important areas of functioning, or warrants medical evaluation.
J. The symptom or deficit is not limited to pain or sexual dysfunction, does not occur exclusively during the course of a somatization disorder, and is not better accounted for by another mental disorder. (pp. 453–457)

The *DSM-IV* criteria for a factitious disorder are

A. Intentional production or feigning of physical or psychological signs or symptoms.
B. The motivation for the behavior is to assume the sick role.
C. External incentives for the behavior, such as economic gain, avoiding legal responsibility, or improving physical well-being, as in malingering, are absent.

As described in this definition, the factitious disorders are separated from conversion reactions by the fact that factitious disorders are intentional. In the author's opinion, there may be some overlap with these diagnoses. For example, an injured worker with persistent low back pain, who has previously demonstrated organic findings by the physician, may often embellish signs and symptoms for numerous reasons. Perhaps the individual continues to have pain and compensation has been delayed, creating extreme financial stress. Does the patient now have a factitious disorder, or should we determine that there are "psychological factors affecting physical condition"? The question of malingering may be entertained. The patient may have a combination of signs, symptoms, and behaviors that have the potential to overwhelm the treating physician.

The assessment of pain should include an integrated observation of physical, psychological, and social/legal. Malingering is not always distinguishable from factitious disease. Concrete motivation for gain is often tied to a wish for care, support, and compensation. The basic issue is that of "abnormal illness behavior" and a wish for care. Evaluation of patients who have complicated pain associated with medical, social, and legal issues requires a biopsychosocial model of assessment.

ASSESSMENT OF TREATMENT OUTCOME

A growing interest has been placed on measurement of treatment outcome, partially driven by insurance authorization and reimbursement requirements. A number of instruments are available that measure an individual's pain and health status, and quality-of-life issues have become very important in the delivery of health care services and health care costs. As an example, the Health Status Questionnaire 2.0 (HSQ) (26) was designed to be used in various settings. The instrument measures the patient's self-perceived health status before, during, and after treatment. The test allows for comparison of treatment results across settings and has been standardized on a normative sample of patients and "nonpatients." The HSQ provides eight specific health attributes, including overall evaluation of health, functional status, and well-being. Multiple psychological and physical status measures are recommended for demonstration of progress and treatment effectiveness. Health care professionals are now held accountable for effectiveness of medical, surgical, and behavioral interventions. Pain and functional status measures not only are required by insurance providers and Medicare, but also help to document objectively specific criteria for diagnosis and treatment. This type of assessment improves referral activity for the health care provider and increases the likelihood of reimbursement. A combination of pretreatment assessment measures with repeated measures for improvement is recommended.

CONCLUSION

The psychological and behavioral assessment of pain should include multidimensional measures, provide estimates of motivational factors, and address the psychological and social influences on the pain syndrome. Specific populations of individuals with pain, such as children and

the elderly, require unique methods for accurate evaluation by an experienced clinician. Several instruments have been developed for evaluating pain in individuals who have communication problems and are available through the Agency for Health Care Policy and Research, U.S. Department of Health and Human Services, Public Health Service, 1994. Evaluation of pain requires specialized training and experience. Psychologists and other health care providers should have demonstrated expertise in pain management through professional organization membership and devotion to this population in practice settings. The Joint Commission for the Accreditation of Healthcare Organizations has now passed requirements for pain management in hospitals and other health care facilities.

REFERENCES

1. Melzack RN, Wall PD. Pain mechanisms: a new theory. *Science* 1965; 150: 971–979.
2. Melzack RN. From the gate to the neuromatrix. Pain supplement 6 S121–S126. Pain. International Association for the Study of Pain. Elsevier Science BV, 1999.
3. American Psychiatric Association. *Diagnostic and statistical manual of mental disorders*, 4th ed. Washington DC: American Psychiatric Association, 1994.
4. Hinnant D. Psychological evaluation and testing. In: Tollison CD, ed. *Handbook of chronic pain management*. 2nd ed. Williams and Wilkins, 1994:18–35.
5. Ransford AO, Cairns D, Mooney V. The pain drawing as an aid to the psychologic evaluations of patients with low back pain. *Spine* 1976;1: 127–134.
6. Ohnmeiss DD, VanHarnta H, Ekholm J. *Relationship between pain location and disc pathology: a study of pain drawings and CT discography*. Philadelphia: Lippincott, Williams, and Wilkins, 1999:210–217.
7. Butcher JN, Dahlstrom WG, Graham JR, Tellegen AM, Kaemer B. *MMPI-2: manual for administration and scoring,* Minneapolis: University of Minnesota Press, 1989.
8. Fordyce WE. Use of the MMPI in the assessment of chronic pain: clinical notes on the MMPI. In: Butcher J, Dahlstrom G, Gynther W, Schofield W, eds. *Clinical notes on the MMPI*. LaRoche, NJ: Hoffman, 1979.
9. Deardorff WW, Chino AF, Scott DW. Characteristics of chronic pain patients: factor analysis of the MMPI-2. *Pain* 1993;54:153–158.
10. Vendrig AA, DeMey HR, Derksen JL, Akkerveeken PF. Assessment of chronic back pain patient characteristics using factor analysis of the MMPI-2: which dimensions are actually assessed? *Pain* 1998;76: 179–188.
11. Riley JL, Robinson ME, Geisser ME, Wittmer VT, Smith AG. Relationship between MMPI-2 cluster profiles and surgical outcome in low back pain patients. *Journal of Spinal Disorders* 1995;8,3:213–219.
12. National Computer Systems. Minneapolis: National Computer Systems, 2000.
13. Melzack R. The McGill Pain Questionnaire. In: Melzack R, ed. *Pain measurement and assessment*. New York: Raven Press, 1983.
14. Dubuisson D, Melzack R. Classification of clinical pain description by multiple group discriminate analysis. *Experimental Neurology* 1976;51:480–487.
15. Bruns D, Disorbio JM, Copeland-Disorbio J. *Manual for the battery for health improvement*. Minnetonka: NCS Assessments, 1996.
16. Bruns D, Disorbio JM. Hostility and violent ideation: physical rehabilitation patient and community samples. *Pain Medicine* 2000;1(2): 131–139.
17. Millon T, Antoni M, et al. *Millon behavioral medicine diagnostic*. Dicandrien Inc., 2000.
18. Tollison CD, Langley JC. *Pain patient profile manual*. Minneapolis: National Computer Systems, 1995.
19. Hinnant D, Tollison CD. *The Pain Patient Profile (P-3) and its use as a screening instrument with neurosurgery patients*. Unpublished manuscript, 2000.

20. Waddell G, Muculloch JA, Kummel EG, Venner RM. Non-organic physical signs in low back pain. *Spine* 1980;5:117–125.
21. Schofferman J, Anderson D, Hines R, Smith G, White A. Childhood sexual trauma correlates with unsuccessful lumbar spine surgery. *Spine* 1992;17(6):(suppl S138–S144).
22. Block AR. *Pre-surgical psychological screening in chronic pain syndromes: a guide for the behavioral health practitioner*. Mahwah, NJ: Lawrence Erlbaum Associates, 1996.
23. Doleys DM, Olsen K. *Psychological assessment and intervention in implantable pain therapies*. Medtronic, Inc., 1997.
24. Frederick RI. *Manual for the Validity Indicator Profile*. Minneapolis: National Computer Systems, 1997.
25. Weintraub MI. Chronic pain and litigation: what is the relationship? *Neurologic Clinics* May 1995;13(2).
26. Health Status Questionnaire 2.0. Health Outcomes Institute. Available through NCS Assessments. Minneapolis. 2000.

APPENDIX A. *A compendium of tests useful in the assessment of pain*

Test	Source	Format	Summary description	Estimated value pain assessment*
Minnesota Multiphasic Personality Inventory (MMPI) and revision (MMPI-2)	NCS Assessments 5605 Green Circle Dr. Minnetonka, MN 55343 1-800-627-7271	Paper-and-pencil or computer-based true/false inventory MMPI-2 has 567 items Administration time approximately 60–90 minutes Intended for ages 18 years and older	Originally normed on a psychiatric population, the MMPI-2 has been revised and restandardized. In addition to the validity and clinical scales, supplementary scales have been developed. Specifically tailored reports are available, including chronic pain treatment programs.	3
Pain Patient Profile	NCS Assessments 5605 Green Circle Dr. Minnetonka, MN 55343 1-800-627-7271	Paper-and-pencil or computer-based multiple-choice test with 44 items Each item consists of three potential responses rank-ordered in terms of intensity Administration time approximately 15 minutes Intended for ages 17 and older	A new screening instrument with targeted characteristics of relevance to patients in pain, brevity, multidimensional scope, and strong psychometric properties. The P-3 is designed to identify patients who are experiencing emotional distress associated with pain, the degrees of psychological distress, and the influence of psychological functioning on pain symptomatology and complaints. The profile measures validity, somatization, depression, and anxiety. The interpretive report compares each patient's responses to populations of both pain patients and a community sample at large. The P-3 Interpretive report also outlines medical management, and psychosocial and pharmacologic treatment recommendations based on each patient's item responses.	5
West Haven-Yale Multidimensional Pain Inventory (MPI)	Pain Evaluation and Treatment Institute University of Pittsburgh Medical Center 4601 Baum Blvd. Pittsburgh, PA 15213 412-578-3350	Paper-and-pencil inventory with 60 items requiring forced choice on a 7-point Likert scale Administration time approximately 20–30 minutes Intended for adults	Based on a cognitive-behavioral model, the MPI consists of 12 scales designed to measure the impact of pain on a patient's life, communication of the pain experience, and the extent to which patient participates in activities of daily living. The MPI should be utilized with other traditional measures of psychological distress.	5

APPENDIX A. *Continued*

Test	Source	Format	Summary description	Estimated value pain assessment*
Behavioral Assessment of Pain (BAP)	Pendrake, Inc. 3370 Southampton Dr. Reno, NV 89509	Paper-and-pencil self-report instrument with 390 items Most items require forced choice on a 7-point rating scale Administration time approximately 60–90 minutes Intended for adults	A comprehensive multidimensional instrument developed on a bio-psychosocial model, the BAP is divided into 9 scales: demographics, activity, interference, avoidance, spouse/partner influence, physician influence, physician qualities, pain beliefs, perceived consequences, and coping. The BAP is normed on 600 pain patients. The test is exceptionally comprehensive but lengthy. Administration can be discouraging to some patients. The BAP should be utilized with measures of psychological distress and physical capacity.	5
Beck Depression Inventory	The Psychological Corporation P.O. Box 839954 San Antonio, TX 87283 1-800-228-0752	Paper-and-pencil or computer-based multiple-choice test with 32 items Each item consists of 4 potential responses, rank-ordered in terms of depressive intensity Administration time approximately 5–10 minutes Intended for ages 17–80 years	A commonly used screening device for assessing the intensity of depression in psychiatrically diagnosed patients and for detecting depression in normal populations. The BDI was derived from clinical observations of the attitudes, behaviors, and symptoms frequently displayed by depressed psychiatric patients. It is often used throughout psychiatric treatment as a measure of improvement.	1–2
Millon Behavioral Health Inventory (MBHI)	NCS Assessments 5605 Green Circle Dr. Minnetonka, MN 55343 1-800-627-7271	Paper-and-pencil or computer-based test with 150 true/false items Administration time approximately 20–30 minutes Intended for ages 18 years and older	A self-report personality inventory designed to assess the psychological coping factors related to the physical health care of adult medical patients. Interpretation is based on 20 clinical scales collectively summarized under 4 major categories: basic coping style, psychogenic attitudes, psychosomatic correlates, and prognostic indicators. The MBHI is normed on medical patients.	2
McGill Pain Questionnaire	Ronald Melzack, Ph.D. McGill University Dept. of Psychology Stewart Biological Sciences Building 1205 Dr. Penfield Ave. Montreal, QC, Canada H&A 1B1 514-389-6100	Paper-and-pencil self-report test containing 20 categories of verbal descriptors of pain and a pain drawing Each category offers the patient 2–5 responses rank-ordered in terms of severity Administration time approximately 30–45 minutes, depending on reading ability and intelligence Intended for adults	Attempts to assess the sensory (temporal, spatial), affective, and evaluative or intensity dimensions of pain. Scoring requires adding the number of words chosen from the 20 category scales or adding the rank values of the descriptors chosen from each of the pain dimensions to form a Pain Rating Index. The MPQ enjoys excellent content validity but requires patients to have a relatively high level of reading ability and intelligence. Available in several foreign languages. A short form is also available.	3–4

APPENDIX A. *Continued*

Test	Source	Format	Summary description	Estimated value pain assessment*
The Chronic Pain Battery (CPB)	Pain Resource Ctr, Inc. P.O. Box 2836 Durham, NC 27715	Paper-and-pencil multiple-choice and true/false instrument with approximately 200 items Administration time 60–75 minutes	A multidimensional instrument with forms for both nonmalignant and cancer pain. The test includes information on a pain history, medical information, social functioning, and incorporates the SCL-90-R. The CPB should be utilized with other measures of psychological distress. Additional research and psychometric investigation of the CPB are recommended.	3
Symptom Checklist 90-revised (SCL-90-R)	NCS Assessments 5605 Green Circle Dr Minnetonka, MN 55343 1-800-627-7271	Paper-and-pencil or computer-based test with 90 items and a 5-point rating scale Administration time approximately 12–15 minutes Intended for adults and adolescents 13 years or older	A multidimensional instrument with forms designed to screen for a broad range of psychological problems and symptoms or good measure of psychopathology in psychiatric and medical patients. Research suggests the value of the SCL-90-R as a screening instrument, which should be correlated with more traditional instruments. Normative data is available for 4 groups: nonpatient adults, nonpatient adolescents, psychiatric outpatients, and psychiatric inpatients.	3
Clinical Analysis Questionnaire (CAQ)	NCS Assessments 5605 Green Circle Dr. Minnetonka, MN 55343 1-800-627-7271	Paper-and-pencil multiple-choice test with 272 items divided into 2 sections Administration time approximately 100 minutes Intended for adults and adolescents 16 years and older	A multidimensional personality test combining the diagnostic assessment of deviant behavior with the measurement of an individual's normal coping skills. It is intended for general clinical diagnosis and for evaluating treatment progress, as well as for vocational guidance. The CAQ measures the same 16 personality factors measured by the 16-PF, plus 12 pathologic characteristics.	2
Personality Assessment Inventory (PAI)	Psychological Assessment Resources, Inc. P.O. Box 998 Odessa, FL 33556-9901	Paper-and-pencil self-report inventory containing 344 items with each item rated on a 4-point scale from "False, not at all true" to "Very True" Administration time approximately 45–60 minutes Intended for adults 18 years or older	A multidimensional personality test with 22 scales covering a broad range of mental disorders: 4 validity, 11 clinical, 5 treatment, -and 2 interpersonal scales. The test is designed to assess various psychopathologic syndromes and provides information relevant to clinical diagnosis, treatment planning, and screening for psychopathology. Normed on adults in a variety of clinical and community settings but does not include patients with a primary complaint of pain.	2

APPENDIX A. *Continued*

Test	Source	Format	Summary description	Estimated value pain assessment*
Millon Behavioral Medicine Diagnostic (MBMD)	NCS Assessments 5605 Green Circle Dr. Minnetonka, MN 55343 1-800-627-7271	New paper-and-pencil, online test with 165 true/false items Administration time 20–25 minutes (Scoring: by hand, mail in)	Normative sample of 700 medical patients including cancer, heart disease, diabetes, HIV, and pain with 29 content scales: health moderators, treatment prognostics, psychiatric indicators, coping style, modifying indices, lifestyle behavior responses. Reported options: interoperative and profile reports.	
Brief Symptom Inventory (BSI)	NCS Assessments 5605 Green Circle Dr. Minnetonka, MN 55343 1-800-627-7271	Paper-and-pencil audio cassette or online Administration time 3–5 minutes	A brief version of the SCL-90-R measures for depression, anxiety, and somatization with a global severity index. May be used to monitor patient progress and treatment outcomes. The global severity index helps to quantify a patient's severity of the illness and provides a simple composite score for measuring symptom reduction. The test provides an interpretive and progress report.	3
Substance Abuse Subtle Screening Inventory (SASSI)	Professional Alternatives Inc. 320 Conant St. Maumee, Ohio 43537 1-800-347-2774	Paper-and-pencil test faxed in 30 minutes or less Administration time 10–15 minutes	A short psychologically based questionnaire that screens effectively for substance related disorders even when a person attempts to deny or conceal a problem, 96 percent selectivity.	1-2
Health Status Questionnaire (HSQ 2.0)	NCS Assessments 5605 Green Circle Dr. Minnetonka, MN 55343 1-800-627-7271	Paper-and-pencil or online test Administered by self-report, interview, or telephone Ages 14 to adult	The HSQ 2.0 questionnaire contains all the items found on the Sf-36 providing the patients self-reported health status on eight health attributes before, during, and after treatment. The test addresses eight attributes under three major health concepts:health perception, functional status (physical functioning, social functioning, role limitations–physical, role limitations–emotional, bodily pain) and well-being (mental health, energy-fatigue)	3
Battery for Health Improvement (BHI)	NCS Assessments 5605 Green Circle Dr. Minnetonka, MN 55343 1-800-627-7271	Paper and pencil, audio cassette, or computer administration. Administration time 25–40 minutes. 202 multiplechoice items. Ages 18–65	Designed to help identify the psychological factors that may interfere with a patient's normal course of recovery. Measures impact of physical, environmental, and psychological factors. Helpful for assessment of readiness for vocational training. surgery, or job placement. Test report includes scales for: symptom dependency, chronic maladjustment, family dysfunction, job dissatisfaction, muscular bracing, somatic complaints, pain complaints, and perseverance.	5

APPENDIX A. *Continued*

Test	Source	Format	Summary description	Estimated value pain assessment*
Validity Indicator Profile (VIP)	NCS Assessments 5605 Green Circle Dr. Minnetonka, MN 55343 1-800-627-7271	Computer scored Administration time 30 minutes	An empirical measure of malingering and other response styles. Provides broad spectrum of information about a patient's performance during an assessment battery. Contains both verbal and nonverbal subtests. Helps to determine whether further testing will be valid and helpful.	3

CHAPTER **8**

Diagnostic and Therapeutic Injections

Roger W. Catlin

Injecting medication or contrast through a needle into a specific anatomical site is not difficult. Knowing what to inject can, at times, require a little thought. Determining when to perform a precision injection, where to perform the injection, and what to do with the collectable information from that process can be difficult and is the "work" of the pain medicine physician.

Pain medicine, as amorphous as that label is, is a new medical specialty. A physician who practices pain medicine is not practicing anesthesiology, neurology, orthopedics, physiatry, neurosurgery, or any other specialty. Granted, knowledge and specialty techniques of any or all other specialties can and do bleed over into this new field; however, the sibling is *not* the parent. Until the physician performing injections doffs the mantle of his or her earlier training and moves forward under the new mantle of "pain medicine doctor," the result of his or her injections and the potential power of those results will be mediocre at best. Pain medicine is a new specialty, a new religion of medicine, and diagnostic and therapeutic injections are not just an appendage of the discipline but part of its heart.

Often injections are discussed and performed as if the very act has essential value and beauty in and of itself, rather like listening to Mozart or Elton John. However, without a real, alive person/patient to dart that needle into, no "beauty" can exist. Therefore, each and every injectionist must be sure that what we do with "the needle" has purpose and at least potential value, or truly we are guilty of assault and battery and have failed our Hippocratic oath.

This chapter, if only by virtue of its brevity, cannot survey all of injection therapy in pain medicine. I will attempt to deal with a collage of concepts, facts, attitudes, policies, guidelines, and so forth, that affect all of a pain medicine doctor's/injectionist's work. The inclusion of some personal anecdotes and beliefs will be unavoidable. There are several excellent texts (1–9) that describe the "how-to" of injections a pain doctor could master and perform. While

reading/studying those texts and other "how-to" references available is valuable and important, there is no replacement for the guidance of a knowledgeable mentor standing at your side the first time you perform a specific injection. While many physicians can perform some of the injections due to the training of their primary specialty, few physicians can perform a majority of all possible injections without additional education and practice. Only with time and conscious effort by the pain medicine doctor can a full repertoire be developed. On the one hand, the physician needs to learn only those tools that will be used reasonably frequently in his or her practice. However, in accordance with the well-known saying "If the only tool you own is a hammer, then everything looks like a nail," the pain medicine physician's injection repertoire of procedural skills must be big enough to meet the needs of the majority of diagnostic and therapeutic challenges. Even so, he or she should be humble and wise to be able to recognize and admit an area of knowledge deficit. The best care he or she can provide may be to refer patients to physicians learned in the most beneficial technique.

The following text discusses those other topics less often discussed, but so very germane to the use of injections. I believe these considerations are the backbone of tying together the utilization of injections.

INJECTION FOR DIAGNOSIS

Diagnosis by injection is demanding. The goal is to stop or otherwise modify nerve transmission, be it a single nerve root (e.g., L-5 on the left) or plexus (e.g., inferior cervical sympathetic chain, the stellate ganglion), and compare the patient's report of pain before and after the "nerve block."

The requirements for injections for diagnosis include:

1. *Perform an appropriate history and physical examination of the patient before the diagnostic injection.* Note the

exact (as possible) distribution of the pain, its character, and its intensity. Clearly document *function* of the involved body part or area, including strength and sensation. Observe and record the patient's gait and balance, if appropriate. Be able to reexamine the patient after the injection, comparing your postinjection findings to the preinjection state, thereby developing impressions and diagnoses.

2. *Chose a local anesthetic appropriate for the study.* While 0.25% to 0.5% Marcaine or 0.5% to 1% Xylocaine may be appropriate for sympathetic chemical blockade (small and slow A-delta, B, and C fibers), 0.75% Marcaine or 2% Xylocaine is needed for a somatic motor blockade (large and fast A-alpha and A-beta fibers) (6). Autonomic nerve blockade (e.g., stellate ganglion) is performed with 4 cc to 10 cc of injectate; therefore, the effective concentration of the local anesthetic placed on the nerve tissue is similar to the medication injected. However, to selectively interrupt a single spinal nerve root and prevent transforaminal flow of local anesthetic on to other nerves close by with the subsequent generation of a more extensive epidural blockade, the volume injected should be limited to 0.5 cc to 1 cc. Because intercellular and intracellular fluid may be mobilized rapidly due to hydrostatic pressure and osmotic effects and because the molecules of the effective anesthetic chemical must penetrate into the nerve to create the physiological block, the concentration of anesthetic molecules is decreased from around the nerve. The effective concentration of the small volume of injectate falls rapidly after injection. Additionally, some contrast is usually in the perineural tissue due to its use to identify the needle tip location prior to local anesthetic injection and acts to dilute the injectate. Usually steroid is added to the already small volume of injectate before injection, thereby diluting the concentration of local anesthetic before injection. Consequently, the effective concentration is markedly reduced. For example, while placing as much as 1 cc to 1.5 cc of pure 0.75% Marcaine directly on a segmental lumbar nerve root (e.g., L-3, Fig. 8-1) can cause some tingling in that nerve distribution, I have never known a person not able to walk at the time of maximum anesthetic effect following a diagnostic injection that was preceded by the injection of contrast and diluted with steroid. Utilization of higher anesthetic concentrations, which are available if sought by the clinician (e.g., 5% Xylocaine), can increase the specificity by allowing the utilization of a decreased volume of injectate.

3. *Know where the injectate flows.* Fluid flow follows the path of least resistance. In tissue the pathway of least resistance may be between two fascial layers where the thickness of the "river of flow" is tiny. One cc can travel several inches on occasion. The effect of a small volume flowing a relatively long distance can be seen when per-

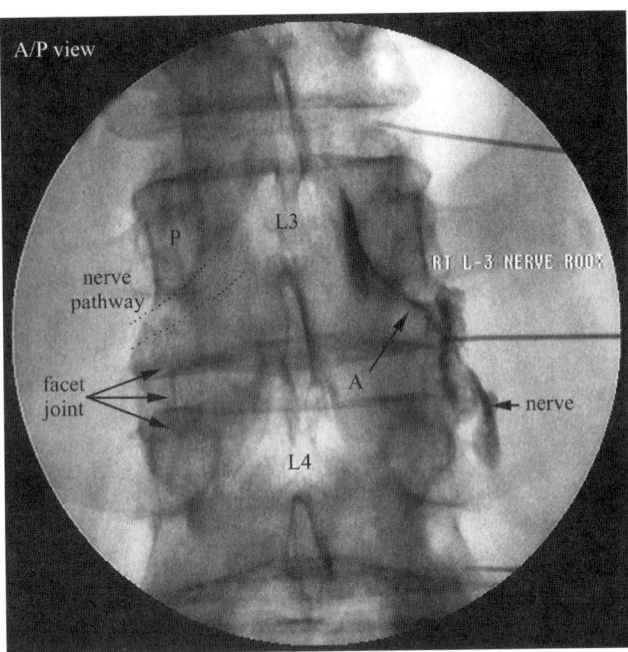

FIG. 8-1. Selective Nerve Root Blocks. Approximately 0.2 cc of contrast is injected into the segmental nerve root, nicely outlining the neurolemma. When injecting for diagnosis, care must be taken not to unduly force the local anesthetic into the spinal canal due to the use of too much volume. The inadvertent epidural effect can produce false diagnostic information/results. (A = probable pathologic nerve root compression at the dorsal root ganglion; P = pedicle)

forming intercostal nerve injections under fluoroscopy. With the needle tip accurately placed in the neurovascular bundle under a rib, 3 cc of injectate can literally flow half way around the chest wall. Therefore, fluoroscopy *must* be utilized (10–12) in all diagnostic injections to determine accurate injectate placement and the volume to be used. Often the needle tip placement will need to be modified to achieve proper injectate placement (Fig. 8-2).

Learning correct injectate placement is a matter of knowledge, injection principles, and practice. For example, the familiar stellate ganglion sympathetic plexus extends from C-4 to T-2 anatomically. If the injectate flow does not stretch from the mid-body of C-4 to at least the cephalic edge, or lower, of T-2 and stay anterior to the cervical vertebral bodies (Fig. 8-3A), the injection is not adequate and cannot be considered diagnostic. If, by fluoroscopy, the contrast mixed with local anesthetic passes posteriorly more than one-third of the cervical vertebral body (Fig. 8-3B), the probability of cervical segmental nerves being partially anesthetized with local anesthetic is great. While such an injection is adequate for therapy (to be discussed), it is not adequate to determine the presence or absence of sympathetic mediated, modulated, or maintained pain. To rely on information from an ill-performed block is

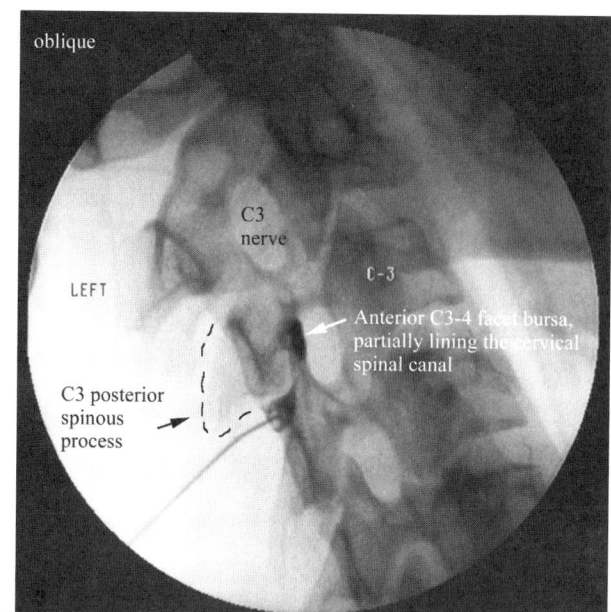

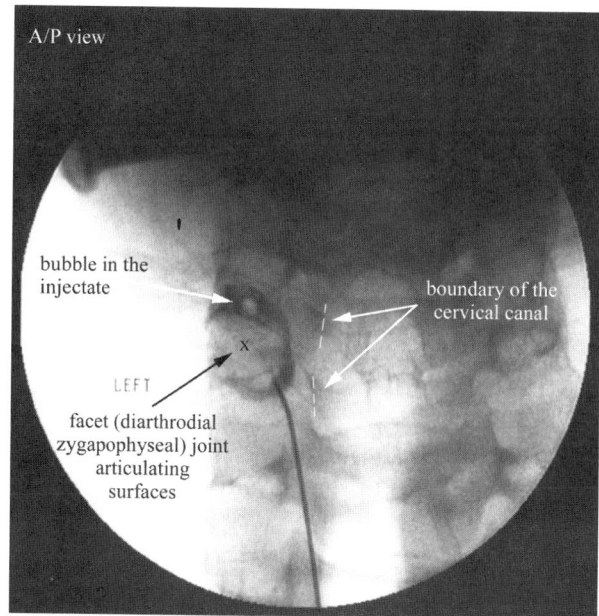

FIG. 8-2. Right C-3–C-4 Facet Joint Injection. With the patient prone, this modestly oblique view (with the C-Arm about 25° from horizontal) is used to visually separate the facets from one side to the other. The 23-gauge needle was placed from a direct posterior approach into the edge of the C-3–C4 facet joint capsule. The 0.10 cc of Isovue 370 has been injected, outlining the capsule and intra-articular space (**A**). The contrast flowed through the facet joint, filling the capsule anteriorly. The A/P image (**B**) is used to align the needle with the cervical pillars (i.e., avoid the canal space) and demonstrates the roundness of the cervical zygapophyseal diarthrodial joint face and bursa.

an error. Such a block would simply need to be repeated. A small amount of contrast (e.g., Isovue 370) is injected before the local anesthetic (and steroid) is injected. If the contrast flow is aberrant and if the contrast then obstructs the ability to "see" where to properly place the needle, the procedure will need to be aborted and performed another day. Although a nuisance with respect to the injectionist's day's work and the patient taking the time to be present for care, it is the correct thing to do. Usually patients are understanding and appreciative of your desire to obtain reliable and accurate results. With an appropriate explanation, very few patients become angry or upset. The precision injectionist must know the target (anatomy) and accept only accurate injections for diagnosis.

4. *Make observations at the appropriate time.* Although it is often convenient to wait for the patient's return visit to evaluate the response, usually this is inappropriate. Patients forget the specifics of their response. Even if they keep a pain diary, they usually do not know the questions that need to be answered. Therefore, the pain doctor must have an environment where patients can be evaluated at the time of expected maximum response to the injectate. Some injections should be evaluated more than once, if only to attempt to determine response authenticity of the known duration of the local anesthetic effect. For example, after diagnostic lumbar facet (diarthrodial zygapophyseal) joint injection (Fig. 8-4), a

patient can be evaluated by repeating forward flexion/posterior extension exercises literally as soon as he or she can step off the procedure table and onto the floor. However, following a trans-discal (L-5–S-1) hypogastric plexus injection for pelvic pain (e.g., 8 cc of 0.75% Marcaine mixed with 3 cc of Isovue 370, and 1 cc of triamcinolone, a total of 12 cc), the sympathetic block may not be maximally effective for 20 to 40 minutes. Even then the patient should be called or asked to call the office the next day to report the later effects of the injection. That information should be added to the patient's records. Only in this way, by the disciplined recording of actual patient responses, can the most valuable and useful information be gathered.

5. *Be as objective as possible.* If there is a way to document that, pharmacologically, the injection affected the nerve or neural plexus targeted, do so. For example:

A. Most effective stellate ganglion blocks cause the ipsilateral eyelid to droop and pupil to constrict (miosis), the same half of the face to warm, the sclera to become reddened, and the superficial veins of the arm to dilate (Horner's response). Observe and record those findings if they occur. Negative findings are also important. Again, after a stellate ganglion injection (as an example), the patient should *not* develop any arm weakness nor should there be any dulling of tactile perception. Evaluate the patient with simple resistant strength testing and

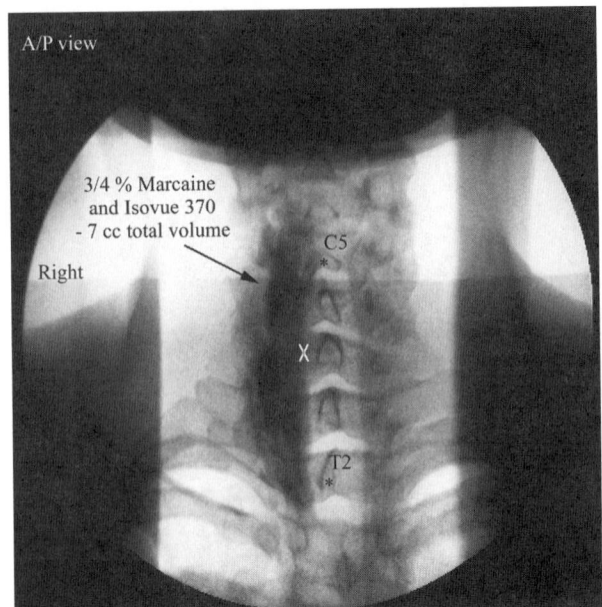

A

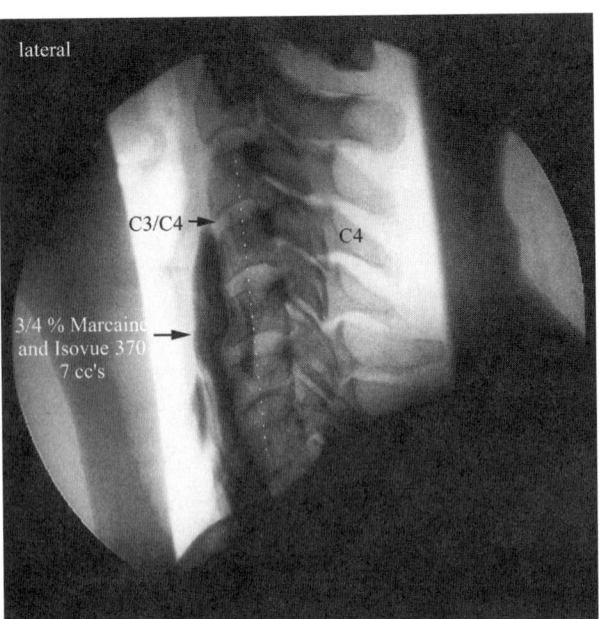

B

FIG. 8-3. Stellate (inferior cervical sympathetic) Ganglion Injection, Diagnostic. To completely "block" the stellate ganglion, local anesthetic must flow cephalad to C-4 and caudad to T-2 (**A**). On the lateral view (**B**) the local anesthetic must *not* pass more than one-third to one-half way posterior on the cervical vertebral body or the cervical and thoracic segmental nerve(s) may be affected. The local anesthetic may be mixed with contrast and steroid as long as the final concentration of local anesthetic is sufficient to stop sympathetic plexus function. The distribution of contrast depicted in these fluoroscopic images is correct for the neural blockade of the right sympathetic ganglion.

In addition to specifically observing (and stating in the procedural report) that the sensation of light touch and coolness were *not* diminished and muscle strength was *not* compromised, radiographically imaging the distribution of injectate is mandatory to guarantee a clean and complete sympathetic blockade. If properly placed 6 to 8 cc is plenty of injectate for the procedure, even in the largest of people. Utilizing more volume invites unwanted spill onto somatic nerve roots.

NOTE: The posterior spinous process images can be misleading when injecting on the "front" (anterior surface) of the cervical vertebral body because we are so used to seeing the anatomy from "behind." Therefore, be careful when thinking about where your needle tip is. A needle tip placed within 2 to 3 mm of the midline often results in at least some bilateral injectate flow because there is no natural "raphe" to restrict fluid movement.

FACT: A diagnostic stellate ganglion block cannot be performed adequately without the utilization of radiographic contrast and fluoroscopic imaging.

(* = posterior spinous process; X = needle was placed on the anterior vertebral body of C7, approximately 4–5 mm to the right of the anatomical midline.)

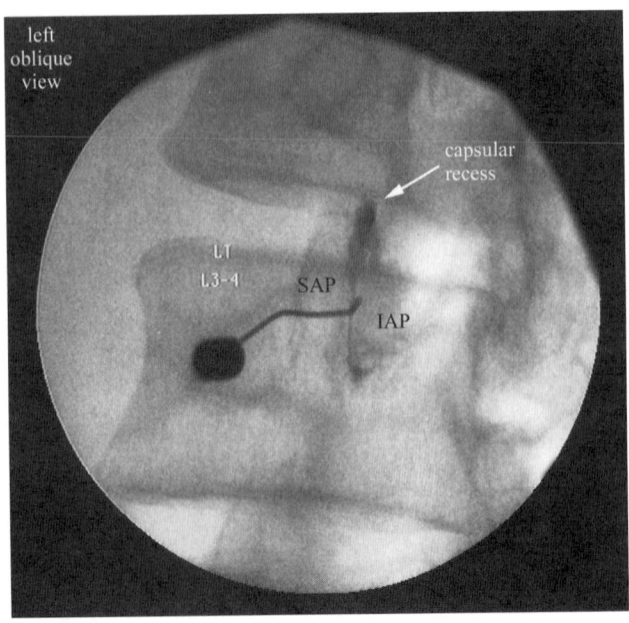

FIG. 8-4. Lumbar Intra-articular Facet Joint Injection. The tip of a 23-gauge 3.2" needle has been placed in the edge of the L-3–L4 left facet joint. The 0.10 cc of Isovue 370 outlines the facet joint internal surfaces and fills small superior and inferior capsular recesses. Excess volume will often tear the capsule. The bursa recesses may be naturally perforated at each end or may tear during injection. The volume necessary to fill lumbar facet joints is generally less than 1 cc. (SAP = superior articulating process of L4; IAP = inferior articulating process of L3)

tactile responses with a pin, and clearly and routinely record these negative findings in your postoperative note. A patient who develops a partially anesthetized arm cannot be said to have a diagnostic stellate ganglion block. Conclusions from such injections are misleading and often result in erroneous diagnoses and therefore inappropriate therapy.

B. Except in patients with severe peripheral vascular disease, a well-performed diagnostic paravertebral lumbar sympathetic block is followed by warming of the ipsilateral extremity. Placing electronic skin temperature probes between any two toes of both feet and watching for temperature change provides an excellent objective, documentable finding to dictate into your record that quantifies the patient's response and signifies the quality of the injection (your work). It also documents the ability, or lack of it, of the patient's vascular bed to respond to sympathetic blockade. Preinjection, allow both lower extremities to cool by being exposed to air at room temperature. Apply the temperature probes before the injection to document preinjection temperatures and continue to measure the temperature for at least 45 minutes after the injection or until there is no doubt that vasodilation on the treated side has selectively occurred. Usually the skin temperature will rise to above 33°C. *Do not* rely on simple subjective tactile monitoring with your own hand. The actual temperature is objective, easy to measure, and important to document. Without the actual skin temperature, the report following a diagnostic percutaneous lumbar sympathectomy is incomplete. The procedure report should contain the results of strength and sensory testing, like that following a stellate ganglion block.

C. Cutaneous selective tissue conductivity may be helpful. Almost all motor and sensory nerves run with some autonomic fibers. Injecting a single root or a peripheral nerve, as well as a sympathetic nerve or plexus is usually followed by a change in skin moisture and conductivity (13,14). Therefore, testing skin conductivity before and after a neural blockade can give an objective finding to document the effect of the injection. However, much work has yet to be done with this technique to substantiate its validation.

6. *Use "none" to "minimal" patient sedation and analgesia* when performing a diagnostic neural blockade. For the patient to be able to accurately evaluate the effect of the diagnostic injection, his or her mental functioning and ability to sense the body's response should not be blunted by a systemic analgesic or sedative. Although easy to say (write) this is often difficult to accomplish. Most patients do not understand the concept of a diagnostic injection, even after it has been explained to them in detail. Many patients want to be "knocked out."

The process of performing the precision diagnostic injection begins with your first encounter with a patient and possibly his or her significant other. If this encounter is in your office when plans are being made, you have an opportunity and an advantage. A warm staff, careful exam, logical reasoning, reasonable explanation, perhaps utilizing anatomical pictures and a skeleton, whether actually understood or not understood by the patient, can win the patient's confidence and cooperation before "the day." However, if the patient has been referred to you, perhaps by an orthopedic surgeon or a neurologist who is requesting that you perform a specific injection for diagnosis, you must be extra smooth in the procedure room's holding area. Again, the comfort of your support staff will quickly be reflected in the patient's anxiety level. A thorough, truthful explanation of the procedure risks and alternatives is mandatory (and also required for informed consent). Often the information is better received from a nurse, physician assistant, or nurse practitioner than from "the doctor" who is usually shorter on time, uses bigger words, and intimidates the patient all too easily and often unknowingly. However, the physician should greet the patient outside the procedure room, make some form of appropriate physical contact (warm handshake, etc.), and ask for final questions and concerns. Be genuine and the patient's confidence will usually come quickly. And, be truthful. If some part of the procedure will be unavoidably painful, such as sliding the needle along the L-2, L-3, L-4, vertebral periosteum during a lumbar sympathetic chain injection, or pressurizing the disc during a discogram, tell the patient, both in the holding area and in the procedure room just before it happens. The average patient will be accepting and cooperative if you do so. Praise the patient for being cooperative after the procedure. Everybody likes a reward. In this way you can then test the patient after the injection and gather the best data on a routine basis.

NOTE: Frequently after the diagnostic procedure is performed and after all testing is complete, when systemic sedation will not interfere with evaluation of the injection, I will order the patient to receive a modest amount of intravenous sedation and analgesic (e.g., Toradol 30 mg IV, Demerol 25 mg to 50 mg IV, and Versed 0.5 mg to 1 mg IV). Often what patients remember is how they felt when they left the facility, and not all the specifics of what they experienced during the procedure. If they are comfortable when on the way home their memory of the procedure will be less unpleasant. (Therefore, do not let the nursing staff remove the IV ASAP, but leave it in until your patient care is complete.)

Some patients simply are not able to be injected without "something." ("Doc, I gotta' have something!") There are many variables. A single deft needle placement for a stellate ganglion injection or supraorbital injection may be acceptable, while a three-level bilateral facet joint injection is not. The injectionist then must make the judgment call of how much the postinjection testing will be compromised by systemic sedation and analgesia administered at the beginning of the procedure and whether to proceed. Often, if the potential pain generator is significantly inflammatory (e.g., facet osteoarthropathy), or if the pain symptom is truly allodynic (e.g., neurogenic etiology), either a very meaningful result can be obtained by patient questioning in the 1- to 3-day period postinjection (for injection of the inflamed facet), or even a significant amount of systemic analgesic will not block the allodynic state (neurogenic pain), while a solid sympathetic neural blockade will. In those cases, some systemic analgesic is acceptable.

When systemic sedation is utilized for a diagnostic injection (or a therapeutic injection), often a true analgesic (e.g., narcotic) is the best first choice. Barbiturates (e.g., Pentothal) and Diprivan (propofol) create a patient with full sensory perception, but with decreased ability to logically reason and with markedly decreased inhibition. These patients can become uncontrollable. Narcotics (e.g., fentanyl) administered intravenously act quickly and decrease the patient's perception of the needle-induced pain, usually leaving the patient able to reason and function rationally. If apprehension is the biggest obstacle, I believe benzodiazepines (e.g., Valium and Versed) are the best class of drugs to lower anxiety and produce an "I don't care" attitude and still leave the patient in control. A wonderful "add-on" drug, if used in small amounts, is droperidol (Inapsine), although droperidol prevents most reasonable immediate postinjection evaluations. The biggest and most vigorous of patients will usually settle down with an appropriate ratio of the above three drug groups. Of course, as always, to use such depressing and sedating systemic-acting medications, the physician should be skilled in airway control and supportive resuscitative equipment and medications. The maximal sedative effect may not be seen for 8 to 10 minutes, and then on occasion, *after* the procedure is completed and the stimulation of the injection is gone. Therefore, resuscitation drugs and equipment, including reversal agents, must be available in the operating room should an inadvertent overdose occur. Appropriate postprocedure observation by trained postanesthetic recovery room nurses is essential.

Last, most patient protests can be circumvented by the quick, accurate placement of small (23 gauge or less), sharp needles with or without skin local. If local is used (e.g., 1 percent Xylocaine), its "burn" at injection can be markedly reduced by buffering with sodium bicarbonate (e.g., 1 cc of sodium bicarbonate mixed with 10 to 30 cc of local anesthetic). Remember, speed, accuracy, and a warm, supportive atmosphere mixed with patient praise goes a long, long way to allow the patient to cooperate fully and remember your care as being "wonderful." Most patients want to be cooperative and want to do their part in their medical care. It is our responsibility as physicians to provide a way for them to do so.

INJECTION FOR THERAPY

If performed appropriately, *all* injections are performed for both diagnosis and therapy. The difference is more a matter of planning, emphasis, and expectation than a procedure being performed in a substantially different manner. Many procedures are naturally diagnostic, whereas others are naturally therapeutic. For example, a selective nerve root injection performed with 1 cc of injectate is more diagnostic, whereas a transforaminal epidural steroid injection (ESI) performed at the same foramen (Fig. 8-5) with 5 to 10 cc of injectate is more therapeutic. A lumbar sympathetic block performed with 3 cc of local anesthetic placed at the anterolateral aspect of the vertebral bodies of L-2, L-3, and L-4 is diagnostic, whereas the same amount of sympathetic blockade achieved via epidural catheter placed with fluoroscopic guidance and left for several days or weeks and injected frequently, if not daily, avoiding daily needle punctures, is therapeutic. Alternately, radiofrequency thermocoagulation (RFT) of the lumbar sympathetic chain is therapeutic. Precision injection of the atlanto-occipital (C0-1) (Fig. 8-6) and atlantoaxial (C1-2) joint capsules for osteoarthritic pain or steroid injection of the occipital nerves (Greater, 3rd, and Lesser occipital nerves) is both diagnostic and therapeutic, whereas partial rhizolysis with RFT of the C-2 and C-3 dorsal root (sensory) ganglion does more definitively to treat pain in the same anatomical area and is definitely therapeutic. Therefore, injecting for therapy does not mean the injectionist can be less disciplined in any manner. It does mean: know the anatomy, know the parameters of the "job to be done" and of the injection to be utilized, and employ that knowledge appropriately and accurately.

A few generalities:

1. Sedation and analgesia can be utilized more liberally with therapeutic procedures because an immediate postinjection response is *not* being sought. When utilizing RFT or any procedure that requires electrical stimulation for accurate needle placement, the patient must be awake and rational.

   NOTE: Patient's wakefulness is your *friend!* Although the patient may prefer to be less aware and not feel the sticks and stings of the injections, it is the patient's response/paresthesia that will help prevent you from performing interneural injections or warn you of an impending vascular toxic reaction or of a profound sudden CNS depression and respiratory arrest. General anesthesia or anything close to it is very strongly discouraged when performing any pain-related injections.

2. Therapeutic injections are often performed in a series. The infamous "series of three" lumbar ESIs is the best example. A series of any kind must be pursued only

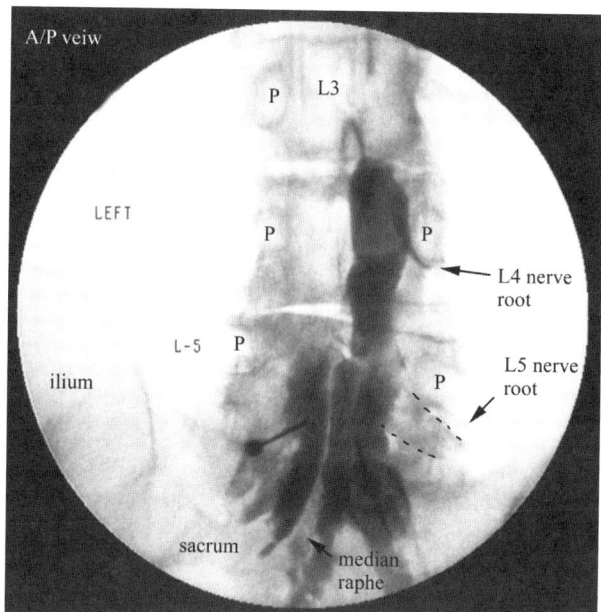

A

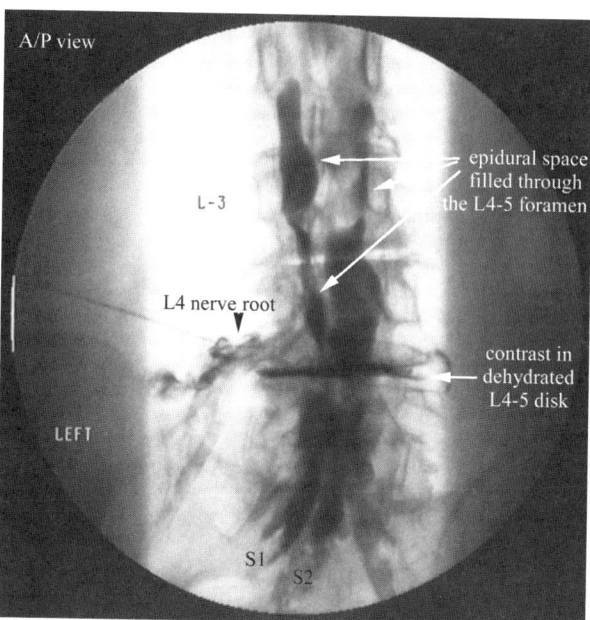

B

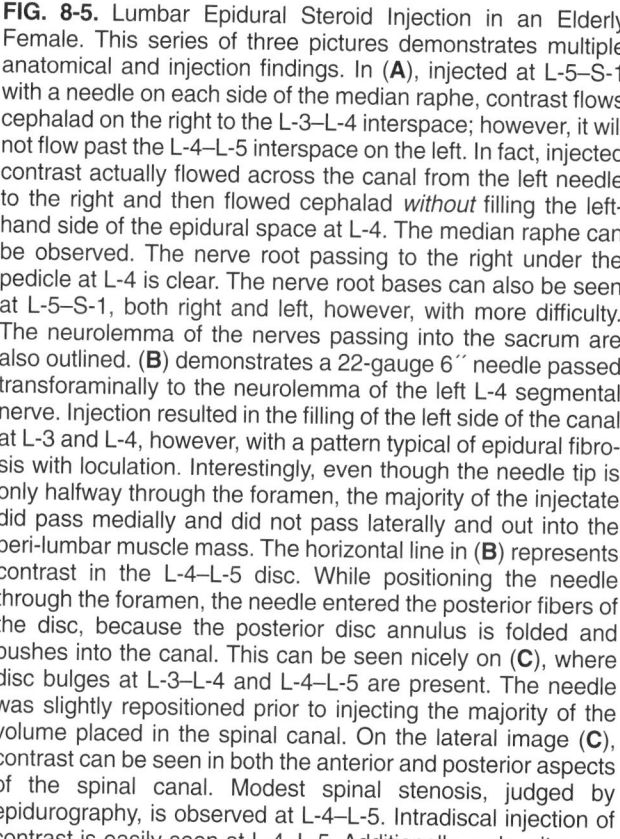

FIG. 8-5. Lumbar Epidural Steroid Injection in an Elderly Female. This series of three pictures demonstrates multiple anatomical and injection findings. In (**A**), injected at L-5–S-1 with a needle on each side of the median raphe, contrast flows cephalad on the right to the L-3–L-4 interspace; however, it will not flow past the L-4–L-5 interspace on the left. In fact, injected contrast actually flowed across the canal from the left needle to the right and then flowed cephalad *without* filling the left-hand side of the epidural space at L-4. The median raphe can be observed. The nerve root passing to the right under the pedicle at L-4 is clear. The nerve root bases can also be seen at L-5–S-1, both right and left, however, with more difficulty. The neurolemma of the nerves passing into the sacrum are also outlined. (**B**) demonstrates a 22-gauge 6″ needle passed transforaminally to the neurolemma of the left L-4 segmental nerve. Injection resulted in the filling of the left side of the canal at L-3 and L-4, however, with a pattern typical of epidural fibrosis with loculation. Interestingly, even though the needle tip is only halfway through the foramen, the majority of the injectate did pass medially and did not pass laterally and out into the peri-lumbar muscle mass. The horizontal line in (**B**) represents contrast in the L-4–L-5 disc. While positioning the needle through the foramen, the needle entered the posterior fibers of the disc, because the posterior disc annulus is folded and pushes into the canal. This can be seen nicely on (**C**), where disc bulges at L-3–L-4 and L-4–L-5 are present. The needle was slightly repositioned prior to injecting the majority of the volume placed in the spinal canal. On the lateral image (**C**), contrast can be seen in both the anterior and posterior aspects of the spinal canal. Modest spinal stenosis, judged by epidurography, is observed at L-4–L-5. Intradiscal injection of contrast is easily seen at L-4–L-5. Additionally, a density con-

C

sistent with a blood vessel full of contrast leading away from the injected disc is also observed. Occasionally these vessels can be large enough that if unobserved, the entire volume of the injectate will be deposited intravascularly and not reach the intended anatomical target. (P = pedicles; S1 & S2 = segmented nerve roots)

with respect to the result of each injection and without fear or hesitation to modify the plan. Three examples:

• If the injection in the first "series of three lumbar ESIs" completely relieves the patient of pain, why do a second injection? Wait and watch.

• If the first and second lumbar ESIs performed a respectful 2 to 3 weeks apart have not been followed by a decrease in the patient's pain, carefully consider the probable value of a third injection. Unless the manner in which the third injection is to be performed

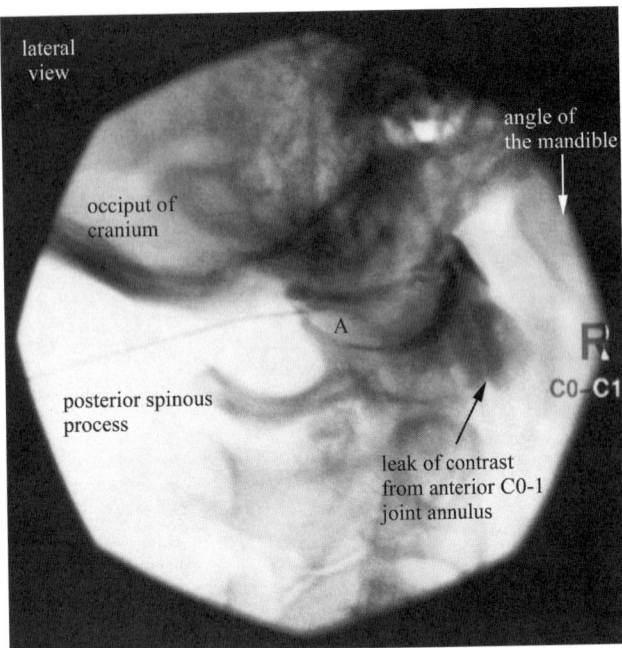

lateral view

occiput of cranium

angle of the mandible

A

R

C0-C1

posterior spinous process

leak of contrast from anterior C0-1 joint annulus

FIG. 8-6. C-0–C-1 Cervical Joint Bursa Injection. When a patient's pain is located in the posterior aspect of the occiput and neck and exacerbated by head motion, upper cervical spine arthritis can be a cause. With care, the cervical bursa/joints of C-0–C-1, (atlanto-occipital joint) and C-1–C-2 (atlantoaxial joint) can be injected with precision. The picture represents 0.15 cc of Isovue 370. Injected posterolaterally to avoid the vertebral artery, the Isovue has flowed around and through the joint, appearing anteriorly in the bursa. (A = annulus of the C0-1 joint)

is different from the first two, the result will probably be identical with the first two. This is the time to be a physician (by reevaluating and revising your plan), not simply a robot on a predetermined course.

- If each ESI seems to build on the results of the previous ESI, achieving a progressively better result, "go for it" and do them all. Consider a fourth injection.

3. Sympathetic blocks are utilized to treat RSDS (Reflex Sympathetic Dystrophy Syndrome), now included in the designation CRPS-I (Complex Regional Pain Syndrome). Often 8 to14, or possibly more, sympathetic blocks (e.g., stellate ganglion injections) may be useful to "break" the sympathetic maintained process. However, this large a series is talked about a lot more than it actually happens. Discussion of the treatment of RSDS is not a goal of this chapter; however, as a general rule the sympathetic blocks should be performed at least three per week, and preferably closer together, depending on symptoms, history, and patient response. The concept is that after about the third sympathetic block, the pain-free interval should be getting longer and longer after each injection. (Adjunctive therapies such as physical therapy are also necessary.) Therefore, although the insurance company may approve a series of 10, if, after the sixth injection, it is obvious clinical

progress is not being achieved, abort! Rethink the process. For example, consider a clinical path toward spinal cord stimulation.

4. All medical care has risks. As an oral examiner told me during my senior surgical exam in medical school, after I had made a modestly snide remark about a surgical complication I had witnessed on the clinical rotation, "Doctor, the only physician who does not have any complications is the physician who does not do anything!" While that admonition is not an excuse, it is a warning and we should all heed it —*daily!* Therapeutic injections and good intentions can cause increased pain and damage. Know it! Pneumothorax may follow intercostal nerve injections. Neuralgia and sympathalgia may follow neurolytic procedures. Weight gain, fluid retention with edema, steroid psychosis, insomnia, and congestive heart failure, to name a few, can occur after a single or repetitive steroid injection.

With respect to therapeutic injections of steroid into an epidural scar, the steroid can seemingly act like a long-lasting local anesthetic and provide 24 to 72 hours of pain relief. This phenomenon has been noted by others and is not simply associated with an intense antiinflammatory effect. If steroid is hydraulically forced into fibrous tissue around lumbosacral nerve roots, bothersome perineal numbness and urinary (and less frequently rectal) incontinence can occur. If and when this happens, cautiously reassure the patient. The problem will usually resolve in 1 to 2 days, and often the patient's pain will be remarkably improved thereafter. Be prepared to be a doctor.

As previously stated, being an excellent physician injectionist in pain medicine is not easy. Be prepared to be diligent, thoughtful, careful, medically appropriate, and make a constant effort to increase your injection skills and knowledge.

The Steroid Test Dose

Many a physician has proudly taken the praise and responsibility for a patient having less pain in the days following a diagnostic or therapeutic injection. However, how can it be known whether the patient's improvement was due to *where* the physician placed the steroid or due to the simple fact the steroid was systemically absorbed and effective (i.e., that the patient received it)? *Simple.* Administer intramuscularly (IM) a similar dose of the same steroid to be used at the time of the therapeutic/diagnostic injection several days before the scheduled injection therapy. Then document the patient's response to that test IM injection. The "risk" is the patient will be so improved from the general systemic effect of the steroid that it will be clinically indicated to cancel the injection therapy. That, however, will give you another kind and level of objective patient information to factor into your evaluation and decision about medical care. Thereafter, academically/

objectively, whatever the patient's response after diagnostic/therapeutic injections utilizing steroid, you will know how much of the response to the precision injection is due to where you put the steroid versus the simple fact that steroid caused a systemic response.

The downside of this test is the "nuisance factor." It may delay the actual diagnostic injection and/or slightly increase the cost of the patient's medical care. Steroids in the doses most injectionists use (e.g., triamcinolone 40 to 120 mg) can cause wakefulness, psychological irritation, slight increase in body temperature, and cutaneous warmth and redness, not unlike a sunburn. Even worse (and mostly in slightly overweight women), steroids can cause fluid retention and markedly increased appetite. Too many times I have heard "I have put on 20 pounds since you started giving me these blocks." Occasionally the patient's response to a steroid dose pack given to them by their family doctor will help you to know the patient's

response to systemically administered steroids without actually having performed an IM test injection, so be sure to ask. However, without this knowledge, errant diagnoses and treatments may be devised.

FLUOROSCOPY

Fluoroscopy is the key to precision diagnostic injections and accurate therapeutic injections. British clinicians were utilizing fluoroscopy for needle placement in the 1970s to perform procedures such as percutaneous cervical cordotomy and gasserian ganglion partial rhizolysis to treat severe pain from cancer and Tic Douloureux, respectively. Hatten (15) discussed lumbar epidurography in *Radiology* in 1980, and Luyendijk (16) studied the "plica mediana dorsalis" (median raphe) (Fig. 8-7) in *Neurology* in 1976. The use of fluoroscopy to "guide injections" grew in popularity slowly throughout the 1980s. An excellent paper by

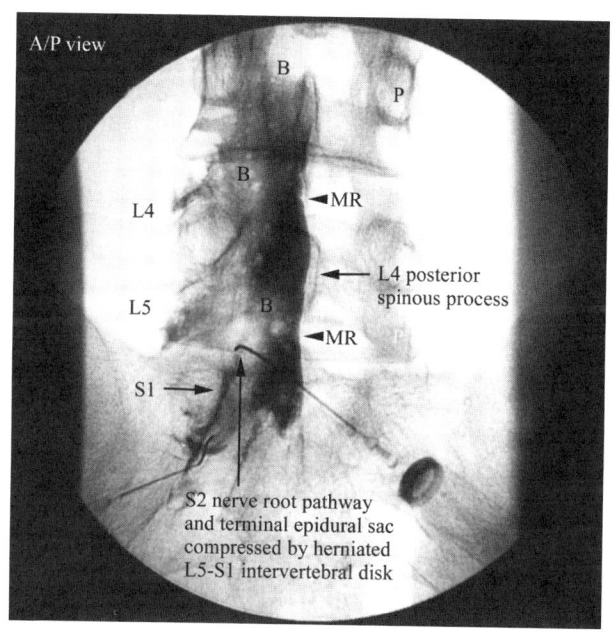

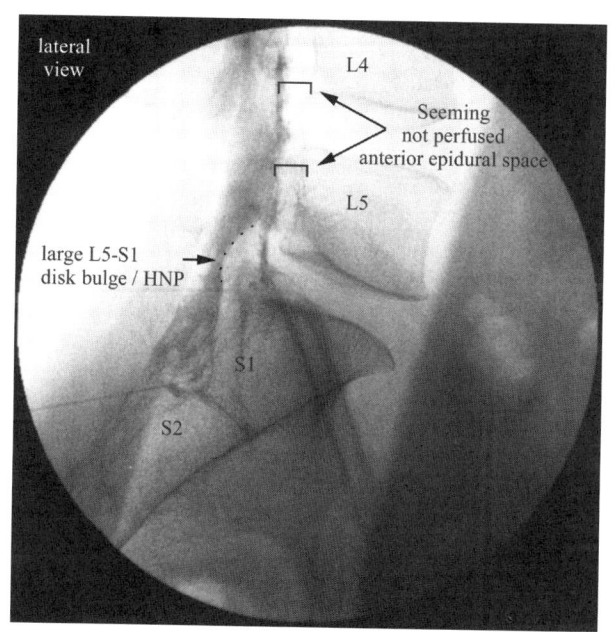

FIG. 8-7. Unilateral Epidural Steroid Injection. The median raphe can be significantly complete in many patients, specifically from the mid-body of S-1 cephalad to the superior endplate of L-4. Cephalad to the L-3–L-4 interspace the raphe usually breaks down and injectate flows across the canal. This A/P fluoroscopic image (**A**) generated by an epidural steroid injection in a 42-year-old gastroenterologist with left low back pain is a good example of the completeness of the raphe. Additionally, the nerve roots of L-4, L-5, and S-1 are nicely demonstrated. Had this procedure been performed "blind" (i.e., without benefit of fluoroscopy), there is a significant chance that the therapeutic steroid would have been confined to the side opposite of this physician-patient's pain. Note the bubbles in the injectate. They are extremely typical and almost a requirement to confirm that the injectate is "epidural." Bubbles are formed by gas coming out of the cool solution injected into the patient's body, then flattened to appear large. On the lateral image (**B**) the patient's L-5–S-1 disc is nicely demonstrated by the displaced contrast, which outlines the bulging annulus seen as a curva-linear density posterior to the L-5–S-1 disc space. The tip of the needle placed into the S-1 foramen can be seen located between the posterior sacral plate and the larger, more dense anterior sacral vertebral segments. Additionally, the lateral view also demonstrates that the majority of the contrast resides in the posterior 50 percent to 65 percent of the vertebral canal posterior to L-4 and L-5. This pattern is frequently seen and is an argument for performing transforaminal epidural steroid injections instead of intra-laminar injection on a regular basis to ensure the posterior aspect of the intervertebral disc annulus and nerve structures in the anterior third of the canal are bathed with a high concentration of steroid. (P = pedicle; B = bubbles; MR = median raphe; L-4, L-5, & S-1 = nerve roots)

El-Khoury (10) was published in *Radiology* in 1988, espousing the advantages of using fluoroscopy for the common lumbar epidural steroid injection performed trans caudally (Fig. 8-8). The use of fluoroscopic-guided injections exploded in popularity throughout the 1990s. Lutz et al. (17) recorded in 1998 the importance of fluoroscopy used in transforaminal lumbar epidural steroid injections (Fig. 8-1). The International Spinal Injection Society (ISIS) was started late in the 1980s to study and teach the use of proper techniques and skills for fluoroscopic guided injections. Since then, many mercenary teaching programs have appeared that, with variable quality, teach spinal anatomy and injection skills using fluoroscopy. Needle companies have produced an ever-widening selection of products such as double needle sets and small bore "Tuohy" (epidural) needles. Radiological equipment companies now offer fluoroscopic C-arms, the one device mandatory to all fluoroscopic-guided procedures, not only with more "bells and whistles" (e.g., picture storage with greater memory, easier image labeling, image printers), but also with markedly improved image clarity and reduced radiation exposure. As of 2000, the AMA CPT Codes and Medicare (HCFA) (18) now recognize fluoroscopy as a valuable skill and mandatory technique and include codes

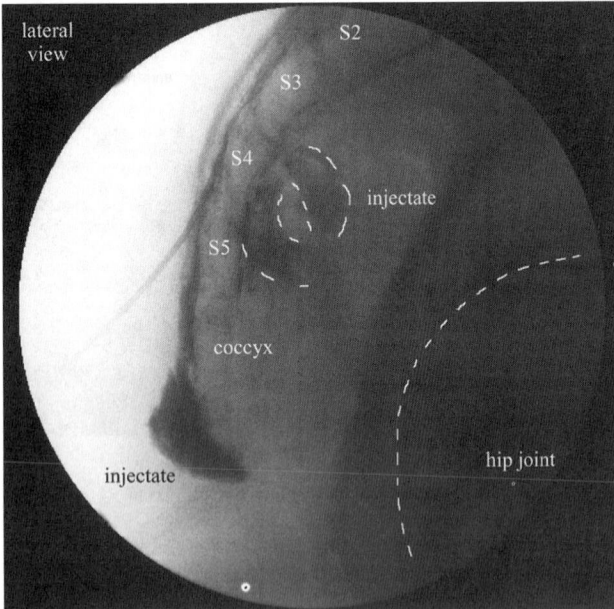

FIG. 8-8. Trans Sacral Caudal Epidural Steroid Injection. Contrast has been injected through the sacral hiatus into the sacral epidural space. Because of incompetent foraminal rings and an open sacral hiatus, contrast has flowed into the pelvis through the S-3 and S-4 foramen, as well as distally out of the sacral hiatus. While some contrast does flow cephalad, resistance to injection builds as the epidural space fills, and more and more contrast will flow through the anterior foramen and sacral hiatus. Therefore, medication intended for the lumbar spine will *not* be delivered there.
POINT: Fluoroscopy and contrast are required for accurate diagnostic and therapeutic injections.

(e.g., Code 76005) that specifically indicate the use of fluoroscopic guidance during injection procedures. Yes, fluoroscopic-guided injections are here to stay (19).

But why? Why spend the money to buy an expensive fluoroscope (Fig. 8-9) (approximately $150,000), employ the support staff and repair services (approximately $30,000 per year), and expose yourself and other staff to radiation while performing injection procedures [e.g., lumbar ESI (Fig. 8-7) and C0-1 (Fig. 8-6) joint injections] when all of the "other physicians" continue to perform (ostensibly) many of these injections in less time and without all "that stuff." Well, you should do so for the following reasons:

1. Fluoroscopy allows the clinician to be able to determine exactly where the needle tip should be placed for the injection and how to get it there. When performing a "simple" low lumbar epidural injection (Figs. 8-7 and 8-5) the lamina can be identified and the needle percutaneously aimed between them and on the side of the patient's pain. When performing a lumbar disc injection (Fig. 8-10) at L-5–S-1 (especially on a person with a high iliac crest), the positioning is a bit more difficult. The needle passes medially to the iliac crest, under the transverse process of L-5, beside the S-1 superior facet process, and in between the L-5–S-1 intervertebral joint endplates. All those structures are at different depths. For ESIs, the ultimate needle depth is still determined most often by loss of resistance. However, the needle tip location is determined by an A/P image, and the depth accurately estimated with a lateral image for both ESIs (Fig. 8-11) and discography (Fig. 8-10). With fluoroscopy the clinician is able to place the needle tip quickly (in fact) and accurately for the easy injections. Fluoroscopy enables him or her to perform procedures not otherwise performable without the ability to "see" the bony anatomy (e.g., in grossly obese patients, injections with small anatomical windows, or selective nerve root blocks and gasserian ganglion injections in any size patient).

2. By injecting contrast, either before injecting the steroid or with it, the clinician can determine where the injectate will flow. Epidurally the injectate may loculate in the spine of an 80-year-old (Fig. 8-12) but will flow smoothly with seemingly minimal resistance in a 40-year-old (Fig. 8-7). *If you do not watch, you cannot know.*

NOTE: The spines of older and less-active people, including paraplegics and quadriplegics, develop what I call *epidural sclerosis* (i.e., fibrous obliteration of the epidural space).

Therefore, to adequately treat the lumbar (T-12–S-1) epidural space (e.g., for the symptoms of spinal stenosis) in the 60-, 70-, or 80-year-old person may require injecting in two to six (or more) spaces, and then perhaps both intralaminarly (Fig. 8-5A) and transforaminally (Fig. 8-5C). This is one reason why the goal of the

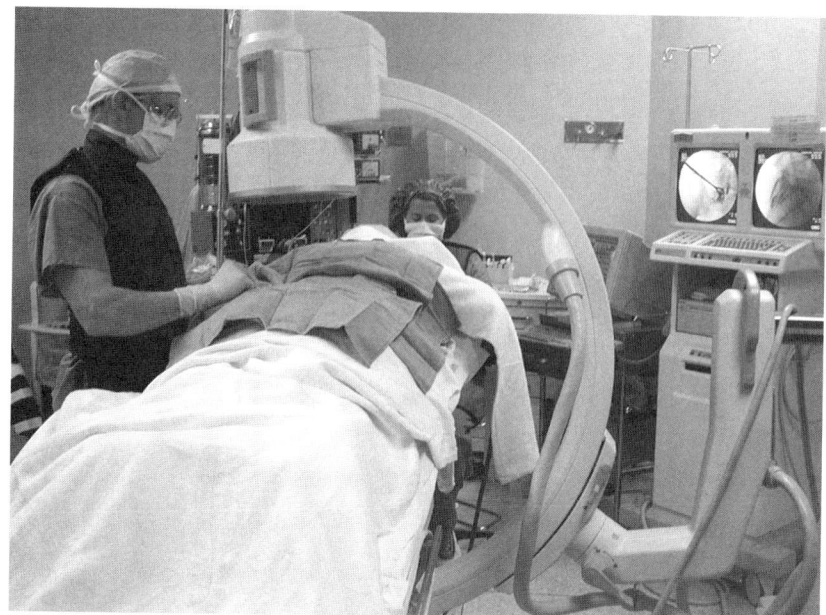

FIG. 8-9. The injectionists' Procedure Room. The chapter's author at work.
NOTE: Procedure rooms can vary significantly from very simple "Fluoro Suites" to complex and cluttered operating rooms. The procedure room pictured is an operating room in an outpatient surgery center. In addition to an appropriate procedure table (cantilevered and without side rails), an adequate C-arm with image storage and reproduction capabilities, support staff, and resuscitative equipment must be readily available.

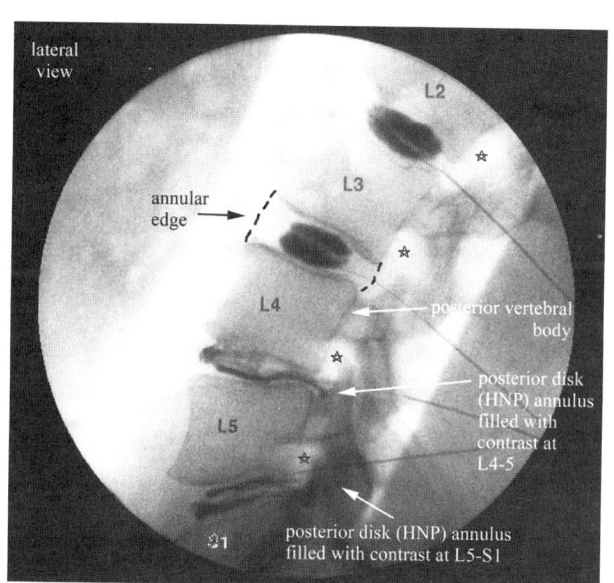

A

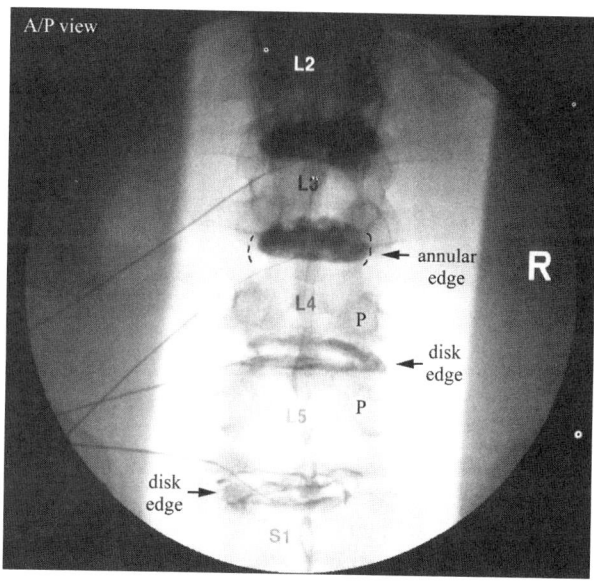

B

FIG. 8-10. Four-Level Lumbar Discogram. In an otherwise healthy 38-year-old, stocky male, this study is performed with a double needle technique (i.e., a 6" 25-gauge injection needle passed through a 3.2" 20-gauge introducer needle). The introducer needle is placed just lateral to the superior articulating facet process of the inferior vertebral body obliquely, aimed at the disc. The 25-gauge needle with the tip bent approximately 15 to 20° is navigated into the central 25% of the disc space. The contrast injected at L-2–L-3 and L-3–L-4, demonstrates a normal round intradiscal pattern and does not touch any aspect of the disc annulus. The disc nucleus is bi-lobed with a light thin bar through the middle. The abnormal discs at L-4–L-5 and L-5–S-1 are degenerated and desiccated. On the A/P view (**B**), contrast can be seen passing to the edge of the disc fibers laterally at L-4–L-5 and to a lesser extent at L-5–S-1. On the lateral image (**A**) contrast can be seen posterior to the posterior aspect of the vertebral body *in* the annulus of the disc which is folded and jutting out into the spinal canal. The disc has lost integrity and volume, bringing the disc endplates closer together. The annular protrusion can be painful due to nerve fibers in the annulus rim (perhaps being literally pinched by the posterior edge of the L-4–L-5 or L-5–S-1 vertebra) and the folded edge can compress on neural tissues. In this discogram pressurization of the L-4–L-5 disc created a very concordant right iliac crest pain while pressurization of the L-5–S-1 disc created concordant posterior low back pain with some right-sided symptomatology. (A = neural foramen; P = pedicles)

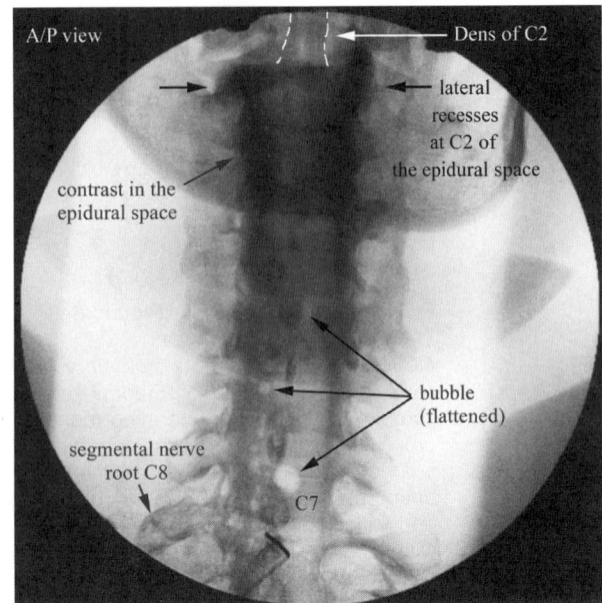

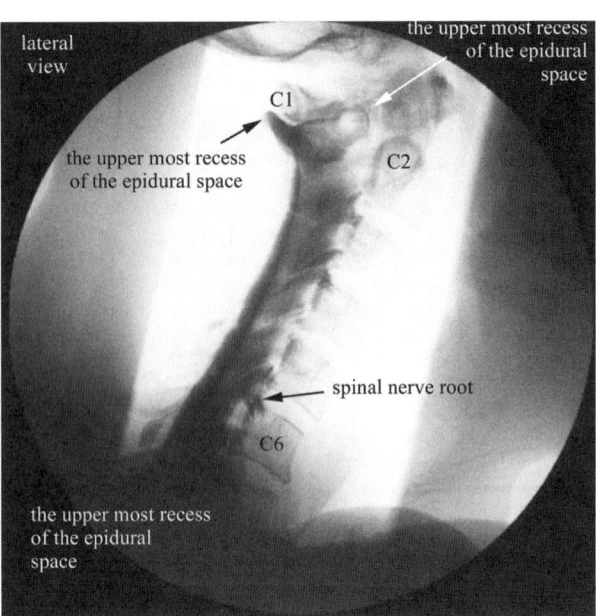

FIG. 8-11. Cervical Epidural Steroid Injection. The cervical epidural space is seen as high as C-1 as the lateral recesses are filled with contrast (**B**). The epidural space often is not "open" this cephalad. Care should be taken when injecting more than 3 to 4 cc of volume epidurally, because if the downward caudal flow of contrast is blocked, sufficient pressure can be exerted on the cord circumferentially to damage it, with the injury occurring at the center of the cord. Obstruction in the epidural space most frequently occurs after cervical spine surgery, especially posterior laminectomies. (C1 = posterior spinous process of C1; C2 = vertebral body of C2 and base of the dens)

injection should be as well defined as possible before the procedure is begun.

As Dr. El-Khoury pointed out, "If the epidural venous plexus is opacified, the needle should be repositioned" (Fig. 8-5C), (10,20). Dr. El-Khoury recognized the vascularity of the intraspinal/peri-spinal anatomy and stated that not infrequently the needle tip can be placed inadvertently into vascular structures (Fig. 8-13). A medication injected intravascularly would not reach the anatomical target. This is at least one explanation for failed "blind" (performed without fluoroscopic guidance) epidural steroid injections. Intravascular injection can occur *any place* except perhaps in the intrathecal space. And the veins in the epidural plexus are valveless. Injection of particulate matter in this venous system could be channeled to the basic vertebral system and the cerebral venous sinus leading to mini-infarcts and central nervous system effects/deficits. Zygapophyseal diarthrodial joints, sympathetic plexus (all of them), intra-articular joint injections (e.g., shoulder, hip, knee, etc.), and atlantoaxial joint (which is not a true zygapophyseal joint) can have venous plexi, and injections can be intravascular. If the targeted anatomical area has been the site of previous surgery (e.g., L-5–S-1 laminectomy and discectomy), the chance of an intravascular injection is greater (e.g., SI joint injection or discogram) than if the patient has not had prior surgery.

Additionally, if the contrast injected simply will not flow to (or into) the target (e.g., into a facet joint), in spite of a well-placed needle, functionally we can assume the joint is fibrosed and perhaps arthrodesed due to arthritis, surgery, or other cause. Spinal epidurography (21,22), mentioned earlier, is an obvious extension of this concept and will be dealt with in greater depth elsewhere.

3. Specifically, with respect to lumbar epidural steroid injections, the needle should be placed on the side of the spine consistent with the patient's symptoms. The "plica mediana dorsalis" or "median raphe" is a membrane (23–25) in the anterior and posterior epidural space that is a barrier to cross-canal flow (Fig. 8-7A) from L-3 caudally, into the sacrum, in approximately 80% of patients, especially patients under 60 years of age. As most discal and spinal canal pathology occurs at L-4–L-5 and L-5–S-1, it seems intuitively obvious it would be important to place the steroid into the epidural space on the same side as the patient's pain, or on both sides if the patient has pain on both sides. (I do not know of any study, peer review or otherwise, that addresses this assumption, however). Injectionists that use fluoroscopy know that contrast (perhaps mixed with steroid) injected through the sacral hiatus often flows out the anterior sacral foramen and into the pelvis (Fig. 8-8), never reaching the lumbar epidural space, especially if a small volume of injectate is utilized.

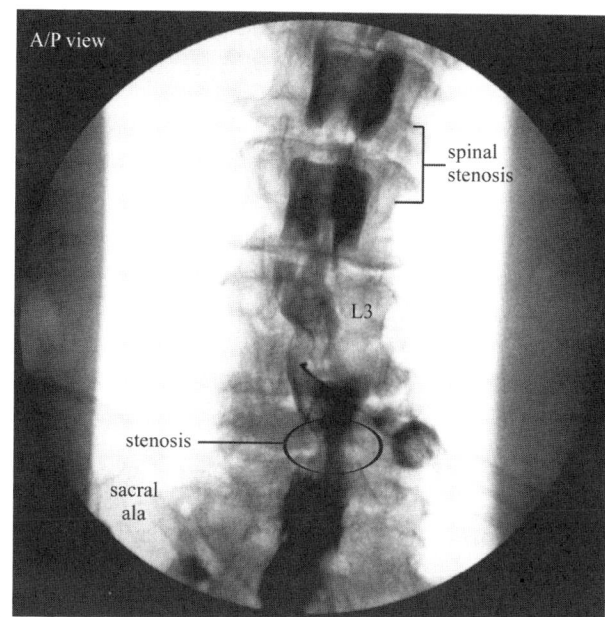

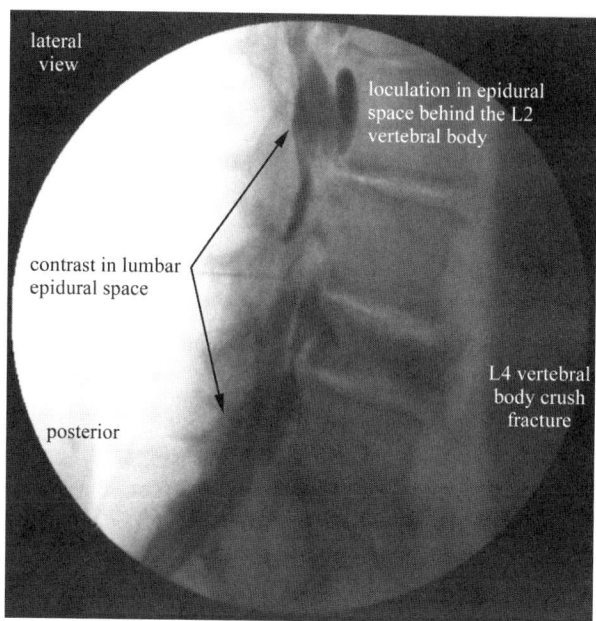

A

B

FIG. 8-12. Pan-Lumbar Epidural Steroid Injection in an Elderly Female. Many believe that placement of steroid in the aged stenotic spine can be quite therapeutic. Note on the lateral image (**B**) the vertebral crush fracture of L-4. The intervertebral disc spaces are shortened, and the disc material is desiccated and striated. These vertebral bodies are probably essentially immobile. The epidural space becomes tight and "sclerotic." Injected contrast loculates and puddles, a phenomenon seen on both the lateral (**B**) and A/P images (**A**). Because the posterior disc annulus is bulged into the canal (in addition to facet hypertrophy posteriorly and thickening of the other spinal ligaments, which cannot be seen on this radiograph), spinal stenosis results and is demonstrated nicely on the A/P image. The patient suffered some discomfort during the injection, however, felt considerably improved within 4 to 5 days after injection of steroid.

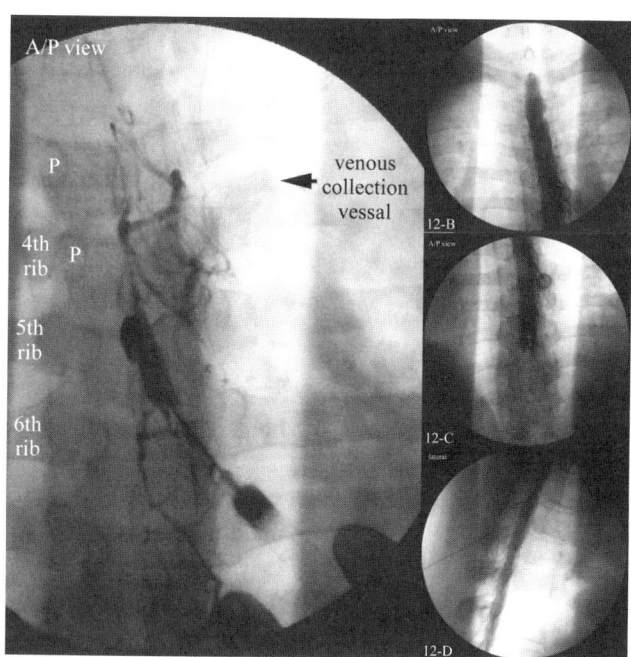

FIG. 8-13. Intra-vascular Injections. While performing a thoracic epidural steroid injection, profound loss of resistance was encountered at a reasonable needle depth considering the location of the injection and the size of the patient. However, injection of contrast resulted in the venogram demonstrated in (**A**). Note that contrast flows only to the right, flows cephalad and caudad, and flows into a larger venous "collection vessel," which is vaguely seen at the tip of the arrow in the right upper quadrant. Subsequently, the 20-gauge Tuohy needle was advanced and solid resistance was quickly reencountered, followed again by profound loss of resistance. Repeat injection of contrast resulted in epidural flow and in the distribution seen in (**B**), (**C**), and (**D**). If this injection had been performed without fluoroscopy, or even with fluoroscopy and without contrast, the injectionist (in this case the author), could not have known of the intravascular needle tip location and would have failed to achieve the thoracic epidural steroid injection intended.

Point: Fluoroscopy and contrast must be utilized to accurately perform diagnostic and therapeutic injections.

Therefore, performing caudal and lumbar epidural steroid injections without fluoroscopic guidance is *"therapy by chance."*

Only because a large number of unknowing referring physicians and unknowing procedural physicians—usually anesthesiologists using anesthesia techniques and experiences—continue to perform lumbar (and cervical) epidural steroid injections without fluoroscopic guidance does it remain an acceptable standard of practice to do so. However, admittedly, the statistical benefits (financial and clinical) of using fluoroscopy, based on a large series of randomly treated patients and reported in peer review journals, have not yet appeared in the literature.

MORE ON THE VALUE OF FLUOROSCOPY

In addition to placing the injectate in the correct location, utilizing fluoroscopy may add a *functional value* to performing injection procedures. Discography (Fig. 8-10), the stressing of one intervertebral disc at a time by pressurizing by injection each disc studied and then analyzing the patient's response to determine if the discomfort created is similar (concordant) to their usual pain, *is* a functional test.

Until the AMA/CPT Guide Book 2000 (18) labeled it as such, epidurography was called "epidural myelography" or "canalography" by many injectionists. In addition to telling the doctor if and when the injectate has reached the targeted location, the pattern of injectate flow may be meaningfully diagnostic. Stewart (26), in 1987, took plain film x-rays after blind caudal epidural injections. Although he appropriately documented various patterns of contrast deposition, he concluded "regrettably we could not demonstrate any prognostic value of epidurography." (One result of the paper was demonstration that 14 percent of the time 30 cc of caudally injected contrast did not reach the lumbar epidural space, either because the medication was not injected in the caudal canal or because it flowed into the pelvis through the anterior sacral foramen (Fig. 8-8).

With a modern fluoroscope, obstruction to epidural contrast flow is easily seen and documents occlusion of the epidural space (Fig. 8-5). On the lateral view, an indentation of the epidural space may correlate with a bulging or herniated disc (Fig. 8-7). A "filling defect" (popular term with injectionists) may coincide with a free disc fragment if the fragment is large enough. The canal anatomy around a level of spondylolisthesis is nicely demonstrated. Luyendijk and Van Voorthuisen (25) previously categorized some of these defects. Additionally, if contrast injected on a segmental nerve root stops abruptly in the foraminal canal, a physical obstruction to flow is suggested. How equivalent is this, if at all, to the root cut-off sign of traditional intrathecal myelography? A distinctive hourglass shape of the intraspinal epidural contrast in an unoperated back surely is consistent with tight spinal stenosis (Fig. 8-12A).

However, what does resistance to contrast flow on one side of the median raphe at L-4 mean in an unoperated back? Some would casually surmise a previous phospholipase A-2 leak has occurred at that level and caused a permanent epidural scar, referred to as fibrosis. Proof is slim. Although several papers have appeared over the last two decades approaching this topic (27,28), in agreement with Stewart's conclusion noted above, epidurography has not been demonstrated to be consistently useful as a diagnostic tool.

A high concentration of contrast is necessary to truly see the details of the epidural space. If the physician chooses to use only enough contrast to determine the needle tip location and grossly demonstrate the extent of contrast flow, detail cannot be appreciated. This is especially true in a large-bodied patient, as the *contrast* (total differential density) of the "contrast" (nonionic water-soluble radiopaque media, such as Isovue or Omnipaque) with the surrounding tissue is reduced and small amounts of the less-concentrated contrast are more difficult, if not impossible, to see. In most body areas, especially the epidural space (any level) and the intercostal space, the injected contrast is rapidly diluted by the interstitial fluids (by hyperosmotic draw and blood flow). Within minutes the differential density perceptibly decreases. Therefore, it is necessary to utilize a state-of-the-art fluoroscope with image-saving capability, and preferably the ability to print permanent pictures/images of the contrast distribution to see, record, and study patterns of contrast injected.

Special Comment: The author abhors the use of the word *dye* for *contrast.* Dye is the color pigment a cobbler uses to modify shoe color or your mother uses to look younger to "wash away the gray." Physician injectionists use a high-grade medical material to modify absorption of x-ray energy in specific anatomical locations. *The Manual of Contrast Media* (28), produced by the American College of Radiology, never once uses the word *dye* as an acceptable synonym for *radiographic contrast.* Are we physician professionals who are supposed to know what we are doing? If the answer is "yes," then we should sound that way when we talk about our work. I implore all who may read these words to be as accomplished with your vocabulary as our radiological colleagues if you expect to receive the same respect as they do when you use the tools developed largely through their specialty. Help yourself and help our new developing specialty to earn respect, appreciation, and understanding of what physician injectionists and pain medicine physicians have to offer in the evaluation and treatment of people (called patients) suffering from pain. It is a simple thing. Refer to *radiographic contrast* by its proper name.

Discography (Fig. 8-10) cannot be performed without fluoroscopy. It is usually considered a skill of the more advanced injectionist. The distribution of contrast within the annulus provides an opportunity not afforded by any other imaging technique, specifically to evaluate the internal anatomical architecture of the disc. Formats such as the Dallas Discogram Score (29) have been developed to record the results of discography verbally. However, the old saying of "a picture is worth a thousand words" is not any less true for discography. Save images, print images, and *include those images with your discogram reports!*

Similar to discography and preserving discogram images, it is *functionally valuable* to save permanent images of all the injections to record the medical event to demonstrate and prove your work. Does your Department of Radiology keep x-ray files and MRI images for several years after the radiologists have interpreted them? Why? Does the general surgeon want the intraoperative cholangiogram films retained after the cholecystectomy? Why? Does the spine surgeon want the intraoperative films that demonstrate his probe is at the correct disc level after the operation is finished? Why? Since it *is* important to be able to demonstrate that the correct interpretation was made of the images and the correct operation performed, if the actual clinical result is not the expected result, or if another medical decision depends on the radiographic interpretation, I believe there is no difference between the above-listed examples of our colleague radiologist, general surgeon, and spine surgeon, and a physician's injections and subsequent interpretations. Weeks and months after the injection procedure, diagnostic or therapeutic, the injectionist should be able to demonstrate exactly where the needle was placed and where the injectate flowed. How else can the results of the injectionist be reinterpreted and substantiated? Why should the dictated results be respected and utilized by other doctors in the multidisciplinary medical care process if injectionists cannot demonstrate the basis of their reports and conclusions? The answer is: the results *cannot* be depended on (to the extent that our brethren specialists substantiate their professional care) without maintenance of proof. Therefore, the injectionist should obtain and maintain good images that record their injection result on every case.

RADIOGRAPHIC CONTRAST MEDIA

That people experience allergic reactions to contrast media is well known. People die every year due to contrast reactions. The fact that greater concern does not generally permeate the medical community when a patient is referred for a contrast study (e.g., myelography or cardiac angiography) is the first indication of the overall safety of utilizing radiographic contrast. Minimal, if any, mention is made of contrast allergies in the references reviewed for this chapter. Why?

According to the American College of Radiology, *Manual on Contrast Media*, 4th edition (28), the incidence of adverse side effects to all intravenous injections with ionic high osmolality contrast media is 5% to 12%, and nonionic contrast media is 1% to 3%. All reactions, from slight flushing to severe anaphylactic reaction and death, are included; however, most reactions are mild. The keys to comparing the diagnostic radiologist's and cardiologist's use of contrast to our use (the injectionist) are:

1. Where the contrast is injected, and therefore the speed of the intravascular appearance.
2. The fact that essentially all contrast used by pain medicine physicians is nonionic, water-soluble media, or should be.

Lesser considerations are:

1. Generally, pain medicine–related injections require a lesser amount of contrast than intravascular studies.
2. A steroid, the first drug of defense used by radiologists to prevent contrast reactions, is almost always included with the pain medicine injectate.

However, with nonionic media used in modest to medium amounts, even in intravascular applications, the recorded incidence is estimated at 0.16 per 1,000 exams. Use of the same drugs in pain medicine studies would logically produce an incidence of reaction rate far less. Contrast reactions usually occur within 20 minutes of injection. Although there are rare delayed reactions that are severe, delayed reactions are usually mild rashes and itching. Delayed reactions are often associated with a patient's other diseases such as arteriosclerotic cardiovascular disease, headache, bronchospastic tendencies, fatigue, etc. Iodine "mumps" (salivary gland swelling) in a syndrome of acute polyarthralgia may occur. Patients treated concurrently or previously with interleukin-2 immunotherapy can develop reactions like those of the drug itself.

The literature documents that most reactions are not true "allergies." Reactions are often multifactorial and related to modifications of substances or medications such as histamine release, compliment activation, and plasma contact system activation (factor XII, prekallikrein, kallikrein, bradykinin). Likewise, acute osmo-toxicity plays a part for intravascular use, however, not for epidural or even intrathecal use. Additives such as calcium-chelating substances or contaminants of latex due to stoppers and syringes can be troublesome. Therefore, the American College of Radiation divides the type of reactions into:

A. Anaphylactoid.
B. Nonanaphylactoid.
   a. Chemotoxic.
   b. Vasovagal.
   c. Idiopathic.
C. Combined.

Vasovagal reactions, or the sudden inappropriate preponderance of vagal (parasympathetic) tone, is common in pain medicine procedures. It seems to occur most frequently in large, young, macho males, less in females, and rarely in the elderly. Early symptoms include sweating and the complaint of feeling hot, becoming apprehensive, feeling nauseated, and developing bradycardia, hypotension, unresponsiveness, and finally loss of bowel and bladder control. This is *not* a contrast allergy reaction. Typically, this neurologically mediated response is easily, rapidly, and effectively treated in 90 seconds by the IV bolus administration of 0.6 mg to 0.8 mg of atropine. Unless the patient is tachycardic and hypertensive, it is better to err on the high side with the first dose of atropine. The use of 0.4 mg of atropine is usually too small a dose to be rapidly and decisively effective, although patient size must be considered. Occasionally a repeat dose is necessary; therefore, do not be surprised and do not wait more than about three circulation times, (e.g., 2 to 4 minutes) to give a second dose to control symptoms.

However, when a patient reports "I'm allergic to dye" and tells you a story to convince you of that fact, what do you do? First, take a careful history and determine the type of preceding events. Remember that a history of other allergies and atopic (skin) reactions increase the likelihood of all allergies and increases the probability of a serious reaction if one does occur. According to the American College of Radiology, the predicted value of specific minor reactions, such as those to shellfish or dairy products, previously thought to be helpful, is now recognized to be similar to other food allergies. A patient with wheezing, hypertension, and lower extremity edema may not be in the best possible condition for an elective contrast reaction challenge. Consider modifying the injectate to minimize the amount of contrast used. The severity and frequency of contrast media reactions are directly related to the amount of contrast load administered. However, a nerve root injection, discogram, or even a simple lumbar epidural steroid injection cannot be performed properly without some, in fact enough, contrast.

Double-check that you and your resuscitative equipment are ready for a contrast reaction emergency. Does your support staff understand the possibility and appropriate reactions?

Preoperative medications recommended to block contrast reactions, including allergies, are:

1. Systemic steroids.
   A. Prednisone 50 mg by mouth, 13 hrs, 7 hrs, and 1 hr before contrast exposure.
   B. Methylprednisilone (Solu-medrol) 120 mg to 250 mg or
   C. Hydrocortisone (Solu-cortef) 100 mg to 200 mg IV, immediately preinjection.
2. An H_1 antihistamine.
   A. Benadryl (diphenhydramine) 25 mg to 50 mg IV.
   B. Atarax (hydroxyzine) 25 mg IV.
   C. Vistaril (hydroxyzine pamoate) 25 mg IV.
   D. Phenergan (promethazine) 25 mg IV.
3. An H_2 antihistamine.
   A. Tagamet (cimetidine) 100 mg to 300 mg IV.
   B. Zantac (ranitidine) 50 mg to 100 mg IV.

The H_2 antihistamines are controversial. Initially included in the prevention program for allergic reactions to the mucoproteolitic enzyme used to dissolve intravertebral discs (chymopapain) (30), its utilization to prevent anaphylactic reactions is not specifically recommended by the American College of Radiology at this time.

If this regimen is utilized, all but the very worst allergic reactions will be blocked. Notably, postoperative continuation of prophylactic medications is not discussed in patients with renal compromise or renal failure. Continuation of prophylaxis postprocedure should at least be considered.

A final consideration is due to the possibility some injectate may be placed into the cerebrospinal fluid (CSF). Certainly only water-soluble, nonionic contrast media should be used in any event. Some contrast preparations are not universally approved for intrathecal use. Standard label Isovue (iopamidol) is not approved while the midrange concentrations of standard Omnipaque (iohexol) (e.g., 180, 240, and 300) are approved for intrathecal use. Isovue has an intrathecal preparation, special label Isovue-M; however, it is a bit more costly.

Interestingly, Bracco Diagnostics, the company that produces and markets Isovue, specifically has stated in writing the standard and intrathecal preparations are chemically *identical*, and the only thing different between the two is the packaging and labeling (personal communication from Bracco via faxed letter).

Other nonionic contrasts are also available. With this information you are encouraged to investigate them for yourself, should you have the need to do so. Most injectionists that I know use either Isovue (standard) or Omnipaque contrast. Some authors propose that, by vascular channels or direct transdural portals, any substance placed in the epidural space can gain access to the intrathecal space. Therefore, although many injectionists have utilized various standard, nonionic contrast media such as Isovue (including the author) for thousands of cases (31), from a legal perspective today (January 2001) the best choice for contrast to be used in and about the spine for diagnostic and therapeutic injections is Omnipaque (iohexol) in the 240 and 300 concentrations.

The total allowable volume of Omnipaque 300 in cerebrospinal fluid is 10 cc, and Isovue-M 200 is 15 cc. Used intravascularly, the allowable volumes of mid-concentration of Omnipaque and Isovue are in the 20 cc to 50 cc range, more than enough to perform pain-related procedures, including epidural lysis of adhesions and larger volume ESIs. Common adverse events after intrathecal injections include convulsions, death, cerebral hemorrhage, and arachnoiditis. It is recommended that the physician read and become familiar with the full package insert of the contrast media that he or she chooses to utilize. Therefore, purposeful injection into the cerebrospinal fluid should be as minimal as needed to achieve the desired result.

Finally, contrast media can have interactions with other drugs. Consideration of those reactions is not within the scope of this text. The reader is referred to the *American College of Radiology Manual* (28) for further information (www.acr.org).

EPIDURAL STEROID INJECTIONS

In this chapter I have already said a lot about epidural steroid injections (ESIs) to demonstrate various points and principles. Because ESIs are such a large percentage of any injectionist's practice, I feel compelled to address this one technique more completely than any other.

1. Whether performing cervical, thoracic, or lumbar ESI, a minimum of sedation and analgesia is necessary. I believe "total sedation" (e.g., propofol anesthesia) is not only ill advised, but also *contraindicated*, especially when injecting above the conus medullaris (the end of the spinal cord at T-12). If the dura is punctured and the needle touches the spinal cord, a mildly sedate patient will complain vigorously. If the patient is anesthetized, the needle may actually enter the cord. If injected, neural damage may be made significantly worse, in fact, catastrophic. (And, malpractice insurance companies are becoming aware of this fact.)

2. By using fluoroscopy to ensure the needle position, there is no need to utilize a local anesthetic in the injectate if the goal is to inject steroid. The development of anesthesia/analgesia postinjection is not necessary to "prove" the medication was placed epidurally. A local anesthetic-induced sympathectomy that results in hypotension and/or extremity weakness, and therefore prolonged recovery room stays, serves no purpose and may frighten the patient.

3. If the injectionist is certain of the target, keep the volume of the injectate small and inject directly on the nerve root or at that spinal level. Remember that, almost always, the injectate flows more cephalad than caudad after an intralaminar ESI. Therefore, an injection at the level of concern may not appear to adequately treat that level. It is generally a good rule of thumb to inject one vertebral space lower. If the exact nerve root utilized is known, consideration should be given to a transforaminal ESI at that level.

4. Unless the ESI is performed transforaminally, often an intralaminar injection appears to flow cephalad posteriorly in the canal. Fibrous septation and metamerically distributed compartments have been described (23). A larger volume of injectate often overcomes the resistance to posterior-anterior canal flow. Below L-3–L-4, added volume is less likely to "push" across the midline, due to the well-formed median raphe (16) (Fig. 8-7A). Therefore, if the patient has bilateral pain and the goal is to treat both sides of the canal, a double-needle technique is advantageous. An epidural needle is intentionally placed on both sides of the median raphe at L-5–S-1 or at L-4–L-5. Then, sufficient volume of contrast, mixed with steroid (and Fentanyl), is utilized to push the injectate to the targeted level.

5. The lumbar epidural space may "hold" a lot of injectate. In one patient, 6 cc will fill three vertebral levels. In the next patient, 12 to 14 cc will barely fill two levels.

And, often the outward size of the individual does not correlate with the size of the epidural space in the low lumbar region. Fluoroscopy allows you to adjust the injectate volume to achieve steroid flow in the canal being injected. Except for a one-sided ESI, or a very targeted one- or two-level ESI, rarely is 10 cc total volume sufficient. *Let fluoroscopy be your guide!*

6. In general, we probably use far more steroid than we need. Eighty mg of triamcinolone over a four-vertebral level is a huge dose. When injecting diabetic patients who have had laminectomies and utilizing Dr. Racz's lysis of adhesions techniques (32,33) (modified), I decrease the triamcinolone dose from 80 mg to 10 or 20 mg, and notice no change in outcome. However, the steroid side effects are markedly reduced. (Only habit keeps me utilizing the larger doses of steroid in nondiabetic patients.) Dose requirement for epidural steroid injection needs to be studied in a disciplined fashion.

WHICH STEROID AND DOSE IS THE BEST

While the FDA has yet to approve the use of deposteroid preparations in the epidural space, the apparent paucity of untoward side effects, in the short and long run following hundreds of thousands (in fact probably millions) of uses worldwide, attests to the safety. No peer review evaluation of various steroid preparations is available.

Three steroids currently popular and equally well accepted are: DepoMedrol (methylprednisolone acetate 40 mg/cc or 80 mg/cc), Aristocort (triamcinolone diacetate 40 mg/cc), and Celestone Soluspan (a 50:50 combination of betamethasone acetate 3 mg/cc and betamethasone sodium phosphate 3 mg/cc). The choice seemingly is based on price, availability, and physician habits. However, the characteristic of eventual/long-term solubility should be considered.

The purpose of a deposteroid preparation is to achieve a long effect, measured in days and weeks. The DepoMedrol preparation never completely dissolves and our spine surgeon colleagues find the "white snow" remaining in the epidural space many months and years after an ESI. Aristocort (triamcinolone), while having a particulate size of about 20 microns, can be initially trapped by most IV filters; however, it seemingly dissolves with time and adequate diluent. However, its pharmacological effect is adequately long to achieve the effect intended for epidural or peripheral applications.

Celestone is soluble in water, and while, arguably, possibly a bit quicker in onset, probably not enough so to give up any significance of action. The preparation called Celestone chronodose has been utilized at the Adelaide Spine Clinic in Adelaide, Australia, for the last 15 years "with no reported ill effects or complications" (34). This is a major safety and support statement for Celestone chronodose used intraspinally. None of the three are "recommended" for intrathecal use. That notwithstanding, most, if not all, busy injectionists have inadvertently injected steroid from time to time into the cerebrospinal fluid (CSF), at least in small amounts. I do not know of any minor or major complications from doing so. To my knowledge most of the academic mavens that I know currently use Aristocort, a fact that may provide some legal defense if such were ever needed. Therefore, for medical, practical, and legal reasons, I recommend the utilization of Triamcinolone or Celestone for deposteroid applications.

The proper dose of deposteroid is also a question with little agreement. Pharmaceutical houses tend to package drugs, if possible, in small vials wherein 1 cc is 20% to 100% of one dose aliquot, or one bottle is a convenient dose size. (For example, 1 cc or 0.4 mg of Narcan is found in a single crack top vial and 1 percent Xylocaine is typically found in a 10 cc to 30 cc vial, be it crack top, pop-off top, or rubber stopper container.) Other sizes are available but not popular. This dose allows us to open a new bottle for each patient. This is good pharmaceutical practice. Where did the dose of 80 mg to 160 mg of DepoMedrol or 40 mg to 80 mg of triamcinolone for injection into the epidural space come from? Simply accepted convention? Nonetheless, these they are. If more than those doses are utilized, the incidence of short-term side effects, such as skin blushing and insomnia (with extra energy), markedly increases. However, when I reduce the therapeutic dose by 50% to 90%, when injecting a patient with diabetes mellitus (because steroid causes a dose-related hyperglycemia), the therapeutic result of the injection is about the same as if a "full dose" of steroid had been utilized. Therefore, while waiting for a published study of deposteroid dose, decide for yourself. But on average, most injectionists, myself included, use much more than our patients need just to make sure we use enough, and it was convenient.

One last note about safety, there are authors (35) who would have us believe that any and all deposteroid preparations and particularly DepoMedrol have "the principle cause of adhesive arachnoiditis in the western world." While quoting multiple, seemingly respectable authors and reasonable text and having significant appropriate facts in her report, in comparison to the massive amount of apparent benefit achieved by the utilization of these drugs when appropriately administered, her case seems grossly overstipulated. However, with such semi-scientific editorial reports in mind, I believe we do have an enhanced responsibility to utilize the minimum amount of drug needed to create the effect desired. Therefore, choosing appropriate doses should not be a thoughtless process.

PLACEBO RESPONSE

The *placebo response* is real, and it can affect the results of any diagnostic injection. Often considered when discussing and performing differential blocks and trials of intraspinal narcotics, the phenomenon also occurs with diagnostic stellate ganglion blockade, selective nerve root blocks, as well as many other diagnostic procedures. Patients who hurt want relief and frequently any reason to feel better for a while will be utilized. Because a "big fuss" has been made to perform the procedure (i.e., plans made days ahead, preoperative lab testing, admission to a facility with a block room, placement of an IV, sterile prep, use of fluoroscopy, the pain from the injection needle—maybe more than once, then special attention after the injection), patients often think, *"Gee, shouldn't I feel better?"* Most patients want to please their doctor and live up to their doctor's hopes and expectations—as well as their own. They know it costs a lot. Additionally, if they do not feel better, then they may have to return and do "all this" over again. Yes, there is a tremendous psychological pressure for the patient from within themselves to create a positive response.

What are some ways to reduce the pressure in order to obtain a more accurate, authentic report? I do these things:

1. Talk about the placebo response from the start. Let the patient know that placebo response is very human and is likely to occur in any of us. Include the description of the response in the description of the procedure. With the informed consent, make the patient aware of the possibility.
2. Take away the *guilt* of a negative response. Let the patient know that he or she is going through the process to find the correct diagnosis and not simply achieve a positive result. "I am not feeling any better" *is* the best response if it is truthful and accurate. Tell the patient and any family members that you and your staff will not be angry with them, and they will not be valued any less as a person, if they do not feel pain relief after your injection.
3. Do all that you can to know that your injection was accurate and that the targeted nerves were treated and "blocked" appropriately. Maybe that means watching the signs of a Horner's response develop. Maybe that means seeing the foot temperature rise from 24°C to 33°C. It could mean measuring an appropriate change in selective tissue conductivity or seeing the patient's tachycardia and mild hypertension resolve. A limp may resolve, especially when the patient is distracted. These changes should occur in a time frame that is reasonable for the medication injected. In short, your observation of the patient can be as important in determining whether a patient's pain resolves meaningfully as what the patient tells you.
4. Family members and significant others often are valuable jurors. They can tell if the mom is faking it, willfully or unwillfully. Again, they also should be taught the concept and importance of the placebo response.
5. If all looks good, the signs of the neural blockade are present, etc., however, the heart rate does not drop, the patient's behavior does not change, and even increases

with testing while the patient says "I am somewhat better," forget it. Do not let yourself be a wishful thinker.

6. Simply repeat the examination. Repeating the diagnostic injection is a little like a prolonged intrathecal infusion. Personally, I believe it is rare that a patient will provide a positive placebo response twice in a row.

If you are unsure if the patient's response is a placebo response, it is not worth pursuing the wrong therapy on a guess. The wrong therapy could simply mean a half dozen therapeutic sympathetic blocks when the patient's pain was really due to a neuroma and the pain is therefore somatic in etiology. An unrecognized placebo response after a selective nerve root block or discogram could mean a discectomy and fusion at the wrong level by your trusting spine surgeon. Perhaps a strange admonition to put in a major pain textbook, but *BE TRUTHFUL!* You will be more trusted and more respected over time if you do not hesitate to use the simple phrases of "I do not know," "I am not sure," and "I made a mistake."

As an aside, remember that a pure sympathetic blockade will reduce somatic pain by 20% to 30%. For example, performing a perfect stellate ganglion block on a patient with a crushed wrist or an upper abdominal sympathectomy after an open cholecystectomy will reduce the patient's pain perception 20% to 30% for the duration of the sympathetic blockade. Therefore, when a patient with chronic foot pain due to a "heister accident," followed by an ORIF of the ankle, with some preblock, quasi signs of sympathetic mediated pain reports a moderate (e.g., 20% to 30%) reduction in pain after a well-performed paravertebral lumbar sympathetic blockade, *do not* believe that pain is sympathetic maintained or even mediated. It is not! Such a "call" is a physician-induced placebo response. Unless or until pain is at least 70% resolved with a "clean" sympathetic block, and only somatic sensation remains, the pain is *not* sympathetic in origin.

HYALURONIDASE

Hyaluronidase is a mucolytic protein that breaks down hyaluronic acid, a component of connective tissue and scar tissue. By doing so, it increases the "spread" of whatever it is mixed with. Hyaluronidase has had many medical applications, including retrobulbar, intraventricular subarachnoid, and peri-subcutaneous infiltration (37,38). One use is to reduce tissue irritation by injection into areas of extravascular infiltration. Another use, popularized by Gabor Racz (32,33), is its inclusion with the injectate when performing the procedure of *percutaneous epidural neuroplasty*, better known as *lysis of lumbar epidural adhesions*, in an attempt to "spread" (39) the steroid into areas around the scar-bound nerve roots. The binding and encapsulating tissue may be due to postlaminectomy epidural fibrosis (surgical scar), the spread of lipophos-

phatase A2 from a ruptured disc annulus, or other inflammatory etiology (40). A dose of hyaluronidase, up to 1,500 units, is recommended. Reconstituted lyophilized hyaluronidase powder is combined with steroid, local anesthetic, hypertonic saline, and contrast (although not necessarily all at one time), and typically placed through a spun wire (Racz Cauda-cath, by Epimed) catheter while it is impaled against the fibrotic tissue in the epidural space of the spinal canal. Hyaluronidase is believed to be more effective about enzymatic activity on pathological tissue than nonpathological tissue. Racz, Heavner, and Raj (32) have demonstrated improved results (reference Interventional Pain Management, 1996), with a reduced failure rate of the lysis procedure from 18% to 6% with hyaluronidase. Adverse reactions of acute hypersensitivity are estimated at less than 1%. These reactions can be treated in the usual fashion with steroids, H_1 and H_2 antihistamines, etc. Although not studied with specific outcome data, this author/injectionist has not had good experience with hyaluronidase as an adjunctive agent (41).

PROCEDURE REPORT

It is extremely important to write/dictate/create an excellent report of the procedure you performed.

This may sound like an inanely simplistic and ridiculous statement to make in a major textbook. However, too often excellent procedure reports are not created even after a well-performed injection.

The reasons to produce an excellent report are as follows:

1. To be able to generate an excellent report, you have to have performed the procedure with excellence. Therefore, knowing the requirements of an excellent report and intending to dictate one, the procedural dictation "pulls" you to do an excellent injection. In other words, knowing that you are going to dictate with excellence, as prerequisite, you must perform the procedure with excellence to be able to do so.

2. After the procedure, the procedural description and the saved fluoroscopic images are what remain. As an analogy, the pictures of the Grand Canyon that are in the photo album and your verbal story are what you have left of a trip there. Because others cannot see into your mind, you need to have taken excellent photographs and have excellent stories. Likewise, you need to dictate excellent reports. As a legal document that memorializes the medical care that you delivered, the value of the procedure, diagnostic or therapeutic, is "held" in the report of it.

NOTE: It may be argued that the value of the procedure is not the report, but the response of the patient over time. Certainly the patient's response the next day and the next week after the procedure is performed is important; however, that response will be recorded in yet another document to be created when the patient is evaluated in your office or the office of the referring physician who ordered the procedure to be performed.

Therefore, for the injection procedure that was performed, the above statement is accurate. Whether the information recorded is utilized to document a successful treatment, to help you or some other (referring) physician decide what medical step to take next (e.g., perform a two-level fusion with anterior and posterior instrumentation), or to provide substantiation for your defense in a courtroom, the recorded data is only what it is at the time you create it. Unlike red wine in a tightly corked bottle, over time it will *not* get better (i.e., more complete, etc.) on its own after you dictate it. Therefore, you *must* do an excellent job in the first place.

3. The report is what other people see of *you!* How many times have you read a letter or paragraph of anything—noting the misspelled words, poor sentence structure, inadequate grammar, missing detail, etc.? Immediately you form an opinion about the writer. If you want respect (and referrals) as a physician injectionist/pain medicine physician, create reports of your work that memorialize procedural excellence, medical analytical observation and thought, and achievement as a communicator.

Writing/dictating an excellent report is work and takes effort. Like most work that you do well, excellent dictation is a developed skill and habit. It takes practice to achieve, and once achieved, it takes continuing effort to perform well. So, how is excellence of dictation accomplished?

1. Before the procedure, delineate as completely as possible what goal you will be achieving by performing the procedure. For instance, are you attempting to determine if a patient's right leg pain is sympathetic mediated? Will a compressed left C-5 painful segmental nerve root respond to steroid injection, or need to be surgically decompressed?
2. Collect and roughly record the basic information needed to achieve the injection's goal (e.g., measure the leg's temperature and evaluate the left upper extremity pain before and after the injection).
3. Record the information in a rigorous style similar to any reputable operative report. Be complete.

The ingredients I include in my procedure notes are the following:

Location

Most injectionists work in several different locations. Usually, if transcription is performed on site, the location of the procedure will be automatic. If it is not, this information must be included in your report.

Title of Report

There are many types of medical reports, from history and physical to discharge summaries. Every medical report needs a title.

Patient Name

This is self-evident. It is excruciatingly important that the information you are about to record is accredited to the proper individual.

Patient Number

Most institutions assign a number to a patient, be it an admission number at an outpatient surgery center, a patient number in a private office, or a medical records number at a hospital. Dictating this number is added ensurance that the report you are about to give will be accredited to the proper individual.

Procedural Physician

That is you, if you are the injectionist/surgeon for the day. *Procedural* is used because on some occasions you may want to be seen as an injectionist only. (Of course, the title *injectionist* could be used instead of procedural.) At other times, if you are performing a "cutting and tying" procedure, such as a spinal cord stimulator implant, you would identify yourself as a *surgeon*.

Day of Week

On occasion, retrospectively, it is valuable to know on what day of the week your procedure was performed. Although this can be determined without too much trouble, if recorded at the time of the procedure performed then there is no question.

Preoperative Impression/Diagnosis

The rational for performing the procedure is considered part of every procedural report. In some instances, what is entered on this line will determine whether an insurance company will pay for the work that you have performed. It is mandatory that you identify, as discretely and distinctly as possible from the information that you have available to you, the impression, if not the diagnosis, that is causing the procedure to be performed. Additionally, it is not only good practice, but in many hospitals and surgery centers it is now required that the procedural physician dictate the ICD-9 code of the impressions/diagnosis justifying and explaining the procedure. The purpose is two-fold: accurate record keeping and unification of billing to maximize reimbursement.

Postoperative Impression/Diagnosis

All reasons as recorded above.

NOTE: If your observations and thought processes during the procedure modify the diagnosis, it is important for the sake of later interpretation to record them accurately.

Operation/Procedure Performed

Delineate each portion of the procedure as carefully and clearly as possible. If the same procedures were repeated at several different levels or both sides, record each level and side distinctly.

> *NOTE:* Follow each procedure part by the appropriate CPT code that delineates the procedure performed. Not only is this good practice to assist your own Billing Department to maximize your reimbursement, it will also help the institution in which you are working, and may be required by that institution.

Interim Report

One to three sentences about the patient that are appropriate to the procedure being performed can be included anywhere among the ingredients discussed, prior to the procedural description. Interim report may include a statement of how the patient responded after a previous procedure if the patient has not been seen in the physician's office since the previous procedure (e.g., between the first and second epidural steroid injections in a series). It may include a note about the patient's physical status (i.e., a BP control) that is a consideration for the current procedure and you would like to have recorded in close proximity to the procedural description. However, if included, this note should be very brief and succinct.

Complications

Procedural dictations should note complications and/or unintended results before delineating the procedural results. An unexpected event that may modify either what was actually done during the procedure or modify interpretation of the results, therefore should be known first. For instance, if the dura was punctured unintentionally, contrast (and steroid) may subsequently appear intrathecally. The fact that a patient's blood pressure rose to 220/120 and the patient began to report chest pain during a caudal lysis of adhesions or selective nerve root injection would explain why the procedure was terminated before completion and subsequently evaluated in the recovery room. If the injectionist miscounted initially and injected at a wrong level, and subsequently corrected the mistake, it should be noted appropriately. Otherwise, "No complications noted at the time of the procedure" is a good statement to make.

Estimated Blood Loss

Although blood loss is usually none or nil, mention of it is one of those items that makes the report complete and gives the report the impression of a bonafide surgical record. Additionally, by including estimated blood loss (EBL) in every report, when it is an important fact to record (i.e., status postimplant of an intrathecal catheter

and creation of subcutaneous pocket for a medication infusion pump), it will not be forgotten.

Medications

1. Medication utilized for skin anesthesia.
2. Medication utilized for injection (e.g., steroid, local anesthetic, narcotic, and contrast).
3. Systemic sedation, kind, and possibly the amount (e.g., Fentanyl and Versed).

It should be obvious that an accurate record of the medication used is mandatory for a complete report of the procedure performed.

Results

1. Results due to operation Part I.
2. Results due to operation Part II.
3. Results due to operation Part III.

While it may seem redundant to list each part of the operation performed, it is important for clarity. This section should also include in addition to the fact that (for example) the epidural space was injected, a brief description of how contrast flowed within the epidural space (e.g., cephalad, caudad, irregularities noted by epidurography). Salient observational comments of the patient's bony anatomy may be appropriate (e.g., "severe osteoarthropathy of the L-5–S-1 facet joint," or "occult spinal bifida of the posterior L-5 lamina").

Procedure Description

The description of the procedure should be relatively temporal (i.e., should flow in a fashion that depicts the order in which the procedural parts were performed). The contents of this section should include considerations such as:

1. The fact that patient consent was obtained.
2. Whether an IV was started.
3. What type of monitoring was utilized.
4. Specification of systemic sedation utilized (if none, state there was none).
5. The position the patient was placed in for performance of the procedure, and whether the patient was placed on a standard operating table or special procedure table, thereby indicating potential limitations of patient position in imaging.
6. The area of the body prepped and medications utilized for the prep.
7. The equipment (e.g., the length, gauge, and type of needles used for injection).
8. Other equipment utilized (e.g., radiofrequency lesion generators and nerve stimulators).
9. Technique utilized to perform the procedure (e.g., loss of resistance, double needle, transdiscal).

10. The approach utilized with the needle (e.g., paravertebral, paramedian, or midline, and the angle of the needle introduced).
11. Observations made with the fluoroscope.
12. Where the contrast flowed that was injected and how that flow was interpreted.
13. Anatomical flow of the injectate.
14. Changes in patient sensorium throughout the procedure.
15. Changes in patient response and behavior, if significant, throughout the procedure.
16. Patient's disposition at the procedure's termination (e.g., taken to the recovery room or observation area).
17. Response to the procedure performed, if appropriate (e.g., development of Horner's Syndrome and resolution of upper extremity pain).

Disposition of Patient/Postprocedure

Although this paragraph does not need to be specifically labeled, how the patient left the facility where the injection was performed and who they left with is important. Did they go on their own, or were they in the company of a responsible adult? Unless recorded elsewhere in the chart, this is a good location to identify special instructions (e.g., patient is instructed to keep a pain diary and follow-up in 2 weeks).

Make a statement as to who interpreted the fluoroscopic images and who takes responsibility for those interpretations. Although this seems intuitively simple, I feel it is important to make the statement so there can be no question. The statement I use is, "I interpreted all the fluoroscopic images and utilized the information for clinical care." If you plan to charge for providing those services, I suggest you do the same or something similar. If you medically guide conscious sedation (CPT code 99161), be sure to record the fact that you did so.

Additionally, if the institution where you are working requires any additional statements, they can be made at this point. For instance, "I certify that the identification of the principle and secondary diagnoses and the procedures performed are accurate and complete to the best of my knowledge."

Signature Line and Below

List the individuals and/or institutions that are to receive a copy of this report in addition to yourself. Typically, this includes the referring physician, if any, and if appropriate. Additionally you may want to list a physician to whom you are going to refer the patient to receive a copy of the procedure report.

Record your work with fluoroscopic images.

Fluoroscopic images should be saved, printed, and considered part of the operative report. If the institution does not keep a copy, then you should keep copies in your office. (I actually keep a copy of each fluoroscopic image saved in the patient's chart in my office, so I can review them when the patient returns for follow-up care.) As discussed in the section on fluoroscopy, as the images can now be printed out on thin and inexpensive Mylar-type paper, this is easy to do and is of immeasurable value.

Whether the procedure is performed in a large hospital or the physician's office, the components of this report should be identical. The report should be dictated as soon as possible after the procedure has been performed and transcribed shortly thereafter. It is a good rule to either dictate immediately after the procedure, or within 24 hours, to be able to preserve detail and accuracy. If specific portions of some procedures are essentially always performed in the same manner (e.g., the radiofrequency lesioning [RFL] cannula placement, stimulation testing, injection of local anesthetic and steroid, and heating of the RFL needles for lumbar facet denervation), those sections may be standardized and used from dictation to dictation. However, each report should accurately reflect the actual procedure performed and be unique to the patient treated. Therefore, in most instances, in addition to the name and date, there will be something clinically different about each report generated. And, of course, each report should be, in total, truthful.

The procedure reports are a golden opportunity to demonstrate to others the quality of your work. Do not fail to take advantage of this opportunity.

INFORMED CONSENT

The doctrine of informed consent was substantially established by a California court in 1957 (42). Today, the principles of informed consent include:

1. Patients are generally persons unlearned in the medical sciences, and therefore except in rare cases, courts may safely assume the knowledge of the patient and physician are not in parity.
2. An adult who is competent has the right to exercise control over what medical treatments are personally rendered.
3. To be effective, a patient's consent to treatment must be an informed consent.
4. The patient has an abject dependence on and trust in the physician for the information that is relied on during the decision-making process.

As clear as these four principles seem to be, it is not always easy to determine how much a reasonable person needs to know to make an informed decision. Therefore, all reasonable risks and the nature of the process and procedure should be reviewed until the patient can reasonably understand and expresses that understanding. The five elements generally deemed necessary to achieve an informed consent include:

1. The nature and purpose of the proposed treatment.
2. The expected outcome and likelihood of success.
3. The material risks.
4. The alternatives and supporting information regarding those alternatives.
5. The effect of no treatment, including the effect on the prognosis and the material risks associated with no treatment.

In pain medicine, especially with respect to injections for diagnosis, many patients have trouble understanding that a procedure is not being performed to help them, however, primarily to make a diagnosis to be able to know how to help them. All guarantees should be avoided; however, reasonable assurances, when truthful and appropriate, are certainly permitted. An area commonly overlooked is the result of not undergoing the procedure suggested, specifically the consequence of not doing so. A physician should always remember the first item in a list of possible therapeutic options is to "do nothing." A patient may choose that option.

Finally, idealistically, the legal instrument that documents informed consent should itemize the following:

1. What information was given to the patient.
2. Whether anyone else was present during that discussion.
3. That an opportunity was given to the patient to ask questions.
4. The indication of understanding by the patient.
5. The amount of time spent discussing the proposed treatment with the patient.
6. Whether any materials were used in providing the information, such as videos, anatomical drawings, or reading materials.
7. Whether further discussions with the patient seem warranted before a decision is to be made.

In a busy medical practice complete informed consent is difficult to achieve, if only because it is so time consuming if done in a single encounter. Therefore, the process is best started with the first patient encounter. Begin early to build the patient/physician, patient/practice trust. Involve your staff, who the patient often understands a lot better than the doctor, to discuss the issues involved. Document when teaching materials are utilized in the office or in the procedural facility holding area and the level of understanding that the patient demonstrates. Always ask if the patient has any additional questions and then ask the patient to make and remake the decision to proceed. Utilize an appropriate witness, a person unemployed by you or your practice, and preferably a family member, who can attest to:

1. The legality and authenticity of the consent.
2. The patient's capacity to give consent at that time.
3. The fact that consent is being given freely, voluntarily, and without coercion.
4. A reasonable belief that the patient has been informed.

Write the procedural description in terms that are easily understood by the patient. Often this is best done in addition to utilizing the most accurate and complete medical jargon. For instance, a medical description may read: "diagnostic bilateral C4-5 and C5-6 facet joint injection with local anesthetic and steroid, and utilizing fluoroscopic guidance." In common terms for the patient the procedure may be expressed as "While I am fully awake, by x-ray guidance, place a thin needle through anesthetized skin at two places on both sides in the back of my neck to numb four small joints and fill them with steroid. I will need to hold very still. All my questions about this procedure have been answered" (42).

In addition to the legal value inherent in achieving and obtaining good and adequate informed consent is the clinical value generated. An informed consent should be seen as a process, not as an event. The patient/physician, patient/practice relationship grows by performing the very steps needed to obtain an informed consent. If the patient is regularly seen in your office, document the steps of teaching, explaining, answering questions, discussing alternatives and expected results—visit by visit—in your patient's chart. However, if you meet the patient for the first time, after they have been undressed, lying on the stretcher, with their IV started, often cold in the outpatient surgery center holding area, the process must be compressed in time, however, not slighted because of the situation. Knowledgeable staff who can discuss the procedure with the patient, describing the details and expected results in an unhurried fashion, are extremely important. However, you, the visiting physician, as stated previously in this chapter, must take the time to stop, have a few minutes of intense person-to-person contact, and ask if the patient has any further questions for you. Then give the patient the opportunity to express the fact he or she would like to proceed with the injection.

Patients can feel respect. They know when you and your practice staff are honestly interested in them as a person. In addition to the steps listed above, if that feeling is projected to the patient, trust and consent will come naturally. You must then document the patient's permission.

CLOSING

Injection for diagnosis and therapy in a chronic pain patient is a demanding discipline that cannot be treated lightly. Knowing that many texts are available to instruct a curious and learning physician how to perform specific injection procedures, I attempted to address those topics less commonly covered. Remember that in addition to being knowledgeable and technically skilled, a real determinate of the success of an injectionist is treating patients like sensitive, needy, hurting human beings and not just another number (i.e., acting as a thoughtful, caring physician and not just a technician). Not only will you be financially and clinically successful with a multitude of appreciative patients and staff, but you will like yourself better also.

REFERENCES

1. Waldman SD. *Atlas of interventional pain management*. Philadelphia: WB Saunders, 1998.
2. Waldman SD. *Atlas of pain management injection techniques*. Philadelphia: WB Saunders, 2000.
3. Brown DL. *Atlas of regional anesthesia*. Philadelphia: WB Saunders, 1992.
4. Katz J, Renck H. *Handbook of thoraco-abdominal nerve block*. Orlando: Grune & Stratton, Inc., 1987.
5. Waldman SD. *Interventional pain management*. Philadelphia: WB Saunders, 2001.
6. Raj PP. *Practical management of pain*. St. Louis: Mosby, Inc., 2000.
7. Lennard TA. *Physiatric procedures in clinical practice*. Philadelphia: Hanley & Belfus, Inc., 1995.
8. Moore DC. *Regional block*. Springfield: Charles C. Thomas Publisher, 1973.
9. Doherty M, Hazleman BL, Hutton CW, et al. *Rheumatology examination and injection techniques*. Philadelphia: WB Saunders, 1993.
10. El-Khoury GY, Ehara S, Weinstein JN, et al. Epidural steroid injection: a procedure ideally performed with fluoroscopic control. *Radiology*, July–Sept 1988;168:554–557.
11. Derby RD, Bogduk N, et al. Precision percutaneous blocking procedures for localizing spinal pain. *Pain Digest* 1993;3:89–100.
12. Broadman, LM. The style and efficacious use of portable C-Arm equipment to facilitate pain clinic block placements. *Epimed Int* December, 1998. Available at: http://www.epimedint.com/articles/dec_article.html.
13. Longmire D, 13150 Hwy. 43 S.E., Suite 4, Russellville, AL 35653 (personal communication)
14. Welcome to the World of EMGs. Available at: http://www.semg.org/intro.htm.
15. Hatten, HPJ. Lumbar epidurography, *Radiology* 1980.
16. Luyendijk W. The plica mediana dorsalis of the dura mater and its relation to lumbar peridurography (candography). *Neuroradiology* 1976;11:147–149.
17. Lutz GE, Vijay BV, Wisneski RJ. Fluoroscopic transforaminal lumbar epidural steroids: an outcome study. *Arch Phys Med Rehabil* 1998;79:1362–1366.
18. Kirschner CG, Anderson, CA, Beebe M, et al. *Current Procedural Terminology CPT 2001*, Prof. ed., 4th ed., 22 rev. Chicago: AMA, 2000.
19. Dreyfuss F. Epidural steroid injections. A procedure ideally performed under fluoroscopic control and with contrast media. *International Spinal Injection Society Newsletter* 1993;1(5).
20. Renfrew DL. Correct placement of epidural steroid injections: fluoroscopic guidance and contrast administration. *Am J Neuro,* 1991;12:1003–1007.
21. Hatten HP Jr. Lumbar epidurography with metrizamide. *Radiology* 1980;137:129–136.
22. Roberson GH, Hatten HP Jr, Hesselink JH. Epidurography: selective catheter technique and review of 53 cases. *Am Roentgen Ray Society* Jan–June 1979;132:787–793.
23. Bloomberg R. The dorsomedian connective tissue found in the lumbar epidural space in humans. *Anesthesia & Analgesia* 1986;65:747–752.
24. Hogan GM. Lumbar epidural anatomy: A new look by cryomicrotome section. *Anesthesiology* 1991;75:767–775.
25. Luyendijk W, VanVoorthuisen AE. Contrast examination of the spinal epidural space. *Acta Radiol [Diagn] (Stockh)* 1966;5:1061–1066.
26. Stewart HD, Quinnell RC, Dann N. Epidurography in the management of sciatica. *Br J Rheum,* 1987;26:424–429.
27. Mattew N, Songer WR, Carson EW, et al. Analysis of peridural scar formation and its prevention after lumbar laminotomy and discectomy in dogs. *Spine* 1995;20(5):571–580.
28. [Multiple Authors] *Manual on Contrast Media*, 4th ed. *Am Coll Radio* 1998;
29. Sachs BL, Vanharanta H, Spivey MA, et al. Dallas discogram description. A new classification of CT/discography in low back disorders. *Spine* 1987;12:287–294.
30. Micromedex, Inc. 2000, Healthcare Series Vol. 106, reference to Chymopapain. Available at: http://memmicro/mdxcgi/display.exe.
31. Gupta RC, Gupta SC, Dubey RK. An experimental study of different contrast media in the epidural space. *Spine* 1984;9(1):778–781.
32. Heaver JE, Racz, et al. Percutaneous epidural neuroplasty. *Regional Anesthesia and Pain Medicine* 1999;24(3):202–207.
33. Racz GB, et al. Lysis of epidural adhesions utilizing the epidural approach. In: Waldman SD, Winnie AP, eds. *Interventional pain management text*. Philadelphia: W.B. Saunders Company, 1996:339–351.
34. Available at: http://www.spine.com.au/epidural-injection.htm.
35. Smith, S. Available at: http://www.backtalk.mildram.co.uk/arach.htm.
36. Gourie-Devi M, Satish P. Hyaluronidase as an adjuvant in the treatment of cranial arachnoiditis (hydrocephalus and optochiasmatic arachnoiditis) complicating tuberculous meningitis. *Acta Neurol Scandinav,* 1980;62:368–381.
37. Hyaluronidase protocol, Children's Hospital of Los Angeles. Young & Mongum, Neo Fax 55.
38. Zank,K.E. Treating IV Extravasations with Hyaluronidase, *ASHP Signal* 1986;10:25–29.
39. Borg PA, Krijnen HJ. Hyaluronidase in the management of pain due to post-laminectomy scar tissue. *Pain* Aug. 1994;58(2):273–276.
40. Payne JN, Rupp NH. The use of hyaluronidase in caudal block anesthesia. *Anesthesilology,* 1951;12:164–172.
41. Fibuch EE. Editorial, percutaneous epidural neuroplasty: cutting edge or potentially harmful management? *Regional Anesthesia and Pain Medicine* May–June 1999;24(3):198–201.
42. Raj PP. Organization and Function of the Nerve Block Facility. In: *Practical management of pain,* 3rd ed. St. Louis: Mosby, Inc., 2000:552–553.

SECTION III

Therapeutic Modalities

CHAPTER 9

Manipulative Therapy in the Management of Pain

John J. Triano

Nociceptive pain of mechanical origin, initially, is a response to tissue failure, or pending failure, under loading conditions. For joint pain, the causative mechanisms are linked to local stress concentration from extremes or repeated positions and loads. Inflammation may occur if stress is sufficiently intense. Manipulative therapy (MT) uses controlled forces and moments to change the behavior of joint structures with the intent of altering local stress distribution. Activity restrictions, staged reactivation with exercise, and lifestyle modifications are introduced to encourage repair and rehabilitate normal function.

Manipulation is recommended, or is an option, for a number of disorders, including acute and chronic low back pain (1,2), radicular pain (1,3), neck pain (4–6), and some types of headache (7). In practice, manipulation also is used in the management of extremity joint disorders (8–10) for complaints such as carpal tunnel syndrome, scapholunate dysfunction, and shoulder, ankle, knee, and hip pain. Historically, claims have been made for manipulation in various other complaints; however, only in the case of infantile colic has there been any reasonable scientific evidence. This chapter will review the evidence of pain relief from the use of manipulation therapy, particularly for the spine, and discuss its theoretical basis.

MANIPULATION AS PLACEBO

Discourse on manipulation usually raises the question of placebo effect. A frequent observation is that chiropractic patients are more satisfied by their treatment experience than when they are attended by other providers (11,12). A number of elements contribute to this popular contentment, including physician–patient interaction. MT often requires several encounters involving physical contact and direct physician attention over a focused time interval. Can these factors be responsible for the perceived clinical benefits?

At least two controlled clinical trials have addressed the question of placebo effect directly (13,14). Using a stratified design, Hadler, Curtis, and Gillings (13) compared two forms of MT: high-velocity, low-amplitude thrusting procedures versus mobilization techniques. A single treatment intervention was administered randomly to patients suffering from acute low back pain. Patients were assessed by one physician and treated by the other. Physicians gave their time to both groups equally and included back educational material and assurance. Triano and colleagues (14) studied treatment effects for patients with low back pain persisting longer than 7 weeks. Subjects were randomly assigned to back education program; high-velocity, low-amplitude (HVLA) manipulation; and sham/mimic treatment procedure groups for a series of ten treatment sessions. Sessions were scripted to balance for physical contact, attention, intervention frequency, and duration. Sessions involved a consistent time commitment and direct one-on-one attention from the physician either in the form of teaching about spine anatomy and function or in assessment and delivery of the sham/HVLA procedures. In both studies, all treatment groups showed improvement over time. However, the patients receiving thrusting procedures demonstrated significantly greater and more rapid rates of improvement from their symptoms and in their ability to function.

These results suggest that physician attention, in any form, appears to benefit patients with back pain. The data also show that, at least for thrusting techniques of manipulation, there is a treatment-specific advantage beyond the nonspecific effects. Attributing patient response and satisfaction from health care encounters with MT to placebo alone is unjustifiable based on the clinical data.

THE LESION

Manipulation is used as a means to treat a functional joint abnormality believed responsible for symptoms. The term generally used to describe the lesion is *joint dysfunction.* Complaints in the spine may be referred to as functional spinal lesions (FSLs) or subluxations. Conceptually, the mechanical behaviors of the affected motion segments have reduced load-bearing capacity and flexibility. Local stress concentrations increase, resulting in symptoms. With the lingering controversy over MT, particularly of the spine, it is somewhat surprising that there is not more information about the lesion and its pathomechanics. The art of diagnosing the FSL is, in many ways, analogous to that for diabetes mellitus research in the early 20th century. Clinicians understand the presentation of symptoms needing treatment, but final confirmation relies on response from a trial of therapy. More recently, a new, evidence-based theory has emerged (15). It is compatible with the variable nature of clinical presentations of patients who seem to benefit from manipulation. The evidence derives from biomechanical data on the behavior of spinal and wrist structures from both *in vitro* and *in vivo* studies.

FSLs may exist as isolated disorders, solely accountable for the patient's complaints. They may also be subcomponents of other pathoanatomical conditions that contribute to the symptomatic picture. Table 9-1 lists common disorders found as a part of the clinical presentation among patients who may benefit from MT. Several of these, including degenerative disease and disc abnormalities observed on imaging, are known to be painful under some circumstances and pain free in others. The confluence and overlap of the conditions, at times, may mask the identity of the actual pain-generating mechanism. As a result, chiropractic use of traditional diagnosis achieves a different purpose than in the standard medical model. Diagnosis serves not so much to drive the treatment plan, but to iden-

tify the lesion site and provide an understanding of the clinical characteristics of the patient presentation that may limit or require modification to therapy. A skilled physician, in his or her administration of procedures, can accommodate age-related and pathoanatomical complications to provide maximum therapeutic benefit where treatment is indicated.

The FSL is a disturbance in joint function of the functional spinal unit (FSU) that is conformable to specific forces and moments appropriately applied. FSU buckling, a biomechanically demonstrable phenomenon, may be the link among clinical observations, biomechanical events, and biochemical events associated with pain. In its simplest form, buckling behavior represents a local, uncontrolled mechanical response to a joint load. When a constituent tissue of the joint may become stressed beyond its injury threshold, the symptoms that result depend on the tissue that has been affected.

Buckling behavior was first observed by Wilder (16) for cardinal planes of motion in individual motion segments. Similar performance has been observed over the entire lumbar region (17). Under biomechanical loading of an FSU at the balance point, disproportionate intersegmental displacements may occur for normal, incremental physiological loads or tasks (17–19). Analogous biomechanics have been observed in the wrist with "zigzag" collapse (20–23) of the carpal articulations under joint compression. Both the wrist and the vertebral motion segment are examples of multimuscular, biarticular joints that rely, in part, on small intersegmental muscles or ligaments for functional integrity. Ill-timed or insufficient muscle activation may leave the joint unguarded and susceptible to sudden, local, disproportionate displacement and tissue strain.

Conditions that potentiate buckling include prolonged static posture perturbed by an incremental load, rapid loads approximating 500 lb/sec, and vibration (16,24–26). Disc damage may decrease the buckling threshold and result in maximum displacement under lower total loads (17). Cholewicki and McGill (27) observed painful buckling in a young subject during fluoroscopic monitoring of spine kinematics of heavy weight lifting effort. Symptoms are produced based on how the peak forces and moments are distributed intrasegmentally and where injury threshold is reached.

TYPES OF MANIPULATION

Effective manipulation uses controlled forces and moments seeking to change the functional lesion behavior (28–32). Treatment is intended to alter tissues' stress distribution and relieve symptoms. The ability to sustain beneficial effects depends on the extent of tissue damage and the residual capacity to accommodate and repair. Skilled manipulation may result in complex procedures to achieve clinical effectiveness under a wide variety of circumstances (33).

TABLE 9-1. *Common disorders that may coexist with functional spinal lesions (FSLs) and that may benefit from manipulative therapy*

Costovertebral joint syndrome
Carpal tunnel syndrome
Degenerative spondylosis
Disc bulge/protrusion/herniation
Instability
Facet syndrome/arthrosis
Radiculopathy
Sprain/strain
Stenosis
Synovitis/capsulitis
Whiplash-associated disorder

Curtis and colleagues (34) attempted to train family practice physicians to perform manipulative techniques using a continuing medical education format. While participants gained additional confidence in working with back pain patients and interacting with local chiropractors (35), they were unable to improve patient outcomes with the level of skill they had developed. Earlier work reported by Cohen and colleagues (36) demonstrated that even professionals familiar, but unpracticed, in a procedure were no better than novice manipulators in their performance. The evidence thus far suggests that skill development requires apprenticeship and consistent practice for maximum skill and safety. To be effective, the physician must be adept in control strategies. Patients display different attitudes and fears that can influence their muscular tension and spinal stiffness (37) in response to manipulative efforts. Underlying or coexisting pathology and a variety of patient statures must be accommodated. Ability to match provider load amplitudes, direction, speed, and procedure type to patient need requires significant experience and practice (33,38,39).

Various systems of manipulation have been developed for both the spine and peripheral joints (40,41). Procedure classification is simplified, and becomes more descriptive, when they are grouped according to biomechanical characteristics (33,39) (Table 9-2). Procedures fall into three basic categories: those that are performed with manual, mechanical, or mechanically assisted methods. Manual methods generally consist of regular, periodic oscillations defined under the term *mobilization* or using high-velocity, low-amplitude (HVLA) thrusting procedures. Mobilization is performed at slow speeds, cycling at 0.5 to 2.0 Hz with low-amplitude forces at approximately 150 N. HVLA, on the other hand, uses a single transient load and reaching peak magnitudes in 80 to 150 msec. HVLA amplitudes commonly range upward to several hundred Newtons force depending on the joint conditions to be treated. Mechanical procedures involve mechanisms to independently move the body segments through specified ranges of motion at prescribed speeds. Originally developed by Salter (42) for postoperative knee rehabilitation, continuous passive motion (CPM) imposes joint loads and displacements as a function of the acceleration of body segment mass. Like mobilization, motion is cyclical at frequencies that can range from being much lower to equivalent with manual methods. Mechanically assisted methods combine manual and mechanical means. Combining CPM with HVLA provides wide flexibility that algebraically sums the inertial joint loading from the CPM with impulse loads. Combinations can be made that provide excellent control of load vector amplitude and direction in both the forces and moments that are transmitted through the target joint (33,39). Impulse hammers are another form of mechanically assisted method (43,44). They hold the advantage of permitting the physician to effect the highest degree of control on applied force direction while eliminating applied moments. These instruments provide the shortest duration of load (< 20 msec) at peak forces comparable to the lower limits of manually applied HVLA (15). Together, these techniques allow for wide versatility in matching treatment method to patient needs.

THE EVIDENCE

Manipulative therapy has been the subject of over 50 clinical trials, several metaanalyses, and formal consensus conferences. Most reports have focused on the more common forms of HVLA procedures. They have been contrasted

TABLE 9-2. *Classification of manipulative procedures may be arranged according to biomechanical characteristics*

Loading mode	Classification	Characteristic
Manual		
	Mobilization	Cyclic, low-speed (0.5–2.0 Hz), low-force (~150 N), insignificant relative intersegmental displacements, complex load vectors (sagittal, frontal, axial) possible.
	High-velocity, low-amplitude (HVLA) manipulation	Single, high-speed (4.0–6.0 Hz), high-impulse loads (<560 N, <84 Nm), significant relative intersegmental displacements (linear and angular), complex load vectors (sagittal, frontal, axial) possible.
Mechanical		
	Continuous passive motion (CPM)	Cyclic, very low speed (0.0+ –0.5 Hz), low-load (<20% BW*, <5% BMI**), large multisegmental displacements (angular), complex load vectors (sagittal, frontal, axial) possible.
Mechanically assisted		
	CPM + HVLA	CPM augmented HVLA
	Impulse hammers	Single, short-duration impulse (~50 Hz); low force (<150 N), significant intersegmental displacements (linear and angular), uniaxial load vectors.

*BW = body weight
** BMI = body mass index
(From 15, 37, 43, 81, 97–108.)

TABLE 9-3. *Clinical effect sizes defined in terms of percent clinical change. According to Cohen (45), a minimum effect size of clinical value is 0.4*

Effect size (ES)	Mean change in pain Scores
Small (0.2)	~5%
Medium (0.5)	~10%
Large (0.8)	~15%

against watchful waiting, sham manipulation procedures, education programs, mobilization, detuned ultrasound, diathermy, physical therapy, medication, and exercise. Comparisons have held up well, generally favoring manipulation. In like manner, a number of different outcomes have been used that include immediate, short-term, and long-term pain relief; activities of daily living; and work time loss. The differences in research formats in connection with clinical studies and the difficulty caused in comparing results from among them are well known. Effect size (ES) (45,46) has been used as a tool to give quantitative values that can be contrasted between studies. For the purpose of simplifying review of the literature, ES as calculated by Bronfort (46) for main outcomes are used here where adequate information is available from the original studies. Table 9-3 provides the definitions for effect sizes with respect to clinically important changes. In its simplest form, effect size is given by the equation:

$$ES = (X_b - X_a) / (Weighted\ SD)$$

The value X_b represents the mean value of the outcome measure for the manipulation group and X_a is the value for the contrasting therapy. The difference between them is divided by the weighted standard deviation (SD), representing both groups and their individual SDs, which typically are unequal. Effect sizes greater than 0.3 represent clinically important differences (45,46).

Low Back and Leg Pain

Several studies have examined the effects of single and multiple session MT on patients with low back pain during the initial weeks following onset of symptoms. Figure 9-1 shows the range extremes for effect sizes observed in studies of acute low back and leg pain. In Hadler's study (13), manipulation achieved 22 percent greater reduction in low back disability after 3 days following a single treatment with HVLA versus mobilization. Glover (47) used detuned ultrasound as a control for a single intervention with HVLA, showing similar results to Hadler in the acute subgroup. Acute sciatica may also respond to manipulation (48). Mathews et al. (49) found a more extensive improvement in the group treated by manipulation at 2 weeks follow-up. Back education programs (ES = 0.7) (50) as well as combinations of exercise, diathermy, and lifestyle modification (ES = 1.0) (51) were all less effective than manipulation.

Bronfort (52), using a mixed sample of acute and chronic patients, found manipulation to hold greater advantage over general practitioner management at 3 and 6 months with significant reduction in work time loss (ES = 0.7). Physiotherapy, corsets, pain relievers (53) (ES = 0.4), and exercise (54) (0.4 < ES < 0.8) also underperformed manipulation.

Several groups from around the world have conducted formal consensus review of the literature. The consensus suggests a preponderance of evidence supporting manipulation to relieve pain from acute low back and leg pain (1–4,55,56).

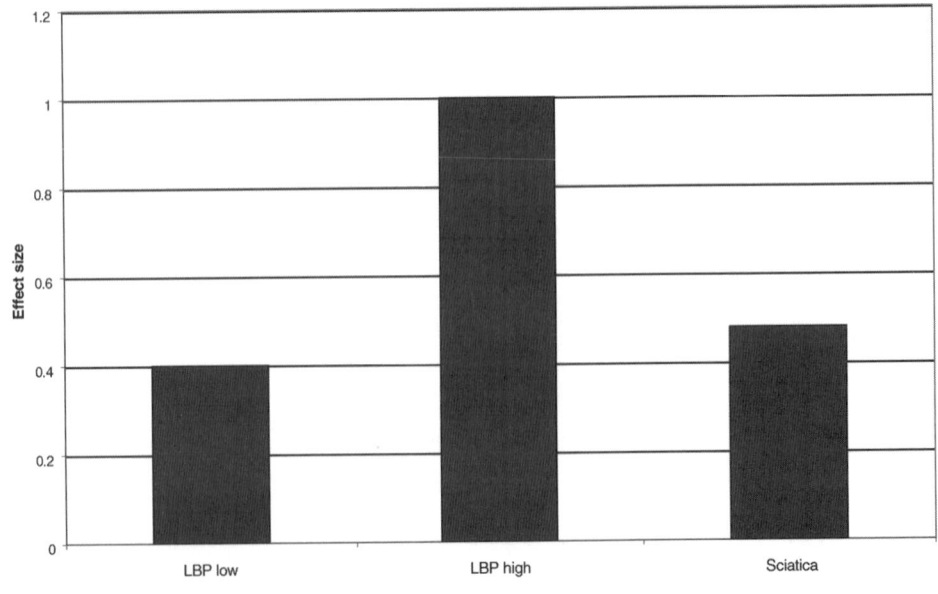

FIG. 9-1. Range limits (low, high) for effect sizes in studies of treatment for acute low back pain and sciatica.

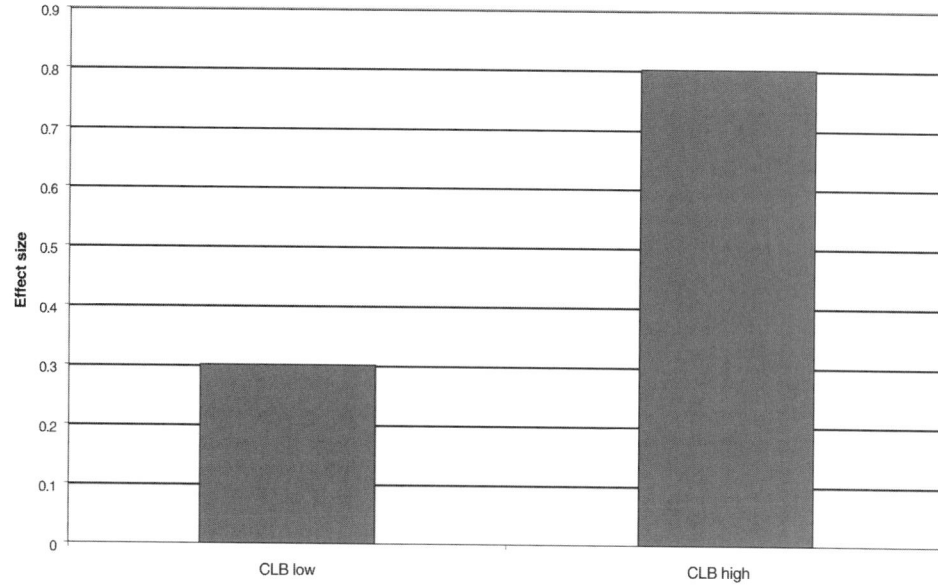

FIG. 9-2. Range limits (low, high) for effect sizes in studies of treatment for chronic low back pain.

Chronic lower back pain has received less attention from investigators testing the effects of manipulation. Figure 9-2 shows the range of effect size observed in three studies (14,57,58) and the subgroup analysis of Koes and colleague (59,60) data by Bronfort (46). Standard physical therapy, traction, exercise, corset, massage, medical management, back education programs, sham manipulation, and watchful waiting have all been contrasted with MT. Van Tulder and colleagues (2) performed extensive meta-analysis. They concluded that there is stronger evidence for use of manipulation for chronic back pain than there is for acute disorders.

Neck Pain

Figure 9-3 gives the ranges for effect size in treatment of neck pain. Mobilization for acute neck pain was studied by Nordemar and Thorner (61). They were unable to show any significant benefit over use of transcutaneous nerve stimulation. When combined with other treatment modalities (62), however, the results were more favorable (ES = 0.6). In contrast, mobilization faired better than massage or analgesic use (ES = 0.7) in a mixed group of acute and chronic neck pain subjects (63). In more homogeneous samples of chronic pain, the advantages appear

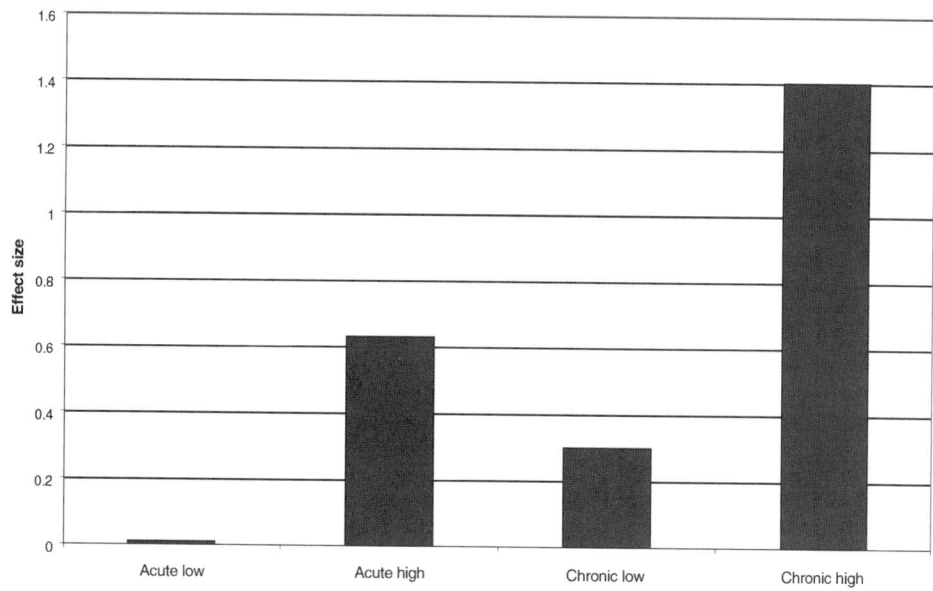

FIG. 9-3. Range limits (low, high) for effect sizes in studies of treatment for acute and chronic neck pain.

clearer. Results range from 0.3 to 1.7 ES (30,59,60, 62,64,65).

Like treatment of back pain, manipulation for neck-related pain has also been a subject of formal consensus review of the literature (4–6) with opinion favoring a trial of therapy.

Headache

Several types of headache pain are treated with MT. Effect sizes for treatment as to both type of headache and control group are given in Figure 9-4. Comparisons in tension, cervicogenic, and posttraumatic headache have included amitriptyline (66), massage and placebo laser (7), cryotherapy (66,67), mobilization, and wait listing (68). Migraine was treated by Parker and colleagues (69) with groups consisting of mobilization, manipulation, standard physical therapy, and medical management. Somewhat surprisingly, it is the course of tension headache that seems most refractory to manipulation treatment (70). While pain may be relieved in the short term, the pattern of recurring pain remains. This may reflect the hypothesis that tension headache is an interaction with the patient's environment rather than being solely a function of cervical, muscular, or vascular factors.

Duration of Effects

Important features of any treatment include the abilities to create enduring benefits and minimize accommodation that reduces the dosage effectiveness. Few studies have included data on these questions. In the study by Triano and colleagues (14), treatment was withdrawn and a final follow-up evaluation was performed after 4 weeks. Bene-fits persisted among the HVLA-treated patients but appeared to begin deteriorating for those in the sham manipulation group. Boline and colleagues (66) demonstrated similar effects on treatment of chronic tension-type headache. After withdrawing all treatments, head pain frequency and severity increased in the amitriptyline group but not for the manipulation group.

Theoretically, repeated use of any treatment may result in accommodation where the benefits require increasing dosage to be achieved. Immediate pain relief was tested at the end of a sequence of treatments for chronic low back pain (14). Comparable immediate pain relief was achieved on the first and the tenth treatment sessions, indicating that accommodation may not be a significant problem.

Nonspinal Conditions

The documented uses of manipulation are nearly all musculoskeletal, more specifically spinal. Only 1 percent of cases treated (71) are outside of the musculoskeletal system. Anecdotes have long circulated about the use of manipulation for other conditions that have pain. Few investigations of these claims have been made. Migraine is one type that is not classically considered a spinal disorder. Evidence showing the use of HVLA in treatment of these headaches has been covered previously. Other conditions that have received scientific attention include carpal tunnel syndrome (10), dysmenorrhea (72,73), and infantile colic (74).

The evidence has found no difference in the treatment of carpal tunnel syndrome with manipulation over conventional night bracing and therapy (10). Preliminary study of women with primary dysmenorrhea suggested a decrease in pain severity when treated with HVLA (72).

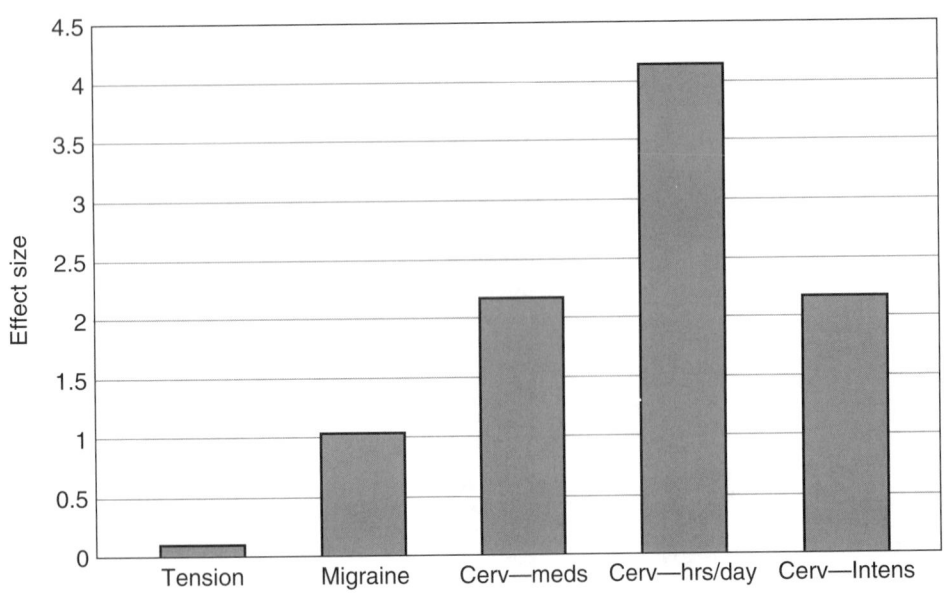

FIG. 9-4. Range limits (low, high) for effect sizes in studies of treatment for types of headaches. Cervicogenic headache outcomes are broken out according to comparison groups.

However, on full-scale randomized trial (73) no beneficial effects could be found. Infantile colic remains the only nonmusculoskeletal pain, other than migraine, with good evidence to support a benefit from spinal manipulation (74). A multidisciplinary team of investigators found that manipulation of the spine resulted in significant reduction in hours of infantile colic behavior after the fifth day in a 2-week series of treatment (ES = 4.0) versus simethicone administration.

THEORETICAL BASIS OF PAIN RELIEF

Pain is a complex perception that incorporates peripheral and central mechanisms as well as physical and psychological elements. Manipulation itself is a mechanical procedure that acts mechanically on the body. To achieve pain relief, it must interrupt the nociceptive component of pain. No direct evidence exists as to how pain is relieved with use of MT. Indirect evidence points to several mechanisms. However, the core feature is the restoration of normal joint behavior intended to alter local tissue stress and allow healing to occur. Figure 9-5 diagrams a cascade of events that are believed to occur as a result of the mechanical overload that occurs with a buckling event. Pain may be activated through two pathways, including the release of neurogenic and nonneurogenic agents (75,76). During the acute phase, joint use is altered in response to the nociceptive reaction. Over time, the joint becomes sensitized to motion, evoking perception of pain even with normal, nonstressful use. Central sensitization, from prolonged painful stimulation, may set up reverberating neural systems that perpetuate pain and muscular spasm. The patient's perception is a reduced threshold for pain and an exaggerated response to sensory input. Cavanaugh reviewed in detail the experimental evidence for these mechanisms (77,78).

Experimental evidence shows that manipulation has local and peripheral physiologic effects. They manifest, for example, as changes in range of motion, muscle spindle responses (79), moderation of reflex actions, paraspinal and peripheral myoelectric activity (80–83), and circulating factors (84,85).

Improved range of motion, associated simultaneously with pain relief, implies an alteration of mechanical joint behavior and distribution of joint loads following manipulation. The work of Nansel and colleagues (28,29) as well as Cassidy and colleagues (30) shows reduced asymmetry of spinal motion immediately following treatment. Figure 9.6 demonstrates the effect of simulated HVLA procedure on the muscle spindle activity of the cat multifidus muscle (79). Impulse loads were applied to the L-6 spinous process in a direction parallel to the long axis of the spine, causing distraction of the L6-7 facet joint. The ramped increase in activity is associated with preloading of the spinous process. At the impulse, the muscle spindle rapidly increases firing rate (inset of Fig. 9-6) followed by full sus-

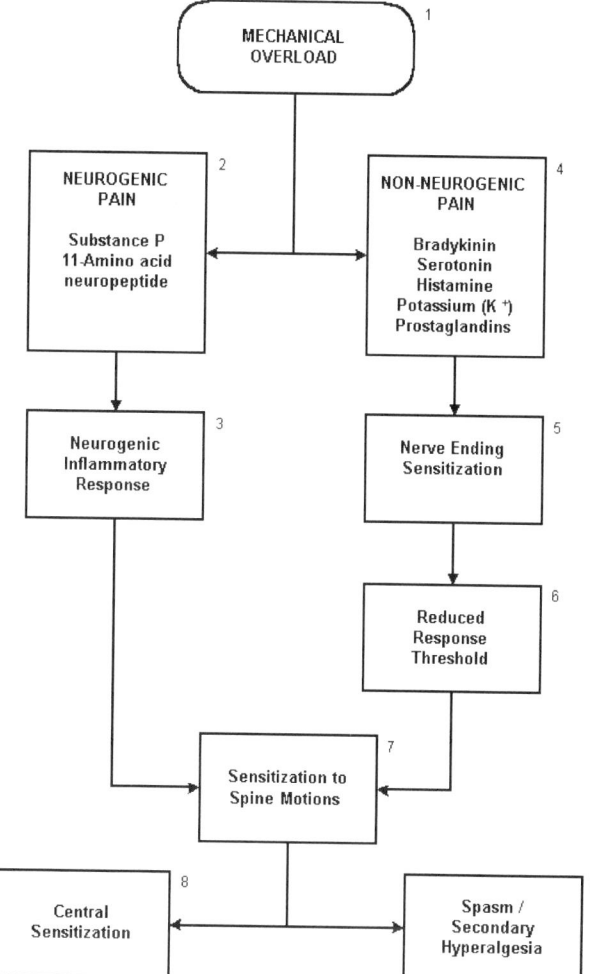

FIG. 9-5. Pathomechanisms of mechanical tissue overload in producing nociceptive and nonnociceptive pain. (From Triano JJ. Biomechanics of manipulation. In: Herzog W, ed. *The clinical biomechanics of spinal manipulation.* St. Louis: Mosby, 2000, page 112, with permission.)

pension of activity. After a 4-second interval, activity is then reset below the initial resting levels.

The action of manipulation has the ability to influence central spinal cord function as evidenced by changes in H reflex behavior in healthy subjects (86) and in patients (87,88). For healthy subjects, a transient suppression of the H reflex amplitude is observed following HVLA or mobilization. Different effects are seen when radicular pain is present. Patients with discogenic S-1 radiculopathy, associated with suppressed H reflex amplitude and prolonged latency, showed improvement in both parameters after HVLA procedure (87). In a separate study, the effect of cutaneous afferent stimulation during manipulation was assessed (88). Asymptomatic volunteers received manipulation to the sacroiliac joint. One group was pretreated topically with an anesthetic cream prior to the procedure. H reflex suppression was noted only in the group

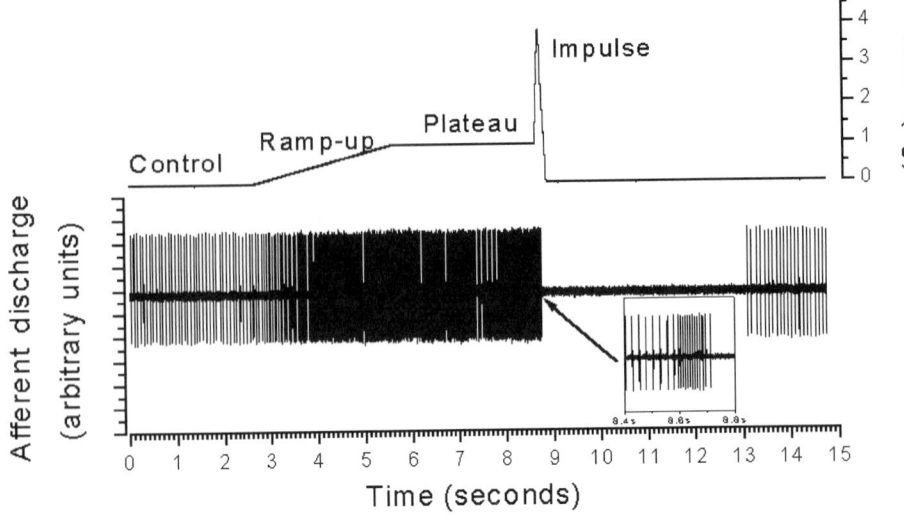

FIG. 9-6. A single unit recording from the muscle spindle of a cat multifidus muscle obtained from a filament in the L-6 dorsal root. The spinal manipulation mimic load was applied parallel to the long axis of the spine, distracting the L6–7 facet joint. The inset shows the spindle's discharge on an expanded time scale immediately before and during the impulse. (From Pickar JG. Response of muscle proprioceptors to spinal manipulative-like loads in the anesthetized cat. *J Manip Physiol Ther* V24, 2001, with permission.)

that was not pretreated and only on the side receiving the HVLA procedure.

Myoelectric activity also responds to spinal manipulation (80,81,83). Figure 9-7 is the record of paraspinal muscle in the thoracic spine of a patient receiving HVLA treatment while in a prone posture. The arrow indicates the timing of the impulse. Muscle activation was reset by the procedure to the expected normal electrical silence.

Finally, the physiologic markers of manipulation effects can be observed systemically. Respiratory burst from circulating polymorphonuclear leukocytes (PMNs) and monocytes has been monitored before and after spinal manipulation (14,84,85). Respiratory burst rates of cells isolated from peripheral blood before and after HVLA were significantly higher after treatment than before. These responses

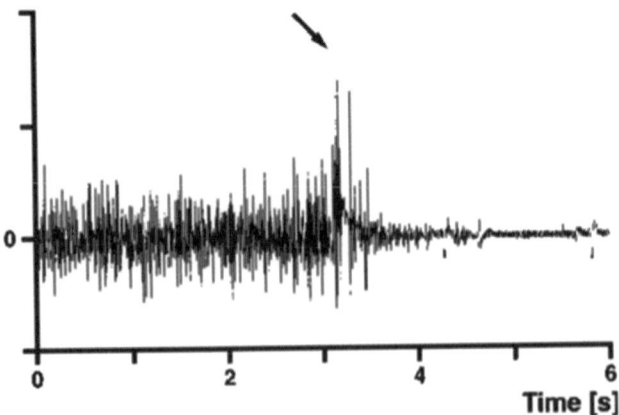

FIG. 9-7. EMG-time history of a hypertonic muscle before, during, and after a chiropractic HVLA procedure. EMG activity high before treatment, increased during the procedure (*arrow*) and then became silent afterward. (From Herzog W. The mechanical, neuromuscular and physiologic effects produced by the spinal manipulation. In: Herzog W, ed. *Clinical biomechanics of spinal manipulation.* New York: Churchill Livingstone, 2000:191–207, with permission.)

show a threshold effect requiring peak HVLA forces of approximately 400 N. Control groups consisted of sham manipulation and soft tissue treated subjects. Additional work (unpublished data) further demonstrates that peripheral joint manipulation fails to generate circulating cell reactions.

SAFETY

Over the years, controversy has surrounded the use of manipulation procedures, particularly for the spine. Systematic studies of complications have been reported (89–93). Approximately one in seven patients can expect minor, self-limiting symptoms in the form of new, local pain or local symptom exacerbation. These tend to resolve within 24 hours. Severe complications yielding permanent damage are on the order of 0.000001 percent (91,92) or less and involve cauda equina syndrome in treatment of the lumbar spine and vertebrobasilar syndrome for the cervical spine. Contrasting this with the risk of many standard medical procedures shows that manipulation risk is extremely small. For example, the risk of intestinal bleed leading to hospitalization and even death from use of NSAIDs in older patients is approximately 1 in 1,000 (91,94).

When incidence data is analyzed to evaluate the relative frequency of serious complications in proportion to the frequency of use according to training, a disturbing trend is observed. There is a disproportionate number of cases of severe complication when HVLA procedures are carried out by those with little training and experience (95,96). The proportion associated with manipulation administered by those other than chiropractors is alarmingly high. In the United States, chiropractic physicians perform 94 percent of procedures (48). One would expect, then, that approximately 94 percent of serious complications also are associated with their treatment and only 6 percent by others. Examination of the literature shows this assumption to be false (95). In Terrett's data, 20 percent are from others. In an additional 30 cases of complication incorrectly attributed to Chiropractors, 13 percent were actually caused by therapists attempting manipulation. Similarly, Hufnagel and colleagues (96) report injuries from "chiropractic" procedures that were actually performed by orthopedists and others.

CONCLUSION

The glare of scientific scrutiny over the past quarter century has stripped away much of the myth and controversy surrounding manipulative therapy. Manipulation is recommended or is an option for acute and chronic low back pain, radicular pain, neck pain, and some forms of headache. Placebo effect is insufficient to explain the therapeutic benefits that are observed.

A theory of the functional spinal lesion (FSL) or subluxation has emerged that is evidence based and accounts for clinical observations. These disorders appear in isolation and in conjunction with other pathoanatomical disorders and may explain why some pathology observed on imaging is symptom free while others are not. The FSL is itself conformable to the application of specific forces and moments. Uses of these procedures are more complex than generally appreciated and skillful application is important. The risk of this method of treatment is very small and well within the bounds of acceptable medical uncertainty when performed by physicians who are adequately trained and experienced.

REFERENCES

1. Bigos S, Bowyer O, Braen G. Acute low back problems in adults. Rockville, MD: 1994. Clinical Practice Guideline, No. 14.
2. van Tulder MW, Koes BW, Bouter LM. Conservative treatment of acute and chronic nonspecific low back pain. a systematic review of randomized controlled trials of the most common interventions. *Spine* 1997;22(18):2128–2156.
3. Poulsen PB. *Low back pain—frequency, management and prevention from an HTA perspective.* Poulsen PB, ed. 1[1]. Copenhagen: Danish Institute for Health Technology Assessment, 1999.
4. Coulter ID, Shekelle PG, Mootz RD, Hansen DT. Use of expert panel results: the RAND panel for appropriateness of manipulation and mobilization of the cervical spine. *Top Clin Chiro* 1995;2(3): 54–62.
5. Coulter ID, Hurwitz EL, Adams AH. The appropriateness of manipulation and mobilization of the cervical spine. RAND/MR-781-CCR. Santa Monica, CA: RAND, Inc., 1996.
6. Coulter ID, Adams AH. The appropriateness of spinal manipulation and mobilization for cervical spine conditionsi and ratings of a multidisciplinary expert panel. Santa Monica, CA: The RAND Corporation, 1996.
7. Nilsson N, Christensen HW, Hartvigsen J. The effect of spinal manipulation in the treatment of cervicogenic headache. *J Manip Physiol Ther* 1997;20:326–330.
8. Bonebrake AR, Fernandez JE, Marley RJ, et al. A treatment for carpal tunnel syndrome: evaluation of objective and subjective measures. *J Manip Physiol Ther* 1990;13:507–520.
9. Bonebrake AR, Fernandez JE, Dahalan JB, Marley RJ. A treatment for carpal tunnel syndrome: results of a follow-up study. *J Manip Physiol Ther* 1993;16:125–139.
10. Davis PT, Hulbert JR, Kassak KM, Meyer JJ. Comparative efficacy of conservative medical and chiropractic treatments for carpal tunnel

syndrome: a randomized clincal trial. *J Manip Physiol Ther* 1998;21(5):317–326.
11. Cherkin D, Hart LG, Rosenblatt RA. Patient satisfaction with family physicians and general internists: is there a difference? *J Fam Pract* 1988;26(5):543–551.
12. Carey TS, Garrett J, Jackman A. The outcomes and costs of care for acute low back pain among patients seen by primary care practitioners, chiropractors, and orthopedic surgeons. *New Engl J Med* 1995;333(14):913–917.
13. Hadler NM, Curtis P, Gillings A. Benefit of spinal manipulation as adjunctive therapy for acute low back pain: a stratified controlled trial. *Spine* 1987;12:703–706.
14. Triano JJ, McGregor M, Hondras MA, Brennan PC. Manipulative therapy versus education programs in chronic low back pain. *Spine* 1995;20(8):948–955.
15. Triano J. The mechanics of spinal manipulation. In: Herzog W, ed. *Clinical biomechanics of spinal manipulation.* New York: Churchill Livingstone, 2000:92–190.
16. Wilder DG, Pope MH, Seroussi RE, et al. The balance point of the intervertebral motion segment: an experimental study. *Bull Hosp Jt Dis Orthop Inst* 1989;49(2):155–169.
17. Crisco JJ III, Panjabi MM, Yamamoto I, Oxland TR. Euler stability of the human ligamentous lumbar spine. Part II experiment. *Clin Biomech* 1992;7:27–32.
18. Cholewicki J, Mcgill SM, Norman RW. Comparison of muscle forces and joint load from an optimization and EMG assisted lumbar spine model: towards development of a hybrid approach. *J Biomecs* 1995;28(3):321–331.
19. Cholewicki J, Mcgill SM. Mechanical stability of the in vivo lumbar spine: implications for injury and chronic low back pain. *Clin Biomech* 1996;11(1):1–15.
20. Landsmeer JMF. *Atlas of the anatomy of the hand.* New York: Churchill Livingstone, 1976.
21. Kauer JMG. Functional anatomy of the wrist. *Clin Orthop* 1980;149:9.
22. Kaptchuk TJ, Landsmeer JMF. Functional anatomy of the wrist. In: Tubiana R, ed. *The hand.* Philadelphia: W.B. Saunders, 1981.
23. Kauer JMG. The mechanisms of the carpal joint. *Clin Orthop* 1986;202:16.
24. Cyclic loading of the intervertebral motion segment. March 15–16; Institute Electrical and Electronic Engineers, 1982.
25. Wilder DG, Pope MH, Frymoyer JW. The biomechanics of lumbar disc herniation and the effect of overload and instability. *J Spinal Disord* 1988;1:16–32.
26. Pope MH, Wilder DG, Krag MH. Biomechanics of the lumbar spine A. Basic principles. In: Frymoyer JW, ed. *The adult spine—principles and practice.* New York: Raven Press, 1991:1487–1501.
27. Cholewicki J, Mcgill SM. Lumbar posterior ligament involvement during extremely heavy lifts estimated from fluoroscopic measurements. *J Biomech* 1992;25(1):17–28.
28. Nansel D, Cremata E, Carleson R, Szalazak M. Effect of unilateral spinal adjustments on goniometrically-assessed cervical lateral-flexion end-range asyummetries in otherwise asymptomatic subjects. *J Manip Physiol Ther* 1989;12(6):419–427.
29. Nansel D, Peneff A, Cremata E, Carlson J. Time course considerations for the effects of unilateral lower cervical adjustments with respect to the amelioration of cervical lateral-flexion passive end-range asymmetry. *J Manip Physiol Ther* 1990;13(6):2997–3004.
30. Cassidy JD, Lopes AA, Yong-Hing K. The immediate effect of manipulation versus mobilization on pain and range of motion in the cervical spine: a randomized controlled trial. *J Manip Physiol Ther* 1992;15(9):570–575.
31. Osterbauer PJ, Long K, Ribaudo TA. Three-dimensional head kinematics and cervical range of motion in the diagnosis of patients with neck trauma. *J Manip Physiol Ther* 1996;19:231–237.
32. Nelson N, Christensen HW, Hartvigsen J. Lasting changes in passive range of motion after spinal manipulation: a randomized, blind, controlled trial. *J Manip Physiol Ther* 1996;19:165–168.
33. Triano J. Biomechanics of spinal manipulation. *Spine* 2001;1(1):In press.
34. Curtis P, Carey T, Evans P, et al. Training primary care physicians to give limited manual therapy for low back pain: patient outcomes. *Spine* 2000;22(15):2954–2959.
35. Carey T. 1998 (personal communication).

36. Cohen E, Triano JJ, McGregor M, Papakyriakou M. Biomechanical performance of spinal manipulation therapy by newly trained vs. practicing providers: does experience transfer to unfamiliar procedures? *J Manip Physiol Ther* 1995;18(6):347–352.
37. Triano JJ. *Biomechanical analysis of motions and loads during spinal manipulation.* University of Michigan, 1998.
38. Biomechanical parameters of skill in lumbar SMT. 94 Jun; Arlington, VA: FCER, 1994.
39. Vernon HT. *Effects of changing lumbar posture on spine loads during SMT.* Oct 21; Toronto, Ontario, Canada: Canadian Memorial Chiropractic College, 2000.
40. Bergmann TF, Peterson DH, Lawrence DJ. *Chiropractic technique principles and practice.* New York: Churchill Livingstone, 1993.
41. Edmond SL. *Manipulation & mobilization: extremity and spinal techniques.* St. Louis: Mosby-Year Book, Inc, 1993.
42. Salter RB. The biologic concept of continuous passive motion of synovial joints. The first 18 years of basic research and its clinical application. *Clin Orthop* 1989;242:12–25.
43. Keller TS. Engineering–in vivo transient vibration analysis of the normal human spine. In: Fuhr A, Collaca CJ, Green JR, Keller TS, eds. *Activator methods chiropractic technique.* St. Louis: Mosby, 1997:431–450.
44. Fuhr AW, Colloca CJ, Green JR, Keller TS. *Activator methods chiropractic technique.* St. Louis: Mosby Books, 1997.
45. Cohen J. *Statistical power analysis for the behavioral sciences.* 2nd ed. 1988.
46. Bronfort G. *Efficacy of manual therapies of the spine.* Vrije Universiteit, EMGO Institute, 1997.
47. Glover JR. Back pain: a randomized clinical trial of rotational manipulation of the trunk. *Br J Ind Med* 1974;31:59–64.
48. Shekelle PG, Adams AH, Chassin MR, et al. Spinal manipulation for low-back pain. *Ann Intern Med* 1992;117:590–598.
49. Mathews JA, Mills SB, Jenkins VM. Back pain and sciatica: controlled trials of manipulation, traction, sclerosant and epidural injections. *Br J Rheumatol* 1987;26(416):423.
50. MacDonald RS, Bell CM. An open controlled assessment of osteopathic manipulation in nonspecific low-back pain. *Spine* 1990;15:364–370.
51. Farrell JP, Twomey LT. Acute low back pain. Comparison of two conservative treatment approaches. *Med J Aust* 1982;1:160–164.
52. Bronfort G. Chiropractic versus general medical treatment of low back pain: a small scale controlled clinical trial. *Am J Chiro Med* 1989;2:145–150.
53. Doran DM, Newell DJ. Manipulation in treatment of low back pain. *Br Med J* 1975;2:161–164.
54. Zylbergold RS, Piper MC. Lumbar disc disease: comparative analysis of physical therapy treatments. *Arch Phy Med Rehabil* 1981;62:176–179.
55. Shekelle PG, Adams AH, Chassin MR. *The appropriateness of spinal manipulation for low-back pain: project overview and literature review.* R-4025/1CCR/FCER. Santa Monica, CA: The RAND Corporation, 1991.
56. Shekelle PG, Adams AH, Chassin MR. *The appropriateness of spinal manipulation for low-back pain.* Indications and ratings by an all chiropractic expert panel. R-4025/3-CCR/FCER. Santa Monica, CA: The RAND Corporation, 1992.
57. Coxhead CE, Inskip H, Meade TW, et al. Multicentre trial of physiotherapy in the management of sciatic symptoms. *Lancet* 1981;1:1065–1068.
58. Pope MH, Phillips RB, Haugh LD, et al. A prospective mechanized three-week trial of spinal manipulation, transcutaneous muscle stimulation, massage and corset in the treatment of subacute low back pain. *Spine* 1994;19:2571–2577.
59. Koes BW, Bouter LM, Van Mameren H, et al. The effectiveness of manual therapy, physiotherapy, and treatment by the general practitioner for nonspecific back and neck complaints: a randomized clinical trial. *Spine* 1992;17(1):28–35.
60. Koes BW, Bouter LM, Van Mameren H, et al. Randomised clinical trial of manipulative therapy and physiotherapy for persistent back and neck complaints: results of one year follow up. *BMJ* 1992;304:601–605.
61. Nordemar R, Thorner C. Treatment of acute cervical pain—a comparative group study. *Pain* 1981;10:93–101.
62. Gross AR, Aker P, Quartly C. Manual therapy in the treatment of neck pain. *Rheum Dis Clin North Am* 1996;22(3):579–598.
63. Brodin H. Cervical pain and mobilization. *Manuelle Medizin* 1982;20:90–94.
64. Koes BW, Bouter LM, Van Mameren H, et al. A randomized clinical trial of manual therapy and physiotherapy for persistent back and neck complaints: subgroup analysis and relationship between outcome measures. *J Manip Physiol Ther* 1993;16(4):211–219.
65. Sloop PR, Smith DS, Goldenberg E, Dore C. Manipulation for chronic neck pain. A double-wind controlled study. *Spine* 1982;7:532–535.
66. Boline P, Kassak KM, Bronfort G, et al. Spinal manipulation vs. amitriptyline for the treatment of chronic tension-type headaches: a randomized clinical trial. *J Manipulative Physiol Ther* 1995;18(148):154.
67. Nilsson N. A randomized controlled trial of the effect of spinal manipulaton in the treatment of cervicogenic headache. *J Manip Physiol Ther* 1995;18(7):435–440.
68. Bitterli J, Graf R, Robert F, Adler R, Mumenthaler M. [Objective criteria for the evaluation of chiropractic treatment of spondylotic headache (author's trans.)]. [German]. *Nervenarzt* 1977;48:259–262.
69. Parker GB, Tupling H, Pryor DS. A controlled trial of cervical manipulation for migraine. *Aust N Z J Med* 1978;8:589–593.
70. Bove G, Nilsson N. Spinal manipulation in the treatment of episodic tension-type headache. *JAMA* 1998;280(18):1576–1579.
71. Hurwitz EL, Coulter ID, Adams AH, et al. Use of chiropractic services from 1985 through 1991 in the United States and Canada. *Am J of Public Health* 1996;88(5):771–776.
72. Kokjohn K, Schmid DM, Triano JJ, Brennan PC. The effect of spinal manipulation on pain and prostaglandin levels in women with primary dysmenorrhea. *J Manip Physiol Ther* 1992;15(5):279–285.
73. Hondras MA, Long CR, Brennan PC. Spinal manipulative therapy versus a low force mimic maneuver for women with primary dysmenorrhea: a randomized, observer-blinded, clinical trial. *Pain* 1999;81(1-2):105–114.
74. Wiberg JMM, Nordsteen J, Nilsson N. The short-term effect of spinal manipulation in the treatment of infantile colic: a randomized controlled clinical trial with a blinded observer. *J Manip Physiol Ther* 1999;22(8):517–522.
75. Saal JS. The role of inflammation in lumbar pain. *Spine* 1995;20(16):1821–1827.
76. Stein C, Millan MJ, Shippenberg TS. Peripheral opiod receptors mediating antinociception in inflammation: evidence for involvement of mu, delta, and kappa receptors. *J Pharmacol Exp Ther* 1989;248:1269–1275.
77. Cavanaugh JM. Neural Mechanisms of Lumbar Pain. *Spine* 1995;20(16):1804–1809.
78. Cavanaugh JM, Ozaktay AC, Ymashita HT. Lumbar facet pain: biomechanics, neuroanatomy and neurophysiology. *J Biomechanics* 1996;29(9):1117–1129.
79. Pickar JG. Response of muscle proprioceptors to spinal manipulative-like loads in the anesthetized cat. *J Manip Physiol Ther* V24, 2001; In press.
80. Suter E, Herzog W, Conway PJ, Zhang YT. Reflex response associated with manipulative treatment of the thoracic spine. *J Neuromusculoskel Syst* 1994;2:124–130.
81. Herzog W. Mechanical and physiological responses to spinal manipulative treatments. *J Neuromusculoskeletal Syst* 1995;3:1–9.
82. Herzog W, Conway P, Zhang Y, Gal J, Guimaraes ACS. Reflex responses associated with manipulative treatments on the thoracic spine: a pilot study. *J Manip Physiol Ther* 1995;18(4):233–236.
83. Herzog W. The mechanical, neuromuscular and physiologic effects produced by the spinal manipulation. In: Herzog W, ed. *Clinical biomechanics of spinal maniuplation.* New York: Churchill Livingstone, 2000:191–207.
84. Brennan PC, Kokjohn K, Kaltinger CJ, et al. Enhanced phagocytic cell respiratory burst induced by spinal manipulation: potential role of substance P. *J Manip Physiol Ther* 1991;14(7):399–408.
85. Brennan PC, Triano JJ, McGregor M, et al. Enhanced neutrophil respiratory burst as a biological marker for manipulation forces: duration of the effect and association with substance P and tumor necrosis factor. *J Manip Physiol Ther* 1992;15(2):83–90.
86. Dishman JD, Bulbulian R. Spinal reflex attenuation associated with spinal manipulation. *Spine* 2000;25(19):2519–2525.

87. Floman Y, Liram N, Gilai AN. Spinal manipulation results in immediate H-reflex changes in patients with unilateral disc herniation. *Eur Spine J* 1997;6:398–401.

88. Murphy BA, Dawson NJ, Slack JR. Sacroiliac joint manipulation decreases the H-reflex. *Electromyogr Clin Neurophysiol* 1995;35:87–94.

89. Haldeman S, Rubinstein SM. Cauda equina syndrome in patients undergoing manipulation of the lumbar spine. *Spine* 1992;17(12):1469–1473.

90. Haldeman S, Rubinstein SM. The precipitation or aggravation of musculoskeletal pain in patients receiving spinal manipulative therapy. *J Manip Physiol Ther* 1993;16(1):47–50.

91. McGregor M, Haldeman S, Kohlbeck FJ. Vertebrobasilar compromise associated with cervical manipulation. *Top Clin Chiro* 1995;2:63–73.

92. Haldeman S, Kohlbeck FJ, McGregor M. Risk factors and precipitating neck movements causing vertebrobasilar artery dissection after cervical trauma and spinal manipulation. *Spine* 1999;24(8):785–794.

93. Senstad O, Leboeuf-Yde C, Borchgrevink C. Frequency and characteristics of side effects of spinal manipulative therapy. *Spine* 1997;22(4):435–441.

94. Adelizzi RA. Clinical implications of NSAID pharmacokinetics: special populations, special considerations. *J Am Osteopath Assoc* 1994;94(5):396–398.

95. Terret AGJ. Misuse of the literature by medical authors in discussing spinal manipulative therapy injury. *J Manip Physiol Ther* 1995;18(4):203–210.

96. Hufnagel A, Hammers A, Schonle PW, et al. Stroke following chiropractic manipulation of the cervical spine. *J Neurol* 1999;246:683–688.

97. Kawchuk GN, Herzog W. Biomechanical characterization (fingerprinting) of five novel methods of cervical spinal manipulation. *J Manip Physiol Ther* 1993;16:573–577.

98. Kawchuk GN, Herzog W, Hasler EM. Forces generated during spinal manipulative therapy of the cervical spine: a pilot study. *J Manip Physiol Ther* 1992;15:275–278.

99. Gal JM, Herzog W, Kawchuk GN, Conway P, et al. Forces and relative vertebral movements during SMT to unembalmed post-rigor human cadavers: peculiarities associated with joint cavitation. *J Manip Physiol Ther* 1995;18(1):4–9.

100. Conway PJW, Herzog W, Zhang Y. Forces required to cause cavitation during spinal manipulation of the thoracic spine. *Clin Biomech* 1993;8:210–214.

101. Herzog W. Biomechanical studies of spinal manipulative therapy (invited review paper). *J Can Chiro Assoc* 1991;35:156–164.

102. Herzog W, Conway P, Kawchuk G, Zhang Y, Hasler E. Forces exerted during spinal manipulative therapy. *Spine* 1993;18:1206–1212.

103. Hessel B, Herzog W, Conway PJW, McEwan MC. Experimental measurement of the force exerted during spinal manipulation using the thompson technique. *J Manip Physiol Ther* 1990;8:448–453.

104. Lee M, Kelly D, Steven G. A model of spine, ribcage and pelvic responses to a specific lumbar manipulative force in relaxed subjects. *J Biomechanics* 1995;28(11):1403–1408.

105. Lee R, Evans J. Load-displacement-time characteristics of the spine under posteroanterior mobilization. *Aust J Physio-ther* 1992;38(2):115–123.

106. Triano J, Schultz AB. Loads transmitted during lumbosacral spinal manipulative therapy. *Spine* 1997;22(17):1955–1964.

107. Triano JJ. Studies on the biomechanical effect of a spinal adjustment. *J Manip Physiol Ther* 1992;15(1):71–75.

108. Osterbauer PJ, Fuhr AW, Keller TS. Description and analysis of activator methods chiropractic technique. In: Lawrence D, Cassidy JD, McGregor M, et al, eds. *Advances in chiropractic*. Chicago: Mosby, 1995:471–511.

109. Triano JJ. Biomechanics of manipulation. In: Herzog W, ed. *The clinical biomechanics of spinal manipulation*. St. Louis: Mosby, 2000.

CHAPTER 10

Rehabilitation Therapies in Pain and Disability Management

An Activity Driven Biopsychosocial Model of Practice

Maureen J. Simmonds and Jacqueline H. Peat

Pain and disability management is central to rehabilitation. Physical therapists (PTs) and occupational therapists (OTs) play complementary and collaborative roles in the interdisciplinary management of patients with pain and disability. Over the last couple of decades, significant changes have occurred in the way pain and disability are conceptualized and managed within health care. Recognition of a broad biopsychosocial model of health (and ill health), the positive role of activity on health and healing, and an emphasis on function and evidence have transformed practice. The primary purpose of this chapter is to discuss the state of the art and state of the science of musculoskeletal pain and disability management with physical and occupational therapies. In addition, attention will be paid to the influence of the health care provider on outcome. Possibly the biggest single influence on patient outcome (positive or negative) is the therapists themselves and the ability they have to engage, educate, and empower the patient to adopt a long-term lifestyle of health and well-being through activity.

Historically, the management of disease and injury often involved long periods of hospitalization, bed rest, and convalescence. Rest until recovery was the basic tenet on which traditional health care practice was based. Health care practitioners used a narrow disease/impairment-based health care model and worked within a hierarchical system. Physicians inevitably headed the hierarchy, therapists assumed the role of "physician's helpers," and patients were dependent, passive recipients of this "care." Therapists working within such a "rest for recovery" framework developed and utilized skills and techniques that were based on the disease/impairment model. Many of these therapies were passive and some may have encouraged dependence (e.g., mobilizations, modalities, and use of adaptive equipment). Most treatments continued for long periods and providers were reimbursed on a fee-for-service basis with few questions asked. Finally, because conservative therapies were—indeed, still are—perceived as either helpful or harmless, untested therapies were/are developed, adopted, and widely practiced with few (if any) questions regarding their biologic plausibility and minimal scientific scrutiny of their efficacy or effectiveness.

In recent years, the theoretical framework of rehabilitation has expanded, and this has helped reshape clinical practice. Assessments now focus on the person rather than the painful part and on function rather than impairment. They are more holistic with consideration given to psychological, sociological, and environmental factors that potentially contribute to persistent pain and to dysfunction. Therapies incorporate cognitive-behavioral principles and promote activity. Such treatment approaches have replaced or at least supplement hands-on passive treatments. Passive treatments (e.g., mobilizations and modalities) still have a role, but the role is limited to short-term symptom management during an acute flare-up of symptoms, and specifically *if* their use promotes exercise and activity or occupation. Client centered practice has evolved (1), and patients/clients are now expected to take an active and responsible role in the management of their problem. Thus, it is now the therapists' role and responsibility to ensure that patients have the knowledge, skills, and confidence to assume this responsibility. So patient education plays a significant role in therapies that have become goal oriented and time limited rather than symptom focused and symptom limited. Finally, although the emphasis on evidence-based assessments and treatment regimens is overdue in therapy, as it is in medicine, the application of evidence-based practice is expected to further change and improve therapies for pain and disability.

The roles of therapists depend somewhat on the setting. PTs and OTs work in a variety of different community and clinical settings and work with individuals of all ages and in all stages of health, injury, and disease. In the community (e.g., health and wellness centers), the primary role of therapists is that of an educator. Therapists help teach healthy individuals how to exercise and participate in activities to maintain their health and well-being. In work environments (e.g., industrial occupational), therapists are involved in educating workers, supervisors, and managers about safe and healthy work environments to prevent injury, and if necessary, to prevent prolonged incapacity should an injury occur. For example, in the UK, a recent "Welfare to Work" strategy proposes that therapists conduct an employability assessment of individuals 3 months after a work absence with the aim of reducing permanent incapacity (2).

In clinical settings (primary, secondary, or tertiary), the major role of a therapist remains that of an educator and helper rather than healer. A problem-solving approach helps patients solve functional difficulties and improve their activity level that may be limited by a variety of factors including actual pain, anticipated pain, or fear of pain.

In primary care, therapists must ensure that their educational information and actions promote self-management and reduce patient's dependence on the therapist. The majority of patients with musculoskeletal problems have chronic problems that are managed rather than cured. And most patients are well able to manage their own physical problems if empowered to do so. Croft (3) reported that although an episode of low back pain (LBP) may resolve quickly, recurrence rates are approximately 50 percent in the following 12 months. Wahlgren et al. (4) showed that in a cohort of 76 individuals, who had a first episode of LBP, 78% still experienced pain at 6 months and 26% were disabled by LBP. He also reported that at 12 months 72% still experienced pain and 14% were disabled by LBP. Thus, a high percentage of individuals have persistent pain that they self-manage. A minority become significantly disabled.

Identification of individuals with pain at risk for disability is crucial. But clinical care of complex patients can be problematic. It is disconcerting to note that of 89 patients referred to a tertiary pain-management center, only 3 had *not* received some sort of inappropriate advice or treatment (5). Gallagher (6) has advocated for the development of pain medicine specialists to support primary care physicians, therapists, and behavioral clinicians in community centers. This is particularly important given that the

pain knowledge of most health care practitioners who are not pain specialists has been found inadequate (7,8).

Thus, primary care practitioners have the responsibility of providing appropriate and clear explanations of the problem and ensuring that the patient understands that explanation. Finally, in addition to providing appropriate advice and appropriate care, primary care practitioners have the responsibility of identifying patients at risk for chronic incapacity. Presently, psychosocial factors are stronger predictors of chronic disability than biological factors. Thus, primary care practitioners have to incorporate some psychosocial measures into standard clinical assessments.

In tertiary care settings, therapists usually work within an interdisciplinary team that includes physicians and psychologists and may include exercise physiologists, social workers, and others. When individuals have pain, activities are affected and many factors mediate pain and activity (9). The role of therapists in pain management is to increase the purposeful activity of patients. Both OTs and PTs have similar goals (i.e., promotion of movement and function), but the strategies while complementary are distinct. OTs have a grounding in theory and practice of group work, activity analysis, and goal setting that is linked to increasing occupation. Therefore, they frequently stress the importance of occupation (work and leisure) to enable individuals to maximize their abilities and enhance their quality of life (10). PTs focus on movement and exercise to promote and improve physical function and thereby quality of life. In that role they identify and address barriers to activity and physical function. These may be physical impairments, such as restricted range of motion, reduced muscle strength, or pain that may be addressed through specific exercise regimens, modalities, or joint mobilizations. Other barriers may be psychological (e.g., fear of activity) and may be addressed through graded exposure to the specific activity (11).

Therapeutic objectives in clinical settings usually include the reduction of pain and restoration of function. These are global objectives, and whether they are achieved for an individual patient depends on several factors. For example, who is asked (patient or practitioner), what is asked (reduction of pain or restoration of function), when it is asked (short term versus long term), what outcome measures are used (self-report versus performance tests), and what criteria are acceptable (magnitude of change versus percent change). In tertiary care, the *emphasis* is on the restoration of function rather than the reduction of pain.

RATIONALE FOR A BIOPSYCHOSOCIAL FRAMEWORK OF PRACTICE

Impairment and disability are terms that were defined by the World Health Organization in 1980 (12) as follows. Impairment is any loss or abnormality of psychological, physiological, or anatomical structures or functions (e.g., decreased range of motion or strength). Disability is any

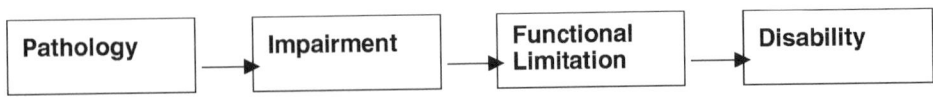

FIG. 10-1. The Nagi Model of Disablement

restriction or lack (resulting from an impairment) of ability to perform an activity in the manner or within the range considered normal (e.g., the inability to work). Nagi (13), a sociologist, was among the first to question the appropriateness of the traditional disease-based medical model as an explanation for disability. He recognized the need for a concept that bridged impairment and disability, and he proposed the term *functional limitation*. Functional limitation is defined as compromised ability to perform a level of activity within the range of "normal" (13; Fig. 10-1)

Although Nagi's model implies a unidirectional and linear progression from pathology through impairment and functional limitation to disability, this is not entirely accurate. Rather, each of the constructs (pathology, impairment, functional limitation, and disability) is complex and each is influenced by a myriad of factors. Thus, depending on when and how the different constructs are measured, and on the influence of different mediating factors (e.g., psychosocial factors), the relationships among the constructs may be trivial. For example, degenerative changes noted on a plain x-ray in a 55-year-old individual (pathology measure) may be surprisingly poor at predicting range of motion or pain (impairment measures). Such a pathological measure is even less likely to predict the individual's ability to climb stairs (functional ability) or work (disability). Better predictors of work include the physical demands of the occupation, the unemployment rate, and

the level of flexibility and satisfaction in the work environment. These factors are external to the individual and the arthritic changes on x-ray are incidental.

Impairment is also a poor predictor of disability. For example, many individuals with chronic back pain continue an active and productive life and never seek professional health care. Others with an apparently similar level of impairment (e.g., pain and reduced spinal range of motion) enter the health care system episodically and for relatively short periods during symptom exacerbation. A minority with an apparently similar level of impairment enter the health care system and begin a downward spiral of distress, disability, and despair. Individuals at risk for chronic disability or poor treatment outcome are better identified by psychosocial than biomedical (impairment) factors. This is why practitioners must use an expanded biopsychosocial conceptual framework to appropriately understand and identify patients at risk of chronic disability and tailor treatment (including no treatment) appropriately.

Another issue with Nagi's model is the implied unidirectional progression from pathology through to disability. Although it is difficult to separate pathological processes (e.g., arthritis) from pathological consequences (disability), there is clearly a bidirectional interaction (Fig. 10-2). For example, osteoarthritis was long thought to cause joint stiffness, muscle weakness, and obesity. It is now evident that these problems are consequences of inactivity

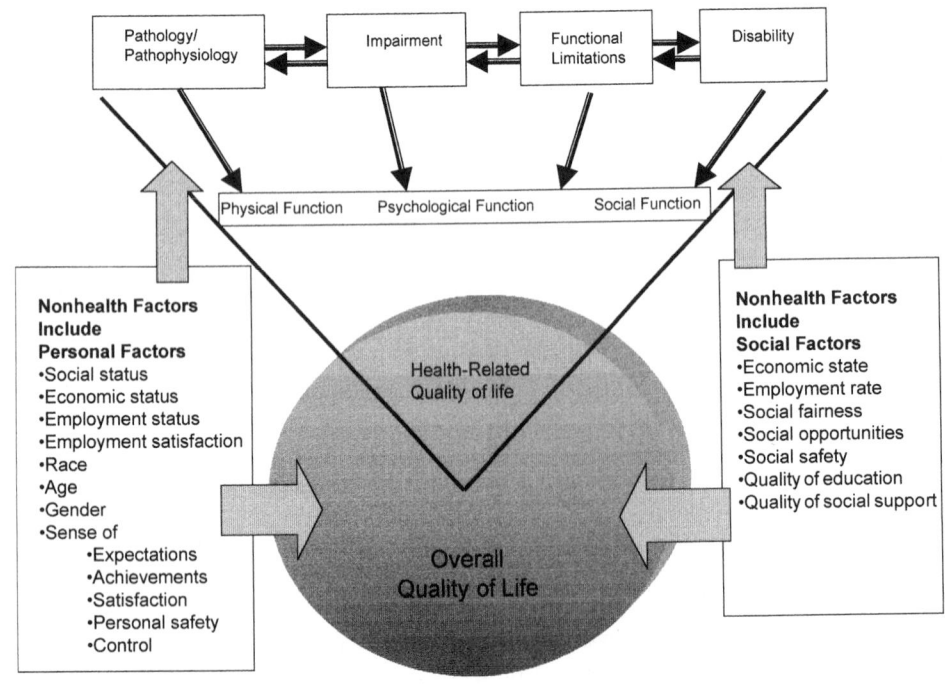

FIG. 10-2. An Expanded Model of Quality of Life (Adapted from American Physical Therapy Association Guide to Clinical Practice. *Phys Ther* 2001,81:1,pS25, with permission.)

Traditional Biomedical Model			Contemporary Biopsychosocial Model	
Nagi model	**Pathology**	**Impairment**	**Functional limitation**	**Disability**
Example measures	Diagnosis Spinal stenosis	Loss or abnormality ROM, pain	Task performance Walking speed	Role in society Ability to work or care for dependents
Assessment level and emphasis	Impact on part	Impact on part of person	Impact on whole person's ability	Impact on whole person in society
Management emphasis	Mobilize or strengthen part (e.g., back)	Activate and exercise person	Identify and address societal barriers	

FIG. 10-3. A Biopsychosocial Conceptual Model of Assessment. This model builds on Nagi's model of disablement and illustrates the conceptual basis for an expanded functional method of assessment.

secondary to arthritis rather than due to the disease process per se (14). More importantly, judicious exercise and activity is not harmful to joints and can promote health and wellness. Finally, it is worth remembering that although pathological processes, abilities, and disabilities contribute to health and quality of life, health-related constructs only represent a component of quality of life. Nevertheless, embedded within an expanded (health and nonhealth related) concept of quality of life, Nagi's disablement model provides a core framework on which to assess and manage patients with pain and dysfunction in a holistic manner (Fig. 10-3).

BIOPSYCHOSOCIAL ASSESSMENT

Pain is a complex, almost chaotic problem. The complex nature of pain mechanisms is well established at multiple levels—genetic to environmental (15). Moreover, an exponential increase in complexity is evident from the molecular level through the systems (e.g., neural, immune, psychological, and musculoskeletal) to the societal level, because the number of factors that can influence the pain experience is so much greater. For example, at the person level, the patient's personal experiences, attitudes, and beliefs influence the meaning and predict the consequences of the pain he or she perceives (albeit the meaning and predicted consequence may be inaccurate). At the societal level family, friends, co-workers, employers, and health care professionals respond to the individual with pain and further shape that person's pain experience.

In the therapeutic environment, health care practitioners add to the levels of complexity. They have a set of beliefs and attitudes about pain and patients with pain that they bring to the therapeutic encounter and thereby influence the therapeutic milieu. These beliefs may or may not be accurate and the attitudes may or may not be appropriate. Regardless, the complex nature of the pain, the patient, the practitioner, and the bidirectional interactions among them represent a challenge to understand, let alone manage. Assessment is the first step in understanding the problems of pain and of the person with chronic pain.

Rehabilitation Assessment

Pain and physical dysfunction are the primary reasons that patients present for therapy. They may also be angry, anxious, frustrated, and have little confidence in their physical ability. Improvement of physical function, reduction of pain, and correction of any catastrophic misconceptions about pain and injury are fundamental aspects of treatment.

Pain and physical dysfunction are both sources of psychosocial distress (16). Improvement in function can improve mood and thereby reduce the negative impact of pain. However, it is vital to separate the notions of pain, the behavior of the pain in relation to movement or mood, and the behavior (or lack thereof) of the individual with pain. Treatment decisions are based on the results of a clinical assessment. So, it is essential that the assessment measures are psychometrically sound (reliable, valid, and responsive) and useful in guiding and refining treatment. The measures must have clinical utility, be simple to use and interpret, and be meaningful to patient and practitioner.

Given that the goals of therapy in tertiary care focus on function, the primary purpose of the assessment is to characterize the functional status of the patient and then identify and address barriers (biological, psychological, or sociological) to functional improvement. The barriers should be identified through the clinical interview and assessment.

Clinical Interview

The clinical interview is standard practice and so will not be presented in detail. Discussion will focus only on specific aspects of the interview that are directly relevant to the management of patients with chronic disabling pain.

For example, individuals with pain have a variety of personal theories for their pain that are shaped by personal experience, culture, and education. These theories should be elicited during the clinical interview. Some of the theories or beliefs may be more appropriate than other ones, but complex beliefs about pain (right or wrong) may be difficult to change regardless of who holds them (practitioner or patient). Also, although all individuals hold beliefs about pain that include notions of blame and responsibility, the beliefs of patients and practitioners (alternative and traditional) tend to differ (17). Thus, therapists must explicitly elicit patient's pain beliefs because their own assumptions about the patient's beliefs are probably different from those of the patient.

Pither and Nicholas (5) found that patients' erroneous beliefs about pain and activity were shaped in part by unclear and incomplete explanations and advice given by health care practitioners. For example, patients with low back pain who are told that they have "disintegrating disks" may conjure such a worrisome image of their spine that they are fearful of any activity. In contrast, patients who are told that there "are no abnormalities observed" or (in the case of back pain) that range of motion is "normal" may be distressed because they think the practitioner is implying that there is nothing wrong with them. They are unlikely to know that pain can't be observed and the range of "normal" is highly variable and often has little to do with chronic pain. Unhelpful (possibly exaggerated) pain behaviors can result when distressed patients have to prove that they have pain.

Incomplete medical advice may also contribute to unhelpful behaviors. Patients may be told to "rest," but never told when or how to resume activity. Neher (18) neatly describes 12 guidelines for any health professional for assisting return to function with limited resources and limited time frame within an interdisciplinary team (Fig. 10-4). It is important to find out what a patient thinks about his or her problem and what the source of that information is. Apparently contradictory medical advice can add to feelings of distress and anxiety.

In addition to eliciting patients' pain beliefs, it is also worthwhile eliciting their treatment beliefs. Treatment beliefs of both patients and practitioners are shaped by a variety of factors, including past experience. Current treatment beliefs and expectations of outcome (both therapists' and patients') have a significant effect on actual outcome through nonspecific (placebo) means (19). *All* treatments have a nonspecific (placebo) effect. Only the magnitude of this effect varies and it may be 100% (20). Patients who are skeptical or fearful about the type of treatment offered are unlikely to benefit regardless of the specific physiological effect of the treatment. Given that treatment outcome is influenced by patients' expectations, it is well worth inquiring in this regard to reduce the frustrations of dealing with "failed treatments."

Clinical Assessment of Pain and Function

Despite the fact that patients' primary presenting problem is pain, it is the consequence of pain on function that is usually addressed through therapy in tertiary care. Although the level of pain alone will not dictate the type or the progression of therapy, it is important that pain is measured at assessment and outcome using standardized measures that are reliable and valid. Pain is a subjective phenomenon and, therefore, self-report is the primary form of assessment. Assessment should include a measure of pain intensity, pain affect, and pain distribution.

Pain

Pain intensity and pain affect can easily be measured using numeric rating scales (NRS) or visual analogue scales (VAS). Research studies provide support for the reliability, validity, and responsiveness of these measures (21). For a measure of pain intensity using the NRS, the individual is asked to select a number between 0 and 10 that best describes the intensity of the pain (i.e., 0 = no pain and 10 = most severe pain imaginable). The VAS consists of a 10 cm line with descriptors at the endpoints (e.g., 0 = no pain and 10 = most severe pain imaginable). The individual places a mark on this line and a level of pain intensity score is computed by measuring the distance from the 0 point to the mark made by the individual.

Twelve guidelines for health professionals working with patients with chronic pain (Neher, 1997).

1. Make clear the goal of therapy is to improve function, not reduce pain.
2. Increase the client's perception of control to reduce perceived helplessness.
3. Impact (emphasize and change) the client's attitudes and beliefs toward illness rather than focusing on symptoms.
4. Utilize an interdisciplinary team.
5. Avoid placing arbitrary physical limitations on the person that are not physiologic.
6. Encourage physical activity.
7. Simulate as closely as possible the types of occupations to which the individual hopes to return.
8. Eliminate high-tech equipment.
9. Decrease the use of analgesics, narcotics, and sedatives.
10. Encourage clients to discuss their pain only with people in a position to help.
11. Involve family and significant others.
12. Be mindful of the individual needs of the client.

FIG. 10-4. Twelve guidelines for health professionals working with patients with chronic pain. (From Neher BC. Chronic pain intervention: Promoting return to function. *Work* 1997;163–175, with permission.)

A second important dimension of the pain experience is pain affect. Pain affect refers to the unpleasantness of pain. It can be measured at the same time as pain intensity using 0 to 10 NRS or 10 cm VAS with different endpoint words. Endpoints for pain affect are 0 cm = not at all unpleasant and 10 cm = most unpleasant pain imaginable. Pain intensity and affect are related but some treatments can contribute to a reduction in pain affect rather than pain intensity (22, 23). Pain location is most easily assessed using a body map (i.e., an outline of a human figure) on which the individual is asked to shade the painful area.

Tests of Function

Traditionally, function was inferred from clinical tests of impairment. Recognition of the limited value of impairment in predicting function, especially in the case of chronic pain (24), led to a surge of interest in alternative and more direct methods of measuring function. These include equipment-intensive tests, physical performance batteries, and patient self-report measures.

Functional performance measures have complemented standard clinical assessments in specialized centers (e.g., functional restoration and pain management centers). However, many of these assessment batteries are center specific and equipment intensive (25). Moreover, the psychometric properties of the test batteries either are not known or are problematic. For example, isokinetic (constant velocity) and isoinertial (constant resistance) testing devices measure trunk strength and movement velocity and can provide information about muscle strength, endurance, power, and coordination in a dynamic manner. However, the constrained manner of testing is functionally unrealistic, implying that the relationship between the test results and functional activities is questionable, at best. Also, although the devices can accurately and reliably measure applied load from calibrated weights and velocity of movement, human performance on such devices is much less stable, especially in patient groups (26,27).

Sincerity of Function?

It is unfortunate that instability in patient performance has been misinterpreted as "insincerity of effort." The notion that variability in patient performance can be used as a "physical lie detector" persists in clinical practice despite the dearth of credible evidence supporting the simplistic view and some evidence that refutes the notion (28). Tasks that require high-velocity, dynamic performance are inherently less reliable (29). This is an interesting observation and important point. Variability in performance during a repeated movement is a characteristic of the task itself and not an indication of questionable patient motivation. In a controlled trial, Simmonds et al. (29) tested the reliability and validity of a battery of physical performance tasks for use as assessment and outcome measures in individuals with low back pain. Examination of the reliability results revealed an interesting phenomenon. The two tasks that involved repeated movements (repeated flexion and sit-to-stand) had relatively low levels of stability, especially in the patient group, suggesting that performance changed during the task. Physiological warm up is the most likely explanation because the speed of performance increases with repetitions, and the change is much more marked in those with back pain. However, it is also possible that performance improves because patients become less fearful of pain or reinjury.

Similar arguments hold regarding the misinterpretation and overinterpretation of the results of functional capacity evaluations. These evaluations have not received sufficient unbiased scrutiny by independent investigators. Yet they form the basis of clinical judgments of patients performing with "submaximal effort" or "insincere effort." These are egregious, value-laden terms that are unhelpful, indeed inappropriate, in a "therapeutic" environment. They can do the individual patient harm and leave him or her with no clear route back into work. They are seductive to practitioners because of their simplicity and because they can be used to "justify" and confirm a clinical bias. They don't consider the patient's previous experiences with attempted activity. And they don't consider psychosocial factors that mediate activity. Arguably, their use reveals more about the practitioner's sincerity than that of the patient. Watson (30) asserts that the evaluations don't necessarily predict success in return to work nor do they identify the most suitable occupation for the individual. Velozo (31) suggests that the focus should be on the actual work environment and the meaning of work to the person. Occupational therapy has an important role in linking work evaluations to psychosocial and environmental variables.

Physical Performance Tests. Nonetheless, as part of a multidimensional assessment battery, standardized performance protocols can provide information that can be useful in tailoring treatment appropriately. Performance batteries help identify what tasks or components of tasks are difficult. A more detailed assessment using valid measures can then help to identify why the tasks are difficult. The primary reason could be physical (e.g., weakness, stiffness, endurance), psychological (e.g., beliefs and concerns about activity and reinjury), or sociological (e.g., employment environment). Identification of the major problem areas should lead toward more appropriate management of problem. It is worth considering that the initiation, coordination, and successful completion of even the simplest of physical tasks is the result of a complex and dynamic interaction of neuromuscular, cardiovascular, cognitive, and emotional factors.

A useful approach to determining function in general clinical practice involves the use of a range of standardized tests of physical function that essentially sample the physical function construct. The tests must be simple, everyday tasks that are easy for the patient to perform so that motor learning is minimized. They must be easy to teach to patients, easy to measure, and easy to interpret. Useful clinical tests should require minimal equipment and the tasks must include those that are fundamental to day-to-day activity and that are compromised by the patient's problem. A myriad of activities can be sampled (e.g., lifting, bending, reaching, walking, rising from sitting, picking up small or large objects). The tests can be measured using the time taken to complete the set task or the distance walked or reached in the set time. Velocity and acceleration of motion is compromised in individuals with pain or other medical conditions (e.g., cancer and HIV/AIDS). In the case of back pain, individuals have difficulty controlling and adjusting to a constantly changing system of external and internal forces applied to the lumbar spine. Thus time taken or distance moved during a given time are simple measures that provide quantitative interval data. Depending on the patient's problem and on the research or clinical question, patients can be tested on one key task or on a battery of tasks.

A few investigators have examined the psychometric characteristics of simple physical performance batteries for patients with pain (29,32). In a series of studies, Simmonds and colleagues developed and tested a task battery of performance measures for patients with back pain that needs no special equipment (29,33–35). The battery has also been modified and used for patients with cancer and with AIDS. The tasks are described in Table 10-1 and shown in Figs.10.5A to 10.5D. The reliability (intra-, inter-rater, and day to day) is good to excellent for all tasks. The simplicity of the task (for the patient) and the method of measurement (for the therapist) clearly contribute to the high level of reliability. Validities (face, discriminative, convergent, construct) of the task battery have also been established (29,33–35). The battery has clinical utility because it is quick and simple to use and is acceptable to patients. Patients are simply asked to complete the task as quickly as possible, or to walk or reach as far as they can. There are no ceiling or floor effects with the battery.

Occupational therapists also use the Canadian Occupational Performance Measure (COPM) as an assessment tool, which allows patients to identify their own problems and later indicate their perceived progress (36). Other methods of testing specific task capacity include the Progressive, Isoinertial Lifting Evaluation (PILE). PILE is a standardized lifting protocol that is a fairly simple method of assessing a person's lifting capability, using relatively inexpensive and nonsophisticated equipment (a variety of weights, weight boxes, and shelves). The PILE protocol requires individuals to lift progressively increasing loads from floor to waist and waist to shoulder. Lifting continues until the subject stops due to pain or fatigue, or the subject reaches a specific aerobic goal or a predetermined "safe load" goal (26). Results are expressed as maximum weight lifted endurance or total time taken and final heart rate. Calculations of work and power consumption can also be made and normalized to body weight.

Self-report Measures of Function. Physical performance tasks essentially sample and measure a component of function. However, it is important to understand the functional problem from the patient's perspective. Thus, patient self-report measures are extremely important components of assessment and outcome. Moreover, everyday life involves the completion of a plethora of required and desired tasks. It would be impossible to test performance on all tasks in the clinical environment. Thus, standardized self-report questionnaires (SRQs) complement performance tasks and can address these issues. SRQs can sam-

TABLE 10-1. *Performance battery for patients*

Task	Procedure	Measure
Repeated Sit-to-Stand (Figure 5a)	Subjects rise to standing and return to sitting as quickly as possible five times. After a brief pause the task is repeated.	The average of the two task times is recorded.
Repeated Trunk Flexion (Figure 5b)	Subjects are timed as they bend forward to the limit of their range and return to the upright position as fast as tolerated five times. After a brief pause the task is repeated.	The average of the two task times is recorded.
Loaded Reach (Figure 5c and d)	Subjects stand next to a wall on which a meter rule is mounted horizontally at shoulder height. They hold a weight that is 5% of their body weight (up to maximum of 5kg) at shoulder height and close to the body and then reach forward.	Maximum distance reached in centimeters is recorded.
50-Foot Walk	Subjects walk 25 feet, turn around and walk back to start as fast as they can.	Time taken is recorded.
5-Minute Walk	Subjects walk as far and as fast as they can for 5 minutes.	Distance walked is recorded.
360° Rollover	Subjects lie supine on a treatment bed. They roll over 360° as fast as they can. After a brief pause, they roll 360° in the opposite direction.	The time to complete a rollover in both directions is summed and recorded.

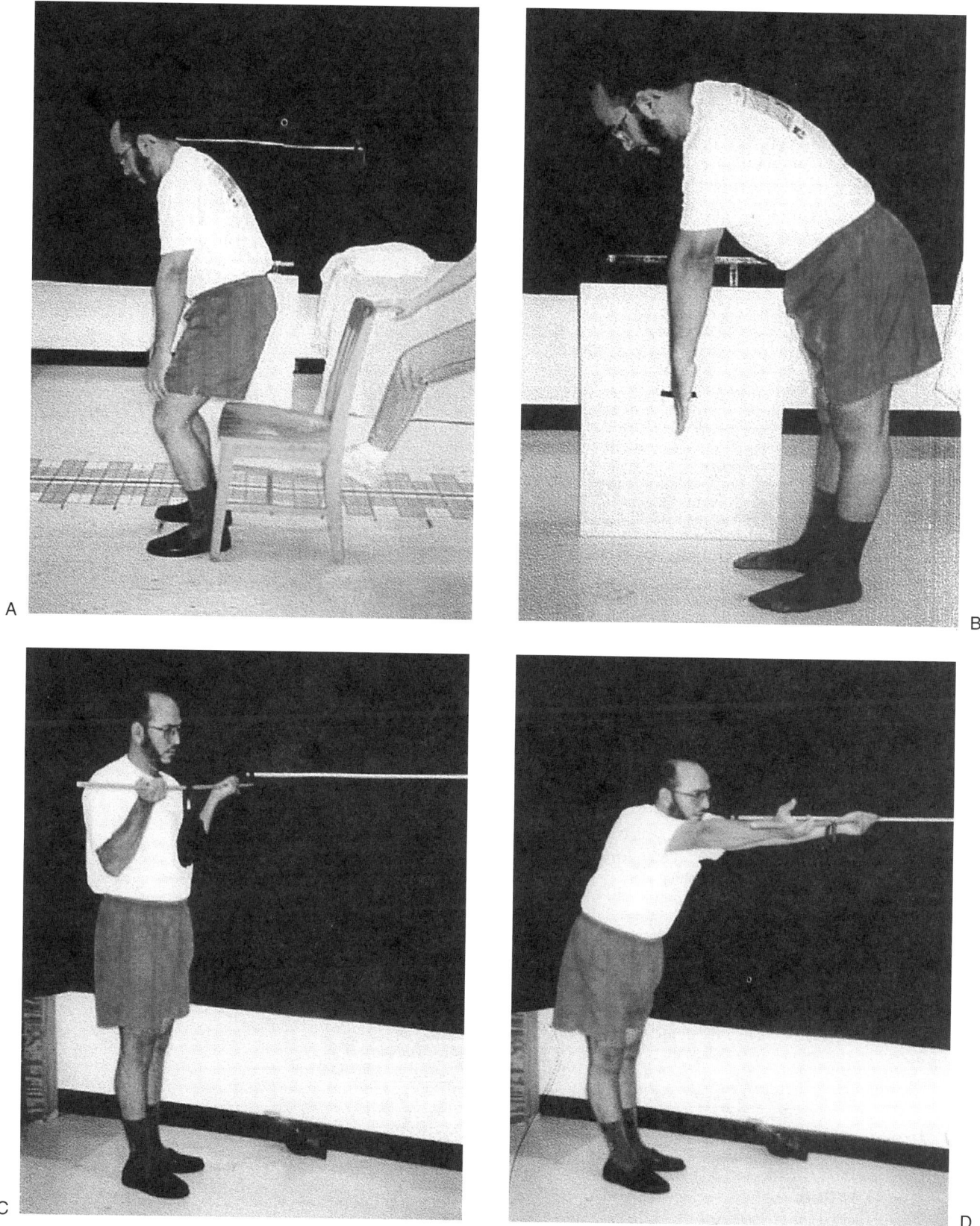

FIG. 10-5. Physical performance tests. **A.** Timed repeated sit-to-stand; **B.** Timed repeated trunk flexion; **C.** Loaded reach starting position; **D.** Loaded reach end position.

ple a range of different activities, including self-care, mobility, the performance of household chores, and other work-related activity. They can be relatively quick, simple, and practical to administer and score. They have been widely used, norms are available, and clearly they have superior face validity when compared to health professionals' *estimates* of function. Ideally objective outcome measures are employed in conjunction with self-report instruments to provide a multimethod assessment of clinical outcome (37).

Self-report of function may not be a valid reflection of a patient's actual functional status if an external reference is unavailable. Deyo and Centor (38) found the sickness impact profile (SIP) and the Roland and Morris scales to be more closely associated with other self-report measures of

functioning than with physical capabilities observed by clinicians. Also, despite its usefulness, self-report of physical function at best assesses only what the patient is conscious or aware of. Individuals have reporting biases, are likely to be reactive to situational demands, and vary in their memory and verbal ability (39). Semantics, physical need, and physical preferences also influence the estimate of function based on SRQ. For example, "Can you do (a specific activity)?" versus "Do you do (a specific activity)?" There may also be a mismatch between an individual's perception and therefore report of his or her activity and the actual activity. Sanders (40) demonstrated a poor correlation of self-report measures of uptime with more objective monitoring with mechanical recording devices. However, this inaccuracy of reporting is not purposeful exaggeration of

---

Guidelines for assessing the effect of pain on activity

1. Find out what activities have stopped or become limited because of pain. Prompt individuals to consider areas such as self-care, social, leisure, home duties, and work. Listen to determine if the individual reports difficulties with basic components of activity such as sitting, standing, walking, lying down, concentration, gripping, etc., and if the individual links these basic components to their problems with activities.
2. Ask individuals to keep a diary of all their activities for a week. This can be specific to home activities or just to work activities depending on the goal of treatment. Examine this diary for patterns of activity and rest, and for balance of activities, e.g., work, rest, and play.
3. Identify "innacurate cognitions" and beliefs such as pain controlling activity level, fear of doing harm through specific activities, a view of the future as the situation just getting worse. Listen for individuals rationalization for their pain problem, e.g., my pain was caused by keyboarding; it's my fault because . . .
4. Listen for hints as to how the family help and hinder the individual in managing their pain. Consider whether the family is unwittingly reinforcing pain and pain behaviors through overly solicitous behaviors.
5. Inquire about previous medical professionals' "explanations" of the problem (and unfulfilled promises of cures). What was the individual told and what was their interpretation of the "explanation," e.g., "I was told I was going to end up in a wheelchair," "I think something is stuck (in my back). They said it's degenerative but what good is that as I've only just turned 50 and have the rest of my life to lead."
6. What strategies does the individual now use to manage a level of activity and is it appropriate? For example, do they do tasks one day and rest the next, do they frantically do tasks in the morning when the pain feels at a relatively low level and then recline all afternoon and evening? Have they downgraded their expectation of what they can manage and in this way 'adjusted' to a life as a 'disabled person'?
7. Is the individual having difficulty with sleep? Likewise does that affect daytime activities and do they sleep (nap) during the day?
8. Does the individual have a frequent exacerbation of pain? What provokes it, e.g., activity, mood, or the "alignment of the stars"? What strategies does the individual use to manage the exacerbation? Are the strategies helpful, e.g., long periods of rest are usually detrimental?
9. Throughout any interaction with the individual notice but "ignore" inappropriate "pain behaviors." Be careful not to reinforce pain beliefs or behaviors by your own reactions, i.e., use "neutral" body language when individuals are describing effects of pain on activities. *Be aware that not all pain behaviors are inappropriate at all times and in all individuals.* Consider whether the "behavior" facilitates activity or function and whether it is a physical adaptation to impairment, e.g., an antalgic gait in individuals with sciatic pain.
10. Does the individual "wear" their pain and is it part of their identity? E.g., do they use corsets outside their clothes, collars, walking sticks, or use special cushions and seats in public places? Do they introduce their pain problem before their name?

FIG. 10-6. Guidelines for assessing the effect of pain on activity.

the problem. It has been shown that health care practitioners also have difficulties with such judgments of distance and time (Fig. 10-6).

Sharrack and Hughes (41) asked 100 physicians and 100 patients to estimate the dimensions of a hospital ward and the distances between five familiar sites. These estimates differed from the measured distance up to 14.6 fold, and the maximum estimates were up to 62.5 times greater than the minimum estimates. Time is also not easily estimated, and people find it difficult to say how long it took them to perform an activity or predict how long it will take them. This has implications for concurrent validity of self-report measures of function.

The two methods (performance and SRQ) measure different components of function so both should be used in clinical practice (33). SRQs can sample a wide range of tasks. In this regard, they can be exhaustive but also exhausting to complete. They can also be unnerving for individuals who don't read and write well. There are essentially three types of SRQ: global health, disease specific, and patient specific.

A global health survey such as the SF-36 is a multidimensional measure in common use and provides information related to physical and emotional health and bodily pain (42). Other SRQs are the Oswestry Disability Questionnaire (43) and the Roland and Morris Questionnaire (44); both are specific to individuals with back pain. Both the SF-36 and its shorter version, the SF-12, and the Roland and Morris Questionnaire have received extensive psychometric evaluation. The idiosyncrasy of patients' needs formed the basis for the development of an individualized method of measurement—individual patient preference questionnaires. A Patient Specific Functional Measure allows a person to identify one or more specific tasks that he or she is having difficulty performing. The patient grades his or her current ability to perform the desired task(s) at various points during the course of treatment, allowing the examiner to track progress. Preliminary work by Chatman et al. (45) has shown promising measurement properties. Patient Specific Functional Measures are particularly useful if there is a unique physical demand required of the patient, such as atypical occupational or sports-related tasks. It is important to note, however, that Patient Specific Functional Measures are intended for within-patient comparisons only and are not appropriate for comparing scores between different patients or groups of patients.

REHABILITATION THERAPIES

Properly conducted and interpreted, the assessment (clinical interview and performance and self-report measures) should identify what patients believe and what they know about their pain, what they can physically do, and what they have difficulty with and why. This information should direct treatment. And the assessment measures will provide standardized baseline measures that can be used to evaluate the effectiveness of treatment and help refine further treatment. *The overarching aim of therapy must be to encourage independence and self-management by the patient.* Therapists must engage, educate, and empower the patient to adopt a long-term lifestyle of health and well-being through activity. Passive treatment (modalities and mobilizations) may encourage dependence. If there is a specific indication for their use, they should be used on a time-limited basis. Also modalities such as heat can be applied by the patient him/herself.

Rehabilitation strategies must be individualized to optimize improvement in physical function, but there are many common elements especially in regards to increasing activity. *The single best rehabilitation exercise/activity is that which is done.* Patients must participate actively in the education process, in the decision-making process, and in physical activity.

Education

Chronic pain and disability is managed, not cured. Education can empower patients to cope with and better manage their pain and physical dysfunction. Patients require good information to assist them in making decisions, overcoming unhelpful beliefs, and initiating or resuming an active lifestyle. Therapists must address concerns that the patient has that may inhibit rehabilitation. These include:

1. Lack of a specific diagnosis or the meaning of explanations such as "wear and tear" or "no observable abnormality."
2. An inability to relate a tissue-based diagnosis to a multifactorial persistent, distressing, and disabling problem.
3. Misunderstanding about the influence of psychological factors on pain.
4. Misunderstandings about the relationships among tissue injury, pain, and activity level.

Goal Setting

Rehabilitation goals and expectations must be discussed and mutually agreed upon between therapist and patient. The patient should participate actively in negotiating goals that are given priority and are at the center of the assessment, intervention, and evaluation (1). The goals must be appropriate and achievable and should be set in areas of social and recreational activity, self-care, occupation, and even psychological functioning. The use of goal-setting charts can be helpful so that progress (which may be slow) can be seen.

Goal setting allows development of a sense of purpose and gives a baseline for reviewing progress (46). Schmitz et al. (47) describe two types of goal setting for coping with chronic pain. These are *flexible goal adjustment* and *tenacious goal pursuit*. The former protects patients with chronic pain from pain-related distress and helps them maintain a positive life perspective. Flexible goal adjustment involves periodic downgrading of aspirations, positive reappraisal, and self-enhancing comparisons. Tenacious goal pursuit is a less successful strategy. It involves active attempts to alter unsatisfactory life circumstances and situational constraints in accordance with personal preference. Unfortunately, some of life's circumstances are beyond personal control, so the strategy is destined to lead to frustration.

Establishing specific, challenging, but attainable, goals can actually facilitate task performance. An outcome tool useful for the measurement of qualitative change and low levels of achievement through goal setting is Goal Attainment Scaling (GAS), which was first developed in 1968 (48). It requires the selection of observable and repeatable goals, the specification of conditions under which performance is measured, criteria for success stated in measurable terms, and goals achieved within specified time limits (49). One advantage of the GAS is in the gradation of five possible outcomes, rather than a simple dichotomous "success or failure" option for each goal (48).

Improvements in task performance result from self-confidence in one's ability to meet expectations. Self-confidence (efficacy) may be the most potent determinant of change during rehabilitation (50). Individuals can be taught to identify specific obstacles to each goal and set measurable, realistic, achievable, and time-limited short-term goals toward a larger long-term goal. Confidence is often low when tackling new goals or returning to previously abandoned activities. However, if patients can be helped to attempt an activity that was previously feared and complete the activity, this can reinforce their self-efficacy.

Poor task performance, decreased motivation, and a sense of failure can result from repeatedly failing to achieve unrealistic goals. Thus, it can be useful to break down large goals into smaller components that are achievable in the short term. Group settings can be useful as problem solving can be encouraged. In this setting it is important that therapists don't provide answers to individuals in this process. Rather, they should lead the discussion around problems and allow individual patients to experience successful problem solving.

Activity Pacing

Individuals with chronic pain often have a history that includes a pattern of over- and underactivity cycles. Pacing of activity is aimed to even out the peaks and troughs of activity that are controlled by pain (36,50). Pacing requires that activities be structured and regulated by a factor other than pain (e.g., time or the introduction of exercise/activity quotas). It is anticipated that a gradual and controlled increase in activity will help prevent a sudden increase in pain and consequent reduction in activity. Individuals can record their progress for specific activities and improvements can be reinforced with contingent praise or self-reinforcement (e.g., an achievement diary). Regular review of goals and achievements should be conducted. Individuals are encouraged to develop their own set of activity pacing principles, for example:

1. Break tasks up into smaller amounts.
2. Take regular short rests.
3. Change position regularly.
4. Plan and prioritize activities.
5. Set a baseline for a specific activity and gradually increase it.

Finally, pacing is a means of achieving a goal of increased activity. It should not be separated from efforts to increase activity in a measured way (51).

Exercise and Activity

Patients with chronic pain and disability are assumed to be deconditioned and thus reconditioning exercise and activity programs make perfect rehabilitation sense. Recent experimental evidence has questioned the veracity of this clinical assumption (52). Moreover, the majority of individuals in the United States are deconditioned but are not disabled by pain. Thus, physical condition, pain, and disability are separate problems. There may or may not be a strong relationship let alone a causal relationship between these constructs. Nevertheless, physical exercise and activity provides health benefits and improves mood and function, so its extensive use in rehabilitation of patients with chronic pain is justified.

Physical activity is an umbrella term that includes concepts such as fitness, exercise, training, and conditioning. Essentially, any bodily movement that increases energy expenditure above the resting level is physical activity. Exercise is frequently used interchangeably with physical activity. However, exercise and exercise training is purposeful activity specifically designed to improve or maintain a particular component of physical fitness (e.g., flexibility, strength, or endurance—cardiovascular or musculoskeletal).

A variety of different forms of exercise and exercise regimens are used and each have their supporters. However, the scientific evidence supporting the rationale or effectiveness of specific regimens, especially in chronic pain, is weaker than the assertions of the proponents. The problems are that patients are heterogeneous; exercise varies in type, intensity, and duration; patient's adherence to exercise is problematic especially in the long term; and a variety of different outcome measures are used.

The general types of exercise include aerobic exercise, specific strengthening and mobilizing exercise, and exercise to promote specific activation and reeducation of key muscle groups. Exercise programs often combine strength training, stretching, and/or fitness. But perhaps *the most effective exercise or activity regimen is that which the patient does.* In that regard, patient preference is one of the most important considerations. Exercise regimens, regardless of the type, should be regular and should gradually increase in intensity and duration. Adherence is greatest if the exercise/activity is easily incorporated into the patient's lifestyle and is an activity that he or she enjoys.

It is interesting that for individuals with chronic back pain, barriers to, and motivators of, physical activity are similar to those in the general population and probably similar to those of most health care providers (e.g., lack of time, inclement weather, and family commitments) (52). It is also interesting that chronic back pain problems are identified as both barriers to, and motivators of, activity. Some individuals believe that being more physically active helps ease their back pain and makes them feel better. They worry about stopping exercise for fear that their back pain will return. Some patients do not exercise on a regular basis but resume exercise when reminded to by their backache. Still others avoid physical activity for fear of an aggravation of back pain (53). Although all subjects identified the avoidance of some physical activity (e.g., lifting and gardening), not all were fearful or anxious about such activity. It appears that those individuals not fearful or anxious about physical activity reported that their confidence was restored over time through reassurance and advice from health professionals; modifying the way an activity was done (e.g., less vigorous); and a progressive exercise program (53). It also appears that a change in behavior can lead to a change in belief about the ability to be active.

Exercise behavior is difficult to change but motivation and counseling can help. Friedrich and colleagues (54) conducted a double-blind, randomized study and evaluated the effect of a motivation program on exercise adherence and disability. Ninety-three patients with low back pain (LBP) were randomly assigned to either a standard exercise program (n = 49) group or a combined exercise and motivation group (n = 44). The exercise program consisted of an individual, submaximal, gradually increased training session. Each patient was prescribed ten sessions that each lasted about 25 minutes. The specific exercises were aimed at "improving spinal mobility, as well as trunk and lower limb muscle length, force, endurance, and coordination." The motivation program consisted of five sessions that included counseling, providing information about LBP and exercise, reinforcement, and forming a treatment contract between patient and practitioner. The combined exercise and motivation group increased the rate of exercise adherence and reduced disability and pain in the short term (4 and 12 months). However, there was no difference in exercise adherence in the long term. Long-term adherence to exercise is an acknowledged problem in the general population and is no different in those with pain.

In the case of chronic pain, exercise benefits may not be immediate or even apparent, and recurrence of pain is inevitable, so it is hardly surprising that adherence to exercise is problematic. For some individuals, encouraging and facilitating them to have a more active lifestyle may be more useful than prescribing exercises that aren't done. For example, individuals can be encouraged to avoid using "drive through" services and walk into the business facility instead; walk across the car park rather than drive around looking for the closest parking space; and use stairs rather than an elevator when going up one flight of stairs. General activity that is done is much more beneficial than a specific exercise regimen that is not.

A number of studies have shown that individuals in exercise programs do better than control subjects. However, there is really no clear indication of the superiority of any specific exercise regimen facilitating resumption of normal activity, and whether the specific mechanisms of effects are biological, psychological, sociological, or all of the above. Certainly, the wide variability in treatment regimens and treatment effects makes it difficult to tease out the mechanisms of effect. For example, the Paris Task Force (55) reviewed ten scientifically rigorous randomized controlled trials of exercise for chronic back pain. They reported that patients in the exercise group had improved function in seven of the ten trials. However, the regimens were characterized by variability of type, intensity, and duration, and some regimens also included education and/or behavior modification.

For example, Frost et al. (56) tested a supervised general fitness program. Eighty-one individuals with chronic LBP were randomized to a fitness program or a control group. Both groups were taught exercises and attended an educational program on LBP. The exercise group also attended eight sessions of a supervised fitness program that extended over 4 weeks. Cognitive behavioral principles and a normal model of human behavior, rather than a disease model, was followed. Participants were encouraged to compare themselves to a sports participant who had been laid off from training and who needed to get back to previous activity level. They were also reminded that unaccustomed exercise might lead to muscle aches, and that pain and injury (hurt and harm) was not synonymous. Finally, participants were encouraged to improve their own performance record (not compete with others) and to complete an activity diary. A mean reduction of 7.7% (pain and disability) was obtained in the exercise group compared to a 2.4% reduction in the control group. This difference was statistically significant and was maintained at the 2-year follow-up. However, the authors note that the confidence interval of the differences between groups was large, indicating a wide variation in treatment effect.

It is not surprising that in studies comparing relatively active to relatively passive interventions, the active intervention appears more effective. However, in a recent study, Mannion and colleagues (57) compared three active therapies for chronic LBP. One hundred and forty-eight subjects were randomly assigned to an active physiotherapy program, a muscle-reconditioning program using training devices, or a low-impact aerobics program. Subjects attended their program twice a week for 3 months. All programs led to a reduction in pain and disability that were maintained at 6 months. There were no differences among groups, suggesting a lack of treatment specificity.

In summary, it appears that the specific type of exercise or exercise regimen is much less important than once thought. Although the notion may be an anathema to therapists entrenched in a structurally focused biomedical (impairment) model, it is less surprising to those who recognize the biopsychosocial nature of chronic LBP. Exercises targeted at a specific musculoskeletal impairment may affect changes in impairment but the actual impairment may contribute relatively little to the individual's problem of pain and disability. Although speculative at present, it is plausible to suggest that exercise is beneficial for those with chronic pain because it reduces psychosocial distress (40), leads to improvement in mood, reduces anxieties about the chronic pain, and changes the perception of self as disabled. Thus, the primary benefits of exercise or activity for individuals with chronic pain may be central rather than peripheral or structural.

Modalities

Modalities are defined as the use of physical energy or agents for therapeutic effect. Physical modalities commonly used include heat, ice, massage, ultrasound, electrical stimulation, mobilization, and manipulation. Physical modalities have a long history of use in rehabilitation. They are primarily used in pain management to provide symptomatic relief. Electrical (neuromuscular stimulation) modalities may be used to help reeducate muscle activity. Within the professional education of physical therapists, pain is most commonly taught within the context of a modalities course (8). The implied message, therefore, is that modalities are appropriate treatments in pain management. In the case of acute pain, or in acute flare-ups of chronic pain, that may be true. However, the long-term use of passive modalities in chronic pain is less useful, though not necessarily useless, and not necessarily harmful either.

In a recent review of physical therapy and physical modalities for the control of chronic pain of musculoskeletal origin, Feine and Lund (58) found no evidence that any specific therapy was more effective, in the long term, than placebo treatment. Yet, they also reported that placebo treatments were usually more effective than no treatment. And, patients who had more treatment did better than those who had less treatment. So how is this "nontreatment" helpful and what are the mechanisms of this effect?

Modalities, especially heat, ice, massage, and transcutaneous electrical nerve stimulation (TENS) may decrease pain in the short term. They are associated with patient satisfaction, indeed expectation, they do have nonspecific (placebo) effects, and may have additional specific physiological effects.

The problem is, placebo treatments are not bereft of effects and these effects may be malevolent as well as benevolent. For example, the individual may become more dependent on the therapist and may be financially exploited when they are at their most vulnerable. Moreover, repeated treatment failures or inappropriate treatments can compound the patients' distress, anxiety, anger, and frustration (19). Wall (59) argues that it is not appropriate to use placebo treatments. He suggests that when patients chose a faith healer they expect treatments based on faith. If, however, they seek help from traditional medicine they expect those treatments to have a rational,

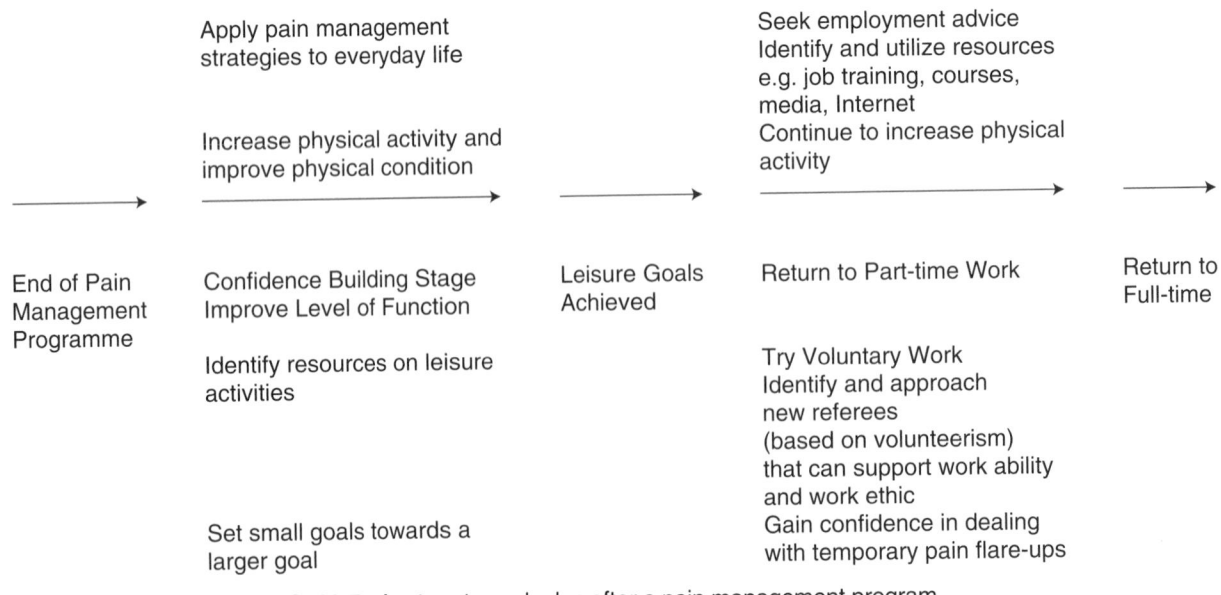

FIG. 10-7. A return to work plan after a pain management program.

tested, scientific basis. Thus, if practitioners utilize placebo treatments, they are capitalizing on patients' expectations, created by the reputation and successes of traditional medicine.

In a recent review of the evidence on exercise and modalities, Nordin and Campello (60) conclude that there is no evidence of efficacy, but high patient satisfaction, with their use. They suggest that one way to resolve the dilemma is to teach the patient self-application of modalities for short-term pain relief. They also suggest that patients should be informed that modalities have low efficacy and that a more active treatment leads to better long-lasting effects. This solution essentially addresses the main position within this chapter. That is, the importance of providing accurate information to patients, educating and empowering them to make decisions about their health (and ill health), and managing their pain and disability (Fig. 10-7).

CONCLUSION

Changes in rehabilitation practice have resulted from the recognition that activity has positive effects physiologically, psychologically, and socially. Therefore, there is now a much greater emphasis on activity in rehabilitation regimens. In this regard, the therapist's role is primarily to work with the client to identify and address perceived and actual barriers to activity. It is noteworthy that potential and actual barriers to activity are plentiful and are used regularly by able-bodied physicians and therapists. Patients with pain simply have to deal with additional pain-related barriers and may need more help in overcoming them.

Finally, and in common with many medical practices, critical appraisal of the evidence supporting many therapies has revealed quite large gaps in knowledge, some erroneous assumptions, and a lack of evidence of effectiveness of some therapies despite their widespread use and strong clinical assertions of effectiveness. Critical appraisal has been perceived as a threat. However, a threat is also a challenge and an opportunity to change and improve therapeutic practices. The practice of evidence-based rehabilitation has begun and is expected to impact and improve therapists and therapies and foster a better understanding of how, why, and when therapists and therapies are effective for patients with pain and dysfunction.

REFERENCES

1. Sumison T. A revised OT definition of client-centred practice. *Br J Occup Ther* 2000;63(7):304–308.
2. Howard M. *Investing in disabled people: a strategy from welfare to work.* Disablement Income Group: Joseph Rowntree Foundation, 1997.
3. Croft P. *Editorial low back pain.* Oxford: Radcliffe Medical Press, 1997.
4. Wahlgren DR, Atkinson JH, Epping-Jordan JE, et al. One-year follow-up of first onset low back pain. *Pain* 1997;73:213–221.
5. Pither CE, Nicholas MK. The identification of iatrogenic factors in the development of chronic pain syndromes: abnormal treatment behavior? In: Bond MR, Charlton JE, Woolf CJ, eds. *Proceedings of the VIth world congress on pain.* Elsevier Science Publishers, 1991. BV.429–434.
6. Gallagher RM. Primary care and pain medicine. *Medical Clinics of North America* 1999;83(3):555–583.
7. Strong J, Tooth L, Unruh A. Knowledge about pain among newly graduated occupational therapists: relevance for curriculum development. *Can J Occup Ther* 1999;66(5):221–228.
8. Scudds RJ, Scudds RA, Simmonds MJ. Pain in the physical therapy curriculum: a faculty survey. *Physiother Theory and Practice.* In Press.
9. Jensen MP, Romano JM, Turner JA, Good AB, Wald LH. Patient beliefs predict patient functioning: further support for a cognitive-behavioural model of chronic pain. *Pain* 1999;81:95–104.
10. Mayers CA. The Casson memorial lecture 2000: reflect on the past to shape the future. *Br J Occup Ther* 2000;63(8):358–366.
11. Vlaeyen JW, de Jong J, Geilen M, et al. Graded exposure in vivo in the treatment of pain-related fear: a replicated single-case experimental design in four patients with chronic low back pain. *Behav Res Ther* 2001 Feb;39(2):151–166.
12. World Health Organization. International classification of impairments, disabilities and handicaps. WHO: Geneva, 1980.
13. Nagi SZ. Disability concepts revisited: implications for prevention. In: Pope AM, Tarlov AR eds. *Disability in america: toward a national agenda for prevention.* Washington, DC: Division of Health Promotion and Disease Prevention, Institute of Medicine, National Academy Press 1991:309–327.
14. Jordan J, Kington R, Lane N, et al. Systemic risk factors for osteoarthritis. In: Felson DT, osteoarthritis: new insights. Part 1: The disease and its risk factors. *Ann Intern Med* 2000;133:637–639.
15. Gifford L. The patient in front of us: from genes to environment. In: Gifford L, ed. *Topical issues in pain 2.* Physiotherapy Pain Association CNS Press: Falmouth 2000:1–12.
16. Simmonds MJ, Kumar S, Lechelt E. Psychosocial factors in low back pain: causes or consequences? *Dis Rehab* 1996;18:(4)161–168.
17. Eccleston C, Williams CdeC, Stainton R W. Patients' and professionals' understandings of the causes of chronic pain: blame, responsibility and identity protection. *Soc Sci Med* 1997;45(5):699–709.
18. Neher BC. Chronic pain intervention: promoting return to function. *Work* 1997;9:163–175.
19. Simmonds MJ. Pain and placebo: the benevolent lie? *Phys Ther* 2001; 86:631–637.
20. Simmonds MJ, Kumar S. Pain and the placebo in rehabilitation. *Dis Rehab* 1993;16:(1) 13–20.
21. Jensen MP, Karoly P. Self-report scales and procedures for assessing pain in adults. In: Turk DC, Melzack R, eds. *Handbook of pain assessment.* New York: Guilford Press, 1992:135–151.
22. Simmonds MJ, Claveau Y. Measures of pain and physical function in patients with low back pain. *Physiotherapy Theory and Practice* 1997: 13:53–65.
23. Marchand S, Charest J, Chenard JR, et al. Is TENS a placebo effect? A controlled study on chronic low back pain. *Pain* 1993;45: 99–106.
24. Waddell G. A new clinical model for the treatment of low back pain. *Spine* 1987;12:632–644.
25. Mayer TG, Gatchel RJ. Functional restoration for spinal disorders: the sports medicine approach. Philadelphia: Lea and Feibiger, 1988.
26. Pope MH. A critical evaluation of functional muscle testing. In: Weinstein JN, ed. *Clinical efficacy and outcome in the diagnosis and treatment of low back pain.* Raven Press: New York 1992:101–113.
27. Newton M, Thow M, Somerville D, et al. Trunk strength testing with Iso-machines. Part 2: Experimental evaluation of the Cybex II back testing system in normal subjects and patients with chronic low back pain. *Spine* 1993;18(7):812–824.
28. Lechner DE, Bradbury SF, Bradley L. Detecting sincerity of effort: a summary of methods and approaches. *Phys Ther* 1998;78:867–888.
29. Simmonds MJ, Olson SL, Jones SC, et al. Psychometric characteristics and clinical usefulness of physical performance tests in patients with low back pain. *Spine* 1998;23(22):2412–2421.
30. Watson P. Maintenance of change and skill enhancement. In: Main CJ, Spanswick CC, eds. *Pain management.* Churchill Livingstone: Edinburgh 1999:329–333.
31. Velozo CA. Work evaluations: critique of the state of the art of functional assessment of work. *Am J Occup Ther* 1993;47(3)203–209.

32. Harding VR, Williams ACdeC, Richardson PH, et al. The development of a battery of measures for assessing physical functioning of chronic pain patients. *Pain* 1994;58(3):367–375.

33. Lee CE, Simmonds MJ, Novy DM, Jones SC. A comparison of self-report and clinician measured physical function among patients with low back pain. *Archives of Physical Medicine and Rehabilitation* 2001; 82:227–231.

34. Novy DM, Simmonds MJ, Olson S, Lee CE. Gender differences in physical performance in individuals with and without low back pain. *Archives of Physical Medicine and Rehabilitation* 1999;80: 195–198.

35. Novy DM, Simmonds MJ, Lee CE. Physical performance tasks: what are the underlying constructs? *Arch Archives of Physical Medicine and Rehabilitation* 2001; In press.

36. Strong J. *Chronic pain—the occupational therapist's perspective*. Edinburgh: Churchill Livingstone, 1996.

37. Klapow JC, Slater MA, Patterson TL, et al. An empirical evaluation of multidimensional clinical outcome in chronic low back pain patients. *Pain* 1993;55: 107–118.

38. Deyo RA, Centor RM. Assessing the responsiveness of functional scales to clinical change: an analogy to diagnostic test performance. *J Chron Diseases* 1986;39:897–906.

39. Craig KD, Prkachin KM, Gruneau RVE. The facial expression of pain. In: Turk DC, Melzack R, eds. *Handbook of pain assessment*. Guilford Press, 1992:257–276.

40. Sanders SH. Automated versus self-monitoring of 'up-time' in chronic low-back pain patients: a comparative study. *Pain* 1983;15: 399–405.

41. Sharrack B, Hughes RAC. Reliability of distance estimation by doctors and patients: cross sectional study. *BMJ* 1997;315:1652–1654.

42. Ware J, Sherbourne C. The MOS 36-item short form health survey (SF-36). *Med Care* 1992;30:473.

43. Fairbank JCT, Couper J, Davies JB, O'Brien JP. The Oswestry low back pain disability questionnaire. *Physiotherapy* 1980;66:271–273.

44. Roland M, Morris R. A study of the natural history of back pain. Part I: development of a reliable and sensitive measure of disability in low-back pain. *Spine* 1983;8:141–144.

45. Chatman AB, Hyams SP, Neel JM, et al. The patient-specific functional scale: measurement properties in patients with knee dysfunction. *Phys Ther* 1997;77:820–829.

46. Sutton J. *Problem solving and goal setting*. Romsey: JPS Publishing, 1995.

47. Schmitz U, Saile H, Nigles P. Coping with chronic pain: flexible goal adjustment as an interactive buffer against pain-related distress. *Pain* 1996;67(1):41–51.

48. Stanley B. Evaluation of treatment goals: the use of goal attainment scaling. *J Adv Nur* 1984;9:351–356.

49. Palisano RJ. Validity of goal attainment scaling in infants with motor delays. *Phys Ther* 1993;73(10):651–658.

50. Harding V, Simmonds MJ, Watson P. Physical therapy for chronic pain. *Clinical Update, International Association for the Study of Pain*. 1998;6:3,1–4.

51. Nielson WR, Jensen MP, Hill ML. An activity pacing scale for the chronic pain coping inventory: development in a sample of patients with fibromyalgia syndrome. *Pain* 2001;89:111–115.

52. Wittink H, Hoskins MT, Wagner A, et al. Deconditioning in patients with chronic low back pain: fact or fiction? *Spine* 2000;25:2221–2228.

53. Keen S, Dowell AC, Hurst K, et al. Individuals with low back pain: how do they view physical activity? *Fam Prac* 1999;16:39–45.

54. Friedrich M, Gittler G, Halberstadt Y, et al. Combined exercise and motivation program: effect on the compliance and level of disability of patients with chronic low back pain: a randomized controlled trial. *Arch Phys Med Rehabil* 1998 May;79(5):475–87.

55. Abenhaim L, Rossignol M, Valat JP, et al. The role of activity in the therapeutic management of back pain. Report of the International Paris Task Force on back pain. *Spine* 2000 Feb 15;25(4 Suppl): 1S–33S.

56. Frost H, Lamb SE, Klaber-Moffett JA, et al. A fitness programme for patients with chronic low back pain: 2-year follow-up of a randomized controlled trial. *Pain* 1998;75:273–279.

57. Mannion AF, Muntener M, Taimela S, Dvorak J. A randomized clinical trial of three active therapies for chronic low back pain. *Spine* 1999;24:2435–2448.

58. Feine JS, Lund JP. An assessment of the efficacy of physical therapy and physical modalities for the control of chronic musculoskeletal pain. *Pain* 1997;71:5–23.

59. Wall PD, The placebo and placebo response. In: Wall PD, Melzack R, eds. *Textbook of pain 3rd ed*. New York: Churchill Livingstone, 1994

60. Nordin M, Campello M. Physical therapy. Exercises and the modalities: when, what and why? *Neurologic Clinics* 1999;17:76–89.

CHAPTER 11

Neuroaxial Opioid Therapy

Y. Eugene Mironer

Neuroaxial opioids were introduced into practice in 1979, when Wang et al. (1) demonstrated pain relief with an intraspinal bolus of morphine. Since that time this modality of pain treatment has achieved widespread recognition and popularity around the world (2). Neuroaxial opioids have been successfully used to treat pre-, intra-, and post-operative pain, as well as chronic malignant and nonmalignant pain (3).

Despite vast clinical experience and data there is no firm scientific proof that neuroaxial opioids provide analgesia superior to systemic opioids (2–4). There are, however, some indisputable advantages of the neuroaxial route of delivery: It lacks motor, sensory, or sympathetic effects with analgesia and uses significantly lower doses, which lead to a lower incidence of side effects than with conventional therapy (3,5). Some of the opioids also provide significantly longer pain relief when administered epidurally or intrathecally (2).

Epidural and subarachnoid methods of drug delivery have their advantages and disadvantages (3). Unfortunately, currently used, totally implantable systems are designed primarily for intrathecal delivery because the epidural route requires significantly higher doses, which translate into frequent refills of the reservoir. Externalized devices, epidural or intrathecal, should be limited to a relatively short duration of therapy due to the increased possibility of infection. For practical purposes we will discuss intrathecal opioid therapy because it is a more prevalent method of treating chronic pain.

PATIENT SELECTION

Patient selection is the key to success in neuroaxial opioid therapy. It is imperative to remember that this modality is part of a pain treatment continuum and occupies a specific place in the analgesic ladder (6,7). Only patients who have been tried previously with strong opioids should be considered for neuroaxial opioid therapy. The use of destructive neuroablative procedures should be utilized only after failure of neuroaxial opioids in patients with chronic nonmalignant pain (4,8), whereas in cancer patients they may sometimes precede it.

There is only one indication for the trial of neuroaxial opioids: chronic intractable pain that has failed conventional opioid treatment due to lack or loss of efficacy and/or intolerable side effects from systemic opioids. There are relatively few contraindications—coagulopathy, sepsis, infection of the CNS or the operative area, and obstruction to CSF circulation. There are certain important considerations that play a role in the decision for neuroaxial opioid therapy. In cancer patients, a life expectancy of less than 3 months is not a contraindication to this modality as is often stated (9), but rather an indicator for the use of externalized devices instead of a totally implantable system. The reason for this is the cost concerns (10). The same decision sometimes has to be made due to extreme cachexia, preventing implantation of the reservoir.

In chronic nonmalignant pain, psychological evaluation is extremely important in successful selection of candidates for neuroaxial opioid therapy (6,11). There are no firm guidelines as to the type of psychological tests that need to be applied to pain patients. Neither are there stringent psychological selection criteria for patient selection for implantation of drug delivery systems (12). The majority of research in this area, for some reason, is concentrated mainly around implantation of spinal cord stimulators rather than intrathecal pumps. There are, however, a few clear suggestions pertaining to testing that are applicable to any potential candidate for implantation: It should be performed by an experienced pain psychologist, and excessive depression, somatization, or secondary gains should be ruled out (12,13). Some of the existing psychological tests, such as the MMPI-2, are not oriented toward chronic pain patients (14). Others, such as the Beck

Depression Inventory or Multidimensional Pain Inventory, lack validity scales (14). In our practice we successfully use the Pain Patient Profile (P-3) (14,15). It not only is pain patient oriented and has validity scales, but also it is fairly short, taking only about 15 minutes for completion (14). Close correlation of P-3 results with the MMPI-2 has been shown (16).

TRIAL

There are several ways of performing the preimplant trial: single injection versus infusion and epidural versus intrathecal. The single-injection method is unfortunately very popular, and more than half of all trials are performed with this method (17). In our opinion, this method is significantly less reliable than continuous infusion. First, a placebo response can interfere with the reported results of a single injection much more than with a more prolonged trial. Second, with a single injection trial patients do not have a chance to be exposed to different types of daily activities such as sleeping, resting, walking, standing, walking up the stairs, etc. Finally, there is no opportunity for titration of the dose, which can be inadequate with a single injection. We suggest that all candidates for neuroaxial treatment of chronic pain should receive a trial infusion of the opioid that has been selected for long-term use.

There is no clear consensus as to the advantage of using the epidural or intrathecal route for the infusion trial (6,9). If the planned treatment will be by the epidural route, then obviously the trial should also be by epidural infusion. For planned intrathecal delivery, both trial methods are acceptable. Epidural infusion reduces the risk of postdural puncture headache, and it is easier to titrate. The intrathecal route more closely reproduces future treatment and is easier technically. In certain cases, i.e., multiple spine surgeries, intrathecal infusion is the only available option. In our practice we are using both methods of testing: epidural and intrathecal infusion. Some authors empirically suggest a higher incidence of adverse effects with the epidural route (9). Our experience does not support this suggestion. Of interest, in two cases in our practice, patients did not have pruritus during epidural infusion of morphine but experienced it after morphine started to be delivered intrathecally via the implanted pump. A recent study showed no difference between the two methods, except cost effectiveness, which was better for the intrathecal trial (18).

Duration of the trial ranges from one day to months and is being performed both as an inpatient or outpatient procedure (6,9,12,19). Ambulatory settings reduce the cost but increase the risk due to lack of continuous observation of the patient. Lengthy outpatient trials eventually will be even more expensive than a relatively short trial in the hospital setting. Some authors even use a control placebo infusion (19). Neither increased length of the trial, nor

have additional attempts at "blinding" it ever been proven more efficacious or more selective (6,12). In our practice we use a 24–48-hour trial on an inpatient basis. If side effects are noted and a change in trial medication is necessary, the duration of the trial can be extended.

TECHNOLOGY

As discussed earlier all currently used systems for long-term epidural drug delivery are not totally implantable because the medication reservoir is located outside of the body. The reason for that is the higher requirements for dose and, possibly, volume for epidural infusion. Even the most capacious implantable pumps will have to be refilled every 10–15 days if used for epidural opioid therapy.

Three of the most popular systems for permanent epidural access used in contemporary pain management are the Du Pen catheter, the Port-A-Cath system, and the Arrow Low Profile Titanium Port with Flextip epidural catheter. The Du Pen catheter is a two-piece externalized catheter (Fig. 11-1), whereas the other two are totally implantable catheters with subcutaneous ports. In our practice, we prefer to use the Arrow Low Profile Titanium Port (Fig. 11-2) with Flextip epidural catheter (Fig. 11-3). The port is very compact, the catheter can withstand about any stress due to reinforcement with a titanium coil, and the locking system is very convenient. The Arrow port system is not yet FDA approved for epidural or intrathecal use.

The Du Pen catheter is made of radiopaque silicon-rubber and consists of an epidural catheter, tunneled catheter connector, and tunneled catheter with a Dacron cuff for subcutaneous tissue ingrowth. The system is fairly easy to use and implant (Fig. 11-4). Detailed description of the implantation technique is presented elsewhere (20). In brief, a needle is placed in the epidural space via a small paramedian incision. After the epidural catheter has been placed, the tunneled catheter is passed subcutaneously from the selected exit site to the incision on the back. Both catheters are connected using a connector and fixed with

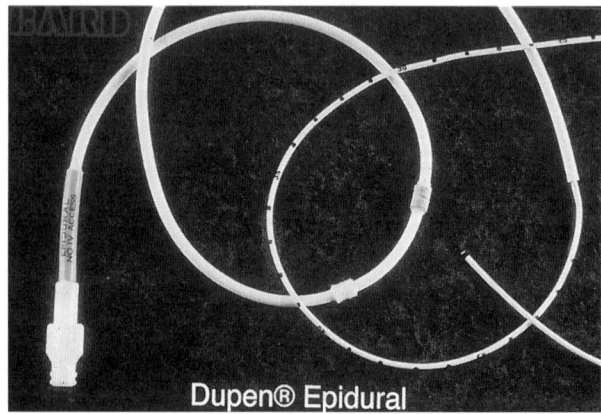

FIG. 11-1. The Du Pen Catheter (C R Bard, Inc., Salt Lake City, UT).

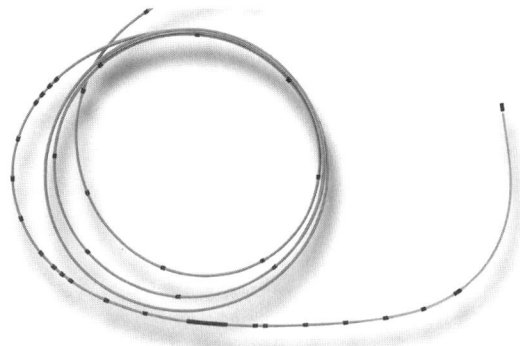

FIG. 11-2. Flextip Epidural Catheter (Arrow International, Inc., Reading, PA).

two silk ties. There are a few modifications that I would suggest in addition to the original technique. First, the spinal incision should be made in a vertical, not transverse, direction and should be not more than 1 cm in length. No pocket formation is necessary because there is no object that will be implanted. The only purpose of the incision is to facilitate connection of the two catheters. Both ends should be pulled out through the incision, and all connections should be made outside and then, by pulling the distal end of the tunneled catheter, the connection site will be internalized. The small size and the direction of the incision will allow better healing and obviate the need for a drain.

The Port-A-Cath II consists of a polyurethane catheter and titanium port with connector. The Arrow system used in our practice has a titanium port, polyurethane connecting catheter, and Flextip polyurethane epidural catheter reinforced with a titanium coil. The function of these systems is simple (Fig. 11-5), although implantation is a little more complicated than for the Du Pen catheter. A detailed description of the surgical technique for Port-A-Cath system implantation is presented by Cherry and co-authors (21). It requires four or more separate incisions.

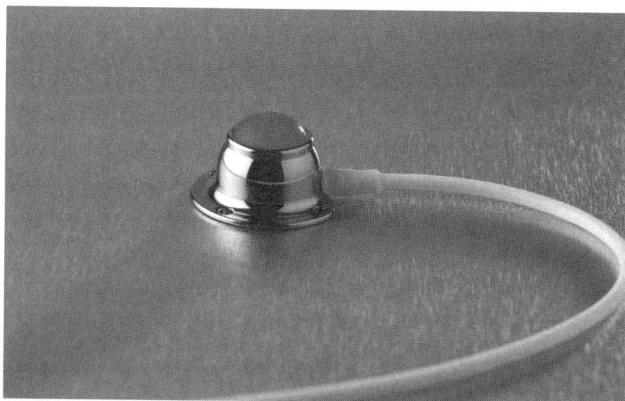

FIG. 11-3. Low Profile Titanium Port (Arrow International, Inc., Reading, PA).

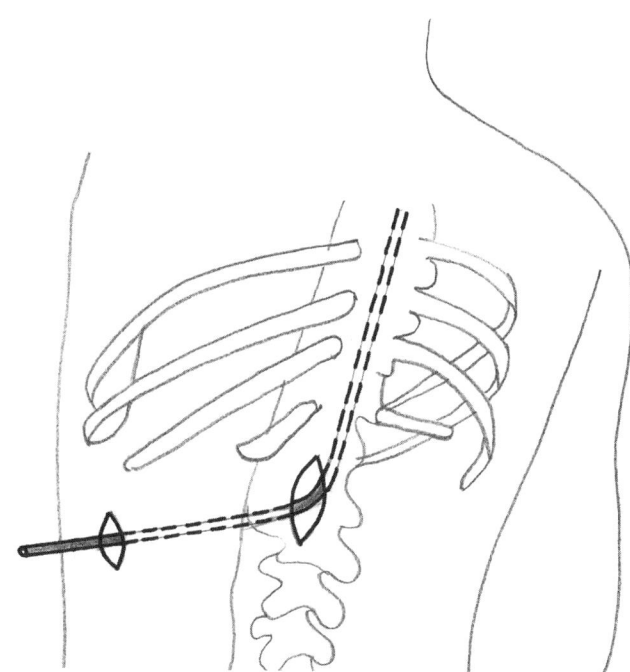

FIG. 11-4. Implanted epidural drug delivery system: transcutaneous tunneled epidural catheter.

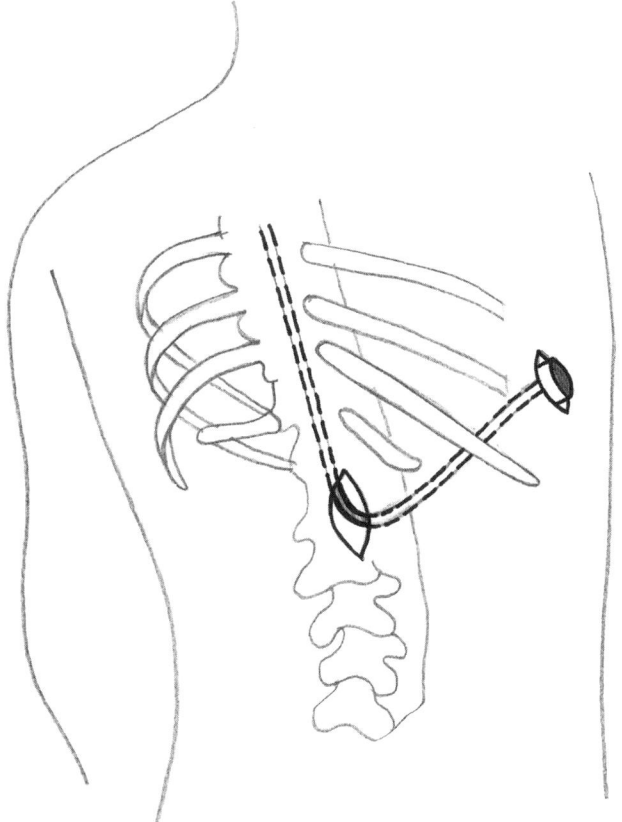

FIG. 11-5. Implanted epidural drug delivery system: epidural catheter with subcutaneous port.

I use a somewhat modified technique with the Arrow system that will limit surgery to two incisions. Initially, through a small paramedian incision, a needle is placed in the epidural space. The catheter is advanced to the desired level. Then a 3-cm transverse incision is performed at the anterior axillary line about 4 cm above the rib margin, and a small pocket is formed just below the incision with the external intercostal membrane serving as the posterior wall of the pocket. The catheter is tunneled between the two incisions, trimmed and connected to the 2–3 cm length of connecting catheter. The latter is attached using a twist-lock connector to the port. An extra 2–3 cm length of the catheter is gently pulled back through the spinal incision. A small loop is formed with the extra length of the catheter, and a suture is put through the fascia and tied around the loop to provide additional protection from dislodgment of the catheter. The port then is positioned in the preformed pocket and anchored to the external intercostal membrane through the four loops using four silk sutures.

Implantation for both systems is quick and minimally invasive. They can be performed under straight local anesthesia in very sick patients. Injection of contrast via the catheter after placement to verify position in the epidural space is absolutely essential (20). Choice of the infused drug will be discussed later. Possible complications are essentially the same as those for implantable intrathecal pumps and will be addressed later.

No differences in efficacy or rate of complications between externalized catheters and implanted port systems have been demonstrated (22). We prefer the latter system because it can easily be made totally implantable by disconnecting the external infusion device. This makes it convenient for many temporary activities: bathing, undergoing surgery, etc. Unfortunately, even though very effective, epidural delivery of opioids is mostly restricted to cancer patients. The reason for this is denial by the majority of insurers of coverage for drugs delivered from outside of the body for nonmalignant pain. If this situation could change, a significant number of patients with different nonmalignant chronic pain syndromes, such as compression vertebral fractures or complex regional pain syndrome, could benefit from an epidural infusion of intermediate duration.

The previously described systems, especially those with implanted ports, can also be used for intrathecal infusion (22). As with epidural delivery of opioids this modality should be restricted to short or intermediate duration of therapy. Long-term neuroaxial drug administration should be performed with totally implantable systems utilizing implanted infusion pumps (23). There are two major groups in this category: programmable and nonprogrammable. The only programmable pump on the market is the Medtronic SynchroMed system. It comes with or without the additional catheter access port (Fig. 11-6). In the nonprogrammable category there are more options: the Medtronic IsoMed System (Fig. 11-7), the Arrow Model

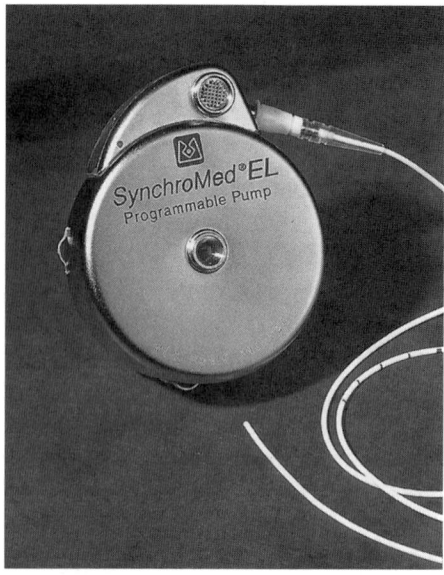

FIG. 11-6. Programmable SynchroMed Pumps (Medtronic, Inc., Minneapolis, MN).

3000 Series (Fig. 11-8), and the Advanced Neuromodulation Systems pump, which is currently used only in Europe. Nonprogrammable pumps come in different volumes (from 16 mL to 60 mL) and with a variety of preset infusion rates (from 0.3 mL to 4.0 mL). Both types have their advantages and disadvantages. Programmable pumps allow prompt and frequent fine adjustments of the rate of infusion but are more expensive and require battery

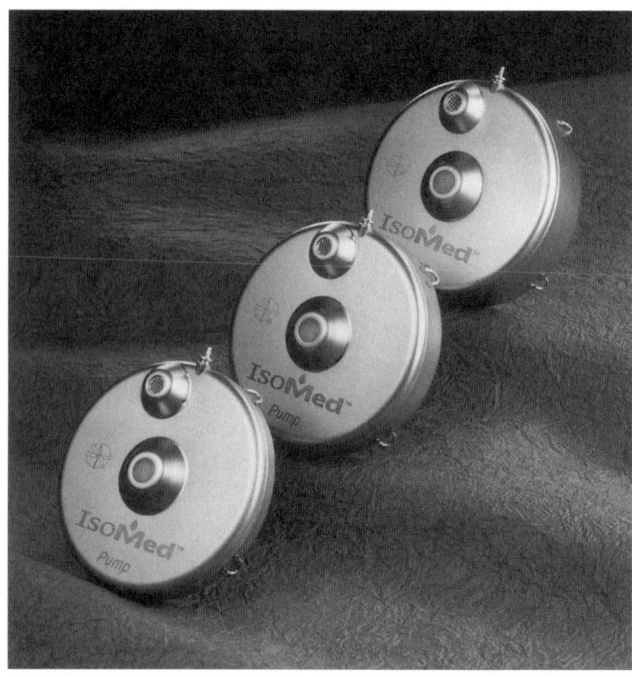

FIG. 11-7. Nonprogrammable IsoMed Pumps (Medtronic, Inc., Minneapolis, MN).

Arrow Model 3000 Series Constant Flow Implantable Pumps

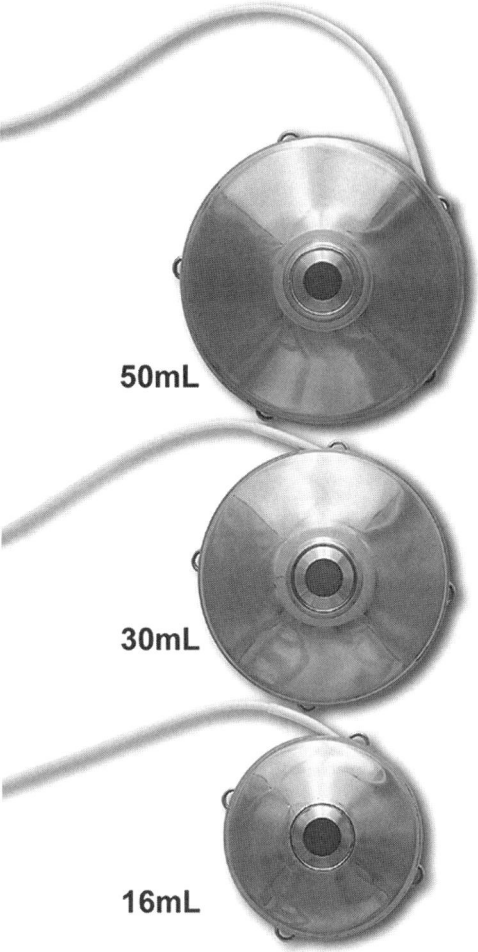

50mL

30mL

16mL

FIG. 11-8. Nonprogrammable Arrow Model 3000 Series Pumps (Arrow International, Inc., Reading, PA).

change (read: the whole pump) every few years. Nonprogrammable pumps do not require repetitive surgeries for battery change and are less expensive but are difficult to fine-tune because complete refill of the pump with a new medication concentration is required to change the infusion rate. The Arrow Model 3000 Series pumps allow a bolus to be performed with a special needle without changing the rate or the medication. The Medtronic IsoMed system has an additional catheter access port that can also be used for giving a bolus. The decision about the type of pump to be used should be made individually in each case. In my opinion, for the initiation of treatment, a programmable pump is the device of choice. On the other hand, in a vast majority of patients with programmable pumps, after expiration of the battery, they can be substituted with a nonprogrammable one. By this time (3–5

years after initiation of the treatment) patients are usually stable enough not to require frequent adjustments of the daily dose.

IMPLANTATION TECHNIQUE

Implantation of the pump can be carried out under either local anesthesia with sedation or general anesthesia and even spinal anesthesia via the implanted catheter (Jeffery Faaberg, personal communication). No advantage of one method over the other has been proven. Proponents of sedation cite possible unnoticed spinal cord damage during catheter insertion under general anesthesia, whereas their opponents claim safety, convenience, and patient comfort. I personally prefer general anesthesia but more than once have had to resort to local anesthesia due to the general health concerns of the patient.

One important part of a successful procedure is a well-determined place for pump implantation. This should be discussed with the patient before surgery. The side of implantation depends on anatomical factors such as scars from previous surgeries, the presence of a colostomy, hernias, etc., as well as the patient's request, i.e., the patient's favorite resting position should preferably be on the contralateral side from the implanted pump. A suggestion that the choice of the side should be done based on the right- or left-handedness of the surgeon does not look sound to me (24). Persons performing implantation should be comfortable with any position or situation. For example, at the request of a young female patient I once had to implant a pump through an existing scar after a low midline laparotomy. The position of pump implantation should be marked on the skin before surgery with the patient in the standing position. If this is performed on an anesthetized patient in the decubitus position, the pump could eventually be a long way from the desired area when the patient starts ambulating. The pump should be sufficiently far away from the rib margin and iliac crest, as well as away from the belt line, if a belt is routinely used. From my experience, female patients are usually more comfortable with the pump positioned somewhat lower and more medially than male patients.

The patient is positioned in the lateral decubitus position, and skin preparation and draping are performed, including the lower back, flank, and one-half of the abdominal wall. This can be achieved either with split drapes or with laparotomy drapes with the opening enlarged in the transverse direction with scissors.

The first step is the placement of the introducing needle in the spinal space. This is performed in the lower lumbar levels, usually L4–5 or L3–4. Placement of the needle can be performed after the skin incision, but it is more practical to do it prior to incision. If the operator has a problem advancing the needle at the selected level, he will have to extend the existing incision for at least another inch. This situation is avoidable if the needle is placed prior to mak-

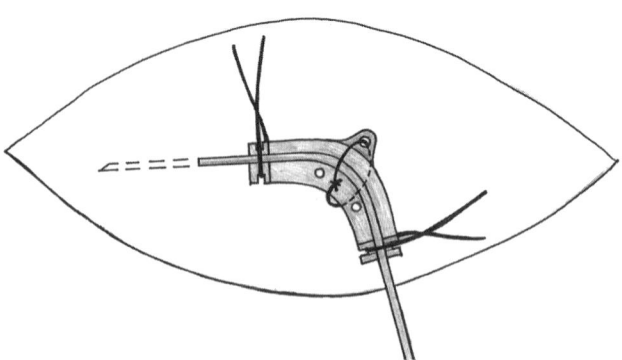

FIG. 11-9. Implantation of intrathecal pump: fluoroscopic control of the direction of the intrathecal catheter.

ing the incision. The needle should be inserted in a paramedian fashion on the ipsilateral side of the planned pump placement and advanced in a cephalad direction with the hub of the needle facing up. This prevents retrograde insertion of the catheter. After free flow of CSF is observed, the catheter is passed under the control of C-arm fluoroscopy. The final level of the tip of the catheter should be 2.5–3 vertebral levels above the site of insertion. Direction can be easily confirmed by placing one of the instruments, i.e., clamp, on the skin of the patient with the handle facing in the caudad direction (Fig. 11-9). Occasional upside-down imaging of the back during fluoroscopy can lead to inadvertent implantation of a retrograde-placed catheter. Whether the tip of the catheter should be advanced to the dermatomal level of pain, as suggested by some authors (24), remains controversial (3). On one hand, even hydrophilic agents lose around half of their concentration from low to high levels of the spine (25) and lipophilic agents do it much more dramatically. On the other hand, some increase in the rate of infusion can compensate for this difference, and practically all known opioid agents have been used successfully without adjustments of the catheter position. Some of the lipophilic opioids, i.e., sufentanil, quickly enter the spinal cord, whereas the others, i.e., fentanyl, rather move to epidural space (26). This makes correct positioning of the catheter difficult without knowing the exact drug that will be used. Infusion of hydrophilic agents via a fairly high-positioned catheter will lead to quicker and more extensive rostral spread with increased sedation and other CNS side effects (25). Adjustment in position is definitely not necessary for hydromorphone, even though it was proposed by some authors (27). Lumbar epidural injection of equianalgesic doses of hydromorphone and morphine produced proportionally equal concentrations of opioids in the cervical CSF (28). Additionally, manipulation of the intrathecal catheter from the lumbar to a high thoracic or cervical level really increases the risk of neural damage in patients under general anesthesia.

After the catheter is positioned, a vertical incision is made through the site of needle insertion for a distance

from 1 to 2 inches, depending on the amount of subcutaneous fat tissue. This incision is deepened to the supraspinous ligament and paraspinal muscle fascia. The operator should make sure that the length of the incision at the ligament is the same or even wider than the skin incision. A tapering or "well-like" wound creates unnecessary technical difficulties and leads to excessively long skin incisions. A pursestring suture with 2-0 silk is placed through the fascia around the needle to prevent CSF leak around the catheter (Fig. 11-10). The needle and stylet are removed, the pursestring is tightened, and continued free flow of CSF via the catheter is confirmed. If no CSF is coming out of the catheter it is advisable to gently aspirate the catheter using a small syringe and 25-gauge needle. To prevent CSF loss and contamination of the catheter the external catheter tip should be fixed to the drape with a clamp (the damaged portion will be trimmed later anyway).

The next step is anchoring of the catheter to the supraspinous fascia. Different types of anchors are available (Fig. 11-11), but in my opinion the elbow-type is the optimal choice. Straight anchors, especially the new

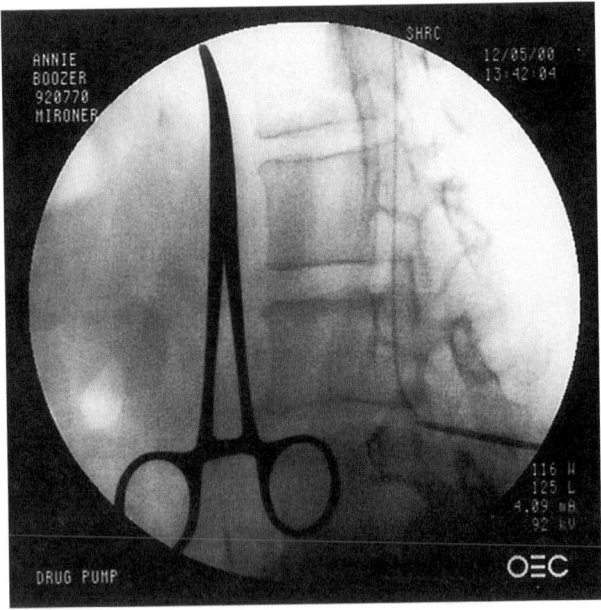

A

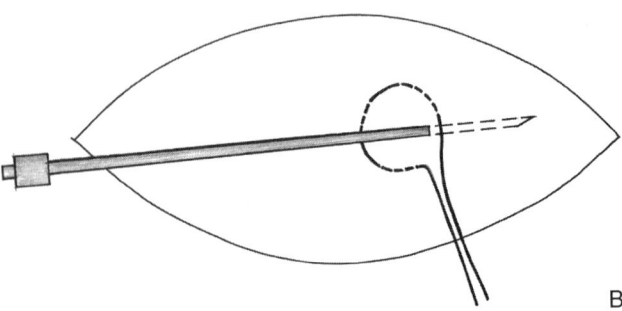

B

FIG. 11-10. Implantation of intrathecal pump: placement of pursestring suture.

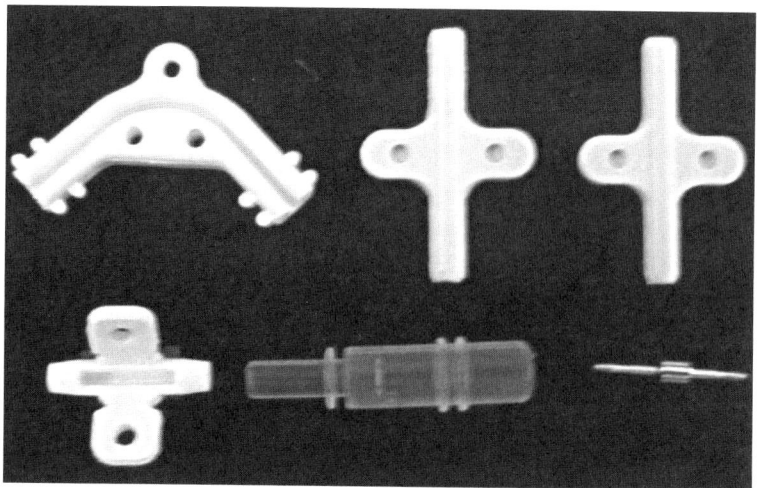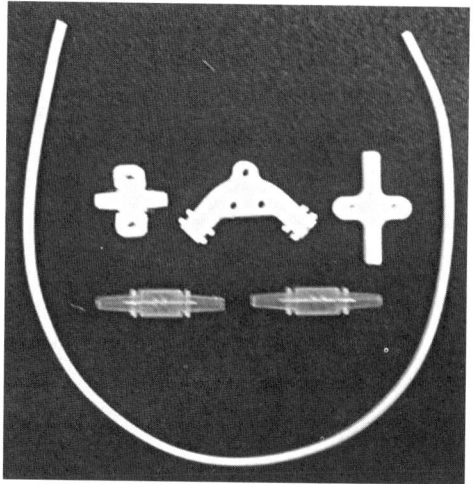

FIG. 11-11. Anchors for intrathecal catheter fixation (Medtronic, Inc., Minneapolis, MN).

shorter type, create a higher risk for catheter kinking because tunneling is done under a nearly straight angle.

The anchor should be placed very close to the site where the catheter exits the fascia (but not over it) to prevent any kinking in this segment. The angle of the elbow should follow the natural curving of the catheter toward the subcutaneous tunnel to the pump. In my opinion the anchoring process described in the Medtronic manual (Medtronic, Inc., 1996) is, on one hand, too complicated and, on the other hand, insufficient. There is no tension that requires five sutures, especially when each one increases the risk of perforating the catheter. At the same time, if only two sutures on the side are holding the catheter within the groove in the anchor, then the middle portion can come out and cause problems. A slightly sim-

plified way of anchoring with just three 2-0 silk sutures that reduces the risk of puncturing the catheter or dislodging it from the anchor is demonstrated (Fig. 11-12).

After this step is finished, the wound is tightly packed with dry gauze. This is, in 99% of the cases, sufficient to completely stop any bleeding in the wound. The chances of hematoma formation in this incision are negligibly small due to the size of the incision and tight suturing of the wound in layers. Unnecessary chasing of "large bleeders" right after the incision is made can cause not only damage to the catheter but also necrotic burned tissue that will produce an inflammatory reaction and eventually formation of a seroma. Irrigation of the wound with antibiotic in "clean" surgical cases after the patient already received a preoperative intravenous dose of

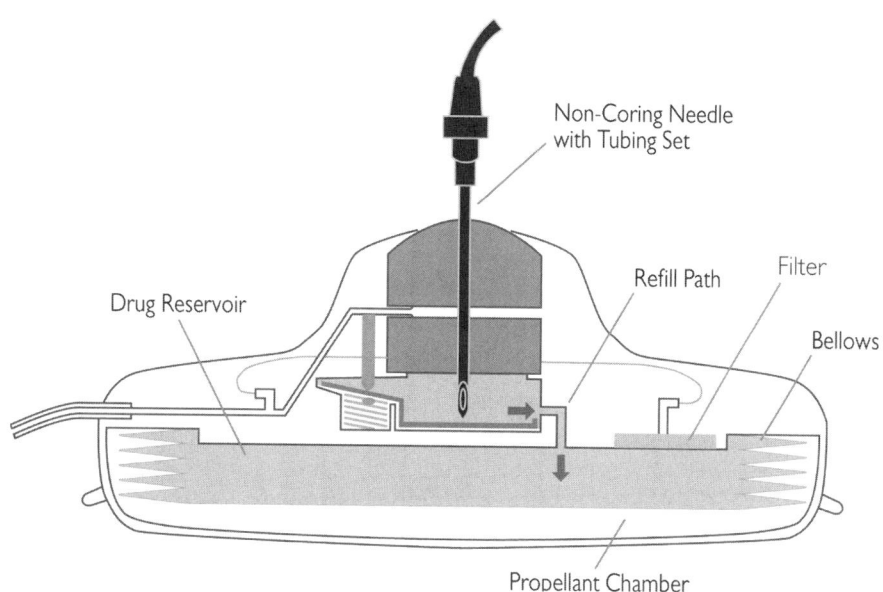

FIG. 11-12. Implantation of intrathecal pump: suturing of the anchor to the supraspinous fascia.

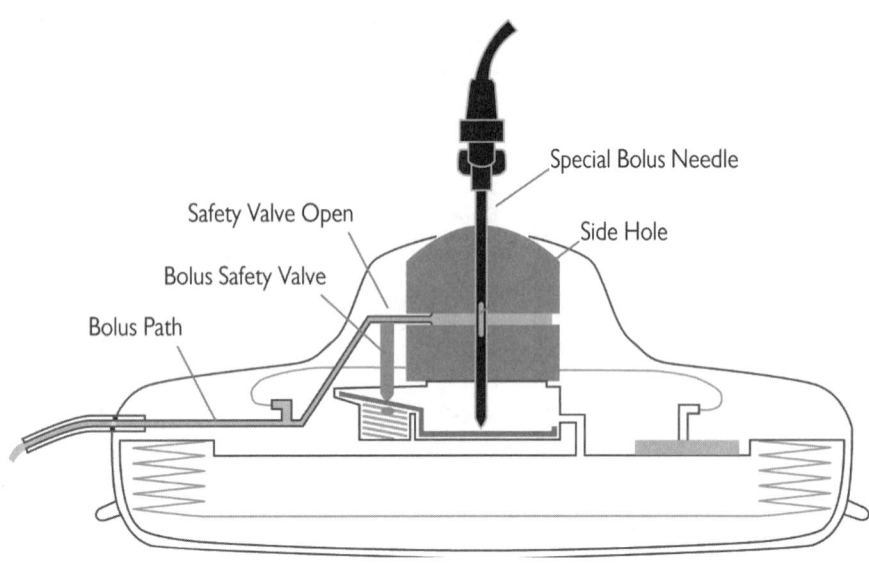

FIG. 11-13. Implantation of intrathecal pump: position of the pump in the pocket.

antibiotic, in my opinion, provides no additional protection from infection.

At this point, a skin incision is performed at the premarked pump pocket site. The pump will be located predominantly or completely below the incision to prevent accessing the pump for refills through the scar (Fig. 11-13). The incision should be slightly smaller than the pump diameter (elasticity of the skin will allow easy placement of the pump in the pocket) and should extend to the aponeurosis or to the superficial fascia in obese individuals. If the proper depth is reached, it is usually very easy to form a pocket with just blunt dissection. Alternatively, one should use a combination of sharp and blunt dissections. The size of the pocket should not significantly exceed the size of the pump to prevent pump movement after surgery and formation of a seroma. The pocket is tightly packed with a sponge (see comments earlier), and tunneling of the catheter is started.

Tunneling of the catheter should be performed differently, depending on the type of catheter used: single piece or dual piece. The connection between the two pieces of catheter adds another "weak" area that can cause problems in the future. The single-piece catheter provides a higher level of safety from catheter-related complications (see "Personal Experience") and in my opinion is the system of choice. Tunneling from the incision in the back is a better technique. The abdominal wall skin and subcutaneous fat are more mobile than in the back. This difference allows easier passage of the end of the tunneling device through the abdominal wound by manipulating the tunneling rod with one hand and abdominal wall with the other. The operator should always maintain control over the position of the sharp end of the tunneling rod. "Disappearance" of the tip of the rod in the depth of the soft tissue is a dangerous sign that should prompt retracting it and restarting the tunneling process anew. Bending the tunneling rod in order to pass the fairly sharp turn from

the back to the abdominal wall makes safe passage easier. As soon as the turn is made, rotate the rod 180 degrees and advance it, simultaneously pulling the abdominal wall incision toward and "over" the sharp end of the tunneling device. The catheter is advanced through the tunneling device, and the latter is pulled out (which is also much more easily done through the abdominal wound than through the incision in the back). CSF flow out of catheter should be checked one more time, and the catheter is then trimmed, leaving an extra 1–2 inches length to prevent excessive tension. The silastic boot is slid over the catheter, the catheter is connected to the connector, and the boot is placed over the connection and fixed in place with two 2-0 silk ties.

The pump is prepared for implantation and filled with the desired drug according to the manufacturer's instructions. The connector is pushed into place over the catheter port tip on the pump and fixed with a 2-0 silk tie. Depending on the choice of the operator the pump is placed in a Dacron pouch, which will hold it in place by facilitating scar formation. Alternatively the pump may be fixed in place by sutures through the surgical loops on certain pump models. For practical purposes I always position the pump in the pocket with catheter port facing in the same direction (i.e., toward the umbilicus) to simplify proper position of the template during refills. It is compulsory to verify one last time that the refill port is facing up (toward the skin); accidental rotation of the pump during its placement is not an impossible event. After placing the pump in the pocket and positioning the excess catheter in a wide-curved loop under the pump, both wounds are closed with 2-0 or 3-0 vicril sutures and skin sutures or staples.

Prophylactic antibiotics are useful in clean surgeries when a foreign body is implanted. To be effective, parenteral antibiotics must be given during the period of time within 30 minutes before the operation begins (29). Multiple studies showed equal efficacy of a single preoperative dose and multiple doses in the perioperative period (29). I would recommend neither postoperative prophylactic antibiotics nor antibiotic irrigation of the clean wound.

MANAGEMENT

The initial dose to be infused after implantation should be the same as during the trial (converted if necessary from epidural to intrathecal). The patient will also benefit from additional oral opioids, not only for postoperative pain or breakthrough pain, but also for prevention of possible withdrawal if he or she was on a high dose prior to implantation. The oral opioids should be tapered down as the intrathecal infusion rate is being adjusted. We always allow patients on neuroaxial opioid therapy to have a small amount of breakthrough oral opioid. Titration of intraspinal opioid should be tailored to each individual, but in general, especially in the early stages, increases of 10% to 20% are safe and appropriate. The highest dose of intrathecal opioid, at which it should be considered ineffective and the plan for treatment should be changed, is arguable and will be discussed later. It is important, though, to remember that lack of response to an increase in the rate of infusion is not always a sign of an ineffective drug. Sometimes it is a warning symptom suggesting malfunction of the implanted system, which needs to be evaluated.

DRUGS

Morphine

Spinal morphine is the only opioid approved by the FDA for use in the implantable pumps, so not surprisingly it is the drug of choice in contemporary pain management (6,30). Two out of every three patients were managed on morphine alone in a 1996 study (17). That did not change significantly 3 years later (31). The starting dose for intrathecal morphine is usually about 1–2 mg/day, whereas the high end varies significantly (31). Some physicians consider 20 mg/day to be the limit, whereas others go as high as 55–60 mg/day (31, Iva Chapple, personal communication). No detrimental effects of high doses of morphine have been proven, but the dose response curve definitely flattens at such levels. If adequate pain control is not achieved at a high infusion rate of morphine, then another drug or drug combination should be substituted. One study showed that around 30% of the patients required such changes (32). It is important to remember that morphine can cause side effects such as nausea, pruritus, and sedation possibly more than many of the other opioids (5,28,33,34). According to different sources, from 30% to 100% of all patients have side effects with intrathecal morphine (35,36). This can be more prominent with increasing daily dose. Morphine can even cause paradoxical hyperalgesia if it is

metabolized into morphine-3-glucuronide instead of morphine-1-glucuronide (37). In order to resolve these problems physicians should either substitute another opioid or nonopioid drug or add an adjuvant drug to morphine, which will improve analgesia, reduce the dose of opioid, and eliminate side effects.

Hydromorphone

Hydromorphone is one of the commonly and successfully used alternative opioids and at the same time one of the most unappreciated; 13.5% of all pump patients were receiving hydromorphone in 1996 (17); this stayed about the same in a 1999 study (31). Nevertheless, short of a suggestion of the drug efficacy in review articles (38,39,40), there are few studies dedicated to spinal hydromorphone (32). It is even more surprising because of the numerous resources proving not only the high success of epidural hydromorphone (28,41,42), but also a lower incidence of side effects than with epidural morphine (33,41,42). Coombs et al. first described a case of successful intrathecal hydromorphone use for intractable cancer pain (43). Mironer and Grumman were first to present the use of intrathecal hydromorphone in a group of patients with nonmalignant intractable pain (32). Thirteen out of 16 patients in this study achieved better results than they did with morphine. Results of the study also raised a question of an adequate conversion rate from intrathecal morphine to hydromorphone. Previously it was suggested that the ratio should be the same as for intravenous use—1:5 (38,40,44). More than that, the starting dose of hydromorphone was only 10% of the last morphine dose (44). Meanwhile, results of clinical observations on a group of patients showed a strength ratio of about 1:2.5 (32). Practically, a majority of physicians are using hydromorphone at about half of the morphine dose (31). Even though the intravenous/intraventricular activity ratio is practically similar between hydromorphone and morphine, the relative strength of epidural hydromorphone was shown to be only 2–3 times higher than parenteral, whereas this ratio equals nearly 10 for morphine (45,46). The difference in intrathecal efficacy, which seems to follow the epidural potency pattern, cannot be explained by diminished spread of the somewhat more lipophilic hydromorphone in the CSF (28). Hydromorphone proved to be an effective intrathecal agent with a side-effect profile that seems to be better than morphine. It also does not have a documented record of producing hyperalgesia as often as morphine. One "expert panel" made a suggestion of using hydromorphone as only "the second line of defense," placing it in a group with other questionable drug combinations (39). In my opinion, this opioid is a candidate to substitute for morphine as a drug of choice. We suggest starting hydromorphone at one-half to one-third of the last morphine dose. Doses in excess of 20 mg/day have been used without any noticeable problems (32).

Fentanyl, Sufentanil, Alfentanil, Buprenorphine

Nearly 8% of pump patients in the 1996 study were receiving one of the opioids from this lipophilic group (17). Nearly 20% of pain clinicians have used either fentanyl or sufentanil in intraspinal pumps (31), whereas buprenorphine has fairly wide usage in Europe (9,47). Unfortunately there are no well-documented results of their use. Some researchers question any additional efficacy from the neuroaxial use of lipophilic opioids versus parenteral infusion (2,48). Indeed, the relative epidural strength of this group is only 1–3 times higher than intravenous (26,48). Some studies failed to show any increased efficacy with their epidural use (3,49). The question about intrathecal infusion is still open. When using one of these opioids, a proper calculation of their dose is required. Maintaining the systemic equianalgesic ratio with morphine, as suggested in some articles and tutorials (40,44), will be a serious mistake because the neuroaxial potency is in a reverse relationship to lipophilia (26). Practical experience confirms this without any doubt (31). The relative strength of neuroaxial opioids is presented in Table 11-1. The group of lipophilic opioids also raises a question of adequate positioning of the catheter tip. Only a few studies prove any increased efficacy of lipophilic opioids delivered directly at the dermatomal level of the pain (3). This notion was primarily born from the ability of these drugs to be quickly absorbed without spreading in the epidural or intrathecal space (2). Nevertheless, a comparison of analgesia produced by lumbar or thoracic epidural fentanyl for thoracic pain did not show any difference (50). Route of absorption of different lipophilic opioids can vary, i.e., sufentanil quickly enters the spinal cord, whereas fentanyl moves to the epidural space (26). This makes the decision regarding correct positioning of the catheter even more difficult. Taking this into account, as well as the negative side effects of high placement of the catheter (see earlier) and the predominant use of hydrophilic opioids in current practice (17,31), it seems reasonable to continue, at least for now, with the "traditional" lumbar placement of the catheter.

Meperidine

Slightly less than 1% of the patients in the study by Paice and co-authors were receiving meperidine (17). In a recent survey, approximately 9% of all participating doctors cited use of this opioid (31). Despite these numbers, meperidine continues to be a mysterious drug. Successful use of single-dose intrathecal meperidine has been well documented (40,52). There were only two reports in the literature on the use of meperidine in the intrathecal pump. Harvey et al. (53) presented one case of chronic nonmalignant pain managed with meperidine, and our study (32) described success in two patients, who had failed multiple other intrathecal drugs. Lack of reports or studies produced speculations in the literature ranging from incompatibility with pumps (40) to an alleged large group of successfully treated patients (4). The highest number of patients in one practice currently receiving intrathecal meperidine that I was able to track down is 12 (John Oakley, personal communication). The interest in meperidine is understandable because it possesses local anesthetic properties on one hand but has the additional specter of side effects in comparison to "standard" opioids. As with a majority of other opioids, direct projection of systemic equianalgesic dose ratio with morphine is not applicable. According to the current standard, neuroaxial morphine is 7–10 times more potent than meperidine (38,40,44). In reality, the intrathecal dose of meperidine should be 25–30 times higher than morphine to maintain equianalgesia (48). In our experience doses up to 60 mg/day appeared to be safe. According to the literature, a single intrathecal dose of 100 mg of meperidine inevitably causes grave complications (54).

Methadone

No mention of methadone was made in the 1996 survey (17), whereas in the latest survey it was one of the "other" drugs used by 2% to 4% of the survey respondents (31). Some researchers advise that it is impractical to use methadone for neuroaxial delivery (48). That opinion was based on the shorter duration of analgesia and higher dose requirements for methadone. Nevertheless, the literature is full of examples of successful use of neuroaxial methadone for acute pain management (55–58). Methadone has a very short half-life in the CSF (59). It does not produce noticeable migration to higher levels of the CNS (59) (which means less sedation), and it is not accumulated in the plasma after the first 24 hours of infusion (60). Methadone is an NMDA-receptor antagonist as well as an

TABLE 11-1. *Relative potency and starting intrathecal doses of commonly used opioids*

Opioid	Parenteral Relative Strength (Morphine = 1)	Neuroaxial Relative Strength (Morphine = 1) (References)	Suggested Starting Intrathecal Dose
Morphine	1	1	1 mg
Hydromorphone	6	2–3 (32,45,46)	0.5 mg
Meperidine	0.125	0.03 (51,104)	25 mg
Methadone	1	0.5 (66,105)	2.5 mg
Fentanyl	100	10–15 (51,106)	50 mcg
Sufentanil	1000	82–100 (51,107)	10 mcg

inhibitor of norepinephrine and serotonin reuptake (61). These qualities allow methadone the broadest coverage of pain of all currently used opioids (62). A group of researchers has demonstrated the ability of methadone to control neuropathic pain in experimental animals (63) and in clinical studies on patients (64). The D-isomer of methadone has been shown to prevent development of tolerance to morphine (65). With all of this in mind it is surprising that no attempts at using methadone for chronic pain via intrathecal pumps have been performed. Our clinic was the first to study the use of methadone in the programmable intraspinal pump for chronic nonmalignant pain (66). Twenty-four patients, who failed multiple other intrathecal drugs, received an infusion of methadone. Fifty-one percent of them reported improved analgesia, and 37.5% continued on this regimen with good pain control and high satisfaction. No side effects related to methadone were noted, and a majority of the patients noticed decreased sedation. As with other lipophilic opioids, traditional calculation of the equianalgesic dose of methadone is not appropriate (48). It requires doses that are at least two times higher than that of morphine (48,66). Doses up to 36 mg/day were used in our study. We believe that methadone is a very promising intrathecal agent and definitely does not deserve to be listed with the last-resort drugs (39).

Local Anesthetics

Local anesthetics have been used for neuroaxial delivery for many years to provide intraoperative anesthesia and postoperative analgesia (3,4). They are of the most common adjunct drugs used in intrathecal pumps. In a 1996 survey, 19.8% of all patients were receiving bupivacaine (17), whereas in a recent study more than 20% of patients had a local anesthetic in their pump (31). Sixty percent of all responding physicians used a morphine/bupivacaine combination (31). This modality of treatment is so popular that an article has been published dedicated to calculating the right proportions of the opioid/bupivacaine mixture (67). This option was proposed to be the "second-line approach" (39). The theoretical application of local anesthetics with opioids for neuroaxial treatment is clear. Meanwhile, the practical situation with opioid/local anesthetic mixtures is far from being as straightforward as suggested (27,39). When epidural opioids were combined with bupivacaine, not only were good results observed (68), but also lack of any improvement was noted in multiple studies (3,69). Short of anecdotal reports only one study showed improved analgesia or decreased opioid use in 10 out of 13 patients with chronic nonmalignant pain receiving intraspinal opioid/bupivacaine infusion (68). A study of cancer patients showed a somewhat slower escalation of morphine dose when bupivacaine was added (70), but this research project used a very small population of patients and had significant design problems.

On the other hand our study showed a lack of positive effect of bupivacaine addition in all 12 patients (32). More than that, 75% of them reported the onset of new side effects. Our group is currently performing a double-blind randomized crossover study of intrathecal opioid/bupivacaine mixtures that will hopefully shed some light on its efficacy. Starting bupivacaine doses of 3 mg/day seem to be appropriate. The average doses according to a recent survey were around 8 mg/day (17). Some researchers suggest that no side effects are observed with doses of bupivacaine below 15 mg/day (30). In our study side effects such as numbness, muscle weakness, and urinary retention were observed at doses ranging from 4.2 mg/day to 14 mg/day (32).

Clonidine

The ability of intrathecal clonidine, an alpha-2 adrenergic agonist, to provide analgesia has been demonstrated in experimental neuropathic pain in animals (71,72). Three studies also showed a decrease in pain levels in patients receiving epidural clonidine, although this effect was compared only to placebo and not to other analgesics (73,74,75). Other studies of the epidural or intrathecal use of clonidine or clonidine/opioid mixtures are just case reports ranging from single patients to the largest group of 32 patients (30). In this group, 56% reported improved pain control. It seems that clonidine is more effective in neuropathic pain, although our personal experience was not very favorable. Clonidine produces hypotension in a significant percentage of patients and requires careful titration (76). Its use increased from 0% in 1996 (17) to 14% of the patients in 1999 (31). In the last survey more than 50% of pain clinicians used clonidine (31). Nevertheless, less than half of those surveyed believe that morphine/clonidine is an effective drug combination, and that number drops to only 21% if the same question was asked about clonidine alone. That makes it even more surprising that some authors would suggest using morphine/clonidine as a "second-line approach" in competition with well-researched hydromorphone and ahead of other opioids (39). More studies are necessary before such decisions can be made. The starting dose of clonidine, mixed with opioid, should be around 50 mcg/day, with the usual effective range between 100 and 200 mcg/day. Doses up to 900 mcg/day have been reported (30).

Experimental Drugs

SNX-111, a calcium channel blocker, has been shown to produce analgesia when delivered intrathecally to patients with neuropathic pain (77). This effect has been compared so far to placebo only. Multiple side effects were noted, including dizziness, confusion, nausea, and others. From personal experience, this drug can be effective in a very narrow category of patients and is very difficult to titrate.

Octreotide, a somatostatin analog, provided improved analgesia in a small group of cancer patients (78). Insufficient data are currently available to give any recommendation regarding this drug.

Intrathecal neostigmine, an acetylcholinesterase inhibitor, produced antinociception in animal studies as well as in human volunteers and postoperative patients (79,80, 81). Preliminary data show a high level of side effects, including weakness, sedation, nausea, and vomiting (79).

Intrathecal use of the NMDA-receptor antagonist ketamine with morphine in cancer patients allowed a decrease in the morphine dose but did not improve pain control (82). Besides, the issue of ketamine neurotoxicity is not resolved (83). Other NMDA-receptor antagonists—memantine, dextrorphan, and dextromethorphan—have been shown to be neurotoxic in animal studies when delivered in the spinal canal (84). Hopefully, the use of methadone, a natural mixture of opioid and NMDA-receptor antagonist, will prove to be successful.

Midazolam, a GABA agonist, has been shown to provide analgesia intrathecally for nonmalignant pain (alone and in combination with clonidine) (85). More research is needed to determine the possibility of future use of neuroaxial midazolam. Anecdotal reports claim that another GABA agonist—baclofen—usually used for spasticity, can provide pain relief in other conditions as well, especially in combination with opioids (27,86).

A number of other drugs have been tried in animals or humans for intrathecal analgesia. Experience with them is so isolated that, currently, no practical applications exist.

OUTCOMES

Numerous reports in the literature describe successes with the neuroaxial treatment of chronic intractable malignant and nonmalignant pain. The majority report 70% to 90+% of patients achieving good to excellent results (7,36,87). Patients received significant improvement in pain control and an increase in activities of daily living (87). They also reported general satisfaction with this modality of treatment, improvement in their mood, and reduced withdrawal from social life (88). Cost-effectiveness and safety of neuroaxial therapy for chronic pain have been established (89,90). For practical purposes we will not repeat the well-published list of results from previous studies (87), but at the end of the chapter we will briefly present some statistics on personal experiences with intrathecal programmable pumps.

COMPLICATIONS, PROBLEMS, SIDE EFFECTS

With all of the positive features of this modality of treatment there are a fairly significant number of side effects (36,91). Every implanter should be able to promptly recog-

nize and treat possible complications during and after surgery and during subsequent use of the devices.

Surgical Complications

Bleeding

Superficial bleeding is an extremely rare problem during pump implantation because neither the lumbar area nor the lateral abdominal wall is heavy vascularized. Most of the time, temporary tamponade of the wound while proceeding with the next step of the surgery will resolve the problem. Aggressive cauterization is unnecessary and can lead to excessive necrotic tissue producing a seroma or creating the perfect substrate for infection. Epidural or intrathecal bleeding is fairly rare but a much more serious problem. Screening patients with bleeding disorders, cancer patients with clotting abnormalities, as well as patients receiving anticoagulant therapy helps to prevent this potentially grave complication. It is not necessary that every patient undergo extensive laboratory testing if a careful collection of medical history is obtained. The question regarding use of NSAIDs is still controversial and should be decided by the surgeon depending on his views and experience. Gentle manipulation of the needle and styleted catheter will help to avoid any trauma to the deep tissues that can cause bleeding. Every patient should undergo routine neurological examination before and after surgery. If bleeding is suspected, this process should become continuous with involvement of a neurosurgeon and radiologist for possible MRI and/or CT.

Hematoma, Seroma

A collection of blood in the superficial wound could lead to formation of a hematoma. Seroma, a collection of serum in the wound, usually the pump pocket, can be the result of an organized hematoma or excessive tissue trauma. These complications are being reported with variable frequency by different authors but are far from being rare occurrences. Most of the cases are benign and resolve spontaneously. Wearing an abdominal binder can expedite this process. Puncture and aspiration are inadvisable, except in cases of significant volume collection. Refills should be delayed as long as possible, but if necessary, simultaneous aspiration of the seroma and continued use of an abdominal binder are recommended. The binder will increase pressure in the pocket, preventing fluid from reaccumulating. If the problem is persistent, surgical revision of the pocket is recommended, the goal of which is to diminish the space between the pump and the walls of the pocket.

Local Infection

Infection is not a very common complication of implantation but has been reported to occur in 2% to 6% of all foreign body implants (92). If the only sign of infection is cellulitis in the area of the pump pocket, but no fluctuance is noted, aggressive parenteral antibiotic treatment can reverse the course. In our experience in two such cases, the consulting infectious disease specialist advised removal of the implant. Because the process was localized to abdominal wall cellulitis, a decision was made to continue conservative treatment. After 3 weeks all signs of infection completely disappeared. On the other hand, any signs of infection inside the pocket, i.e., abscess, or spreading of the process along the course of the catheter toward the wound in the back, should prompt removal of the implant without any hesitation. It has been suggested by some authors to aspirate the pocket (35). However, aspiration of the pocket will not treat an abscess in the presence of a foreign body and can cause only generalization of the infectious process.

Epidural Abscess, Meningitis

The clinical picture of epidural abscess is similar to epidural hematoma with associated symptoms of infection. It requires immediate neurosurgical treatment. Meningitis usually produces a clinical picture of a generalized infectious process with signs of meningeal irritation. Neurological and infectious disease specialists should be involved, CSF samples obtained, and hardware removed without delay.

CSF Leak

CSF leak after placement of the catheter is a common development but usually is a self-limited problem. It requires either no treatment or conservative measures like hydration and analgesics for a few days after surgery if postdural puncture headache develops. In cases of persistent headache, an epidural blood patch is the next step. I would recommend delaying this procedure more than after simple dural puncture because of the increase in infection risk and the possibility of catheter damage. To avoid the latter, epidural puncture should be performed under fluoroscopy or, at least, distinctly a level below the entry of the catheter. Continuous CSF leak with development of a fistula will lead either to drainage through the incision or the formation of a hygroma. Suggested aspiration of the hygroma (35) not only increases the risk of infection, but also predisposes to continuous CSF leak due to decreased pressure in the pocket and the tract that was balanced with spinal CSF pressure. Alternatively, wearing an abdominal binder will increase pressure in the pocket, reduce CSF leak, and can facilitate healing of the dura. If no progress is noted this condition requires surgical closure with removal or repositioning of the catheter. Placement of a silk pursestring suture through the supraspinous ligament around the catheter entry site helps somewhat to reduce the extent of CSF leak around the catheter.

"Reaction" to the Pump

This is a rare condition described just recently (93). A similar clinical picture was better known with pacemakers (93). It resembles an allergic reaction and is possibly more prevalent in patients who have had previous titanium implants.

Change in Pump Position

The presence of a seroma or a rapid change in weight can cause increased mobility of the pump, which usually moves lower and can cause unpleasant pressure on the iliac bone. In extreme cases, mobility is so great that the pump actually flips over. That not only makes refills impossible but can also cause obstruction of the catheter. In such cases, the pump pocket should be revised, pump repositioned, and a new Dacron pouch should be used (even if the original method of fixation was surgical loops).

Implanted Device Complications

The current literature indicates that more than 20% of patients experience delivery system problems (35). The vast majority of equipment failures are related to the catheter (35). Pump malfunctions are extremely rare with the newer generation of delivery devices. Inaccurate dose delivery is practically nonexistent with current programmable pumps. Battery failure is an easily diagnosable and correctable event. Other pump-related complications are iatrogenic in nature and will be discussed later.

Catheter problems, on the other hand, are not unusual and can be divided into loss of patency, loss of continuity, and dislocation. They are, to a certain extent, applicable to all types of drug delivery systems, both epidural and intrathecal.

Loss of Patency

This most commonly occurs due to kinking of the catheter or obstruction with a "slipped" surgical tie. The most common site of occurrence is at the metal connector between the intrathecal (epidural) section and connector and at the site of anchoring. Both areas have ties or sutures that can "migrate" as well as "firm-soft" connections that could be the site of kinking. Use of the angled anchor and modified sutures, as described earlier, as well as positioning of the anchor close to the ligament puncture site, decreases the possibility of technical problems.

The development of a one-piece catheter (Model 8709, Medtronic, Inc., Minneapolis, MN) dramatically reduced the incidence of loss of patency and continuity by eliminating a "weak" area—the metal connector site. The only published testing of the one-piece catheter did not confirm its indisputable advantages, in my opinion, only due to improper design of the study (94). In our practice, since we started to use the single-piece catheter no kinking or disconnection of the catheter has been noted in more than 70 consecutive patients during the last 2 years.

Kinking of the catheter in the pump pocket is rare and can be easily prevented by trimming the catheter and carefully positioning the extra length in a gentle curve behind the pump.

Loss of Continuity

This is usually the result of disconnection of the catheter at one of the connection sites or, less often, breakage of the catheter. Again, the most common site is the metal connector, so the single-piece catheter, as mentioned, reduces this complication significantly. Disconnection at the pump site is not common but can occur if there is increased mobility and/or rotation of the pump.

Dislocation of the Catheter

This commonly presents as dislodgment of the catheter out of the intrathecal or epidural space. An exception to this is perforation of the dura by the tip of the epidural catheter with subsequent intrathecal delivery (92). This is the only condition that can cause symptoms of opioid overdose. All other catheter complications produce an increase in pain that more commonly is acute and dramatic. Sometimes it can be more gradual and subtle, for example, if kinking initially produces only partial obstruction to the flow of medicine.

A single case has been described in which with gradual dislodgment of the catheter from the spinal space a large fistula was formed (95). The patient continued to have communication between the tip of the catheter and the intrathecal space despite a significant distance between both structures. The existence of the fistula was discovered only during surgery for pump replacement.

Residual volume in the pump during refill that is substantially larger than the volume calculated by the computer indicates loss of catheter patency. Some of the catheter complications can be diagnosed with plain radiography, but as a general rule, it requires injection of contrast. Pump models with a side-port to bypass the main chamber make this an easy diagnostic procedure. Before injection of contrast media, at least 0.4 mL (volume of the catheter) of fluid should be aspirated to prevent pushing an excessive amount of opioid into the spinal fluid. Inability to aspirate fluid indirectly suggests a catheter complication. After this procedure if no catheter problems were discovered, the pump should be programmed to deliver a quick bolus equal to the catheter volume. If the pump has no second port, all of the medicine should be aspirated from the reservoir, and it should be filled with contrast media, and, if possible with this model, a bolus injection should be programmed. In such cases CT is necessary for

an accurate picture because only a very small amount of contrast will advance via the catheter.

All cases of catheter complications described here require surgical revision and correction. In the majority of these patients, except the simplest cases of disconnection, one should proceed with replacement of the malfunctioning part of the catheter rather than trying to correct it.

Iatrogenic Complications

Iatrogenic complications are related to errors in refilling and reprogramming of the pump and should either be avoided or quickly diagnosed and treated.

Introduction of infection during pump refill should be prevented by strictly following aseptic rules during the procedure.

Mistakes related to the use of the wrong medication or wrong concentration of the drug should be avoided by double-checking the prescription and label on the injected drug. The same precautions will help to eliminate programming mistakes.

Checking of the reservoir pressure after each refill will eliminate overfilling of the pump, which can lead to overdose.

Administration of refill medications outside of the pump reservoir (in the subcutaneous pocket) is a potentially grave complication if it goes unrecognized. Absorption of extremely high doses of opioid from the subcutaneous tissue will lead, in 1–3 hours, to opioid overdose. In some patients localization of the port can be difficult, and sliding of the needle along the surface of the pump can be mistakenly misinterpreted as entering the port. It is important to always expect to feel the firm "end-point" when the needle enters the refill port.

We suggest a rule of three signs, which will confirm the correct refill procedure:

1. The ability to aspirate clear liquid, the volume of which is equal to the residual volume indicated by computer.
2. Initial negative pressure in the reservoir during refill that lets the plunger move by itself after attachment of the refill syringe.
3. The ability to easily aspirate the injected medicine during refill. It is mandatory to do this after the first 1–2 mL of solution is injected, especially if one of the first two signs raises any question.

If subcutaneous injection has been diagnosed, the patient should be transferred to an emergency room in the presence of medical staff and with naloxone readily available. The patient should be monitored for respiratory rate, pulse oximetry, and mental status. There is usually at least an hour after the injection before the onset of symptoms. In our experience, one case of subcutaneous injection of 240 mg of morphine sulfate (4 mL) required 12 hours of observation without any pharmacological management.

Another area of potential confusion is calculation of the "bridge bolus"—programming of the pump when the nature or the concentration of the drug is changing. The existing formula is complicated and usually just mechanically copied by personnel performing the procedure. Making any error in mathematical calculation or pushing the wrong button on your calculator can lead to devastating results. The author has witnessed more mistakes with the "bridge bolus" than with any other refilling and reprogramming activities. Here is an easy way to calculate the "bridge bolus" or to at least recheck your results from the standard "formula" calculations:

Two variables that should be programmed in the computer are the amount of the bolus (in mg or mcg) and the time over which the bolus should be given. The amount of the bolus should equal the volume of the catheter, where the "old" drug is still present after refill. This is always equal to 0.4 mL (with variations from 0.38 to 0.42 mL, this eventually can produce a maximal error of not more than 10%, which is completely benign). Unfortunately, the computer will accept only the amount but not the volume of the drug. To make the pump produce a bolus of 0.4 mL you should order a bolus equal to the new concentration of the drug multiplied by 0.4. It is important to remember that in reality the drug in the catheter is the "old" drug with the "old" concentration, so the real amount you will give is equal to the "old" concentration multiplied by 0.4. This bolus should go at the rate that you have used before or are planning to give now. To figure out the duration of the bolus you should divide the amount of medicine in the catheter by the desired rate. This number should be entered as the duration of the bolus.

This is the full sequence of these easy calculations:

1. New concentration multiplied by 0.4. Enter this as the amount of bolus.
2. Old concentration multiplied by 0.4.
3. Result from step 2 divided by the desired speed of infusion. Enter this as the duration of the bolus.

The following is a sample calculation of the "bridge bolus" after refill of the pump, when the old concentration was 10 mg/mL and the new concentration is 25 mg/mL. The desired speed of infusion is 5 mg/day.

1. 25 mg/mL × 0.4 mL = 10 mg. Amount of the bolus entered as 10 mg.
2. 10 mg/mL × 0.4 mL = 4 mg. "Real" amount of the bolus.
3. 4 mg : 5 mg/24 hours = 19.2 hours = 19 hours 12 minutes. For all practical purposes duration of the bolus entered as 19 hours.

One more trick of the trade is the ability to maintain a very low rate of delivery without turning the pump off. If necessary, this can be achieved by using the intermittent bolus program instead of a continuous infusion.

Drug-related Side Effects

Gastrointestinal

Gastrointestinal symptoms are the most common neuroaxial opioid-related side effects (35,36).

Constipation

Even though the incidence of constipation is often less than with systemic opioids, it can be fairly significant (36). Standard measures, such as increased intake of fluid and fiber, stool softeners, and, if needed, stimulant laxatives, should be used. Additionally, decreasing the opioid dose or using an alternative drug can help in resolving the problem.

Nausea and Vomiting

This is not an infrequent side effect but is usually not as much of a problem in the majority of patients as with high-dose systemic opioids. Mild symptoms are usually transient and can be temporarily dealt with by using standard antiemetics. More persistent or severe symptoms should be addressed by a change of the opioid. In our experience all but two cases of intractable nausea related to intrathecal morphine were resolved by substituting with hydromorphone (32).

Urinary

Urinary Retention

This is related to spinal opioids and is a fairly common problem during the initial 24–48 hours of treatment. In the vast majority of cases this resolves spontaneously as the treatment continues. Because the stress from surgery and anesthesia can also play a role in development of initial urinary retention, it sometimes helps to turn the pump off for a few days. As the problem resolves itself, infusion should be restarted at a lower rate and then the rate slowly titrated up. If there are persistent symptoms and urological pathology was ruled out, a change of opioid may alleviate urinary retention. Both hydromorphone and methadone have been shown to cause a lower rate of urinary retention than morphine (33,34).

Cutaneous

Pruritus

Pruritus with neuroaxial opioids is fairly common, although the frequency of this side effect is much higher in opioid-naive patients than in the typical candidates for implantation of epidural or intrathecal delivery systems. Symptoms will usually be picked up during the trial, and a change of opioid should be done at this time. The frequency of pruritus is lower with hydromorphone than with morphine (28,33). In the vast majority of cases, the use of hydromorphone instead of morphine resolved pruritus completely. Twice in our practice, patients had no pruritus during the epidural trial but developed it with intrathecal infusion. I do not find it helpful to use any additional drugs to counteract the problem, contrary to some statements in the literature (35). One of the possible future modalities of treatment can be the use of opioid antagonists or partial antagonists in the pump mixed with the opioid. Use of those combinations was described in the literature for treatment of acute pain. We described one case of successful use of a mixture of hydromorphone and nalbuphine in the programmable intrathecal pump (32). The patient did not have any pruritus and maintained the same level of analgesia on 0.5 mg/day of hydromorphone and 0.02 mg/day of nalbuphine.

CNS

Sedation, Dizziness, Memory Problems

These are not unusual, even though less common than with high doses of systemic opioids. These symptoms are related to the rostral spread of the intrathecal opioid and will improve if an opioid with a lesser ability to migrate rostrally is used. Methadone practically does not show any spread to high spinal levels, so it is of no surprise that in our study of intrathecal methadone, all patients noticed a decrease in sedation.

Respiratory Depression

Respiratory depression is a rare complication in the treatment of chronic pain patients due to their tolerance to opioids. I purposefully decided to skip discussions of the higher occurrence in opioid-naive patients (35) because they should not be candidates for neuroaxial opioids. The most common time of occurrence is during the trial, if an inappropriately high dose of neuroaxial opioid was chosen. In a patient who is already receiving intrathecal opioid, respiratory depression can be caused by inadvertent mistakes in reprogramming of the pump, use of wrong drug concentration, too aggressive titration, or use of adjunct medication, affecting respiratory function.

Sexual and Endocrine Dysfunction

The presence of sexual dysfunction with chronic neuroaxial opioid treatment has attracted the attention of researchers only recently, even though its prevalence seems to be surprisingly high (36,96). A pilot study suggested that it can be a result of decreased levels of serum testosterone (97).

New research has indicated significant endocrine consequences of neuroaxial opioids (98). Out of 73 patients the majority had hypogonadotropic hypogonadism, 13% developed central hypocorticism, and 17% growth hormone deficiency. These changes significantly affected sexual function in this group of patients.

Edema of the Lower Extremities

Developing pedal edema with systemic opioids is not unusual. As a result of multiple communications with pain clinicians and from my own experience I feel that this problem is much more prevalent in patients receiving neuroaxial opioids than previously suggested (36). For reasons unknown, this side effect has been completely ignored in reviews and textbook chapters dedicated to neuroaxial opioid therapy. The use of diuretics and elastic stockings usually provides mild to minimal improvement. Recent attempts to use oral aldactone produced good results in one group of patients. More attention to this side effect will hopefully bring a better understanding of the problem that eventually will lead to the development of treatment algorithms.

Tolerance

Reduction in the level of analgesia with the same dose of opioid is the result of the development of tolerance and is a physiological process. The initial solution to the problem is titration of the infusion rate higher. If this approach fails, the use of alternative opioids or nonopioid drugs is the next step. I want to refer the reader to the section describing the various drugs because no special recipes exist. D-methadone has been shown in animal models to prevent the development of tolerance to intrathecal morphine. That makes methadone a front-runner in a group of future medications that possibly will resolve this problem.

New Neurological Symptoms

The appearance of new neurological symptoms or complaints, i.e., increase in pain, new distribution of pain, or new weakness or paresthesia, can be the sign of advancement of disease, onset of new disease, or complications of the implanted system. Any of the preceding complaints should warrant thorough examination and testing, possibly including MRI. The controversy about using MRI with implantable drug delivery devices is over. The only precaution should be to check the programmable pump settings after the procedure to verify that no accidental reprogramming occurred.

As with any invasive procedure involving the epidural or intrathecal space, implantation can cause arachnoiditis. Clinical symptoms, MRI picture, and CSF testing via the catheter port can help with the diagnosis. No specific measures exist in dealing with this complication. In two cases of severe arachnoiditis I removed the catheter for a few months, keeping the pump on (delivering a minuscule amount of water subcutaneously). That caused the disappearance of the symptoms and normalization of the CSF. Reimplantation of the catheter did not produce a new inflammatory reaction, but I still periodically perform CSF sampling.

The catheter can exert pressure on the spinal cord or nerve roots, especially when it angles or loops in the spinal space. MRI or myelography via the catheter will help with the diagnosis. Clinical symptoms should coincide with the anatomical site of irritation by the catheter. In one case I had to replace a catheter that formed a loop in the spinal space with pressure on a nerve root, causing the new onset of radiculopathy. All symptoms disappeared immediately after surgery.

The formation of granuloma-type masses in proximity to the tip of the intrathecal catheter is a serious, though not very common, complication (35,99–102). A few reports show that this is more prevalent in long-term treatment with high doses of morphine (99,103). The nature of the mass formation is not completely clear, although it seems that a reaction to the drug is the most plausible explanation. Symptoms suggestive of this complication are new or increased pain, numbness, weakness, or abnormalities of bladder and bowel control. An MRI will help with final confirmation of the diagnosis. It is important to remember that even though the symptoms can initially be restricted to the lumbar sensory and motor levels, the affected site is at the tip of the catheter, possibly at the thoracic level. Specific instructions to include this area during MRI study are necessary. Removal of the catheter and surgical decompression, if necessary, are appropriate steps of treatment. I have personally encountered three cases of mass formation at the tip of the catheter in my patients and one case as an expert reviewer. One patient underwent surgical removal without any consequences. Two others, despite prompt surgery, still have residual weakness of the lower extremities. The fourth patient is in the process of testing and treatment as this is being written. All patients had received relatively high doses of intrathecal morphine for more than 24 months.

PERSONAL DATA

In the 24-month period from January 1998 to January 2000, I implanted 66 programmable intrathecal pumps for chronic intractable pain. All of the data presented are as of September 2000.

Only three patients had a malignant source of pain, the rest were suffering from chronic nonmalignant pain; 26 patients were male, and 40 were female. The ages ranged from 19 to 91.

Five patients died from either their primary disease or concurrent medical problems. Three patients moved out of the area and were lost to followup. In three cases the pump was explanted for different reasons: infection, lack of effect, new CNS pathology.

The drugs delivered via the pump at the time of data collection were as follows: 27 patients received morphine, 16 hydromorphone, 5 mixture of opioid and adjuvant drug, 4 methadone, 2 meperidine, 1 SNX-111.

Four patients (6%) developed infection of the pump pocket area, one of them about a year after surgery. Two were successfully treated conservatively, the other two underwent removal of the implant. One of those was reimplanted without any complications.

Two patients (3%) required revision of the catheter. In one case, the two-piece catheter was disconnected at the metal connector site. The other patient developed pressure on a nerve root that was successfully eliminated by replacing the catheter. Again I want to stress that none of the patients with the one-piece catheter (majority in this group) had loss of patency or continuity of the catheter.

Two patients developed granuloma-type masses at the tip of the catheter; one underwent surgery, the other is still continuing workup.

SUMMARY

Neuroaxial drug delivery is an important part of a continuum of managing chronic intractable pain. It is hard to imagine contemporary pain management without this modality of treatment. Very effective and relatively safe, it still poses a lot of questions and problems as we are becoming more acquainted with it and use it more widely. Significant efforts in research of new drugs are needed. Unfortunately, most of the effort so far has been aimed at data collection and retrospective reviews of clinical experience. Prospective randomized studies are necessary to answer many questions. Recent attention to some previously ignored problems indicates that we are moving from the initial period of excitement and fascination to a period of serious and critical analysis and a more scientific approach.

Acknowledgment

The author gratefully acknowledges Katherine Mironer for her assistance in providing the illustrations for this chapter.

REFERENCES

1. Wang JF, Nauss LA, Thomas JE. Pain relief by intrathecally applied morphine in man. *Anesthesiology* 1979;50:149–151.
2. Sinatra RS. Spinal and epidural opioids. In: Rogers MC, Tinker JH, Covino BG, et al. eds. *Principles and practice of anesthesiology*. St. Louis, MO: Mosby Year Book. 1993:1425–1443.
3. Rawal N. Current status of epidural and spinal opioids. In: Waldman SD, Winnie AP, eds. *Interventional pain management*. Philadelphia: W.B. Saunders, 1996:431–442.
4. Walia K, Mitchell V, Staats PS. Intrathecal analgesics as we approach the new millennium. *Pain Digest* 2000;10:34–50.
5. Chaney MA. Side effects of intrathecal and epidural opioids. *Can J Anaesth* 1995;42:891–903.

6. Krames ES, Olson K. Clinical realities and economic considerations: patient selection in intrathecal therapy. *J Pain Symptom Manage* 1997;14:S3–S13.

7. Krames ES. Spinal administration of opioids for nonmalignant pain syndromes: a U.S. experience. In: Waldman SD, Winnie AP, eds. *Interventional pain management.* Philadelphia: W.B. Saunders, 1996: 443–446.

8. Krames ES. Intraspinal opioid therapy for chronic nonmalignant pain: current practice and clinical guidelines. *J Pain Symptom Manage* 1996;11:333–352.

9. Deer T, Winkelmuller W, Erdine S, et al. Intrathecal therapy for cancer and nonmalignant pain: patient selection and patient management. *Neuromodulation* 1999;2:55–66.

10. Bedder MD, Burchiel K, Larson A. Cost analysis of two implantable narcotic delivery systems. *J Pain Symptom Manage* 1991;6:368–373.

11. Monsalve V, de Andres JA, Valia JC. Application of a psychological decision algorithm for the selection of patients susceptible to implantation of neuromodulation systems for the treatment of chronic pain. A proposal. *Neuromodulation* 2000;3:191–200.

12. Doleys DM. Psychological assessment for implantable therapies. *Pain Digest* 2000;10:16–23.

13. Kidd DH, North RB. Spinal cord stimulation: an effective and cost saving treatment in management of chronic pain. In: Pain treatment centers at crossroads: a practical and conceptual reappraisal. Cohen MJM and Campbell JN, eds. *Progress in Pain Research and Management.* Seattle: IASP Press, 1996;7:174.

14. Tollison CD, Hinnant DW. Psychological testing in the evaluation of the patient in pain. In: Waldman SD, Winnie AP, eds. *Interventional Pain Management.* New York, Philadelphia: W.B. Saunders. 1996: 119–128.

15. Tollison CD. The comprehensive diagnosis of spinal pain: a new psychodiagnostic instrument. *Orthopaedic Review* 1993;22:335–340.

16. Willoughby SG, Hailey BJ, Wheeler LC. Pain patient profile: a scale to measure psychological distress. *Arch Phys Med Rehabil* 1999;80: 1300–1302.

17. Paice JA, Penn RD, Shott S. Intraspinal morphine for chronic pain: a retrospective, multicenter study. *J Pain Symptom Manage* 1996;11: 71–80.

18. Anderson VC, Burchiel KJ, Cooke B. *Randomized screening trial of intraspinal morphine for selection of patients for chronic opioid therapy.* Presented at the Worldwide Pain Conference, San Francisco, CA. July 2000.

19. Maeyaert J, Kupers RC. Long-term intrathecal drug administration in the treatment of persistent noncancer pain: a 3-year experience. In: Waldman SD, Winnie AP, eds. *Interventional pain management.* Philadelphia: W.B. Saunders. 1996:447–456.

20. Du Pen SL, Williams A. Tunneled epidural catheters: practical considerations and implantation techniques. In: Waldman SD, Winnie AP, eds. *Interventional pain management.* Philadelphia: W.B. Saunders. 1996:457–472.

21. Cherry DA, Gourlay GK, Cousins MJ, et al. A technique for the insertion of an implantable portal system for the long-term epidural administration of opioids in the treatment of cancer pain. *Anaesth Intens Care* 1985;13:145–152.

22. Dahm P, Nitescu P, Appelgren L, et al. Efficacy and technical complications of long-term continuous intraspinal infusions of opioid and/or bupivacaine in refractory nonmalignant pain: a comparison between the epidural and the intrathecal approach with externalized or implanted catheters and infusion pumps. *The Clinical Journal of Pain* 1998;14:4–16.

23. Brazenor GA. Long term intrathecal administration of morphine: a comparison of bolus injection via reservoir with continuous infusion by implanted pump. *Neurosurgery* 1987;21:484–491.

24. Krames ES. Implantation techniques for totally implantable drug administration systems. In: Waldman SD, Winnie AP, eds. *Interventional Pain Management.* Philadelphia: W.B. Saunders. 1996:473–482.

25. Kroin JS, Ali A, York M, et al. The distribution of medication along the spinal canal after chronic intrathecal administration. *Neurosurgery* 1993;33:226–230.

26. Ummenhofer WC, Arends RH, Shen DD, et al. Comparative spinal distribution and clearance kinetics of intrathecally administered morphine, fentanyl, alfentanil, and sufentanil. *Anesthesiology* 2000;92: 739–753.

27. Krames E, Buchser E, Hassenbusch SJ, et al. Future trends in the development of local drug delivery systems: intraspinal, intracerebral, and intraparenchymal therapies. *Neuromodulation* 1999;2: 133–148.

28. Chaplan SR, Duncan SR, Brodsky JB, et al. Morphine and hydromorphone epidural analgesia: a prospective, randomized comparison. *Anesthesiology* 1992;77:1090–1094

29. Nichols RL. Bacteriology in surgery. In: Nyhus LM, Baker RJ, eds. *Mastery of surgery.* Boston: Little, Brown and Company. 1992:83–94.

30. Hassenbusch SJ, Garber J, Buchser E, et al. Alternative intrathecal agents for the treatment of pain. *Neuromodulation* 1999;2:85–91.

31. Hassenbusch SJ, Portenoy RK. Current practices in intraspinal therapy—a survey of clinical trends and decision making. *J Pain Symptom Manage* 2000;20:S4–S11.

32. Mironer YE, Grumman S. Experience with alternative solutions in intrathecal treatment of chronic nonmalignant pain. *Pain Digest* 1999;9:299–302.

33. Goodarzi M. Comparison of epidural morphine, hydromorphone and fentanyl for postoperative pain control in children undergoing orthopaedic surgery. *Paediatric anaesthesia* 1999;9:419–422.

34. Evron S, Samueloff A, Simon A, Drenger B, Magora F. Urinary function during epidural analgesia with methadone and morphine in post-cesarean section patients. *Pain* 1985;23:135–144.

35. Naumann C, Erdine S, Koulousakis A, et al. Drug adverse events and system complications of intrathecal opioid delivery for pain: origins, directions, manifestations, and management. *Neuromodulation* 1999;2:92–107.

36. Paice JA, Winkelmuller W, Burchiel K, et al. Clinical realities and economic considerations: efficacy of intrathecal pain therapy. *J Pain Symptom Manage* 1997;14:S14–S26.

37. Smith MT, Watt JA, Cramond T. Morphine-3-glucuronide—a potent antagonist of morphine analgesia. *Life Sci* 1990;47:579–585.

38. Krames ES. Intrathecal infusional therapies for intractable pain: patient management guidelines. *J Pain Symptom Manage* 1993;8: 36–46.

39. Bennett G, Burchiel K, Buchser E, et al. Clinical guidelines for intraspinal infusion: report of an expert panel. *J Pain Symptom Manage* 2000;20:S37–S43.

40. Krames ES, Schuchard M. Implantable intraspinal infusional analgesia: management guidelines. *Pain Review* 1995;2:243–267.

41. Goodarzi M. Comparison of analgesic potency of epidural fentanyl, hydromorphone and morphine for postoperative analgesia in children. *Anesthesiology* 1997;87:A1049.

42. Brodsky JB, Chaplan SR, Brose WG, et al. Continuous epidural hydromorphone for postthoracotomy pain relief. *Ann Thorac Surg* 1990;50:888–893.

43. Coombs DW, Saunders RL, Fratkin JD, et al. Continuous intrathecal hydromorphone and clonidine for intractable cancer pain. *J Neurosurg* 1986;64:890–894.

44. Schuchard M, Krames ES, Lanning R. Intraspinal analgesia for nonmalignant pain. *Neuromodulation* 1998;1:46–56.

45. Parker RK, White PF. Epidural patient-controlled analgesia: an alternative to intravenous patient-controlled analgesia for pain relief after cesarean delivery. *Anesth Analg* 1992;75:245–251.

46. Liu S, Carpenter RL, Mulroy MF, et al. Intravenous versus epidural administration of hydromorphone. *Anesthesiology* 1995;82:682–688.

47. Winkelmuller M, Winkelmuller W. Long-term effects of continuos intrathecal opioid treatment in chronic pain of nonmalignant etiology. *J Neurosurg* 1996;85:458–467.

48. Chrubasik J, Chrubasik S, Friedrich G, et al. Long-term treatment of pain by spinal opiates: an update. *The Pain Clinic* 1992;5:147–156.

49. Loper KA, Read LB, Downey M, et al. Epidural and intravenous fentanyl infusions are clinically equivalent after knee surgery. *Anesth Analg* 1988:13:15.

50. Coe A, Sarginson A, Smith MW, et al. Pain following thoracotomy. *Anaesthesia* 1991;40:918–921.

51. Van den Hoogen RHWM, Colpaert FC. Epidural and subcutaneous morphine, meperidine (pethidine), fentanyl and sufentanil in the rat: analgesia and other in vivo pharmacologic effects. *Anesthesiology* 1987;66:186–194.

52. Thi TV, Orliaguet G, Liu N, et al. A dose-range study of intrathecal meperidine combined with bupivacaine. *Acta Anaesth Scand* 1992; 36:516–518.

53. Harvey SC, O'Neil MG, Pope CA, et al. Continuous intrathecal meperidine via an implantable infusion pump for chronic nonmalignant pain. *Ann Pharmacother* 1997;31:1306–1308.
54. Ong B, Segstro R. Respiratory depression associated with meperidine spinal anesthesia. *Can J Anaesth* 1994;41:725–727.
55. Jacobson L, Chabal C, Brody MC, et al. Intrathecal methadone and morphine for postoperative analgesia: a comparison of the efficacy, duration, and side effects. *Anesthesiology* 1989;70:742–746.
56. Chung KS, Sinatra R, Fermo L, Paige D, Weinstock A. Perioperative efficacy of intrathecal methadone-bupivacaine for cesarean section: comparison with fentanyl. *Anesthesiology* 1993;79:A1026.
57. Boutte JN, Martindale ML, Ramanathan J. Comparison of intrathecal methadone and fentanyl for labor analgesia. *Anesthesiology* 1992; 77:A993.
58. Jacobson L, Chabal C, Brody MC, et al. Intrathecal methadone: a dose-response study and comparison with intrathecal morphine 0.5 mg. *Pain* 1990;43:141–148.
59. Max MB, Inturrisi CE, Kaiko RF, et al. Epidural and intrathecal opiates: cerebrospinal fluid and plasma profiles in patients with chronic cancer pain. *Clin Pharmacol Ther* 1985;38:631–641.
60. Shir Y, Eimerl D, Magora F, et al. Plasma concentrations of methadone during postoperative patient-controlled extradural analgesia. *Br J Anaesth* 1990;65:204–209.
61. Gorman AL, Elliott KJ, Inturrisi CE. The d- and l-isomers of methadone bind to the non-competitive site on the N-methyl-D-aspartate (NMDA) receptor in rat forebrain and spinal cord. *Neurosci Lett* 1997;223:5–8.
62. Morley JS. New perspective in our use of opioids. *Pain Forum* 1999; 8:200–205.
63. Shimoyama N, Shimoyama M, Elliott KJ, Inturrisi CE. d-Methadone is antinociceptive in the rat formalin test. *J Pharmacol Exp Ther.* 1997;283:648–652.
64. Mironer YE, Haasis JC, Chapple IT, et al. Successful use of methadone in neuropathic pain: a multicenter study by the National Forum of Independent Pain Clinicians. *Pain Digest* 1999;9:191–193.
65. Inturrisi CE, Davis AM, Shimoyama N, et al. *d-Methadone has NMDA receptor antagonist activity and prevents the development of tolerance to morphine.* Presented at the 16th American Pain Society Annual Scientific Meeting, New Orleans, LA, October 1997.
66. Mironer YE, Tollison CD. Methadone in the treatment of chronic nonmalignant pain resistant to other neuroaxial agents: the first experience. *Neuromodulation* 2000;4. In press.
67. Atlas G. Calculating mixtures of local anesthetic and morphine for implantable intrathecal pumps. *Pain Digest* 1996;6:232–236.
68. Krames ES, Lanning RM. Intrathecal infusional analgesia for nonmalignant pain: analgesic efficacy of intrathecal opioid with or without bupivacaine. *J Pain Symptom Manage* 1993;8:539–548.
69. Parker RK, Sawaki Y, White P. Epidural patient-controlled analgesia: influence of bupivacaine and hydromorphone basal infusion on pain control after cesarean delivery. *Anesth Analg* 1992;75:740–746.
70. Van Dongen RTM, Crul BJP, van Egmond J. Intrathecal coadministration of bupivacaine diminishes morphine dose progression during long-term intrathecal infusion in cancer patients. *The Clinical Journal of Pain* 1999;15:166–172.
71. Puke MJC, Xu XJ, Wiesenfeld-Hallin Z. Intrathecal administration of clonidine suppresses autotomy, a behavioral sign of chronic pain in rats after sciatic nerve section. *Neurosci Lett* 1991;133:199–202.
72. Puke MJC, Weisenfeld-Hallin Z. The differential effects of morphine and the a2-adrenoreceptor agonists clonidine and dexmedetomidine on the prevention and treatment of experimental neuropathic pain. *Anesth Analg* 1993;77:104–109.
73. Filos KS, Goudas LC, Patroni O, et al. Dose-related hemodynamic and analgesic effects of intrathecal clonidine administered after cesarean section. *Reg Anesth* 1993;18:S18.
74. Rauck RL, Eisenach JC, Jackson K, et al. Epidural clonidine treatment for refractory reflex sympathetic dystrophy. *Anesthesiology* 1993;79:1163–1169.
75. Eisenach JC, Du Pen S, Dubois M, et al. Epidural clonidine analgesia for intractable cancer pain. *Pain* 1995;61:391–399.
76. Filos KS, Goudas LC, Patroni O, et al. Hemodynamic and analgesic profile after intrathecal clonidine in humans. *Anesthesiology* 1994;81:591–601.

77. Staats P, Charapata S, Presley R. *Chronic, intractable neuropathic pain: marked analgesic efficacy of ziconotide.* Poster presentation at the 4th International Congress of the International Neuromodulation Society; September 20th, 1998; Lucerne, Switzerland.
78. Penn RD, Paice JA, Kroin JS. Octreotide: a potent new no-opiate analgesic for intrathecal infusion. *Pain* 1992;49:13–19.
79. Klamt JG, Slullitel A, Garcia IV, et al. Postoperative analgesic effect of intrathecal neostigmine and its influence on spinal anaesthesia. *Anaesthesia* 1997;52:547–551.
80. Bouaziz H, Chuanyao T, Eisenach JC. Postoperative analgesia from intrathecal neostigmine in sheep. *Anesth Analg* 1995;80:1140–1144.
81. Hood DD, Eisenach JC, Tuttle R. Phase I safety assessment of intrathecal neostigmine methylsulfate in humans. *Anesthesiology* 1995;82:331–343.
82. Yang CY, Wong CS, Chang JY, et al. Intrathecal ketamine reduces morphine requirements in patients with terminal cancer pain. *Can J Anaesth* 1996;43:379–383.
83. Beltrutti DPC, Coletta P, Di Santo S, et al. The spinal administration of ketamine: lights and shadows. *Pain Digest* 1997;7:127–135.
84. Hassenbusch SJ, Satterfield WC, Gradert TL, et al. Preclinical toxicity study of intrathecal administration of the pain relievers dextrorphan, dextromethorphan, and memantine in the sheep model. *Neuromodulation* 1999;4:230–240.
85. Borg PAJ, Krijnen HJ. Long-term intrathecal administration of midazolam and clonidine. *Clin J Pain* 1996;12:63–68.
86. Taira T, Kawamura H, Tanikawa T, et al. A new approach to control central deafferentation pain: spinal intrathecal baclofen. *Stereotact Funct Neurosurg* 1995;65:101–105.
87. Winkelmuller W, Burchiel K, Van Buyten JP. Intrathecal opioid therapy for pain: efficacy and outcomes. *Neuromodulation* 1999;2:67–76.
88. Tutak U, Doleys DM. Intrathecal infusion systems for treatment of chronic low back and leg pain of noncancer origin. *South Med J* 1996;89:295–300.
89. Mueller-Schwefe G, Hassenbusch SJ, Reig E. Cost effectiveness of intrathecal therapy for pain. *Neuromodulation* 1999;2:77–84.
90. Hassenbusch SJ, Paice JA, Patt RB, et al. Clinical realities and economic considerations: economics of intrathecal therapy. *J Pain Symptom Manage* 1997;14:S36–S48.
91. Patt RB, Hassenbusch SJ. Implantable technology for pain control: Identification and management of problems and complications. In: Waldman SD, Winnie AP eds. *Interventional pain management.* Philadelphia: W.B.Saunders. 1996:483–499.
92. Erdine S, Yucel A. Complications of drug delivery systems. *Pain Reviews* 1995;2:227–242.
93. Mironer YE, Flandry RE, Grumman S. Local erythema and edema of soft tissue after intrathecal morphine pump implant: an unusual complication. *Pain Digest* 1998;8:171–172.
94. Follett KA, Naumann CP. A prospective study of catheter-related complications of intrathecal drug delivery systems. *J Pain Symptom Manage* 2000;19:209–215.
95. Somerville JJ, Mironer YE, Beattie C. *Cerebrospinal fluid fistula between the dislodged catheter and intrathecal space: an unusual complication of implantable pump.* Presented at the Worldwide Pain Conference, San Francisco, CA, July 2000.
96. Doleys DM, Dinoff BL, Page L, et al. Sexual dysfunction and other side effects of intraspinal opiate use in the management of chronic non-cancer pain. *AJPM* 1998;8:5–11.
97. Paice JA, Penn RD, Ryan WG. Altered sexual function and decreased testosterone in patients receiving intraspinal opioids. *J Pain Symptom Manage* 1994;9:126–131.
98. Verhelst AR, Maeyaert J, Van Buyten JP, et al. Endocrine consequences of long-term intrathecal administration of opioids. *J Clin Endocrinol Metab* 2000;85:2215–2222.
99. Cabbell KL, Taren JA, Sagher O. Spinal cord compression by catheter granulomas in high-dose intrathecal morphine therapy: case report. *Neurosurgery* 1998;42:1176–1181.
100. Sjoberg M, Karlsson PA, Nordbog C, et al. Neuropathologic findings after long term intrathecal infusion of morphine and bupivacaine for pain treatment in cancer patients. *Anesthesiology* 1992; 76:173–186.
101. Blount JP, Remley KB, Yue SK, et al. Intrathecal granuloma complicating chronic spinal infusion of morphine: report of three cases. *J Neurosurg* 1996;84:272–276.

102. Schuchard M, Lanning R, North R, et al. Neurologic sequelae of intraspinal drug delivery systems: results of a survey of American implanters of implantable drug delivery systems. *Neuromodulation* 1998;1:137–148.

103. Anderson SR, Racz G, Raj PR. *Intrathecal granuloma in patients receiving high-dose intrathecal morphine therapy: a report of two cases.* Presented at the Worldwide Pain Conference, San Francisco, CA, July 2000.

104. Tamsen A, Hartvig P, Fagerlund C, et al. Patient-controlled analgesic therapy: clinical experience. *Acta Anaesthesiol Scan* 1982; 74(Suppl):157–160.

105. Eimerl D, Magora F, Shir Y, et al. Patient-controlled analgesia with epidural methadone by means of an external infusion pump. *Schmerz/Pain/Douleur* 1986;7:156–160.

106. Chrubasik J, Wust H, Schulte-Monting J, et al. Relative analgesic potency of epidural fentanyl, alfentanil and morphine in treatment of postoperative pain. *Anesthesiology* 1988;68:929–933.

107. Van der Auwern A, Verborgh C, Camu F. Analgesic and cardiorespiratory effects of epidural sufentanil and morphine. *Anesth Analg* 1987;66:999.

CHAPTER **12**

Neurostimulation Techniques

Y. Eugene Mironer

In the ever-expanding and constantly changing field of chronic pain management, neurostimulation is a very important, if not "trendy," modality of treatment. The transcutaneous use of electrical current has been around for a very long time. The beginning of the modern era started with the first spinal cord stimulation by an intrathecally placed lead in 1967 (1). Over the next 30 years this modality underwent significant transformation and expansion in both use and variety of technologies. In the beginning of the 21st century it is a very popular mode of treatment (2,3). Our knowledge in this field has increased tremendously. At the same time this improvement in our scope of knowledge has demonstrated that we still have more questions than answers. This is true for mechanisms of stimulation, selection of patients, selections of hardware, or modes of stimulation, etc. The goal of this chapter is to give an overview of new developments in the field as well as provide some detailed practical knowledge of certain aspects of neuroaugmentation. One of the applications—deep brain stimulation—will be discussed in a separate chapter.

MECHANISMS OF NEUROSTIMULATION

Multiple theories have been offered to suggest possible mechanisms of action of spinal cord stimulation (4,5). Current data support multiple mechanisms participating in the final effects produced by stimulation of the spinal cord. A brief overview of the current theories of mechanisms of SCS will be presented here; more detailed information can be obtained from review articles dedicated to the subject (4,6).

Spinal cord stimulation was developed in response to the gate control theory (7). It seems, though, that this mechanism is not directly applicable because no evidence has been produced to show that SCS influences nociceptive pain (4,6). It has been shown to have no effect on acute pain or experimental pain (8,9,10). Also, simple spinothalamic conduction block, proposed as an explanation of SCS effect (11,12), does not explain the fact that the duration of the stimulation effect lasts some time after stimulation has been discontinued. Animal studies indicate that SCS affects abnormal, but not normal, function of A-beta fibers (13,14). This effect was preserved even in animals with transected spinal cords (14). Several animal studies have confirmed that SCS suppresses hyperexcitability of wide-dynamic-range neurons in the dorsal horn (15,16). Activation of supraspinal structures has been demonstrated as well (17,18), but the exact mechanisms of it and its role in SCS responses are not yet clear.

SCS causes multiple biochemical changes in spinal and supraspinal neural structures (6). Neurochemical mechanisms without any doubt are involved in the dorsal horn modulation of SCS inhibitory action. The most notable dorsal horn effects are an increase in the release of inhibitory transmitters—GABA and glycine (19,20)—and a decrease in the release of excitatory amino acids—aspartate and glutamate (21). Another possible central neuromodulator of the SCS action is adenosine (22).

Somewhat different mechanisms are involved in the beneficial effects of SCS on ischemic pain. In peripheral vascular disease it increases blood flow with or without modulation of the sympathetic outflow (23,24), whereas in coronary ischemia it also reduces tissue oxygen demand (6). In ischemic heart disease this ultimately increases anginal threshold (25). Researchers have shown that this is the result of vasodilation produced by an antidromic activation of dorsal root structures as well as an inhibitory effect on sympathetic function (26,27).

Our knowledge of SCS mechanisms is not only incomplete but also constantly changing. A better understanding of the neurophysiology and neurochemistry of CNS function during neurostimulation will lead to an improvement in technology and eventually better outcomes of this modality of treatment.

ANATOMICAL AND PHYSIOLOGICAL CONSIDERATIONS IN SCS

The main target for SCS is the dorsal columns, containing large-diameter sensory fibers. The initial terminology, *dorsal column stimulator,* is not correct because a multitude of structures are activated with SCS. The position of the lead relative to different structures of the spinal space proved to provide variable results of stimulation. Specific anatomical and physiological (mainly electrical) properties of different structures in the spinal space are extremely important in our understanding of this phenomenon.

The initial, somewhat simplistic, outlook on the relationship between lead position and the area of stimulation was one-dimensional. The level of the electrode was considered the single determinant of the recruited area. For example, to stimulate the anterior thigh, the lead should be at T-11–T-12, posterior thigh at T-11–L-1, foot at L-1 (28). The only other requirement was not to put the lead too lateral. The contemporary scope of knowledge indicates that we should look at positioning of the lead in its full, three-dimensional complexity.

The lead is positioned in the epidural space so that the current travels through the epidural space, dura mater, CSF, and spinal cord (29). Besides, the current is not moving in one direction, so it involves other structures besides the dorsal columns, i.e., dorsal roots or ventral roots. The nerve roots have much lower excitation thresholds than the dorsal columns (29). This is the result, not only of the larger diameter of the dorsal root fibers, but also of their transverse position and curved shape (30).

The conductivity of CSF is significantly higher than that of any other involved structures, so the distribution of the current predominantly depends on the thickness of the CSF layer (29). He and co-authors (31) showed a close correlation between the dorsal CSF space thickness and the threshold for SCS. That means that with a thinner CSF space, lower current is necessary to produce dorsal column stimulation. This is very important because the excitation threshold for the dorsal columns is significantly higher than for dorsal root fibers. An increase in current, required to stimulate the dorsal columns in the areas with high CSF thickness, will produce recruitment of the dorsal root fibers, causing stimulation at the segmental level as well. This property of SCS creates "better" areas for cephalo-caudal placement of the lead: C-5–T-1 and below T-10 (29). The "worst" position is at the midthoracic level (Fig. 12-1). Based on these data it seems logical that success with stimulation, in general, is in reverse proportion to the CSF thickness (32).

Electrode position in the horizontal plane turns out to be very important as well. Studies have shown that there is a noticeable decrease in the area covered with stimulation and perception threshold in laterally placed electrodes versus near-midline placement (28,29). This is the result of preferential recruitment of dorsal root fibers by lateral electrodes versus activation of the dorsal column by medial electrodes. Successful stimulation can be produced by the stimulation of the 2–3-mm area on each side of physiological midline (28,29).

Another maneuver that can improve capture during SCS is the use of a "guarded" cathode or cathode surrounded by anodes. This is the most successful array of electrodes (33,34).

The anatomical picture gets even more complicated when one takes into consideration the laminar composi-

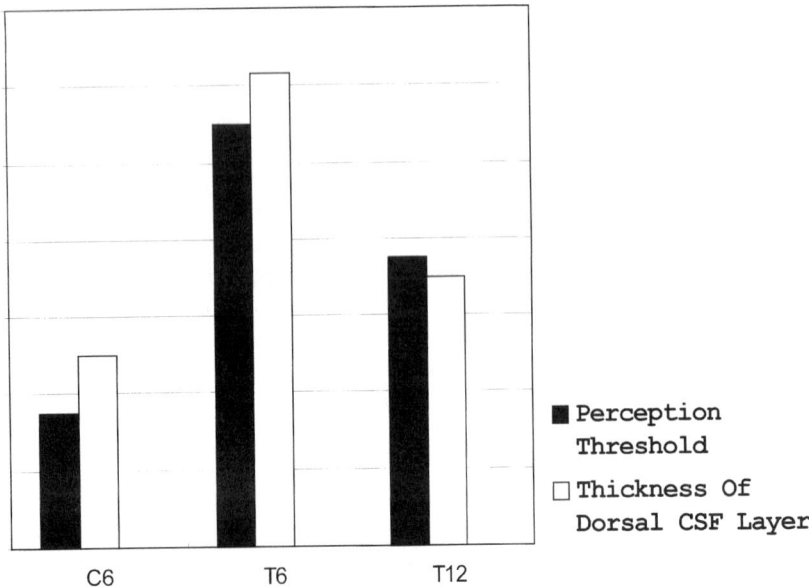

■ Perception Threshold

□ Thickness Of Dorsal CSF Layer

FIG. 12-1. Relationship between thickness of the CSF layer and threshold for dorsal column stimulation. (Adapted from Barolat G. Epidural spinal cord stimulation: anatomical and electrical properties of the intraspinal structures relevant to spinal cord stimulation and clinical correlations. *Neuromodulation* 1998;1:63–71.

tion of the dorsal column. More caudal areas are represented by more medially located laminae, whereas the segmental fibers are entering the dorsal columns as the most lateral layer (35). The significance of this will be discussed later.

TECHNOLOGY

Current technology offers multiple options for spinal cord stimulation. All systems consist of the epidural lead, some type of connector, and a generator.

The major difference in the leads depends on the method of insertion: percutaneous through the needle or surgical through a laminotomy. The percutaneous lead electrode arrays can be quadripolar or octapolar and can be positioned with increased or decreased spacing on the lead (Fig. 12-2). Surgical lead electrode arrays can be quadripolar or octapolar with a single or dual row of electrodes (Fig. 12-3).

The most important factor in generator design is if it is totally implantable or if the only part that is implanted is a receiving device while the pulse generator is external (Fig. 12-4). The other characteristic is the ability of the generator to produce two or more independent pulses.

The right choice of technology is not straightforward and can, in numerous cases, depend, not only on the patient, but also on the level of comfort of the physician. Nevertheless, I will try to review some basics of this process.

Computerized models of SCS show that the electrodes should be about 1.5 mm in length with 2–2.5 mm spacing between the edges (36). Increased distance between electrodes reduces the chance of covering large areas of the body (37). The ability to use bipolar or tripolar arrangements is a must for successful stimulation. A transverse tripolar lead is being investigated currently; it will allow

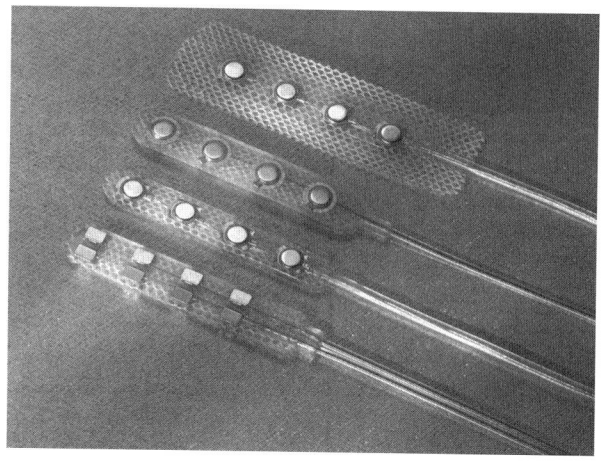

A

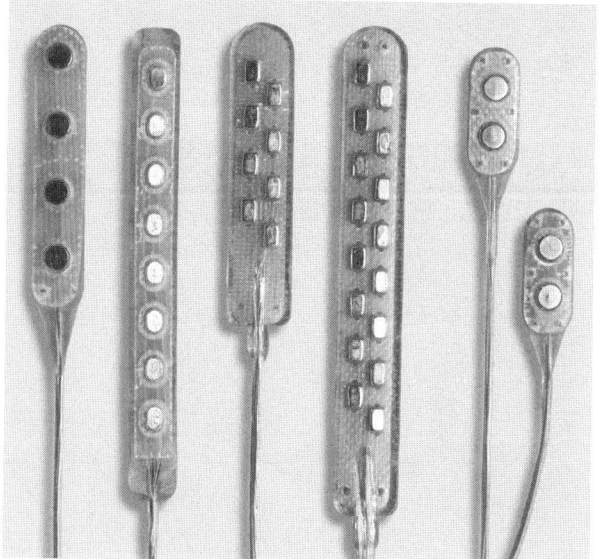

B

FIG. 12-3. **A.** Laminotomy leads (Medtronic, Inc., Minneapolis, MN). **B.** Laminotomy leads (ANS, Plano, TX).

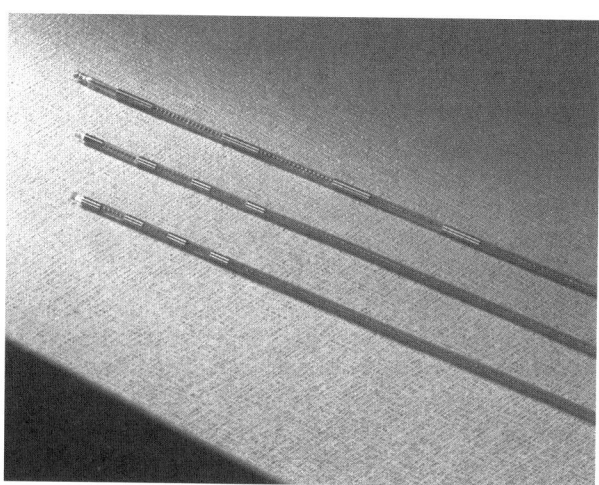

A

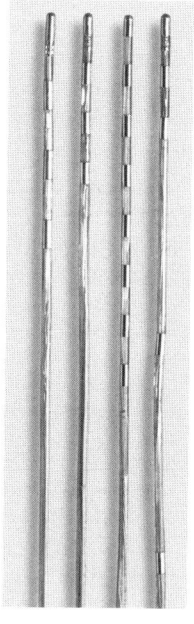

B

FIG. 12-2. **A.** Percutaneous leads (Medtronic, Inc., Minneapolis, MN). **B.** Percutaneous leads (ANS, Plano, TX).

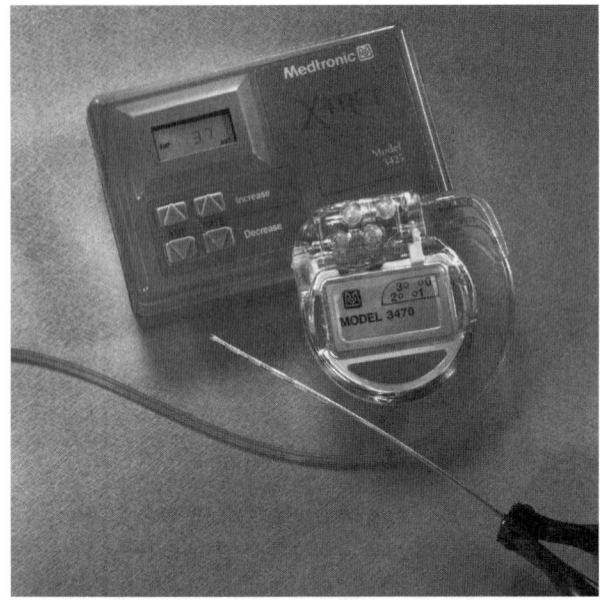

A

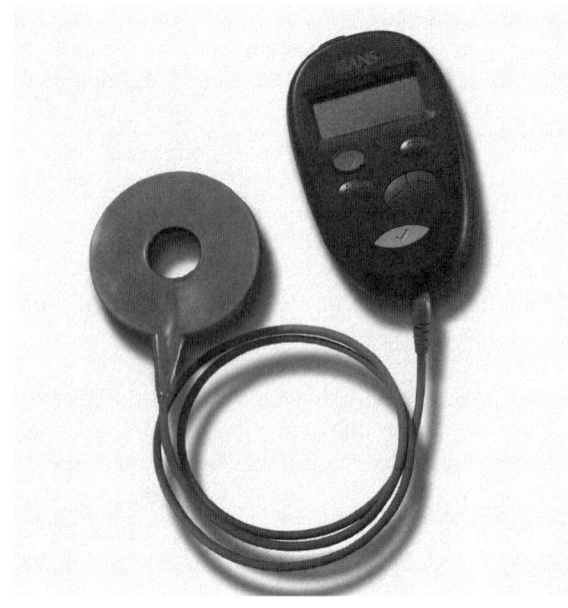

B

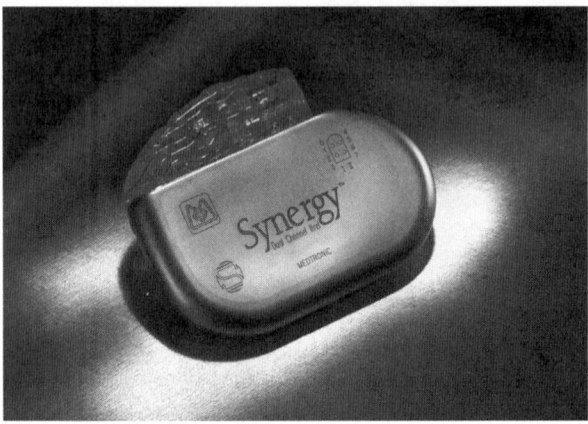

C

FIG. 12-4. A. External generators (Medtronic, Inc., Minneapolis, MN). **B.** External generators (ANS, Plano, TX). **C.** Internal generators (Medtronic, Inc., Minneapolis, MN).

"steering" of the paresthesia in the horizontal plane at one specific level (36,38).

The advantage of an octapolar versus quadripolar lead is subject to debate (39,40). The majority of the current reports are anecdotal or are the result of inadequately designed studies (41,42). In actuality, the only significant difference is familiarity with and level of comfort of the implanter with the chosen electrode. This also applies to the extended length lead (Pisces-Quad Plus, Medtronic, Inc., Minneapolis, MN) and more compact leads (Pisces-Quad Compact, Medtronic, Inc., Minneapolis, MN). The ability of one to better cover a larger area (43) and the other to produce more precise coverage has not been proven scientifically.

The benefit of a totally implantable generator versus an external radio-coupled device is also questionable and a matter of patient and physician preference (44). There is no doubt that totally implantable generators are somewhat more bulky and require surgical intervention for depleted battery replacement. On the other hand, they eliminate the restrictions related to the necessity of constantly wearing

an external device, skin irritation from the antenna, etc. The choice should be left to the patients, many of whom do not like the external system (44,45). In my opinion, younger, potentially more active patients are better candidates for a totally implantable system, even though they are facing future battery replacements. Patients with restricted mobility will be more comfortable wearing the antenna and external device. The other consideration would be generator settings during the trial. Patients requiring a high amplitude and pulse width should be advised regarding possible rapid battery depletion with frequent replacements. In this situation I would proceed with an external radio-coupling device.

Finally, one more decision that determines, to a certain extent, the type of hardware used is whether to implant one lead or two. Even the "simple" Itrel IPG (Medtronic, Inc., Minneapolis, MN) will allow the use of two leads (with a Y-connector), but the requirements are too stringent: Amplitude, pulse rate, and width should be identical for both leads. For the vast majority of patients this is impossible, so the use of other generators is necessary for multiple lead implantation. This topic is a subject for heated debates and speculations and is so controversial that we decided to discuss it separately (see "One versus Two Leads").

PATIENT SELECTION

Patient selection is the key to success in neurostimulation therapy (44). It is imperative to remember that this modality is part of a pain treatment continuum and occupies a specific place in the analgesic ladder (42,46). The use of destructive neuroablative procedures should be utilized only after failure of neuroaxial therapy in patients with chronic nonmalignant pain. In patients who can be candidates for both neurostimulation and neuroaxial opioids, in general, neurostimulation is the first in the sequence of therapy trials.

The list of pain conditions that can be amenable to neurostimulation is constantly growing. The following is a generalized list of pathological states that can qualify the patient for neurostimulation:

- Failed back surgery syndrome (including epidural fibrosis, arachnoiditis, radiculitis)
- Chronic intractable radiculopathy
- Complex regional pain syndrome
- Neuropathy (mono- and polyneuropathy) and plexopathy
- Spinal cord and nerve root injury
- Postherpetic neuralgia
- Occipital neuralgia
- Peripheral vascular insufficiency (including Raynaud's phenomenon)
- Inoperable angina
- Pelvic pain due to interstitial cystitis

Another possible but currently controversial indication is mechanical back pain due to degenerative disc disease or failed back surgery syndrome.

There are relatively few contraindications to SCS therapy: coagulopathy, sepsis, infection of the CNS or the operative area, pathology of the epidural space in the operative area due to disease or previous surgery. One contraindication is relative—the presence of a pacemaker. The manufacturers should be contacted to determine the types of the devices and the possibility of safe operation of both implants.

In chronic nonmalignant pain, psychological evaluation is extremely important in successful selection of candidates for spinal cord stimulation (47,48,49). There are no firm guidelines as to the type of psychological tests that need to be applied to pain patients (50). Neither are there stringent psychological selection criteria for patient selection for implantation of SCS (47,50). There are, however, a few clear suggestions pertaining to testing that are applicable to any potential candidate for implantation: It should be performed by an experienced pain psychologist, and excessive depression, somatization, or secondary gains

should be ruled out (47,51). On the other hand, standard psychological evaluation does not add much to the opinion of an experienced physician (38).

Some of the existing psychological tests, such as the MMPI-2, are not oriented toward chronic pain patients (52). Others, such as the Beck Depression Inventory or Multidimensional Pain Inventory, lack validity scales (52). In our practice we successfully use the Pain Patient Profile (P-3) (52,53). It is pain patient-oriented and has validity scales and also is fairly short, taking only about 15 minutes for completion (52). Close correlation of P-3 results with the MMPI-2 has been shown (54).

TRIAL

After the patient is determined to be a suitable candidate for SCS, a trial is in order. There are a few ways to proceed with the trial. The lead can be inserted using surgical laminectomy or a percutaneous approach. I agree with the notion that there is no justification for laminectomy surgery for a trial procedure (55) unless the technical situation prevents percutaneous placement or unless previous attempts at one failed due to the inability to properly place the lead or obtain stimulation covering the affected area.

With a percutaneous trial, the lead can be left emerging through the original insertion site or anchored and internalized with a temporary extension. In the first case the lead should be removed within 3–5 days due to the risk of infection. After internalization the lead can be kept in place for a significantly longer period of time, measured in weeks. The dispute about preference of one method over the other is unresolved (2,38,42,56). The proponents of leaving a "permanent" lead during the trial are citing the following advantages: longer trial period and elimination of repetitive lead reinsertion, which means that a successfully placed lead will keep its position plus decrease the cost by eliminating the use of an additional lead. The disadvantages of this method are as follows: necessity of surgery to remove the lead in a failed trial, necessity of surgery in the event of suboptimal coverage of the pain area during the trial. Claims that outpatient percutaneous trial carries an increased risk of infection (57) in my opinion reflect unfortunate personal experience rather than general rule. I have not seen any infection in more than 200 consecutive percutaneous trials.

Based on different sources the success of trials ranges from 40% to 80% (58–60). Even with the most optimistic statistical data at least every fifth patient will fail SCS trial. In my opinion it is inconceivable to perform two surgeries on every fifth patient (if not more often) with an unsuccessful trial. A comparison of the cost of the lead and the price of surgery to remove it plus an increase in the cost of the trial with an internalized lead produce a very rough estimated ratio of 1 to 4 (Medicare of South Carolina, personal communication). That leads to, at best, equal spending, based on the numbers of failed trials.

Besides, the validity of a shortened percutaneous trial seems to show no difference from longer periods (61). I would not recommend anchoring of the trial lead in the vast majority of cases. One possible exception to the rule can be an extremely technically difficult placement with excellent coverage and at least an initial positive response by the patient. Another possible exception is an inadequate initial trial due to certain technical problem, i.e., lead migration, with initial positive results. Instead of complete implantation of the SCS, I usually proceed with a more prolonged retrial using an anchored lead.

The trial should be performed under local anesthesia with fairly light sedation. The ability of the patient to clearly communicate with the physician is crucial for successful placement of the lead.

The physician should always personally perform an assessment of the results of the trial. Not only the extent of the pain relief, but also overall patient satisfaction are important in making any decision regarding permanent implantation. Small details can be extremely important, including areas with inadequate coverage or excessive stimulation in areas without pain. As far as pain relief is concerned, the majority of physicians use 50% improvement as a threshold of success (2,50,38,55), but some researchers reported using more stringent criteria (2). I use 60 percent or better pain relief as a sign of successful SCS trial in my practice.

NEW DISCOVERIES IN MEASUREMENTS OF TRIAL RESULTS

Currently, short-term as well as long-term trials rely on the patient's report of pain relief to determine a successful trial. Psychological testing helps to decrease the number of "false-positive" results, but by no means is it an objective measure. This "gap" in the selection of patients for implantation of permanent SCS is responsible for the significant number of "failed" cases. Because the exact mechanisms of analgesia with spinal cord stimulation are still not fully known, there are difficulties in finding reliable criteria for a successful trial. Lack of objective selection criteria leads to the high rate of failure after SCS implantation: between 22% and 44% (62,60).

Attempts at assessing the influence of SCS on tactile and vibratory sensation and on nociceptive function as possible objective criteria for selection of adequate candidates for SCS implantation were made by Lindblom and Meyerson (8,9). They showed some decrease in sensory threshold to tactile and vibratory stimulation, whereas pain threshold was not influenced by SCS, except in patients with abnormally low threshold. Some other studies showed contradictory results of SCS influence on pain threshold (63,64). No specific predictors of a successful SCS trial were discovered.

In our recent study on 44 patients who underwent SCS trial, a close correlation was found between outcome of the trial and pain tolerance threshold, but not pain perception threshold (65). That gives us some hope in finding an objective measurement of the SCS trial results.

IMPLANTATION TECHNIQUE

The implantation of the permanent percutaneous lead starts exactly the same way as the trial. The patient is put in the prone position with pillows under the upper abdominal area for improved flexion of the spine. In the case of cervical SCS implantation a pillow is positioned under the upper chest, and the neck is flexed by using a small "donut" as a headrest. Sedation should be extremely light at this point. The back is prepared and draped so that the midline and the upper quadrant of the buttock are exposed. Using the C-arm a site of entry is determined. I prefer L-1–L-2 for lower extremity pain, T-12–L1 for higher levels of pain, and C-7–T-1 for cervical positioning. The site of entry of the epidural space should be at an area between two laminas easily recognizable under fluoroscopy as the more radiolucent area between two spinous processes (Fig. 12-5A). I always introduce the needle at an angle to the midline to avoid contact with the spinous process. That also allows improved maneuverability because a midline position allows adjustments of the needle angle only in one plane, whereas the paramedian allows two. Placement of a 16- or 18-gauge hypodermic needle on the skin will help delineate the desired angle to the right target site (Fig. 12-5B). A shallower angle will make steering of the lead a much easier task. After local anesthesia, a 15-gauge Tuohy needle is advanced into the epidural space using loss-of-resistance technique. Use of intermittent fluoroscopy enhances this process significantly.

I do not see any advantages of epidurography during lead placement. On top of delaying the procedure and making it even more expensive, it can alter "normal" stimulation by changing the conductivity of the epidural space. I would also discourage the use of the guide-wire, suggested by some authors (43). Not only does it increase the chances of perforating the dura, but also it creates a pathway in the epidural fat that sometimes prevents any steering of the lead off the guide-wire "track." In cases where, despite all standard maneuvers, problems with needle advancement are encountered, I would advise reintroducing the needle at a different angle or level. Multiple attempts to "squeeze" the lead are not only a waste of time, but also could lead to perforation of the dura or neurological injury.

The lead is advanced under real-time imaging and positioned at the intended level. At this point, stimulation with the external source should be initiated to determine the area of coverage. Very often I start with lead settings "0" negative and "3" positive to get a rough idea of the stimulation paresthesia location. The next decision is usually whether the lead should be advanced or retracted. This can be checked by subsequent stimulation with lead set-

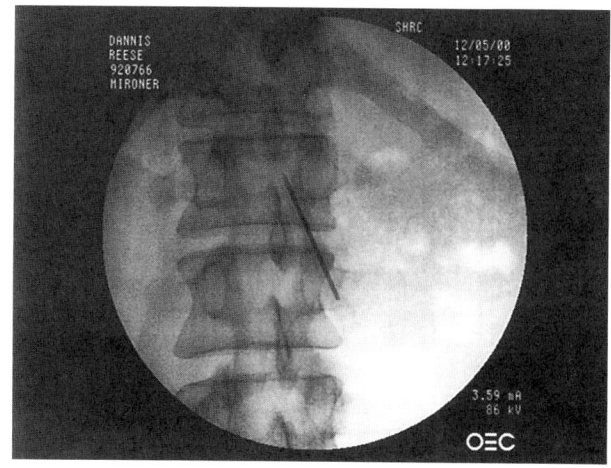 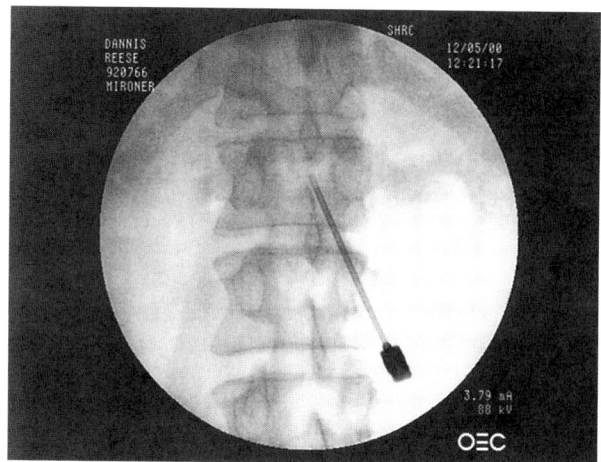

FIG. 12-5. SCS implantation. **A.** Marking the needle entry target. **B.** Position of the insertion needle.

tings "0" negative "1" positive and "3" negative "2" positive. Fine-tuning can be done by changing the polarity of the electrodes, adding or deleting "active" electrodes, or using a "guarded" cathode. The final step is to adjust the amplitude, pulse rate, and especially pulse width. Increases in the latter usually broaden the area of coverage, more so in the distal areas. After the desired coverage is obtained I recommend repeating stimulation after the stylet has been removed. Because the tip of the stylet is bent, the lead not infrequently changes its position slightly after stylet removal, which causes alterations in stimulation pattern.

Placement of the surgically implanted lead is performed through a small laminotomy access. This lead is placed in the same position as the trial percutaneous lead, and after that the process in general is not much different than for the percutaneous implant.

Additional local anesthesia should be administered and an incision made after the desired coverage with initial stimulation is achieved. The incision should not, in most cases, exceed 3 cm in length. It should be deepened to the supraspinous ligament. Attention must be paid to keeping the length of the incision at the fascial level the same or wider than at the skin to prevent the formation of a "well-like" wound. If not, a bigger skin incision will be required to achieve the same operative conditions.

The next step is anchoring of the lead. A few different types of anchors are available currently. By far the best one, in my opinion, is the plastic twist-lock anchor (Medtronic, Inc., Minneapolis, MN). It is the only anchor that practically eliminates the possibility of any movement of the lead in the cephalocaudad direction. The only drawback of the new anchor is its increased size, which makes suturing it more difficult without enlarging the incision. A modified technique of anchoring was introduced in our clinic that makes the process easier, even in a very small wound (66).

After the incision has been made and a clear view of the supraspinous ligament is achieved, two silk sutures are placed through the ligament. One is positioned just posterior to the epidural needle, the other, a half centimeter posterior to the first one (Fig. 12-6A). Both sutures are then threaded through the bilateral small holes in the plastic anchor (Fig. 12-6B). A clamp is placed, holding both ends of each suture, to prevent inadvertent tying of the wrong ends. The epidural needle is then withdrawn, and the lead is threaded through the anchor. The anchor is then moved down the lead all the way to the ligament, and the sutures are securely tied. After the anchor is locked, one more suture is placed around its distal end and secured, making sure that the suture is lying in the bilateral grooves on the sides of the anchor (Fig. 12-6C). This technique allows an unobstructed view of the supraspinous ligament during suture placement because the anchor is out of the wound for the entire process.

Test stimulation should always be performed after removal of the epidural needle. This maneuver can frequently cause movement of the lead. Another step that can alter the position of the electrodes is locking the anchor. I usually maintain the stimulating current throughout the process until the anchor is securely locked.

When dual leads are being implanted I try to choose close entry sites for both leads so that only one incision will be required for anchoring. All of the other steps of the procedure remain essentially the same.

After this part is finished I tightly pack the wound with dry gauze. In 99% of the cases, this is sufficient to completely stop any bleeding in the wound. The chance of hematoma formation in this incision is negligibly small due to the size of the incision and tight suturing of the wound in layers. Unnecessary chasing of "large bleeders" right after the incision can cause not only damage to the electrode but also necrotic burned tissue that will produce an inflammatory reaction and eventually the formation of a seroma. In my opinion, irrigation of the wound with antibiotic in "clean" surgical cases after the patient has

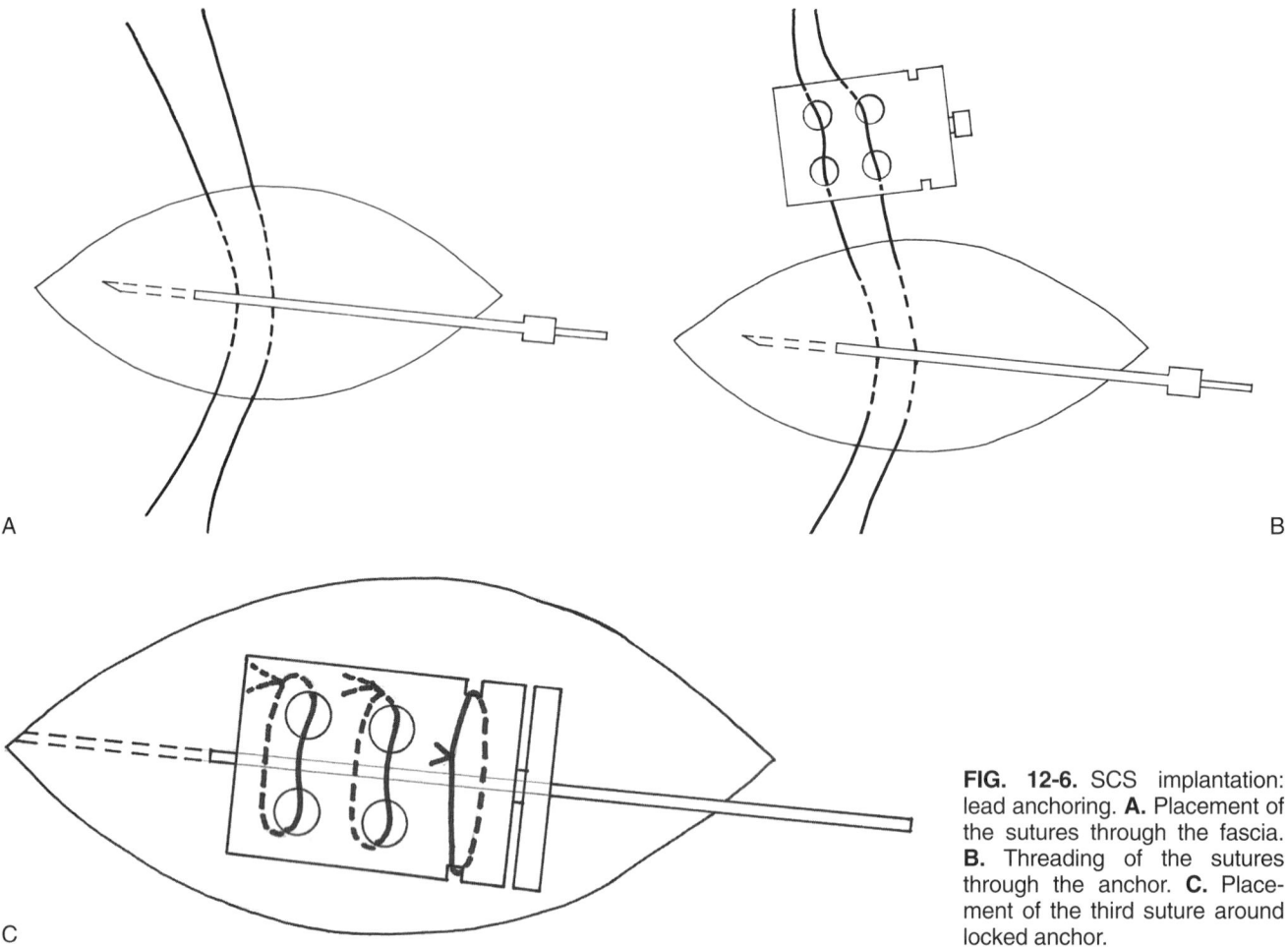

A

B

C

FIG. 12-6. SCS implantation: lead anchoring. **A.** Placement of the sutures through the fascia. **B.** Threading of the sutures through the anchor. **C.** Placement of the third suture around locked anchor.

already received a preoperative intravenous dose is absolutely unnecessary, providing no additional protection from infection.

After the lead is anchored, sedation should be increased and local anesthesia performed at the site chosen for the generator (or receiver, in the case of a radio-coupling device). In general, there are two commonly used sites: the abdominal wall and on the border of the lower lumbar area and upper external quadrant of the buttock. Some physicians use the lateral thoracic wall for generator implantation in cervical SCS. In my experience, a fair number of patients do not like the last option due to some discomfort and awareness of the implant's presence during regular daily activities. An abdominal wall pocket, even though a comfortable site of implantation, poses difficulties for the operator, requiring changing of the patient's position during surgery. In my practice, I use the lumbar site for implantation in a vast majority of patients. A transverse incision should be made. If it is equal to or just shorter than the largest parameter of the generator, the operator will not have any trouble inserting the implant. A pocket is then formed from a half centimeter to a centimeter deep in the subcutaneous fat tissue. The size of the pocket should not significantly exceed the size of the implant to prevent generator movement after surgery or the formation of a seroma. The pocket is tightly packed with a sponge (see earlier comments), and tunneling of the connecting cable is started.

Local anesthesia is performed in a linear fashion between the two incisions. Using the appropriate tunneling device, the connecting cable is pulled through. I bend the tunneling rod slightly and keep the sharp tip facing toward the skin. This effectively prevents "disappearance" of the tip in the depths of the lumbar and gluteal muscles.

The connecting cable should then be connected to the lead and the generator. The screws are tightened with the small screwdriver included in the kit. A "plastic boot," fixed in place with two silk ties, should cover the connection between the lead and the cable. This theoretically will prevent exposure of the contacts to body fluids.

Placement of the connection between the lead and the cable is another step that provides different options. The original location suggested by the manufacturer was at the midline incision to the side or on top of the anchor. The only advantage of this location is the proximity of both crucial sites during revision of the SCS. There are some disadvantages as well. First, it requires a bigger incision. Second, in patients without excessive subcutaneous fat tissue it often produces bulging that can cause long-lasting discomfort. Third, due to significant scar formation, it is not unusual to damage the lead coiled above the anchor during a revision procedure. Placement of the connection site in the generator pocket eliminates all of these problems but will require two incisions if revision becomes necessary. Because our rate of revisions dramatically dropped (the reasons will be discussed later) I usually use the last option.

After placing the generator in the pocket, the wounds are closed with 2-0 or 3-0 vicril sutures and skin sutures or staples.

Prophylactic antibiotics are useful in clean surgeries when a foreign body is implanted. To be effective, parenteral antibiotics must be given during a short period of time, within 30 minutes before the operation (67). Multiple studies showed equal efficacy between a single preoperative dose and multiple doses in the perioperative period (67). I would recommend neither postoperative prophylactic antibiotics nor antibiotic irrigation of the clean wound.

OUTCOMES

Multiple articles dedicated to the outcomes of SCS have been published since the classic 5-year followup article by North and co-authors (68). The results vary significantly depending on the length of observations, type of pathology, methods of testing, and expertise of researchers (62,69, 70). Systematic review of the literature, performed by Turner and co-authors (2), showed that an average of 59% of patients continued to experience relief equal to or exceeding 50%. The wide range of 15% to 100% in my opinion is just a confirmation of the subjectivity and poor reliability of a significant number of these studies.

At least for failed back surgery syndrome, use of SCS was proven to have a superior outcome in comparison to reoperation (71). Cost-effectiveness of this procedure for the same patient population was established as well (3).

It is outside of the scope of this chapter to provide detailed coverage of all outcome studies. For those readers who want more information on the topic, a superb article on the subject exists (2).

USE OF SCS FOR PERIPHERAL VASCULAR DISEASE (PVD) AND CARDIOVASCULAR DISEASE (CVD)

SCS has been used in the treatment of PVD for about 20 years. Whereas it is the number one indication for all SCS implantations performed in Europe (72), it is much less frequently used for this purpose in the United States. Patients with unreconstructable, chronic, critical limb ischemia are candidates for this procedure (24,72,73). The trial, as well as

surgical technique for implantation, is not different from those used for the treatment of chronic pain (74,75). Mechanisms of action of SCS for PVD were briefly discussed earlier. Results are very encouraging (24): Pain relief was achieved in 60% to 90% of the patients, whereas limb salvage rate was 60% to 80% (72). SCS also improved healing of the ischemic foot ulcers (75).

Since the first implantation of SCS for chronic refractory angina (76), this field of SCS application has been growing (25). Patients suffering from severe refractory angina pectoris, who could not have revascularization, are candidates for SCS (25,77,78). Mechanisms of action of SCS for coronary artery disease (CAD) were briefly discussed earlier. Surgical technique is standard, although a one-stage procedure was proposed as an optimal approach (77). Safety and efficacy of SCS for CAD have been shown by a number of studies (25,77,79). Around 60% of the patients still have positive results 5 years after implantation (80), whereas during a shorter period of time this number was as high as 80% (81).

PROBLEMS AND COMPLICATIONS

Multiple studies in the literature discuss the complication rate after SCS implantation. The frequency of complications varies from a few percent to more than 50% of all implantations, with the average being around 42%, according to a systematic literature review (2).

Surgical Complications

Bleeding

Superficial bleeding is an extremely rare problem during SCS implantation because neither the posterior thoracic wall, the lumbar area, nor the lateral abdominal wall is heavily vascularized. Most of the time, temporary tamponade of the wound while proceeding with the next step of the surgery will resolve the problem. Aggressive cauterization is unnecessary and can lead to excessive necrotic tissue, producing a seroma or creating the perfect substrate for infection. Epidural bleeding is fairly rare but a much more serious problem. Screening patients with bleeding disorders, cancer patients with clotting abnormalities, as well as patients receiving anticoagulant therapy helps to prevent this potentially grave complication. It is not necessary that every patient undergo extensive laboratory testing if a careful review of the medical history is obtained. The question regarding use of NSAIDs is still controversial and should be decided by the surgeon depending on his views and experience. Gentle manipulation of the needle and styleted lead will help to avoid any trauma to the deep tissues, which can cause bleeding. Every patient should undergo routine neurological examination before and after surgery. If bleeding is suspected, this process should become continuous, with involvement of a neurosurgeon and radiologist for possible CT scan.

Hematoma, Seroma

A collection of blood in the superficial wound could lead to formation of a hematoma. Seroma, a collection of serum in the wound, can be the result of an organized hematoma or excessive tissue trauma. These complications are reported with variable frequency by different authors but are very rare occurrences after SCS implantation because the pocket size is much smaller than for pump implant. Most of these are benign and resolve spontaneously. Wearing an abdominal binder can expedite this process. Puncture and aspiration are inadvisable, except in cases of significant volume collection. The binder will increase pressure in the pocket, preventing fluid from reaccumulating. If the problem is persistent, surgical revision of the pocket is recommended, the goal of which is to diminish the space between the generator and the walls of the pocket.

Local Infection

Infection is not a very common complication of implantation but has been reported to occur in around 5% of all implants (2,3,60,70). The infection rate is usually lower for SCS implants than for pump implants. If the only sign of infection is cellulitis in the area of the generator pocket, but no fluctuance is noted, aggressive parenteral antibiotic treatment can reverse the course. On the other hand, any signs of infection inside the pocket, i.e., abscess, or spreading of the process along the course of the cable toward the epidural entry wound, should prompt removal of the implant without any hesitation.

Epidural Abscess, Meningitis

The clinical picture of epidural abscess is similar to epidural hematoma with associated symptoms of infection. It requires immediate neurosurgical treatment. Meningitis usually produces a clinical picture of a generalized infectious process with signs of meningeal irritation. Neurological and infectious disease specialists should be involved, CSF samples obtained, and hardware removed without delay.

CSF Leak

Dural puncture with CSF leak during placement of the lead is not an uncommon development. The best mode of action is reinsertion of the needle at a new level or angle to avoid intrathecal placement of the lead. The latter is easily recognizable by the larger area of coverage at extremely low amplitude. CSF leak is usually a self-limited problem. It requires either no treatment or conservative measures

like hydration and analgesics for a few days after surgery if postdural puncture headache develops. In cases of persistent headache, an epidural blood patch is the next step. I would recommend delaying this procedure more than after simple dural puncture because of the increase in infection risk and the possibility of lead damage. To avoid the latter, epidural puncture should be performed under fluoroscopy or, at least, distinctly a level below the entry of the lead. Continuous CSF leak will lead either to drainage through the incision or the formation of a hygroma. Both conditions require surgical closure with removal of the SCS.

Implanted Device Complications

Lead Migration

This is the most common complication of SCS implantation (2,44,60). Needless to say, the occurrence of this problem is significantly higher with percutaneous lead placement than with surgical lead placement. The rate of percutaneous lead migration is around 20% (2,3,44, 60). More often this is observed fairly recently after the surgery or as a consequence of trauma. Restriction of certain types of activity after surgery in order to let the lead "scar in" probably helps somewhat. Development of the plastic twist-lock anchor practically eliminated movement of the lead along the cephalocaudad spinal axis. The majority of migrations are in the horizontal plane, causing the lead to move laterally to the other side of physiological midline or to the anterior epidural space. This presents itself as a change in the area of coverage or the appearance of unpleasant sensations during stimulation, frequently described as "drawing." The new area of stimulation is often either in the contralateral extremity or the segment representing the location of the electrodes (nerve root stimulation). Lateral and AP radiographic images of the spine will help to confirm changes in position of the lead. This is a good reason to obtain permanent x-ray documentation of final lead placement at the time of surgery.

Occasionally, changing the lead polarity and the pattern of coverage may restore coverage of the desired area. In the majority of cases, revision of the lead is necessary. From my experience, use of the existing lead can cause repetitive problems. It can possibly be explained by the development of some curvature in the lead and a congruent "track" in the epidural space that will allow the lead to move again. I would advise either proceeding with implantation of a new percutaneous lead or substituting it for a surgical lead.

New developments, which may aid in the reduction of the incidence of this complication, are discussed later.

Hardware Malfunction

The most probable cause of hardware failure is lead fracture and current leakage. According to the literature, the frequency of these events is low, somewhere around 5% to 7% (2,3,60,70). Amazingly enough, one recent report showed that 19% of all the patients in the study developed lead fractures or current leakage (82). Judging from the literature and my own experience (described later), I would be inclined to think that the authors somehow may have mishandled the hardware.

A plastic boot covers the connection site to prevent its exposure to fluid. Unfortunately, if the body fluid finds its way inside the boot it works as a fluid "trap," causing shorting of the electric circuit. In this case, the patient would experience a burning sensation at the connection site with or without complete loss of stimulation in the desired area. One of the suggested remedies is to create a longitudinal cut in the boot. After two ties are secured around the boot, no space will be left to allow fluid collection. The other remedy is to leave the connection site without any cover.

Disconnection of the wires or cable is described in the literature but is extremely rare.

New Neurological Symptoms

The appearance of new neurological symptoms or complaints, i.e., increase in pain, new distribution of pain, or new weakness or paresthesia, can be the sign of advancement of disease, onset of new disease, or complications of the implanted system. Any of the previously mentioned complaints should warrant thorough examination and testing. The controversy about using MRI with SCS still exists. According to the manufacturers, MRI is contraindicated for patients with SCS, although their explanations do not sound plausible from an engineering point of view. A significant number of patients had MRI by accident after implantation, and none of them had any complications or hardware malfunction (John Oakley, personal communication).

Across Midline Lead Positioning: A Novel Approach

Migration of the percutaneous leads keeps plaguing outcomes of SCS implantation. In the opinion of Law and Miller, "electrode movement caused at least 30% of the failures" (83).

Our clinic has developed a new approach to positioning of the SCS lead that provides some advantages (84). Approximately 80 patients underwent SCS trial using this technique, and about 40 patients had SCS implanted with the lead placed using an across-the-midline position.

Theoretical Mechanisms

As discussed earlier, lead migration with loss of proper pain coverage still plagues percutaneous SCS implantation. The rates of SCS revision are in the 14% to 24% range (2,3), which translates into significant cost, not to

mention increased patient dissatisfaction. With the new twist-lock anchor, movement of the lead is usually in the lateral direction, the most extreme version of which is migration to the anterior epidural space. With conventional placement of the lead there is nothing (except scar tissue) that prevents this shift. Even worse is the situation when the lead is positioned in the "physiological" midline to provide bilateral stimulation. Any horizontal movement can produce loss of stimulation on one side.

The new method is based on stabilizing the lead using the plica mediana dorsalis, a well-described band of connective tissue in the epidural space (85–88), as an additional point of "fixation" to enhance stability of the lead. The direction of the forces acting on the lead should prevent lateral movement of the tip (Fig. 12-7). In cases of bilateral stimulation, the presence of the electrode on both sides will preserve bilateral coverage.

Technique

The lead is inserted contralaterally to the side of pain and advanced to the anticipated level of stimulation (Fig. 12-8A). The stylet is removed and bent manually, then reinserted with the tip facing the midline (Fig. 12-8B). The lead is advanced through the midline (plica mediana dorsalis) (Fig. 12-8C), then rotated with the tip again facing midline and moved slightly farther in the cephalad direction (Fig. 12-8D). The stylet is removed and the lead pulled back (that always brings the tip closer to midline) (Fig. 12-8E). At this point stimulation is initiated and necessary adjustments in position are made (Fig. 12-9).

Results

In a published study, results of midline "anchoring" in 20 patients with failed back surgery syndrome were compared with a group of 20 similar patients who received conventional implantation (84). Change in stimulation pattern was observed in one patient in the study group and in eight patients in the control group. Reprogramming of the SCS did not amend the situation in five patients (all in

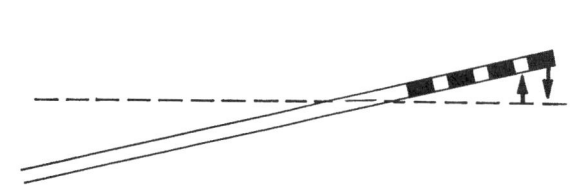

FIG. 12-7. Midline "anchoring" of the SCS lead: opposing forces prevent lateral lead migration.

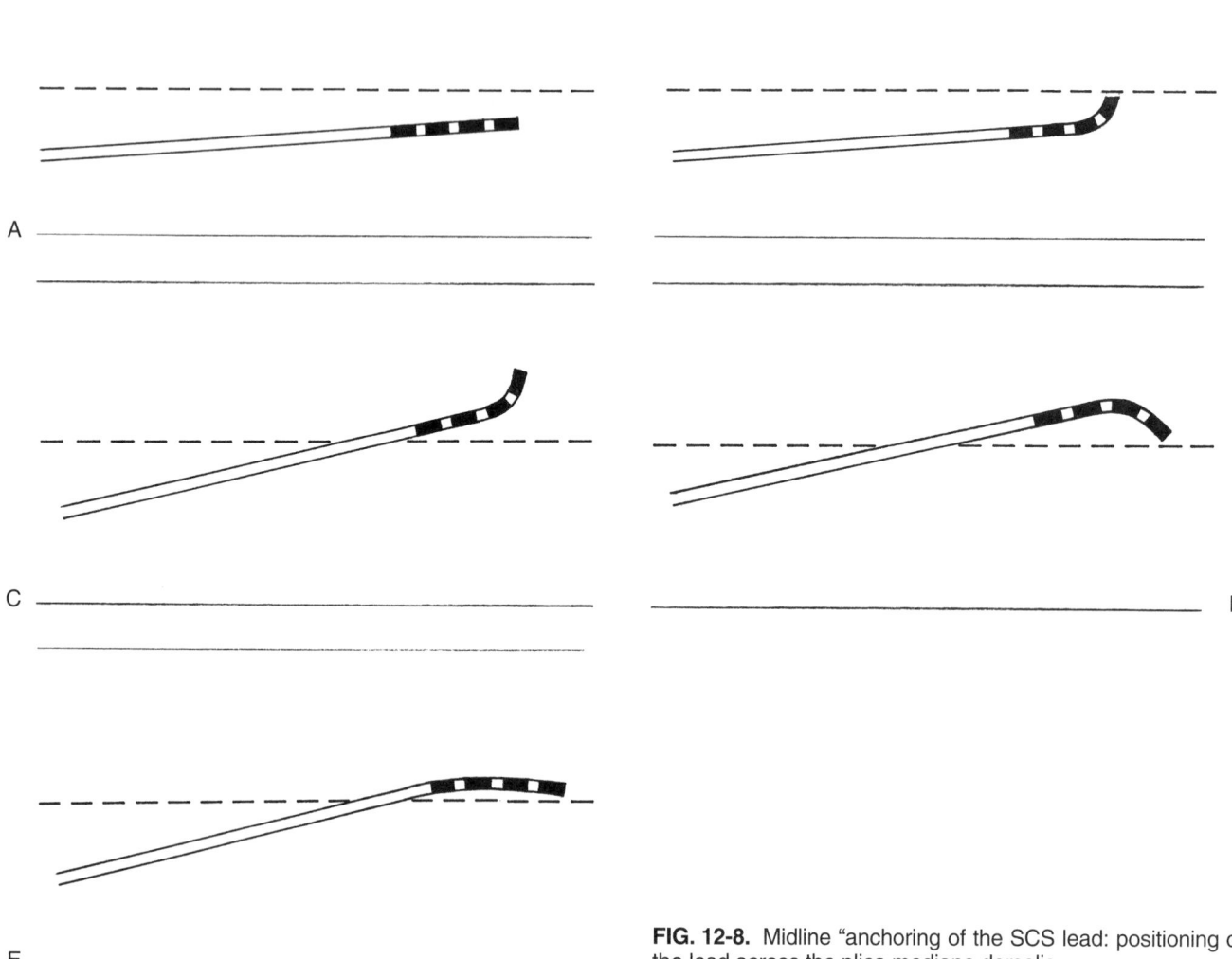

FIG. 12-8. Midline "anchoring of the SCS lead: positioning of the lead across the plica mediana dorsalis.

the control group). After the lead migration was documented, surgical revision with reposition or replacement of the lead was performed in three patients, whereas the rest underwent replacement with a Resume lead. In an unpublished observation, a stunning decrease in the incidence of changes in stimulation pattern during the trial was also observed when this technique was used.

Use of the plica mediana dorsalis to stabilize the lead resulted in a dramatic reduction in the frequency of lead migration and subsequent surgical revision. The midline "anchoring" technique produced an increased lead stability with a decreased incidence of lead migration.

A pleasant surprise was improved coverage of axial pain at a lower level of electrode position with the new technique (89). The majority of researchers agree that higher position of the electrodes, somewhere above T-10, is necessary (13). It has been postulated that the closer the lead is positioned to the midline, the better is the stimulation coverage due to recruitment of the dorsal column fibers (29). Improved stimulation should theoretically be produced at a lower level (below T-10) due to the lower perception threshold (29). In a retrospective review of electrode position in all patients with low back pain who had single-lead placement across the midline, out of 26 patients 62% had the tip of the lead located below the T-10 vertebral body, whereas in 27% of the cases it was placed below the T-11 vertebral body (89). These results constitute a very significant difference from the results suggested by the current literature. The implication of this finding is discussed later.

Drawbacks

Unfortunately, not all patients have a plica mediana dorsalis that is well enough developed to allow successful use of the midline "anchoring" technique. This is well documented by our current knowledge of epidural space anatomy (85,88). As soon as free movement of the lead across the midline is recognized a change in the initial plan is in order.

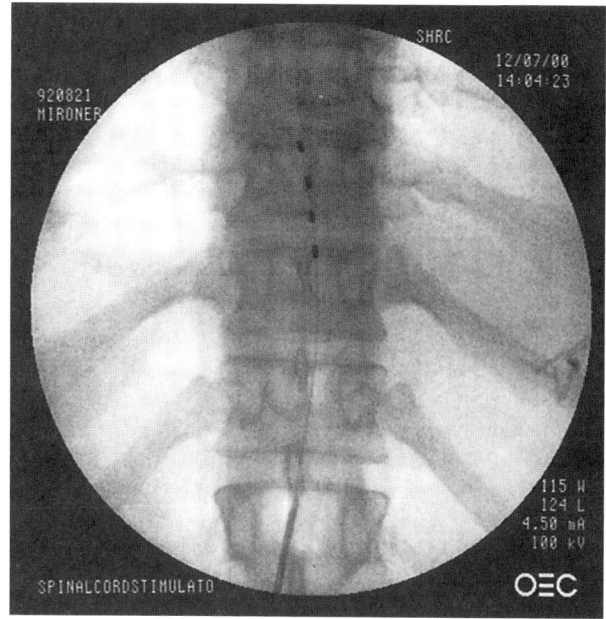

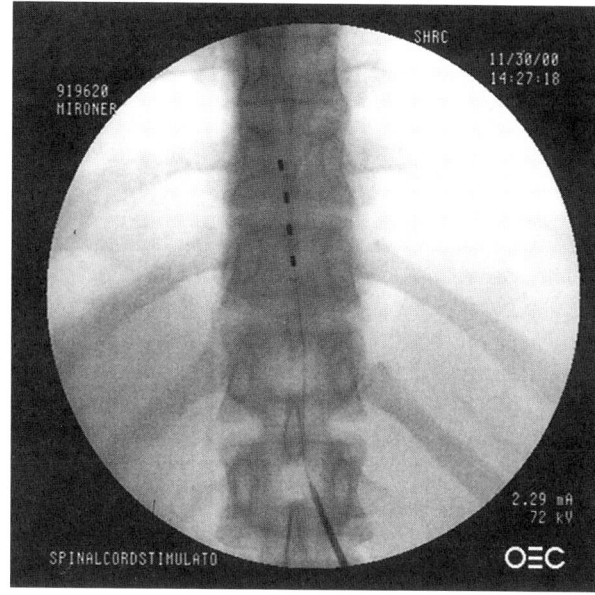

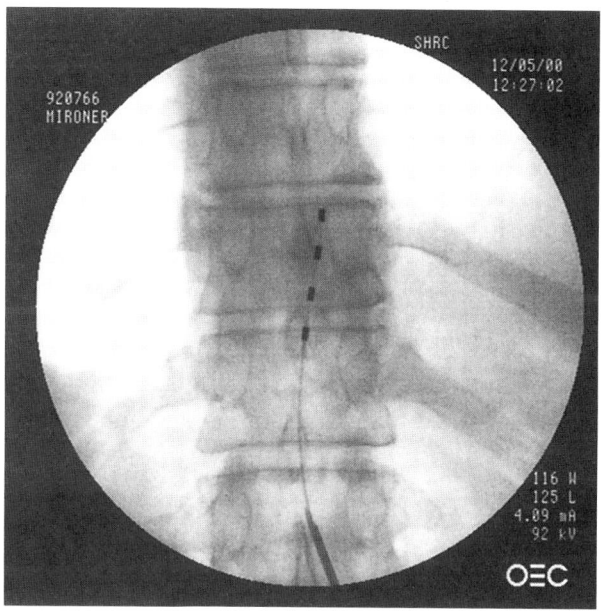

FIG. 12-9. Midline "anchoring" of the SCS lead: final position of the lead across the midline.

Percutaneous Lead versus Laminotomy Lead

In my opinion, there is no doubt that during the trial only a percutaneous lead should be used if at all possible. As far as permanent implantation is concerned, the question of superiority remains open. Obviously an excessively mobile lead during the trial should indicate the need for laminotomy. The same is true for the patient undergoing repetitive revisions due to lead migration. In all other cases the jury is still out. A couple of observations suggested an advantage of the laminotomy lead (38,90). Because both came from neurosurgeons and were based on small numbers of compared cases, no definite conclusions can be made at this time.

One versus Two Leads

The dispute about the use of one versus two percutaneous leads is still very heated and unresolved (39,45). Unfortunately, it has produced many poorly conducted, tendentious studies and unproven statements (50,91). This is partially the result of heavy promotion of the dual-lead systems by both manufacturers. In order to briefly review this subject I want to divide the applications of SCS into three groups: unilateral pain, bilateral pain, and axial back pain.

In my opinion, there are no compelling reasons to use dual leads in unilateral pain. No serious studies have supported dual leads for this purpose.

Bilateral pain in the majority of cases requires placement of the dual-lead system. Even if coverage can be achieved with a single lead, the danger of its migration is too high. This notion possibly will change in view of the success with the across-midline positioning, described earlier. Not only does it afford bilateral coverage in a majority of cases, but also it produces the necessary stability to a single lead.

The most difficult decision is in cases of axial low back pain. This type of pain is much more difficult to cover and relieve with SCS in general (28), so it is not surprising that no consensus on the subject exists. For a period it seemed that the majority of indirect evidence supported use of the dual-lead system for low back pain (45,92). More than that, the old notion of "the more, the merrier" started to be applied not only to the number of leads but also to the number of electrodes. Surprisingly enough, the latest developments make this position less than certain. First, North (93) demonstrated in a prospective, controlled study of SCS for axial low back pain that all measured parameters (including overlap of pain area by stimulation) were slightly better with a single versus dual leads. Then Holsheimer (35) showed that the so-called summation effect, beneficial for low back coverage, does not exist. Computer models suggest an advantage of a single lead as well as a negative effect of overlap of two electric fields from bilateral symmetrical electrodes (94). In the opinion of Holsheimer, "a single, carefully placed midline lead will generally perform better than a dual lead" (35). I completely agree with this notion (95). That is when our technique of across-midline lead positioning can play a positive role. Not only does it allow capture of low back stimulation at a lower, more favorable level (see "Anatomy Related to Neurostimulation"), but also it assures the sta-

bility of the lead, capturing the axial low back area. Future studies will hopefully help to create the optimal approach to stimulation for axial low back pain.

Personal Experience

In the 18-month period from January 1999 to June 2000 I performed SCS trials on 84 patients, 39 of whom underwent implantation of the permanent percutaneous SCS. An additional three patients were referred for implantation of a lead via laminotomy. All of the data presented are as of September 2000.

Of those implanted by me, 24 were female and 15 were male. The ages ranged from 22 to 87.

Four patients were implanted with a dual-lead system, whereas all the rest had a single-lead system. One patient had the SCS removed 14 months after initial surgery due to inadequate analgesia. He was eventually implanted with an intrathecal drug delivery system.

Six patients required revision of the implant: three due to spontaneous migration of the lead, two due to traumatic migration, and one due to current leakage. None of this group had an across-the-midline implantation technique. Out of this group, two had replacement with a laminotomy lead, the other four had successful revision.

Two of 39 patients were lost to followup. One patient, as mentioned, was explanted. All of the other 36 patients continue to use their SCS regularly and report at least 50% relief of pain.

Nerve Root Stimulation

The use of this relatively new modality of neurostimulation is associated with the treatment of voiding disorders

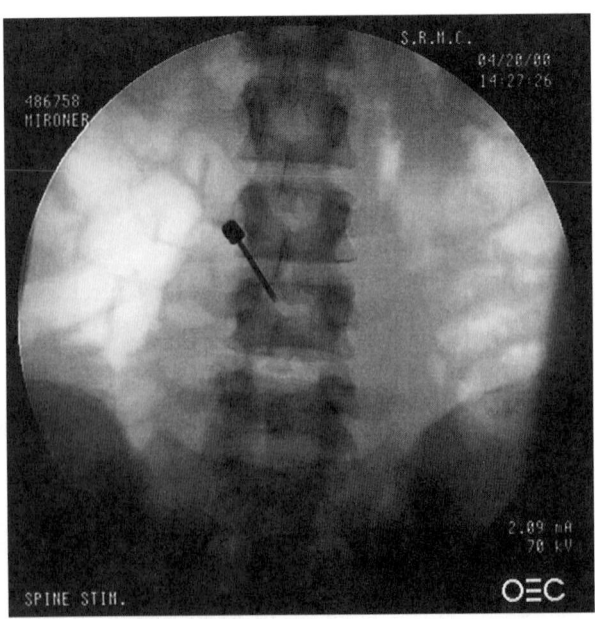
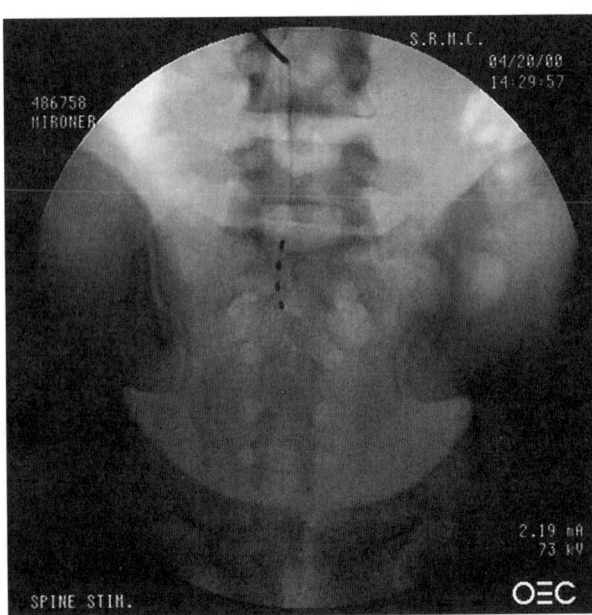

FIG. 12-10. Retrograde SCS lead insertion. **A.** Position of the needle. **B.** Advancement of the lead.

refractory to conventional treatment. Stimulation of the sacral nerves produces "somatic afferent inhibition of sensory process" (96). Patients with urinary urge incontinence, urgency/frequency syndromes, and voiding difficulties can be candidates for sacral nerve implantation (97). Implantation of the Interstim (Medtronic, Inc.) leads is carried out via the sacral foramina after surgical incision has been made. Either the trial is performed during the implantation process, or the procedure is done in two stages.

An increasing amount of data supports the efficacy of nerve root stimulation for chronic pelvic pain due to interstitial cystitis as well as other pathology. The most common approach is retrograde lead positioning, although placement of surgical leads was used as well (97). The best level for insertion of the needle is L-3–4 or L-4–5. The patient is put in the prone position with maximum possible flexion of the lumbar spine (I usually use two pillows under the lower abdomen). At a slightly caudad angle with a paramedian approach, the needle is inserted with the bevel facing caudally (Fig. 12-10). The lead is advanced to the S-2–S-3 foraminal level aiming to position at least the distal electrode through the foramen. Bilateral leads are usually required to produce adequate coverage (Fig. 12-11). In certain cases placement of the leads in the lateral recess will be enough to produce good coverage and pain relief. Some other described approaches include percutaneous transforaminal placement of the leads (98) and placement via the sacrococcygeal ligament (99).

Retrograde placement of the leads with stimulation of more cephalic nerve roots (L-5 or S-1) can also be used successfully for a better or an exclusive capturing of a smaller pain area, i.e., foot.

Peripheral Nerve Stimulation (Including Occipital Nerve Stimulation)

Peripheral nerve stimulation (PNS) is a fairly well-researched area of neurostimulation, though, by far, less popular than SCS. Patients with damage or disease of a single large- or medium-size nerve can be candidates, although it has also been used for the treatment of reflex sympathetic dystrophy (100). Some authors advocate the use of a nerve block or TENS as a trial for possible implant, whereas others perform a two-stage procedure (101). The electrodes are placed directly over the nerve, separated by a flap of fascia. The vast majority of these procedures are performed on the upper or lower extremities. The safety and efficacy of PNS were proven to be good (100,101). Improvement in the trial process is necessary to make this modality more commonly used in the contemporary practice of pain management.

Of interest, we reported a case of successful percutaneous trial stimulation of the ilioinguinal nerve (102). Other superficially located nerves with well-defined landmarks could also be the target of percutaneous stimulation in the future. One example, the occipital nerve, is a new popular target of stimulation with a relatively easy percutaneous trial.

Occipital Nerve Stimulation

This modality of treatment, first described by Weiner (103), is quickly gaining widespread acceptance as an effective method of treatment of intractable refractory occipital neuralgia.

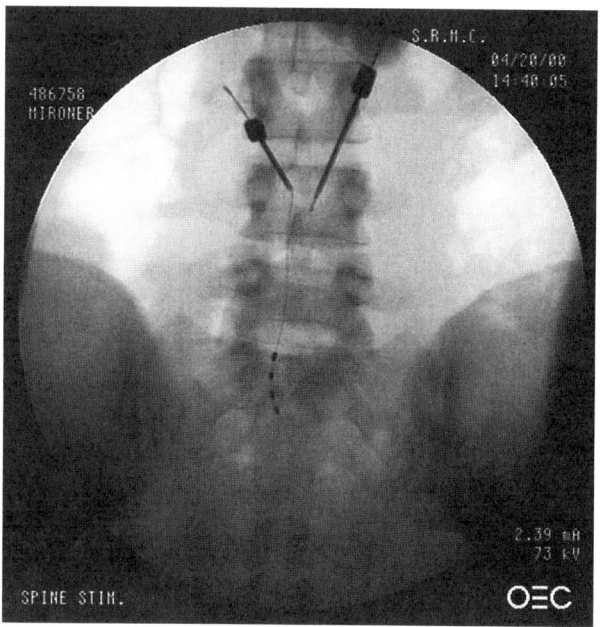
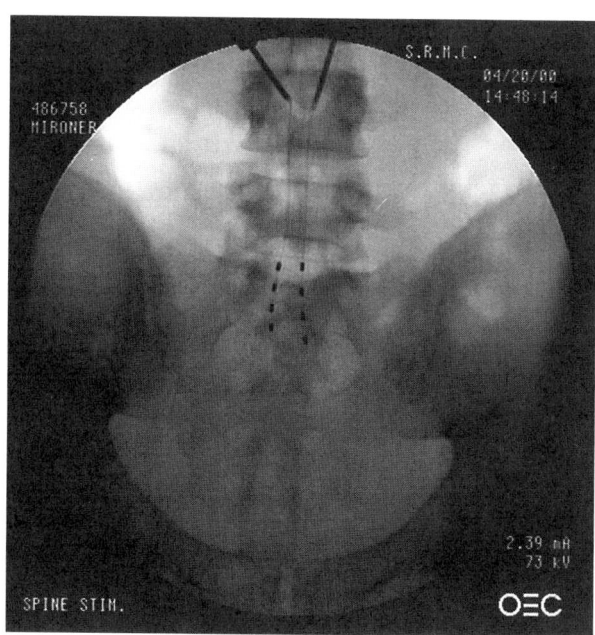

A   B

FIG. 12-11. Retrograde SCS lead position. **A.** Bilateral needle position. **B.** Bilateral lead advancement.

Patient selection should be very careful because the nature of the headache is very often mixed, and this syndrome is very commonly accompanied by overt psychological pathology. I am categorically opposed to a growing trend of implantation without trial stimulation (103,104). The only patient in our clinic who underwent surgery without a trial had to be explanted 2 months later.

Trial

The patient is positioned laterally with the affected side up. After preparation and draping, using fluoroscopy, a line is drawn perpendicular to spinal axis at the level of the C-1 spinous process. A small skin wheel is raised with local anesthetic just posterior to the mastoid process on the drawn line. A skin nick is performed with the tip of a knife blade, and sedation is deepened, usually with a bolus of propofol. The SCS insertion needle is slightly bent. After insertion under the skin, the needle is advanced subcutaneously along the drawn line toward midline. A lead is inserted to the tip of the needle, and the needle is gently withdrawn. Intermittent use of fluoroscopy will help in the correct positioning of the lead (Fig. 12-12).

At this point, after communication with patient is reestablished, trial stimulation is performed. The settings are usually somewhat different from those used in SCS, i.e., a significantly higher pulse rate (150–200 Hz) and lower pulse width (90–120 msec) are preferable for occipi-

tal nerve stimulation. After good coverage with paresthesia is established, the lead is fixed with one 2-0 silk skin suture. Four to five days later it can be easily removed in the office setting. For bilateral occipital neuralgia I usually repeat the same procedure on the other side, leaving the midline intact for possible future implant.

Implantation

The initial steps for implantation are not different from those in the trial if unilateral implantation is planned. For bilateral implants the patient is placed in the prone position. After the C-1 level line is marked and the patient is under local anesthesia, a midline incision is performed. Two leads are positioned as described during the trial process, but they are advanced from the midline to both sides (Fig. 12-13). After satisfactory testing the leads are anchored in the standard fashion to the trapezius fascia.

I usually use the upper buttock for the generator implantation (see preceding discussions). Due to the long distance from the insertion site and traumatic passing of the regular tunneler through the neck and upper thoracic wall I use the straw tunneler, provided in the kit for the trial implantation. That makes the procedure easier and less traumatic. A small skin incision is made in the lateral thoracic wall, and after the lead is connected to the connecting cable, the connection site is placed in the wound, which is closed with a couple of skin sutures.

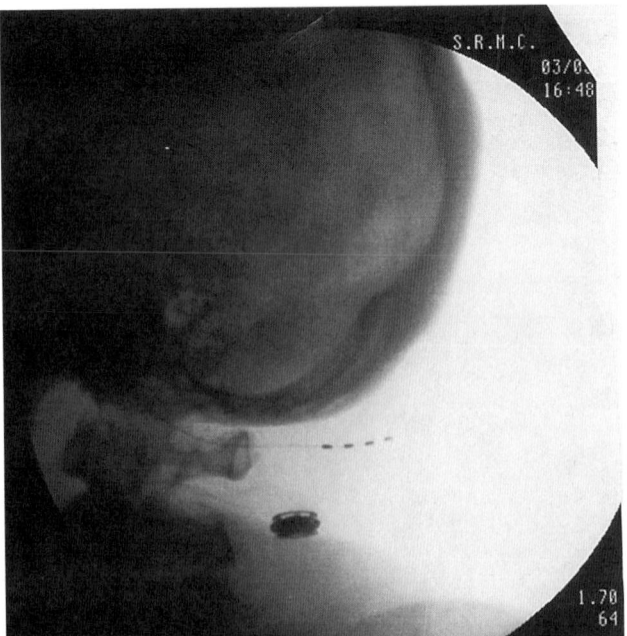

FIG. 12-12. Occipital nerve stimulation: position of unilateral lead.

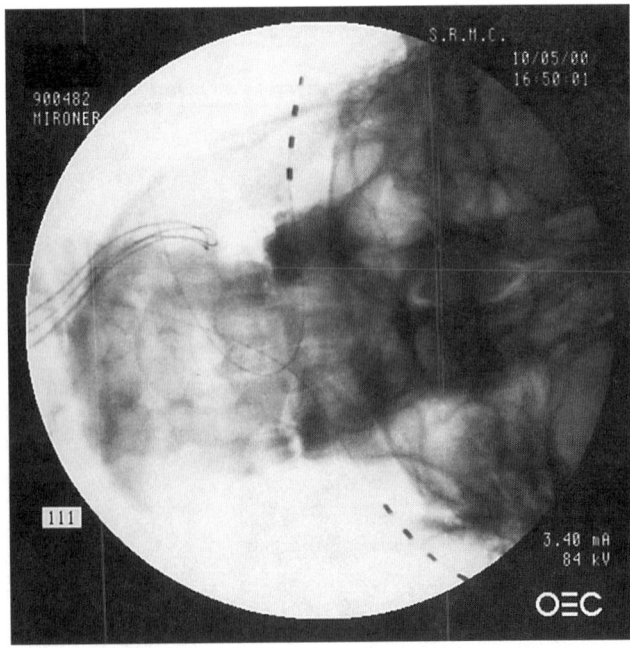

FIG. 12-13. Occipital nerve stimulation: position of bilateral leads.

Outcomes

With careful selection of candidates and proper technique, results of occipital nerve stimulation are promising (103). Larger studies involving a significant number of patients are needed to confirm initial experience.

Problems

The biggest problem with occipital nerve stimulation is a high risk of migration due to its location in a mobile area and subcutaneous position. Leaving extra length of the lead or creating a loop can help to reduce this problem. More advanced design of the occipital nerve stimulator will hopefully allow complete elimination of this problem in the future.

In cases of occipital neuralgia associated with cervical radiculopathy, full coverage can be achieved with "paddle" laminotomy leads, placed bilaterally at C-1–C-2. Alternatively, successful combined use of cervical SCS and occipital stimulation has been demonstrated (105).

SUMMARY

Neurostimulation is an important part of the continuum of managing chronic intractable pain. It is hard to imagine contemporary pain management without this modality of treatment. Very effective and relatively safe, it still poses a lot of questions and problems as we are becoming more accustomed to it and use it more widely. Significant research regarding the reliable selection of patients based on mechanisms of SCS is needed. Neurophysiological studies will help to determine the optimal configuration of SCS systems for different applications. Unfortunately, most of the effort so far has been aimed at data collection and retrospective review of clinical experience to prove advantages of one type of product over the other. Serious scientific research is necessary to answer many of the existing questions. Recent attention to some previously ignored discrepancies indicates that we are moving from the initial period of excitement and fascination to a period of serious and critical analysis and a more scientific approach.

Acknowledgment

The author gratefully acknowledges Katherine Mironer for her assistance in providing the illustrations for this chapter.

REFERENCES

1. Shealy CN, Mortimer JT, Reswick JB. Electrical inhibition of pain by stimulation of the dorsal columns: preliminary clinical report. *Anesth Analg* 1967;46:489–491.
2. Turner JA, Loeser JD, Bell KG. Spinal cord stimulation for chronic low back pain: a systematic literature synthesis. *Neurosurgery* 1995; 37:1088–1096.
3. Bell GK, Kidd D, North RB. Cost-effectiveness analysis of spinal cord stimulation in treatment of failed back surgery syndrome. *J Pain Symptom Manage* 1997;13:286–295.
4. Meyerson BA, Lynderoth B. Mechanisms of spinal cord stimulation in neuropathic pain. Neurol Res 2000;22:285–292.
5. Krames ES. Mechanisms of action of spinal cord stimulation. In: Waldman SD, Winnie AP, eds. *Interventional pain management.* W.B. Saunders, Philadelphia, 1996:407–411.
6. Linderoth B, Foreman RD. Physiology of spinal cord stimulation: review and update. *Neuromodulation* 1999;2:150–164 .
7. Melzack R, Wall PD. Pain mechanisms: a new theory. *Science* 1965; 150:971–978.
8. Lindblom U, Meyerson BA. Influence on touch, vibration and cutaneous pain of dorsal column stimulation in man. *Pain* 1975;1: 257–270.
9. Lindblom U, Meyerson BA. Mechanoreceptive and nociceptive thresholds during dorsal column stimulation in man. Advances in Pain Research and Therapy, ed. Bonica JJ, Albe-Fessard, Raven Press, NY, 1976;1:469–474.
10. Price DD. The use of experimental pain in evaluating the effects of dorsal column stimulation on clinical pain. *Pain* 1999;45:225–226.
11. Larson SJ, Sances A, Riegel DH, et al. Neurophysiological effects of dorsal column stimulation in man and monkey. *J Neurosurg* 1974; 41:271–223.
12. Campbell JN, Davis KD, Meyer RA, et al. The mechanism by which dorsal column stimulation affects pain: evidence for a new hypothesis. *Pain* 1990;5:S228.
13. Meyerson BA, Ren B, Herregodts P, et al. Spinal cord stimulation in animal models of mononeuropathy: effects on the withdrawal responce and the flexor reflex. *Pain* 1995;61:229–243.
14. Ren N, Linderoth B, Meyerson BA. Effects of spinal cord stimulation on the flexor reflex and involvement of supraspinal mechanisms: an experimental study in mononeuropathic rats. *J Neurosurg* 1996;84: 244–249.
15. Sotgiu ML, Biella G, Riva L. Poststimulus after discharges of spinal WDR and NS units in rats with chronic nerve constriction. *NeuroReport* 1995;6:1021–1024.
16. Yakhnitsa V, Linderoth B, Meyerson BA. Spinal cord stimulation attenuates dorsal horn neuronal hyperexcitability in a rat model of mononeuropathy. *Pain* 1999;79:223–233.
17. Stiller CO, Linderoth B, O'Connor WT, et al. Repeated spinal cord stimulation decreases the extracellular level of gamma-aminobutyric acid in the periaqueductal gray matter of freely moving rats. *Brain Res* 1995;699:231–241.
18. DeJongste MJL, Hautvast RVM, Ruiters MHJ, et al. Spinal cord stimulation and the induction of c-fos and heat shock protein in the central nervous system of rats. *Eur Heart J* 1994;15:284.
19. Linderoth B, Stiller CO, Gunasekera L, et al. Gamma-aminobutyric acid is released in the dorsal horn by electrical spinal cord stimulation: an in vivo microdialysis study in the rat. *Neurosurg* 1994;34:484–489.
20. Simpson RD, Robertson CS, Goodman JC. Glycine: a potential mediator of electrically induced pain modification. *Biomed Lett* 1993;48:193–207.
21. Cui JG, O'Connor WT, Ungerstedt U, et al. Spinal cord stimulation attenuates augmented dorsal horn release of excitory amino acids in mononeuropathy via a GABAergic mechanism. *Pain* 1997;73:87–95.
22. Cui JG, Sollevi A, Linderoth B, et al. Adenosine receptor activation suppresses tactile hypersensitivity and potentiates effect of spinal cord in mononeuropathic rats. *Neurosci Lett* 1997;223:173–176.
23. Croom JE, Foreman RD, Chandler MJ, et al. Reevaluation of the role of the sympathetic nervous system in cutaneous vasodilation during dorsal spinal cord stimulation: are multiple mechanisms active. *Neuromodulation* 1998;1:91–101.
24. Claeys LGY. Epidural spinal cord stimulation: an effective treatment for ischemic pain. *Pain Digest* 1997;7:10–12.
25. DeJongste MJL. Spinal cord stimulation for ischemic heart disease. *Neurol Res* 2000;22:293–298.
26. Linderoth B, Fedorcsak I, Meyerson BA. Is vasodilatation following dorsal column stimulation mediated by antidromic activation of small diameter afferents? *Acta Neurchir* (Suppl) 1989;46:99–101.
27. Linderoth B, Gunasekera L, Meyerson B. Effects of sympathectomy on skin and muscle microcirculation during dorsal column stimulation: animal studies. *Neurosurgery* 1991;29:874–879.

28. Barolat G, Massaro F, He J, et al. Mapping of sensory responses to epidural stimulation of the intraspinal neural structures in man. *J Neurosurg* 1993;78:233–239.

29. Barolat G. Epidural spinal cord stimulation: anatomical and electrical properties of the intraspinal structures relevant to spinal cord stimulation and clinical correlations. *Neuromodulation* 1998;1:63–71.

30. Struijk JJ, Holsheimer J, Boom HB. Excitation of dorsal root fibers in spinal cord stimulation: a theoretical study. *IEEE Trans Biomed Eng* 1993;40:632–638.

31. He J, Barolat G, Holsheimer J, et al. Perception threshold and electrode position for spinal cord stimulation. *Pain* 1994;59:55–63.

32. Holsheimer J, Barolat G. Spinal geometry and paresthesia coverage in spinal cord stimulation. *Neuromodulation* 1998;1:129–136.

33. Holsheimer J, Struijk JJ, Tas NR. Effects of electrode geometry and combination on nerve fiber selectivity in spinal cord stimulation. *Med Biol Eng Comp* 1995;33:676–682.

34. North RB, Nigrin DJ, Fowler KR, et al. Automated "pain drawing" analysis by computer-controlled, patient-interactive neurological stimulation system. *Pain* 1992;50:51–57.

35. Holsheimer J. Does dual lead stimulation favor stimulation of the axial lower back? *Neuromodulation* 2000;3:55–57.

36. Holsheimer J, Struijk JJ, Wesselink WA. Analysis of spinal cord stimulation and design of epidural electrodes by computer modeling. *Neuromodulation* 1998;1:14–18.

37. Barolat G, Zeme S, Ketcik B. Multifactorial analysis of epidural spinal cord stimulation. Stereotact Funct *Neurosurg* 1991;56:77–103.

38. Espinosa F, McKean JDS, Burchiel KJ, et al. Spinal cord stimulation using new transverse tripole lead and steering of field with two simultaneous, non-equal pulses. Presented at the Worldwide Pain Conference, San Francisco, CA, July 2000.

39. Krames ES. Overview of spinal cord stimulation: with special emphasis on a role for dual spinal cord stimulators. *Pain Digest* 2000;10:6–12.

40. Mironer YE. Letter to the editor. *Neuromodulation* 1998;1:160–162.

41. Alo KM, Yland MJ, Kramer DL. Computer assisted and patient interactive programming of dual octrode spinal cord stimulation in the treatment of chronic pain. *Neuromodulation* 1998;1:30–45.

42. Stanton-Hicks M. Spinal cord stimulation for the management of complex regional pain syndromes. *Neuromodulation* 1999;2:193–201.

43. Bedder MD. Implantation techniques for spinal cord stimulator. In: Waldman SD, Winnie AP(eds.). *Interventional pain management*. W.B. Saunders, Philadelphia, 1996:419–422.

44. Augustinsson LE. Avoiding difficulties in spinal cord stimulation. In: Waldman SD, Winnie AP(eds.). *Interventional pain management*. W.B. Saunders, Philadelphia, 1996:427–430.

45. Van Buyten JP, Zundert JV, Milbouw G. Treatment of failed back surgery syndrome patients with low back and leg pain: a pilot study of a new dual lead spinal cord stimulation system. *Neuromodulation* 1999;2:258–265.

46. Krames ES, Olson K. Clinical realities and economic considerations: patient selection in intrathecal therapy. *J Pain Symptom Manage* 1997;14:S3–S13.

47. Doleys DM. Psychological assessment for implantable therapies. *Pain Digest* 2000;10:16–23.

48. Monsalve V, de Andres JA, Valia JC. Application of a psychological decision algorithm for the selection of patients susceptible to implantation of *Neuromodulation* systems for the treatment of chronic pain. A proposal. *Neuromodulation* 2000;3:191–200.

49. Ruchinskas R, O'Grady T. Psychological variables predict decisions regarding implantation of a spinal cord stimulator. *Neuromodulation* 2000;3:183–189.

50. Bennett DS, Alo KM, Oakley J, et al. Spinal cord stimulation for complex regional pain syndrome I (RSD): a retrospective multicenter experience from 1995 to 1998 of 101 patients. *Neuromodulation* 1999;2:202–210.

51. Kidd DH, North RB. Spinal cord stimulation: an effective and cost saving treatment in management of chronic pain. In: *Pain treatment centers at crossroads: a practical and conceptual reappraisal, Progress in Pain Research and Management. Vol.7*, MJM Cohen and JN Campbell, eds. Seattle: IASP Press, 1996:174.

52. Tollison CD, Hinnant DW. Psychological testing in the evaluation of the patient in pain. In: Waldman SD, Winnie AP, eds. *Interventional Pain Management*. New York, Philadelphia: W.B. Saunders, 1996:119–128.

53. Tollison CD The comprehensive diagnosis of spinal pain: a new psychodiagnostic instrument. *Orthopaedic Review* 1993;22:335–340.

54. Willoughby SG, Hailey BJ, Wheeler LC. *Pain* patient profile: a scale to measure psychological distress. Arch *Phys Med Rehabil* 1999;80:1300–1302.

55. Bedder MD. Spinal cord stimulation and intractable pain: patient selection. In: Waldman SD, Winnie AP(eds.). *Interventional pain management*. W.B.Saunders, Philadelphia, 1996, pp.412–418.

56. Segal R, Stacey BR, Rudy TE, et al. Spinal cord stimulation revisited. *Neurol Res* 1998;20:391–396.

57. Hsu FPK, Israel Z, Limonadi F, et al. Is outpatient trial for spinal cord stimulation more cost-effective than inpatient trial? Presented at the Worldwide Pain Conference, San Francisco, CA, July 2000.

58. North RB, Kidd DH, Zahurak M, et al. Spinal cord stimulation for chronic, intractable pain: two decades' experience. *Neurosurgery* 1993;32:384–395.

59. De La Porte C, Siegfried J. Lumbosacral spinal fibrosis (spinal arachnoiditis): its diagnosis and treatment by spinal cord stimulation. *Spine* 1983;8:593–603.

60. Kumar K, Toth C, Nath RK, et al. Epidural spinal cord stimulation for treatment of chronic pain - some predictors of success. A 15–year experience. *Surg Neurol* 1998;50:110–121.

61. Mironer YE. Efficacy and selectivity of short-term percutaneous spinal cord stimulator trial. Presented on APM 17th Annual Scientific Meeting, San Diego, CA, November 1998.

62. Barolat G, Ketcik B, He J. Long-term outcome of spinal cord stimulation for chronic pain management. *Neuromodulation* 1998;1:19–29.

63. Doerr M, Krainick JU, Thoden U. *Pain* perception in man after long term spinal cord stimulation. *J Neurol* 1978;217:261–270.

64. Marchand S, Bushnell MC, Molina-Negro P, et al. The effects of dorsal column stimulation on measures of clinical and experimental pain in man. *Pain* 1991;45:249–257.

65. Mironer YE, Somerville JJ. *Pain* tolerance threshold: a pilot study of an objective measurement of spinal cord stimulator trial results. *Pain Medicine* 2000;1:110–115.

66. Mironer YE. Improved technique of spinal cord stimulator anchoring using plastic twist-lock anchor. Presented at 19th APS Annual Scientific Meeting, Atlanta, GA, November 2000.

67. Nichols RL. Bacteriology in surgery. In: Nyhus LM, Baker RJ (eds.). *Mastery of surgery*. Boston: Little, Brown and Company, 1992:83–94.

68. North RB, Ewend MG, Lawton MT, et al. Failed back surgery syndrome: five-year follow-up after spinal cord stimulator implantation. A prospective, randomized study design. *Neurosurgery* 1991;28:692–699.

69. Wetzel ET, Hassenbusch S, Oakley JC, et al. Treatment of chronic pain in failed back surgery patients with spinal cord stimulation: a review of current literature and proposal for future investigation. *Neuromodulation* 2000;3:59–74.

70. Burchiel KJ, Anderson VC, Brown FD, et al. Prospective, multicenter study of spinal cord stimulation for relief of chronic back and extremity pain. *Spine* 1996;21:2786–2794.

71. North RB, Kidd DH, Lee MS, et al. Spinal cord stimulation versus reoperation for the failed back surgery syndrome: a prospective, randomized study design. Sterotact Funct *Neurosurg* 1994;62:267–272.

72. Huber SJ, Vaglienti RM, Huber JS. Spinal cord stimulation in severe, inoperable peripheral vascular disease. *Neuromodulation* 2000;3:131–143.

73. Claeys LGY. Effects of spinal cord stimulation on nutritional skin flow in patients with ischemic pain. *Neuromodulation* 2000;3:123–130.

74. Claeys LGY. Spinal cord stimulation in the treatment of chronic critical limb ischemia: review of clinical experience. *Neuromodulation* 2000;3:89–96.

75. Claeys LGY, Horsch S. Effects of spinal cord stimulation on ischemic inflammatory pain and wound healing in patients with peripheral arterial occlusive disease Fontaine stage IV. *Pain Digest* 1997;7:200–203.

76. Murphy DF, Giles KE. Dorsal column stimulation for pain relief from intractable angina pectoris. *Pain* 1987;28:365–368.

77. Chester MR. Spinal cord stimulation for the treatment of refractory angina. *Pain Digest* 2000;10:13–15.

78. DeJongste MJL. Efficacy, safety and mechanisms of spinal cord stimulation used as an additional therapy for patients suffering from chronic refractory angina pectoris. *Neuromodulation* 1999;2:188–192.

79. Jessurun GAJ, Ten Vaarwerk IAM, DeJongste MJL, et al. Sequelae of spinal cord stimulation for refractory angina pectoris. Reliability and safety profile of long-term clinical application. *Coronary Artery Dis* 1997;8:33–38.
80. Bagger JP, Jensen BS, Johannsen G. Long-term outcome of spinal cord electrical stimulation in patients with refractory chest pain. *Clin Cardiol* 1998;21:286–288.
81. Sanderson JE, Ibrahim B, Waterhouse D, et al. Spinal cord stimulation for intractable angina—long-term clinical outcome and safety. *Eur Heart J* 1994;15:810–814.
82. Heidecke V, Rainov NG, Burkert W. Hardware failures in spinal cord stimulation for failed back surgery syndrome. *Neuromodulation* 2000;3:27–30.
83. Law JD, Miller LV. Importance and documentation of an epidural stimulating position. *Appl Neurophysiol* 1982;45:461–464.
84. Mironer YE. A new technique of the spinal cord stimulator midline "anchoring" prevents lead migration. Presented at the Worldwide Pain Conference, San Francisco, CA, July 2000.
85. Luyendijk W. The plica mediana dorsalis of the dura mater and its relation to the lumbar peridurography (canalography). *Neuroradiology* 1976;11:147–149.
86. Blomberg R. The dorsomedian connective tissue band in the lumbar epidural space of humans: an anatomical study using epiduroscopy in autopsy cases. *Anesth Analg* 1986;65:747–752.
87. Blomberg RG, Olsson SS. The lumbar epidural space in patients examined with epiduroscopy. *Anesth Analg* 1989;68:157–160.
88. Savolaine ER, Pandya JB, Greenblatt SH, et al. Anatomy of the human lumbar epidural space: new insights using CT-epidurography. *Anesthesiology* 1988;68:217–220.
89. Mironer YE. Spinal cord stimulator lead positioned at the lower level across midline covers axial pain. Presented at the Worldwide Pain Conference, San Francisco, CA, July 2000.
90. Gorecki JP, Rose A, Rubin L, et al. A retrospective comparison of laminotomy lead placement to percutaneous lead placement in 41 patients undergoing spinal cord stimulation for chronic pain. Presented at the Worldwide Pain Conference, San Francisco, CA, July 2000.
91. Barolat G. A prospective multicenter study to assess the efficacy of spinal cord stimulation utilizing a multi-channel radio-frequency system for the treatment of intractable low back and lower extremity pain. Initial considerations and methodology. *Neuromodulation* 1999; 2:179–183.
92. Law JD. Spinal cord stimulation in the "failed back surgery syndrome": comparison of technical criteria for palliating pain in the leg vs. in the low back. *Acta Neurochir* 1992;117:95.
93. North RB. Spinal cord stimulation for axial low back pain: single versus dual percutaneous electrodes. *International Neuromodulation Society Abstracts*, Lucerne, Switzerland 1998:212.
94. Holsheimer J, Wesselink WA. Effect of anode-cathode configuration on paresthesia coverage in spinal cord stimulation. *Neurosurgery* 1997;41:654–659.
95. Mironer YE. Letter to the editor. *Neuromodulation* 2000;4:209.
96. Chancellor MB, Chartier-Kastler EJ. Principles of sacral nerve stimulation (SNS) for the treatment of bladder and urethral sphincter dysfunctions. *Neuromodulation* 2000;3:15–26.
97. Feler CA, Whitworth LA, Brookoff D, et al. Recent advances: sacral nerve root stimulation using a retrograde method of lead insertion for the treatment of pelvic pain due to interstitial cystitis. *Neuromodulation* 1999;2:211–216.
98. Lou L, Racz G, Raj PP, et al. Sacral stimulation for the treatment of chronic intractable pelvic pain. Presented at the Worldwide Pain Conference, San Francisco, CA, July 2000.
99. Palmer P, Johnson-Harvey D, Lee DJ, et al. Placement of neurostimulator electrode lead via sacrococcygeal ligament for treatment of sacral neuropathic pain; case report. Presented at the Worldwide Pain Conference, San Francisco, CA, July 2000.
100. Hassenbusch SJ, Stanton-Hicks M, Schoppa D, et al. Long-term results of peripheral nerve stimulation for reflex sympathetic dystrophy. *J Neurosurg* 1996;84:415–423.
101. Shetter AG, Racz GB, Lewis R, et al. Peripheral nerve stimulation. In: North RB, Levy RM (eds.). *Neurosurgical management of pain*. New York: Springer-Verlag, 1997:261–270.
102. Mironer YE. Transcutaneous placement of the peripheral nerve stimulator trial lead for post-herniorrhaphy pain. *Pain Insider*, Summer 1999.
103. Weiner RL, Reed KL. Peripheral neurostimulation for control of intractable occipital neuralgia. *Neuromodulation* 1999;2:217–221.
104. Weiner RL. The future of peripheral nerve stimulation. *Neurol Res* 2000;22:299–304.
105. Mironer YE. Combined use of cervical spinal cord stimulator and occipital nerve stimulator. AAPM Abstracts. *Pain Medicine* 2000; 1:193.

CHAPTER **13**

Neurosurgical Options for the Management of Intractable Pain

Richard K. Osenbach

The modern neurosurgical armamentarium for the treatment of chronic intractable pain is considerable. Indeed, the contemporary neurosurgeon currently has a wide array of surgical options for treating chronic pain that becomes debilitating and refractory to the customary multimodality, less "invasive" nonoperative therapies. Procedures such as cordotomy and some of the other brainstem ablative procedures have been utilized for many decades and have a rich history unto themselves. More contemporary techniques such as spinal cord stimulation, spinal infusion therapy, and various forms of brain stimulation have largely replaced many of the destructive procedures that were once commonplace. Although many of these destructive procedures are now infrequently used, they still have a role in properly selected patients.

Obviously, a comprehensive discussion of all of the various neurosurgical techniques for the management of chronic pain is beyond the scope of this discussion, and the interested reader is referred to several excellent comprehensive texts that discuss some of these procedures in greater depth (1,2). The main purpose of this chapter is to present a procedurally oriented overview of the neurosurgical management of chronic pain, the major emphasis focusing on indications, clinical decision making, and efficacy.

GENERAL PRINCIPLES OF SURGICAL TREATMENT OF CHRONIC PAIN

Management of patients with a chronic pain condition is often a complex and difficult challenge, both for the patients and the health-care provider. Successful management of these patients requires a thorough understanding of the pain problem along with a careful and contempla-

tive approach in developing an effective treatment algorithm. Failure to obtain a complete and meticulous history regarding the details of a patient's pain and previous treatment not uncommonly leads to poor patient selection and failure of the treatment employed. It simply cannot be emphasized sufficiently that careful patient selection represents the cornerstone of successful surgical management of chronic pain. Additionally, one should remember that chronic pain is a multidimensional biopsychosocial problem and in a sense really represents a disease entity. Consequently, it *must* be understood that effective management of most patients with long-standing pain requires a multidisciplinary approach, utilizing all modalities and specialists at one's disposal. Indeed, the belief on the part of the patient and/or physician that a surgical procedure alone such as implantation of a spinal cord stimulator or intrathecal drug pump will provide a "cure" is a foolish thought and will nearly always result in treatment failure and a dissatisfied patient. The successful treatment of chronic pain should follow a logical algorithm, beginning with the most simple and least interventional therapies and progressing to more complex invasive modalities.

SURGICAL PROCEDURES

The surgical procedures for the treatment of chronic pain can be divided into two general categories: modulatory and ablative (Table 13-1). In general, taking into consideration the underlying cause, location, and type of pain, attempts at neuromodulation should almost always be considered before moving on to destructive procedures. Neuromodulation procedures are particularly attractive because they are nondestructive and reversible. Moreover, most can be tested with *some* degree of certainty as to

TABLE 13-1. *Neuromodulation and ablative procedures for chronic pain*

Neuromodulation
  Spinal cord stimulation (a.k.a. dorsal column stimulation)
  Peripheral nerve stimulation
    Major extremity nerves (median, ulnar, radial, sciatic, peroneal, tibial)
    Occipital nerve stimulation
    Spinal nerve root stimulation
    Trigeminal nerve stimulation (peripheral)
  Spinal drug infusion
  Intraventricular opiates
  Deep brain stimulation
    Endogenous opiate system (PAG, PVG)
    Lemniscal system (medial lemniscus, sensory thalamus, internal capsule)
  Motor cortex stimulation

Ablative Procedures
  Peripheral Procedures
    Peripheral neurectomy
    Excision of painful neuromas
    Sympathetic ganglionectomy
    Trigeminal system procedures
      Retrogasserian radiofrequency thermal rhizotomy
      Percutaneous glycerol rhizolysis
      Balloon microcompression
  Spinal Procedures
    Dorsal root ganglionectomy
    Dorsal rhizotomy
    Anterolateral cordotomy
    Midline (commissural) myelotomy
    Percutaneous high cervical cordotomy (C-1–2)
    Dorsal root entry zone lesion
  Brainstem and Thalamic Procedures
    Caudalis DREZ
    Medullary tractotomy
    Pontine tractotomy
    Mesencephalic tractotomy
    Medial thalamotomy
    Pulvinotomy
  Other Procedures
    Cingulotomy
    Pituitary ablation
    Hypothalamotomy
    Stereotactic radiosurgery

1960s based on the seminal work of Melzak and Wall, who developed the gate control theory of pain transmission. Although the gate control theory helps to explain some of the effects of SCS, a substantial body of evidence over the past 3 decades has shown that multiple mechanisms are likely responsible for the analgesic effects of SCS. Spinal cord stimulation has improved considerably since its inception more than 30 years ago. This evolution can be linked to a number of factors, including a better understanding of the mechanisms of SCS, improvements in equipment and technology, the use of novel electrode placements, and a greater appreciation of the indications and efficacy of SCS. All of these factors have contributed to improved patient selection outcomes.

Spinal cord stimulation is currently used for a wide variety of painful conditions (Table 13-2) (3–8). In the United States, the most common applications of SCS are for patients with so-called failed back surgery syndrome (FBSS) and patients with complex regional pain syndromes (CRPS). Over the past several years SCS has been applied to other painful conditions, including refractory angina pectoris, ischemic limb pain, and interstitial cystitis, to name a few. Indeed, the future of SCS is likely to include all of the conditions mentioned plus new applications outside the central nervous system, such as treatment of neurogenic bladder in patients with spinal cord injury.

Spinal cord stimulation should be considered for pain that is primarily neuropathic in nature when more conservative approaches have failed to achieve satisfactory pain relief. Ideally, SCS is most effective for pain that is mostly confined to an extremity. Predominantly axial pain in the lower back or pain that involves other midline regions (e.g., perineum) can be very difficult to treat. This discrepancy in therapeutic effect of SCS for axial and extremity pain is believed to be due to a differential ability to drive stimulation-induced paresthesias into these areas. However, with multiple electrodes placed and programmed in novel ways even these difficult areas can sometimes be effectively stimulated.

whether they will produce effective long-term pain relief. In fact, a screening trial for analgesic efficacy should always precede implantation of a permanent system, whether it is for electrical stimulation or spinal drug infusion. For example, a drug pump for delivery of intrathecal opiates should never be implanted without an adequate screening trial of spinal narcotics that demonstrates efficacy.

NEUROMODULATION PROCEDURES

Spinal Cord Stimulation (SCS)

Spinal cord stimulation (SCS), formerly known as dorsal column stimulation (DCS), was introduced in the late

TABLE 13-2. *Current applications of spinal cord stimulation*

Postlaminectomy pain syndrome, a.k.a. failed back surgery syndrome (FBSS)
Complex regional pain syndromes (CRPS)
  Type I (a.k.a. reflex sympathetic dystrophy)
  Type II (a.k.a. causalgia)
Peripheral nerve injury pain
Postthoracotomy pain or intercostal neuralgia
Ilio-inguinal neuralgia
Ischemic limb pain secondary to peripheral vascular disease
Intractable angina pectoris
Interstitial cystitis
Coccyxodynia
Vulvodynia

For SCS to be successful, it is critical that the patient be able to perceive paresthesias in the distribution of the pain. It is relatively easy to produce paresthesias in both the upper and lower extremities but more difficult to effectively stimulate axial regions (3,4). For example, an electrode positioned in the lower thoracic-upper lumbar region has a greater than 70% chance of producing stimulation in the foot; this probability approaches nearly 100% if the cathode (negative electrode) is located around L-1 (3,4). Similarly, there is a high likelihood of producing effective stimulation in the hand with electrodes placed all the way from C-1 to C-7. In contrast, stimulation of the lower back is more difficult, especially if chest wall or abdominal stimulation is to be avoided. This may be related to anatomical and physiological factors related to the size and relative position of low back fibers within the spinal cord. The lower back is best captured with either a single perfectly midline electrode or closely placed parallel dual electrodes with closely spaced contacts placed between T-8 and T-10 (3,4).

Every patient selected for SCS should have a screening trial performed before implantation of a permanent system. There is no general consensus as to the ideal duration for a trial, which can last anywhere from 24 hours to several weeks. The author's protocol is to usually perform a 1-week trial using what will be the permanent electrode(s) and temporary extensions. The major disadvantage of this method is that if the trial is *unsuccessful,* a second, albeit short, procedure is required to remove the electrode(s). In general, 70%–90% of patients who are selected for screening will obtain sufficient pain relief to justify a permanent implant (5). For better or worse, the benchmark of analgesia is at least a 50% reduction in baseline pain.

There are several principles of screening that are central to obtaining accurate information that will eventually lead to a successful permanent implant. With few exceptions, one should select the type of electrode configuration for the screening trial that one anticipates will be required for an effective permanent implant. For example, if a dual-electrode system is considered necessary to achieve optimal paresthesia coverage, then dual electrodes should be used for the trial. It is crucial that an optimal stimulation pattern, i.e., 100% coverage of the pain topography, be achieved with the trial in order to make an accurate judgment as to the therapeutic benefit. Lastly, to the greatest extent possible, one should avoid overdriving a given area in order to get stimulation into a different area. For example, if a patient has pain that is restricted to the foot and first perceives stimulation in the thigh, one should avoid simply ramping up the amplitude in order to drive the stimulation more caudally. This may produce painful stimulation in an area that is not part of the pain topography and may cause the patient to dislike the sensation and effectively produce a "false negative" trial.

Although numerous published series in the literature detail the results of SCS, most are retrospective and vary significantly in their methods of data collection and reliability. Indeed, prospective series, in general, and randomized trials, in particular, are lacking. One of the major problems in assessing the efficacy of SCS, based on the available literature, is a lack of uniformity on the definition of a successful outcome and the manner in which outcomes are reported in general.

The overall long-term results of SCS vary considerably. The percentage of patients who continue to maintain more than 50% reduction in pain ranges from less than 20% to as high as 75%, depending on the clinical series, underlying pain conditions, and length of followup (5). Traditionally, the most common indication for SCS in the United States has been patients with FBSS. Although early success rates as high as nearly 90% have been reported in this population, the long-term analgesia has not been as durable as one would desire. Indeed, a gradual decline in efficacy tends to occur over time such that long-term outcomes are considerably less. Kumar et al. summarized the overall results of 16 series of SCS reported in the literature (5). Pooled data from 8 of these series, including all types of pain syndromes, indicated that of 1261 patients who were screened, 894 (71%) received a permanent implant. Long-term pain relief (i.e., > 50%) was achieved in 530 (59%) patients. The results for the group of patients with FBSS are less impressive. Collated data from 10 series showed that the implantation rate was higher in the group with FBSS; 860 (88%) patients were implanted out of 972 who were initially screened. However, in examining the long-term efficacy, only 42% of patients continued to maintain more than a 50% reduction in pain.

Although the reasons are not clear, it would indeed appear that different pain syndromes respond more or less favorably to SCS. High degrees of success, in some cases exceeding 80% to 85%, have been achieved for patients with intractable angina (7), ischemic pain from peripheral vascular disease (8), and reflex sympathetic dystrophy (5,6). Long-term studies of SCS for intractable angina carried out in Europe demonstrate that more than 80% of patients enjoy lasting effects in terms of reduction in angina frequency and severity, reduction in the intake of short-acting nitrates, increased exercise tolerance, and overall improved quality of life (7). Similarly, satisfactory pain relief has been reported in 67% to 93% of patients with ischemic pain related to peripheral vascular disease (8). Additionally, a limb salvage effect has also been suggested in this group of patients.

Peripheral Nerve Stimulation (PNS)

The analgesic mechanisms of peripheral nerve stimulation (PNS) may be quite similar to those of SCS, and for all practical purposes PNS represents a spinoff of SCS. Traditionally, PNS was thought of only in the context of stimulation of major peripheral nerves in the extremities (e.g., median, ulnar, peroneal, etc.), but more recently other applications have evolved, including occipital nerve stimulation (ONS), spinal root stimulation, and even stimulation of the peripheral trigeminal system. For the most part, applications of PNS are restricted to patients with neuropathic pain that is essentially limited to the distribution of a single peripheral nerve. For example, there is a subgroup of patients with RSD or peripheral nerve injury (i.e., causalgia) with pain limited to a single peripheral nerve territory; some of these patients may be effectively treated with PNS (9). This technique can be applied to most of the major nerves in the upper or lower extremity. As with SCS, a screening trial is necessary to evaluate the potential efficacy of a long-term implant.

One of the more promising applications of PNS is ONS. Occipital nerve stimulation has been utilized for treatment of neuropathic pain in patients with refractory occipital neuralgia and even in selected patients with cervicogenic headaches. For occipital neuralgia, a percutaneous electrode is introduced just beneath the skin and positioned transversely at the C-1 level. A test period of stimulation is conducted to determine efficacy. If the trial is successful, a permanent system with a programmable pulse generator can then be implanted.

Deep Brain Stimulation (DBS)

Nearly 50 years ago during the course of performing various intracranial neurosurgical procedures, a serendipitous observation was made: that electrical stimulation of various anatomical structures within the brain could produce analgesia. Beginning in the 1960s and continuing into the 1970s several authors reported that stimulation of the lemniscal pathways, including the ventrocaudal (Vc) thalamic sensory relay nucleus (a.k.a. ventral posterolateral [VPL] and ventral posteromedial [VPM] nuclei) and internal capsule, could effectively relieve neuropathic pain. In 1969, Reynolds discovered that stimulation of the periaqueductal gray (PAG) area in rats produced such a profound analgesia that surgical procedures could be performed without any evidence of pain (10). This resulted in a large number of animal studies further investigating stimulation produced analgesia (SPA). Subsequently DBS was carried out using a variety of targets, including PAG, periventricular gray (PVG), VPL, and VPM.

Deep brain stimulation has been performed for a variety of pain conditions, including FBSS, brachial plexus avulsion, painful peripheral neuropathy, refractory trigeminal neuropathic pain, spinal cord injury pain, and thalamic pain syndromes (11,12). Deep brain stimulation should be considered a procedure of last resort for patients with intractable pain in whom multiple, more conventional therapeutic modalities have failed.

There are several major considerations in patient selection for DBS. First, one should seek a clear organic basis for the pain. Clearly, patients with vague diffuse pain complaints without a clear underlying cause should be ex-cluded from consideration. As with most other types of "pain surgery," patients should be evaluated by a multidisciplinary team. Preoperative psychological evaluation should be routinely performed, although many of these patients will have already undergone such an evaluation prior to other treatment modalities. Most, if not all, patients with chronic pain of such severity in whom DBS is being given serious consideration harbor mild psychological disturbances such as depression and anxiety that influence their pain but are not so significant as to exclude them from surgical consideration. A second major consideration is the location of the pain. Patients with pain in the upper half of the body and pain in the head and face may be good candidates for DBS. Patients with poorly defined diffuse pain in the pelvis, rectum, and perineum of unclear etiology should not be considered for DBS. Because there are multiple target sites that may be selected, it is important to determine if the pain is primarily nociceptive or neuropathic because this will influence target selection. In general, nociceptive pain that is opiate responsive responds best to PAG or PVG stimulation, whereas neuropathic pain responds most favorably to stimulation of VPL/VPM (11).

Deep brain stimulation is performed using stereotactic guidance under local anesthesia. For unilateral pain that is purely neuropathic, an electrode is stereotactically placed in the contralateral Vc (VPL or VPM); of course, if the pain is bilateral, then bilateral electrode placement is obviously necessary. The location of Vc is initially determined with stereotactic anatomical coordinates and then confirmed using physiological mapping (13). The goal is to identify the area where stimulation-induced paresthesias are perceived in the area of pain. After the optimal target has been localized a permanent electrode is placed and connected to a temporary extension for a trial period that may last anywhere from a few days to a week. Generally, at least a 50% reduction in baseline pain is required to justify implantation of the permanent system that is then implanted as a second stage under general anesthesia.

In patients with primarily nociceptive pain that is opiate responsive, the preferred target is the PVG. The specific target coordinates vary between authors. Richardson selects his PVG target 8 to 10 mm behind the midcommissural (MC) point, approximately 5 mm from the midline, and places the tip of the electrode on the commissural plane (12). Stimulation is again performed, although the responses obtained from PVG and/or PAG stimulation are not as discrete as those from stimulation in Vc. At this target location, a good indicator of correct electrode placement is a sensation of either heat or cold in the contralateral face (12). Other sensations that have been reported include a sensation of bodily warmth, floating, dizziness, or general well-being. Again, after the target is confirmed permanent electrodes are introduced and connected to temporary extensions that are externalized for a trial period of stimulation. Although PVG or Vc stimulation is preferred for pure nociceptive or neuropathic pain, respectively, in fact, many patients have mixed nociceptive and neuropathic pain. In these patients it has become a common practice to place electrodes at both targets and permanently implant the electrode that produces the best analgesia. In some cases, both electrodes are implanted for chronic stimulation (11). More than 1000 patients have been treated using DBS. Various measures of long-term efficacy have been employed, including greater than 50% reduction in baseline pain, continued use of the stimulator, and pain relief reported using descriptive terms such as "excellent," "good," "fair," and "poor." The overall long-term success rate for DBS has been reported to average 60% (range 19% to 79%). Bendok and Levy performed a metaanalysis of DBS for chronic pain that encompassed all studies that included more than 15 patients (11). Thirteen series were identified with 1114 patients for whom long-term outcome data were available. Long-term successful pain relief was reported in 561 (50%) patients. Nearly 700 patients underwent DBS for neuropathic pain, with an average long-term success rate of 42%. Both initial and long-term success rates were quite variable, ranging from 29% to 78% and 26% to 84%, respectively. For patients who underwent DBS for nociceptive pain, the long-term efficacy was somewhat better, averaging 61% (272 out of 443 patients). Again, initial and long-term success rates were variable, ranging from 0% to 98% and 0% to 81%, respectively.

There appears to be a relatively clear relationship between efficacy, type of pain (nociceptive vs. neuropathic), and target selection (VPL/VPM or PVG/PAG). Treatment of nociceptive pain with sensory thalamic stimulation (i.e., VPL/VPM) is uniformly unsuccessful. Indeed, not a single patient (n = 51) with nociceptive pain, in whom VPL/VPM stimulation was used, achieved long-term pain relief. On the other hand, PAG/PVG stimulation produced long-term success in 59% of patients with nociceptive pain. In contrast, VPL/VPM stimulation for patients with deafferentation pain was successful in 56%. For patients with nociceptive pain, VPL/VPM stimulation was successful in only 23%.

Ten to 15 years ago, the FDA reclassified DBS (previously an approved procedure) as experimental, citing a lack of safety and efficacy data. There are certainly sufficient safety data from the literature on thalamic stimulation for tremor. However, the device used is not approved for pain applications. Deep brain stimulation is presently performed under the auspices of a physician investigational device exemption (IDE) or at the discretion of the physician with the consent of a well-informed patient in whom no other viable treatment options exist. However, on the basis of the available data, it would appear that DBS is indeed a safe and effective treatment option for carefully selected patients.

Motor Cortex Stimulation (MCX)

Motor cortex stimulation (MCX) represents a novel approach to the treatment of patients with deafferentation pain (14–17). Deafferentation pain develops when sensory information is either partially or completely interrupted at any point within the neospinothalamic system. The presence of deafferentation pain necessarily implies the presence of either partial or complete sensory loss, most notably related to pain and temperature. Common examples of this type of pain include pain following brachial plexus root avulsion, pain following either bulbar or thalamic infarction, phantom limb pain following amputation, and pain following spinal cord injury. Deafferentation pain may also be iatrogenic and may occur after destructive pain procedures that target the spinothalamic system, such as cordotomy or peripheral destructive procedures of the trigeminal system, such as retrogasserian radiofrequency rhizotomy that may occasionally result in anesthesia dolorosa.

There is physiological evidence suggesting that at multiple levels of the central nervous system, nociceptive neurons are subject to inhibitory influences exerted by the somatosensory system, which mediates nonnoxious sensation such as light touch (14,15). This concept is supported by the observation that PNS, SCS, and thalamic sensory stimulation can attenuate nociceptive responses. However, in many patients with partial sensory preservation, peripheral nonnoxious stimulation *within* the area of sensory loss may actually evoke pain that can spread over the entire area of sensory loss, implying dysfunction of the pain inhibitory function of the sensory system mediating nonnoxious sensation. It has been observed that stimulation at a site *rostral* to the level of deafferentation may provide better pain relief, implying a functional somatosensory pain inhibitory system rostral to the site of deafferentation. Based on these considerations and their own observation that stimulation of the precentral rather than postcentral gyrus sometimes produced profound pain inhibition, Tsubokawa and colleagues pioneered the concept of MCX for deafferentation pain (14,15). The exact mechanism(s) through which MCX produces analgesia is not clear. However, there are known to be reciprocal connections between the primary motor and sensory areas. Based upon the proposed mechanism of deafferentation pain described previously, it is believed that MCX produces its effect by restoring inhibitory fields that would normally surround primary sensory neurons but that have been lost as a result of deafferentation.

MCX has been most effectively utilized in patients with deafferentation pain following thalamic or bulbar stroke and in patients with refractory trigeminal neuropathic pain. It has been suggested that response of the patient's pain to intravenous (IV) opiates, barbiturates, or ketamine may provide prognostic information regarding the potential response to MCX. Yamamoto et al. performed IV infusions of morphine, thiamylal (barbiturate), and ketamine in 39 patients with central poststroke pain (hemibody pain with dysesthesias) (16). Definite pain reduction occurred in 22 of 39 (56%) patients with barbiturate infusion, 11 of 23 (48%) patients with ketamine infusion, and only 8 of 39 (21%) patients with morphine infusion. Comparison of long-term results demonstrated that patients whose pain responded favorably to barbiturates or ketamine and was resistant to morphine displayed long-lasting pain reduction with MCX.

MCX is performed through a small craniotomy that exposes the dura overlying the motor cortex *contralateral* to the side of pain. The motor cortex can be localized using a variety of methods, including framed-based as well as frameless stereotactic techniques, somatosensory evoked potentials, or direct cortical stimulation mapping and also using either functional magnetic resonance imaging (MRI) or magnetoencephalography. Functional MRI and magnetoencephalography are particularly exciting and intriguing because the possibility now exists for the "functional" images to be imported into a variety of frameless intraoperative stereotactic navigation systems that can then be used for precise localization of the primary motor cortex.

A four-contact insulated plate electrode, identical to that used for SCS, is placed *epidurally* over the area of the motor strip, from which motor contractions can be elicited in the painful area. The electrode is then tunneled and connected to a temporary extension, and a trial period of stimulation is conducted. Stimulation is performed and analgesia obtained at stimulation amplitudes that are well below the motor threshold, implying that the mechanism of action is unrelated to activation of primary motor neurons. If at least a 50% reduction in baseline pain is achieved, the electrode is then connected to a permanently implanted pulse generator during a second stage. Stimulation is intermittent and is usually performed several times per day for approximately 20 minutes.

MCX, using the devices described, is not FDA approved, and therefore the application of this technique should be dictated by the same principles outlined for DBS. Notwithstanding these limitations and the paucity of long-term efficacy data in large numbers of patients, MCX is emerging as a promising tool for the treatment of deafferentation pain. Yamamoto et al. performed chronic MCX on 28 patients with central pain and reported the results after one year of therapy (16). Overall, MCX was judged to be effective in 13 of 28 (46%) patients. However, when the results were analyzed based on the preoperative response to IV infusion, the results were quite interesting. Of the 18 patients who responded to either barbiturate or ketamine, 12 (67%) were considered successful. In contrast, out of 10 patients whose pain was not responsive to barbiturate or ketamine infusion, only 1 (10%) had a successful result.

Nguyen et al. reported the results of chronic MCX in 32 patients with refractory neuropathic pain of either central or peripheral origin (17). Long-term mean VAS scores fell from 86 to 40 (p = 0.001), and medication intake as measured by the medication quantification scale (MQS) was reduced (17.9 preop to 12.3, p = 0.001). Overall, 24 of 32 (75%) experienced either a "good" (pain reduced by 70% to 100%) or satisfactory (pain reduced by 40% to 69%) result in terms of pain reduction. Ten of 13 (77%) patients with central pain had pain reduction; 9 of 12 (75%) patients with trigeminal neuropathic pain also enjoyed a definite benefit. Interestingly, one patient with postherpetic neuralgia had a positive response, and this may represent at least one alternative for the treatment of this dreadful condition for which few treatments are effective. Several patients experienced loss of effect over the first few months of therapy. In most cases, this was related to migration of the electrode, which, when repositioned correctly, resulted in restoration of analgesia.

Spinal and Intraventricular Drug Delivery

Over the past 20 years, intraspinal drug delivery has assumed an increasingly important role in the management of intractable pain. Although the initial application of this therapy was restricted to patients with refractory cancer pain, the use of spinal opiates for nonmalignant pain has now become the primary indication for this therapy. Chronic intrathecal (IT) drug infusion has been shown to be effective and has clearly been accepted in patients with cancer pain who cannot gain effective analgesia without significant side effects with systemic narcotics. In this group of patients, the treatment generally has a defined end point and can produce substantial improvements in quality of life. Even though chronic spinal drug infusion is now well accepted for noncancer pain, there continues to be an element of controversy surrounding its long-term use in this particular patient population.

Intrathecal opiates should be considered only after less invasive and complex modalities have failed. Again, patient selection, particularly with nonmalignant pain, plays a central role in the success of this therapy. It must be appreciated, by the treating physician, other members of the pain treatment team, and the patient, that the decision to implant a drug pump represents a huge commitment on the part of all parties. Indeed, for patients with nonmalignant pain, chronic spinal drug infusion is a labor-intensive therapy that has no definitive end point.

Several factors should influence the clinician in considering spinal drug infusion, including pain topography, type of pain (nociceptive vs. neuropathic), pain response to long-acting oral opiates, prior history of drug abuse, psychological screening, response to a screening trial, and patient access to care. In general, spinal drug infusion, particularly using narcotics, is *most* ideally suited to patients with nociceptive pain that has a more diffuse pattern (e.g., patient with FBSS with primarily diffuse axial lower back pain). Classically, it has been taught that neuropathic pain does not respond to opiates, but this is not true in many instances. There are clearly patients with pure neuropathic pain who do, in fact, respond to opiates, albeit perhaps at higher doses than might be required for nociceptive pain. This is actually true for both oral as well as IT opiates. Although spinal infusion may be effective for head and neck pain in selected patients, because of drug properties and factors related to drug distribution in the CSF, this therapy is best suited to pain that occurs below the upper thoracic dermatomes. In general, the pain should be opiate responsive, although, again, patients whose pain has a significant neuropathic component may show a relative resistance to opiates even at reasonable dose levels that are devoid of systemic side effects.

Prior to implantation of a permanent pump for chronic therapy, *all* patients should undergo a screening trial. Screening can be performed in a variety of single- or multiple-intrathecal boluses, continuous epidural or intrathecal infusion. Screening can be performed either with or without placebo control. There are advantages and disadvantages of each technique, and there is currently no consensus as to which method best predicts long-term response to therapy. The author's preference is to perform a continuous intrathecal trial over 3 to 4 days using a tunneled IT catheter. For patients who are opiate tolerant, the daily opiate dose is reduced by half at the beginning of the trial, and a short-acting oral agent is prescribed as needed for breakthrough pain. This method most closely replicates the effect that will be derived from a pump and may, in theory, at least partially eliminate the potential placebo response that can occur with a single IT bolus. Moreover, this method allows dose escalation during the trial, which may be important in opiate-tolerant patients who have been receiving exceedingly high doses of oral narcotics. The trial should be conducted using the drug that one plans to deliver with the implanted pump. For example, it is not rational to screen a patient with a combination of morphine and clonidine and then begin chronic therapy with morphine alone. Also, catheter position is important depending on the drug chosen. With hydrophilic drugs, such as morphine, catheter position is not critical because the drug will distribute over the entire spinal axis. However, when using drugs such as clonidine or fentanyl, which are more lipophilic, the catheter tip must be positioned within several segments of the dermatomal level of the pain.

In the past, IT drug infusion was synonymous with IT opiates. Even presently, morphine is still the only drug approved by the FDA for intrathecal delivery using a programmable pump. Notwithstanding, other opiates (hydromorphone, fentanyl, sufentanil, meperidine, methadone) as well as a number of nonopiate agents such as bupivacaine and clonidine are currently being used. Indeed, the concept of polyanalgesia has become quite popular in so far as IT drug delivery is concerned. There is a substantial body of literature detailing the efficacy of many of these alternative agents and drug combinations, and it would appear based on clinical series that many of these agents and combinations are in fact safe for long-term use. However, one should be cautious about utilizing agents for which animal toxicity data are lacking and/or that have not been shown at least over time to be safe.

In 1999, the Polyanalgesic Consensus Conference was convened in an effort to address some of the crucial issues in the field of spinal drug delivery. A panel, consisting of 17 internationally recognized experts in the field of spinal drug delivery, critically reviewed the literature on the use of opioids, local anesthetics, adrenergic agents, N-methyl D-aspartate (NMDA) antagonists, somatostatin analogs, calcium channel blockers, and various other agents (18); developed standardized clinical guidelines for spinal analgesia (19); and suggested future directions for research and development of alternative agents for IT analgesia (20).

Intraventricular drug administration may occasionally be indicated in patients with craniocervical pain due to head and neck cancer with limited survival (usually less than 3 months) who either fail to respond to intraspinal opioids or who had an initial favorable response but subsequently developed tolerance to the intraspinal infusion (21). The drug may be administered by an implanted infusion pump or by intermittent injection through an Ommaya reservoir. The usual daily dose of morphine for intraventricular delivery is between 50 and 700 micrograms per day. Intraventricular administration of morphine produces a potent analgesia in excess of that provided by intraspinal infusion (epidural or intrathecal) that appears to be mediated through supraspinal pathways. The side-effect profile of intraventricular morphine appears similar to that of intraspinal delivery except that the risk of respiratory depression appears to be minimal after the first several days of therapy.

Lazorthes and colleagues, over a 10-year period, treated 82 patients with terminal cancer, all of whom were opiate tolerant, using intraventricular opiates (21). The authors employed a subcutaneous access port attached to a ventricular catheter. The initial dose to determine efficacy and minimize the occurrence of side effects was around 0.1 mg of morphine. Depending on the degree of analgesia, the dosage was later increased. The average followup for these patients was 65 days (range 12–443 days). The mean initial daily intraventricular morphine dose required for analgesia was 0.3 mg (0.1–2.0 mg); the final mean dose was 2.5 mg (0.1–60 mg). Overall, during a followup period of around 2.5 months, 66 (80%) patients achieved good or excellent pain relief, 14 (17%) achieved moderate relief, and there were 2 (3%) failures. Relatively minor morphine side effects such as nausea, vomiting, drowsiness, urinary retention, and constipation were common during the trial and titration phase but were almost always transient. In fact only six patients (7%) experienced chronic side effects (nausea and vomiting 5, drowsiness 1). Only three patients (3.5%) experienced major central side effects; two patients developed drowsiness and respiratory depression, and a single patient experienced visual hallucinations and behavioral problems. All of the central side effects were immediately reversed by systemic naloxone administration with minimal effects on analgesia.

Although IT opiates delivered chronically with an implanted pump have proven highly effective, this therapy does in fact have its drawbacks, including cost, requirements for ongoing refills and pump maintenance, and the risk of bacterial contamination with refills. Consequently, there have been a number of preclinical studies to determine the feasibility and efficacy of IT adrenal medullary transplants for the management of chronic pain. The theory is that chromaffin cells that are grafted into the CSF will produce analgesic substances such as catecholamines (which are known to be involved in the descending inhibitory system) and opioid peptides, which reduce pain in a synergistic manner. Along those lines, Lazorthes et al. recently published their results of a phase II trial of IT chromaffin cell grafts in 15 patients with cancer pain (22). Pain had previously been controlled in all patients with IT morphine. Twelve patients with an average followup of 4.5 months were judged to benefit from enhanced analgesia. Seven patients were able to either eliminate (n = 5) or significantly decrease (n = 2) their requirements for IT morphine; five patients were able to remain at a stable IT morphine dose without the need for dose escalation. In most of the patients, a relationship was noted between analgesic response and CSF metenkephalin levels. Although this represents a small series of patients, the results suggest that this therapy may be beneficial and that it should perhaps be tested and confirmed in a larger controlled group of patients.

NEUROABLATIVE PROCEDURES

Destructive neurosurgical techniques have a long and rich history. Indeed, these techniques have been used for many years, primarily for the treatment of cancer pain and to a lesser extent for nonmalignant pain syndromes. However, with the evolution of IT opiates, there has been a radical trend away from the use of ablative procedures. This is rather unfortunate because some of these techniques, such as percutaneous cordotomy and midbrain tractotomy, can be very beneficial in properly selected patients. Indeed, improvements in imaging, stereotactic localization, electrode design, and lesioning techniques have created the potential to make these techniques safer and more effective than ever.

There are certainly both positives and negatives to destructive pain procedures. On the negative side, destructive procedures are obviously irreversible and carry the risk of neurological morbidity. Also, the analgesic efficacy of most of the destructive procedures cannot be tested

with the degree of certainty that is present with augmentative procedures such as electrical stimulation and/or spinal drug infusion. On the positive side, many of these techniques can be performed as a single-stage procedure that often results in immediate analgesia. An effective ablative procedure often allows the patient more freedom because it can often eliminate the requirement of continuous interactions with health-care providers that is necessary in the case of spinal drug pumps that require periodic refilling and sometimes frequent reprogramming in order to achieve effective pain control. Moreover, the overall cost of ablative procedures is probably less because the high costs of an implant are avoided. Consequently, this author, as well as other neurosurgeons who are familiar with these techniques, believes that they should probably continue to play an important role in the management of patients with cancer-related pain. For patients with nonmalignant pain syndromes, with some exceptions (e.g., trigeminal neuralgia), whenever feasible, one of the neuroaugmentative approaches should generally be attempted because these are more likely to result in long-term success than are destructive procedures for which the analgesic effects often fade with time. The various ablative procedures are summarized next, beginning with peripheral procedures and progressing farther rostrally in the nervous system.

Peripheral Neurectomy

Pain is a common symptom following peripheral nerve injury as well as some diseases of the peripheral nerve, such as diabetic neuropathy. Indeed, injury to a major nerve trunk may result in a devastating pain syndrome known as causalgia, a.k.a. CRPS Type II. Painful nerve injuries are often complex problems that necessitate commitment and perseverance from the physician. Many pathophysiological mechanisms that have been proposed to explain nerve injury pain, including sensitization of peripheral nerve terminals, abnormalities in primary afferent fibers, abnormal electrical communication between adjacent axons, and alterations in the circuitry and neurochemistry of the dorsal horn. Much work has been focused on the pathophysiology of neuromas, which have been shown to produce abnormal single-unit electrical discharges, although neuroma formation is not necessary to produce abnormal electrical activity within a nerve.

Peripheral neurectomy is sometimes beneficial in carefully selected patients with peripheral nerve pain. The pain may be related to a traumatic injury (e.g., painful neuroma) or a compressive problem (e.g., meralgia paresthetica or tumor invasion of the brachial plexus), or may be idiopathic (e.g., occipital neuralgia). Another group of patients for whom peripheral neurectomy may be beneficial includes those with trigeminal neuralgia who because of significant comorbidity may not be candidates for more standard therapies such as microvascular decompression or any of the percutaneous retrogasserian procedures.

Neurectomy of the supra- and infraorbital nerves for first and second division pain, respectively, can be performed quite readily under local anesthesia. Even inferior alveolar neurectomy for third division pain is feasible, although it is necessary to expose this nerve through a small opening in the mandible. Although peripheral trigeminal neurectomy is infrequently indicated, it should be remembered as a viable alternative in selected patients (23).

Assuming that all appropriate conservative measures have been exhausted and psychological screening reveals no contraindications, surgical therapy may be considered. Obviously, peripheral neurectomy can be performed only on pure sensory nerves or on mixed nerves in which there has been complete loss of function (e.g., painful amputation neuroma) without the hope of any return. Neuromas that involve pure sensory nerves, including the dorsal cutaneous ulnar branch, superficial radial sensory branch, antebrachial cutaneous nerves, and the sural and saphenous nerves, are usually best managed with excision without repair (24). The sensory territories supplied by these nerves are of low functional importance, and numbness in their distribution is usually preferable to pain, dysesthesias, hyperalgesia, and allodynia. Also, recurrent pain and paresthesias are all too frequent if regeneration occurs. The potential for regeneration and recurrent neuroma formation can be minimized by burying the proximal nerve stump in either muscle or bone.

One of the major prerequisites of peripheral neurectomy is *complete* relief of pain following repetitive nerve blocks. It is important that these blocks be performed using local anesthetic *without epinephrine* because injured peripheral nerves and neuromas abnormally express adrenergic receptors that, when activated, produce pain and can therefore produce a "false negative" response. There are several other factors that seem to have prognostic value in predicting a successful result. Ideally, the pain should be related to a traumatic injury; the pain should be restricted to the territory of a *single* peripheral nerve; and a Tinel's sign should be present with percussion over the neuroma. Even adhering to these criteria, the overall success rate for excision of painful neuromas is probably not higher than 60% (25).

Dorsal Rhizotomy and Dorsal Root Ganglionectomy

Dorsal rhizotomy for the relief of pain is based on the law of Bell and Magendie, which states that the dorsal roots subserve afferent and ventral roots efferent function, respectively. Intuitively, then, destruction of the dorsal roots should eliminate the entry of segmental nociceptive information that normally would enter the spinal dorsal horn at these levels. Unfortunately, the results of dorsal rhizotomy have been variable at best and often unrewarding. Two factors likely contribute to the poor outcomes associated with dorsal rhizotomy. First, dorsal rhizotomy depends on denervation of the area from which the pain is believed generated. However, the ability to completely denervate a particular region with this procedure is limited by the high degree of sensory innervation between adjacent dermatomes. In other words, complete denervation of a single thoracic dermatome requires that afferent input be interrupted *at least* two dermatomal levels above and below the dermatome of interest. Second, a substantial body of literature now indicates that as much as 30% of nociceptive afferent fibers enter the spinal cord through the ventral root. Consequently, dorsal rhizotomy fails to completely interrupt the nociceptive afferent input. In animal studies, it has been shown that removal of the dorsal root ganglion (DRG) leads to degeneration of most of these small, unmyelinated high-threshold fibers that enter through the ventral root, and horseradish peroxidase labeling studies have confirmed the origin of these fibers to be the DRG. Based on these observations and the large number of failures with dorsal rhizotomy, dorsal root ganglionectomy is now generally the preferred technique that is expected to produce the best results. Aside from improved efficacy, dorsal root ganglionectomy offers several other advantages over intradural dorsal rhizotomy (26). Ganglionectomy obviates the need for a laminectomy and an intradural exposure and therefore reduces the anesthetic time to which a debilitated patient must be exposed. It also significantly reduces the risk of CSF leak. Additionally, each DRG is associated with its corresponding neural foramen, making localization somewhat easier.

Dorsal root ganglionectomy may be indicated for pain in the neck, trunk, or abdomen. It is *contraindicated* for extremity pain because the extent of denervation required to produce the desired effect would result in near complete loss of tactile and proprioceptive function, thereby rendering the extremity useless. Therefore, the procedure can be applied to the following roots: C-1–4, T-1–12, and L-1–2 (26). Although dorsal root ganglionectomy is infrequently performed, it is indicated and has been effective in a selected number of pain conditions. Prior to surgery selective nerve root blocks that result in 100% pain relief may *suggest* but not unequivocally prove that ganglionectomy may be effective. On the other hand, failure to derive any pain relief from local anesthetic blockade may indicate that there is a central component to the pain that will not be helped by ganglionectomy.

Dorsal root ganglionectomy may be effective in the following conditions: intractable occipital neuralgia that has not responded to electrical stimulation (either occipital nerve stimulation or high cervical [C-1–2] SCS) or peripheral neurectomy; postthoracotomy or postlaparotomy pain; chest wall pain related to pleural-based malignant tumor invasion; and perineal pain secondary to pelvic malignancy. In patients with perineal pain, bilateral interruption of the sacral roots is necessary. Because this may produce a sensory neurogenic bladder, this procedure should be limited to either patients who have already lost control of urinary and rectal sphincter function or patients who have undergone colostomy and urinary diversion (26). For patients with preserved sphincter function, midline myelotomy (see following) may be a reasonable alternative.

Dorsal Root Entry Zone (DREZ) Lesions

Dorsal root entry zone (DREZ) lesioning was developed by Nashold based on the theory that in some patients, deafferentation pain develops and is sustained due to lesions that isolate afferent input from the second order neurons whose cell bodies reside within the dorsal horn, brachial plexus avulsion being a classic example. Isolation or deafferentation of these second order neurons is believed to result in abnormal electrochemical signals, thus producing pain. Consequently, it was proposed that destruction of this abnormal neuronal pool in the dorsal horn might produce pain relief, which indeed was the case for certain conditions.

Several techniques can be used for performing DREZ lesions, the details of which have been extensively published (27). Suffice it to say that central to all of these techniques is surgical exposure of the DREZ and destruction of the superficial five layers of Rexed's laminae. The DREZ operation has been employed and the results evaluated for a number of deafferentation pain conditions. Probably the best single indication for the DREZ lesioning is pain that follows brachial plexus avulsion injuries. Pain relief following DREZ lesioning is usually immediate but in some patients may occasionally be delayed for a short time following surgery. Long-term pain relief in excess of 5 years has been reported in approximately 70% of patients who have undergone the DREZ procedure for brachial plexus avulsion (28). DREZ lesioning may also be performed following avulsion injuries of the lower lumbosacral nerve roots, although this injury is far less common than brachial plexus avulsion. Pain relief is similar to that achieved with brachial plexus avulsion. Another good indication for the DREZ procedure is in patients with spinal cord injury who suffer from "end zone" pain. Other conditions in which DREZ has been used, albeit less successfully, have included phantom limb pain, diffuse spinal cord injury pain, and postherpetic neuralgia.

The nucleus caudalis DREZ operation is really an offshoot of the spinal procedure. The nucleus caudalis represents the origin of the second order afferent neurons that carry nociceptive information from structures of the head and face. The nucleus caudalis receives afferent nociceptive input from not only the trigeminal but also the facial, glossopharyngeal, and vagus nerves. This structure corresponds to lamina II or the substantia gelatinosa in the spinal cord. The procedure is performed through a small suboccipital craniotomy and C-1 laminectomy. A series of radiofrequency lesions is made from the level of the C-2 dorsal root to the obex in order to destroy the second order neurons originating in the nucleus caudalis and ascending rostrally to connect with the thalamus and retic-

ular formation. The operation is in some respects similar to the trigeminal tractotomy described by Sjoquist, except that the latter is designed to interrupt the descending spinal trigeminal fibers. The major complication associated with caudalis DREZ lesioning is ipsilateral ataxia due to injury to the spinocerebellar tract, which covers the entire length of the nucleus caudalis. A caudalis DREZ operation can be considered in patients with intractable recurrent trigeminal neuralgia who have failed multiple previous operations, postherpetic neuralgia, and anesthesia dolorosa. It has also been recommended for selected patients with refractory atypical facial pain, although in the author's opinion destructive procedures in general should be avoided in this particular condition.

Anterolateral Cordotomy

A number of procedures destroy nociceptive afferent information that is carried by the spinothalamic pathway in the spinal cord. These include open or percutaneous cordotomy and commissural or midline myelotomy. Given the relative advantages of percutaneous cordotomy, the open procedure is rarely if ever performed in the United States. In considering a patient for cordotomy or myelotomy, for that matter, the severity of the pain should be sufficient to justify the procedure and the attendant risks. In this sense, it is important to attempt to segregate physical pain (biological) due to the underlying cancer and the emotional suffering related to depression and other socioeconomic and secondary gain issues (psychosocial). Also, as with any destructive procedure, all reasonable noninvasive methods for pain control should have been attempted and failed to provide adequate pain relief.

The most common indication for percutaneous cordotomy is in the patient with opiate-resistant or opiate-tolerant cancer pain. Indeed, most candidates for cordotomy have failed to respond adequately to high doses of long-acting oral opiates and/or intraspinal opiates. In some patients, for a variety of reasons, intraspinal opiates may not be a practical or viable option for pain management, in which case percutaneous cordotomy remains an excellent alternative. Percutaneous cordotomy has also been utilized in other pathologic conditions such as spinal cord injury pain, radiation plexitis, postamputation stump pain (phantom pain does not respond to cordotomy), pain from tabes dorsalis, and even intractable pain from failed back surgery (30).

Another important consideration in patient selection is the pathophysiology of the pain. In general, cordotomy is more effective for nociceptive than for neuropathic pain syndromes. Pain generated from continuous activation of peripheral nociceptors, such as that produced by involvement of a long bone by cancer and pain from direct compression or infiltration of nerve plexuses, represents the two conditions that respond best to percutaneous cordotomy. Central pain and evoked pain with hyperpathia or allodynia *may* respond to cordotomy but less predictably than the conditions listed previously. Location of the pain is another important consideration. A properly performed high cervical percutaneous cordotomy will reliably produce analgesia through the C-5 dermatome (30). Therefore, pain that is consistently rostral to C-5, as well as pain in the head, is not effectively treated by cordotomy. Also, unilateral localized pain is much more effectively treated than is bilateral or midline pain, which requires a bilateral procedure. Unilateral cordotomy is a *relatively* low risk procedure, whereas a bilateral C-1–2 cordotomy carries a significantly higher rate of complications.

Patients considered for cordotomy should have a limited life expectancy, generally less than 6 months, because the analgesic effects of cordotomy are not permanent. Indeed, the analgesia produced by cordotomy tends to fade with time, and pain concomitantly recurs. Additionally, patients may develop mirror pain, which may be difficult to manage. Finally, there should be no medical contraindications to the procedure. Assessment of baseline pulmonary function is important in this regard because percutaneous cordotomy at C-1–2 may damage the ipsilateral reticulospinal pathway that lies adjacent to the cervical fibers in the spinothalamic tract. This pathway originates in the respiratory center of the medulla and mediates unconscious or automatic respiration. If both lungs are normal, unilateral damage to this pathway is not clinically significant. However, if there is underlying pulmonary insufficiency, especially of the lung on the side contralateral to the cordotomy or loss of unconscious respiration from underlying disease such as a Pancoast tumor, then loss of the reticulospinal pathway may lead to life-threatening respiratory compromise and even fatal sleep apnea (Ondine's curse).

It is difficult if not impossible to correlate and compare the results of different authors due to variability in selection criteria and definitions of outcome in terms of pain relief. Tasker reviewed and collated data from 21 published series of unilateral percutaneous cordotomy, including his personal series (30). Complete pain relief was reported in between 63% and 90% of patients; significant pain relief occurred in 59% to 96% of patients. In a series of 136 patients at the last followup, 72% and 84% of patients had either complete or significant relief of their target pain, respectively. Thus, 28% of patients in Tasker's personal series had persistent pain in the target area.

Ischia et al. reviewed the outcome in terms of pain relief of 69 patients who underwent cordotomy for neoplastic vertebral bone pain (31). Seventy-one percent of the patients were felt to have benefited from the surgery, obtaining either complete pain relief or a significant reduction in pain amenable to control by analgesics. Ischia et al. later reported the results of unilateral percutaneous cordotomy in a group of 119 patients with cervicothoracic and thoracic pain secondary to lung cancer who were followed up until death (32). Approximately one-third of the patients

enjoyed complete pain relief up to the time of death. However, 81% of patients achieved complete pain control with cordotomy and the addition of analgesic medications. Nathan reported satisfactory pain relief (complete or partial relief) in 76% of patients who underwent unilateral cordotomy and in 80% of those who had bilateral procedures (33). Amano et al. compared the results of unilateral to bilateral cordotomy in a series of 221 patients (34). Unilateral high cervical cordotomy was performed in 161 patients, with bilateral procedures in 60. Complete or nearly complete pain relief was reported in 95% and 82% of patients who underwent bilateral or unilateral procedures, respectively. Overall, percutaneous cordotomy failed to produce even tolerable pain relief in only 5% of all patients. Finally, Kanpolat et al. performed CT-guided percutaneous cordotomy in 67 patients with pain due to malignancy (35). Complete pain control was achieved in 97% of patients. In just over two-thirds of the patients, the authors were able to perform a selective cordotomy, meaning that analgesia was produced in an area limited to the distribution of pain.

There are a number of explanations for persistent pain following unilateral cordotomy. In general, postcordotomy pain can be classified into three categories: (a) original pain that is not relieved, (b) original pain that disappears only to recur, and (c) new pain (30). Cordotomy has been shown to consistently reduce nociceptive pain. Therefore, failure to relieve pain may indicate that the pain for which the procedure was done had a significant neuropathic component that is not consistently relieved by cordotomy. Alternatively, the original pain may have been bilateral or had a significant midline component, in which case a bilateral procedure must be considered. Often, the original pain will be relieved only to recur anywhere from several days to several months following cordotomy. In many cases, this is due to regression of the level of analgesia, in which case the procedure may need to be repeated. Some patients will also develop new pain following cordotomy. For new pain located on the same side above the level of analgesia produced by cordotomy, one must be suspicious that there is progression of the underlying disease. Progression of disease may also lead to development of a new neuropathic pain syndrome. The third cause of new pain is the development of postcordotomy dysesthesias. The development of pain on the side of the body *opposite* the original pain may also signal progression of disease or the development of mirror pain.

Commissural Myelotomy

Midline or commissural myelotomy is a procedure in which the decussating fibers of the spinothalamic tract are interrupted as they cross in the anterior white commissure of the spinal cord. The lesion is usually created over several spinal cord segments at the lower thoracic level, although lesions at C-1 have also been reported. Midline myelotomy is most effective for pain in the lower portion of the body, especially midline or bilateral pain for which cordotomy or other ablative procedures may not be as applicable (21). The overall efficacy of midline myelotomy has been reported to be on the order of 70%.

Broager reported his results of midline myelotomy in 44 patients, followup information regarding outcome being available for 33 (36). Forty-one (93%) suffered from malignant pain. An excellent result (pain eliminated, no side effects) was initially achieved in 25 patients. Pain recurrence occurred between 1 and 6 months in nine of these patients. Cook and Kawakami summarized their results of midline myelotomy in 24 patients (37). Most patients achieved initial pain relief. However, in the group of patients with nonmalignant pain related to lumbar arachnoiditis, the procedure was ultimately a total failure as pain uniformly returned. These authors also concluded that pain from pelvic metastases does not respond particularly favorably to myelotomy. Several authors have recently introduced the concept of a more limited midline myelotomy, particularly for patients whose pain may be more visceral than somatic in nature (38,39). It is thought that a rather large component of visceral pain is carried in the medial aspect of the dorsal columns. Therefore, in a limited myelotomy, rather than dividing the crossing fibers of the spinothalamic tract in the anterior white commissure, these procedures are designed to interrupt visceral nociceptive pathways that lie in the deep aspects of the medial dorsal columns. Kim et al. performed limited high thoracic (T-1–2) myelotomy on eight patients with gastric cancer who suffered from intractable visceral pain (39). Five of these patients were either pain free or had residual pain that was adequately managed, either with a weak opiate (i.e., codeine) or even nonopiate analgesics. Limited myelotomy has been reported to have a number of advantages over the more classic midline myelotomy. There is a better chance of alleviating visceral pain, the risk of bothersome dysesthesias seem to be less, and the risk of neurological dysfunction such as loss of proprioception, transient motor weakness, etc., albeit relatively small, is less. Because neither classical nor limited myelotomy is performed with any frequency, more studies are needed to determine the role, particularly of limited myelotomy.

Brainstem and Diencephalic Procedures

Midbrain Tractotomy

Mesencephalic or midbrain tractotomy (a.k.a. mesencephalotomy) is not commonly used in the United States. The procedure depends on destruction of the spinothalamic and/or trigeminothalamic fibers that ascend in the brainstem. The primary indication for midbrain tractotomy is pain in the head, face, neck, or arm that is refractory to pharmacological management, including intraspinal narcotics. Intrathecal opiates are generally best for

pain that is located below the T-3 to T-4 dermatomal level, although in selected patients upper extremity pain and occasionally even pain in the head and neck can be effective managed with this therapy. Although C-1–2 percutaneous cordotomy may be effective for upper extremity pain, effective analgesia is difficult in patients whose pain is in the shoulder and neck region, and cordotomy is ineffective for pain in the head and face.

Midbrain tractotomy was first performed as an open procedure in the late 1930s, and around a decade later stereotactic midbrain tractotomy was introduced by Spiegel and Wycis. Presently, improvements in imaging techniques, stereotactic localization, and electrode design have made this procedure much easier and probably safer. Following imaging and target selection, stereotactic midbrain tractotomy is performed under local anesthesia. The midbrain target, namely the spinothalamic and/or quintothalamic pathway, cannot be directly visualized from the MRI but is calculated based on standard landmarks used for functional neurosurgery. The customary target is located 5 mm behind and 5 mm below the posterior commissure, and 5 to 10 mm lateral to the midline (40). The target is roughly in line with the inferior border of the superior colliculus. The target is confirmed with intraoperative physiological testing, i.e., macrostimulation before the lesion is made. A lesion or series of lesions is then made; the lesion parameters depend to some extent on the electrode configuration. The major complications associated with midbrain tractotomy include ocular disturbances and injury to the lemniscal tract, which can produce bothersome dysesthesias. Midbrain tractotomy appears to be of significant benefit in the treatment of patients with cancer pain, in whom 75% pain relief has been reported on both a short- and a long-term basis (40,41). Based on the available literature, it is difficult to assess the efficacy of midbrain tractotomy for pain related to nonmalignant conditions.

Thalamotomy

The multiple connections between the sensory pathways that terminate in the thalamus have made this structure a natural target for the treatment of pain. Discriminative somatotopically arranged sensory information carried by spinothalamic fibers along with the sensory input of the lemniscal pathways project to and terminate in the main sensory relay nucleus of the thalamus or Vc (VPL and VPM) nucleus. The nociceptive information that terminates in Vc is considered to be part of the neospinothalamic pathway. Nociceptive information is also diffusely projected from the reticular formation through a more medial paleospinothalamic system that has more diffuse projections to nonspecific nuclei (centrum medianum [CM], parafascicular [PF], intralaminar, centrolateral, nucleus submedius). A nociceptive relay, the ventral parvocellular nucleus (VCpc), has also been identified at the most caudal margin of Vc (42).

Although Vc thalamotomy has been performed in the past, it is not currently recommended because it is accompanied by a high complication rate such as loss of contralateral sensory modalities and pseudoparesis. Indeed, lesions in Vc are associated with a high incidence of dysesthesias and may even produce a full-blown thalamic pain syndrome. It has been reported that selective lesions of VCpc may offer pain relief by producing a dissociative sensory loss, i.e., interruption of nociceptive information with preservation of lemniscal input. However, the results of selective lesions of this nucleus have produced wide discrepancies in success.

There is no consensus as to which nuclei are included in medial thalamotomy (42,43). Medial thalamotomy targets the nuclei described earlier, and although specific nuclear targets have been described, it is somewhat difficult to conceive that, with the current technology, lesions can be produced that respect the physiological borders of these individual nuclei. In general, medial thalamotomy is generally centered around the CM-PF-intralaminar nuclei, an area in which a lesion produces no detectable neurological deficit (42,43). Intraoperative stimulation in this area likewise produces no characteristic response except at very high intensities where stimulation may produce paresthesias. The degree of pain relief afforded by medial thalamotomy appears to be superior to that achieved with Vc or VCpc thalamotomy (42). Nociceptive pain seems to be treated more effectively than neuropathic or deafferentation pain, and pain in the upper body appears to respond better than that in the lower body and legs.

The results of medial thalamotomy vary widely. However, comparison of results is difficult because of the heterogeneous nature of the clinical series, the nonuniformity of how the procedure is performed (exact target, unilateral vs. bilateral lesions), and variable methods by which results are conveyed (42,43). Young and Rinaldi suggested that 65% to 85% of patients with cancer pain whose life expectancy is less than one year should obtain lasting pain relief with medial thalamotomy (44). The authors suggested that for nonmalignant pain, medial thalamotomy carries a 20% immediate failure rate and that pain relief occurs in only 50% to 60% of patients for more than one year. More recently with the evolution of radiosurgical techniques, there has been a renewed interest in medial thalamotomy. Several groups have reported pain relief in 40% to 50% of patients with cancer-related pain, although there was a latency of 1 to 6 weeks before a positive benefit was achieved (42).

Cingulotomy for Intractable Pain

Surgical interruption of limbic pathways has traditionally been employed in patients with intractable psychiatric illness such as obsessive-compulsive disorder, major refractory depression, bipolar disorder, and even patients with Gilles de la Tourette syndrome. However, in patients with intractable pain due to widespread cancer, especially those who also have a component of anxiety that is intolerable, bilateral cingulotomy can provide effective relief of pain and suffering for patients with relatively limited life expectancy (45). Indeed, cingulotomy can sometimes provide impressive results in patients for whom more traditional therapies have been ineffective.

Cingulotomy is indicated and is most effective for nociceptive pain related to diffuse musculoskeletal metastases, in patients whose life expectancy is less than 6 to 9 months. These patients usually have exhausted all other forms of conventional therapy, including surgical resection, radiation, chemotherapy, systemic and/or spinal narcotics, as well as other interventions such as nerve blocks, etc. The cingulum is an integral part of the medial limbic loop or Papez circuit and is believed to play an integral role in pain perception that is still not clearly understood. The procedure is performed stereotactically under local anesthesia and is usually well tolerated, even by very debilitated patients. The center of the cingulate gyrus can be located stereotactically 24 mm posterior to tip of the frontal horn of the lateral ventricle, 1.5 mm lateral to the midline, and 15 mm above the roof of the lateral ventricles (45). The object of the procedure is to produce a lesion, usually by radiofrequency thermocoagulation, in as large an area of the cingulate gyri as possible without impinging on surrounding structures. Cingulotomy is contraindicated in patients with intracranial vascular anomalies that would be in the path of the electrode trajectory and in patients with an active calvarial or intracranial infection. The operation is also probably ill advised in patients with epilepsy, prior stroke, previous craniotomy, or untreated hydrocephalus (45).

The pain relief from cingulotomy is usually immediate and can be dramatic. However, the pain relief is not generally durable over a long period, and therefore patients with life expectancy much more than 9 months are probably not good candidates. Most patients are able to significantly reduce their intake of oral narcotics and increase activity levels. Several clinical studies of MRI-guided cingulotomy have reported that at least 50% of patients have moderate to complete pain relief 3 months following the procedure (46). Notwithstanding any ethical or technical concerns, for this reason alone, cingulotomy is probably not indicated for the treatment of benign pain conditions. Although repeat lesioning is possible and has been performed for psychiatric applications, there is little data to support the use of repeat cingulotomy for pain. Interestingly, some patients report only modest pain reduction in spite of dramatic reduction in narcotic usage and increased levels of activity. Moreover, these patients respond appropriately to new sources of pain, indicating that there may be a discrepancy in discriminative pain sensation and pain perception.

Pituitary Destruction for Cancer Pain

Destruction of the pituitary gland for the relief of pain is not new. In fact, pituitary ablation has been employed for several decades (47). There appears to be a clear association between the pituitary gland, pain, and analgesia. However, the exact mechanism(s) by which hypophysectomy produces analgesia remains unclear. The initial and most obvious logic was that there is some type of endocrine effect because the treatment is primarily effective for patients with breast or prostate carcinoma. It was believed that the degree of pain relief should correlate with the extent of hormonal depletion. However, there is a well-recognized discrepancy between pain relief, the hypopituitarism produced by the procedure, and tumor regression, and in fact some authors report a complete absence of correlation between hormonal depletion and analgesia (48). Consequently, other mechanisms have been proposed, including a stress analgesic effect, as well as a neurolytic effect because there are known to be connections between the pituitary gland and regions of the hypothalamus that are known to be involved in pain processing. Indeed, there have been reports of stimulation-produced analgesia when electrical stimulation has been applied to the pituitary gland.

Whatever the mechanism, pituitary ablation is indicated for patients with very advanced malignancy with intractable pain secondary to widespread metastases. Pituitary destruction can be performed in a variety of ways: (a) transcranial hypophysectomy, (b) transsphenoidal hypophysectomy, (c) radiation-induced hypophysectomy, (d) radiofrequency thermal coagulation, (e) cryogenic hypophysectomy, and (f) chemical hypophysectomy using alcohol. Open procedures such as transcranial or transsphenoidal hypophysectomy are major surgical procedures and would now be rarely indicated given the other options available. Radiation-induced pituitary destruction was previously performed by either transsphenoidal implantation of an yttrium screw or external radiation. Although there is little, if any, data, it might be feasible to now consider stereotactic radiosurgery for this purpose. High doses of radiation can be focused in the pituitary fossa without injuring surrounding structures. The one potential problem with this technique is that pain relief may be delayed, as it commonly is when radiosurgery is used for the treatment of trigeminal neuralgia. This is potentially significant in this population of patients who are suffering, have a limited life expectancy, and thus for whom immediate pain relief is highly desirable.

Perhaps the most useful technique for pituitary ablation is by transsphenoidal injection of absolute alcohol into the pituitary fossa. The procedure can be performed under light general anesthesia using an intravenous neuroleptic and/or inhalation agent. The procedure is performed using C-arm fluoroscopy and involves placing a special cannula with sharp obturator through the anterior wall of the sella and into the pituitary gland. After confirming that the tip is within the pituitary gland by injection of a small amount contrast agent (0.1–0.2 mL), absolute alcohol is injected at a rate of 0.1 mL per minute. During the injection period one is able to track the ascent of the contrast up the pituitary stalk into the hypothalamus and third ventricle. Customarily a total of 1–2 mL of alcohol is injected. During injection, pupillary size and reaction are carefully observed because there is a risk of damage to the optic pathways. In the event that pupillary changes are observed, Miles has advocated immediate subarachnoid injection of corticosteroids via a C-1–2 puncture. Because the degree of hypopituitarism is unpredictable, all patients should routinely receive pituitary replacement therapy.

The pain relief achieved with pituitary destruction is variable, most authors reporting pain relief on the order of 70% to 90%, with nearly two-thirds of patients having complete pain relief (47). Patients with hormonally independent tumors achieve pain relief at the lower end of the spectrum, whereas those with breast or prostate cancer enjoy pain relief nearer to 90%. The duration of pain relief is somewhat variable but tends to fade rather quickly. Around 65% of patients will experience pain relief for 3 months or less, although long-term relief in excess of a year has certainly been reported. Notwithstanding the more successful cases, it would seem that pituitary destruction is therefore primarily indicated for patients with a life expectancy of perhaps 3–6 months. Aside from damage to the visual system, other complications include diabetes insipidus (as high as 50% with large volumes of alcohol), ocular palsies, CSF leakage, and meningitis.

SUMMARY

From the preceding discussion it should be clear that we now have at our disposal more options for the surgical treatment of pain than ever. Indeed, in qualified hands any of these may be highly effective depending on the clinical situation. However, along with the opportunities provided comes a responsibility to utilize these techniques in a careful, thoughtful, and rational manner. This begins with a thorough assessment of the biological, psychological, and social aspects of each patient's pain and knowledge of the indications for, advantages, and limitations of the various surgical approaches. It is the firm belief of the author that when it comes to the surgical treatment of pain, one should take very seriously the philosophy of Hippocrates to "*do no harm.*" Unfortunately, not every patient with pain can be helped with surgery, in which case alternative or complementary nonoperative approaches must be recommended. Indeed, the philosophy that one "just has to do something" for the desperate patient with intractable pain is, at its best, misguided and, at its worst, potentially harmful. However, on a more optimistic note, it should be clear that surgical treatment of pain can be highly effective and when used in a thoughtful way can dramatically change the lives of many patients for the better.

REFERENCES

1. Gildenberg PL, Tasker RR. *Textbook of stereotactic and functional neurosurgery*, New York: McGraw-Hill, 1998.
2. Burchiel K. *Pain surgery*, Thieme (in press).
3. Barolat G. Current status of epidural spinal cord stimulation. *Neurosurg Quarterly* 1995;5:98–124.
4. Barolat G, Sharan A. Future trends in spinal cord stimulation. *Neurol Res* 2000;22:279–284.
5. Kumar K, Toth C, Nath R, et al. Epidural spinal cord stimulation for treatment of chronic pain—some predictors of success. A 15-year experience. *Surg Neurol* 1998;50:110–121.
6. Kemler M, Barendse G, Kleef M, et al. Spinal cord stimulation in patients with chronic reflex sympathetic dystrophy. *N Engl J Med* 2000;343:618–624.
7. Eliasson T, Augustinsson L, Mannheimer C. Spinal cord stimulation in severe angina pectoris—presentation of current studies, indications, and clinical experience. *Pain* 1996;65:169–179.
8. Augstinsson L, Linderoth B, Mannheimer C, et al. Spinal cord stimulation in cardiovascular disease. *Neurosurg Clinics North Amer* 1995; 6:157–165.
9. Hassenbusch S, Stanton-Hicks M, Schoppa D, et al. Long-term results of peripheral nerve stimulation for reflex sympathetic dystrophy. *J Neurosurg* 1996;84:415–423.
10. Reynolds D. Surgery in the rat during electrical analgesia induced by focal brain stimulation. *Science* 1969;164:444–445.
11. Bendok B, Levy R. Brain stimulation for persistent pain management. In: Gildenberg PL, Tasker RR, eds. *Textbook of stereotactic and functional neurosurgery*. New York: McGraw-Hill, 1998:1539–1546.
12. Richardson D. Deep brain stimulation for the relief of chronic pain. *Neurosurg Clinics North Amer* 1995;6:135–144.
13. Tasker R, Kiss Z. The role of the thalamus in functional neurosurgery. *Neurosurg Clinics North Amer* 1995;6:73–104.
14. Tsubokawa T, Katayama Y, Yamamoto T, et al. Chronic motor cortex stimulation for the treatment of central pain. *Acta Neurochir Suppl (Wien)* 1991;52:137–139.
15. Tsubokawa T, Katayama Y, Yamamoto T, et al. Chronic motor cortex stimulation in patients with thalamic pain. *J Neurosurgery* 1993;78:393–401.
16. Yamamoto T, Katayama Y, Hirayama T, et al. Pharmacological classification of central post-stroke pain: comparison with the results of chronic motor cortex stimulation. *Pain* 1997;72:5–12.
17. Nguyen JP, Lefaucheur JP, Decq P, et al. Chronic motor cortex stimulation in the treatment of central and neuropathic pain. Correlations between clinical, electrophysiological, and anatomical data. *Pain* 1999;82:245–251.
18. Bennett G, Serafini M, Burchiel K, et al. Evidenced-based review of the literature on intrathecal delivery of pain medication. *J Pain Symptom Manage* 2000;20(Suppl):S12–S36.
19. Bennett G, Buchser E, Burchiel K, et al. Clinical guidelines for intraspinal infusion therapy: report of an expert panel. *J Pain Symptom Manage* 2000;20(Suppl):S37–S43.
20. Bennett G, Deer T, Du Pen S, et al. Future directions in the management of pain by intraspinal drug delivery. *J Pain Symptom Manage* 2000;20(Suppl):S44–S50.
21. Lazorthes Y, Sallerin B, Verdie J. Intracerebroventricular administration of morphine for control of irreducible cancer pain. In: Gildenberg PL, Tasker RR, eds. *Textbook of Stereotactic and Functional Neurosurgery*. New York: McGraw-Hill, 1998;1477–1482.
22. Lazorthes Y, Sagen J, Sallerin B, et.al. Human chromaffin cell graft into the CSF for cancer pain management: a prospective phase II clinical study. *Pain* 2000;87:19–32.
23. Osenbach R. Trigeminal neurectomy. In: Burchiel K, ed. *Pain Surgery*, Thieme, (in press).
24. Kline D, Hudson A. *Nerve injuries*. Philadelphia: W. B. Saunders, 1995.
25. Burchiel K, Johans K, Ochoa J. Painful nerve injuries: bridging the gap between basic neuroscience and neurosurgical treatment. *Acta Neurochirurgica* 1993;58(Suppl):131–135.
26. Arguelles J, Burchiel K. Ablative neurosurgical procedures for the treatment of pain: peripheral. In: Tindall G, Cooper P, Barrow D, eds. *The Practice of Neurosurgery*. Baltimore: Williams and Wilkins, 1996:3153–3174.
27. Nashold BS, Pearlstein R, eds. *The DREZ operation*, The American Association of Neurological Surgeons Publications Committee, 1996.
28. Ostdahl R. DREZ surgery for brachial plexus avulsion pain. In: Nashold BS, Pearlstein R, eds. *The DREZ operation*, The American Association of Neurological Surgeons Publications Committee, 1996: 105–124.
29. Nashold B, El-Naggar A, Gorecki J. The microsurgical trigeminal caudalis nucleus DREZ procedure. In: Nashold BS, Pearlstein R, eds. *The DREZ Operation*, The American Association of Neurological Surgeons Publications Committee, 1996:159–188.
30. Tasker RR: Percutaneous cordotomy for persistent pain. In: Gildenberg PL, Tasker RR, eds. *Textbook of stereotactic and functional neurosurgery*, New York: McGraw-Hill, 1998:1491–1505.
31. Ischia S, Luzzani A, Ischia A, et al. Role of unilateral percutaneous cervical cordotomy in the treatment of neoplastic vertebral pain. *Pain* 1984;19:123–131.
32. Ischia S, Ischia A, Luzzani A, et al. Results up to death in the treatment of persistent cervico-thoracic (Pancoast) and thoracic malignant pain by unilateral percutaneous cervical cordotomy. *Pain* 1985; 21:339–355.
33. Nathan PW. Results of antero-lateral cordotomy for pain in cancer. *J Neurol Neurosurg Psychiatry* 1963;26:353–362.
34. Amano K, Kawamura H, Tanikawa T., et al. Bilateral versus unilateral high cervical percutaneous cordotomy as a surgical method of pain relief. *Acta Neurochir (Wien)* 1991;52(Suppl):143–145.
35. Kanpolat Y, Akyar S, Caglar S, et al. CT-guided percutaneous selective cordotomy. *Acta Neurochirurgica* 1993;123:92–96.
36. Broager B. Commissural myelotomy. *Surg Neurol* 1974;2:71–74.
37. Cook A, Kawakami Y. Commissural myelotomy. *J Neurosurg* 1977; 47:1–6.
38. Nauta H, Hewitt E, Westlund K, et al. Surgical interruption of a midline dorsal column visceral pain pathway. *J Neurosurg* 1997;86: 538–542.
39. Kim Y, Kwon S. High thoracic midline dorsal column myelotomy for severe visceral pain due to advanced stomach cancer. *Neurosurgery* 2000;46:85–92.
40. Gorecki J. Stereotactic midbrain tractotomy. In: Gildenberg PL, Tasker RR, eds. *Textbook of stereotactic and functional neurosurgery*. New York: McGraw-Hill, 1998:1651–1660.
41. Frank F, Tognetti F, Gaist G, et al. Stereotaxic rostral mesencephalotomy in treatment of malignant faciothoracobrachial pain syndromes. *J Neurosurg* 1982;56:807–811.
42. Gorecki J. Destructive central lesions for persistent pain. Part I, An Overview.In: Gildenberg PL, Tasker RR, eds. *Textbook of stereotactic and functional neurosurgery*. New York: McGraw-Hill, 1998:1417–1424.
43. Gorecki J. Thalamotomy for cancer pain. Part I. An overview. In: Gildenberg PL, Tasker RR, eds. *Textbook of stereotactic and functional neurosurgey*. New York: McGraw-Hill, 1998:1431–1441.
44. Young R, Rinaldi PC. Stereotactic ablative procedures for pain relief. In: Wilkins R, Rengechary S, eds. *Neurosurgery*, 2nd ed. New York: McGraw-Hill, 1996:4061–4065.
45. Hassenbusch SJ. Surgical management of cancer pain. *Neurosrg Clin North Am* 1995: **6**;127–134.
46. Hassenbusch S, Pillay P, Barnett G. Radiofrequency cingulotomy for intractable cancer pain using stereotaxis guided by magnetic resonance imaging. *Neurosurgery* 1990;27:220–223.
47. Miles J. The pituitary gland and pain relief. In: Gildenberg PL, Tasker RR, eds. *Textbook of stereotactic and functional neurosurgery*. New York: McGraw-Hill, 1998:1457–1461.
48. Williams N, Miles J, Lipton S, et. al. Pain relief and pituitary function following injection of alcohol in to the pituitary fossa. *Ann Coll Surg* 1980;62:203–207.

CHAPTER **14**

Cognitive Behavioral Therapies and Beyond

Albert L. Ray and Albert Zbik

> If you are distressed by anything external,
> the pain is not due to the thing itself,
> but to your estimate of it.
> This you have the power to revoke at any time.
> *Marcus Aurelius,* circa AD 180

Patients suffering chronic pain are often overwhelmed psychologically and emotionally. The toll taken upon these individuals includes changes in lifestyle, mood, interpersonal and family interactions, and generally a sense of being out of control of one's own life and destiny.

Psychological treatments for chronic pain, both in the past and present, have centered on offering patients validation for their pain problem and attempting to reestablish a sense of control over one's own life. Dynamically oriented psychotherapy had shown equivocal results in its applications to chronic pain management. Specifically, one study found that although the level of function of the person was increased, the pain awareness was also increased. Over the past 20 years, cognitive behavioral therapies have come to the forefront as one of the most effective psychological treatments for chronic pain management.

The 1990s was officially the Decade of the Brain, and fortunately for pain management, much information has been learned in terms of acute versus chronic pain, memory, learning, and perception. This research has generated newer understanding and hypotheses of nociception and the psychological ramifications of chronic pain, and this newer understanding is now being applied to psychological methods in pain management.

This chapter will discuss some of the newer research in terms of central sensitization, how memory is made and stored, concepts of learning, and perception in general. We will then attempt to place these newer concepts in perspective for their application to pain management, reviewing both cognitive behavioral treatments and more recently developed approaches, including eye movement desensitization and reprocessing (EMDR).

PAIN

Price has introduced a new definition of pain. He proposes that pain is "a somatic perception containing: 1) a bodily sensation with qualities like those reported during tissue-damaging stimulation, 2) an experienced threat associated with this sensation, and 3) a feeling of unpleasantness or other negative emotion based on this experienced threat" (1). This suggested definition of pain distinguishes somatosensory sensations from unpleasantness and requires nociceptive sensation and unpleasantness in order to produce pain. It links integrally the affective dimension of pain to the cognitive-evaluative dimension of pain. By linking the three components in his new definition of pain, Price aligns this definition with the experience of pain or the resultant holistic perception. According to Price, this new definition "helps justify using the term 'pain' for persons whose pain is *not* objectively or subjectively associated with tissue injury. Nevertheless, the definition retains the idea that painful sensations have at least a putative relationship to tissue injury because the sensations are *like* those that result from tissue injury" (1).

Pain has been categorized, with difficulty, over the years. Earlier efforts attempted to differentiate pain as acute or chronic and also as Category I or Category II types of pain. Category I (acute pain) pain represents a symptom of underlying illness or injury. Category I pain is considered a warning, and its purpose is to alert the person that something is wrong and needs to be investigated and treated at the site of primary pathology. Category II pain, on the other hand, has no value to the person in terms of its message and reflects pain resulting from a neurobiological change within the nervous system. These changes in

TABLE 14-1. *The experience of pain*

	Immediate pain (Eudynia, acute pain, Category I)	Long-term pain (Maldynia, Category II)
Primary Quality	"Ouch"; primary stage of pain affect	Suffering ("yuck"); secondary stage of pain affect
Meaning of Pain	Physically based; sudden intrusion; possible harm	Interference; difficulty in enduring; ultimate consequences
Felt Sense	Fear; shortly followed by anxiety, anger	Despair; frustration; hopelessness; depression
Dimensions of the Experience	Desire to avoid harm; expectation of avoiding harm; threat to self	Desire to avoid or terminate the interference; burden of enduring pain; expectations whether desires can be fulfilled
Psychophysical Attributes	Highly reliable pain thresholds; minimal adaptation of pain intensity in the presence of maintained nociceptive stimulation; slow temporal summation; spatial summation; and radiation of perceived areas of pain sensation at suprathreshold levels of nociceptive stimulation	Exaggerations or abnormal triggering of same mechanisms

the central nervous system result in a central sensitization that tends to affect the sensory system in general, which includes the nociceptive and limbic systems as well as special senses perception. The American Academy of Pain Medicine has officially adopted the term *eudynia* (good pain; i.e., normal pain, warning pain) for Category I. Category II represents *maldynia* (bad, destructive pain). Some ongoing painful disorders can actually represent a combination of eudynia and maldynia concurrently.

Most definitions of pain, including Price's new definition, include both a sensory nociceptive component and an emotional component. However, it is important to understand that the emotional component adds the affective dimension to pain and unpleasantness and is not a separate issue from the painful experience. The emotional experience is based on desire and expectation, which incorporate both cognitive appraisal (2) and physiological activation or arousal. The extent of physiological arousal generally increases with the significance of the desire factor and early stimulation (3,4), and the patterns of that arousal are often codetermined by the nature of attitudes, expectations, and intentions (1). How expectation and desire factor into the experience of pain differs for immediate pain (Category I) and long-term pain (Category II). These are summarized in Table 14-1, based upon the work of Price (1).

The affective dimensions of pain also differ between immediate pain and long-term pain. Table 14-2, again based on Price's work (1), summarizes these differences.

PAIN AND GENDER

Although there has been a great deal of interest regarding sex differences and pain perception, the issue remains largely unanswered. Fillingim (5) points out the discrepant research findings, with some indicating that sex differ-

TABLE 14-2. *Affective dimensions of pain*

	Immediate affective dimension	Secondary affective dimension
Unpleasantness	Moment to moment	More reflective cognitions
Orientation	Present or short-term future	Past and long-term future
Affect	Closely linked with the intensity of painful sensation and associated arousal	A component of the pain itself
Meaning of the pain	Attentional shift to bodily area of concern and motor orientation to this area; autonomic responses	Interruption of function; burden; permanency of damage or harm
Neuroticism (high emotionality and arousability)	Contributes mild influence	Can contribute significant influence
Age	No effect	Decreased negative emotional feelings with increasing age

ences in pain are robust, and others indicating only mild to moderate differences. Mogil (6) reports that genetic pain-related differences may relate to species as well as biological sex and that they may be interrelated. For example, in some species of rats males demonstrated a greater pain threshold than females, whereas other species of rats showed the reverse condition. Robinson et al. (7) indicate that as the psychosocial factors affecting pain reporting and pain response are stripped away, there seems to be less and less sex difference (biological) in humans than gender difference. The increased reporting of pain by women is felt to be strongly psychosocial in humans.

Much of the discrepancy regarding pain, sex, and gender remains because of the complexity of research strategies and identified criteria in this area. Most of the work has focused on the sensory discriminative portion of acute pain, with less research being done on the affective dimension of chronic pain. Thus, there are no clear-cut answers for this issue.

CENTRAL SENSORY DYSFUNCTION

Central sensitization seems to occur at different levels within the central nervous system. Studies have shown sensitization of the spinal cord, brainstem, and possibly at the cortical level as well (1,8–14). This sensitization of the central nervous system seems to result either from repetitive timed stimulations or an overwhelming single stimulation resulting in long-term potentiation. It has been known for many years from animal studies that sensitization can result in seizures through kindling (11,15). There are three stages to kindling. In the early stage, repetitive subthreshold stimulation results in an occasional seizure in the animal. In the complete stage, each subthreshold stimulation will result in a seizure, and in the automatic phase, seizure occurs without further stimulation. In addition to seizure itself, behavioral and nociceptive sensitization has been demonstrated in animals and is strongly postulated in humans (16). Repetitive timed stimulation has been shown to promote kindling, whereas continuous stimulation has been shown to inhibit it. In addition, animal studies have shown that recruitment and convergence are important in the development of sensitization. Through recruitment and convergence, nonrelated (nonnociceptive) neurons are drawn into action, so that seemingly innocuous stimulation can now result in the sensitized behavior. For example, in rats that have reached the complete stage of sensitization, a seizure can be produced from the resultant stimulation of the hand touching the rat hair by simply picking the animal up (17,18).

Central sensitization has been implicated in multiple painful syndromes, including complex regional pain syndrome (CRPS) (19), phantom pain (19), myofascial syndrome and fibromyalgia (20), chronic headache (11) and rebound headache (21), chronic visceral painful syndromes (especially irritable bowel syndrome) (22), and

chronic dysphoria (depression) (23). Central sensitization is also considered to be heavily involved with posttraumatic stress disorder (PTSD) (24–28). This takes on special importance because it is known that the incidence of psychological traumatization, with or without a full-blown posttraumatic stress disorder clinically evident, is much higher in chronic pain patients than it is in the general population (29–31).

Because of the strong correlation between posttraumatic stress disorder, psychological trauma, and chronic pain, let us take a more in-depth look at posttraumatic stress disorder. Kardiner has described the five cardinal features of human response to trauma as (32,33):

1. The persistence to the startle response and irritability
2. A proclivity to explosive outbursts of aggression
3. A fixation on the traumatic event
4. A constriction of the general level of personality function
5. An atypical dream life

The clinical symptoms that we see as described by Sonenberg (33) include intrusiveness (having thoughts, having dreams, and feeling the event again), diminished interests, detachment, constriction of affective responses, hyperalertness, cognitive dysfunction (including memory/concentration problems), avoidance of activities that arouse recollections, intensification of symptoms by exposure to similar events, autonomic lability, headaches, and vertigo.

Van der Kolk (34) has described the difficulty with modulating the intensity of affect as secondary to the hyperarousal seen in these patients. He quotes a patient as saying, "You can never feel just a little bit: it is all or nothing." According to van der Kolk (35), it is common for the dichotomy of mature intellectual growth and emotional immaturity to coexist in adults who were traumatized as children. As one patient expressed it, "The head keeps growing, but the body keeps count." Van der Kolk (25,34, 36) has examined the concept of intrinsic vulnerability to PTSD and has found that individuals with a high internal locus of control (those who have previously successfully overcome adversities) appear to be more stress resistant. Spiegel (37) has pointed out that part of the locus of control is inborn, and part is also affected by early trauma. Inescapable shock studies in animals show that those animals that previously had exposure to escapable shock are more stress resistant (26,34). Rauch (38) points out that MRI studies of PTSD patients show an increase in the cavum septum pellucidum (a small midline cerebrospinal fluid-filled variant of normal anatomy) and that this increase may represent the notion of preexisting vulnerability. Hence, there may be both constitutional and learned determinants to vulnerability.

Rauch also postulates that PTSD patients exhibit hypersensitivity within the amygdala and a failure of the medial frontal cortex to exert governance over the amygdala. He asserts that hippocampal damage results in amnesia, learning problems, and memory decrease. Hence, there is clear evidence for involvement of the limbic system in PTSD.

Shalev (39) demonstrated with auditory stimulation that there is a neuronal sensitization involved with PTSD. In this study, loud noise was shown to produce a more severe and exaggerated effect in persons with PTSD compared to normal controls, supporting the findings for lowered thresholds to actually cause a reaction, in addition to augmentation of the reaction itself. (A separate but similar study looking at hypervigilance in fibromyalgia also supports the same kind of response. In fact, in that study, it was suggested that fibromyalgia patients have a perceptual style of amplification and prefer lower levels of external stimulation than do controls [40].)

MEMORY

We will look further at how sensitization is involved in painful syndromes and their concomitant emotional states later. Now we will explore newer concepts in memory.

Memory is made for all events in our lives. It is in our "hard drive." This memory is permanent on a cellular level but does not necessarily remain in our conscious awareness. For example, van der Kolk found that the victims of early (before age 6 to 7 years) sexual abuse are generally amnestic to it, unless the memory has been revived by a more recent event (28,34,35,41,42).

Recent research on memory has concluded that memory is made and stored according to events and patterns. The magnitude of the activation in the left prefrontal, temporal, and parahippocampal cortices predicted whether events would be remembered or forgotten (43,44). The hippocampus and amygdala (45) are heavily involved with emotional memory and the evaluation of emotional stimuli through a complex chemically modulated system, including NMDA (N-methyl-D-aspartate) receptors and dopamine (12,46–48). Long-term potentiation in the hippocampus may underlie learning and memory (12).

Memory can be declarative or procedural. Working memory is short-term and operates over a period of seconds but is integrally related in behavior, language, and thinking. This memory can be declarative or procedural. The prefrontal cortex seems to be quite significant for object identity, spatial locations, memory and coding, and analysis of the meaning of items (2,49,50). Different parts of the prefrontal cortex are involved in different types of memory. The middorsolateral and midventrolateral frontal cortical areas make distinct functional contributions to spatial working memory. Imaging studies show increased prefrontal cortex activity as the complexity of semantic processing rises (43,44,46,50).

Contrary to earlier precepts, it is now understood that memory is made in mnemonics and not pictures. This mnemonic-type memory involves both the memory traces of the actual event as well as the memory traces of the affective and emotional components of that event. Memory is stored according to like associations, whether they be actual events or their affective components (43,44, 46,50). It is now postulated that memory to sensory discriminative nociceptions (lateral pain pathways) is made separately, but in parallel, with memories for the affective dimensions (medial pain pathways) of those nociceptive events (10,51).

Based on this understanding of dual and parallel memories, we can then begin to understand how memory made to two seemingly disparate actual events, which may have a similar emotional or psychological meaning to the patient, will then create memory storage of like mnemonics (associations) for the affective or emotional component but separate remembrances for the actual events. Recall of events then consists of drawing upon the storage compartment for the actual events as well as the storage compartment for the affective component. But if the mnemonic storage compartment of the affective component is heavily loaded because of other affectively similar (linked) events in that person's life, the recall of the actual event may then be burdened with an affective response disproportionate to what one might expect (52).

PAIN AND MEMORY

This affective augmentation in relationship to pain perception is best explained by the hypothesis of Rome and Rome (10). They have titled this hypothesis "Limbically Augmented Pain Syndrome (LAPS)." This syndrome is characterized by chronic pain often disproportionate to physical findings, with associated disturbances of mood, sleep, energy, concentration/memory, libido, behavior, and stress tolerance.

According to the LAPS hypothesis, a central sensitization takes place through kindling of both nociceptive and nonnociceptive systems. Rome and Rome postulate that through the lateral and medial pain systems, a sensitization occurs in vulnerable individuals, which results in an augmented pain response to future stimuli, which may not even be nociceptive in nature.

The lateral pain system has projections from the spinothalamic tract to the ventral posterolateral and posteromedial thalamic nuclei. The cortical projections go from there to the primary and secondary ipsilateral somatosensory cortices and result in contralateral, highly discriminative nociception. This lateral system provides the "ouch" portion of our pain consciousness, or the sensory discriminative component.

On the other hand, the medial pain system has projections from the spinal reticular and spinothalamic tracts to brainstem nuclei (including periaqueductal gray, locus coeruleus, and raphe nuclei) and medial thalamic nuclei (including parafascicular and central lateral nuclei). These thalamic and extrathalamic pathways go to the limbic and paralimbic regions and continue rostrally to the prefrontal and motor cortices. There are direct and indirect nociceptor projections to the hypothalamus, central nucleus of the amygdala, nucleus accumbens, infralimbic cortex, ventral pallidum, and globus pallidus. The medial pain system can represent one or both sides of the body, can be both ipsilateral and contralateral, is nondiscriminative, and provides the affective coloration or the "yuck" component to our pain consciousness.

Especially important to the Romes' LAPS hypothesis are the concepts of behavior sensitization, long-term potentiation, and time-dependent sensitization. These are all considered related mechanisms of neuroplasticity and share a premise that a neurobiologic mechanism or sets of mechanisms that occur preferentially within the limbic system serve as an amplifier for biologic reactivity to repetitive/low intensity stimuli.

Rome and Rome draw upon the work of Price (1), Harkins (53), as well as Gracely (54) to develop a tiered system of pain perception, involving a primary pain affect (which is related to the current nociceptive signal) and a secondary affect (which can include both pain-related and nonpain-related affects). This tiered system allows for secondary affects (pain related and nonpain related) to serve as a gain mechanism to amplify the affective (and possibly the nociceptive) component of our conscious perception of pain, which is consistent with the understanding of memory storage for like associations being linked together (52). This emotional memory is processed through the amygdala (45).

There is support for the LAPS concept in both animal and human research. In their work with animals, Weiss and Post (55) have identified six common features in response to repeated stimuli:

1. There are shorter latency and increased magnitude of response (sensitization).
2. Effects are dose related and persist for weeks or months.
3. Intermittent stimulation facilitates sensitization.
4. Genetic factors may influence sensitization.
5. Sensitization is highly context-dependent and conditionable.
6. Cross-sensitization occurs between various stimuli.

Human studies have shown that pain-evoked potentials in control subjects show a graded increase in wave amplitude depending on whether the stimulus was above or below pain threshold. However, in chronic pain patients (sensitized individuals) the wave amplitude was high in both stimulus conditions. Studies with deep brain stimulation of the somatosensory thalamus reproduced pain with a strong affective loading in patients who previously had such affectively charged pain, but in those subjects without such a history the induced pain was free of such coloration.

It is this repetitive affective stimulation, according to the LAPS hypothesis, that can lead to sensitization, especially of the medial (limbically connected) pain system. The gain control amplification of the primary pain signal ("ouch") may come about by the extra load then placed on the actual event (the primary signal) by the overloaded affective component ("yuck") as the message passes through the cortex and is finalized in conscious perception.

Thus, we can begin to understand how earlier traumatization(s) may be drawn into the person's conscious perception of current pain. This concept correlates with what we see clinically in the syndromes associated with central sensory dysfunction. There can be augmentation of the affective component of a pain signal in a person with previous like-mnemonic memory traces, even if there is no full-blown posttraumatic stress syndrome present in that person.

LEARNING

Learning theory also has benefited from the Decade of the Brain research. New understandings of how we learn show that learning seems to be integrated in the brain through multiple neurochemical channels and is more closely linked with brain circuits and interconnections rather than with any one particular area of the brain or any one neurochemical transmitter. NMDA is highly involved in learning, restorative function for neuronal cell life and growth, as well as cell death, and is also thought to be intricately woven with sensitization-related neurobiological changes (12,13,56–58). As with other areas of cortical functioning, the amount of NMDA involvement is more predictive of better memory (55). The same intensity of synaptic strength underlies long-term potentiation development (12). As cited earlier, dopamine and serotonergic systems are also involved with long-term memory and learning (46,59).

Thus, we are beginning to understand the involvement of the prefrontal cortex in short- and long-term memory development with subsequent involvement of the amygdala and limbic system. In fact, brain-imaging studies have shown that the prefrontal cortex shows sustained activity during the delay period of visual working memory tasks, even in the absence of sensory input (60). This working memory is considered one of the components of conscious perception or awareness of pain.

Perhaps one of the best applications of these new learning concepts in terms of pain management is the placebo response. Studies of the placebo response (1) have shown clearly that the amount and intensity of placebo response are most closely correlated with expectancy than any other phenomenon. Conceptually, we may then begin to understand why many of our patients can be maintained on long-term opioid use without significant increases in dosage, yet with good maintenance of pain relief.

PERCEPTION

Conscious perception is still somewhat of an enigma, in spite of all the recent learning that has taken place about brain function. There does not seem to be any one "perception center" within the brain, but rather conscious perception seems to be a manifest intricate networking of multiple systems coming together through related patterned tracts within the brain to produce our awareness. The eventual consciousness that arises from this construction of perceptions is defined as qualia and represents psychologically projected constructs into the external world. Some of these perceptions may be up to 90% memory (61). Thus, pain perception, per se, is influenced by the lateral pain system with its highly discriminative nociceptive identification, mixed with the medial pain system, including its affective colorations and stored memories, previous memory trace expectancies, and nonnociceptively related (but linked in memory by the brain) inputs.

Although the brain is continually "multitasking," conscious perception is limited to "single tasking" (37). That is, we can have only one image on our screen at a time. This can serve to our advantage in terms of pain management because as we develop ways to keep conscious perception on any issue other than pain, we then defeat the awareness of pain for that amount of time. Indeed, this limitation has been usefully adapted in many techniques, including cognitive behavioral techniques, self-hypnotic techniques, meditative techniques, etc. We are all familiar with the cliche that if your foot hurts, bang your thumb with a hammer, and your foot will no longer hurt. This concept is based upon that single-tasking screen we have for conscious perception. However, that screen can also replace nociception with anything pleasant.

APPLICATIONS OF BRAIN RESEARCH TO PAIN MANAGEMENT

The LAPS hypothesis, as mentioned, can help us understand an augmented affective component, or increased emotional intensity, to painful syndromes. This concept can apply to any painful syndrome where sensitization has occurred. In addition to emotional augmentation, we can see the effects of central sensitization resulting in a central sensory dysfunction for the nonemotional (sensory discriminative) component of painful syndromes. Let's review some common painful conditions representing this central sensory dysfunction, including fibromyalgia, chronic fatigue syndrome (CFIDS), visceral pain, headache, complex regional pain syndrome (CRPS), phantom pain, and dysphoria.

Fibromyalgia

In studying fibromyalgia, Vecchiet (20) found hyperalgesia of the skin, subcutis, and muscles in both tender points and nontender points, and Graven-Nielsen (62) found lower pain thresholds in patients with fibromyalgia. Both of these findings seem to be indicative of a spinal level of sensitization. Graven-Nielsen also found larger areas of

referred pain, which are attributed to a supraspinal central sensitization.

Bradley et al. (63) found decreased regional cerebral blood flow (rCBF) to the caudate nucleus and thalamus in patients with fibromyalgia syndrome, who concurrently also demonstrated a decreased pain threshold and increased CSF substance P. They postulate that "central sensitivity is the final common pathway for the development of abnormal pain in fibromyalgia syndrome."

Chronic Fatigue Syndrome (CFIDS)

In chronic fatigue syndrome (CFIDS), a related problem apparently also reflecting central sensitization, Goodnick and Klimas describe myalgias, arthralgias, cognitive difficulties, depression, and concentration/memory problems among the associated symptoms in addition to fatigue (64). Goodnick indicates that in their patient series, 80% had complaints of depression, and 74% had a diagnosis of fibromyalgia (65). Hence, CFIDS may represent another variant of central sensory dysfunction.

Visceral Pain

Giamberardino (9) has described early visceral pain as a poorly defined sensation that is always in the same location (usually midline abdomen or thorax) and accompanied by marked autonomic signs and emotional reactions. Subsequently, pain is referred to somatic structures (skin, subcutis, and muscle) and may or may not be accompanied by hyperalgesia to that referred area. At that stage the pain becomes sharper and better localized and no longer has the autonomic signs. She describes three forms of visceral hyperalgesia: primary, that is, hyperalgesia of the involved organ; secondary, which involves the referred site; and viscero-visceral, which is hyperalgesia of a noninvolved visceral organ that shares afferent innervation with the involved organ. That same author found that patients with irritable bowel syndrome developed pain to smaller bowel distention and had larger areas of referred pain than normal controls. There was also evidence of hypervigilance, inducible visceral hyperalgesia, and lower rectal sensory threshold in these patients. In healthy persons, acute rectal pain was associated with activation of the anterior cingulate cortex (ACC), but there was no ACC response in patients with irritable bowel syndrome. Instead, there was activation of the left prefrontal cortex during both painful rectal distention and during the anticipation of it. The lack of ACC response in patients with irritable bowel syndrome is felt to possibly represent a failure of descending pain inhibition. Studies in rats show a supraspinal descending influence for visceral hyperalgesia in the brainstem rostral ventrum medial medulla, and this includes a facilitatory component (which is NMDA-mediated) and an inhibitory component (which is non-NMDA-mediated). Selective block of either component unmasks the other. Trophic changes in the referred areas reveal an increase in subcutis thickness and a decrease in muscle thickness.

Giamberardino showed that it is the perceived visceral pain and not the visceral pathology that determines the occurrence of referred hyperalgesia, its degree, and its duration. The extent of muscle hyperalgesia was also a function of the pain experienced. In studies of renal calculosis, for example, patients passing stones had higher levels and longer-lasting episodes of visceral hyperalgesia than those who underwent lithotripsy because of the repetitive pain experience (with resultant sensitization) of the former as the stone passed through the ureter. Pain thresholds in renal calculosis were also normal for naive patients, but lowered in those with a previous history of this pain. Based on her research, Giamberardino has proposed that visceral hyperalgesia is the result of a peripheral sensitization that first occurs, causing a lowered pain threshold. Through recruitment, this process then leads to a central (supraspinal) sensitization, which results in increased spontaneous activity of central neurons, enlarged receptor field areas, and an increased response of large and small primary afferent fibers. This central sensitivity is also mediated through NMDA.

Headache

The headache literature reveals substantial evidence to support peripheral and central sensitization concepts. Silberstein et al. (11) have stated that "sensitization of the nucleus caudalis neurons can cause normal, nonpainful stimuli to become painful, producing trigger spots, and overlap of the symptoms of migraine and tension headache, and activation of the trigeminal vascular system." Rapoport and Sheftell (66) have stated that the blood vessels of migraineurs show a greater sensitivity to serotonin and have more extreme reactions to tyramine and adrenaline than do controls. Burstein and Strassman (67) found that following chemical irritation of the dura, 66% of the neurons became hypersensitive and reacted to subthreshold stimulation. Hence, they feel that this peripheral sensitization of the mechanosensitive meningeal nociceptors might explain how small increases in intracranial pressure during routine activities, such as bending over, coughing, etc., can aggravate headache pain. These same authors also describe central sensitization and in their research showed that sensitization of the trigeminal mechanosensitive meningeal primary afferent neurons can lead to activation and sensitization of second order trigeminal brainstem neurons. In fact, following chemical irritation of the dura, 95% of the animals showed increased sensitivity to mechanical indentation, decreased pain thresholds, and a two- to fourfold increase in intensity and magnitude of

response. Because the second order nociceptive neurons receive convergent input from cerebral blood vessels, meninges, and facial skin, the clinical implication of central sensitization is the development of intra- and extracranial hypersensitivity through convergence and recruitment. There was also evidence for autonomic augmentation.

Srikiatkhachorn et al. (21) studied analgesic rebound headache. They found a role of central 5-hydroxytryptamine (5HT)-dependent neurons in response to paracetamol. Chronic administration of paracetamol produced a down-regulation of 5HT2A receptors by causing an increase in 5HT release, followed by depletion. More specifically, 15 days of paracetamol administration resulted in a down-regulation of 5HT2A receptors and an up-regulation of 5HT transporters in the frontal cortex. However, 30 days of paracetamol administration resulted in normalization of 5HT levels, and this occurs simultaneously with a decreased efficacy of the drug. The up-regulation of 5HT2A receptors may result in a hyperalgesic state and facilitate the headache because there appears to be an inverse relationship of 5HT levels and headache. They postulate that because there is already 5HT suppression in migraine, this further suppression via these neuroplastic changes may result in an increase in headache frequency. What is interesting is that the neuroplastic changes they describe are mainly in the cortex, not the brainstem, and seem to be reversible after the paracetamol is withdrawn.

Complex Regional Pain Syndrome (CRPS)

Complex regional pain syndrome (CRPS) has been postulated to represent a central sensitization with significant autonomic involvement as well (19). Certainly the allodynia seen with CRPS represents not only sensitization, but also recruitment and convergence. Here, clearly nonnociceptive neuronal transmission is perceived as painful.

Phantom Pain

Likewise, phantom pain is most likely another example of central sensitization (19), felt to result from a one-time overwhelming nociceptive input as peripheral nerves are severed in the process of the amputation or alternatively from the release of previously inhibited afferents. The concept of so-called preemptive anesthesia, as utilized in elective amputations, is designed to prevent this barrage of nociceptive input and thereby prevent the chance of phantom pain.

Dysphoria

The dysphoria seen so frequently in patients with maldynia is often labeled as depression. However, many of these mood problems do not run the same clinical course when left untreated and do not show the same treatment response to antidepressants that more classical major depressions do. In fact, this type of dysphoria seems to clinically fit better with the limbically augmented emotions described by Rome and Rome.

Mayberg et al. have argued that "the associated impairment of cognitive, motor, and somatic functions in patients with dysphoria suggests that depression is a composite disorder affecting discrete but functionally interconnected limbic, paralimbic, and neocortical circuits" (23). Metabolic and rCBF flow studies consistently show decreases in the prefrontal cortex of patients with depression. Less consistently seen are changes in the limbic (amygdala) and paralimbic (cingulate gyrus) systems and may represent different subgroups of depression. Positron emission tomography (PET) studies show changes of two pathways of regional localization: (a) orbital frontal → striatal → thalamic circuits and (b) basotemporal limbic circuits. Mayberg suggests that these changes may be explained by "disease specific disruption of converging pathways to the paralimbic frontal and temporal cortices" and could account for "the presence of indistinguishable depressive symptoms in patients with distinctly different pathologies." Recent neuroimaging studies have placed particular emphasis on the prefrontal cortex, anterior cingulate gyrus, parietal cortex, and amygdala as critical components of dysfunctional circuitry involved in both depression and anxiety (59).

This cluster of apparently divergent syndromes (fibromyalgia, headache, CRPS, phantom pain, visceral painful syndromes including irritable bowel, and dysphoria), which we feel represents central sensory dysfunction, has similar overlapping associated symptoms (decreased energy, decreased concentration with its consequent memory dysfunction, decreased motivation, decreased libido, decreased tolerance to stress, disrupted sleep patterns, and magnified behavioral responses to stimuli, including nociception) with different "target organs." There is also similarity in the brain areas involved, as demonstrated anatomically and by functional studies (imaging, rCBF, etc.), by the neurochemistry involved, by the neuroplastic changes that occur resulting in sensitization at both the spinal cord and supraspinal levels, and by effective treatments.

Rauch (38) has pointed out that limbic system dysfunction results in hyperresponses affectively, with poor ability of the frontal cortex to exert governance, and a resultant decrease in memory and learning. The paralimbic system serves as a conduit from the motor, sensory, and associative cortex to the limbic system and plays a role in prioritizing the flow of information within the brain and in coding the information based on its importance within the brain. The anterior cingulate gyrus (AC) integrates cognitive, affective, and sensory motor functions. The dorsal AC connects with motor centers; the rostral AC connects with the affective centers, including limbic and paralimbic; and the ventral AC connects with deep brain regions that monitor and mediate visceral motor functions. The rostral AC regulates the prioritization between cognitive and affective processing. Thus, the rostral AC and the paralimbic system form a feedback loop for affective intrusions on cognition and for cognitive modulation of emotional information processing.

Thus, we may be seeing in central sensory dysfunction syndromes one "genotype" (central sensitization) with various "phenotypic" (target organ) presentations. Further support for this genotype-phenotype analogy comes from the positive results of treatments that seem to alter the conscious perceptions that are the result of the "genotype" rather than the "phenotype." In fact, the portions of the phenotypes that are apparently due to peripheral sensitization seem to respond differently. For example, the work by Srikiatkhachorn on analgesic rebound headaches showed that the decrease in the headaches when the offending agent is removed is due to the peripheral sensitization of the dura. But the affective component and intense reactions to future headaches, which are represented by the central sensitization, continue. Similarly, Giamberardino has demonstrated that the subcutis and muscle changes of referred pain areas, due to central sensitization and not the peripheral sensitization portion of visceral hyperalgesia, continue indefinitely beyond the instigating event of visceral pathology.

Marcus Aurelius also said,

> As for pain, a pain that is intolerable carries us off;
> But that which lasts a long time is bearable;
> The mind maintains its own tranquility
> By retiring into itself,
> And the ruling faculty is not injured.
> As for the parts which are hurt by the pain,
> Let them, if they can, give their opinion of it.

Marcus Aurelius clearly seems to be relating how a nontraumatized or noncentrally sensitized individual could handle chronic pain. Is there a way to help sensitized individuals do the same?

COGNITIVE BEHAVIORAL THERAPIES (CBT) AND PAIN

Cognitive behavioral therapies have evolved over the past 35 years as a result of early animal research on patterns of behavior. Early studies of extinction gave rise to behavioral and cognitive approaches to humans with painful conditions. Since about 1985, cognitive behavioral therapies have come to the forefront of the treatment armamentarium for chronic painful conditions.

Multidimensional Aspects of Pain

The multidimensional aspects of pain have been described in the literature over the last 25 to 30 years. Fordyce (68,69) was among the earliest writers to elucidate the importance of cognition and behavior in chronic pain. Since then, much has been written about the cognitive dimension of chronic pain. The cognitive aspects of pain and the relationship to pain behaviors as a learned mechanism have been reviewed extensively (70–72). Ciccone and Grzesiak found specific patterns of dysfunctional thinking, including "awfulizing," low frustration tolerance, self-downing, and overgeneralizing, as important in accounting for major symptoms of chronic pain. Turk and Rudy (73) have even suggested a multiaxial assessment of pain (MAP), classifying patients into three subgroups, and this system was applicable across multiple pain syndromes, including low back pain, headache, and temporomandibular disorders. This work was based on the assessment scale of the Multidimensional Pain Inventory developed by Turk, which was derived initially from the West Haven-Yale Multidimensional Pain Inventory (WHYMPI) (74).

Brands (75) described the importance of learning processes in the persistence behavior of chronic pain patients in the face of acute pain stimulation. Chronic pain patients were found to demonstrate poorer acute pain tolerance and to report higher levels of acute pain than controls. Richard (76) studied the relationship of pain behaviors in chronic pain patients in relationship to their children and families. Their study demonstrated a higher frequency of behaviors in the children of pain patients—behaviors that are thought to be learned through observation of and interaction with the parent in pain—than was found in children of control groups or children of patients with diabetes mellitus.

This multidimensional approach to chronic pain has certainly led to the development of multidisciplinary treatment of chronic pain, with an emphasis on addressing cognitive, affective, behavioral, and social factors in addition to physical pathology (77). The success of the multidisciplinary approach has been reviewed elsewhere and is nicely demonstrated by Flor et al. (78). That metaanalysis demonstrated that multidisciplinary treatment is superior to single-discipline treatments, such as standard medical or surgical approaches, with resultant improvement in pain, mood, and interference in life activities, including return to work and decreased use of the health-care system. Moreover, these effects were stable over time.

COGNITIVE BEHAVIORAL APPROACHES

Because of the complex multidimensional nature of chronic pain, the cognitive behavioral therapies have evolved over the past 35 years as a result of early animal research on patterns of behavior. Early studies of extinction gave rise to behavioral and cognitive approaches to humans with painful conditions as well. Cognitive behavioral therapy focuses on bringing about changes in attitudes, judgments, and values; correction of distorted thinking; reexamination of core assumptions; correction of behaviors; and involves validation, remotivation, and resocialization; increasing coping skills; increasing prob-

lem-solving abilities; increasing self-esteem; and increasing a sense of personal control (79). This form of psychological treatment has been applied to multiple disorders, including addictive behaviors, especially problem drinking (80), depression (81), chronic psychotic disorders, including hallucinations and delusions (82), insomnia secondary to chronic pain (83), compulsive hoarding (84), infertility (85), pathological gambling (86), noncardiac chest pain (87), and terminal illness (88). Interestingly, the use of cognitive behavioral treatment in terminal illness by Fishman (88) emphasized two ideas: Pain and suffering are not the same, and patients can exercise substantial control over their thoughts, feelings, and behavior. In this study, patients were taught to separate suffering (as a feeling of pervasive personal destruction) from pain, the sensory stimulus (the affective dimension of pain vs. the sensory discriminative dimension). These patients were able, even in advanced stages of their terminal illness, to experience themselves as active agents who could reduce their own suffering and enhance their sense of well-being.

CBT and Age

Cognitive behavioral therapy also seems to be efficacious across age groups (89). Children have been especially successful using cognitive behavioral interventions during painful procedures (90–93), including such procedures as bone marrow aspirations and burn wound debridements. Treatments included breathing exercises, relaxation and distraction techniques, imagery, cognitive coping skills, videotaped modeling, behavioral rehearsal, and active coaching. Humphreys and Gevirtz (94) describe the use of cognitive behavioral biofeedback-assisted treatments combined with fiber for treating recurrent abdominal pain in children. Cognitive behavioral interventions for pain have been used as an effective adjunct to pharmacologic interventions with juvenile rheumatoid arthritis (95).

The elderly also are able to utilize cognitive behavioral techniques effectively. Manetto and McPherson (96) showed that noncognitively impaired elderly pain patients can benefit as well as younger populations from the use of behavioral cognitive techniques with emphasis on concreteness, high organization in terms of format, and brief sessions. Luskin et al. (97) reviewed geriatric literature regarding musculoskeletal disorders in the elderly and found that multiple mind-body practices, including cognitive behavioral therapy, were effective as complementary treatments for these musculoskeletal disorders. They do point out the need, however, for good randomized controlled studies. Cook (98) found that elderly residents of a nursing home who received cognitive behavioral training reported less pain and less pain-related disabilities and that these treatment effects were maintained at 4-month followup, despite an overall increase in reported pain.

Thus, the cognitive behavioral therapies are useful in multiple disorders, both pain related (see the following) and nonpain related, and they are useful across all age groups, from pediatric through geriatric.

Characteristics of CBT

Cognitive behavioral therapies are problem oriented and practical, emphasize real-life and living skills, and offer concrete viewpoints and techniques (99). These characteristics enable the wide application as mentioned and allow for usefulness both by professionals and by nonprofessionals. For example, many cognitive behavioral programs for pain also educate families in appropriate cognitive behavioral interventions toward their loved ones in pain. Keijsers (100) and others point out that cognitive behavioral therapy is also characterized by a more active and directive stance on the part of the therapist and higher levels of emotional support than are found in insight-oriented psychotherapies. These relationship factors between therapist and patient have a moderate, yet consistent, impact on outcome of cognitive behavioral techniques. Dobson and Khatri (101) also discuss the art of psychotherapy and the impact of "nonspecifics" of therapy in addition to the specific techniques used on the outcome. Other differences between psychodynamic psychotherapy and cognitive behavioral therapy reveal that the latter tend to promote control of negative affect through the use of intellect and rationality combined with vigorous encouragement, support, and reassurance from the therapists. Dynamic psychotherapy, on the other hand, emphasizes the evocation of affect by bringing troublesome feelings into awareness and integrating these with previous life experience.

Caudill (102) has pointed out that cognitive behavioral therapies in the treatment of pain tend to improve functioning while decreasing pain perception. These findings are consistent with the earlier understanding of the affective dimension of pain as described by Price (1) and Rome and Rome (10), where the goal of therapeutic intervention would be to use the cognitive abilities of the patient to decrease limbic arousal as much as possible.

CBT and Learning

As cognitive behavioral therapies have gained importance in the treatment of chronic pain, the role of learning in chronic pain has been emphasized in the literature (72, 103–108). Tan (109) recently reviewed cognitive behavioral therapy as 1 of 25 empirically validated or supported psychological treatments for chronic pain and other disorders.

Brands and Schmidt have shown that chronic low back pain patients demonstrate poorer acute pain tolerance and report higher acute pain (75,110). Jensen et al. (111) have demonstrated that patients' beliefs predict their level of functioning. In the Jensen study, patient beliefs were compared with patient-reported functioning and family-reported functioning and association of pain behaviors. Significant associations between patient beliefs and pain behavior were

found. A significant hindsight-effect (112) has been demonstrated in a chronic pain population and was found to be significantly higher in this group than in a control group. Hindsight bias is considered a universal cognitive mechanism; and relates to the concept that information processing is in part uncontrolled, automatic, and pre-attentive; and that information available at any given time will change the memory of prior judgments, predictions of future events, and resultant behavior. Indeed, anticipation of pain and fear-avoidance beliefs predicted variation in a spinal isometric strength test (113). Wegner et al. (114,115) have demonstrated the effects of thought suppression and disruption of memory sequence on current cognition and perception.

The power of learned pain beliefs and behaviors is such that it affects not only patients, but also their families. Children of chronic low back pain patients exhibit higher frequency of behaviors felt to be learned through observation or interaction with the parent in pain (76), as we have pointed out.

Goals of CBT

Cognitive approaches to chronic pain focus on the way the person perceives, interprets, and relates to pain rather than on elimination of pain per se (70). The goals of cognitive behavioral therapy are to help patients restructure their view of their pain and what it means to their life. Additionally, in view of the concepts of kindling of pain (1,10), it is also important to prevent chronicity from developing. As soon as possible an attempt should be made to prevent eudynia from becoming maldynia. Chronic low back pain patients have shown an inability to habituate the pain, and this inability is now considered a significant risk factor for the development of chronic pain (75,110). Hasenbring et al. (116) have shown the usefulness of cognitive behavioral interventions in acute sciatic pain. They demonstrated in a group of patients with "acute sciatica" and "psychosocial high risk factors for chronicity" that both electromyographic (EMG) biofeedback and cognitive behavioral approaches were effective in reducing pain and preventing chronicity. The cognitive behavioral interventions were superior to the EMG biofeedback, and 90% of their patients showed a clinically significant reduction in pain comparable to the psychosocially low-risk patients, 83% of whom experienced pain reduction. Patients who refused such intervention had poorer outcomes in pain reduction, disability, and work performance.

Cognitive behavioral techniques incorporate multiple strategies and can be administered individually to the person in pain and to groups and can be taught to families as well. Puder (89) found cognitive behavioral group therapy to be successful in decreasing the degree of pain interference with activities, increasing ability to cope with pain, and decreasing use of medications and other physical treatments. There was, however, little effect on perceived pain intensity. These gains were maintained at a 6-month followup as well. The ultimate goal of cognitive behavioral therapy is to teach patients coping strategies that can be used over time by the patients, supporting their ability to regain control over their lives (107,108,117).

The actual techniques of cognitive behavioral therapy are at the discretion and creativity of the therapist. Davison et al. (118) demonstrate the usefulness of having patients articulate their thoughts while engaging in a task or situation. They point out the immediacy of the effect of this technique, as opposed to being retrospective. Rosenstiel and Keefe (119) have described techniques for diverting attention, reinterpreting pain sensations, offering coping self-statements, eliminating catastrophizing, and increasing activity levels as ways of intervening. Likewise, Blinchik and Grzesiak (120) emphasize having patients conceptualize their pain by becoming aware of their thoughts prior to and during their experience of pain and then training the patients in replacing those thoughts and relabeling their pain experience.

CBT and Painful Disorders

Cognitive behavioral therapies have been shown to be useful in multiple painful syndromes (71,107,121–126). Johansson et al. (127) employed cognitive behavioral therapies, including educational sessions, goal setting, graded activity training, pacing, relaxation techniques, cognitive restructuring, social skills training, medication reduction techniques, contingency-based pain behavior management, and planning of work return, in a multidisciplinary pain program. This program was effective at up to 1-year followup in improving occupational training and nonvocational activity level, decreasing catastrophizing, and decreasing pain behaviors. Measures of sick leave, pain interference, control over one's life, pain intensity, suffering and affective distress, physical fitness, medication reduction, and increased avocational activities all improved.

There is rather extensive literature on the usefulness of cognitive behavioral therapies for treatment of soft tissue pain, pain of arthritis, and chronic low back pain. Bradley (128) has discussed cognitive behavioral therapy for treating the pain of fibromyalgia. Similarly, Haldorsen et al. (129) used a cognitive behavioral 4-week program to treat "musculoskeletal pain" in patients who were sick-listed in Norway. Although the group receiving cognitive behavioral therapy had no higher return-to-work rate than the control group at 1-year followup, their work potential, quality of life, suffering, and ergonomic behaviors showed significant improvement.

Treatment of rheumatoid arthritis-related pain has shown mixed results. Bradley et al. (63) demonstrated clinically and statistically significant improvement in pain behavior and anxiety, for up to 6 months, and a short-term beneficial effect on pain and disease activity in patients with rheumatoid arthritis who were treated with a cognitive behavioral program. Likewise, Leibing et al. (130)

found an effect of cognitive behavioral treatment in slowing the progression of rheumatoid arthritis in their patients. The more significant effects, however, were in stabilizing emotion, improving coping, and reducing impairment more than pain level. They found reduction in emotion-focused coping, helplessness, depression, anxiety, and pain unpleasantness. Keefe and Van Horn (105) reviewed the role of cognitive behavioral therapy in managing pain in patients with rheumatoid arthritis and found variable results in pain and disability reduction and found, as did Bradley et al. (63), a significant dropoff of maintenance of pain coping skills with time.

The literature is more supportive of effectiveness for cognitive behavioral techniques in the treatment of chronic low back pain, even though that term can be representative of multiple pain-producing factors. Patients with chronic low back pain in which the pain and symptomatology are incongruent with physical pathology have shown a poorer outcome in response to treatment and excessive use of health-care resources in the past (131). These patients have been found to have more maladaptive and dysfunctional cognitions. They have been viewed as overwhelmed and ineffective in their attempts to cope and as more physically disabled as a result of their pain. Burns et al. (124) explained low back pain according to the manner in which noxious stimuli are attended to and interpreted, the degree to which certain behaviors become conditioned stimuli for fear responses, and how environmental contingencies increase and decrease the frequency of maladaptive and adaptive behaviors. They have found cognitive behavioral therapies to be effective in reducing pain, decreasing disability, and improving mood. Other authors likewise have found significant improvement in affect, higher activity tolerance, decreased pain behaviors, better coping, and better pain control (122,123,126). Slater et al. (125) found that 47% of patients in their program receiving behavioral treatment evidenced clinically significant improvements in at least one of the dimensions of the pain, disability, and/or depression associated with chronic low back pain. However, it was rare for patients to show improvement on all three measures. Sullivan et al. (81) also found success with cognitive behavioral approaches in conjunction with antidepressants in treating depression-related chronic low back pain. Nicholas et al. (132) found significant improvement in self-efficacy beliefs, decreased medication usage, improved active coping strategies, and other-rated functional impairment. Interestingly, at 6-month followup, the patients receiving the cognitive behavioral treatment program were continuing to do their physical exercise as well as relaxation, maintaining an increased activity level, and cognitive coping strategies on a regular basis of 1 to 3 days per week.

Thus, cognitive behavioral therapies have been shown to be useful in a variety of painful conditions. The positive effects also seem to be ongoing and long lasting. These cognitive behavioral therapies seem to effect change in patients with chronic pain by improving the ability of the prefrontal cortex to alter cognition and thereby have a downward effect on the brain pathways involved with nociceptive perception, including the limbic system, the descending inhibitory pathways, and motor output.

HYPNOSIS

The role of hypnosis in pain management, even today, remains controversial (133). Turner and Chapman (107) have emphasized that clinical research on the use of hypnosis for pain "has been sparse, and quite poor methodologically." Recently, however, better studies have shed more light on the role of hypnosis in pain management and how it may be working (1). Montgomery et al. (134) examined the effectiveness of hypnosis in pain management, comparing studies of hypnoanalgesia in healthy volunteers versus pain patients, and also comparing hypnoanalgesic effects in participants' hypnotic suggestibility. Metaanalysis of 18 studies revealed a moderate to large hypnoanalgesic effect for both clinical and experimental pain reduction. Likewise, Edelson and Fitzpatrick (135) showed improvement on the McGill Pain Questionnaire in patients treated with cognitive behavioral techniques or hypnosis relative to patients treated with only attention control. They found superiority in the cognitive behavioral treatment on behavioral measures, but equivalence between cognitive behavioral and hypnotic treatment on subjective measures. These results were also sustained on a 1-month followup. Eimer (136) had success with hypnoanalgesia coupled with development of individualized pain-coping strategies through trance, including such constructs as direct suggestion, cognitive reframing, hypnotic metaphors, and pain-relief imagery. In addition, that author used psychodynamic reprocessing of emotional factors during the trance state. Spira and Spiegel (137) emphasized that success with hypnosis for pain control depends upon the hypnotizability of the patient, the patient's particular cognitive style, the patient's specific motivation, and the patient's level of cognitive functioning. They did find success with hypnoanalgesia through individual sessions and group sessions and found hypnoanalgesia useful even for hospice patients confined to bed. Spiegel and Spiegel (37) have correlated the degree of hypnotizability and learning style for usefulness in hypnoanalgesia. Specifically, highly hypnotizable subjects are able to create anesthesia through the use of hypnosis, whereas lowly hypnotizable subjects are better able to utilize distraction as a hypnotic technique.

Liossi and Hatira (138) found both hypnosis and cognitive behavioral coping skills effective in preparing pediatric oncology patients for bone marrow aspiration. They found that both techniques resulted in lowered pain and lowered pain-related anxiety compared to controls and compared to patients at baseline.

Alden and Heap (139) view hypnoanalgesia as part of cognitive and behavioral interventions. They view hypnosis as a set of skills deployed by the individual rather than as a state in and of itself. Factors common to a trance, however, that facilitate management of pain include a sustained focus of attention, an absence of judgment and censorship, a suspension of time, the experiencing of one's own responses as automatic, and a feeling of relaxation (1,37). These factors allow for facilitation of new ideas or cognitions, which may or may not contain accepted inconsistencies, and heighten the suggestibility of the patient. Hypnosis, through these mechanisms, is then available to target both the affective-motivational dimension of pain as well as the sensory-discriminative dimension through such mechanisms as reinterpretation or dissociation. For example, one of our patients, who was suffering from a severe electric-type painful peripheral neuropathy secondary to snake venom toxicity, was taught to place a mental rheostat switch between himself and his electric-type pain and turn the switch down until the pain was lowered to a bearable intensity. He was then taught to alter that minor electrical feeling into a pleasant one from an unpleasant one.

Rainville et al. (140) demonstrated that hypnotic suggestions can selectively modulate the affective dimension of pain but that when it is used to modulate the sensory discriminative dimension, the affective dimension is modulated in parallel with it. This work also supports the work of Spiegel and Spiegel (37) in using hypnotic susceptibility to target different dimensions of pain.

Price (1) suggests that hypnoanalgesia works through three general mechanisms: The first is related to spinal cord descending mechanisms; the second relates to prevention of awareness of pain at higher centers by dissociation; and the third is a selective reduction in the affective dimension of pain by reinterpretation of meanings. He further substantiates these mechanisms by citing brain activity in the anterior cingulate cortex, as related to pain unpleasantness, with no change in neural activity of the somatosensory cortex. However, when hypnotic suggestions were targeted toward pain sensation, there was change in activity within the primary somatosensory cortex. Price concludes that "hypnotic modulation of pain is both psychologically and neurophysiologically multidimensional; that is, different mechanisms target different pain dimensions." He concludes that hypnosis may be more useful than had been formerly thought in pain management. He suggests that utilization of suggestions for "reducing both sensory and affective dimensions of pain experience may more effectively optimize the capacities of individuals to alter the overall experience of pain by changing any one of several aspects of their experience. . . . It is important to consider that the efficacy of attempts to induce hypnotic analgesia may differ somewhat depending on susceptibility, the hypnotic approach used, the relationship between the hypnotist and the patient, the pain dimensions assessed, and the level of pain. The observed magnitude of hypnotically-induced analgesia, in both clinical and experimental contexts, must be considered in terms of all of these factors."

PSYCHOTHERAPEUTIC DETERMINANTS

Thus far, several psychotherapeutic modalities have been discussed, i.e., cognitive behavioral therapy, etc. Although such approaches are indeed helpful to many patients suffering from chronic pain, there are inherent limitations. Cognitive therapy, by its very nature, relies on dealing with a given patient's cognitive structure relative to his or her intellectualized beliefs about pain and challenging such beliefs in favor of achieving a reorganization of the belief system, leading to different conclusions about the patient's situation. Although virtually anyone can engage in rational thought and enter into a therapeutic dialog about his or her painful situation, not everyone approaches his or her world initially through logic and reason. Many patients view their world initially through their emotions. The notion of how they "feel" may be much more important to them than what they "think." Herein lies a long-held belief by many mental health professionals that they must first psychologically evaluate patients in order to ascertain their inherent personality characteristics and then tailor the manner of psychotherapy so as to be consistent with patients' orientation to their own existence. By contrast, other clinicians, by virtue of their training and adherence to a particular theoretical orientation—i.e., psychoanalysis, psychodynamic psychotherapy, cognitive-behavioral therapy, etc.—apply the same "brand" of therapy to all patients, regardless of a patient's personal style of relating to the world.

The issue of "matching" the style of psychotherapeutic intervention to the personality of the patient has been considered quite important relative to maximizing the level of treatment outcome. Spiegel and Spiegel (37) have looked at the relationship between personality type and hypnotic trance capacity and found a modest statistical correlation. In effect, there is an inverse relationship between personality style and inherent trance capacity. Persons who are more cognitively oriented tend to have a lower potential to enter a deep hypnotic trance, whereas more affectively oriented individuals tend to have a higher trance capacity. Accordingly, applying hypnotherapy to all patients suffering from chronic pain will be only partially helpful, insofar as only certain personality types will have a higher biological potential to benefit from such an intervention. It is arguable that a highly motivated patient can still benefit from hypnotherapy. However, patients with the personality characteristics that correlate with lower biological trance capacity can still achieve a positive result, albeit to a probable lesser degree. Applying hypnotherapy to all pain patients would be both clinically ineffective and inefficient.

As with all aspects of the field of medicine, the treatment should fit the needs of the patient.

Although the foregoing implies the inherent limitations of hypnosis, it has been previously noted that Price (1) has concluded that hypnosis may be more clinically useful than previously thought in the area of pain management. He suggests that the procedure focus more on "reducing both sensory and affective dimensions of the pain experience." His justification relates to the relationship of hypnoanalgesia to neurophysiological processes, as previously discussed. However, once again, the personality of the individual must be taken into account relative to his or her inherent trance potential based on the patient's basic personality structure. A similar rationale can be applied to providing such modalities as cognitive behavioral therapy, or perhaps biofeedback to all patients as well.

As previously stated, cognitive behavioral therapy attempts to challenge an individual's belief system and modify the thought processes engaged in by the individual. However, in a chronic pain population, a differentiation must be made between "pain intensity" and "suffering." In comparing two patients with the same diagnosis and the same reports as to pain intensity, one may differentiate one patient to be in more pain by virtue of the degree to which he or she is suffering. This implies that the individual's emotions and attitudes toward pain play a greater role in the production and maintenance of the painful experience. To have any particular treatment modality serve the intellectual needs of the patient at the expense of his or her emotional well-being will ultimately fail to achieve positive results. Treatment will not generalize from the office setting to daily life experiences. An example might be a patient who achieves excellent clinical results utilizing thermal biofeedback in the office, demonstrating a peripheral body temperature of 95 degrees. The patient has learned to "master" the machine; however, after having left the office, the patient will revert to his or her typical manner of relating to pain, that is to say, with negative cognitions and emotional suffering, unless these specific issues are addressed. Generalization of clinical effect will tend to occur only in those patients who take consistent personal responsibility for "practicing" their newly learned strategies outside the office setting. This implies that even in those cases where such modalities as hypnotherapy and/or biofeedback are learned skills by the patient, the clinical effect of the procedure is inherently time limited. This requires the patient to repeatedly incorporate the procedure one or more times during daily activities in order to minimize pain. Such procedures generally do not produce a permanent reduction or elimination of pain and/or suffering.

In addition, some patients have difficulty relating to the technology associated with biofeedback machinery, again lowering their potential to benefit from the procedure. In order to be maximally effective, it is suggested that any treatment modality take into account the patient's cognitive and affective functioning, with the need to alter both. Within today's managed care environment, the need for effective and highly efficient treatment takes on even added importance.

EYE MOVEMENT DESENSITIZATION AND REPROCESSING (EMDR)

Given the more recently published knowledge regarding memory, perception, learning, and particularly central sensory dysfunction and the role of the limbic system in augmenting pain intensity and suffering, as previously discussed, more advanced psychotherapeutic procedures must be brought into the treatment. One such procedure is eye movement desensitization and reprocessing (EMDR) (52). EMDR is to a large degree a rapid information-processing system in which the patient "internally" processes traumatic or dysfunctional thoughts and/or feelings. Many of the components of EMDR in its current form have been developed over the past 13 years or so, based on extensive research on patients suffering from posttraumatic stress disorder (PTSD), with refinements made and expanded to include an increasingly wide variety of clinical populations. Although EMDR is a very precise procedure, it is clearly compatible with a variety of theoretical orientations, i.e., cognitive behavioral, psychodynamic, etc.

Shapiro (52) draws an analogy of EMDR with the emotional processing effects of rapid eye movement (REM), with the procedural portion of EMDR found to be equally efficacious when also incorporating other sensory modalities, i.e., auditory and tactile stimulation. The key feature in "activating" the brain to engage in rapid informational processing appears to be the initiation of bilateral alternating brain stimulation. In this sense, the old adage of "all roads lead to Rome" clearly applies. However, it is not meant to be suggested that EMDR is a "simple" procedure by which the clinician activates the brain for the purpose of processing information, with an automatic result ensuing. Rather, EMDR is a sophisticated and complex procedure that requires a highly skilled and knowledgeable mental-health professional. The goal of EMDR is to disengage affective memories that are neurophysiologically linked through various perceived similarities, thereby reducing the affective dimension of painful memory to a situation-appropriate level. As in all clinical work, one should not entertain a particular treatment modality until a differential diagnosis has been rendered, which most importantly applies to EMDR.

A standard protocol for EMDR intervention requires eight phases (see Table 14-3), with a differential diagnosis based on a detailed history being the first phase. The second phase of treatment relates to preparing to begin the procedure, which requires the establishment of rapport with the patient, explaining the procedure to the patient, allaying any concerns and developing safety procedures. The third phase relates to assessment. This phase focuses on identifying the particular components or "targets" that will be addressed during treatment, as well as establishing a baseline level of disturbance that is operating at cognitive, affective, as well as somatic levels. The fourth phase is desensitization, in which an attempt is made with specific EMDR interventions to alter the patient's cognitive, affective, and somatic symptoms or distress, regardless of whether the intensity of such symptoms is increasing, decreasing, or remaining stationary. The fifth phase is an installation phase. Whereas the fourth phase serves to decrease, or eliminate, the negative or dysfunctional aspects of the patient's presenting problems, the fifth phase attempts to "install" a positive replacement to the negative or dysfunctional aspects. An example of comparing phases 4 and 5 might relate to desensitizing the patient in phase 4 regarding a negative thought and feeling that his/her level of pain and the associated suffering will never improve. Phase 5's focus would be to insert a "positive cognition" that the patient **does** have power over his or her pain. Here, it is important to note that one of the differentiating characteristics of EMDR compared to most other forms of clinical intervention is the emphasis on using the patient's own perceptions as to thoughts and feelings to generate exactly what will be targeted in the treatment process in terms of the initial desensitization, as well as on the patient's articulating his or her own internally derived source that would be needed to obtain clinical relief. This procedure is felt to contrast with psychotherapeutic approaches such as hypnosis or biofeedback, in which the clinician is typically required to generate the components of intervention, i.e., creating the correct posthypnotic suggestion to alleviate pain and suffering, or asking the patient to "think of something" that will result in increas-

TABLE 14-3. *Phases of EMDR treatment*

Phase 1	Establish differential diagnosis based on obtaining a detailed history
Phase 2	Preparation: establish rapport; explanation of procedure to patient; allay concerns; develop safety procedures
Phase 3	Assessment: identification of specific targets that will be focus of intervention; establish baseline of disturbance
Phase 4	Desensitization: specific EMDR intervention to alter cognitive, affective, and somatic disturbances
Phase 5	Installation: install a positive replacement to the dysfunctional symptoms
Phase 6	Body scan: identification of any residual somatic symptoms that had been associated with previously identified negative cognitions and emotions
Phase 7	Closure: ensure equilibrium at the close of a treatment session
Phase 8	Reevaluation: reassessment of the patient's clinical status at the outset of the next treatment session

Adapted from Shapiro (52).

ing peripheral body temperature or decreasing EMG activity during a biofeedback session. Phase 6 is identified as the body scan, in which, after a positive cognition has been installed and the patient has been desensitized to the target event, a review of the entire body is conducted in order to identify any somatized residual symptoms that had been associated with the previously identified negative cognitions and emotions. The seventh phase relates to closure. In this phase, the clinician ensures that the patient is left with a state of equilibrium (cognitive and emotional stability) at the termination of a treatment session. The eighth and final phase of the EMDR protocol relates to reevaluation, in which the clinician reassesses the patient's clinical status at the beginning of the next treatment session.

Whereas research on the uses and effects of EMDR continues to proliferate, in the area of chronic pain, a paucity of data is available. However, as the clinical efficacy of this procedure regarding the treatment of chronic pain becomes more recognized, particularly within the field of pain medicine and pain management, increasing application of this procedure is predicted to occur, thereby leading to a corresponding increase in the needed research. To date, there have been a number of case reports that support EMDR's role in facilitating pain relief (141–144).

Despite limited controlled studies of EMDR to date, its importance to the future of effective and efficient pain management relates to its presumed consistency with what we now believe relative to neurophysiological mechanisms of pain, particularly in terms of the involvement of the amygdala, hippocampus, and prefrontal cortex (145). With regard to EMDR's similarity with processes associated with REM sleep in humans, research has demonstrated that "the pattern of activation in the amygdala and the cortical areas provides a biological basis for the processing of some types of memory during REM sleep" (146).

Chronic pain patients are indeed a difficult clinical population to treat for a variety of obvious reasons. For the medical practitioner, this task is made more difficult when a patient presents not only with emotional trauma associated with the illness or injury that defines his or her chronic pain, but also with a traumatic premorbid history that serves to exacerbate his or her perception and complaints of pain and suffering. The physician cannot be expected to separate the emotional from the organic; rather, the physician must treat the patient as a whole. Accordingly, in more traditional terms, it is incumbent on the mental-health professional to identify and deal with the "functional" aspects of the patient's presenting pain, so as to reduce or eliminate the "nonorganic aspects," leaving the patient more available for appropriate treatments of the sensory discriminative portion of his or her pain. In this regard, a procedure such as EMDR can be of invaluable assistance.

One of the most important theoretical constructs associated with EMDR relates to what Shapiro (52) refers to as "memory networks." She hypothesizes about the "brain's innate information-processing system which metaphori-

cally reflects a series of channels where related memories, thoughts, images, emotions, and sensations are stored and linked to one another" (52). Although Shapiro's conceptualization is theoretical, emerging information about the function of the brain, as previously discussed, is providing compelling evidence as to the neurophysiological validity of the model.

When a patient presents with a traumatic injury that results in chronic pain, the original injury can be viewed as a traumatic event. The chronicity of the pain and the associated limitations frequently imposed by the sequela serve to maintain the trauma. When the patient has a traumatic premorbid history, there is a significant probability, according to Shapiro's model, that both the premorbid traumatic event(s) and the trauma associated with the chronic pain situation are stored in the same "channel." Clinically, the patient may not be aware of any relationship between previous and current traumas. Nevertheless, the effects are believed to be both intertwined and cumulative by virtue of the manner in which memories are stored at a neurophysiological level. In the past, traditional training would have caused the mental-health practitioner to look for hysteroid or perhaps hypochondriacal tendencies as a theoretical construct that would potentially account for the patient's intensity of clinical presentation. However, if one takes into account what has recently emerged in the area of brain research, there are now neurochemical explanations, i.e., kindling, neuroplasticity, limbically augmented pain syndrome, etc., that can properly account for much of a patient's degree of suffering. No one would argue that there are a significant number of patients who do present with underlying characterological disorders or other forms of psychopathology that are of long-standing duration that predate their presenting complaints. However, given the role and importance of brain function relative to the emotional expression of the chronic pain experience, it is quite important to restore the integrity, the respect, and most importantly, the credibility of those patients who have emotionally decompensated for reasons of neurological etiology.

Case Illustration

It is believed that EMDR is an important tool that can facilitate the processing of emotional trauma that is linked in memory to present pain complaints. A specific case report illustrates this importance. A 36-year-old female presented to a multidisciplinary pain treatment program a lifting injury suffered one year earlier in an industrial accident. MRI scan revealed evidence of a small central herniated disc at L-5–S-1, with no clinical evidence of lumbar radiculopathy or cauda equina syndrome. There was also a very mild diffuse annular bulge at the level of L-4–5. Further radiological studies revealed straightening of the lumbar lordosis and a diagnosis of lumbosacral strain. Multiple physicians who examined this patient consistently reported a strong "functional overlay." Vegetative functioning was positive for a sleep continuity disorder, with recurrent nightmares. Appetite was decreased, although she experienced a 20-pound weight gain due to physical inactivity associated with her injury. Sexual performance was decreased secondary to pain. Mood was noted to be significantly depressed, with frequent crying episodes and passive suicidal ideation. Energy level was decreased, with a corresponding decrease in her functional routine activities. Historically, the patient married at the age of 17, had five children (one of whom was autistic and rarely left her presence, largely for reasons of safety), and was divorced. During her marriage she had been the victim of verbal, emotional, and physical abuse. Subsequent relationships with boyfriends were also reported to have been abusive for the patient. Academically, she reported a seventh-grade education, with her premorbid medical history having been negative. Clinically, the patient ambulated very slowly with a markedly antalgic gait. Prior to her industrial accident, the patient was an avid jogger and cognizant of engaging in regular exercise, all of which had been aborted since her injury. Baseline exercise performance on admission to the program and prior to EMDR intervention was: treadmill: 20 minutes @ 1.5 mph; health rider: 5 minutes @ 30 rpm; stationary bicycle: 10 minutes.

During the patient's involvement in a multidisciplinary pain treatment program, the patient entered into psychotherapy. Given that the patient was unable to work, she had been experiencing pronounced financial strain, making it increasingly difficult to support her family, this having been identified as a significant source of her depression, notwithstanding her ongoing pain. Despite the patient's limited educational background, she was able to articulate a metaphor characterizing how she felt about her situation. She felt "as if she were stuck in mud filled with earthworms, with all of her children." Subjectively, she was feeling a very strong need to "save them" but could not as long as she could not work. Following is a transcript of a single EMDR session comprised of 13 "sets," which dealt with the preceding traumatic content:

Set 1   I'm with my kids in the mud . . . they're gonna get sick and die . . . I have to get them out . . . I can't move, I'm stuck.

Set 2   (Patient begins to cry) I'm stuck, I can't move . . . I'm telling them to move. I can't reach any of them. I'm going under, the mud is reaching my chin.

Set 3   (Patient continues to cry) I'm a bad parent . . . I'm not doing enough for my kids. I'm gonna die and who's gonna take care of them?

Set 4   (Patient continues to cry) I just want to die 'cause I can't take care of my kids. My kids would be better off without me (At this point the patient admitted to a recent suicide gesture 1 month prior to this session in which she took a knife into the bathroom and contemplated cutting her wrists).

Set 5   I'm in mud up to my neck. I feel like I'm being pulled under . . . feel like I'm losing my breath. Don't like it!

Set 6   I feel worms crawling on my legs (Patient becomes short of breath and complains of having no more strength).

Set 7   I can't raise my hands to remove the worms from my head or nose. I can't get out of the mud . . . the mud is too thick.

Set 8   The mud is very thick and heavy (The patient is asked to think of something that would soften the mud).

Set 9   It's raining and I hear thunder. The mud now feels like a pool of dirty water. The kids help each other get out of the mud.

Set 10   I see the kids on the porch. They look like their clothes are dry and clean, but I'm still in the mud.

Set 11   I found some stairs under the mud. Climb out of the mud hole. Shaking off the worms, but I'm still dirty standing on the porch (Patient is asked how she could become clean).

Set 12   Patient leaves the protection of the porch and walks out into the rain. Patient smiling, stating that the rain water is cleansing her and spontaneously states "I'm free." Patient states that she sees the sun and a rainbow and sees that her children are laughing.

Set 13   Patient is laughing that she and the children are "all wet." Patient is asked what she could do to become dry. Patient and children begin playing in the sun until completely dry.

The preceding reflects a patient who not only was experiencing chronic pain, but also by virtue of having been unable to work and thereby financially provide adequately for her children was severely depressed with suicidal features. The magnitude of her depression was sufficient to impede her motivation and energy levels regarding her physical involvement in the various somatic therapies. Accordingly, treatment of the depression became the priority regarding her overall treatment plan. It is believed that traditional verbal psychotherapy, regardless of the clinician's theoretical orientation, i.e., psychodynamic, cognitive behavioral, etc., might have been clinically effective over the course of time. Also presumed is that the clinician would have developed a particular thematic focus in treating the previously described depression that would have alleviated the problem. By comparison, within an EMDR framework, the patient was able to arrive at her own metaphor regarding her depression, with EMDR facilitating a rapid and effective amelioration of the depression based on the patient's "internal" perspective, as well as utilize her own cognitive and emotional strategies to effect the needed change. By facilitating the patient's ability to extricate herself from a "mud hole," the patient's level of emotional and physical energy was sufficiently raised so as to result in a dramatically improved response to the somatic therapies offered by the multidisciplinary pain treatment program. For example, her discharge exercise performances were: treadmill: 30 minutes @ 4.2 mph; health rider: 20 minutes @ 55 rpm; and stationary bicycle: 20 minutes. Concurrently, however, it was also important to deal with her pattern of entering into dysfunctional relationships, which had repeatedly served to cause her to view herself as "victimized" in the context of being in another "muddy hole." Despite the patient's medical diagnoses, she was subsequently able to physically improve to the point of returning to work without the need for invasive surgical intervention. Virtually any "brand" of psychotherapy is potentially useful in treating chronic pain patients, although cognitive behavioral approaches have demonstrated the most significant utility in assisting such patients. However, even the most skilled psychotherapist is seen as not as effective as patients' own internal resources in healing themselves. EMDR appears to afford such patients the opportunity of rapidly and effectively accessing their own "power of the mind."

In addition to being a powerful cognitive tool in the treatment of pain, EMDR, by separating the affective dimension of linked memories, with a resultant "appropriate" response rather than augmented affective response, appears to have a direct effect on the limbic system. Thus, this new tool would appear to allow us to access the patient's abilities on a neurophysiological level, through cognitions both in a downward serial system and in a parallel system through precortical intervention. It has also been our experience and that of others (144,147–150) that the limbically "deaugmented" emotions remain this way unless further traumatization takes place. That is, after the patient establishes a more normalized emotional response to pain and stressors, he or she does not revert to a limbically augmented reaction to further pain, without further traumatization. In our experience, this parallel response to EMDR gives this technique an added dimension beyond that of more traditional cognitive behavioral interventions, including hypnosis, cognitive approaches, and biofeedback. Those techniques allow for significant cognitive interventions to help improve a person's perception of pain and quality of life but do not offer a permanent change in the affective dimension of his or her pain experience, as does EMDR.

CONCLUSION

In this chapter we have attempted to bring together the most current knowledge regarding learning, perception, and the interface of these brain functions with the nociceptive system. We find the concepts of Price (1) and Rome and Rome (10) particularly important to this understanding. Price has elegantly described both the sensory discriminative dimension and the affective dimension of pain perception. Rome and Rome have further utilized these concepts in describing the lateral and the medial pain

systems and how limbic augmentation can occur through the neuroplastic changes in the brain in a chronic pain state. Central sensitization is a key feature of many chronic painful disorders, leading to what often becomes a generalized central sensory dysfunction, affecting not only the nociceptive system, but also other sensory systems, as evidenced by the hypervigilance noted in multiple chronic pain disorders.

Peripheral nociceptive stimulation can result in local sensitization in acute pain, and this peripheral stimulation, if repetitive, chronic, or intense enough, can produce spinal level and/or supraspinal level sensitization. This sensitization affects both the sensory discriminative dimension of pain as well as the affective dimension (through the limbic system). Both the affective dimension and the sensory discriminative dimension, one or both of which can be augmented as a result of sensitization, connect to higher cortical areas, thus contributing to the ultimate perception of pain by the person. Depending on which dimension has a greater contribution to that perception of pain, the qualitative experience of the person will vary.

Through cortical feedback in a downward fashion, we are able to utilize cognitions and behavioral modifications to alter both the sensory discriminative and affective dimensions of pain. Changes in cognition result in a change in perceptual awareness; that is, we change the channel on our television screen. In addition, these cognitive changes and the associated motor changes through behavioral interventions have a downward effect on the limbic system and brainstem, modifying the affective experience of the patient and stimulating the thalamospinal nociceptive inhibitory fibers. As Price has pointed out, modifying the sensory discriminative dimension of pain, which works in parallel with the affective dimension, results in a change in the latter as well. However, the opposite is not true, and therefore we have the ability to also utilize cognitive and behavioral changes directed at the affective component without necessarily modifying the sensory discriminative dimension. These cognitive behavioral interventions, including hypnosis, can thus be effective tools directed at modifying the patient's experience of pain.

However, in addition, we have described EMDR as a new and powerful tool in treating chronic pain. Recent research on memory has demonstrated the neurophysiological involvement of the limbic system, with a strong correlation to the areas of the limbic system involved with nociception as well. EMDR is useful in separating linked memories of traumatic and painful associations and allows persons to affectively experience their memories and their consequent motor expressions in behavior to those events more appropriately. It is our belief that EMDR not only works through cognitions, but also seems to have a direct effect on desensitizing the limbically augmented portion of the pain experience. Thus, in effect, it seems to reset the circuit breaker for emotion. It allows a more normal affective response to pain signals and to stressful events posttreatment, and this response seems to be permanent, unless the individual is retraumatized or resensitized. In this way, EMDR adds a dimension to the treatment of pain that is quite different from other cognitive and/or behavioral interventions, including hypnosis.

Traditionally, psychiatric and psychological interventions in chronic painful disorders have frequently been based upon the theoretical orientation of the particular therapist. In regard to treating chronic pain, the modus operandi was based on "a pain is a pain is a pain." However, our current understanding of neurophysiological central nervous system function, especially the nociceptive system, would seem to mandate that psychiatric and psychological interventions for persons with chronic painful conditions be based on these newer understandings, rather than on the orientation of the therapist. It is incumbent upon us as practitioners to develop the understanding and knowledge necessary for the techniques that have shown themselves to work most effectively in helping patients improve the quality of their existence and to be able to do this through the most effective techniques.

The U.S. Congress declared this decade, beginning January 2001, as the Decade of Pain. We can all anticipate a much richer knowledge base about nociception, pain perception, and appropriate physical and psychological treatments as a result. We who practice pain medicine and management have already gained a significant enrichment from the previous Decade of the Brain research. We look forward to the next 10 years in terms of added benefits that further research may help us bring to more successful treatment of our patients.

REFERENCES

1. Price D. *Psychological mechanisms of pain and analgesia.* Seattle: IASP Press, 1999.
2. Damasio AR. On some functions of the human prefrontal cortex. *Ann N Y Acad Sci* 1995;769:241–251.
3. Kagan J, Zentner M. Early childhood predictors of adult psychopathology. *Harv Rev Psychiatry* 1996;3:341–350.
4. Carlson M, Earls F. Psychological and neuroendocrinological sequelae of early social deprivation in institutionalized children in Romania. *Ann N Y Acad Sci* 1997;807:419–428.
5. Fillingim RB. *Sex, gender, and pain: a biopsychosocial framework in sex, gender, and pain.* Seattle: IASP Press, 2000:1–6.
6. Mogil J. *Interaction between sex and genotype in the mediation and modulation of nociception in rodents in sex, gender, and pain: a biopsychosocial framework in sex, gender, and pain.* Seattle: IASP Press, 2000:25–40.
7. Robinson M, Riley J, Myers C. *Psychosocial contributions to sex-related differences in pain responses in sex, gender, and pain: a biopsychosocial framework in sex, gender, and pain.* Seattle: IASP Press, 2000:41–68.
8. Burstein R, Strassman A. Peripheral and central sensitization during migraine. In: Devor M, et al., eds. *Proceedings of the 9th World Congress on Pain.* Seattle: IASP Press, 2000:589–602.
9. Giamberardino M. Visceral hyperalgesia. In: Devor M, et al. *Proceedings of the 9th World Congress on Pain.* Seattle: IASP Press, 2000: 523–550.
10. Rome H, Rome J. Limbically augmented pain syndrome (LAPS): kindling, corticolimbic sensitization, and convergence of affective and sensory symptoms in chronic pain disorders. *Pain Medicine* 2000; 1:7–23.
11. Silberstein S, et al. Neuropsychiatric aspects of primary headache disorders. In: Yudofsky S, Hales R, eds. *Textbook of Neuropsychiatry,* 3rd ed. Washington, DC: Amer Psychiatric Press, 1997:381–412.
12. Malenka RC, Nicoll RA. Long-term potentiation—a decade of progress. *Science* 1999;285:1870–1874.
13. Klintsova AY, Greenough WT. Synaptic plasticity in cortical systems. *Curr Opin Neurobiol* 1999;9:203–208.
14. Coderre TJ, Katz J, Vaccarino AL, Melzack R. Contribution of central neuroplasticity to pathological pain: review of clinical and experimental evidence. *Pain* 1993;52:259–285.
15. Post RM, Weiss SRB, Smith MA. Sensitization and kindling: implications for the evolving neural substrates of post-traumatic stress disorder. In: Friedman MJ, Charney DS, Deutch AY, eds. *Neurobiological and clinical consequences of stress: from normal adaptation to post-traumatic stress disorder.* Philadelphia: Lippincott-Raven, 1995:203–224.
16. Weiss SR, Post RM. Caveats in the use of the kindling model of affective disorders. *Toxicol Ind Health* 1994;10:421–427.
17. Cain DP. The transfer of phenomenon in kindling. In: Wada JA, ed. *Kindling 3.* New York: Raven Press, 1986:231–248.
18. Caggiula AR, Antelman SM, Aul E, et al. Prior stress attenuates the analgesic response but sensitizes the corticosterone and cortical dopamine responses to stress 10 days later. *Psychopharmacology (Berl)* 1989;99:233–237.
19. Wall P, Melzack R. *Textbook of Pain.* Churchill Livingstone, 1994:651–666,685–698.
20. Vecchiet L, Giamberardino M. Muscle pain, myofascial pain, and fibromyalgia: recent advances. *J Musculoskeletal Pain* 1999;7(1/2).
21. Srikiatkhachorn A, et al. Effect of chronic analgesic exposure on the central serotonin system: a possible mechanism of analgesic abuse headache. *Headache* May 2000;40:343–350.
22. Giamberardino M, et al. Referred muscle pain and hyperalgesia from viscera. *J Musculoskeletal Pain* 1999;7(1/2)61–69.
23. Mayberg H, et al. Neuropsychiatric aspects of mood and affective disorders. In: Yudofsky S, Hales R. *Textbook of neuropsychiatry,* 3rd ed. Washington, DC: Amer Psychiatric Press, 1997:883–902.
24. van der Kolk BA. The psychobiology of posttraumatic stress disorder. *J Clin Psychiatry* 1997;58(Suppl)9:16–24.
25. van der Kolk BA, Fisler RE. Childhood abuse and neglect and loss of self-regulation. *Bull Menninger Clin* 1994 Spring;58(2):145–168.
26. van der Kolk B, Greenberg M, Boyd H, et al. Inescapable shock, neurotransmitters, and addiction to trauma: toward a psychobiology of post traumatic stress. *Biol Psychiatry* 1985 Mar 20(3):314–325.
27. van der Kolk B, Greenberg MS, Orr SP, et al. Endogenous opioids, stress induced analgesia, and posttraumatic stress disorder. *Psychopharacol Bull* 1989;25(3):417–421.
28. van der Kolk BA, Pelcovitz D, Roth S, et al. Dissociation, somatization, and affect dysregulation: the complexity of adaptation of trauma. *Amer J Psychiatry* July 1996;153(7) Suppl:83–93.
29. Linton SJ. The population based study of the relationship between sexual abuse and back pain: establishing a link: *Pain* 1997;73:47–53.
30. Schofferman J, Anderson D, Hines R, et al. Childhood psychological trauma and chronic refractor low-back pain. *Clin J of Pain* 1993;9: 260–265.
31. Walker EA, Katon WJ, Roy-Byrne PP, et al. Histories of sexual victimization in patients with irritable bowel syndrome or inflammatory bowel disease. *Amer J of Psychiatry* 1993;150:1502–1506.
32. Kardiner A. *The traumatic neuroses of war.* New York: P Hoeber, 1941.
33. Sonnenberg S, et al. The trauma of war: stress and recovery in Viet Nam Veterans. Washington, DC: Amer Psychiatric Press, 1985.
34. van der Kolk BA. Psychological trauma. Washington, DC: Amer Psychiatric Press, 1987.
35. van der Kolk BA. The body keeps the score: memory and the evolving psychobiology of posttraumatic stress. *Harv Rev Psychiatry* 1994; 1:253–265.
36. van der Kolk BA. Psychology and psychobiology of childhood trauma. *Prax Kinderpsychol Kinderpsychiatr* 1998;47:19–35.
37. Spiegel H, Spiegel D. *Trance and treatment.* New York: Basic Books, 1974.
38. Rauch S, et al. Neuroimaging and the neuroanatomy of PTSD. *CNS Spectrums* 1998;3(Suppl) 2:31–33.
39. Shalev A, et al. Auditory startle response in trauma survivors with PTSD: a prospective study. *Amer J Psychiatry* 2000;157:255–261.
40. McDermid AJ, Rollman GB, McCain GA. Generalized hypervigilance in fibromyalgia: evidence of perceptual amplification. *Pain* 1996; 66:133–144.

41. van der Kolk BA, Perry JC, Herman JL. Childhood origins of self-destructive behavior. *Am J Psychiatry* 1991;148:1665–1671.
42. van der Kolk BA, Hostetler A, Herron N, et al. Trauma and the development of borderline personality disorder. *Psychiatr Clin North Am* 1994;17:715–730.
43. Brewer JB. Making memories: brain activity that predicts how well visual experience will be remembered. *Science* 1998;281:1185–1187.
44. Wagner AD, Schacter DL, Rotte M, et al. Building memories: remembering and forgetting of verbal experiences as predicted by brain activity. *Science* 1998;281:1188–1191.
45. Phelps EA, Anderson AK. Emotional memory: what does the amygdala do? *Curr Biol* 1997;7:311–314.
46. Goldman-Rakic PS. Regional and cellular fractionation of working memory. *Proc Natl Acad Sci USA* 1996;93:13473–13480.
47. Shi SH, Hayashi Y, Petralia RS, et al. Rapid spine delivery and redistribution of AMPA receptors after synaptic NMDA receptor activation. *Science* 1999;284:1811–1816.
48. Engert F, Bonhoeffer T. Dendritic spine changes associated with hippocampal long-term synaptic plasticity. *Nature* 1999;399:66–70.
49. Owen AM, Herrod NJ, Menon DK, et al. Redefining the functional organization of working memory processes within human lateral prefrontal cortex. *Eur J Neurosci* 1999;11:567–574.
50. D'Esposito M, Detre JA, Alsop DC, et al. The neural basis of the central executive system of working memory. *Nature* 1995;378:279–281.
51. Price DD, Harkins SW. The affective-motivational dimension of pain: a two stage model. *APS J* 1992b;1:229–239.
52. Shapiro F. *Eye movement desensitization and reprocessing.* New York: Guilford, 1995.
53. Price DD, Harkins SW. The affective-motivational dimension of pain: a two-stage model. *APS Journal* 1992;1:229–239.
54. Gracely RH. Affective dimensions of pain. How many and how measured? *APS Journal* 1992;1:243–247.
55. Weiss SR, Post RM. Caveats in the use of the kindling model of affective disorders. *Toxicol Ind Health* 1994;10:421–447.
56. Tang YP, Shimizu E, Dube GR, et al. Genetic enhancement of learning and memory in mice. *Nature* 1999;401:63–69.
57. Olsson T, Mohammet AH, Donaldson LF, et al. Glucocorticoid receptor and NGF1-A gene expression are induced in the hippocampus after environmental enrichment in adult rats. *Molec Brain Res* 1994;23:349–353.
58. Torasdotter M, Metsis M, Henriksson BF, et al. Environmental enrichment results in higher levels of nerve growth factor mRNA in the rat visual cortex and hippocampus. *Behav Brain Res* 1992;51:179–183.
59. Davidson RJ, Abercrombie H, Nitschke JB, et al. Regional brain function, emotion and disorders of emotion. *Curr Opin Neurobiol* 1999;9:228–234.
60. Courtney SM, Petit L, Haxby JV, et al. The role of prefrontal cortex in working memory: examining the contents of consciousness. *Philos Trans R Soc Lond B Biol Sci* 1998;353:1819–1828.
61. Gregory R. Brainy mind. *BMJ* 1999;317:1693–1695.
62. Graven-Nielsen T. Central hyperexcitability in fibromyalgia. *J Musculoskeletal Pain* 1999;7(1/2):261–272.
63. Bradley L, Young, LD, Anderson KO, et al. Abnormal regional cerebral blood flow in the caudate nucleus among fibromyalgia patients and non-patients is associated with insidious symptom onset. *J Musculoskeletal Pain* 1999;7(1/2)285–292.
64. Goodnick P, Klimas N. Chronic fatigue and related immune deficiency syndromes. Washington, DC: Amer Psychiatric Press 1993.
65. Goodnick P. Personal Communication, 1995.
66. Rapoport A, Sheftell F. *Headache relief.* New York: Simon & Schuster 1990.
67. Burstein R, Strassman A. Peripheral and central sensitization during migraine. In: Devor M, et al., eds. *Proceedings of the 9th World Congress on Pain.* Seattle: IASP Press, 2000:589–602.
68. Fordyce WE, Fowler RS, Lehmann JF, et al. Operant conditioning in the treatment of chronic pain. *Arch Phys Med Rehabil* 1973;54:399–408.
69. Fordyce WE. *Behavioral methods for chronic pain and illness.* St. Louis: Mosby, 1976.
70. Weisenberg M. Cognitive aspects of pain and pain control. *Int J Clin Exp Hypn* 1998;46:44–61.
71. Turk DC, Okifuji A. Evaluating the role of physical, operant, cognitive, and affective factors in the pain behaviors of chronic pain patients. *Behav Modif* 1997;21:259–280.
72. Ciccone DS, Grzesiak RC. Cognitive dimensions of chronic pain. *Soc Sci Med* 1984;19:1339–1345.
73. Turk DC, Thomas ER. The robustness of an empirically derived taxonomy of chronic pain patients. *Pain* 1990;43:27–35.
74. Kerns RD, Turk DC, Rudy TE. The West Haven-Yale Multidimensional Pain Inventory (WHYMPI). *Pain* 1985;23:345–356.
75. Brands AM, Schmidt AJ. Learning processes in the persistence behavior of chronic low back pain patients with repeated acute pain stimulation. *Pain* 1987;30:328–337.
76. Richard K. The occurrence of maladaptive health-related behaviors and teacher-rated conduct problems in children of chronic low back pain patients. *J Behav Med* 1988;11:107–116.
77. Gardea MA, Gatchel RJ. Interdisciplinary treatment of chronic pain. *Curr Rev Pain* 2000;4:18–23.
78. Flor H, Fydrich T, Turk DC. Efficacy of multidisciplinary pain treatment centers: a meta-analytic review. *Pain* 1992;49:221–230.
79. Blair DT, Ramones VA. Education as psychiatric intervention: the cognitive-behavioral context. *J Psychosoc Nurs Ment Health Serv* 1997;35:29–36.
80. Oei TP, Lim B, Young RM. Cognitive processes and cognitive behavior therapy in the treatment of problem drinking. *J Addict Dis* 1991;10:63–80.
81. Sullivan MJ, Reesor K, Mikail S, et al. The treatment of depression in chronic low back pain: review and recommendations. *Pain* 1991;50:5–13.
82. Haddock G, Tarrier N, Spaulding W, et al. Individual cognitive-behavior therapy in the treatment of hallucinations and delusions: a review. *Clin Psychol Rev* 1998;18:821–838.
83. Currie SR, Wilson KG, Pontefract AJ, et al. Cognitive-behavioral treatment of insomnia secondary to chronic pain. *J Consult Clin Psychol* 2000;68:407–416.
84. Hartl TL, Frost RO. Cognitive-behavioral treatment of compulsive hoarding: a multiple baseline experimental case study. *Behav Res Ther* 1999;37:451–461.
85. Tuschen-Caffier B, Florin I, Krause W, et al. Cognitive behavioral therapy for idiopathic infertile couples. *Psychother Psychosom* 1999;68:15–21.
86. Lopez Viets VC, Miller WR. Treatment approaches for pathological gamblers. *Clin Psychol Rev* 1997;17:689–702.
87. van Peski-Oosterbaan AS, Spinhoven P, van Rood Y, et al. Cognitive-behavioral therapy for non-cardiac chest pain: a randomized trial. *Am J Med* 1999;106:424–429.
88. Fishman B. The cognitive behavioral perspective on pain management in terminal illness. *Hosp J* 1992;8:73–78.
89. Puder RS. Age analysis of cognitive-behavioral group therapy for chronic pain outpatients. *Psychol Aging* 1988;3:204–207.
90. McCarthy AM, Cool VA, Hanrahan K. Cognitive behavioral interventions for children during painful procedures: research challenges and program development. *J Pediatr Nurs* 1998;13:55–63.
91. Chen E, Joseph MH, Zeltzer LK. Behavioral and cognitive interventions in the treatment of pain in children. *Pediatr Clin North Am* 2000;47:513–525.
92. Powers SR. Empirically supported treatments in pediatric psychology: procedure-related pain. *J Pediatr Psychol* 1999;24:131–145.
93. Thurber CA, Martin-Herz SP, Patterson DR. Psychological principles of burn wound pain in children. I: theoretical framework. *J Burn Care Rehabil* 2000;21:376–387.
94. Humphreys PA, Gevirtz RN. Treatment of recurrent abdominal pain: components analysis of four treatment protocols. *J Pediatr Gastroenterol Nutr* 2000;31:47–51.
95. Walco GA, Varni JW, Ilowite NT. Cognitive-behavioral pain management in children with juvenile rheumatoid arthritis. *Pediatrics* 1992;89:1075–1079.
96. Manetto C, McPherson SE. The behavioral-cognitive model of pain. *Clin Geriatr Med* 1996;12:461–471.
97. Luskin FM, Newell KA, Griffith M, et al. A review of mind/body therapies in the treatment of musculoskeletal disorders with implications for the elderly. *Altern Ther Health Med* 2000;6:46–56.
98. Cook AJ. Cognitive-behavioral pain management for the elderly nursing home residents. *J Gerontol B Psychol Sci Soc Sci* 1998;53:51–59.
99. Yamagami T. Psychotherapy, today and tomorrow: status quo of behavior and cognitive therapy and its efficacy. *Psychiatry Clin Neurosci* 1998;52:S236–237.

100. Keijsers GP, Schaap, CP, Hoogduin CA. The impact of interpersonal patient and therapist behavior on outcome in cognitive-behavior therapy. A review of empirical studies. *Behav Modif* 2000;24:264–297.

101. Dobson KS, Khatri N. Cognitive therapy: looking backward, looking forward. *J Clin Psychol* 2000;56:907–923.

102. Caudill M. Decreased clinic use by chronic pain patients: response to behavioral medicine intervention. *Clin J Pain* 1991;7:305–310.

103. Flor H, Turk DC. Etiological theories and treatments for chronic back pain. I. somatic models and interventions. *Pain* 1984;19:105–121.

104. Keefe FJ, Dunsmore J, Burnett R. Behavioral and cognitive-behavioral approaches to chronic pain: recent advances and future directions. *J Consult Clin Psychol* 1992;60:528–536.

105. Keefe FJ, Van Horn Y. Cognitive-behavioral treatment of rheumatoid arthritis pain: maintaining treatment gains. *Arthritis Care Res* 1993;6:213–222.

106. Morley S, Eccleston C, Williams A. Systematic review and meta-analysis of randomized controlled trials of cognitive behaviour therapy and behaviour therapy for chronic pain in adults, excluding headache. *Pain* 1999;80:1–13.

107. Turner, JA, Chapman CR. Psychological interventions for chronic pain: a critical review. II. Operant conditioning, hypnosis, and cognitive-behavioral therapy. *Pain* 1982;12:23–46.

108. Turk DC, Flor H. Etiological theories and treatments for chronic back pain. II. Psychological models and interventions. 1984;19: 209–233.

109. Tan SY, Leucht CA. Cognitive-behavioral therapy for clinical pain control: a 15-year update and its relationship to hypnosis. *Int J Clin Exp Hypn* 1997;45:396–416.

110. Peters ML, Schmidt AJ, Van den Hout MA. Chronic low back pain and the reaction to repeated acute pain stimulation. *Pain* 1989;39: 69–76.

111. Jensen MP, Romano JM, Turner JA, et al. Patient beliefs predicted patient functioning: further support for a cognitive-behavioural model of chronic pain. *Pain* 1999;81:95–104.

112. Ruoss M. Pain patients show a higher hindsight bias. *Z Exp Psychol* 1997;44:561–588.

113. Al-Obaidi SM, Nelson RM, Al-Awadhi S, et al. The role of anticipation and fear of pain in the persistence of avoidance behavior in patients with chronic low back pain. *Spine* 2000;25:1126–1131.

114. Wegner DM, Quillian F, Houston CE. Memories out of order: thought suppression and the disturbance of sequence memory. *J Pers Soc Psychol* 1996;71:680–691.

115. Wegner DM, Schneider DJ, Carter SR, et al. Paradoxical effects of thought suppression. *J Pers Soc Psychol* 1987;53:5–13.

116. Hasenbring M, Ulrich HW, Hartmann M, et al. The efficacy of a risk factor-based cognitive behavioral intervention and electromyographic biofeedback in patients with acute sciatic pain. An attempt to prevent chronicity. *Spine* 1999;24:2525–2535.

117. Neumann W, Kugler J, Pfand-Neumann P, et al. Psychological concepts in pain therapy practice. 2. Behavior therapy, self-management and overview of cognitive interventions. *Z Arztl Fortbild Qualitatssich* 1998;92:107–112.

118. Davison GC, Vogel RS, Coffman SG. Think-aloud approaches to cognitive assessment and the articulated thoughts in simulated situations paradigm. *J Consult Clin Psychol* 1997;65:950–958.

119. Rosenstiel AK, Keefe FJ. The use of coping strategies in chronic low back pain patients: relationship to patient characteristics and current adjustment. *Pain* 1983;17:33–44.

120. Blinchik ER, Grzesiak RC. Reinterpretative cognitive strategies in chronic pain management. *Arch Phys Med Rehabil* 1979;60:609–612.

121. Tan SY. Cognitive and cognitive-behavioral methods for pain control: a selective review. *Pain* 1982;12:201–228.

122. Turner JA. Educational and behavioral interventions for back pain in primary care. *Spine* 1996;21:2851–2857.

123. Laborde JM. Cognitive-behavioral techniques in the treatment of chronic low back pain: preliminary results. *J South Orthop Assoc* 1998;7:81–85.

124. Burns JA, Kubilus A, Michael E. Cognitive-behavioral factors in the management of chronic low back pain: conceptualization and evidence of treatment efficacy. *Curr Rev Pain* 1999;3:300–307.

125. Slater MA, Doctor JN, Pruitt SD, et al. The clinical significance of behavioral treatment for chronic low back pain: an evaluation of effectiveness. *Pain* 1997;71:257–263.

126. Kole-Snijders AM, Vlaeyen JW, Goossens ME, et al. Chronic low-back pain: what does cognitive coping skills training add to operant behavioral treatment: results of a randomized clinical trial. *J Consult Clin Psychol* 1999;67:931–944.

127. Johansson C, Dahl J, Jannert M, et al. Effects of a cognitive-behavioral pain-management program. *Behav Res Ther* 1998;36: 915–930.

128. Bradley LA. Cognitive-behavioral therapy for primary fibromyalgia. *J. Rheumatol Suppl* 1989;19:131–136.

129. Haldorsen EM, Kronholm K, Skouen JS, et al. Multimodal cognitive behavioral treatment of patients sicklisted for musculoskeletal pain: a randomized controlled study. *Scand J. Rheumatol* 1998;27:16–25.

130. Leibing E, Pfingsten M, Bartmann U, et al. Cognitive-behavioral treatment in unselected rheumatoid arthritis outpatients. *Clin J Pain* 1999;15:58–66.

131. Reesor KA, Craig KD. Medically incongruent chronic back pain: physical limitations, suffering, and ineffective coping. *Pain* 1988;32: 35–45.

132. Nicholas MK, Wilson PH, Goyen J. Comparison of cognitive-behavioral group treatment and an alternative non-psychological treatment for chronic low back pain. *Pain* 1992;48:339–347.

133. Schoenberger NE. Research on hypnosis as an adjunct to cognitive-behavioral psychotherapy. *Int J Clin Exp Hypn* 2000;48:154–169.

134. Montgomery GH, DuHamel KN, Redd WH. A meta-analysis of hypnotically induced analgesia: how effective is hypnosis: *Int J Clin Exp Hypn* 2000;48:138–153.

135. Edelson J, Fitzpatrick JL. A comparison of cognitive-behavioral and hypnotic treatments of chronic pain. *J Clin Psychol* 1989;45: 316–323.

136. Eimer BN. Clinical applications of hypnosis for brief and efficient pain management psychotherapy. *Am J Clin Hypn* 2000;43:17–40.

137. Spira JL, Speigel D. Hypnosis and related techniques in pain management. *Hosp J* 1992;8:89–119.

138. Liossi C, Hatira P. Clinical hypnosis versus cognitive behavioral training for pain management with pediatric cancer patients undergoing bone marrow aspirations. *Int J Clin Exp Hypn* 1999;47: 104–116.

139. Alden P, Heap M. Hypnotic pain control: some theoretical and practical issues. *Int J Clin Exp Hypn* 1998;46:62–76.

140. Rainville P, Carrier B, Hofbauer RK, et al. Dissociation of sensory and affective dimensions of pain using hypnotic modulation. *Pain* 1999b;82:159–171.

141. Hekmat H, Groth S, Rogers D. Pain ameliorating effect of eye movement desensitization and reprocessing. *J of Behavior Therapy and Experimental Psychiatry* 1994;25(2):121–129.

142. McCann DL. Post-traumatic stress disorder due to devastating burns overcome by a single session of eye-movement desensitization. *J of Behavior Therapy and Experimental Psychiatry* 1992;23: 319–323.

143. Wilson SA, Becker LA, Tinker RH. A pilot study into the use of EMDR in the treatment of phantom limb pain. Paper presented at the EMDRIA International Conference in San Francisco, 1997.

144. Grant, M. Pain control with eye movement desensitization and reprocessing. J. Lichti, Waterloo, ON, 1998.

145. Bergmann, U. Speculations on the neurobiology of EMDR. *Traumatology* 1998;4:1(2), 1–13.

146. Maquet P, Peters JM, Aerts J, et al. Functional neuroanatomy of human rapid-eye movement, sleep and dreaming. *Nature* 1996;383: 163–166.

147. Shapiro, F. Eye movement desensitization: a new treatment for post-traumatic stress disorder. *J Behavior Ther and Exper Psychiatry* 1989;20:211–217.

148. Carlson JG, Chemtob CM, Rusnak K, et al. Eye movement desensitization and reprocessing (EMDR) treatment for combat-related posttraumatic stress disorder. *Journal of Traumatic Stress* 1998; 11:13–24.

149. Wilson S, Becker L, Tinker R. Eye movement desensitization and reprocessing (EMDR) treatment for psychologically traumatized individuals. *J Consult Clin Psychol* 1995;63(6):928–937.

150. Wilson S, Becker L, Tinker R. Fifteen-month follow-up of eye movement desensitization & reprocessing (EMDR) treatment for posttraumatic stress disorder and psychological trauma. *J Consult Clin Psychol* 1997;65(6):1047–1056.

CHAPTER 15

Alternative Therapies

John C. Haasis

Chronic pain is commonly defined as pain that persists for longer than the expected time for healing, usually long after the tissue damage that initially triggered the onset of pain has resolved (1). Chronic pain is one of the most prevalent and costly health issues known, affecting approximately 50 million Americans annually at a cost of $100 billion per year (2). Because conventional medical treatments for chronic pain diagnoses quite often fail to provide patients with significant pain relief, it is no surprise that "complementary" or "alternative" therapies are becoming increasingly popular (3,4). A growing number of insurance carriers, as well as managed care organizations, are now offering alternative and complementary medicine benefits (5). The mainstreaming of alternative medicine can also be seen at many major U.S. medical schools, where alternative medicine courses are being incorporated into the teaching curriculum (6).

The decision to integrate complementary medicine with conventional therapies can be extremely rewarding. It gives people who have often failed traditional medical care a chance to improve (7). Choosing the right alternative practitioner to provide advice regarding complementary therapies is crucial (8). The success of complementary care is dependent upon both a knowledgeable patient and a care provider with good communication skills and clinical expertise (9).

Complementary medicine offers a wide variety of alternative health techniques (10–12). Some of these address structural and mechanical imbalances (13–15), whereas others address the importance of proper body biochemistry (16,17), emotional balance (18,19), and body energetics (20,21). It is quite apparent that the various alternative techniques differ in their approach to wellness. It is acknowledged, however, that they all share common philosophical ground. Emphasis is placed on the individual, empowering the individual to accept responsibility regarding medical treatment and related health maintenance issues. Proper nutrition, exercise, and a balanced emotional state are stressed. Treating the patient rather than a symptom is emphasized.

BODYWORK

Bodywork is a term that refers to therapeutic treatments designed to encourage the proper structure and functioning of the human body (22,23). The aim of bodywork is to promote an environment that allows the body to restore itself to equilibrium and balance. In all of its focus, the therapeutic benefits of bodywork are undeniable.

For thousands of years, some form of therapeutic touch has been used to treat the sick (24,25). Ancient Greek and Roman physicians used massage as a principal form of relieving pain and suffering. Bodywork can reduce pain by stimulating the release of naturally occurring endorphins (26,27), soothe injured tissue by decreasing spasm and improving circulation (28), and reduce stress by promoting a greater sense of well-being (29,30).

Massage

Therapeutic massage, a form of bodywork, has been shown to be beneficial in a wide variety of musculoskeletal disorders, including muscle spasm and pain, spinal curvatures, headaches, temporomandibular joint syndrome (TMJ), mechanical body pain, and whiplash injuries (14,31). Massage involves systematically stroking, kneading, and/or pressing the soft tissue of the entire body in order to induce a state of total relaxation promoting the body's regenerative capacity and an individual's self-healing ability (32).

Scientific evidence indicates that massage therapy has a sedative effect upon the nervous system promoting muscle relaxation and restoration of normal muscle tone (33). Numerous studies demonstrate the benefit of massage in promoting recovery from fatigue and illness (34). Massage can also help reduce swelling from acute injuries and improve body motion as well as circulation. Additional studies indicate massage is useful in the treatment of chronic inflammatory conditions, including adhesions and tissue fibrosis, which can accompany injury or immobilization. On a mental and spiritual level, massage therapy not only relieves stress and anxiety, but also helps people to become more conscious of their own self-being and be more inclined to take responsibility for their own happiness and health.

Rolfing

Rolfing, the popular name for structural integration, is another form of contemporary bodywork. The philosophy of rolfing is based on the idea that human function is improved when segments of the body are properly aligned (35). Structural integration involves a series of provider-patient encounters during which one person manipulates another's body in a systematic way aimed at evoking a more optimal alignment.

Biochemist Ida P. Rolf, Ph.D., founded the Rolf Institute for Structural Integration in 1970. Her beliefs are based on several assumptions generated from years of observation and experimentation (36). She believes the body functions best when it is in balance. Most people are not aware if and when their bodies are out of balance. If any one segment of the body is in an out-of-balance position, a compensatory change occurs in other segments of the body (head, torso, pelvis, arms, legs, and feet), resulting in impaired movement, decreased function, and emotional stress. Dr. Rolf identified the fascia as the organ of change. In chronic pain states, stress, or trauma, physiological changes occur within the fascia affecting movement of muscles and joints.

Rolfers use deep tissue manipulation techniques by applying pressure with fingers, knuckles, and elbows to release suspected adhesions and restore balance. Research on the effects of structural integration conducted at UCLA's Department of Kinesiology indicate that rolfing has a positive impact on body movement, energetics, and posture (37). Subjective reports of reduced stress, improved self-image, and general well-being are frequently reported (38).

Reflexology

In addition to therapeutic massage and structural integration, reflexology is another system of bodywork used to relieve stress and promote well-being (39). Unlike massage therapy and rolfing, reflexology is an energy-based system of bodywork based on the concept that there are areas or reflex points on the hands and feet that correspond to each organ, gland, and structure in the body. By working these reflex points, there is a stimulating effect on specific body parts, promoting a decrease in congestion, inflammation, and tension (40).

The foundations of modern reflexology grew out of earlier work performed by Dr. William Fitzgerald and a system known as zone therapy. Dr. Fitzgerald discovered that by applying pressure to key points on the extremities, he was able to bring about normal physiological functioning in other parts of the body. He postulated the existence of 10 energy zones ascending longitudinally from the base of the feet to the top of the head. Energy is constantly flowing through channels, which terminate to form reflex points on the hands and feet. When energy flow is decreased or obstructed, congestion develops and manifests itself physically as a disease of the body part or organ system. When the reflexes are treated, blocked energy flows, restoring balance and harmony to the body (41).

Eunice Ingham, a physiotherapist, applied Dr. Fitzgerald's work and developed reflexology into the science it is today. She discovered that the feet are more responsive to pressure than the hands. She mapped organ reflexes on the feet and developed techniques to maximize the healing effect of reflex point stimulation (42).

All of the contemporary systems of bodywork utilize the therapeutic use of touch. For centuries, some form of laying on of the hands has been used to heal and promote well-being (43). Everyone needs to relax and escape from life's daily pressures. Stress management strategies incorporating bodywork techniques enable the body to maintain balance and equilibrium (44). In addition to the physical benefits obtained from bodywork sessions, a heightened spiritual awareness is reached. Bodywork techniques create the environment and circumstance through which self-healing can proceed (45).

HERBAL MEDICINE

A significant portion of alternative medicine practices today focuses on an individual's desire to maintain proper body biochemical balance. Herbal remedies, diet, and nutritional supplements are used by many individuals seeking nontraditional modalities to maintain homeostasis (46).

The medicinal use of herbs, plants, and plant products, referred to as herbal medicine (47), is the most ancient form of health care (48,49). Texts from the ancient cultures of China, Greece, Egypt, and India document the use of many therapeutically active plant products. Today, approximately 80% of the world's population use herbal remedies for healing, protecting, and regulating their body health. Herbal remedies account for a significant portion of alternative medicine practices in the United States (50).

Herbs are derived from flowers, roots, seeds, fruit, bark, or any other plant part. They are used to treat acute and chronic illnesses as well as improve quality of life. The herbal renaissance being experienced in the United States is felt to be due in part to the general public's concern about the high cost of health care, the side effects of many commonly prescribed pharmaceutical drugs, and the ongoing research attesting to the medicinal value of herbal remedies (51,52).

Over 600 medicinal herbs have been comprehensively profiled (53), including common varieties such as aloe vera, cayenne, chamomile, echidna, ephedra, feverfew, garlic, ginger, ginza, ginseng, goldenseal, St. John's wort, saw palmetto, witch hazel, and senna. These medicinal herbs have been shown to be of value in a wide range of physical ailments, including chronic skin disorders, constipation and diarrhea, joint and muscle pain, anxiety and depression, menstrual irregularities, headaches, and circulatory and neurological dysfunctions (54–67).

Herbs contain many naturally occurring chemicals. An herb's mechanism of action or chemical effect may be due to a specific chemical present in the herb or a result of a complex interaction between herb constituents. Given the growing popularity of herbal medicine and the potential adverse interaction with prescribed pharmaceutical agents (68), treating physicians and patients should be well informed.

DIET

As an increasing number of physicians integrate alternative therapies into their practice, proper diet and nutritional supplements are receiving well-deserved attention. Mainstream medicine has acknowledged the central role that diet plays in chronic diseases, including atherosclerosis, hypertension, cerebral vascular disease, diabetes, and cancer (69); however, it has failed to educate the public regarding the omnipresent contamination found in the American food supply (70).

For many years, the Food and Drug Administration (FDA) has allowed the great food conglomerates to grow and process foods with hundreds of questionable chemicals. A balanced diet, such as fruits and vegetables, no longer ensures proper health (71). One must not only be aware of what food to eat, but also pay close attention to where it was grown or raised and what chemical it may have come in contact with (72).

Some suggest that long-term exposure to pesticides, industrial pollutants, dyes, antibiotics, and hormones may play a role in the development of chronic disease (73). In his book *Diet for a Poisoned Planet,* David Steinman writes, "Sometimes it seems that nothing is safe to eat, and that we live in a constant state of food anxiety . . . , but you must not feel helpless. There is plenty of safe, delicious food to eat. And for your own well-being, you need to find it." He suggests eating food as low on the food chain as possible to minimize exposure to food laden with pesticides.

Proponents of both complementary and traditional medicine agree that there are benefits in moving toward a vegetarian-based diet. Published reports show that a vegetarian lifestyle can reduce the risk of colon cancer, obesity, hypertension, heart disease, and diabetes. By also using an

exercise program and stress management strategies, chronic degenerative diseases can also be reversed (74,75).

Nutritional Supplements

Many Americans take nutritional supplements on a daily basis (76). Some believe supplements are part of an increasingly popular trend as more people take a proactive approach to health care (77). Research suggests that diet alone may not provide sufficient nutrients to maintain good health (78,79). Data compiled by the U.S. Department of Agriculture (USDA), as well as by the National Health Survey, indicate a significant number of Americans are not receiving the recommended daily allowance (RDA) of many vitamins and essential minerals (80).

A typical American diet contains significant amounts of fat and refined sugars regarded as having low or no nutritional density. *Nutritional density* is defined as the ratio of nutrients to calories. A diet low in nutritional density, coupled with stressful life patterns (81), can produce mild to moderate deficient states. Subtle nutritional imbalances can result in a variety of symptoms, including insomnia, mood swings, fatigue, nervousness, muscle weakness, and inability to concentrate (82,83). Nutritional supplements can often correct these imbalances (84,85) and promote optimal physical and psychological health.

MIND/BODY MEDICINE

Patients, as well as physicians, are reluctant to acknowledge the profound interconnection of psychological and physical variables (86). For hundreds of years, technological advancements have changed the "art" of medicine. The biomedical model has certainly produced wondrous achievements, but it also has led patients and physicians alike to lose sight of the extraordinary power of the mind and its ability to affect healing (87). *Mind/body medicine* is an umbrella term covering therapies that focus on the interrelationship between mind and body (88,89). The individual is an active player in all forms of treatment rather than a passive recipient of medical intervention.

The goal in most forms of mind/body medicine is stress reduction. A basic tenet in mind/body therapies is that chronic stress and lack of balance result in illness and disease (90). Some major categories of mind/body intervention include meditation, hypnosis, imagery, music therapy, and aromatherapy. Through mind/body techniques, an individual acquires the ability to consciously control involuntary systems.

Meditation

Meditation, broadly defined as an activity that keeps one's attention pleasantly anchored in the present moment, is a type of mental practice that has been shown to elicit the "relaxation response," a complex physiological reaction opposite of the "stress response" (91). Repeated elicitation of the relaxation response can lead to profound psychological and physiological changes (92). Meditation techniques can lead to spiritual growth and be a source of personal insight and self-awareness (93). Physiological benefits include improved stress control and pain management.

Hypnosis

Hypnosis and imagery are additional forms of mind/body medicine that use the power of the mind to evoke positive physiological change. *Hypnosis* can be defined as an altered state of consciousness in which the individual has intense focal concentration coupled with a relative suspension of peripheral awareness (94). The intensity of focus allows the hypnotized person to make maximal use of innate abilities to control perception, memory, and somatic function.

A person experiencing hypnosis routinely describes an altered consciousness or dissociative state (95). Hypnosis requires a skilled therapist to guide the individual through the multiple levels of trance phenomenon. After training, an individual can perform self-hypnosis.

Despite extensive research, the hypnotic mechanism of action is unclear. Ample evidence exists, however, supporting its clinical efficiency in pain management (96). Hypnotic pain control can be easily learned and applied, providing an individual with an additional tool for controlling illness and pain.

Imagery

Visualization techniques, including guided imagery, are a form of distraction. The aim of distraction is to focus one's attention away from a painful event or situation to a pleasant experience (97). Imagery has been shown to affect heart rate, blood pressure, gastrointestinal motility, local blood flow, secretions, neurotransmitters, and immune function (98,99).

Clinically, imagery has been successfully applied in cardiac rehabilitation programs, stress-management clinics, chronic pain programs, and cancer treatment facilities. The healing potential of guided imagery extends beyond its ability to dramatically affect physiology. Being able to relax is a fundamental aspect of self-healing. Arguably, imagery is one of the easiest ways to learn to relax (100).

Music Therapy

Music therapy offers another option when considering mind/body medicine (101). It has been extensively studied in the palliative care setting. Music therapy used in this environment has been shown to raise a patient's pain threshold and alleviate the distress of patients and family members (102). Researchers in the field of music therapy believe music alters the affective, cognitive, and sensory components of the pain experience, resulting in the perception of reduced pain (103).

Aromatherapy

Aromatherapy is a unique brand of mind/body medicine that essentially uses oils extracted from plants for the treatment and prevention of disease (104). Aromatherapy is said to be a holistic therapy in that aromatherapists select an essential oil or combination to suit each individual's symptom and personality (105). Each essential oil is said to contain approximately 100 chemical constituents with a host of pharmacological properties, including antiviral, antibacterial, antispasmodic, and antiinflammatory effects (106).

Aromatherapy is most widely used for stress-related health issues. Some aromatherapists believe aromatherapy can be used quite successfully in a number of medical conditions, including skin infection and respiratory disorders (107). The most common method of essential oil application is massage. At times, however, oils are added to baths, ingested, or inhaled.

Aromatherapists believe that using touch is particularly important in the application and in the treatment of pain. Massage encourages the penetration of essential oils through the skin and into the system circulation, where the analgesic components within essential oils react.

The odor of most essential oils is pleasurable. Aromatherapists believe an oil's smell has beneficial effects on health via stimulation of the olfactory nerves and limbic system, producing a tranquilizing effect and promoting a calmness and sense of well-being (108).

HOMEOPATHY

Unlike conventional medical therapy and allopathic philosophy, many complementary therapies focus on body energetics rather than anatomic concepts when addressing a patient's symptom complex. Two such treatments are homeopathy and acupuncture. Homeopathy is one of the most frequently used complementary therapies worldwide (109). Founded in the last part of the eighteenth century by German physician Samuel Hakneman, homeopathy has been proven to be effective in treating diseases for which traditional medicine has had little to offer (110).

The term *homeopathy* has its origin in the Greek word *homois*, meaning "similar," and *pathos*, meaning "suffering." The basic purpose of homeopathic medicine is "like curves like" (111). Natural substances from plants, minerals, and animals that produce a pattern of illness in large doses stimulate the body's natural healing response when diluted. The FDA acknowledges homeopathic remedies as official drugs.

Controversy exists within the scientific community regarding the therapeutic action of highly diluted homeopathic remedies (112). Prominent researchers believe homeopathic remedies convey a unique electromagnetic "message" to the body that corresponds to the apparent electromagnetic frequency present with illness, promoting the self-healing response (113).

Homeopathy is an energetic-based form of natural medicine. Articles published in the *British Medical Journal, The Lancet,* and *The British Journal of Chemical Pharmacology* attest to the benefits of homeopathic remedies (114–116). The World Health Organization believes homeopathy should be integrated into mainstream medicine worldwide (117).

The trend toward integration of complementary and alternative-based therapies will continue as patients' interest in nontraditional treatments grows.

ACUPUNCTURE

Acupuncture is a popular form of alternative health care. It is an ancient eastern therapeutic technique based on the belief that health is determined by a balanced flow of vital energy termed Qi (pronounced "chee") (118). According to the principles of traditional Chinese medicine, the workings of the human body are controlled by Qi, which circulates between organs and along 12 energy pathways called meridians (119).

The philosophy of acupuncture is quite distinct from that of allopathic medicine. Organs are considered energetic, not anatomic, with realms of influence expanded from their conventional medical physiology (120). The concept of disturbance in Qi as a basic causative factor in disease and illness is a primary tenet. Treatment is based on manipulation of the energy flow by placement of special needles into points along meridian lines to encourage the flow of Qi, relieve blockages, and restore balance.

Acupuncture is considered by many to be a complete system of disease management. The World Health Organization (121) and the National Institutes of Health (122) have identified many conditions that acupuncture can treat, including addiction, nausea, asthma, carpal tunnel, fibromyalgia, headache, low back pain, myofascial pain, osteoarthritis, stroke rehabilitation, and tennis elbow. Proponents of acupuncture not only advocate its use as a first-time treatment, but also note its clinical value when used in an adjuvant role.

As noted earlier, acupuncture can treat a wide range of conditions. Following diagnosis, acupuncture needles are placed in any one of over 1000 accupoints on the body. Although it is still unclear the exact mechanism or mechanisms underlying acupuncture's mode of action, western scientific research has suggested that acupuncture might act by the principle of the gate control theory (123). Other theories include the suggestion that both ascending and descending neural pathways are modulated via the production of endorphins serotonin and acetylcholine within the CNS (124).

CONCLUSION

The barriers between alternative medicine and traditional medical practices appear to be falling. Increasingly, more and more individuals who are unhappy with conventional therapies are utilizing complementary services. It is apparent that the general public is recognizing the effectiveness of alternative medicine's holistic approach to health.

REFERENCES

1. Mersky H, Bogdick N. *Classification of chronic pain,* 2nd ed. Seattle: IASP Press, 1994:1.
2. Bergnir P, et al. The U.S. health care, costs crisis; a crisis of chronic disease. *American Ass. Of Naturopathic physicians* (Sept 1992).
3. Eisenberg DM, et al. Trends in alternative medicine use in the United States, 1990–1997. *JAMA* 1998;280:1569–1575.
4. Asten JA. Why patients use alternative medicine: results of a national study. *JAMA* 1998;279:1548–1553.
5. Pelletier KR, et al. Current trends in the integration and reimbursement of complementary and alternative medicine by managed care, insurance carriers, and hospital providers. *Am. J Health Promot* 1997; 12:112–122.
6. Wetzel MS, et al. Courses involving complementary and alternative medicine at US medical schools. *JAMA* 1998;280:784–787.
7. Kaptchuler TJ, Essemberg DM. The persuasive appeal of alternative medicine. *Ann Intern Med* 1998;129:1061–1065.
8. Essenberg DM. Advising patients who seek alternative medical therapies. *Ann Intern Med* 1997;127:61–69.
9. *Medical Economics* Aug. 7, 2000.
10. Berman B, Larson DB, Suyers JP, eds. Alternative medicine: expanding medical horizons. Bethesda, MD: National Institutes of Health. *NIH publication No. 94-066,* 1994.
11. British Medical Association. *Complementary medicine: new approaches to good practice.* Oxford, UK: Oxford University Press, 1993:138–141.
12. Lewith G, Kenyon J, Lewis P. *Complementary medicine: an integrated approach.* Oxford, UK: Oxford University Press, 1996.
13. The Bodywork Knowledge Base is an abstracted collection of the world literature on massage compiled by Richard Van Wiley, available from the American Massage Therapy Association.
14. Yates J. *A physicians guide to therapeutic massage.* Canada: Massage Therapists Association of British Columbia, 1990.
15. Rolf I. *Rolfing: the integration of human structures.* New York: Harper and Row, 1977.
16. Steinman D. *Diet for a poisoned planet.* New York: Ballantine Books, 1990.
17. Pao EM, et al. Problem nutrients in the United States. *Food Technology* Sept 1981:58–79.
18. Antonio MH, et al. Cognitive-behavioral stress management intervention buffers distress responses and immunologic changes following notification of HIV-I seropositivity. *Journal of Consulting and Clinical Psychology* Dec 1991;59(6):906–915.
19. Shapiro DH, Walsh RN *Meditation: classic and contemporary perspectives.* New York: Aldine 1984.
20. Lange, A, Homeopathy. In: Pezzorus JE and Murray MT, eds. *A textbook of natural medicine.* Seattle WA: John Bostyr College Publications, 1989.
21. Eisenberg D, et al. *Encounters with Qi: exploring chinese medicine,* 2nd ed. New York: Penguin Books, 1987:77.
22. Cherkin DC, Mooty RD, eds. Chiropractic in the United States: training, practice, and research. *Publication no. 98-N002.* Rockville, MD: Agency for Health Care Policy and Research, Dec 1997.
23. Koes BW, et al. Spinal manipulation and mobilization for back and neck pain: a blended review. *BMJ* 1991;303:1298–1303.
24. Ernest E, Fralka V. The clinical effectiveness of massage therapy—a critical review. *Fossel Konplementasmed* 1994;1:226–232.
25. Ernest E. Mechanotherapic. *WMW* 1994;20/21:504–508.
26. Christian GF, et al. Immunoreactive ACTH, beta endorphin and central levels in plasma following manipulative therapy. *Spine* 1998;13:1411–1417.

27. Day JA, et al. The effect of massage on serum level of beta endorphin and beta hypatophic in healthy adults *Physical Therapy* 1987;67:926–930.
28. Wright A. Hypoalgerin port-manipulative therapy: a review of a potential neurophysiological mechanism. *Manual Therapy* 1995;1:11–16.
29. Krieger D. *The therapeutic touch: how to use your hands to help or heal.* Englewood Cliffs, NJ: Prentice-Hall, 1979.
30. Heidt P. Effects of therapeutic touch in anxiety levels of hospitalized patients. *Nursing Research* 1981;30: 32.
31. Quebec Task Force on Spinal Disorders. Scientific zpproach to the assessment and management of activity—related spinal disorders. A monograph for clinicians. *Spine* Sept 12 1982;7(Suppl):51–59.
32. Liedell L, et al. *The book of massage: complete step-by-step guide to eastern and western techniques.* New York: Fireside/Gaia Books, 1984.
33. Beard G. *Beard's massage.* 3d ed. Philadelphia: W.B. Saunders Company, Reprint 1981.
34. Weintraub M. Alternative medical care. Shiatsu, Swedish muscle massage, and trigger point suppression in spinal pain syndrome. *American Journal of Pain Management* 1992;2(2);74–78.
35. Rolf I. *Rolfing: the integration of human structures.* New York: Harper and Row, 1988.
36. Rolf IP. *Structural integration: gravity, an unexplored factor in a more human use of human beings.* Boulder, CO: Rolf Institute, 1962. New ed. San Francisco, CA: Guild for Structural Integration, 1962.
37. Cannolby L. "Ida Rolf." *Human Behavior G* May 1977;5:17–23.
38. Cottingham J, et al. Inclination angle and parasympathetic tone produced by rolfing soft tissue manipulation. *Physical Therapy* Sep. 1988;68(9):1364–1370.
30. Byers DC. *Better health with foot reflexology—the original Ingham method.* 4th ed. St. Petersburg, FL: Ingham Publishing, 1983.
40. Flocco B. *A reflexology and premenstrual syndrome research study.* A paper given at the International Council of Reflexologists Conference: Reflexology Around the World. Virginia Beach, VA: 1991 (the paper is printed in a transcript of that conference): 35–49.
41. Kunz K, Kunz B. *Hand and foot reflexology: a self-help guide.* St. Louis: Fireside Books, 1992.
42. Norman L. *Feet first: a guide to foot reflexology.* St. Louis: Fireside Books, 1988.
43. Johnson D. *Body, spirit, and democracy.* Berkeley, CA: North Atlantic Books, 1993.
44. Downing G. *The massage book.* New York: Random House, 1972.
45. Kabat-Zunn J. *Full catastrophe living: using the wisdom of your body and mind to face stress, pain, and illness.* New York: Dell, 1990.
46. Casper J. *Food—your miracle medicine: how food can prevent and cure over 100 symptoms and problems.* New York: Harper-Collins, 1993.
47. Bensky D, Gamble A. *Chinese herbal medicine: material medicine.* Revised edition. Seattle: Easland Press, 1993.
48. Castleman M. *The healing herbs: the ultimate guide to the curative power of nature's medicines.* New York: Bantam, 1995.
49. Herb Trade Association. *Definition of "herb."* Austin, TX: Herb Trade Association, 1977.
50. Eisenberg DM, et al. Unconventional medicine in the United States—prevalence, cost, and patterns of use. *N Engl J Med.* 1993;328:246–252.
51. Landtrack Report on Public Perception of Alternative Care. *Alternative Therapies* 1998;4:29.
52. Fransworth NR, et al. Medicinal plants in therapy. *Bulletin of the World Health Organization* 1985;63(6):965–981.
53. German Ministry of Health. *Commission E monographs for phytomedicines.* Bonn, Germany: German Ministry of Health, 1984.
54. Henry CJ. Effect of spiced food on metabolic rate. Human Nutrition. *Clinical Nutrition.* Mar. 1986;40(2):165–168.
55. German Ministry of Health. Chamomile flowers. *Commission E. monographs for phytomedicines.* Bonn, Germany. GMH, 1984.
56. German Ministry of Health. Echidna purpurea leaf. *Commission E. monographs for phytomedicines.* Bonn Germany: German Ministry of Health, 1989.
57. Hobbs C. Valerian. A literature review. *Herbal Gram* 1989;21:19-34.
58. Foster S. Garlic. *Botanical series 311.* Austin, TX: *America Botanical Journal,* 1991.
59. Grontved A, et al. *Ginger root against seasickness.*
60. Bone, ME, et al. Ginger root—a new antiemetic: the effect of ginger root on postoperative nausea and vomiting after mason gynecological surgery. *Anesthesia* Aug. 1990;45(8): 669–671.
61. Foster S. Ginkga. *Botanical Series 304.* Austin, TX: American Botanical Counsel, 1991.
62. Yamamoto M, Vemura T. *Endocrinological and metabolic actions of P. ginseng principles* Proceeding 3rd International Ginseng Symposium 1980:115–119.
63. Hobbs C. Hawthorne. *A literature review. Herbal Grain* 1990;21: 19–33.
64. Hoffmann D. *The new holistic herbal.* Rockport, MA: Element, Inc., 1991:204.
65. Suzuki O, et al. Inhibition of monoamine oxidose. *Hypenicin Planta Medica* 1984;50:272–274.
66. Duvia R, et al. Advances in phytotherapy of prostatic hypertrophy. *Med Praxis* 1982; 4:143–145.
67. German Ministry of Health. Senna. *Commission E. monographs for phytomedicines.* Bonn, Germany: German Ministry Health, 1984.
68. Spyker D. Reports of exposure to dietary supplement and traditional remedies to AADCC/AACT: the need for cooperation with the FDA. *J Toxicol Clin Toxicol* 1996;34:618.
69. *The Surgeon General's Report on Nutrition.* U.S. Government Printing Office, 1988.
70. Robbins J. *Diet for a new America.* Walpole, NH: Shellpoint, 1987.
71. Ballentine R. *Transition to vegetarianism: an evolutionary process.* Humalayan Press, 1987.
72. Steinman,D. *Diet for a poisoned planet.* New York: Ballentine Books, 1990:4.
73. Jamisson E. *Medical, environmental, and economic information on: nitrates, nitrates, niboso—compounds. Why American exposure needs to be reduced by more than 50 percent.* Washington, D.C.: National Network to Prevent Birth Defects, Aug. 1, 1987.
74. Ornish D. *Dr. Dean Ornish's program for reversing heart disease.* New York: Random House, 1990.
75. Ornish D, et al. Can lifestyle changes reverse coronary heart disease? *Lancet* July 21, 1990;336:129–133.
76. Yankelovich L, et al. Survey for nutritional health alliance 1992: *Whole Foods Magazine* Mar, 1993;16(3):55.
77. Balch JF, et al. *Prescription for nutritional healing.* Garden City Park, NY: Avery, 1990.
78. Pao EM. Problem nutrients in the United States. *Food Technology* Sep, 1981:58–79.
79. Wenbach M. Common nutritional deficiencies–part 2, *Townsend Letters for Doctors,* Feb.-Mar. 1995:24.
80. Dietary Intake Source Data: U.S. 1976-1980. Data from the National Health Survey, series 11, #231. DHHS Publication (PHS) 8361 (Mar, 1983).
81. Brin M. Drugs and environmental chemicals relation to vitamin needs. In: Hathcoch J, ed. *Nutrition and drug interrelations.* New York: Academic Press, 1978:131–150.
82. Brin M. *Examples of behavioral changes in marginal vitamin deficiencies in the ran and man.* Natural Institute of Health Publication no. 79-1906 Aug, 1979:272–277.
83. Machlin L, et al. Vitamin E. In: Alfin-Slater R, Kritchersky D, eds. *Human nutrition—a comprehensive treatise,* vol. 3, New York: Plenum Press, 1980.
84. Braverman ER, et al. *The healing nutrients within: facts, findings, and new research on amino acids.* New Canaan, CT: Keats Publishing, 1987.
85. Benton D, et al. *Effect of vitamin and mineral supplementation on intelligence of sample of school children.* Lancet 1 no. 8578 Jan, 1988:140–143.
86. Justice B. *Who gets sick: how beliefs, moods, and thought affect your health.* Los Angeles: Jeremy P. Torcher, 1987.
87. Spiegel, D. *Living beyond limits: a scientific mind-body approach to facing life-threatening illness.* New York: Fawcett, 1994.
88. Moyers B. *Healing and the mind.* New York: Doubleday, 1993.
89. Bonysenko J. *Minding the body, mending the mind.* New York: Bantam Books, 1988.
90. Jaffe D. *Healing from within.* New York: Simon and Schuster, 1988.
91. Benson H, et al. The relaxation response, *Psychiatry* 1974;37:37–46.
92. Hoffman JW, et al. Reduced sympathetic nervous system responsivity associated with the relaxation response. *Science,* 1982;215: 190–192.
93. Goleman D. *The meditative mind.* Los Angeles: J.P. Tarcher, 1988.
94. Cheek D. *Hypnosis: the application of ideomotor techniques.* Boston: Allyn, 1993.

95. Murphy M. *The future of the body: explorations into the further evaluation of human nature.* Los Angeles: J.P. Tarcher/Perigie Books, 1993.

96. *Mind-body intervention, in alternative medicine: expanding medical horizons. A Report to the NIH on alternative medical system and practices in the United States,* NIH pub. No. 94-006 Washington, D.C.: US Government Printing Office, 1994.

97. McCarthy AM, et al. Cognitive behavioral pain and anxiety intervention in pediatric oncology centers and bone marrow transplant units. *Journal of Pediatric Oncology Nursing* 1996;13:3–12.

98. Murphy M. *The future of the body.* Los Angeles: J.P. Tarcher, 1992.

99. Sheikh AA, et al. *Psychosomatic and mental imagery. In the potential of fantasy and imagination.* New York: Brandon, 1979.

100. Dienstfrey H. *Where the mind meets the body.* New York: Harper-Collins, 1991.

101. Bassano M. *Healing with music and color: a beginner's guide.* York Beach, Maine: Samual Weiser, 1992.

102. O'Callaghan CC Pain, music creativity, and music therapy in palliative care. *The American Journal of Hospice and Palliative Care* March/April, 1996.

103. Trauger-Quersy B, et al. Balancing the focus: art and music therapy for pain control and symptom management in hospice care. *The Hospice Journal* 1999; 14(1).

104. Joyeux AM. Aromatherapy and healing fragrances. *Pract Nuvs* 1994;5(20):25–26.

105. Tesserand RB. *The art of aromatherapy.* Rochester, Vermont: Healing Arts Press, 1977.

106. Vichers A. *Massage and aromatherapy. A guide for health professionals.* London: Chapman & Hall, 1996.

107. Janssen AM, et al. Antimicrobial activity of essential oils: 1976-1986. Literature review. Aspects of the test methods. *Planta Med* 1987;53:395–398.

108. Dodd GH. *Receptor events in perfumery. The psychology and biology of fragrance.* London: Chapman and Hull, 1985.

109. Ullman D. *Discovering homeopathy: medicine for the 21st century.* Berkeley, CA: North Atlanta, 1991.

110. Leviton R. Homeopathy. *Yoga Journal* no. 85 Mar/Apr 1989:42–51, 97–98, 100, 105.

111. Lange A. Homeopathy. *In a Textbook of Natural Medicine.* Seattle, WA: John Bustyr College Publication, 1989.

112. Rubik,B. Frontiers of homeopathic research. *Frontier Perspectives 2* Philadelphia: Temple University, Center for Frontier Sciences, Spring/Summer 1991;1.

113. Gerber R. *Vibratimal medicine.* Santa Fe, NM: Bear and Company, 1988:84.

114. Kleignen J, et al. Clinical trial of homeopathy. *British Medical Journal* 302 Feb, 1991:316–323.

115. Shipley M, et al. Controlled trial of homeopathic treatment of osteoarthritis. *The Lancet* 1983:97–98.

116. Ferley JP, et al. A controlled evaluation of a homeopathic preparation in the treatment of influenza-like syndromes. *British Journal of Clinical Pharmacology* Mar. 1989;27:329–335.

117. Bannerman RH, et al. *Traditional medicine and health care coverage.* Geneva, Switzerland: World Health Organization, 1983.

118. O'Conner J, et al. *Acupuncture: a comprehensive text.* Shunghai College of Traditional Medicine. Chicago, IL: Easland Press, 1981.

119. Stux G.,et al. *Acupuncture: textbook and atlas.* New York: Springer-Verbag, 1987.

120. Helms JM. An overview of medical acupuncture. *Alternative Therapies* May 1998; 4(3): 35–45.

121. Helms JM. Report on WHO consultation on acupuncture. *Med Acupunct* 1997;7(1).

122. Acupuncture—NIH consensus conference. *JAMA* November 4, 1998;280(17).

123. Melzoch R, Wall PD. Pain mechanism: a new theory. *Science 1965* 150: 971–979.

124. Han JS, et al. Neurochemical basis of acupuncture analgesia. *Ann Rev Pharmacal* 1982;22:193–220.

CHAPTER **16**

Opioid Analgesics

Kenneth C. Jackson, II and Arthur G. Lipman

Opioids remain the most effective analgesics available, yet these drugs remain the most misunderstood of all analgesics. Much of the opioid pharmacology learned by health professionals is based on animal model data or studies in isolated tissues. Such studies cannot simulate the profound impact of cognition on pain and analgesia that so greatly influences opioid treatment outcomes in humans. Confusion about opioids among health-care professionals results from the failure to recognize the great differences between potential acute opioid toxicity and the relative safety of these drugs when used chronically. Incorrect assumptions and beliefs about opioid toxicity, addiction potential, dependence, and tolerance result in suboptimal use of these very effective medications. The result is widespread *opiophobia,* defined as the irrational and undocumented fear that appropriate use of opioids causes addiction (1).

Confusion about opioids stems partly from the terminology used for this group of medications. The terms *narcotic, opiate,* and *opioid* are often incorrectly used interchangeably. For centuries, the term *narcotic*—derived from the Greek word meaning "benumbing"—was used to describe opium derivatives. Today, the word *narcotic* has become a legal term that includes a broad range of sedating and potentially abused substances. Many of the substances labeled "narcotics" are not at all related to opium. As many clinicians know, the word *narcotic* can have very negative connotations, and as such clinicians should not use this term when communicating with patients. Literally, opioids are opium-like substances. In the past, *opioid* was used primarily to describe endogenous opium-like substances, whereas the term *opiate* was used to describe drugs that derived from opium. Today the term *opioid* accurately describes both types of compounds. Thus, *opioid* has become the preferred term in both clinical and scientific dialogs.

HISTORICAL BACKGROUND

Opium is derived from the milky exudate of the opium poppy, *Papaver somniferum.* This natural product is heterogeneous in nature and contains over 20 alkaloids. Opium has been used to treat human discomfort for over 5000 years. The word *opium* actually derives from a Greek word meaning "juice." Opium has been used clinically since the early days of European medicine but fell into disfavor as a consequence of toxic outcomes from a nonstandardized drug that was not used with necessary care. In the sixteenth century Paracelsus repopularized the use of opium, and by the second half of that century opium use was understood and adopted by physicians throughout the continent.

In 1803, the French pharmacist Jean-François Derosne isolated a crystalline precipitate from opium that was a mixture of morphine and narcotine. Three years later the German pharmacist Friedrich Wilhelm Sertürner isolated the alkaloid morphine from opium. Sertürner named this powerful alkaloid drug after Morpheus, the Greek god of dreams. Other opium alkaloids, including papaverine and codeine, were subsequently isolated, and over the next decades purified alkaloids largely replaced crude opium in clinical practice.

By the midnineteenth century, many of the patent medicines sold as panaceas or cure-alls contained opioids. Steadily increasing federal and state control of opioids in the United States began with the passage of the Harrison Narcotic Act in 1914. The federal Bureau of Narcotics was created in the twentieth century to address use of potentially abused drugs. In recent decades, political and law enforcement demands rather than scientific or clinical findings have defined the control system for opioid use in the United States. Creation of the Drug Enforcement Administration (DEA) by the Controlled Substance Act of 1970 assured that control of opioids and other controlled substances would be driven by law enforcement, not a patient care focus. Numerous initiatives, both within and outside of the government, have worked to emphasize that opioids are important—and frequently underused—clinical drugs. These include the 1979 *Report to the White House of the Federal Interagency Committee on New Therapies for Pain and Discomfort* (2), the 1985 report of the federal Interagency Committee on Pain and Analgesia (3), and the 1986 NIH Consensus Development Conference report entitled *The Integrated Approach to the Management of Pain* (4).

When Congress created the Agency for Health Care Policy and Research (AHCPR) (now the Agency for Health Care Research and Quality [AHCRQ]) of the U.S. Public Health Service in 1989, the agency was explicitly charged to develop clinical practice guidelines for areas of health care that were delivered inconsistently. Pain was selected as the first topic to be addressed. This is reflective of the serious concerns that the American public and public health professionals had about the ways in which pain management often was provided. Two federal clinical practice guidelines resulted. *Acute Pain Management* was published in 1992 (5). *Cancer Pain Management* was published in 1994 (6). The full text for both of these guidelines is available in a searchable format on the World Wide Web at www.ahrq.gov. These scientifically based references document serious misconceptions about use and underuse of opioids in the management of both acute and chronic malignant pain.

The use of opioids in chronic nonmalignant pain was considered controversial by many clinicians well into the 1990s. This controversy existed despite the fact that numerous published studies documented the safety and efficacy of opioids in the management of a variety of chronic nonmalignant pain states, i.e., neuropathic, myofascial, arthritic, and osteoporosis pain (7).

In 1997, the American Academy of Pain Medicine and the American Pain Society published a joint consensus statement entitled *The Use of Opioids for the Treatment of Chronic Pain* (8). A year later, the Federation of State Medical Boards of the United Sates published *Model Guidelines for the Use of Controlled Substances in the Treatment of Pain* (9). These two authoritative publications clearly document that opioids have a place in the management of many patients' chronic nonmalignant pain.

Most physicians are far more willing to use opioid analgesics in patients with cancer pain than noncancer pain. The fact that opioids are seriously underused was underscored by a study of opioid prescribing for cancer pain patients that was published in the *Journal of the American Medical Association* in 1998 (10). Researchers evaluated the records of 13 625 cancer patients discharged from hospitals to Medicare- or Medicaid-certified nursing homes during the period 1992 to 1995 in five midwestern states. A

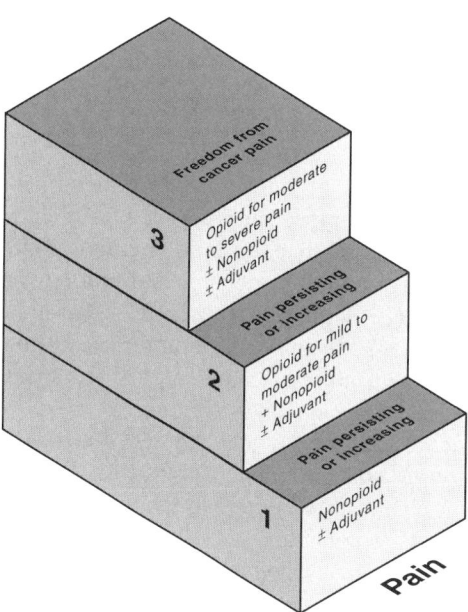

FIG. 16-1. World Health Organization analgesic ladder. A progression of analgesics and doses to be used to manage pain of varying intensities.

total of 4003 patients reported and had multiple factors independently associated with daily pain. Only 26% of these patients received morphine or another opioid considered to be on level 3 of the World Health Organization (WHO) analgesic ladder (11) (Fig. 16-1). Only 32% of the patients received a level 2 analgesic, and 26% received only acetaminophen or an NSAID for analgesia.

The World Health Organization analgesic ladder, which was developed to guide analgesic therapy for cancer patients in developing countries, has been shown to be applicable in most pain management in most societies (WHO 1986). This approach describes three levels of analgesia. It suggests that pharmacological management of mild to moderate pain should include a nonsteroidal anti-inflammatory drug (NSAID) or acetaminophen unless there is a contraindication as a first step. When pain persists or increases, an opioid is added at the second step. The third step consists of increasing the opioid dose to treat persistent moderate to severe pain. At all of the steps, indicated adjuvants are to be used concurrently.

This was never intended to be a stepped approach in which prior steps must be tried before initiating more aggressive therapy. Analgesia should be started at the level appropriate for the patient's pain. Of concern, many managed care monitors have suggested using this three-step ladder as a stepped approach. As a result, future cancer pain management guidelines may not include this useful and effective graphical description of analgesic use.

A fourth step, including palliative radiation and chemotherapy for cancer pain, nerve blocks, more invasive procedures, cognitive-behavioral therapy, and other modalities, is available in developed countries.

MYTHS AND MISCONCEPTIONS

Unnecessary fears of addiction, dependence, tolerance, and toxicity often impede appropriate prescribing and use of these important medications. Inappropriate beliefs about opioids have been documented among physicians (12), nurses, (13), and pharmacists (14). Societal barriers to the use of opioids are now being refuted by many professional organizations (8) and regulatory agencies (9). Nevertheless, many clinicians continue to avoid opioids in their practices to the detriment of their patients. Unlike the use of nonsteroidal antiinflammatory drugs (NSAIDs) and acetaminophen, chronic opioid use rarely causes end organ toxicity. Still, opioids are often underprescribed, underdosed, taken erratically, or even abruptly discontinued.

Misconceptions about addiction may be the most commonly held regarding opioid therapy. *Addiction* is defined as the compulsive use of a substance that results in the physical, psychological, or social harm to an individual *and* continued use despite the harm (15). Drug-seeking behavior does not in and of itself indicate addiction. Until recently, most of what was known about opioid-induced addiction was based on the experience of drug abusers, not patients with pain. Studies of the actual incidence of iatrogenic opioid-induced addiction have shown that this phenomenon is actually quite rare. The Boston Collaborative Drug Surveillance Program study revealed only four cases of iatrogenic opioid-induced addiction among a total of 11 882 patients who had no prior history of substance abuse. These patients received opioids for a broad range of indications and were followed for up to 2 years (16). Similarly, a national survey of over 10 000 burn patients who received opioids over an extended period of time revealed no cases of addiction. None of these patients had a prior history of drug abuse (17). Abuse was also rare in the chronic headache patient population: Only 3 of 2369 patients abused analgesics (18).

Many patients who may appear to have addictive traits may actually suffer from what has been labeled as pseudoaddiction. This phenomenon was defined over a decade ago as an iatrogenic syndrome of drug-seeking behavior resulting from inadequate analgesia, not substance abuse (19). The American Society of Addiction Medicine, in its April 1997 *Public Policy Statement,* said this about pseudoaddiction:

> . . . individuals who have severe, unrelieved pain may become intensely focused on finding relief for their pain. Sometimes, such patients may appear to observers to be preoccupied with obtaining opioids, but the preoccupation is with finding relief of pain, rather than using opioids, *per se.* (20)

Many clinicians conclude that patients are abusing or are addicted to opioids when the patients present with complaints of new pain(s) after the initial pain complaint is controlled. In a study of 955 patients with advanced cancer, 34% experienced two or more types of pain, and an impressive 80% of patients reported pain due to two or more etiologies (21). Similar findings have been reported in the AIDS patient population (22). In most cases, more severe pain masks less intense pains. After the severe pain is effectively treated, the previously masked pain, which may require other treatments, becomes evident. If the new pain complaints are treated effectively aberrant behavior should subside.

In contrast to *addiction, dependence* is defined as a physiological phenomenon characterized by an abstinence syndrome following abrupt discontinuation, substantial dose reduction, or administration of an antagonist (15). *Dependence* is often confused with *addiction,* even to the point that some clinicians consider the terms synonymous. Dependence occurs predictably when patients take opioids on a regular basis for more than a few days. It occurs in almost everyone receiving opioids on a continual schedule for 10 or more days. Dependence also occurs predictably when patients take steroids, beta blockers, and many other commonly prescribed medications. Tapering of the dose over a period of 5 to 10 days, after the medication is no longer needed, can usually prevent signs and symptoms of withdrawal in the opioid-dependent individual (23). Dependence should not be a barrier to use when opioids are indicated.

Tolerance is the reduced effect of a drug after repeated doses of the drug or repeated doses of drugs in the same class. Analgesic tolerance with opioids is widely believed to be a serious limitation to the effective use of these medications. Clinical experience does not support this belief. Although analgesic tolerance has been documented with animal studies, it does not appear to be a clinical problem in humans. The phenomenon does appear to occur with initial dosing in humans but subsides with chronic use. It is believed that this effect results from second-messenger effects and not changes in opioid receptor status.

When analgesic tolerance appears it is typically during the first 2 weeks of therapy. In these cases it is often necessary to increase the opioid dose to find an effective dose. Effective dose titration negates the clinical implications of tolerance. In the cancer patient population, dose requirements normally remain stable over weeks to months unless the disease progresses (24,25). For many advanced cancer patients, dose requirements decrease with resolution of tumor size, decreased anxiety, destruction of nerve endings in painful organs or tissues secondary to disease or treatment, or other comorbidity. When stable opioid doses become ineffective this may signal increasing or new pathology, increased or excessive physical activity secondary to previous pain relief, drug interactions, noncompliance, or other nonpharmacological factors. This phenomenon has been referred to as pseudotolerance (26).

Tolerance to the constipating effects of opioids typically does not occur (27). Activated mu opioid receptors in the colon inhibit peristalsis. Peristaltic stimulants, e.g., senna, bisacodyl, are needed to induce colonic emptying. Stool softeners alone are almost always ineffective. Prophylaxis with stimulating laxatives may be indicated when opioid therapy is started in light of the risks for severe constipation and possible fecal impaction (28). Oral naloxone has been evaluated as a treatment for opioid-induced constipation (29). Although oral naloxone appears to maintain peristalsis by inhibiting opioid effects in colonic receptors, concerns for potential systemic opioid withdrawal exist. There is insufficient data to support the routine use of oral naloxone for prevention of opioid-induced constipation.

Opioids are effective analgesics for most nociceptive and neuropathic pain, but all pain is not responsive to opioids. The underlying cause for all reported pain should be investigated and treated before considering the sole use of opioids as a treatment measure. Examples include neuropathic pain for which tricyclic antidepressants, anticonvulsants, and nerve blocks may be indicated or preferred; painful infectious cysts for which incision and drainage followed by antiinfectives would be indicated; and gastrointestinal spasm for which an anticholinergic medication may be more effective (30).

MECHANISM OF ACTION

It is not logical for the human organism to contain specific receptors for alkaloids derived only from a plant source. The presence of endogenous opioids was postulated to explain the presence of opioid receptors prior to the isolation of these endogenous substances. Three families of endogenous human opioid peptides have been isolated and identified: endorphins, enkephalins, and dynorphins. These peptides can be found within the central nervous system (CNS), adrenal medulla, nerve plexi, gastric exocrine glands, and intestines. These peptides appear to have multiple roles, including pain modulation, neurohumoral transmission, and neurohormonal effects.

Opioid receptors are found in the CNS, gastrointestinal tract, and to a lesser degree in peripheral tissues. Opioid drugs manifest analgesic effects primarily by binding to and activating (agonizing) the opioid receptors located in the CNS. The interaction of exogenous opioids and opioid receptors mimics the interaction seen when endogenous opioid peptides (dynorphins, endorphins, enkephalins) bind with these same receptors (31).

The three generally recognized classes of opioid receptors are mu, delta, and kappa (32–34). Sigma and epsilon receptors were originally classified as opioid receptors because opioids can bind to them. Subsequent research has shown that neither sigma nor epsilon receptors are opioid receptors *per se* because neither of these receptor types is opioid specific (35).

Opioid receptors are comprised of glycoproteins found in cellular membranes and are coupled to G proteins that modulate potassium and calcium ion conduction (36). When opioid agonists occupy either mu or delta receptors, they open a potassium ion channel that permits an increase in potassium conductance. Kappa receptor activation inhibits calcium entry via a calcium ion channel. The hyperpolarization that results subsequently inhibits neuronal activity. Activation of opioid receptors decreases signal transmission from the primary peripheral afferent nerves to the higher CNS centers as well as processing of the pain stimulus (37).

Activation of opioid receptors leads to analgesia and potentially adverse effects. All three of the opioid receptor types have known subtypes (Table 16-1). To date, the two mu subtypes that have been best elucidated are Mu_1, activation of which produces supraspinal analgesia, and Mu_2, activation of which is thought to be responsible for some of the adverse sequelae of opioid administration. Activation of kappa and delta receptors appears to produce spinal analgesia. $Kappa_3$ receptors are also thought to mediate some supraspinal analgesia (38). Activation of delta receptors may enhance mu receptor analgesia. The clinical implications of delta and kappa receptor subtypes have not been fully developed at this time.

The lock-and-key receptor theory describes the interaction between receptors and opioids (39). Opioids can function as full and partial agonists as well as mixed agonists-antagonists. Partial agonists function by occupying only part of an opioid receptor and thereby result in a lesser degree of analgesia than do full agonists. Antagonists prevent opioid agonists from occupying opioid receptors. Clinically useful antagonists bind to the receptors rapidly and have a higher affinity for the receptors than agonists. Similarly, any agonist with a higher affinity for the receptor than one that is already on the receptor may

TABLE 16-1. *Opioid receptors, subtypes, and physiological effects*

Receptor type	Subtype	Effects
Mu	Mu_1	Supraspinal analgesia
	Mu_2	Physical dependence Euphoria Sedation Respiratory depression Constipation Orthostatic hypotension Arteriolar/venous dilation
Delta	$Delta_{1,2}$	Spinal analgesia Euphoria Potentiates mu receptor analgesia
Kappa	$Kappa_{1,2,3}$	Spinal analgesia Sedation Miosis Supraspinal analgesia (K3)

Reprinted from Lipman AG, Jackson KC. Opioids. In Warfield C, Bajwa Z, eds. *Principles and Practice of Pain Management*, 2nd ed. New York: McGraw-Hill, 2001.

displace the drug with lower affinity. If the second agent (agent with higher affinity) produces less activity than the previously administered drug, withdrawal may occur. Antagonists can produce competitive antagonism by direct receptor binding, or they can produce noncompetitive antagonism by binding near opioid receptors. In the case of the mixed agonist-antagonist opioids, agonism occurs at kappa receptors, and mu receptors are antagonized.

The role of peripheral opioid receptors has been described, and it is now believed that mu and kappa receptors in peripheral tissues effect inflammation and produce an antihyperalgesic activity (34). Opioids administered into peripheral tissues (topically or by intraarticular injection) have been used to treat pain in soft tissue and joints with some success (40–42). Most uses of opioids in peripheral tissues remain experimental at this time; however, this may prove to be a useful route of administration in the future for diseases with localized pain foci.

Dose ceiling effects limit the usefulness of kappa agonists and partial agonists. A true dose ceiling results from a lack of additional efficacy after doses exceed some predetermined level while incurring additional adverse effects. Both the mixed agonist-antagonist opioids (butorphanol, dezocine, nalbuphine, pentazocine) and the partial agonist (buprenorphine) exhibit true dose ceilings. Therefore, these drugs should not be used in doses that exceed those listed in the FDA-approved labeling. Additionally, these analgesics can displace pure mu agonists from mu receptor sites and can produce a withdrawal reaction. The functional dose ceiling occurs with only one mu agonist: codeine. This effect is due to unacceptable side effects, i.e., nausea and constipation that occur predictably at higher doses (43). It often occurs with oral doses of codeine administered every 4 hours in excess of 65 to 100 mg. Codeine doses higher than these produce far more incremental adverse effects than any potential analgesia. For the other mu opioid agonists, the effective dose range varies broadly among patients, and unacceptable side effects that last more than a few days are not commonly seen until very large doses are attempted. For most patients, the functional ceiling occurs with doses higher than are used clinically. There is no a priori dose or serum concentration at which this functional ceiling occurs. Opioid doses should be titrated upward until either analgesia or unacceptable side effects occur.

PHARMACOKINETICS

Pharmacokinetic factors can impact the effectiveness of any given route of administration. Four phases of pharmacokinetics are considered: absorption, distribution, metabolism, and elimination. Pharmaceutically formulated controlled-release dosage forms add an element for consideration.

Absorption

Opioids are readily absorbed from the gastrointestinal tract following oral and rectal administration. Oral administration maintains convenience and is simple and is typically less expensive than other routes of administration. Oral opioids are subject to first-pass metabolism because oral administration requires drugs to pass through the liver prior to reaching the systemic circulation. As a consequence, larger doses of oral opioids are needed when compared to the parenteral route. Most immediate-release oral opioids maintain an onset of analgesia of approximately 20 to 40 minutes, with a peak in analgesic effect occurring 45 to 60 minutes after administration. Oral morphine has been reported to require 30 to 45 minutes to reach peak plasma levels, whereas oxycodone peak levels may not occur until 60 to 90 minutes after oral administration (44). Although delayed peak concentrations would appear to make oral opioids less than ideal for managing breakthrough pain, experience has shown that not to be the case (44). Oral opioids can usually be effective in the management of breakthrough pain.

Morphine and oxycodone are currently available in controlled-release formulations that provide extended pain relief without the need for doses every 4 hours. In the near future a controlled-release formulation of hydromorphone will be available. Methadone and levorphanol are additional options for long-acting pain management secondary to their inherently long half-lives.

Many opioids can be administered rectally when access to the oral route is no longer feasible. Proper rectal administration avoids the hepatic first-pass effect. There are three sets of veins responsible for rectal blood return: the superior, middle, and inferior rectal veins. The superior vein is responsible for blood return of the upper portion of the rectal vault (approximately 15–20 cm high) and returns blood to the portal vein for immediate hepatic biotransformation. The middle and inferior rectal veins return blood to the inferior vena cava and avoid first-pass metabolism. Opioid administration into the lower rectal vault allows for larger amounts of the parent drug to reach the systemic circulation without becoming subject to first-pass metabolism (45,46).

Hydromorphone, morphine, and oxymorphone are commercially available as rectal suppositories. Controlled-release morphine tablets have also been used via the rectal route with good results at essentially the same doses used orally (47). There are no data to support such equianalgesic dosing with controlled-release oxycodone tablets.

Lipophilic opioids, e.g., fentanyl, pass across biological surfaces more readily and at a faster rate than do more hydrophilic opioids, e.g., morphine. These surfaces include the skin and oral mucosa. Transdermal fentanyl patches provide a simple and convenient administration vehicle for the drug to enter patients unable to take opioids orally or rectally. The fentanyl is released from a gel matrix in the transdermal patch into the subcutaneous fat layer. This fat layer serves as an *in vivo* drug reservoir from which the drug is released into the serum slowly over a period of 48 to 72 hours. Following patch application, fentanyl serum levels slowly rise. The average time to achieve relative steady-state serum levels following application of trans-dermal fentanyl patches is 15 to 20 hours (48). Upon patch removal, the drug continues to move into the serum compartment from the subcutaneous fat depot. Serum fentanyl levels will slowly decrease, and opioid effects may continue for an additional 12 to 24 hours after patch removal. These factors make transdermal fentanyl a sub-optimal option for patients with rapidly changing opioid requirements.

Oral, transmucosal fentanyl has been available for several years in the form of a lozenge on a handle for both preoperative and preprocedural pain management. Recently another oral lozenge on a handle was approved for the management of breakthrough pain in cancer patients. Approximately 25% of an oral, transmucosal dose is absorbed across the buccal surface of the oral mucosa. Medication that is not absorbed trickles down the throat and is absorbed in the GI tract. An additional 25% (one-third of the remaining 75%) is available for systemic use after metabolism. Systemic bioavailability of oral, trans-mucosal fentanyl is generally considered to be about 50% of the administered dose. Analgesic onset typically occurs within 5 to 10 minutes, with a peak effect in 20 to 40 minutes. Additional opioids, including morphine and methadone, have been administered as concentrated, aqueous solutions via sublingual or buccal administration. In most cases, larger doses are often required for morphine and other hydrophilic compounds when they are administered across the oral mucosa. Table 16-2 lists bioavailability information on the sublingual administration of opioids.

Intravenous (IV) opioids provide 100% bioavailability by definition. Subcutaneous (SC) opioid infusions provide similar drug levels to those achieved with IV infusion (49). Intramuscular (IM) injections provide similar pharmacokinetics as well. Time to peak serum levels for IM- and SC-administered opioids is delayed due to the need for absorption; however, these two routes provide similar levels

TABLE 16-2. *Sublingual opioid bioavailability*

Drug	Percentage absorbed
Morphine	22 %
Methadone	34%
Fentanyl	51%
Buprenorphine	55%

1 mL SL; held for 10 minutes @ pH 6.5
Adapted from Weinberg D, Inturrisi C, Reidenberg B, et al. Sublingual absorption of selected opioid analgesics. *Clin Pharmacol Ther* 1988;44:335–342.

at similar times. As previously discussed with transdermal delivery, more lipophilic compounds like fentanyl act more rapidly after injection. Absorption of opioids from the IM route is a rate-limiting step for which lipophilicity is a major factor. IM injections are generally not recommended due to the pain and possible tissue damage inflicted, as well as erratic absorption.

Distribution

Opioid distribution is a function of plasma protein binding and lipophilicity. Morphine is 30% to 35% plasma protein bound and does not appear to be greatly influenced by displacement. Additionally, morphine does not remain in tissues for an extended amount of time. Fentanyl, by contrast, is both highly protein bound (80% to 85%) and extremely lipophilic. The free fraction of fentanyl increases in acidotic patients. Fentanyl also distributes to fat tissues throughout the body and redistributes slowly into the systemic circulation.

Metabolism (Biotransformation) and Elimination (Excretion)

Opioids that cannot be readily excreted through the kidneys in their parent form are metabolized to form more water-soluble metabolites. The liver metabolizes opioids via numerous processes, including dealkylation, glucuronidation, hydrolysis, and oxidation. Opioids can also be metabolized, to a minor extent, in other body compartments. Examples of tissues that can also metabolize opioids are the central nervous system, kidneys, lungs, and placenta. Metabolism of opioids can impact the selection of an appropriate therapeutic regimen. Some metabolites have been shown to cause untoward neurotoxicity (50) and can displace more active parent compounds from opioid receptor sites. Patients at risk for toxicity from the accumulation of metabolites include patients with impaired renal function (which includes most elderly individuals) and those receiving high-dose or long-term opioid therapy.

A special case of toxicity occurs with meperidine. Accumulation of normeperidine, a metabolite of meperidine, causes neurotoxicity. This can be especially problematic in the elderly or those patients with poor renal function. Use of meperidine should be limited to 1 to 2 days for acute pain in appropriate patient populations and should be avoided in the management of chronic pain.

Morphine-3-glucuronide (M3G) and morphine-6-glucuronide (M6G) are two major morphine metabolites (51). As much as 50% of morphine can be renally excreted as M3G, with an additional 5 percent from M6G (52). Both glucuronides are water soluble and depend on renal elimination for clearance. M3G appears to be antinociceptive and has been associated with hyperalgesia, myoclonus, and other neurotoxicities (50,53). M6G possesses analgesic properties and appears to be significantly more potent than morphine. Accumulation of these metabolites predisposes patients to toxicity as well as poor pain control.

Normorphine, the desmethyl morphine metabolite, may be a minor contributor to the toxic effects seen with high-dose or long-term morphine use. Reports of normorphine accumulation indicate that M6G and M3G were also elevated (54). As a consequence, the contribution of normorphine accumulation toxicity remains unclear. It is also unclear how often metabolites of other opioids may be problematic in renally impaired patients. It has been suggested that caution be exercised with hydromorphone because it has a metabolic fate similar to morphine, including the 3 and 6 glucuronides, and also with fentanyl, which has a desmethyl metabolite (50). The incidence of adverse effects to hydromorphone appears clinically to be less severe and less common than with morphine. Oxycodone has only one active analgesic metabolite, oxymorphone, which may make oxycodone safer for elderly patients and persons with renal impairment.

Renal excretion accounts for approximately 90% of opioid elimination (parent drug and metabolites). Fecal elimination remains a minor pathway, accounting for less than 10% of opioid excretion.

ADVERSE EFFECTS

Opioid use is associated with a number of potentially problematic side effects, principally sedation, constipation, and nausea and vomiting. Many of these effects are mediated by activation of opioid receptors in the CNS (Table 16-1). In addition, adverse effects are controlled through opioid receptors located outside the CNS as well as through nonopioid-related mechanisms. Adverse events may also be the consequence of drug interactions with other medications, e.g., sedative-hypnotics (Table 16-3).

Opioid-induced sedation occurs in a dose-dependent fashion and is commonly seen during the initiation phase of opioid therapy. Sedation may prove beneficial to some patients and indeed is warranted in situations where sedation is beneficial, e.g., prior to some medical procedures. Clinicians should be careful not to confuse sleep after initiation of opioids with the sleep that sleep-deprived individuals attain with pain control. If sedation becomes problematic at doses needed for analgesia, addition of low doses of a central stimulant, e.g., methylphenidate 5 mg morning and noon, may prove beneficial (55).

In addition to sedation, opioids have the potential to impair judgment and psychomotor function when therapy is initiated. As with sedation, mental clouding can occur with dose escalation. These effects diminish markedly in most patients who continuously receive opioids on a regular basis for more than 1 week. In a review of motor vehicle crashes in Finland there was no significant difference between the number of accidents that involved 24 drivers taking opioids on a regular schedule for chronic pain management and the number of accidents that involved the general population (56). If patients are not experiencing any observable opioid-induced impairment, and the opioid dose has been consistent for at least a week, then it appears that these patients should be able to drive or carry out other normal functions safely. Caution must be exercised, however, when doses are increased. These patients should refrain from driving or other potentially dangerous activities for approximately another week or until any impairment due to the increased dose resolves.

TABLE 16-3. *Important opioid drug interactions*

Opioid(s)	Interacting drug(s)	Description
All	Antihistamines, butyrophenones	Increased sedation
	Tricyclic antidepressants	Increased sedation; potentiation of opioid-induced respiratory depression
Controlled-Release Opioids	Metoclopramide	Earlier peak plasma concentration; increased sedation
Codeine	Quinidine	Inhibition of conversion to morphine; decreased analgesia
Meperidine	Monoamine oxidase inhibitors	Excitatory response (including seizures, arrhythmias, hyperpyrexia)
Meperidine, Morphine	Cimetidine	Inhibition of opioid metabolism; increased opioid effects
Methadone	Carbamazepine Erythromycin Phenytoin	Increased opioid metabolism; may induce withdrawal
Methadone, Morphine	Desipramine	Inhibition of desipramine metabolism; toxicity possible
Propoxyphene	Carbamazepine	Increased carbamazepine levels, potential for toxicity
Propoxyphene	Doxepin	Increased doxepin levels, potential for toxicity
Propoxyphene	Metoprolol, propranolol	Increased plasma levels of these beta blockers

Adapted from Maurer P, Bartkowski R. Drug interactions of clinical significance with opioid analgesics. *Drug Saf* 1993; 8:30–48. Quinn D, Day R. Drug interactions of clinical importance. An updated guide. *Drug Saf* 1995;12:393–452. Hansten PD, Horn JR. Drug interactions analysis and management. Vancouver WA, Applied Therapuetics,Inc., updated quarterly.

The major gastrointestinal effect resulting from opioids is decreased intestinal motility leading to constipation. This delay in gastric emptying appears to occur with both systemic and intrathecal opioid administration. Propulsive contractions are decreased in both the small and large intestines. Constipation should be anticipated and prevented in all patients who receive opioids. Treatment should be aggressive and include both increased fluid intake and stimulant laxatives such as standardized senna concentrate or bisacodyl. Other laxatives are of limited usefulness in the narcotized gut, e.g., saline cathartics and stool softeners. Bulk laxatives may prove detrimental by contributing to fecal impaction.

Nausea and vomiting can occur with opioid treatment, primarily during the first few days of treatment. Many patients require concomitant antiemetic therapy during the first few days after the opioid is initiated. Some patients actually report that they would rather suffer from pain than endure continued nausea and vomiting. Effective treatment of this side effect improves patient compliance and pain control. The primary mechanism of opioid-induced nausea results from the action of the opioids on the chemoreceptor trigger zone of the medulla. Therefore, most patients respond well to a centrally acting antiemetic, e.g., prochlorperazine. Motion can also potentiate opioid-induced nausea and vomiting in some patients through a vestibular mechanism. In these cases, a motion sickness antiemetic, e.g., cyclizine, meclizine, can be added to the centrally acting antiemetic. If decreased gastrointestinal motility contributes to the nausea and vomiting, a gastrokinetic antiemetic, e.g., metoclopramide, can be administered orally or by the subcutaneous route to improve symptom control.

Opioids cause urinary retention by increasing sphincter tone. Resulting bladder capacity is increased due to the relaxation of the detrusor muscle. Mu and delta, but not kappa, agonists can inhibit the micturition reflex. Interestingly, this effect occurs more often with spinal opioids than with other routes of administration.

Pruritus usually involves the face and is more common with neuraxial administration. Epidural administration produces itching in less than 10% of patients, whereas approximately 50% of patients receiving intrathecal opioids complain of some pruritus.

Normally, the cardiovascular effects seen with opioids are inconsequential. Indeed, most patients with chest pain benefit from the administration of an opioid for pain control. However, opioids—morphine in particular—can cause vasodilation and histamine release, which can prove problematic in patients who have hypovolemia or who have limited cardiac reserve.

Opioid-naive patients may experience respiratory depression when first exposed to large doses of the drugs. This effect appears to be mediated by mu-2 receptors found in the brainstem. These pulmonary effects normally do not present a clinical problem for patients receiving chronic opioid therapy. Opioids should always be used with caution and titrated to effect in patients with serious pulmonary dysfunction. This class of medications can decrease the cough reflex, and the potential for histamine release could lead to bronchial constriction and possible bronchospasm. Additionally, opioids may promote drying of pulmonary secretions.

CURRENTLY AVAILABLE OPIOIDS

Morphine remains the standard for opioid comparisons. Many equianalgesic dosing tables use parenteral morphine 10 mg every 4 hours as the standard for comparison. Equianalgesic doses are listed in Table 16-4. No equianalgesic table can always apply to all patients because of the great variance of interpatient responses to opioids. These tables can provide an approximation of equally effective doses, but patients should be retitrated to analgesic response after an opioid medication is changed.

Three types of opioids are currently available for clinical use. These include the mu agonists, mixed agonist-antagonists (which are kappa agonists and neutral or antagonistic at the mu receptors), and partial mu agonists. As mentioned, kappa agonists and partial mu agonists exhibit dose ceiling effects that limit their clinical utility. Table 16-5 lists commercially available mu agonist opioids.

Mu agonists may be placed into three categories based on individual pharmacokinetic parameters: short-acting, long-acting, and ultrashort-acting. Morphine and other opioids with short half-lives require frequent administration to maintain analgesia. Immediate-release oral morphine provides about 4 hours of pain relief and should be dosed accordingly. Controlled-release formulations of oral opioids (e.g., MS Contin, Oramorph-SR, Kadian, Oxy-Contin), pharmacologically long-acting oral opioids (methadone, levorphanol), and transdermal fentanyl provide alternatives to the frequent administration of immediate opioids. Controlled-release oral dosage forms of hydromorphone have been developed and are expected to become commercially available in the near future.

The fentanyl series of mu agonists is highly lipophilic, providing certain advantages over other mu agonists. The lipophilicity provides rapid onset of action, which is useful preoperatively. The high lipophilicity of these substances also facilitates transdermal, transmucosal, and subcutaneous administration. When these agents are administered through or under the skin, they tend to depot within the subcutaneous fat layer. This depot function allows the medication to be released from the fat slowly. Conversely, when these highly lipophilic medications are administered transmucosally or sublingually, they are rapidly absorbed due to the lack of the buccal and sublingual fat. Rapid absorption via the transmucosal or sublingual route makes administration of these drugs useful in managing breakthrough pain.

TABLE 16-4. Dosing comparison for some common opioids

Name	Equianalgesic dose (mg) Oral	Parenteral®	Starting oral dose Adults (mg)	Children (mg/kg)	Comments	Precautions and contraindications
a. Morphine-like agonists						
Morphine	30	10	15–30	0.30	Standard of comparison for opioid analgesics. Sustained-release preparations (MS Contin, OramorphSR) release drug over 8–12 hours. Recent addition of once-a-day sustained release formulation (Kadian)	For all opioids, caution in patients with impaired ventilation, bronchial asthma, increased intracranial pressure, liver failure
Hydromorphone (Dilaudid)	7.5	1.5	4–8	0.06	Slightly shorter duration than morphine	
Oxycodone	20	—	15–30	0.30		
Methadone (Dolophine)	20 acute 2–4 chronic	10 acute 2–4 chronic	5–10	0.20	Good oral potency, long plasma half-life (24–36 hours)	Accumulates with repeated dosing, requiring decreases in dose size and frequency, especially on days 2–5
Levorphanol (Levo-Dromoman)	4 acute 1 chronic	2 acute 1 chronic	2–4	0.04	Long plasma half-life (12–16 hours)	Accumulates on days 2–3
Fentanyl	—	0.1	—	—	Transdermal fentanyl (Duragesic) 25 mcg/hour, roughly equivalent to sustained-release morphine, 45 mg/day. Oral transmucosal fentanyl citrate now available for treatment of breakthrough pain in chronic cancer pain patients already taking around-the-clock opioids	Because of skin reservoir of drug, 12-hour delay in onset and offset of transdermal patch; fever increases dose rate
Oxymorphone (Numorphan)	—	1	—	—	5-mg rectal suppository = 5 mg morphine IM	Like IM morphine
Meperidine (Demerol)	300	75	Not recommended	—	Slightly shorter acting than morphine	Normeperidine (toxic metabolite) accumulates with repetitive dosing, causing CNS excitation; avoid in children who have impaired renal function or who are receiving monoamine oxidase inhibitors**
b. Mixed agonist-antagonists						
Nalbuphine (Nubain)	—	10	—	—	Not available orally, not scheduled under Controlled Substances Act	Incidence of psychotomimetic effects lower than with pentazocine; may precipitate withdrawal in narcotic-dependent patients
Butorphanol (Stadol)	—	2	—	—	Like nalbuphine	Like nalbuphine
c. Partial agonist						
Dezocine (Dalgan)	—	10	—	—	Like nalbuphine	May precipitate withdrawal in narcotic-dependent patients; SC injection irritating
Buprenorphine (Buprenex)	—	0.4	—	—	Sublingual preparation not yet available in United States; lower abuse liability than morphine; does not produce psychotomimetic effects	May precipitate withdrawal in narcotic-dependent patients; not readily reversed by naloxone; avoid in labor

*These are standard IM doses for acute pain in adults and also can be used to convert doses for IV infusions and repeated small IV boluses. For single IV boluses, use half the IM dose. IV doses for children > 6 months = parenteral equianalgesic dose × weight (kg)/100.

†Once-a-day formulation (Kadian) available as 20-, 50-, or 100-mg capsules. Sustained-release formulation not destroyed by breaking capsule and sprinkling over food such as applesauce.

**Irritating to tissues with repeated IM injection.

Reprinted from *Principles of Analgesic Use in the Treatment of Acute Pain and Cancer Pain*, Fourth Edition. Glenview, Il: American Pain Society, 1999.

TABLE 16-5. *Commercially available opioids*

Generic (proprietary) name	Dosage forms and strengths available	Comments
Mu Agonists		
Alfentanil (Alfenta)	Injection: 500 mcg/mL	
Codeine (Various)	Injection: 50 mcg/mL Tablets: 15, 30, 60 mg	Also in combination with acetaminophen (Tylenol with Codeine) and aspirin (Empirin)
Fentanyl (Sublimaze, Duragesic, Fentanyl Oralet, Actiq, others)	Injection: 50 mcg/mL Transdermal patch: 25, 50, 75, 100 mcg/hr (Duragesic) Transmucosal: 100, 200, 300, 400 mcg (Fentanyl Oralet) Transmucosal: 200, 400, 600, 800, 1200, 1600 mcg (Actiq)	
Hydromorphone (Dilaudid, others)	Injectable: 1, 2, 3, 4, 10 mg/mL Tablets: 1, 2, 3, 4, 8 mg Oral liquid: 5 mg/5 mL Suppositories: 3 mg	
Levorphanol (Levo-Dromoran)	Injection: 2 mg/mL Tablets: 2 mg	
Meperidine (Demerol, others)	Injection: 10, 25, 50, 75, 100 mg/mL Tablets: 50, 100 mg Oral liquid: 50 mg/mL	Meperidine with Phenergan (Mepergan Fortis) Capsules: 50 mg with 25 mg promethazine
Methadone (Dolophine, others)	Injection: 10 mg/mL Tablets: 5, 10 mg Dispersible tablets: 40 mg Oral liquid: 5 mg/5 mL, 10 mg/5 mL, 10 mg/10 mL Oral concentrate: 10 mg/mL	
Morphine (MSIR, MS Contin, Oramorph SR, Kadian, others)	Injection: 0.5, 1, 2, 3, 4, 5, 8, 10, 15, 25, 50 mg/mL Tablets: 15, 30 mg Soluble tablets: 10, 15, 30 mg Controlled-release tablets: 15, 30, 60, 100, 200 mg (MS Contin) Oral liquid: 10 mg/5 mL, 10 mg/2.5 mL, 20 mg/5 mL, 20 mg/mL, 100 mg/5 mL Suppositories: 5, 10, 20, 30 mg	
Oxycodone (Roxicodone, OxyContin, others)	Tablets: 5 mg Controlled-release tablets: 10, 20, 40 mg (OxyContin) Oral liquid: 5 mg/5 mL Oral concentrate: 20 mg/mL	Also in combination with aspirin (Percodan) and acetaminophen (Percocet, Roxicet, others)
Oxymorphone (Numorphan)	Injectable: 1, 1.5 mg/mL Suppository: 5 mg	
Propoxyphene (Darvon, Darvon-N, others)	Tablets (as HCl): 32, 65 mg Tablets (as napsylate): 100 mg	Also in combination with acetaminophen (Darvocet N-100)
Sufentanil (Sufenta, others)	Injectable (as Citrate): 50 mcg/mL	Solution contains no preservatives
Partial Mu Agonist		
Buprenorphine (Buprenex)	Injectable: 0.3 mg/mL	Sublingual form available in some countries, not the U.S.
Mixed Agonist-Antagonists		
Butorphanol (Stadol, Stadol NS)	Injectable: 1, 2 mg/mL Nasal spray: 10 mg/mL	
Nalbuphine (Nubain, various)	Injectable: 10, 20 mg/mL	
Pentazocine (Talwin NX, Talwin)	Injectable: 30 mg/mL Tablet: 50 mg (with 0.5 mg naloxone)	Also in combination with aspirin (Talwin Compound) and acetaminophen (Talacen)

Adapted from Warren D. Practical use of rectal medications in palliative care. *J Pain Symptom Manage* 1996;11:378–387.

ROUTES OF ADMINISTRATION

Mu agonists can be administered by a variety of routes, including oral, parenteral, rectal, sublingual, transdermal, and transmucosal. The mixed agonist-antagonists are all available in parenteral dosage forms. Pentazocine is also available in an oral tablet and butorphanol as a nasal spray. Oral dosage forms are preferred for most patients on time-contingent opioid therapy. The oral route is effective, easy, relatively inexpensive, and does not signal increasing disease to the patient or family. Incomplete bioavailability should not represent a concern because this limitation is easily overcome by increasing the dose. The only advantage of the parenteral route over the oral route for patients able to take oral drugs is that delivery of the drug to sites of action is more rapid. The time difference to onset and peak levels between oral administration and IM or SC injections is usually negligible.

Patients and clinicians often hold false beliefs regarding potency and the route of medication administration. This seems most problematic when discussing parenteral versus oral administration. Intravenous administration affords quicker onset, but it does not increase potency. Additionally, the psychological advantage of oral administration should not be minimized. The fear of loss of control can become a major cause of depression among chronic and terminally ill pain patients.

The transmucosal route for fentanyl has become a useful method for managing rapidly escalating breakthrough pain. This route can facilitate rapid serum levels of lipophilic opioids and has shown efficacy in both preoperative and preprocedural sedation, as well as analgesia. Oral transmucosal fentanyl provides very rapid onset because there is no submucosal fat layer in the mouth. Transmucosal fentanyl, with its rapid onset of action, may prove to be beneficial as a breakthrough medication for patients who are on time-contingent opioid regimens, regardless of etiology. At this time two oral transmucosal forms of fentanyl are commercially available as lozenges on handles. They do not resemble lollipops and should never be referred to as such to reduce the risk that children will assume that these potentially toxic vehicles are a candy. The two dosage forms differ in appearance and amounts of drug and should not be used interchangeably. The original form (Fentanyl Oralet) is indicated for prevention and management of pain associated with medical and surgical procedures, whereas the newer form (Actiq) is indicated for breakthrough pain in the oncology patient population (Table 16-5).

Sublingual opioid administration has enjoyed extensive use in the palliative care setting for a number of years. Advantages include the relative ease of administration, low cost (using oral solutions), avoidance of the hepatic first-pass effect, and a rapid onset of action (approximately 5–15 minutes). Disadvantages include the relatively low bioavailability, a potential for poor taste acceptance, and the need to avoid oral consumption of food or drink for at least 15 minutes after administration. Simple aqueous solutions are the most appropriate vehicles for this route of administration. The volume of a dose should not exceed 1 mL of fluid to minimize the loss of medication that trickles down the throat. If a larger amount of medication is needed than will readily dissolve in 1 mL of water, it is advisable to use a second dose after 5 to 10 minutes. Not surprisingly, it has been shown that sublingual absorption favors lipophilic compounds. Results from a study on sublingual administration are listed in Table 16-2 (57). Opioids often taste bitter, yet many patients find overly sweet solutions even less palatable. Mild citrus or bland flavors are typically the most pleasing. A number of alterations in the oral mucosa as well as the overall condition of the mouth can influence the absorption from sublingual, buccal, and oral transmucosal administration. Clinicians should be aware of any issue involving the oral mucosa, including stomatitis, increased keratinization, decreased salivary flow, changes in salivary pH, oral disease, trauma, radiation, or chemotherapy regimens.

Patients unable or unwilling to tolerate oral medications often do well with opioids administrated rectally, especially for short time periods or in terminal care. Hydromorphone, morphine, and oxymorphone are commercially available in rectal suppositories. Controlled-release oral morphine tablets have been used effectively via the rectal route (46) (Table 16-6). Mucosal irritation appears to occur in fewer patients with rectally adminis-

TABLE 16-6. *Rectal opioid times to peak and duration of action*

Morphine immediate-release oral tablets	
Peak	1.1 hour
Duration	< 6 hours
Morphine controlled-release oral tablets	
Peak	5.4 hours
Duration	8–12 hours
Morphine oral solution	
Peak	0.5 hours
Duration	4–6 hours
Morphine rectal suppositories	
Peak	1.1 hours
Duration	< 6 hours
Hydromorphone rectal suppositories	
Peak	1 hour
Duration	4–6 hours
Methadone oral tablets	
Peak	not known
Duration	6–8 hours
Oxycodone	oral tablets and solution
Peak	3.1 hours
Duration	8–12 hours

Adapted from Warren D. Practical use of rectal medications in palliative care. *J Pain Symptom Manage* 1996;11:378–387.

tered oral controlled-release morphine tablets than with the commercially available morphine suppositories (47). In one report, no local side effects were reported using controlled-release oral morphine administered rectally (58). Rectal administration of oral liquids may be an option in some patients; however, limitations on acceptable rectal fluid volumes and the obvious aesthetic issues may limit this option.

Fentanyl remains the only opioid available for transdermal administration. Transdermal fentanyl patches are indicated only for the management of chronic pain in patients tolerant to the respiratory depressant effects of opioids. The patches provide for up to 72 hours of clinically effective CNS opioid levels in most cases, but some patients get only about 48 hours of relief from the patches. The patches remain more expensive than oral dosage forms but are a convenient and cost-effective alternative to parenteral opioids. Transdermal fentanyl patches can be a useful option for patients unable or unwilling to use oral or rectal opioids. The patch also appears to be useful for patients who exhibit noncompliant behaviors, e.g., patients who cannot remember to take their opioid.

Subcutaneous (SC) delivery offers a relatively easy and inexpensive parenteral method to deliver opioids yet has not enjoyed universal acceptance in the United States. The pharmacokinetics of SC delivery are similar to IM administration, without the obvious disadvantage of painful IM injections. Subcutaneous delivery is common in terminal care and has shown to provide a good alternative to the intravenous route.

Intravenous (IV) administration of opioids is especially useful after surgery or traumatic events. Intravenous patient-controlled analgesia (IV PCA) has become common in many acute settings, especially for postoperative analgesia. Although IV opioids may be useful when gastrointestinal function is precluded, e.g., postoperative ileus, the IV route can negatively reinforce the sick role for patients with chronic pain and at the end of life. The major advantage for IV PCA is that this mechanism promotes a sense of control for patients. PCA does not offer a pharmacologic advantage over regularly scheduled oral opioids for patients able to tolerate oral medications.

Neuraxial opioid administration may be warranted for a small subset of patients. This route does provide for avoidance of the toxicity associated with the systemic delivery of opioids. The epidural and intrathecal routes each have advantages and disadvantages. Epidural administration allows for opioid placement at any desired dermatomal level and does not require the anesthesiologist to puncture the dura. However, epidural administration requires larger doses than those needed with intrathecal administration. Additionally, systemic effects may occur with epidural administration, increasing the risk of adverse effects. Intrathecal administration does require puncturing of the dura, placing the drug closer to the spinal cord receptors. Intrathecal administration also pro-

vides for an increased potential for meningitis and risk of postdural puncture headaches. Dose-related problems associated with both forms of spinal analgesia include pruritus, urinary retention, and the potential for delayed respiratory depression.

DOSING

Pure mu opioid agonists do not differ pharmacodynamically but do differ in their pharmacokinetic properties. With the exception of codeine, opioids normally provide the same level of analgesia when dosed appropriately. For reasons that remain unclear, certain patients respond better to some opioids than to others. Clinical trial remains the only way to determine a preferred alternative if a patient does not respond as expected to the initial selection. Opioids maintain a relatively straight-line dose response curve over a broad therapeutic range. As such, low doses of opioids may be appropriate when the pain is not advanced. Higher doses of opioids typically become necessary when pain progresses or when pain is advanced. Because tolerance is not a clinical issue, morphine and other potent opioids should be initiated when indicated.

As long as a pain stimulus exists and responds to opioids, these agents should be used on a regular schedule or time-contingent basis. Undertreatment of acute pain can lead to the development of chronic pain syndromes. The use of around-the-clock opioids often breaks the cycle of pain and can decrease or eliminate the centrally mediated processes that complicate pain control. Thus, it may require less drug to prevent the recurrence of pain than would be required to treat recurring pain.

Morphine and the other pure opioid agonists can provide analgesia in most acute and chronic malignant pain patients and many chronic nonmalignant pain patients. There is no *a priori* maximum dose for the pure mu agonists. All patients will require individual titration of their opioid regimen. Morphine doses required for comfort following similar pain stimuli may vary as much as 50 to 100 fold among chronic malignant pain patients (59) and 10 to 20 fold among acute pain patients (60).

In addition to scheduled opioid doses, supplemental doses should be always be available for management of breakthrough pain. *Breakthrough pain* can be defined as the transitory increases in pain that are greater than moderate in intensity and occur in addition to baseline pain of moderate or less intensity (61). Breakthrough pain doses should be based on the scheduled (time-contingent) dose. Sufficient rescue doses of opioids should be made available to the patient in the form of immediate-release dosage forms to provide comfort when breakthrough pain occurs. For breakthrough pain, a typical rescue dose is one-half of the every-4-hours scheduled dose (one-sixth of the every-12-hours scheduled controlled-release dose) administered every 2 hours as needed. When chronic pain patients exhibit breakthrough pain that requires more than two to three rescue doses for more than 2 to 3 days in succession, an increase in the scheduled (time-contingent) dose should be considered.

Another variation of breakthrough pain is incident pain. Incident pain occurs predictably when a patient ambulates, gets tired, or undergoes medical procedures. In these cases an additional dose of an appropriate immediate-release dosage form should be administered prior to the incident to provide effective levels about a half-hour before the anticipated pain increase.

Fear of opioids causes many clinicians to utilize overly conservative dose adjustments that often lead to treatment failure. Opioid doses should be titrated to response. When escalation of a dose is warranted, it is important to increase the opioid dose as a percentage of the current regimen, not a preset number of milligrams. Increases of 33% to 50% should be made as soon as steady-state serum levels are achieved (5 half-lives, which is equal to about 10 hours for morphine). An increase from 30 mg every 4 hours to 45 mg every 4 hours would be appropriate. If the inadequate dose is 300 mg every 12 hours, the increase should be to 450 mg every 12 hours. When patients know that an opioid dose has been increased, yet inadequate analgesia results, anxiety often increases. This anxiety can increase the pain perception and in turn increase future opioid dose requirements. It is often better to err slightly in the direction of too much than too little opioid.

Clinicians should carefully evaluate complaints of increased pain or diminished analgesic efficacy in patients whose analgesia was adequate before simply increasing the opioid dose. Clinical tolerance to opioid analgesia *per se* is rare after comfort has been achieved and maintained for a few days. Ineffective analgesia is almost always the result of factors that increase pain or compromise analgesic efficacy. Factors include progressive disease, new disease, increased or excessive activity, poor compliance, change in medication formulation or brand, drug interactions, and opioid addiction or diversion (26).

Medications with long half-lives, such as methadone and levorphanol, can be useful for managing patients with chronic pain syndromes. These drugs afford analgesia for 8 hours or longer after steady-state serum levels are achieved. Of note, methadone may be required every 4 hours during the first days of analgesic therapy but can usually be administered every 8 to 12 hours in about 4 days. The longer duration of actions for these drugs is often useful for providing time-contingent opioid therapy to chronic pain patients. Due to the long and variable half-lives, clinicians should exercise caution before using these agents. Patients may achieve adequate analgesia initially but with continued use may become toxic due to accumulation of the parent drug or its metabolites. Methadone has little usefulness in acute pain due to its extended half-life.

A World Health Organization (WHO) expert committee has defined five principles for opioid use in the management of cancer pain in developing countries (WHO Cancer Pain Relief 1986, 1996). These principles have been validated in numerous studies in undeveloped, developing, and developed countries including the United States. Recently, the applicability of these principles to both acute pain (5) and chronic noncancer pain has been documented (8). A summary of these principles is as follows:

1. Use the oral (or other noninvasive) routes when possible.
2. Titrate doses to individual response.
3. Utilize analgesics as described on the analgesic ladder.
4. Maintain effective drug concentrations while noxious stimulus is present.
5. Use adjuvant medications when indicated.

The usefulness of the WHO approach has been studied in over 2100 cancer patients over a period of 10 years for a total of 140 478 treatment days. Medications from step 1 of the WHO analgesic ladder provided adequate analgesia for only 11% of the days, step 2 for 31% of the days, and step 3 for 49% of the days. Over half of these patients (56%) received morphine. During the final days of life, 84% of the patients rated their pain as moderate or less (62).

DRUG INTERACTIONS

Opioids have the potential to interact with a variety of medications (Table 16-3). The majority of these interactions are due to additive effects, i.e., pharmacodynamic interactions. Increased sedation is common with opioids, especially when administered with alcohol, benzodiazepines, butyrophenones, phenothiazines, sedative-hypnotics, and tricyclic antidepressants. Midazolam use may decrease the effectiveness of fentanyl (63). Analgesic activity can be impaired by benzodiazepine administration via inhibition of the descending inhibitory control pathways (63).

Methadone withdrawal may be the best elucidated of the pharmacokinetic opioid drug interactions. This withdrawal has been precipitated by a number of agents known to induce microsomal enzymes, resulting in an increase in the metabolism of methadone (64). Inhibition of methadone metabolism has also been shown with several agents, resulting in an increase in methadone levels.

These drug interactions are not a one-way phenomenon. Opioids are capable of inhibiting the metabolism of other agents, leading to increases in serum levels of affected drugs. For example, desipramine levels may be increased during coadministration with methadone or morphine (63, 64).

CONCLUSION

Opioid analgesics continue to provide clinicians with a viable option for treating a variety of painful conditions, both acute and chronic in nature. Unfortunately, many clinicians refuse or feel unable to utilize these valuable and effective medications because of improper knowledge or

TABLE 16-7. *Selected statements and guidelines addressing opioid analgesia*

Organization	Publication	Year	Information source
Agency for Health Care Policy and Research (AHCPR) U.S. Public Health Service	*Clinical Practice Guideline for Acute Pain Management*	1992	www.ahrq.gov
Agency for Health Care Policy and Research (AHCPR) U.S. Public Health Service	*Clinical Practice Guideline for Cancer Pain Management*	1994	www.ahrq.gov
American Society of Addiction Medicine (ASAM)	*Public Policy Statement*	1997	www.asam.org
American Geriatrics Society (AGS)	*Clinical Practice Guideline on the Management of Chronic Pain in the Older Persons*	1998	*JAGS* 1997;46: 635–51
American Pain Society (APS)	*Principles of Analgesic Use in Acute and Cancer Pain*, 4th ed.	1999	www.ampainsoc.org
American Pain Society (APS)	*Clinical Practice Guideline for Sickle Cell Disease Pain*	1999	www.ampainsoc.org
American Medical Directors Association (AMDA)	*Clinical Practice Guideline for Chronic Pain in the Long Term Care Setting*	1999	www.amda.com
American Pain Society (APS)	*Clinical Practice Guideline for Osteo-arthritis and Rheumatoid Arthritis Pain*	2001	www.ampainsoc.org

unfounded and irrational fears. Recent policy statements by the American Pain Society, American Academy of Pain Medicine, and the Federation of State Medical Boards of the United States will hopefully begin to turn the tide and promote the appropriate and rational use of opioids in all patients who have pain that should be treated with opioid analgesics (Table 16-7).

It is important that clinicians differentiate between the pure mu opioid receptor agonists, mixed agonist-antagonists, and partial agonists. Pharmacokinetic differences can be clinically significant and should always factor into decisions regarding opioid selection and dosing. Differences in metabolism and elimination may make some opioids preferable to others, especially in the patient with impaired hepatic or renal function. When in doubt, the WHO analgesic ladder can provide invaluable assistance in designing a regimen in the vast majority of cases.

REFERENCES

1. Morgan J. American opiophobia: customary underutilization of opioid analgesics. *Adv Alcohol Subst Abuse* 1985;5:163–173.
2. The Interagency Committee on New Therapies for Pain and Discomfort: report to the White House. US Department of Health Education and Welfare, Public Health Service, National Institutes of Health May 1979.
3. Pinkert T. Report from the Interagency Committee on Pain and Analgesia: a Public Health Service initiative. *J Pain Symptom Manage* 1986;1:174–177.
4. National Institutes of Health Consensus Development Conference. The integrated approach to the management of pain. *J Pain Symptom Manage* 1987;2:35-44.
5. Acute Pain Management Guideline Panel. Acute pain management: Operative or medical procedures and trauma. Clinical Practice Guideline. AHCPR Pub. No. 92-0032. Rockville, MD: Agency for Health Care Policy and Research, Public Health Service, U.S. Department of Health and Human Services, 1992 (Feb.).
6. Jacox A, Carr DB, Payne R, et al. Management of cancer pain. Clinical practice guideline No. 9. AHCPR Publication No. 94-0592. Rockville,

MD: Agency for Health Care Policy and Research, U.S. Department of Health and Human Services, Public Health Service, 1994.
7. Portenoy RK. Opioid therapy for chronic nonmalignant pain: a review of the critical issues. *J Pain Symptom Manage* 1996;11: 203–217.
8. Haddox JD, Joranson DE, Angarola RT, et al. Consensus Statement from the American Academy of Pain Medicine and American Pain Society. The use of opioids for the treatment of chronic pain. *Clin J Pain* 1997;13:6–8.
9. The Federation of State Medical Boards of the United States. Model guidelines for the use of controlled substances for the treatment of pain, May 2, 1998.
10. Bernabei R, Gambassi G, Lapane K, et al. Management of pain in elderly patients with cancer. *JAMA* 1998;279:1877–1882.
11. World Health Organization. Cancer pain relief and palliative care: report of a WHO Expert Committee. Technical Report Series 804. Geneva: World Health Organization; 1990.
12. Elliot T, Murray D, Elliot B, et al. Physician knowledge and attitudes about cancer pain management: a survey from the Minnesota Cancer Pain Project. *J Pain Symptom Manage* 1995;10:495–504.
13. Rankin M, Snider B. Nurses' perceptions of cancer patients' pain. *Cancer Nurs* 1984;7:149–155.
14. Doucette W, Mays-Holland T, Memmott H, et al. Cancer pain management: pharmacist knowledge and practices. *J Pharm Care Pain Symptom Control* 5:1997;1(17):7–32.
15. Rinaldi R, Steindler E, Wilford B, et al. Clarification and standardization of substance abuse terminology. *JAMA* 1998;259:555–557.
16. Porter J, Jick H, NEJM. Addiction rare in patients treated with narcotics (letter). *NEJM* 1980;302:123.
17. Perry S, Heidrich G. Management of pain during debridement: a survey of U.S. pain units. *Pain* 1982;13:267–280.
18. Medina J, Diamond S. Drug dependency in patients with chronic headache. *Headache* 1977;17:12–14.
19. Weissman DE, Haddox JD. Opioid pseudoaddiction—an iatrogenic syndrome. *Pain* 1989;36:363–366.
20. The American Society of Addiction Medicine. Public Policy Statement on Definitions Related to the Use of Opioids in Pain Treatment. www.asam.org, 1997 (April).
21. Twycross R, Fairfield S. Pain in far-advanced cancer. *Pain* 1982; 14:303–310.
22. Breitbart W, McDonald M, Rosenfeld B, et al. Pain in ambulatory AIDS patients: pain characteristics and medical correlates. *Pain* 1996; 68:315–321.
23. Hare BD, Lipman AG. Uses and misuses of medications in the management of chronic pain. *Problems in Anesthesia* 1990;4:577–594.
24. Twycross RG. Clinical experience with diamorphine in advanced malignant disease. *Int J Clin Pharmacol* 1974;9:184–198.

25. Collins E, Poulain P, Gauvin-Piquard A et al. Is disease progression the major factor in morphine "tolerance" in cancer pain treatment? *Pain* 1993;55:319–326.
26. Pappagallo M. The concept of pseudotolerance to opioids. *J Pharm Care Pain Symptom Control* 1998;6:95–98.
27. Basta S, Anderson D. Mechanisms and management of constipation in the cancer patient. *J Pharm Care Pain Symptom Control* 1998; 6:21–40.
28. Levy M. Pain management in advanced cancer. *Semin Oncol* 1985; 12:394–410.
29. Sykes, NP. An investigation of oral naloxone to correct opioid related constipation in patients with advanced cancer. *Palliative Medicine,* 1996;10:135–144.
30. Lipman AG. Comments on Fitzgibbon and Galer (letter). *Pain* 1995; 63:135.
31. Ferrante F. Principles of opioid pharmacotherapy: practical implications of basic mechanisms. *J Pain Symptom Manage* 1996;11:265–273.
32. Rushton A, Sneyd J. Opioid analgesics. *Br J Hosp Med* 1997;57: 105–106.
33. Singh V, Bajpai K, Biswas S, et al. Molecular biology of opioid receptors. *Recent advances. Neuroimmunomodulation* 1997;4:285–297.
34. Yaksh T. Pharmacology and mechanisms of opioid analgesic activity. *Acta Anaesthesiol Scand* 1997;41:94–111.
35. Franz D. Pharmacology of analgesic receptors. *J Pharm Care Pain Symptom Contr* 1994;2:37–58.
36. Sabbe M, Yaksh T. Pharmacology of spinal opioids. *J Pain Symptom Manage* 1990;5:191–203.
37. Lipman AG, Gauthier M. Pharmacology of opioid drugs: basic principles. In: Portenoy R, Bruera E, eds. *Topics in palliative care. Vol. 1.* New York: Oxford University Press, 1997:137–161.
38. Pasternak G. Pharmacological mechanisms of opioid analgesics. *Clin Neuropharmacol* 1993;16:1–18.
39. Hare B. The opioid analgesics: rational selection of agents for acute and chronic pain. *Hosp Formul* 1987;22:64–86.
40. Back I, Finlay I. Analgesic effect of topical opioids on painful skin ulcers. *J Pain Symptom Manage* 1995;10:493.
41. Stein C, Pfluger M, Yassouridis A, et al. No tolerance to peripheral morphine analgesia in presence of opioid expression in inflamed synovia. *J Clin Invest* 1996;98:793–799.
42. Stein C, Yassouridis A. Periperal morphine analgesia. *Pain* 1997;71: 119–121.
43. Walker D, Zacny J. Subjective, psychomotor, and analgesic effects of oral codeine and morphine in healthy volunteers. *Psychopharmacology (Berl)* 1998;140:191–201.
44. Cleary J. Pharmacokinetic and pharmacodynamic issues in the treatment of breakthrough pain. *Semin Oncol* 1997;24:13–19.
45. Rusho W. Clinical issues and concerns in the use of extemporaneously compounded medications. *J Pharm Care Pain Symptom Control* 1996;4:5–20.
46. Warren D. Practical use of rectal medications in palliative care. *J Pain Symptom Manage* 1996;11:378–387.
47. Kaiko R, Fitzmartin R, Thomas G, Goldenheim P. The bioavailability of morphine in controlled-release 30-mg tablets per rectum com-

pared with immediate-release 30-mg rectal suppositories and controlled-release 30-mg oral tablets. *Pharmacother* 1992;12:107–113.
48. Korte W, Stoutz N, Morant R. Day-to-day titration to initiate transdermal fentanyl in cancer patients: short and long term experience in a prospective study of 39 patients. *J Pain Symptom Manage* 1996;11: 139–146.
49. Moulin D, Kreeft J, Murray-Parsons N, Bouquillon A. Comparison of continuous subcutaneous and intravenous hydromorphone infusion for management of cancer pain. *Lancet* 1991;337:465–468.
50. Pereira J, Bruera E. Emerging neuropsychiatric toxicities of opioids. *J Pharm Care Pain Symptom Control* 1997;5:3–29.
51. Christrup L. Morphine metabolites. *Acta Anaesthesiol Scand* 1997; 41:116–122.
52. Forman W. Opioid analgesic drugs in the elderly. *Clin Geriatr Med* 1996;12:489–500.
53. Sjøgren P, Jensen N, Jensen T. Disappearance of morphine-induced hyperalgesia after discontinuing or substituting other opioid agonists. *Pain* 1994;59:313–316.
54. Glare P, Walsh T, Pippenger C. Normorphine, a neurotoxic metabolite? *Lancet* 1990;335:725–726.
55. Bruera E, Brenneis C, Chadwick S et al. Methylphenidate associated with narcotics for the treatment of cancer pain. *Ca Treatment Rep* 1987;71:67–70.
56. Vainio A, Ollila J, Matikainen E, et al. Driving ability in cancer patients receiving long-term morphine analgesia. *Lancet* 1995;346: 667–670.
57. Weinberg D, Inturrisi C, Reidenberg B, et al. Sublingual absorption of selected opioid analgesics. *Clin Pharmacol Ther* 1988;44:335–342.
58. Maloney C, Kesner R, Klein G, et al. The rectal administration of MS Contin: clinical implications of use in end stage cancer. *Am J Hospice Care* 1989;6:34–35.
59. Twycross R. Morphine and diamorphine in the terminally ill patient. *Acta Anaesth Scand* 1984;74:128–134.
60. Beeton A, Upton P, Shipton E. The case for patient-controlled analgesia. Inter-patient variation in postoperative analgesic requirements. *S Afr J Surg* 1992;30:5–6.
61. Portenoy R, Hagen N. Breakthrough pain: definition, prevalence and characteristics. *Pain* 1990;41:273–281.
62. Zech D, Grond S, Lynch J, et al. Validation of the World Health Organization guidelines for cancer pain relief: a ten year prospective study. *Pain* 1995;63:65–76.
63. Maurer P, Bartkowski R. Drug interactions of clinical significance with opioid analgesics. *Drug Saf* 1993;8:30–48.
64. Quinn D, Day R. Drug interactions of clinical importance. An updated guide. *Drug Saf* 1995;12:393–452.
65. Principles of Analgesic Use in the Treatment of Acute Pain and Cancer Pain, Fourth Edition. Glenview, Il: American Pain Society, 1999.
66. Lipman AG, Jackson KC. Opioids. In Warfield C, Bajwa Z, eds. *Principles and practice of pain management*, 2nd ed. New York: McGraw-Hill, 2001.
67. Hansten PD, Horn JR. *Drug interactions analysis and management.* Vancouver WA, Applied Therapuetics, Inc., updated quarterly.

SECTION IV

Pharmacologic Intervention

Behavioral Issues and Controversies in Opioid Analgesia for Cancer and Nonmalignant Chronic Pain

Leslie J. Heinberg, Lisa M. Yacono Freeman and Marzban Rad

Chronic pain, whether due to malignant or benign etiology, provides a significant challenge not only to patients, but also to their employers, families, and physicians. For many patients with chronic pain, adequate management of their condition requires the long-term use of medications, including opioids. Opioids are potent analgesics that produce an analgesic effect by binding to specific receptors on the spinal cord and in the brain (1). Although there is marginal acceptance of opioid therapy for acute pain management, the longer-term continued use of these medications for patients with cancer and chronic, nonmalignant pain has been highly debated. As a result of medical and psychosocial controversies, there is significant ambivalence on the part of many physicians toward treating malignant and nonmalignant pain with opioids (2). Unfortunately, this has led to a delay in strong empirical clinical research examining the advantages and disadvantages of opioid use that in turn may help elucidate the dilemma.

This chapter will explore the use of chronic or long-term opioid therapy for patients with cancer and nonmalignant pain. Widespread implementation of chronic opioid therapy has been thwarted by concerns regarding efficacy, addiction liability, tolerance to opioid analgesia (3,4), impairment of cognition (5), reductions in physical functioning (6), and beliefs that depression (7,8) may result from chronic opioid treatment. We will discuss controversies, barriers to use, and behavioral management of patients on chronic opioid therapy. Finally, the management of problematic patients will be reviewed.

Overview

In those cases where chronic pain has failed to respond to standard treatment interventions (e.g., nonsteroidal anti-inflammatory medications, tricyclic antidepressants, antiepileptic drugs, physical rehabilitation, psychological interventions, and, if indicated, surgical procedures), opioids can be added or used as a single-drug treatment. In general, more conservative pharmacological and behavioral interventions are offered to patients initially, and only after these interventions fail to provide significant pain relief is chronic opioid analgesia offered (2).

Opioid analgesia is characterized by a dose-response relationship without an apparent "ceiling" dose. That is, the opioid dose is adjusted upward until satisfactory pain relief or unmanageable side effects occur. Often the pain is constant for patients with cancer and nonmalignant chronic pain. Controlled-release opioid preparations (e.g., MS Contin, OxyContin, Duragesic) or opioids with a prolonged half-life (e.g., methadone, levorphanol) are recommended for the treatment of chronic pain (2). The long-acting agents are usually prescribed at regular intervals on an around-the-clock schedule and not on an as-needed basis. This is thought to improve treatment compliance and markedly decrease the daily occurrence of miniwithdrawal symptoms, which are related to blood level fluctuations of the medications. In addition, such medication scheduling helps decrease the reinforcing effects of the drug and may lessen the likelihood of problematic misuse (9).

EFFICACY/USE/UNDERUSE

Pain Treatment

The National Institutes of Health's Agency for Health Care Policy and Research has issued clinical practice guidelines for the management of acute (10) and cancer pain (11). These guidelines identify opioid use as not only acceptable but also frequently mandated. Similarly, the World Health Organization (WHO) has developed guidelines for the treatment of cancer pain (12). These guidelines describe a three-step process of analgesic use that includes nonopioid, weak opioid (e.g., codeine), and strong opioid (e.g., morphine, methadone) medications, plus adjuvants (12–14). However, in spite of these pronouncements regarding nonmalignant and cancer pain, many patients' pain is subtherapeutically managed.

Central to the debate of prescribing opioids for chronic pain is the issue of efficacy. Pain relief is considered the most important goal by pain physicians, with functional improvement an important secondary goal (15). Many anecdotal reports (3), surveys (16,17), uncontrolled studies (18,19), and two clinical controlled studies (20,21) have confirmed opioid efficacy for analgesia, even for the treatment of neuropathic pain. Despite noted efficacy, patients with nonmalignant pain are generally undertreated with opioid analgesia (22). The efficacy of opioid medications for cancer pain, and the belief that pain relief will lead to improved psychosocial functioning, may explain why physicians seem more willing to prescribe opioids for cancer pain than for other types of chronic pain (2,22,23). However, despite apparent acceptance of opioids as an integral part of the treatment of cancer pain, WHO data suggest that approximately 4.3 million cancer victims die annually with suboptimal pain control (12,13). Further, less than half of cancer patients may be receiving pain treatment adequate to alleviate their pain (24–26) due to underdosing by medical providers (27).

In addition to evidence that opioids are helpful for ameliorating cancer (26,28,29) and nonmalignant pain (20,21, 30) there is evidence that pain relief provided by opioid therapy is associated with improved functioning in patients with osteoarthritis pain (31) and nonmalignant neuropathic pain (32), at least to the extent that pain and not the primary disease is the root cause of disability (26). Improvements in functioning may be intimately linked to improvements in mood that have been observed to accompany pain relief (26). Global quality of life may also improve (33).

CONTROVERSIES/BARRIERS

A number of controversies and barriers may explain why potentially effective pain treatment guidelines (10,12) have not translated into effective pain relief for the majority of patients. Perhaps most important among these is that medical personnel are by and large uninformed about the appropriate use of analgesics, including opioids, in non-malignant and cancer pain (22,25,34,36). Mismanagement and undertreatment occur in the treatment of acute cancer and chronic nonmalignant pain, and physicians undertreat patients already dependent upon opioids and withhold opioids despite evidence that the risk of iatrogenic addiction is markedly low (22).

Concerns about the Potential for Misuse

Although the majority of oncologists and pain specialists admit to maintaining some of their cancer and chronic nonmalignant pain patients on long-term opioid therapy, the majority of U.S. physicians are reluctant to prescribe opioids for chronic pain conditions (27), including cancer (37), a phenomenon termed *opiophobia* (6,37,38). Opiophobia results in customary underutilization of opioid analgesics and is fueled by the misperception that chronic opioid therapy is equivalent to or will lead to addiction. This belief is shared by physicians, nurses, and patients alike (26,37,39). Moreover, the societal stigma of drug use, difficulty for the patient locating dispensing pharmacies, family resistance, and patient bias may decrease the likelihood of physicians garnering compliance for such pharmacotherapy. It is important for physicians to recognize the conceptual difference between addiction and physical dependence and the clinical usefulness of chronic opioid therapy. Therefore, we later will discuss the definitions of physical dependence, tolerance, addiction and pseudoaddiction, the pros and cons of the major controversies surrounding the use of opioids for chronic pain, and management of potential side effects. This will be followed by guidelines for the ethical management of chronic pain patients generally and those who may be at risk for opioid misuse or abuse.

Physical dependence involves the occurrence of a withdrawal syndrome when there is a sudden cessation in the use of the medication. This phenomenon is relatively common with the use of opioids as well as with the use of other medications such as those for hypertension, epilepsy, or depression (40). Physical dependence on a prescribed medication does not, in itself, signify addiction (41). Withdrawal syndromes vary in characteristics depending upon the medication taken. When a patient abruptly stops taking an opioid analgesic, symptoms of full withdrawal may start approximately 24–48 hours after the last dose. The opioid withdrawal syndrome is characterized by "flulike" symptoms, such as rhinorrhea, chills, yawning, sweating, aching muscles, abdominal cramps, nausea, and diarrhea. The syndrome is self-limited, usually lasting 3–7 days according to the type of opioid taken (2). Although uncomfortable and unpleasant for the patient, opioid withdrawal is not considered to be life threatening (2). It is imperative, however, that patients be strongly forewarned against sudden discontinuation of the medication as part of informed consent. If the discontinuation of opioids is therapeutically indicated, symptoms of withdrawal can be avoided by gradually tapering the drug (on the average over 2 weeks). Patient education regarding the inevitability of physical dependence and the lack of a necessary correlation between this and addiction should be an essential aspect of the informed consent prior to initiating a chronic opioid therapy trial.

Tolerance is defined as the requirement for a dose escalation to maintain the same drug-related effect. Similarly, analgesic tolerance is characterized by a continued need for dose escalation to maintain the same level of pain relief (2). Contrary to conventional belief, clinical experience indicates that tolerance to opioid analgesia is not a significant problem for the majority of patients. One recent study found the emergence of tolerance in only 1 of 48 patients with neuropathic pain treated with transdermal fentanyl (42). Progression or flareup of the underlying disease, increased physical activity, or occurrence of new pathology, not true analgesic tolerance, is often responsible for the dose escalation (2). Of note, tolerance to most of the opioid-related side effects (but not constipation) occurs much more commonly and quickly than tolerance to analgesia. These side effects include drowsiness, mental cloudiness, nausea, vomiting, dysphoria, and euphoria (although euphoria is very rarely seen in pain patients treated with long-acting oral or transdermal preparations). The development of tolerance to the opioid side effects constitutes a positive phenomenon that often allows upward dose titration to satisfactory pain relief.

Addiction is defined as an abnormal and compulsive use of a substance and continued use in spite of physical, psychological, occupational, or interpersonal difficulties resulting from use. Addicted individuals may spend an inordinate amount of time using the drug and securing its supply and may have a very high relapse rate following withdrawal (43). Often the drug is self-administered, and its use deviates from any approved medical or social patterns. Jaffe (43) defined *addiction* as a term that conveys a "quantitative rather than a qualitative sense" when "the drug use pervades the total life activity of the user" to the point that "drug use controls the user's behavior." Such severe behavioral disturbance is relatively rare in patients with cancer or chronic nonmalignant pain and may be more common in individuals who have a history of alcohol or substance abuse or dependence (2; see following).

Pseudoaddiction describes behaviors that are suggestive of addiction and may be observed in some patients whose pain is poorly managed. Undertreatment of pain leads to patient behaviors that mimic those of addicted patients (2). That is, pseudoaddiction is an iatrogenic effect of ineffective pain management. For example, borderline abnormal drug-seeking or -taking behavior may be observed in undertreated cancer pain patients who return to proper, normal behavior after they are successfully treated for pain (44). Some pain patients exhibit anxiety, frustration, and what may appear to be drug-seeking behavior at the prospect of either treatment discontinuation or discharge from the care of the physician. This behavior has also been called *treatment dependence behavior* (4). These patients can be mislabeled "addicted," leading to anger, frustration, and avoidance in the health-care provider and increasing anger, hopelessness, suspiciousness, and isolation in the patient (1).

The risk of addiction remains the primary concern among the majority of general practitioners, nurses, patients, and their families. However, extensive clinical experience with the treatment of cancer pain and postsurgical pain has indicated that the mere exposure to opioid medications is not sufficient to cause addiction. As further elucidation, whereas addiction is characterized by a desire to "get high," compulsive drug-seeking, declines in psychosocial functioning, and difficulty stopping the drug use, pain patients on opioids, with very rare exceptions, do not exhibit these desires or behaviors, often are able to increase their functioning due to decreased pain, and actually wish they did not need to depend on medications to function (27). Friedman suggests that it is the inadequately treated pain patient who is more likely to exhibit poor functioning (27).

Psychosocial and genetic factors, including a history of substance abuse and antisocial personality disorder, appear to be extremely important in determining the onset of addiction. Nevertheless, addiction was found to be a very rare treatment complication in several uncontrolled and controlled studies, particularly in patients with no history of drug abuse (4). Although the prevalence of addiction was found to be as high as 19% in a series of surveys of pain patients referred to psychiatrically oriented pain clinics (45), figures derived from surveys and clinical studies of pain patients nonselectively referred to specialized pain programs indicate a much lower prevalence rate, as low as 0% to 2% (17,19,20,46–49). For example, only 4 cases of addiction were documented among 11 882 hospitalized patients who were treated with opioids and had no known history of substance abuse (47).

Another important, and related, barrier for physicians with limited knowledge of opioids in cancer pain treatment is the concern that prescribing opioids for a cancer patient is tantamount to assisted suicide (13). However, there is no evidence to support this concern, and, as noted, *untreated* pain is a significant risk factor for suicide in cancer patients.

Implementation Problems

If concerns about opioid abuse (e.g., addiction or use in committing suicide) do not prevent a physician from initiating opioid therapy for pain patients, implementation issues may still hamper the appropriate and effective use of opioids. For example, many physicians continue to use standard dosing guidelines, rather than opioid responsiveness, to determine treatment course, an approach that may be inadequate for severe pain (13). Cancer pain and some types of nonmalignant chronic pain are not static phenomena because the underlying disease is changing.

In addition to dosing issues, there is widespread disagreement about a number of other implementation issues, including the efficacy of opioids for neuropathic pain, the appropriate choice of drugs, and the optimal route of administration (13).

Inadequate Assessment

Another key factor that interferes with appropriate narcotic treatment of pain is inadequate pain assessment (26). Continuous pain assessment is not a routine part of cancer treatment, in part due to time constraints and in part due to lack of knowledge or skill about pain and its treatment. Also, malignant pain assessment is more difficult than is assessment of the typical case of nonmalignant chronic pain due to the progressive nature of the underlying disease and the destructive treatments that accompany its progression (26). Similarly, few physicians treating nonmalignant chronic pain rely upon diaries (30) or other types of continuous assessment devices. Repeated pain intensity measures as well as instruments assessing functioning, side effects, and perceived quality of life should be a standard part of managing any patient on chronic opioid therapy.

Communication barriers between patient and physician also interfere with accurate pain assessment. Because the experience of pain is completely subjective, the patient's pain report is the only appropriate measure of pain (46). However, patient and physician estimates of pain are often disparate, particularly for more severe pain (26). The patient's pain report must be taken at face value if effective pain management is to be achieved. Communication between patients and their physicians about pain also may be hampered by patients' hesitance to fully report the extent of their pain for fear of drawing the physician's attention away from the crucial issue of disease treatment or of facing the possibility that the increased pain signifies a progression of their cancer (26).

Side Effects

Common opioid side effects, for patients with malignant and nonmalignant pain alike, include constipation, nausea, vomiting, drowsiness, dry mouth, and sweating. Fortunately, tolerance to all of these side effects except constipation usually occurs within 2 weeks (14). Persistent side effects such as constipation and nausea are readily treated with additional pharmacological agents or may be alleviated by switching to another opioid medication. Indeed, failure to appropriately manage side effects may lead to unneeded discontinuation of narcotic therapy or underdosing (14). Patients also can be expected to develop tolerance to the respiratory depression associated with opioids, such that respiratory depression rarely presents an obstacle to continuing opioid therapy (14).

Cognitive Functioning

The potential for opioid medications to impair cognition has also contributed to controversy surrounding their chronic use. This controversy is based on experimental subjects without pain or patients with known addiction rather than on a more representational group of chronic pain patients (see Zacny, 1995, for a review). For example, opioids administered acutely to opioid-naive subjects were shown to slow encoding, processing, and recalling of serial verbal information (50). Chronic pain patients classified as drug-dependent or drug-abusing scored lower on measures of attention and motor speed than did patients classified as nonabusing (5). Other studies suggest that patients with nonmalignant chronic pain receiving long-term oral opioid therapy perform worse than normal, pain-free controls on a variety of neuropsychological measures (51). Limited conclusions can be drawn from these studies, however, because of sampling biases and unknown levels of premorbid cognitive functioning.

Studies that compare functioning before and after chronic opioid administration provide more convincing data that the possible long-term cognitive effects of opioid medications are minimal. In recent studies, improved reaction time (52), normal driving ability (53,54), and no impairment in cognition (17), motor coordination, verbal information processing, visual memory, attention, and psychomotor speed (55,56) were found in cancer and non-cancer pain patients undergoing chronic and stable opioid treatment. In a randomized, double-blind, crossover study trial, chronic opioid therapy with controlled-release oral morphine was shown to have no significant negative impact on most measures of mood, functional status, perceived disability, psychiatric symptomatology, and cognition (20). These studies indicate that, although a temporary decline in cognitive function may occur when the opioid dose is acutely increased, only a few nonsignificant cognitive effects are apparent in patients taking chronic and stable doses.

Assessing any potential cognitive effects of opioid therapy for cancer patients is more difficult. Impairment in cognitive functioning is a common problem for patients with advanced cancer, and particularly terminal cancer, although the exact cause of this dysfunction is often unknown (57) and may reflect the disease process itself, increased likelihood of high-dose medication with concomitant side effects, both, or additional factors. Evidence that chronic opioid therapy is directly and primarily responsible for cognitive dysfunction in cancer patients is equivocal at best and based on specific neuropsychological indices rather than complex, real-life tasks (58–61). Cognitive impairment in cancer patients may be better explained by lower psychosocial functioning and the presence of pain, which tend to occur together with opioid use, rather than by opioid use per se (61). Notably, some research has suggested that additional pharmacological agents such as the amphetamine methylphenidate may be useful in attenuating the cognitive effects of chronic high-dose subcutaneous opioid therapy (57).

Depression

It is a common belief that opioid therapy may cause an exacerbation of symptoms of depression and decreased motivation to improve. Distinguishing this putative opioid-related side effect from premorbid depression is critical because of the high coprevalence of depression in patients with chronic pain (62,63). Additionally, depression can negatively affect physical functioning and scores of pain intensity (63). Major depression was found in 60% of noncancer pain patients maintained on oral opioids and referred to a psychiatrically oriented pain clinic (8). Hypochondriasis, depression (64), apathy, and decreased motivation to function were observed in addicts on methadone maintenance (7). However, psychosocial and medical differences between addicts and chronic pain patients make any comparison or generalization inappropriate. Moreover, clinical and controlled studies (20,55,65) argue against the concept that depression is directly induced by chronic opioid therapy. Regardless, because of the high comorbidity of depression in cancer and nonmalignant pain, any complaints of depression should be taken seriously and result in referral to a psychiatrist or psychologist specializing in working with chronic pain or oncology patients. Finally, it should be noted that cognitive dysfunction is often mistaken for depression (57).

Systemic Considerations

The perceived risk by physicians of legal and regulatory sanctions contributes to the underuse of opioids for the treatment of chronic nonmalignant pain. The Drug Enforcement Administration's *Physician's Manual* indicates that narcotic analgesics may be used in the treatment of pain in patients with a terminal illness or chronic disorder. Further, the physician should not hesitate to prescribe, dispense, or administer narcotic analgesics when they are indicated for a legitimate medical purpose (66). However, frequent concerns are common among physicians, including oncologists. Foley (1995) faults several systemic variables, most notably tight regulation and limited availability of opioids, as obstacles to effective treatment of cancer pain. Indeed, many pharmacies are hesitant to keep in stock certain narcotic medications (67).

BEHAVIORAL MANAGEMENT OF CHRONIC PAIN PATIENTS WITH LONG-TERM OPIOID THERAPY

Few specific guidelines have been empirically validated for selecting appropriate patients for long-term opioid therapy. It has been suggested that the ideal candidate is an individual who has been historically medically compliant, is socially stable, is free from psychiatric diagnoses, is not in a chaotic work (disability) environment, and needs a finite drug intake (68). Unfortunately, many patients with chronic cancer or nonmalignant pain are far more complicated, and empirical studies have not been completed to substantiate these guidelines (30). As a result, clinicians are often left attempting to manage a variety of patients with little guidance. The considerations and problems just discussed suggest a number of areas for behavioral management.

Education

Patients, their families, and physicians may require education about evidence supporting the use of opioids to treat chronic pain. Particularly, education about the difference between addiction and physical tolerance may help to diminish negative connotations about the use of opioids for medical conditions. Providing accurate information about the course and appropriate management of common side effects also will help to prevent unnecessary discontinuation of opioid therapy by either physician or patient.

Assessment

As previously stated, pain assessment for pain patients should be continuous and comprehensive in order to ensure that treatment decisions about opioid therapy (e.g., dose changes) are based on the most accurate, current information possible. These regular pain evaluations should measure not only pain severity, but also pain quality, location, pattern, and life impact (e.g., effect on mood, subjective quality of life, functioning, and social activity), which will provide ongoing feedback about the adequacy of pain treatment (26). Written questionnaires may elicit more accurate feedback than verbal questioning because the former do not require the patient to directly confront the caregiver with the "failure" of that caregiver's treatment efforts (26). Psychologists also can play a role in encouraging hesitant patients to give physicians accurate and complete feedback about their pain experience.

Initial and periodic communication with an individual from the patient's environment (a partner or family member) can also be an invaluable help in initial assessment and in monitoring followup efficacy and compliance (68).

Psychological Symptoms and Disorders

For patients with significant depression or anxiety associated with pain and other factors, psychotherapy should be considered. There is substantial evidence that psychological interventions improve emotional well-being and coping in cancer patients and patients with nonmalignant chronic pain (69,70), and preliminary evidence suggests they may even prolong the life of cancer patients (71). Indeed, regardless of level of depression, psychosocial and coping factors may need to be addressed concurrently with chronic opioid therapy in order to ensure that pain reduction translates into improved functioning.

Pain Coping Skills

Psychological factors influence pain perception (72). Patients with a similar extent of tissue damage may report widely varying levels of pain, or no pain. Exaggerated pain perception may be the result of increased somatic focus and a tendency to interpret ambiguous physical sensations as pain or disease, which increases negative affect, which increases pain perception, and so on (72). Relaxation and distraction may be particularly useful for cancer patients to increase their sense of self-control (72) and also to decrease pain perception. Cognitive behavioral interventions, as well as traditional psychotherapy, should be considered as adjuncts, not substitutes, for analgesic therapy (46).

BEHAVIORAL CONSIDERATIONS

Although patients generally respond well to chronic opioids, and many have a long history of utilizing shorter-acting preparations without incident, a protocol for optimal management of these patients *prior* to an opioid trial is strongly recommended and may decrease the likelihood of a negative outcome. As outlined in Pappagallo and Heinberg (2), when patients are considered medical candidates for chronic opioid management, a number of essential agreements and evaluations must take place. Patients should be asked to read, discuss, and sign an informed consent form. This consent form not only educates the patient regarding potential problematic side effects, potential symptoms of withdrawal, and danger of potential overdose, but also outlines a number of patient responsibilities that must be fulfilled in order for the physician to continue to provide prescriptions and/or continue the physician/patient relationship. It is important to note, however, that simply giving a patient a form to read and garnering his or her signature does not ensure true consent or understanding. The health-care provider should verbally discuss the outlined behavioral responsibilities of the patient, including: (a) taking medication only as prescribed and contacting the physician prior to making any self-administered or other-physician-recommended medication changes, (b) not requesting or accepting opioids from any other physician or individual, (c) contacting the physician if the need to see another physician is necessary or if the patient becomes pregnant, (d) agreeing to contact the prescribing physician prior to taking benzodiazepines, sedatives, and antihistamines (and receiving an explanation of potential drug interactions), (e) making regular clinic visits, (f) understanding that as a general rule refill prescriptions cannot be written for longer than 1 month and must be dispensed

by the same pharmacy, shall be made during regular office hours, and will not be made if the patient runs out early, loses a prescription, or spills or misplaces medication, and (g) agreeing to contact the police and obtain a stolen item report if medication is stolen. In addition, patients are required to agree to urine and blood screens at any time as determined by the prescribing physician in order to detect the use of nonprescribed medications (2). Patients should also be informed and strongly encouraged that the goal of such treatment is not simply pain reduction but also improvement in daily function and quality of life. Finally, patients are informed that if they do not follow the aforementioned responsibilities they may no longer receive any type of opioid medication from the provider. If a problem or question arises regarding these responsibilities, patients may make an appointment with the physician to discuss and receive clarification, *prior to the development of a problem or before a crisis arises*. A clearly defined agreement between patient and physician is essential for setting limits, enforcing consequences if problems arise, and encouraging conversations about the patient's role in his/her care prior to emergencies.

It is also recommended that all candidates, but certainly those who do not meet "ideal candidate" criteria, be referred for evaluation to a clinical psychologist specializing in chronic pain. This evaluation has several purposes. It provides a baseline multidimensional assessment of the patient's pain intensity, mood, functioning, and quality of life prior to taking long-acting opioids. In addition, potential behavioral and/or psychological contraindications for chronic opioid use can be identified. Contraindications include current alcohol, illicit drug, or prescription drug abuse or dependence, severe major depression, or antisocial or borderline personality disorder. Other behavioral/psychological factors that may require stepped-up supervision by the physician or concurrent psychiatric care include a history of alcohol, illicit drug, or prescription drug abuse or dependence, a significant family history of chemical dependency, mild to moderate depression, a strong family history of affective illness, personality disorders (e.g., histrionic or dependent personality), a severe level of disability, severe marital or family dysfunction, or other psychiatric illness. Such individuals may do well on opioid therapy but will require closer supervision and may need concurrent mental-health care (2).

Psychological evaluation is also helpful for patients who are concerned with cognitive functioning. Brief screening of intellectual functioning, memory, psychomotor speed, and attention prior to initiation of opioids and following titration to therapeutic doses can demonstrate to patients (and often employers) the lack of or minimal cognitive side effects of opioid medications (2). Indeed, many patients are relieved to find that baseline deficits, likely due to the distracting effects of pain, are ameliorated by chronic opioid therapy.

Finally, brief psychoeducational interventions are helpful in describing the risks and benefits of opioid medications, their mechanism of action, and probable side effects. More pragmatic issues are also addressed, such as informing family members of medications, addressing negative reactions (e.g., friends, pharmacists, primary physicians), and setting goals for improving function and quality of life. Followup treatment is often offered as an adjunct to chronic opioid pharmacotherapy.

Although the majority of patients do remarkably well on long-term opioid therapy and are good candidates, certain individuals may be at markedly higher risk. The following section will discuss patients with current addiction, those with a history of addiction, and those exhibiting problem behaviors.

CHRONIC PAIN PATIENTS WITH CURRENT ADDICTION

In general, current alcohol, illicit drug, or prescription drug addiction is a contraindication for chronic opioid therapy. However, management of acute pain (e.g., postsurgery) may necessitate opioids. Active addicts who also have chronic pain represent a dilemma for treating physicians, particularly when their addiction may have played a role in their current illness (e.g., pancreatitis) (74). Negative emotional reactions often make it difficult for physicians to accept that these patients, like all pain patients, require adequate pain relief. Physicians must also learn to tolerate the possibility of being "duped" by such patients, as the reported pain intensity is the only manner in which the pain experience may be assessed (75). Such patients may be manipulative and verbally abusive. However, it has been suggested that this may be due to the patients' lack of exposure to more appropriate ways of communicating rather than direct hostility toward their physicians (74). Such behaviors require firm and consistent limit setting and assertiveness on the part of all medical caregivers. Clearly, addicted patients with chronic pain are difficult to manage. But chemical dependency does not guarantee that any pain complaints are manipulative or unfounded (75).

In general, initial management of these patients should be conservative and rely upon pharmacological and nonpharmacological interventions that have a low abuse potential. These may include psychological techniques (e.g., cognitive-behavioral interventions, biofeedback, relaxation), physical therapy, and analgesics with no or low abuse potential. In addition, patients should be strongly encouraged to receive treatment for their addiction. However, rehabilitation from addiction is not possible when it is not consistent with the patient's goals. If opioid therapy is deemed necessary, patients should be required to receive concurrent addiction treatment, medications should be prescribed around the clock or in long-acting preparations, and stringent behavioral requirements

should be clarified. Such clarification involves the signing of a contract that outlines the various behaviors that would necessitate the termination of care (e.g., forging of prescriptions) and the guidelines for responsible use (e.g., no self-adjustment of medications). A referral to an inpatient pain or drug rehabilitation program and termination of the physician/patient relationship may be a final step for patients unable to fulfill the contracted necessary behavior for treatment.

CHRONIC PAIN PATIENTS WITH A HISTORY OF ADDICTION

Although prescribing physicians may express wariness regarding the appropriateness of opioid therapy for patients with a history of chemical dependency, such patients are themselves often reluctant to have their chronic pain treated pharmacologically, particularly with opioids. Patients may be frightened that any opioids utilized for pain relief will trigger a relapse, and family members may also be concerned about the potential for abuse. Chronic pain patients involved in recovery programs may fear that they will destroy their record of sobriety and may be fearful of the reaction of their fellowship community. Similarly, physicians may undermedicate such patients because of fear of the development of problems or because of misinterpretation of pain complaints as drug-seeking behavior.

As discussed previously in regard to those patients who are currently addicted, nonpharmacological and other conservative interventions may be the most beneficial (2). However, if such strategies fail and opioid medication is deemed necessary, the following treatment suggestions may be helpful in managing these individuals and reducing any risk of relapse.

1. Although is important for all patients, it is especially important that these patients understand the difference between physiological dependence, which is to be expected, and addiction, which should be avoided. Helping patients identify specific warning signs and problematic behaviors to monitor is necessary.
2. Patients should be strongly encouraged to join or increase involvement in a recovery program or in individual psychological care in order to garner support and develop and bolster relapse prevention strategies.
3. As with all patients, written behavioral contracting should occur to provide patients with a clear definition of problematic use, misuse, and abuse behaviors.
4. Closer supervision by the physician should occur, including frequent followup appointments, the use of only one prescribing physician and dispensing pharmacy and toxicology screenings.
5. Long-acting opioids, around-the-clock dosing, or transdermal preparations may be especially helpful for these patients in reducing any reinforcing quality of the medications.

Some patients in recovery may decline the use of opioid analgesics in spite of their potential treatment efficacy. A patients' decision to decline such treatment should be respected, and all other medical, pharmacological, and behavioral alternatives (e.g., biofeedback) should be offered.

CHRONIC PAIN PATIENTS CURRENTLY MISUSING OPIOID MEDICATIONS

As noted, in rare instances, some patients without a history of chemical dependency will evidence misuse and/or abuse of their medications following the initiation of an opioid trial. In making a diagnosis of addiction, assessing behavioral indicators is far more important than assessing aspects of physical dependence or tolerance (41). A diagnosis of addiction may be made as a result of a number of behaviors, including forging prescriptions, supplementing prescriptions with street drugs, abusing other street drugs, losing control over medication use, or stealing drugs. Additionally, a pattern of less serious, but still problematic, behaviors may be evidence of addiction. These behaviors include experiencing family difficulties related to drug use, "losing" prescriptions, demanding medications with a high street value, receiving prescriptions from more than one physician, and self-adjusting the prescription dose. A concise manner of documenting abnormal behaviors should be part of each patient's chart. The date, physician comments, and evidence for any major abnormal behaviors should be clearly documented, and termination of treatment may be considered at that time (2). Because patients with addiction are likely to deny problematic behaviors and attempt to manipulate their health-care providers, careful documentation is essential. Episodes of major problem behaviors include forging/altering prescriptions, stealing drugs or prescription pads, concurrently abusing alcohol or illicit drugs, or grossly misusing medication. Such individuals should be referred for evaluation of their potential addiction immediately and should subsequently follow the guidelines for chemically dependent patients outlined earlier. If patients are willing to undergo pain and/or chemical dependency rehabilitation and can demonstrate a period of sobriety, their future management should follow the preceding recommendations for persons in recovery.

Similar to major abnormal behaviors, borderline behaviors should be documented with the date, evidence, and any comments. These behaviors include losing prescriptions or medications, receiving narcotics from other physicians, failing to notify the physician of prescription of other sedative medications, using self-administered dose increases, and other manipulative behaviors such as emotional outbursts, bullying of staff, splitting of staff, etc. (2) Although a single episode of borderline abnormal behaviors may be easily redirected by the physician, a continued pattern may suggest the necessity of treatment termination or referral for psychiatric or substance abuse followup.

SUMMARY AND CONCLUSION

This chapter has outlined various controversies and barriers to opioid use in cancer and nonmalignant chronic pain patients with recommendations on behaviorally managing patients on opioids. The prevalence of chronic pain is continuing, and over the past several years there has been a shift toward greater acceptance of opioids as a viable treatment alternative for patients with cancer and nonmalignant chronic pain. However, many physicians, nurses, patients, and employers continue to exhibit significant ambivalence about opioids. This ambivalence is due to such factors as a misunderstanding of addiction; a lack of knowledge that a variety of chronic pain syndromes may respond to opioid therapy; the misconception that chronic opioid therapy can cause depression, personality changes, and a significant impairment of physical and cognitive function; a lack of information about the correct use of opioids (e.g., titration, use of long-acting agents, management of the side effects, etc.); and a lack of knowledge that opioid therapy can be managed ethically in a variety of patients with comprehensive assessment, clear definition of patient responsibilities, and behaviorally and pharmacologically well-structured protocols (2). Clarification of such issues is necessary to reduce suffering from chronic nonmalignant and cancer pain.

REFERENCES

1. Conigliaro DA. Opioids for chronic non-malignant pain. *J Fla Med Assoc* 1996;83(10):708–711.
2. Pappagallo M, Heinberg LJ. Ethical issues in the management of chronic nonmalignant pain. *Semin Neurol* 1997;17:203–211.
3. McNairy SL, Maruta T, Ivnik RJ, et al. Prescription medication dependence and neuropsychologic function. *Pain* 1984;18(2):169–177.
4. Turk DC, Brody MC, Okifuji EA. Physicians' attitudes and practices regarding the long-term prescribing of opioids for non-cancer pain. *Pain* 1994;59(2):201–208.
5. Martin WR, Jasinski DR, Haertzen CA, et al. Methadone—a reevaluation. *Arch Gen Psychiatry* 1973;28(2):286–295.
6. Bouckoms AJ, Masand P, Murray GB, et al. Chronic nonmalignant pain treated with long term analgesics. *Ann Clin Psychiatry* 1992;4:185–192.
7. Portenoy RK. Chronic opioid therapy in nonmalignant pain. *J Pain Symptom Manage* 1990;5(1 Suppl):S46–S62.
8. Portenoy RK. Opioid therapy for chronic nonmalignant pain: current status. In: Fields HL, Liebeskind JC, eds. *Progress in pain research and management.* Seattle: IASP Press, 1994:247–287.
9. Fordyce WE. *Behavioral methods for chronic pain and illness.* St. Louis: Mosby, 1976.
10. Agency for Health Care and Policy Research. Acute pain management: operative or medical procedures and trauma. *AHCPR Publication* 1992.
11. Jacox A, Carr DB, Payne R. Management of cancer pain. *AHCPR Publication No.4-0592* 1994.
12. *Cancer Pain Relief and Palliative Care.* Geneva: World Health Organization, 2000.
13. Foley KM. Misconceptions and controversies regarding the use of opioids in cancer pain. *Anticancer Drugs* 1995;6(Suppl)3:4–13.
14. Von Gunten CF, Ferris FD. Pharmacological management of cancer pain. In: Benzon HT, Raja SN, Borsook DB, et al., eds. *Essentials of pain medicine and regional anesthesia.* New York: Harcourt Brace, 1999: 308–315.

15. Turk DC, Brody MC. What position do APS's physician members take on chronic opioid therapy? *APS Bulletin* 1992;2:1–5.
16. Portenoy RK, Foley KM. Chronic use of opioid analgesics in non-malignant pain: report of 38 cases. *Pain* 1986;25(2):171–186.
17. Pappagallo M, Raja SN, Haythornthwaite J, et al. Oral opioids in the management of postherpetic neuralgia: a prospective study. *Anesth Analg* 1994;1:51–55.
18. Taub A. Opioid analgesics in the treatment of chronic intractable pain of non-neoplastic origin. In: Kitahata LM, Collins D, eds. *Narcotic analgesics in anesthesiology*. Baltimore: Williams and Wilkins, 1982:199–208.
19. Zenz M, Strumpf M, Tryba M. Long-term oral opioid therapy in patients with chronic nonmalignant pain. *J Pain Symptom Manage* 1992;7(2):69–77.
20. Moulin DE, Iezzi A, Amireh R, et al. Randomised trial of oral morphine for chronic non-cancer pain. *Lancet* 1996;347(8995):143–147.
21. Arkinstall W, Sandler A, Goughnour B, et al. Efficacy of controlled-release codeine in chronic non-malignant pain: a randomized, placebo-controlled clinical trial. *Pain* 1995;62(2):169–178.
22. Weinstein SM, Laux LF, Thornby JI, et al. Physicians' attitudes toward pain and the use of opioid analgesics: results of a survey from the Texas Cancer Pain Initiative. *South Med J* 2000;93(5):479–487.
23. Passik SD, Weinreb HJ. Managing chronic nonmalignant pain: overcoming obstacles to the use of opioids. *Adv Ther* 2000;17(2):70–83.
24. Bonica JJ. Treatment of cancer pain: current status and future needs. In: Fields HL, ed. *Advances in pain research and therapy*. 1985:589–616.
25. Cleeland C. Research in cancer pain. What we know and what we need to know. *Cancer* 1991;67(3Suppl):823–827.
26. Cleeland CS, Syrjala KL. How to assess cancer pain. In: Turk DC, Melzack R, eds. *Handbook of pain assessment*. New York: Guilford Press, 1992:362–387.
27. Friedman DP. Perspectives on the medical use of drugs of abuse. *J Pain Symptom Manage* 1990;5(1Suppl):S2–S5.
28. Takeda F. Management of cancer pain—WHO cancer control programme. Tokyo: Diamond Planning Services. 1987;61–69.
29. Ventafridda V, Tamburini M, Caraceni A, et al. A validation study of the WHO method for cancer pain relief. *Cancer* 1987;59(4):850–856.
30. Jamison RN. Comprehensive pretreatment and outcome assessment for chronic opioid therapy in nonmalignant pain. *J Pain Symptom Manage* 1996;11(4):231–241.
31. Roth SH, Fleischmann RM, Burch FX, et al. Around-the-clock, controlled-release oxycodone therapy for osteoarthritis-related pain: placebo-controlled trial and long-term evaluation. *Arch Intern Med* 2000;160(6):853–860.
32. Anderson VC, Burchiel KJ. A prospective study of long-term intrathecal morphine in the management of chronic nonmalignant pain. *Neurosurgery* 1999;44(2):289–300.
33. Grond S, Zech D, Lehmann KA, et al. Transdermal fentanyl in the long-term treatment of cancer pain: a prospective study of 50 patients with advanced cancer of the gastrointestinal tract or the head and neck region. *Pain* 1997;69(1–2):191–198.
34. Ferrell BR, McGuire DB, Donovan MI. Knowledge and beliefs regarding pain in a sample of nursing faculty. *J Prof Nurs* 1993;9(2):79–88.
35. Joranson DF, Cleeland CS, Weissman DE, Gilson AM. Opioids in chronic cancer and non cancer pain: a survey of state medical board members. *Fed Bull Med J Licensure Discipline* 1992;79:15–49.
36. Results of a physician attitude toward cancer pain and its management survey by ECOG. 1991.
37. Zenz M, Willweber-Strumpf A. Opiophobia and cancer pain in Europe. *Lancet* 1993;341(8852):1075–1076.
38. Morgan JP. American opiophobia: customary underutilization of opioid analgesics. In: Stimmel B, ed. *Advances in alcohol and substance abuse*. New York: Haworth, 1986:163–173.
39. Greipp ME. Undermedication for pain: an ethical model. *ANS Adv Nurs Sci* 1992;15(1):44–53.
40. Heinberg LJ. Psychological management of chemically dependent patients with chronic pain. *Straight Forward* 1996;7:4–5.
41. Sees KL, Clark HW. Opioid use in the treatment of chronic pain: assessment of addiction. *J Pain Symptom Manage* 1993;8(5):257–264.
42. Dellemijn PL, van Duijn H, Vanneste JA. Prolonged treatment with transdermal fentanyl in neuropathic pain. *J Pain Symptom Manage* 1998;16(4):220–229.
43. Jaffe JH. Drug addiction and drug abuse. In: Gilman G, Rall TW, Nies AS, Taylor P, eds. *Goodman and Gilman's the pharmacological basis of therapeutics*. New York: Pergamon, 1990:522–573.
44. Weissman DE, Haddox JD. Opioid pseudoaddiction—an iatrogenic syndrome. *Pain* 1989;36(3):363–366.
45. Fishbain DA, Rosomoff HL, Rosomoff RS. Drug abuse, dependence, and addiction in chronic pain patients. *Clin J Pain* 1992; 8:77–85.
46. Von Gunten CF, Ferris FD. Approach to management of cancer pain. In: Benzon HT, Raja SN, Borsoonk DB, et al., eds. *Essentials of pain medicine and regional anesthesia*. New York: Harcourt Brace, 1999:306–307.
47. Porter J, Jick H. Addiction rare in patients treated with narcotics [letter]. *N Engl J Med* 1980;302(2):123.
48. Perry S, Heidrich G. Management of pain during debridement: a survey of U.S. burn units. *Pain* 1982;13(3):267–280.
49. Chapman CR, Hill HF. Prolonged morphine self-administration and addiction liability. Evaluation of two theories in a bone marrow transplant unit. *Cancer* 1989;63(8):1636–1644.
50. Kerr B, Hill H, Coda B, et al. Concentration-related effects of morphine on cognition and motor control in human subjects. *Neuropsychopharmacology* 1991;5(3):157–166.
51. Sjogren P, Thomsen AB, Olsen AK. Impaired neuropsychological performance in chronic nonmalignant pain patients receiving long-term oral opioid therapy. *J Pain Symptom Manage* 2000;19(2):100–108.
52. Lorenz J, Beck H, Bromm B. Cognitive performance, mood and experimental pain before and during morphine-induced analgesia in patients with chronic non-malignant pain. *Pain* 1997;73(3):369–375.
53. Vainio A, Ollila J, Matikainen E, et al. Driving ability in cancer patients receiving long-term morphine analgesia. *Lancet* 1995; 346(8976):667-670.
54. Galski T, Williams JB, Ehle HT. Effects of opioids on driving ability. *J Pain Symptom Manage* 2000;19(3):200–208.
55. Haythornthwaite JA, Menefee LA, Quatrano-Piacentini AL, Pappagallo M. Outcome of chronic opioid therapy for non-cancer pain. *J Pain Symptom Manage* 1998;15(3):185–194.
56. Bruera E, Macmillan K, Hanson J, MacDonald RN. The cognitive effects of the administration of narcotic analgesics in patients with cancer pain. *Pain* 1989;39(1):13–16.
57. Bruera E, Miller MJ, Macmillan K, Kuehn N. Neuropsychological effects of methylphenidate in patients receiving a continuous infusion of narcotics for cancer pain. *Pain* 1992;48(2):163–166.
58. Banning A, Sjogren P. Cerebral effects of long-term oral opioids in cancer patients measured by continuous reaction time. *Clin J Pain* 1990;6:91–95.
59. Banning A, Sjogren P, Kaiser F. Reaction time in cancer patients receiving peripherally acting analgesics alone or in combination with opioids. *Acta Anaesthesiol Scand* 1992;36:480–482.
60. Sjogren P, Banning A. Pain, sedation and reaction time during long-term treatment of cancer patients with oral and epidural opioids. *Pain* 1989;39(1):5–11.
61. Sjogren P, Olsen AK, Thomsen AB, Dalberg J. Neuropsychological performance in cancer patients: the role of oral opioids, pain and performance status. *Pain* 2000;86(3):237–245.
62. Romano JM, Turner JA. Chronic pain and depression: does the evidence support a relationship? *Psychol Bull* 1985;97(1):18–34.
63. Haythornthwaite JA, Sieber WJ, Kerns RD. Depression and the chronic pain experience. *Pain* 1991;46(2):177–184.
64. Haertzen CA, Hooks NT, Jr. Changes in personality and subjective experience associated with the chronic administration and withdrawal of opiates. *J Nerv Ment Dis* 1969;148(6):606–614.
65. Pappagallo M, Campbell JN. The pharmacologic management of chronic back pain. In: Frymoyer JW, ed. *The adult spine: principle and practice*. New York: Raven Press, 1996.
66. Drug Enforcement Administration. *Physician's Manual, An Informational Outline of the Controlled Substances Act of 1970*. 1990.
67. Kanner RM, Portenoy RK. Unavailability of narcotic analgesics for ambulatory cancer pain patients in New York City. *Pain* 1984; Supplement 2.
68. Murphy TM. Chronic opioids for chronic low back pain—solution or problem?. *J Am Board Fam Pract* 1996;9(3):225–228.

69. Andersen BL. Psychological interventions for cancer patients to enhance the quality of life. *J Consult Clin Psychol* 1992;60(4):552–568.

70. Haythornthwaite JA, Heinberg LJ. Coping with pain: what works, under what circumstances and in what ways. *Pain Forum* 1999;8: 172–175.

71. Spiegel D, Bloom JR, Kraemer HC, Gottheil E. Effect of psychosocial treatment on survival of patients with metastatic breast cancer. *Lancet* 1989;2(8668):888–891.

72. Turk DC, Meichenbaum D, Genest M. *Pain and behavioral medicine.* 1983.

73. Bonica JJ. Importance of the problem. In: Bonica JJ, Ventafridda V, eds. *Advances in pain research and therapy.* New York: Raven Press, 1979.

74. McCaffery M, Vourakis C. Assessment and relief of pain in chemically dependent patients. *Orthop Nurs* 1992;11(2):13–27.

75. Heinberg LJ. Psychological management of chemically dependent patients with chronic pain. *Straight Forward* 1996;7:4–5.

76. Macaluso D, Weinberg D, Foley KM. Opioid abuse and misuse in a cancer pain population. *Journal of Pain and Symptom Management* 1988;3:s24.

CHAPTER **18**

Nonopioid and Adjuvant Analgesics

Glen D. Solomon

ANALGESIC MEDICATIONS

There are three general classes of analgesic medications: opioids, which are covered in another chapter; nonopioids, including aspirin, acetaminophen, nonsteroidal antiinflammatory drugs (NSAIDs), and cyclooxygenase-2 (COX-2) specific inhibitors; and adjuvants, which are drugs that are not generally considered as analgesics but that can enhance the efficacy of opioids or nonopioid analgesics or are effective for certain painful conditions. Nonopioid analgesics can be given concurrently with opioids for an additive analgesic effect.

Although opioids are considered the most potent analgesic drugs, adverse effects, including respiratory depression, sedation, nausea, vomiting, dizziness, constipation, and the development of physical dependence with abstinence symptoms with chronic use, limit their utility for patients with mild to moderate pain. In addition, specific pain syndromes such as neuropathic pain and pain from bone metastasis may respond better to nonopioid drugs than to opioids.

ANATOMY OF PAIN

To better understand how analgesics act, it is worthwhile to briefly review the anatomy of pain sensation. Pain is generally thought of as having two components—a fast, localized sensation carried by myelinated A-delta fibers, which respond to mechanical (i.e., sharp) or thermal stimulation, and a slower, more unpleasant, and diffuse sensation carried by unmyelinated C fibers (1).

Mechanical, chemical, or thermal threats to tissue integrity cause nociceptive neurons to increase their discharge rate. The primary afferent nociceptor is a bipolar neuron with its centrally directed process innervating the central nervous system and its peripherally directed process

innervating tissues such as skin and joints. Tissue destruction activates nociceptors and initiates a local inflammatory response sustained by mediators such as monoamines, cytokines, prostanoids, peptides, growth factors, and neurotransmitters. These mediators sensitize functional nociceptors or activate dormant ones. Multiple interacting mediators and receptors allow for sensory integration and amplification of nociceptive input in the periphery (2).

C fibers and A-delta fibers convey nociceptive information from visceral and somatic sites to the dorsal horn of the spinal cord. Many of the same mediators that act in peripheral nociceptive processing function in spinal nociceptive integration. Agents that impair the synthesis, release, or effects of such substances within the dorsal horn include morphine, N-methyl D-aspartate (NMDA) receptor blockers, sodium or calcium channel blockers, alpha-2 adrenergic agonists, gamma-aminobutyric acid (GABA), and antagonists of substance P (2).

The dorsal horn of the spinal cord is the primary processing site of the primary afferent nociceptive information. Nociceptive fibers enter the spinal cord through the dorsal horn, synapse in laminae I, II, and V of the spinal cord, and ascend as the spinothalamic tract. The spinothalamic tract consists of the neospinothalamic and the paleospinothalamic tracts. The neospinothalamic tract ascends to the thalamus, terminates in the ventral posterolateral nucleus, and projects to the somatosensory cortex. The neospinothalamic tract provides information on the quality, intensity, and location of the painful stimulus. The paleospinothalamic tract is polysynaptic, with many interactions with the reticular system and periaqueductal gray. It terminates in the medial, intralaminar, and posterior thalamic nuclei and then projects diffusely to limbic and subcortical areas. The paleospinothalamic tract, unlike the neospinothalamic tract, is not topographically organized and does not project to the somatotopically organized cerebral cortex (3). Thus, pain impulses carried by the paleospinothalamic tract are perceived as diffuse, whereas pain impulses carried by the neospinothalamic tract are highly localized.

The first component of pain—the sharp, localized sensation—is initiated by mechanothermal nociceptors, transmitted to the spinal cord via myelinated A-delta fibers, and carried by the neospinothalamic tract to the thalamus and cortex. The second component of pain—the prolonged, burning, poorly localized "hurt"—is initiated by C-polymodal nociceptors, transmitted to the spinal cord via unmyelinated C fibers, and carried by the paleo-spinothalamic tract to the reticular system, limbus, and subcortex. Because of these projections to the reticular and limbic systems, the second component of pain is associated with the arousal and emotional aspects of pain.

ASPIRIN

Salicylates and salicylic acid are contained in medicinal plants that have been used to treat pain and fever since antiquity; 3500 years ago in ancient Egypt, the Ebers papyrus recommended the application of dried myrtle leaves to treat rheumatic pain. Hippocrates prescribed the juices of the poplar tree to treat eye diseases and those of the willow bark to relieve the pain of childbirth and to reduce fever. In 1763, Reverend Edward Stone read a report to the British Royal Society on the use of willow bark to treat fever (4).

Salicylic acid was chemically synthesized in 1860 in Germany. In 1899, Felix Hoffman, a chemist working for Bayer, synthesized acetylsalicylate, or aspirin, as a more palatable form of salicylate (4).

There are many systemic and a few local uses of salicylates. Salicylates are commonly used to treat inflammation in a wide variety of settings, alleviate the pain of headache, arthritis, dysmenorrhea, neuralgia, and myalgia, and to reduce fever (5). The analgesic and antipyretic dose of aspirin for adults is 325 to 650 mg orally every 4 hours; for children, 50 to 75 mg/kg per day is given in four to six divided doses, not to exceed a total daily dose of 3.6 g. In children with varicella or influenza, aspirin can cause Reye's syndrome, and its use is contraindicated.

Platelet inhibition with aspirin can significantly reduce cardiovascular events for patients with a history of atherosclerotic cardiovascular disease (6). Although some NSAIDs may confer a cardiovascular benefit, aspirin's unique pharmacologic properties (irreversible platelet inhibition) and extensive clinical data support its use in cardiovascular prevention (6,7). Patients requiring NSAIDs or coxibs for pain relief should also be given low-dose aspirin for cardiovascular protection, if clinically indicated.

In high doses, salicylates have toxic effects on the central nervous system, consisting of stimulation (including convulsions) followed by depression. Confusion, dizziness, tinnitus, high-tone deafness, delirium, psychosis, stupor,

and coma may occur. Salicylates stimulate respiration directly and indirectly, leading to respiratory alkalosis in patients treated with intensive salicylate therapy. When toxic doses are ingested, there is a decrease in blood pH, a low plasma bicarbonate concentration, and a normal or nearly normal Pco_2. This reflects a combined metabolic and respiratory acidosis (5).

Aspirin use may result in epigastric distress, nausea, and vomiting. It may cause gastric ulceration, exacerbation of peptic ulcer disease, gastrointestinal hemorrhage, and erosive gastritis. The daily ingestion of 4 or 5 g of aspirin results in an average fecal blood loss of 3 to 8 mL per day as compared with 0.6 mL per day in untreated subjects (5).

Aspirin has a dose-dependent effect on uric acid excretion. At low doses (1 to 2 g per day), urate excretion is decreased, causing an elevation in plasma urate concentrations; at high doses (over 5 g per day), aspirin indices uricosuria and lower plasma urate levels (5).

Ingestion of aspirin causes a prolongation of the bleeding time. The acetyl group of aspirin irreversibly binds to platelet cyclooxygenase, rendering the platelet ineffective for clotting for its entire 7–12-day life span. A single dose of aspirin approximately doubles the mean bleeding time of normal persons for a period of 4 to 7 days.

ACETAMINOPHEN

Acetaminopen is the active metabolite of phenacetin. It is an analgesic-antipyretic agent with weak antiinflammatory activity. Because acetaminophen is generally well tolerated, lacks the common side effects of aspirin and NSAIDs, and is available without a prescription, it is widely used (5).

As an analgesic, acetaminopen is as effective as aspirin, similar in potency, and in single analgesic doses has the same time-effect curve (8). It is thought to be centrally active, producing analgesia by elevation of the pain threshold. At therapeutic doses it does not inhibit prostaglandin synthetase in peripheral tissues, which explains its lack of antiinflammatory activity (9).

Acetaminophen is a suitable substitute for aspirin for analgesic or antipyretic uses. It is most valuable for patients in whom aspirin or NSAIDs are contraindicated, for example, patients with peptic ulcer disease, children with influenza or varicella (due to risk of Reye's syndrome), or patients for whom the prolongation of bleeding time would be a disadvantage (5). The usual dose of acetaminophen is 325 to 1000 mg orally or 650 mg rectally. The total daily dose should not exceed 4000 mg (5).

In 1995, the American College of Rheumatology recommended acetaminophen as first-line therapy for osteoarthritis of the hip or knee (10,11). This recommendation was supported by the results of a randomized, double-blind study demonstrating that acetaminophen at 4000 mg daily was more effective than placebo and as effective as commonly used NSAIDs for relief of joint pain and improvement of function in patients with osteoarthritis (9). Additionally, acetaminophen was preferred because many osteoarthritis patients are elderly and have increased risk of NSAID-related gastropathy and renal adverse effects (9).

In recommended therapeutic dosage, acetaminophen is well tolerated. It causes little or no gastrointestinal irritation and has minimal effects on renal function (9). Skin rash and other allergic reactions occur occasionally (5).

The most serious adverse effect of acute overdosage of acetaminophen is a dose-dependent, potentially fatal hepatic necrosis (5). Patients who are alcoholics, people who are fasting, and those taking isoniazid, zidovudine, or a barbiturate concurrently may develop hepatic injury after modest overdosage or even high therapeutic doses (8).

NONSTEROIDAL ANTIINFLAMMATORY DRUGS

Nonsteroidal antiinflammatory drugs (NSAIDs) are widely used agents for the treatment of musculoskeletal pain, acute and chronic pain, biliary and ureteric colic, dysmenorrhea, and headache. NSAIDs have a major role in the management of acute and chronic pain syndromes associated with inflammation. NSAIDs have been shown to reduce joint pain and stiffness associated with osteoarthritis and to reduce joint pain, stiffness, swelling, and tenderness associated with rheumatoid arthritis (12,13). NSAIDs have also been shown to be effective in the management of seronegative spondyloarthropathies, acute gout, bursitis, tendonitis, and many models of acute and chronic pain, including postsurgical pain (12–14). In general, most NSAIDs provide similar efficacy when given in appropriate doses for the treatment of osteoarthritis and rheumatoid arthritis.

Over 35 million prescriptions and billions of over-the-counter aspirin and other NSAID preparations are sold annually in the United States. Greater than 1% of the U.S. population uses these drugs on a daily basis (15).

The major mechanism of action of NSAIDs is the inhibition of cyclooxygenase (COX) activity and therefore the synthesis of prostaglandins (15) (Fig. 18-1). Inhibition of cyclooxygenase leads to both the therapeutic and toxic effects of NSAIDs (16).

Cyclooxygenase, also called prostaglandin synthase, is the first enzyme in the biosynthetic pathway leading from arachidonic acid to prostaglandin G_2 (PGG_2) and prostaglandin H_2 (PGH_2), precursors of prostanoids that act as local mediators throughout the body (16). The COX enzyme has at least two isoforms—a constitutive isoform (COX-1), which is expressed in most tissues throughout the body and is responsible for maintaining normal function in the gastrointestinal tract, platelets, and kidney, and an inducible isoform (COX-2), which is expressed at low levels in most cells. Expression of COX-2 can be up-regulated in areas of inflammation and in the brain by cytokines and bacterial products such as lipopolysaccharide (15,17).

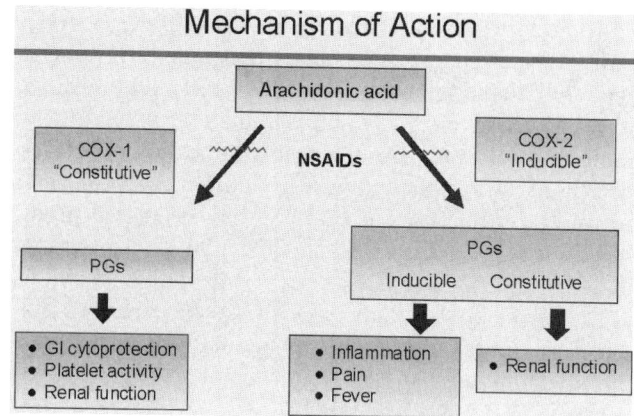

FIG. 18-1. Mechanism of action of NSAIDs and coxibs. NSAIDs inhibit both COX-1 and COX-2, whereas coxibs inhibit only COX-2.

In both the kidney and the stomach, prostanoids synthesized by the action of COX-1 act as vasodilators. In the kidney, these prostanoids help to maintain renal plasma flow and glomerular filtration during periods of systemic vasoconstriction. In the gastric antrum, local vasodilation appears to play a major role in maintaining mucosal defenses. COX-1 in the platelets generates thromboxane, which plays a role in mediating platelet aggregation (16).

In contrast to constitutive COX-1 expression, COX-2 is almost undetectable in most normal resting cells. During inflammation, COX-2 expression in cells such as synoviocytes, macrophages, and endothelial cells increases dramatically. COX-2 can be evoked by inflammatory mediators such as cytokines and growth factors. Induction of COX-2 has been observed in both osteoarthritis and rheumatoid arthritis (16).

Local injury or inflammation increases COX-2 activity, resulting in increased levels of prostanoids, which leads to hyperalgesia. Prostaglandin E_2 (PGE_2) sensitizes pain receptors. Prostanoids may also facilitate pain transmission in the spinal cord, and painful stimuli have been shown to increase COX-2 expression within the central nervous system. Induction of COX-2 has been verified at both local and central sites of pain reception and transmission. COX-2 inhibitors have been shown to act locally and centrally to reduce inflammatory-mediated pain in animal models (16).

Traditional (nonselective) NSAIDs inhibit both COX-1 and COX-2 at therapeutic concentrations (17). It is hypothesized that the unwanted gastrointestinal and platelet side effects of NSAIDs are due to their ability to inhibit COX-1, whereas their antiinflammatory and analgesic effects are due to COX-2 inhibition (4). Selective COX-2 inhibitors (also called coxibs) have recently been developed with the goal of reducing certain NSAID adverse effects while maintaining their antiinflammatory and analgesic benefits.

In addition to their role in inhibiting COX, NSAIDs have other mechanisms of action that may contribute to their antiinflammatory and analgesic effects. These include lowering of superoxide radicals, induction of apoptosis, inhibition of the expression of adhesion molecules, decreased nitric oxide synthase from inhibition of nuclear factor K beta-dependent transcription, decreased proinflammatory cytokine levels, modification of lymphocyte activity, and alteration of cellular membrane functions (18). Some NSAIDs have been shown to have a central analgesic action in animal pain models and in humans when administered by the intrathecal route (18).

NSAIDS AS ANALGESICS

There are at least 20 NSAIDs currently available in the United States, including over-the-counter aspirin, ibuprofen, naproxen, and ketoprofen (Table 18-1). At equipotent doses, the clinical efficacy of the various NSAIDs in patient populations is similar; however, individual responses are highly variable (19). Based on anecdotal reports, it is believed that if a patient fails to respond to one NSAID, it is reasonable to try another NSAID from another chemical class. This belief has not been systematically evaluated in a prospective study (19).

Variability in the efficacy of NSAIDs has been attributed to differences in mechanisms of action (i.e., potency of inhibition of COX-2, central analgesic effect, etc.), variability of the enantiomeric state of the drug, as well as pharmacokinetics, pharmacodynamics, and individual metabolism of specific agents (19).

Unlike opioids, NSAIDs have an analgesic response marked by a ceiling effect, beyond which dosage increments yield no additional analgesia (20). However, NSAIDS have proven utility in many pain models, including postoperative pain, malignancy-related bone pain, orthopedic pain, postthoracotomy pain, dental pain, headache, dysmenorrhea, and diabetic neuropathy (21).

TABLE 18-1. *NSAIDs*

Aspirin
Diclofenac
Diflunisal
Etodolac
Fenoprofen
Ibuprofen
Indomethacin
Ketoprofen
Ketorolac
Meclofenamate
Mefenamic acid
Nabumetone
Naproxen/Naproxen sodium
Oxaprozin
Piroxicam
Sulindac
Tolmetin sodium

Adverse Effects

The adverse effects of nonselective NSAIDs are similar to those of aspirin. NSAIDs can precipitate asthma and anaphylactoid reactions in aspirin-sensitive patients.

NSAIDs inhibit platelet aggregation and prolong the bleeding time, an effect that may be critical to patients undergoing surgery. The acetyl group of aspirin irreversibly binds to platelet cyclooxygenase, rendering the platelet ineffective for clotting for its entire 7–12-day life span. Unlike aspirin, NSAIDs cause reversible inhibition of platelet aggregation; platelet function returns when most of the drug has been eliminated (about five half-lives) (21).

NSAIDs have been estimated to be responsible for up to 100 000 excess hospitalizations and 16 000 deaths per year in the United States (22,23). It has been estimated that serious GI events (perforation, ulceration, and bleeding) caused by NSAIDs occur in 2% to 4% of patients treated for 1 year (22,23). This risk remains relatively constant with longer courses of therapy, increasing the likelihood of such an event. However, even short courses of therapy are not without risk.

Alternative routes of administration do not reduce GI effects (24). Parenteral and rectal NSAID formulations, which bypass direct contact with the UGI mucosa, produce similar GI toxicities as oral formulations (23,25). The lowest dose and shortest duration of NSAID therapy should be sought to minimize the risk of a serious GI event.

NSAID-related dyspepsia is common. Up to 30% of patients in some studies have experienced NSAID-related GI symptoms (22,23). The symptoms often occur early in therapy and can cause patients to discontinue therapy. The mechanism by which NSAIDs cause these symptoms is not understood. Several studies have failed to demonstrate a correlation between GI mucosal damage (erosions and ulcers) and GI symptoms (23,26). The presence of GI symptoms, although worrisome to patients and providers, is not a predictor of a serious GI event (perforation, obstruction, or serious GI bleed) (23,26).

With chronic use, gastrointestinal bleeding, ulceration, and perforation can occur, often without warning (8). Advanced age or a history of complicated peptic ulcer disease creates a fourfold increased risk for upper gastrointestinal tract bleeding in NSAID users (27). Other risk factors for gastrointestinal complications include male gender, high doses of NSAIDs, prolonged use, excessive alcohol intake, and concomitant use of more than one NSAID (8).

When individual NSAIDs were compared for risk of upper gastrointestinal tract bleeding, ibuprofen was associated with the lowest risk (8,27). Following ibuprofen were diclofenac, sulindac, naproxen sodium, indomethacin, and ketoprofen. Piroxicam and apazone had the highest risk of upper gastrointestinal tract bleeding (27).

Renal prostaglandins participate in the regulation of several homeostatic functions in the kidney, including sodium and potassium excretion and renal blood flow

(28,29). COX-1 is widely expressed in the kidney, including the renal vasculature, cortex, medulla, and collecting ducts, whereas COX-2 is expressed in the renal vasculature, glomerulus, and ascending limb of the loop of Henle. Despite the differences in COX-1 and COX-2 tissue expression, NSAIDs and coxibs have very similar clinical renal effects.

In healthy individuals renal prostaglandins do not have a significant role in regulating renal blood flow (28,30). However, patients with decreased actual (blood loss) or effective (congestive heart failure) intravascular volume are dependent on renal prostaglandins (prostacyclin and, to a lesser extent, PGE_2) to maintain renal perfusion. Under these conditions, NSAIDs can decrease renal blood flow and, in rare cases, precipitate acute renal failure (28,29). If this is recognized early and NSAID therapy withdrawn, patients usually recover and return to baseline renal function. Prolonged renal ischemia can lead to acute tubular necrosis. Patients at risk for acute renal decompensation include those with decreased effective circulating volume because of congestive heart failure, hepatic insufficiency, renal insufficiency, or aggressive diuresis. Although elderly patients typically have age-related decreases in renal function, age alone is not a risk factor for NSAID-related acute renal failure (28,30).

Although acute renal decompensation is rare, there is some evidence that elderly patients with risk factors for NSAID-related renal impairment can develop clinically important decrements in renal function with chronic NSAID use (30). Treatment with long-acting NSAIDs (piroxicam and sulindac) in elderly patients with mild renal insufficiency was associated with small decrements in renal function over a 1-month treatment period, whereas treatment with short-acting NSAID (ibuprofen) did not result in renal deterioration (30). Elderly patients with preserved renal function tolerated both long-acting and short-acting NSAIDs. Therefore, elderly patients with mild renal insufficiency (< 70 mL/minute) or with risk factors for NSAID-related renal impairment (heart failure, cirrhosis with ascites, volume depletion) should be routinely monitored during NSAID therapy. Preference should be given to prescribing low-dose, short-acting NSAIDs when necessary in this patient population (30,31).

Fluid retention is the most common renal manifestation of NSAID therapy (28). Renal PGE_2 regulates sodium homeostasis by decreasing sodium reabsorption in the ascending limb of the loop of Henle. NSAIDs inhibit the synthesis of PGE_2, leading to an increase in sodium reabsorption. Although sodium balance is altered during NSAID treatment in most patients, the effects are generally mild and of no clinical consequence (28). A small percentage of patients develop clinical sequelae, including weight gain, peripheral edema, hypertension, and, rarely, pulmonary edema (28,33,35). In most NSAID studies the incidence of these renal effects is 3% to 5% of patients treated (28,33,34). Because changes in sodium balance

occur rapidly, clinical manifestations of sodium retention tend to occur shortly after initiating or increasing NSAID therapy (28).

Clinically significant fluid retention is more likely to develop in patients with underlying renal disease, congestive heart failure, or hepatic insufficiency or in patients receiving diuretics (28). NSAIDs should be used with caution in these patients. It is advisable to monitor body weight when treating high-risk patients with NSAIDs. There is some evidence that longer-acting NSAIDs (t ½ > 4 hours) may be associated with more sodium retention compared with shorter-acting NSAIDs (30,31).

Hyperkalemia is a rare but potentially life-threatening consequence of NSAID therapy (28,29). NSAIDs inhibit renal prostacyclin formation, blunting renin release, aldosterone formation, and potassium excretion. Patients at risk for hyperkalemia include those taking potassium supplements, potassium-sparing diuretics, or ACE inhibitors or those with underlying renal insufficiency (e.g., diabetic nephropathy) (28,29). Hyperkalemia tends to occur early in the course of NSAID therapy and is reversible with discontinuation of the NSAID.

Relative toxicity of NSAIDs was determined for patients with rheumatoid arthritis. Toxic side effects were most frequent for patients taking indomethacin, tolmetin sodium, and meclofenamate. Least toxic were coated or buffered aspirin, salsalate, and ibuprofen (35).

Choice of an NSAID in Clinical Situations

The choice among NSAIDs for the treatment of pain is largely empirical, based on dosing schedule, price, and physician or patient preference. A drug may be chosen and given for a week or more; if the therapeutic effect is adequate, treatment should be continued unless toxicity occurs. A week is generally long enough to determine the effect of a given drug. Side effects usually appear in the first weeks of therapy, although gastrointestinal ulceration may develop later in the course of therapy. If the patient does not achieve therapeutic benefit from one NSAID, another compound should be tried because there is a marked variation in the response of individuals to different but closely related drugs (5).

Ibuprofen and naproxen sodium, the most commonly prescribed NSAIDs in the United States, are very effective analgesics and, in some models, are as effective as mild opiates (12). Other NSAIDs have also been shown to be effective in the treatment of acute pain, including etodolac, diclofenac potassium, ketoprofen, and ketorolac. Indomethacin, one of the most potent NSAIDs, remains the gold standard for the treatment of acute gout. In general, NSAIDs with longer half-lives or delayed absorption are better suited for the treatment of chronic pain.

Propionic acid derivatives represent a group of effective NSAIDs. Agents in this class include ibuprofen, naproxen, flurbiprofen, fenoprofen, ketoprofen, and oxaprozin. They are generally better tolerated than aspirin or indomethacin, although they share the adverse effect risks of the NSAID class. All of these drugs are potent cyclooxygenase inhibitors. All alter platelet function and prolong bleeding time. Propionic acid derivatives do not alter the effects of hypoglycemic drugs or warfarin.

Ibuprofen was the first member of the propionic acid derivative class to come into general use. It is available without a prescription in a 200-mg dose and as a prescription medication as 400-, 600-, and 800-mg tablets. Ibuprofen is rapidly absorbed after oral administration, and peak plasma concentrations are observed after 1 to 2 hours. The plasma half-life is about 2 hours. For mild to moderate pain and for dysmenorrhea, the usual dose is 400 mg every 4 to 6 hours, as needed. For rheumatoid and osteoarthritis, daily doses of up to 3200 mg in divided doses may be given. When individual NSAIDs were compared for risk of upper gastrointestinal tract bleeding, ibuprofen was associated with the lowest risk (8,27). Aseptic meningitis has occurred rarely in patients receiving ibuprofen, most commonly in patients with systemic lupus erythematosus or related connective tissue disease.

Naproxen is available without a prescription in 220-mg tablets (naproxen sodium) and by prescription in 250-, 375-, and 500-mg tablets, 375- and 500-mg enteric-coated tablets, and as a liquid suspension (125 mg/5 mL). It has a half-life of about 14 hours, allowing for twice-daily dosing. Peak plasma concentration occurs within 2 to 4 hours. The sodium salt (naproxen sodium) reaches peak plasma concentrations more rapidly, making it more useful as an analgesic. For relief of mild to moderate pain, the usual initial adult dose of naproxen is 500 mg (550 mg of naproxen sodium), followed by 250 mg (275 mg of naproxen sodium) every 6–8 hours.

Flurbiprofen is a propionic acid derivative related to ibuprofen. It is used for acute and chronic treatment of osteo- and rheumatoid arthritis. Usual doses are 50 to 100 mg twice daily.

Fenoprofen calcium is structurally related to ibuprofen and naproxen. The drug's analgesic effect seems to plateau at a dose of 200 mg.

Ketoprofen is available as an over-the-counter tablet with a dose of 12.5 mg and by prescription as 25-, 50-, and 75-mg capsules and 100-, 150-, and 200-mg extended-release capsules. The usual dosage for relief of mild to moderate pain or dysmenorrhea is 25 or 50 mg every 6–8 hours.

Oxaprozin is administered once daily at 600 to 1200 mg. It is used for the symptomatic treatment of acute or chronic osteoarthritis or rheumatoid arthritis.

Diclofenac, a phenylacetic acid derivative, is available as a conventional tablet (diclofenac potassium), an enteric-coated tablet, and an extended-release tablet. It is also available as a fixed combination of enteric-coated diclofenac sodium with a misoprostol outer shell. The misoprostol inhibits gastric acid and protects the mucosa

from the irritant effects of the diclofenac. For acute pain, the usual dose of diclofenac potassium is 50 to 100 mg, followed by 50 mg every 8 hours.

Indomethacin, an indoleacetic acid derivative, is available orally as a tablet or extended-release capsule and as a rectal suppository. Adverse effects occur in 30% to 60% of patients treated with indomethacin. Headache is the most frequent adverse effect, occurring in at least 10% of treated patients. Adverse effects appear more commonly with indomethacin than with most other NSAIDs (35). Because of the potential for serious adverse effects, indomethacin should not be used as a simple analgesic or antipyretic.

Ketorolac is a potent analgesic but only a moderately effective antiinflammatory drug. It is one of the few NSAIDs approved for parenteral administration. It is used for postoperative pain as an alternative to opioids. The drug is indicated for the management of moderately severe, acute pain. Unlike opioids (but like other NSAIDs), ketorolac is not associated with tolerance, withdrawal effects, or respiratory depression. It inhibits platelet aggregation and promotes gastric ulceration. Typical intramuscular or intravenous doses are 30 to 60 mg, and oral doses are 5 to 30 mg. The dose may be repeated every 4–6 hours. Peak plasma concentrations are reached in 30 to 50 minutes whether given orally or intramuscularly. The half-life of ketorolac is 4 to 6 hours. There is some evidence for dose-related adverse effects, particularly gastrointestinal bleeding. Therapy with ketorolac generally should not exceed 5 days.

Meclofenamate, an anthranilic acid derivative (fenamate), is given as 50–100 mg every 4–6 hours for mild to moderate pain. The most frequent adverse effect with meclofenamate is diarrhea, occurring in 10% to 33% of treated patients.

Nabumetone is a prodrug with little activity until it undergoes oxidation in the liver. The active metabolite is structurally similar to naproxen. It is used for the symptomatic treatment of acute or chronic osteoarthritis or rheumatoid arthritis.

Piroxicam, an oxicam derivative, has a half-life of 50 hours. The long half-life permits once-daily dosing at 20 mg. This property also may lead to a higher rate of gastrointestinal and renal adverse effects.

Sulindac is used for the symptomatic treatment of acute or chronic osteoarthritis, rheumatoid arthritis, or ankylosing spondylitis. The usual dose is 150 to 200 mg twice daily.

Tolmetin sodium is used for the symptomatic treatment of acute or chronic osteoarthritis, rheumatoid arthritis, or juvenile rheumatoid arthritis. The usual adult dose is 400 mg three times daily.

COX-2 INHIBITORS (COXIBS)

Recently, two COX-2 inhibitors (coxibs)—rofecoxib and celecoxib—were approved in the United States (Table 18-2). At therapeutic concentrations both drugs inhibit COX-2

TABLE 18-2. *Coxibs*

Celecoxib
Rofecoxib

but do not inhibit COX-1 (32,33,36). This absence of COX-1 activity, which distinguishes coxibs from standard NSAIDs, can be demonstrated pharmacologically using several assays. The simplest and most common COX-1 assays measure platelet function (32,33,36). In these assays, neither rofecoxib nor celecoxib inhibits serum thromboxane or platelet aggregation, and neither drug prolongs bleeding time at doses that are clinically effective (32–34,36).

Although they share a similar mechanism of action, rofecoxib and celecoxib differ in their chemical structure, metabolism, and pharmacokinetic properties. Rofecoxib, a methyl sulfone, has a 17-hour half-life and is dosed once daily (34,36). Celecoxib, a sulfonamide, has an 11-hour half-life and is contraindicated for patients with a history of sulfonamide allergies (33). Celecoxib is dosed once or twice daily in the treatment of OA and twice daily in the treatment of RA (33). Both compounds are extensively metabolized in the liver. Celecoxib is metabolized through the cytochrome P450 system, specifically cytochrome P450 2C9 (33). Care should be used when administering celecoxib with inhibitors of 2C9 (fluconazole, zafirlukast, etc.) because these drugs could significantly increase plasma concentrations of celecoxib (33). Celecoxib has also been shown to inhibit cytochrome P450 2D6. Therefore, celecoxib may increase the plasma concentrations of drugs metabolized by P450 2D6 (antidepressants, beta blockers, etc.). Rofecoxib's major metabolites are formed by hepatic reduction; a metabolic pathway independent of the cytochrome P450 system (34). Both rofecoxib and celecoxib can interact with warfarin. Anticoagulant activity should be closely followed when initiating or increasing coxib therapy for patients receiving warfarin.

Efficacy in Acute and Chronic Pain

Both rofecoxib and celecoxib are indicated for the treatment of osteoarthritis (33,37,38). Both coxibs were shown to reduce joint pain and stiffness and improve function in patients with osteoarthritis. In both cases maximal benefit was achieved within 1 week of initiating therapy. The celecoxib dose for the treatment of OA is 200 mg daily in single or divided doses (33,38). The rofecoxib dose range for the treatment of osteoarthritis is 12.5 to 25 mg once daily (34,37).

Celecoxib is also indicated for the treatment of RA. Celecoxib was shown to decrease joint pain, swelling, and stiffness in RA patients with efficacy comparable to naproxen 500 mg twice daily (39). Celecoxib dosing in RA is 100 mg to 200 mg twice daily (33).

Rofecoxib is indicated for the treatment of acute pain (34). In several studies of acute postsurgical and oral surgery pain, rofecoxib provided rapid onset of action and peak analgesic efficacy comparable to ibuprofen and naproxen sodium (34,40). Consistent with its long half-life, rofecoxib provided 24-hour pain relief. Additionally, rofecoxib treatment was associated with a reduction in the need for narcotic analgesics following hip surgery. Single-dose trials have found celecoxib 100 or 200 mg more effective than placebo but less effective than naproxen sodium in oral surgery pain. Celecoxib has not been approved by the FDA for analgesic use (8).

The efficacy of coxibs, although matching high-dose NSAIDs, does not offer an advantage over conventional NSAIDs. The benefit of the coxib class is in the improved GI safety and tolerability compared to NSAIDs (39, 41,42).

COX-2 Inhibitor Toxicity

In 1999, two COX-2 inhibitors, celecoxib and rofecoxib, developed as safer alternatives to standard NSAIDs, were approved in the United States. Studies supporting the approval of rofecoxib and celecoxib included surveillance endoscopy studies designed to assess the effects of the coxibs on the integrity of the upper GI mucosa (33,39,42). In these endoscopy trials, both rofecoxib and celecoxib were associated with fewer gastric and duodenal ulcers compared with standard NSAIDs, and, in general, the endoscopic ulcer rates in the coxib-treated patients were similar to placebo-treated patients (39,42).

There are only limited clinical data on the combined use of coxibs and aspirin (33,34). Importantly, it is not known how the addition of low-dose aspirin (for cardiovascular prophylaxis) to a coxib will affect the rate of clinically significant GI events. There are data to suggest that even low doses of aspirin (81 mg daily) result in significant sustained inhibition of gastric prostaglandins (43). It is possible that concomitant use of even low doses of aspirin and a coxib will negate or significantly reduce the GI benefit of the coxib.

Renal effects of the coxibs are similar to those of the NSAIDs. A small percentage of patients develop clinical sequelae, including weight gain, peripheral edema, and hypertension. In most coxib studies the incidence of these renal effects is 3% to 5% of patients treated.

Capsaicin

Substance P causes the degranulation of mast cells, with the subsequent release of histamine, vasodilation, and exudation of fluids into the tissues, resulting in inflammation, swelling, and pain. Substance P is also released from proximal nerve terminals of the nociceptive neurons (type-C fibers) to activate the spinothalamic tract for transmission of the pain impulse to the CNS.

Capsaicin is a white crystalline material found in minute quantities in red pepper and is recognized to impart the pungency to chili and other foods made from hot peppers. When topically applied to peripheral type-C nociceptive nerve fibers, capsaicin induces the initial release of substance P with an excitatory effect. After the initial excitatory effect, substance P is subsequently depleted from the nerve ending, and the neuronal membrane is desensitized to noxious stimuli. Capsaicin depletes substance P throughout the length of the neuron, providing both local and central analgesic effects. Because its effect is limited to type-C nociceptive fibers, capsaicin does not alter sensory modalities other than pain (44).

Capsaicin has been shown to be effective for pain reduction in several pain syndromes, including osteoarthritis (45), rheumatoid arthritis (45), diabetic neuropathy (46), postherpetic neuralgia (47), trigeminal neuralgia (48), and cluster headache (49). It is available as a topical cream containing 0.025% or 0.075% capsaicin. For arthritis and neuralgia, capsaicin is applied topically to the affected area three to four times daily. For cluster headache, it is applied intranasally to the affected side once daily.

Serotonin

Serotonin (5-HT) is a neurotransmitter that plays a role in the endogenous modulation of pain. Decreased central serotonergic function causes increased sensitivity and reactivity to noxious stimuli and partial failure of the analgesic effects of opioids (50). Decreased serotonergic function plays a role in the pathogenesis of depression, and the effects of serotonin on opioid analgesia may explain the increased pain complaints (and decreased efficacy of analgesic medications) in patients with depression. Conversely, increased serotonergic neurotransmission is associated with both analgesia and normalization of the pain threshold.

Pain seems to increase the turnover of serotonin. The cerebral synthesis of serotonin requires the passage of the amino acid tryptophan (unbound to protein) through the blood-brain barrier by carrier-mediated active transport. Increased free-plasma tryptophan is essential to augment central serotonin synthesis.

Intravenous L-tryptophan, 7.5 and 15 mg/kg, has been shown to be effective in the treatment of postoperative (cholecystectomy) pain. Oral L-tryptophan has given good results in patients suffering from deafferentation pain, and oral 5-hydroxytryptophan has benefited patients with acute migraine headache (50). Oral L-tryptophan is no longer available in the United States due to an outbreak of eosinophilic myalgia syndrome attributed to a contaminant produced in the manufacture of the product. The triptan drugs (sumatriptan, zolmitriptan, naratriptan, rizatriptan) are serotonin receptor agonists that are effec-

tive in treating acute migraine, although they have not been shown to have intrinsic analgesic properties (see Chapter 22). Antidepressant drugs probably exert their analgesic effects through the modulation of central serotonin (see Chapter 17).

Anticonvulsants

Gamma-amino butyric acid (GABA) is the major inhibitory neurotransmitter in the central nervous system. Inhibitory neurotransmitters, such as GABA, are thought to have a role in analgesia. THIP (4,5,6,7-tetrahydroisozazole (5,4c) pyridine-3-ol) is an analog of the GABA-mimetic drug muscimol. THIP was shown to be an effective analgesic in patients with chronic pain; however, side effects of dizziness, sedation, and nausea were commonly observed (51).

Valproic acid (sodium valproate) is an anticonvulsant that is a GABA agonist (5). Valproic acid easily crosses the blood-brain barrier and increases the GABA concentration in various areas of the central nervous system, including the hypothalamus (52). It has been shown to be effective in the prophylaxis of migraine (52), cluster (53), and chronic daily (mixed) (54) headache syndromes.

Other anticonvulsants, such as carbamazepine and phenytoin, have been used in specific pain states such as trigeminal neuralgia. These drugs are not analgesics, nor do they possess antiinflammatory properties. These drugs are thought to work by reducing or inhibiting synaptic transmission, interrupting the temporal summation of afferent impulses that set off a painful neuralgia attack (55). Carbamazepine is the treatment of choice in trigeminal neuralgia and is useful in other neuropathic types of pain, such as glossopharyngeal neuralgia, intercostal neuralgia, herpetic and postherpetic neuralgia, phantom limb states, and central pain states. Pain is frequently controlled at dosages lower than used for seizure control. The addition of a low dose of a tricyclic antidepressant along with carbamazepine may improve the analgesic effect (56). Gabapentin has been shown to provide benefit in diabetic neuropathic pain and postherpetic neuralgia.

These agents are covered in greater detail in Chapter 18.

SUMMARY

NSAIDs are among the most commonly prescribed classes of drugs in the world. They are effective in the treatment of mild, moderate, or severe pain and inflammation and can be used to treat a wide variety of conditions. In the treatment of severe pain, the addition of an NSAID can reduce opioid requirements and the side effects of analgesia. NSAIDs are associated with several mechanism-based adverse effects, especially gastrointestinal toxicity, which can limit therapy with chronic use. Coxibs have an efficacy comparable to high-dose NSAIDs but significantly reduce the risk of both common (dyspepsia) and severe GI adverse events compared to NSAIDs. Renal effects, however, are not diminished with coxibs; high-risk patients should be carefully monitored when NSAIDs or coxibs are administered.

Anticonvulsants have a role in specific pain states, particularly neuropathic pain. Capsaicin also provides benefit in the treatment of some neuropathic pain syndromes, particularly postherpetic neuralgia. It is also useful for the management of osteoarthritis pain.

Acknowledgments

I wish to thank Linda Bacher, information scientist, for her help in providing recent articles and a literature search, and Dr. Greg Bell for providing updated data on NSAIDs and the coxibs.

REFERENCES

1. Fields HL. *Pain.* New York: McGraw-Hill, 1987:20–22.
2. Carr DB, Goudas LC. Acute pain. *Lancet* 1999;353:2051–2058.
3. Pasternak GW. Multiple morphine and enkephalin receptors and the relief of pain. *JAMA* 1988;259:1362–1367.
4. Vane JR, Botting RM. Mechanism of action of nonsteroidal anti-inflammatory drugs. *Am J Med* 1998;104(3A):2S–8S.
5. Insel PA. Analgesic-antipyretic and antiinflammatory agents and drugs employed in the treatment of gout. In: Hardman JG, Limbird LE, Molinoff PB, et al. eds. *Goodman and Gilman's the pharmacologic basis of therapeutics,* ed 9, New York: McGraw-Hill, 1996:617–657.
6. Hennekens C. Update on aspirin in the treatment and prevention of cardiovascular disease. *Am Heart J* 1999;137:S9–S13.
7. Fornaro G, Rossi P, Mantica P. Indobufen in the prevention of thromboembolic complications in patients with heart disease. A randomized, placebo-controlled, double-blind study. *Circulation* 1993;87:162–164.
8. Drugs for pain. *Medical Letter* 2000;42:73–78.
9. Schnitzner TJ. Non-NSAID pharmacologic treatment options for the management of chronic pain. *Am J Med* 1998;105(1B):45S–52S.
10. Hochberg MC, Altman RD, Brandt KD, et al. Guidelines for the medical management of osteoarthritis, Part 1: osteoarthritis of the hip. American College of Rheumatology. *Arthritis Rheum* 1995;38:1535–1540.
11. Hochberg MC, Altman RD, Brandt KD, et al. Guidelines for the medical management of osteoarthritis, Part 1: osteoarthritis of the knee. American College of Rheumatology. *Arthritis Rheum* 1995;38:1541–1546.
12. Egbert A. Postoperative pain management in the frail and elderly. *Clinics in Geriatric Medicine* 1996;12(3):583–599.
13. Phillips A, Polisson R, Simon L. NSAIDs and the elderly. Toxicity and economic implications. *Drugs & Aging* 1997;10(2):119–130.
14. Davies N, Wallace J. Selective inhibitors of cyclooxygenase-2. Potential in elderly patients. *Drugs & Aging* 1996;9(6):406–417.
15. Brooks PM, Day RO. Nonsteroidal antiinflammatory drugs—differences and similarities. *N Engl J Med* 1991;324:1716–1725.
16. Lipsky PE. Specific COX-2 inhibitors in arthritis, oncology, and beyond: where is the science headed? *J Rheumatology* 1999;26(Suppl) 56:25–30.
17. Cryer B, Feldman M. Cyclooxygenase-1 and cyclooxygenase-2 selectivity of widely used nonsteroidal anti-inflammatory drugs. *Am J Med* 1998;104:413–421.
18. Moreland LW, St Clair EW. The use of analgesics in the management of pain in rheumatic diseases. *Rheumatic Dis Clin of North Amer* 1999;25:153–191.
19. Simon LS, Strand V. Clinical response to nonsteroidal antiinflammatory drugs. *Arth Rheum* 1997;40:1940–1943.
20. Portenoy RK. Drug treatment of pain syndromes. *Semin Neurol* 1987;7:139–149.
21. Honig SM. Nonsteroidal anti-inflammatory drugs. In: Tollison CD, Satterwaite JR, Tollison JW, ed. *Handbook of chronic pain management,* ed 2. Baltimore: Williams and Wilkins, 1994:165–172.
22. Singh G. Recent considerations in nonsteroidal anti-inflammatory drug gastropathy. *Am J Med* 1998;105(1B):31S–38S.
23. Wolfe M, Lichtenstein D, Singh G. Gastrointestinal toxicity of nonsteroidal anti-inflammatory drugs. *N Engl J Med* 1999;34:1888–1899.
24. Gabriel S, Jaakkimainen L, Bombardier C. Risk for serious gastrointestinal complications related to use of nonsteroidal anti-inflammatory drugs. *Ann Intern Med* 1991;115:787–796.
25. Evans J, MacDonald T. Tolerability of topical NSAIDs in the elderly. Do they really convey a safety advantage? *Drugs & Aging* 19969(2):101–108.
26. Laine L. Nonsteroidal anti-inflammatory drug gastropathy. *Gastrointestinal Endoscopy Clinics of North America* 1996;6(3):489–504.
27. Hernandez-Diaz S, Garcia Rodriguez LA. Association between nonsteroidal anti-inflammatory drugs and upper gastrointestinal tract bleeding/perforation. *Arch Intern Med* 2000;160:2093–2099.
28. Brater D. Effects of nonsteroidal anti-inflammatory drugs on renal function: focus on cyclooxygenase-2-selective inhibition. *Am J Med* 1999;107(6A):65S–71S.
29. Whelton, A. Nephrotoxicity of nonsteroidal anti-inflammatory drugs: physiologic foundations and clinical implications: *Am J Med* 1999;106(5B):13S–24S.
30. Murray M, Black P, Kuzmik D, et al. Acute and chronic effects of nonsteroidal antiinflammatory drugs on glomerular filtration rate in elderly patients. *Am J Med Sci* 1995;310(5):188–197.
31. Page J, Henry D. Consumption of NSAIDs and the development of congestive heart failure in elderly patients. An underrecognized public health problem. *Arch Intern Med* 2000;160:777–784.
32. Boyce E, Breen G. Celecoxib: a COX-2 inhibitor for the treatment of osteoarthritis and rheumatoid arthritis. *Formulary* 1999;34:405–417.
33. Celebrex [package insert]. Chicago, IL: GD Searle & Co. May, 1999.
34. Vioxx [package insert]. West Point, PA: Merck & Co, Inc. 1999.
35. Fries JF, Williams CA, Bloch DA. The relative toxicity of nonsteroidal antiinflammatory drugs. *Arth Rheum* 1991;34:1353–1360.
36. Depre M, Ehrlich E, Van Hecken A, et al. Pharmacokinetics, COX-2 specificity, and tolerability of supratherapeutic doses of rofecoxib in humans. *Eur J Clin Pharmacol* 2000;56:167–174.
37. Cannon G, Caldwell J, Holt P, et al. Rofecoxib, a specific inhibitor of cyclooxygenase 2, with clinical efficacy comparable with that of diclofenac sodium: results of a one-year, randomized, clinical trial in patients with osteoarthritis of the knee and hip. *Arthritis Rheum* 2000;43(5):978–987.
38. Simon L, Lanza F, Lipsky P, et al. Preliminary study of the safety and efficacy of SC-58635, a novel cyclooxygenase 2 inhibitor: efficacy and safety in two placebo-controlled trials in osteoarthritis and rheumatoid arthritis, and studies of gastrointestinal and platelet effects. *Arthritis Rheum* 1998;41:1591–602.
39. Simon L, Weaver A, Graham D, et al. Anti-inflammatory and upper gastrointestinal effects of celecoxib in rheumatoid arthritis. *JAMA* 1999;282(20);1921–1928.
40. Ehrich EW, Dallob A, De Lepeleire I, et al. Characterization of rofecoxib as a cyclooxygenase-2 isoform inhibitor and demonstration of analgesia in the dental pain model. *Clin Pharmacol Ther* 1999;65:336–347.
41. Langman M, Jensen D, Watson D, et al. Adverse upper gastrointestinal effects of rofecoxib compared with NSAIDs. *JAMA* 1999;282(20):1929–1933.
42. Hawkey C, Laine L, Simon T, et al. Comparison of the effect of rofecoxib (a cyclooxygenase 2 inhibitor), ibuprofen, and placebo on the gastroduodenal mucosa of patients with osteoarthritis: *Arthritis & Rheumatism* 2000;43(2);370–377.
43. Cryer B, Feldman M. Effects of very low dose daily, long-term aspirin therapy on gastric, duodenal, and rectal prostaglandin levels and on mucosal injury in health humans. *Gastroenterology* 1999;117:17–25.
44. Hautkappe M, Rozien MF, Toledano A, et al. Review of the effectiveness of capsaicin for painful cutaneous disorders and neural dysfunction. *Clin J Pain* 1998;14:97–106.
45. Deal CL, Schnitzer TJ, Lipstein E, et al. Treatment of arthritis with topical capsaicin: a double-blind trial. *Clin Ther* 1991;13:383–395.
46. Ross DR, Varipapa RJ. Treatment of painful diabetic neuropathy with topical capsaicin. *N Engl J Med* 1989;321:474–475.

47. Bernstein JE, Bickers DR, Dahl MV, Roshal JY. Treatment of chronic postherpetic neuralgia with topical capsaicin. *J Am Acad Dermatol* 1987;17:93–96.

48. Fusco BM, Geppetti P, Fanciullacci M, Sicuteri F. Local application of capsaicin for the treatment of cluster headache and idiopathic trigeminal neuralgia. *Cephalalgia* 1991;11(Suppl 11):234–235.

49. Sicuteri F, Fanciullacci M, Nicolodi M, et al. Substance P theory: a unique focus on the painful and painless phenomena of cluster headache. *Headache* 1990;30:69–79.

50. Ceccherelli F, Diani MM, Altafini L, et al. Postoperative pain treated by intravenous L-tryptophan. *Pain* 1991;47163–172.

51. Jensen LK, Egsmose C, Lund B, Halskov O. Evaluation of the effect of the GABA-agonist THIP in the treatment of chronic pain. *Clin J Pain* 1988;4:51–54.

52. Hering R, Kuritzky A. Sodium valproate in the prophylactic treatment of migraine: a double-blind study versus placebo. *Cephalalgia* 1992;12: 81–84.

53. Hering R, Kuritzky A. Sodium valproate in the treatment of cluster headache: an open clinical study. *Cephalalgia* 1989;9:195–198.

54. Mathew NT, Ali S. Valproate in the treatment of persistant chronic daily headache. An open label study. *Headache* 1991;31:71–74.

55. Dalessio DJ. The major neuralgias, postinfectious neuritis, and atypical facial pain. In: Dalessio DJ, ed. *Wolff's headache*, New York: Oxford University Press, 1987:266–288.

56. Browne TR, Empting L, Lydiard RB, Yerby MS. New uses and old for carbamazepine. *Patient Care* 1990:48–81.

CHAPTER **19**

Pharmacological Management of Chronic Pain: A Review

Gerald M. Aronoff, Rollin M. Gallagher and Jashvant G. Patel

Relief of pain and suffering has been the objective of the medical profession throughout history. Despite advances in treatment technology, however, pain often remains a medical enigma. Traditional management has generally encompassed such options as bed rest, physical therapy, nerve blocks, surgery, and medication. The purpose of this chapter is to discuss the role of medications in the treatment of nonmalignant chronic pain.

As late as 1628, Harvey still believed that the heart is where pain is felt. Descartes in the same period considered pain to be conducted by nerves to the brain directly. This seemed to predate the later specificity theories of Muller (1), Latze (2), and von Frey (3). It was not until the late 1800s that Erb (4), Goldscheider (5), and others proposed the pattern theory of pain. Finally, in the middle of the twentieth century, a modern understanding of pain emerged with the work of Hardy (6), Beecher (7), and Wall and Melzack (8) showing the neurophysiological complexities of the pain experience (9,10). A growing body of evidence indicates that pain itself can be considered as a disease process that is self-perpetuating, causing both morphological and physiological changes in the CNS, and that new systems of classification, based upon this pathology, are indicated (11). Developing pharmacological interventions that specifically target these processes is in the near future of pain medicine (11,12). A solid appreciation of the complex peripheral and central neurophysiology of nociception, pain perception, and pain modulation, which earlier chapters discuss in detail, and of the principles of behavioral pharmacology, forms the basis for the rational and effective use of pharmacological agents for chronic pain.

Pain Perception, Pain Behavior, and Reinforcement

Pain and the relief of pain powerfully modify behavior. Because pain hurts and is unpleasant, people go to great lengths to ablate or minimize pain or to avoid conditions that precipitate pain. Thus, drugs and other treatments that promise to modify pain, even when of unproven or questionable validity, have great salience in human society. When the well-developed desire for pain relief is combined with the natural human tendency to experiment to find solutions to problems, physicians are arguing against powerful human motivations when trying to dissuade a patient from trying new treatments.

Drugs that reduce pain powerfully reinforce drug-seeking behavior (13). These drugs are readily available and historically successful in life experience for our various aches and pains—hence the highly prevalent use of over-the-counter pain remedies such as NSAIDs, which act primarily in the periphery to reduce nociception. Centrally acting remedies abound as well, although they may not be promoted as analgesics per se. Alcohol, marijuana, and opiates are well-known examples of ancient remedies for pain and suffering still used widely today. These drugs powerfully influence emotions and behavior as well as pain perception. Figure 19-1 presents a simplistic model of the interaction of pain perception, pain behavior, and medications (14).

Medications influence this model in several ways:

- By inhibiting prostaglandin synthesis and secondary activation of nociceptors (e.g., the NSAIDs)
- By stabilizing neuronal membranes to reduce ectopic nerve impulse generation and neuropathic pain (e.g., anticonvulsants and probably the tricyclic antidepressants)

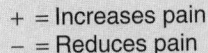

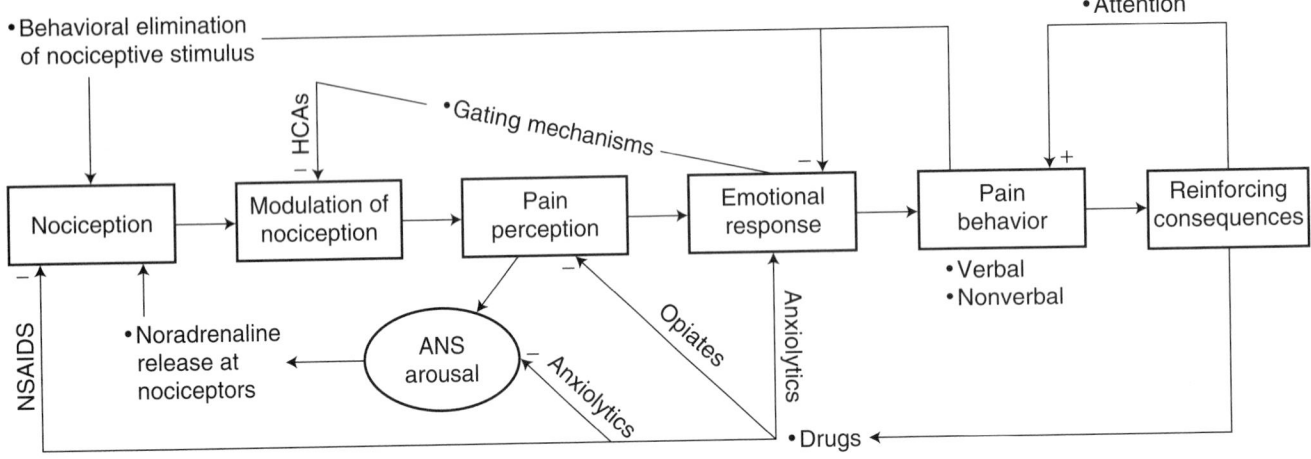

FIG. 19-1. Biobehavioral model (Gallagher and Pasol, 1997, with permission, *Current Therapies*).

- By reducing the suffering from pain (e.g., the opioid analgesics)
- By modifying emotional and behavioral responses to pain that may perpetuate nociception or worsen pain perception (e.g., antidepressants, by treating secondary depression or anxiety, may improve patients' ability to comply with pain management instructions, including regimens in exercise, pacing, relaxation, and medication)

So closely related are pain and emotions that separating the analgesic effects from the emotional and behavioral effects of certain drugs may be difficult. This close relationship forms the basis for the rational use of centrally acting drugs in chronic pain disorders.

THE CLINICAL PHARMACOLOGY OF CHRONIC PAIN: GENERAL PRINCIPLES

The successful use of medications for chronic pain depends upon careful clinical reasoning founded upon a working knowledge of the phenomenology and physiology of pain syndromes and the specific clinical actions of these drugs. Gallagher and Pasol (14) have outlined 10 *general principles* that will guide the practitioner to rational choices when prescribing medication.

1. *Prioritize safety when treating nonmalignant chronic pain.* The principles of efficacy, expediency, and cost follow. Consider drug and disease interactions. Benzodiazepines must be used cautiously, particularly in the elderly or those operating machinery because they increase the risk for falls and accidents. Consider other serious risks such as GI bleed from NSAIDs or liver disease from long-term, high doses of acetaminophen

(Tylenol). Ironically, opioids have fewer deleterious and toxic side effects or drug or disease interactions than most other medications used for pain. The literature does not substantiate the long-held belief that opioids are deleterious for patients in pain, particularly when used judiciously within a comprehensive pain program (15,14,16). Unfortunately, in a misguided effort to avoid exposure to opioids, toxic doses of ineffective drugs may be used in a futile effort to control pain. Undertreatment of pain and suffering may lead to unnecessary impairment, disability, stress, immunological compromise, and secondary medical and psychiatric disorder.

2. *Prioritize efficacy when treating a terminally ill patient with pain.* Physicians and patients together may find that the risk of using combinations of drugs in high doses is acceptable to obtain relief of pain and suffering, enabling a patient to be more functional. However, the physician must continuously reevaluate the risk-benefit ratio of dosing. Unnecessarily high doses in an attempt to ablate pain without regard for untoward physiological, cognitive, emotional, and behavioral effects may worsen outcome in terms of functional losses such as valuable interpersonal time with family and friends and inability to complete one's affairs.

3. *Review potential interactions with medical conditions and with other medications.* The physician should carefully review potential interactions of analgesics with illnesses causing pain (e.g., diabetes with neuropathy, cancer, or rheumatoid arthritis) or comorbid with pain, particularly when treating older patients and those with chronic medical illness. For example, avoid heterocyclic antidepressants in post-A–V node conduction disturbance and use them cautiously in urinary retention.

The plethora of medications taken by chronically ill and elderly populations may interact with analgesics. Changing metabolism and, secondarily, serum levels, may lead to toxicity or alterations in the therapeutic activity of medications.

4. *Selectively choose drugs for pain disorder and comorbid psychiatric disorder based on efficacy and specificity of mechanism.* The efficacy of medication in chronic pain syndromes has been difficult to establish because of methodological problems such as poorly defined populations for study (e.g., low back pain, which can be caused by several mechanisms), longitudinal designs of insufficient duration (e.g., most studies are less than 3 months), and inadequate outcome measures (e.g., subjective pain relief rather than functional improvement). Despite these problems, as we shall discuss, the efficacy of individual drugs in well-defined conditions, many with known receptor-based mechanisms, has been supported in the literature and should help guide psychotropic drug choice.

5. *Balance side-effect profile against efficacy.* For example, in a patient with radicular low back pain in whom weight loss may be critical for functional outcome, amitriptyline or doxepin, which are effective in neuropathic pain, also may cause considerable weight gain. Choose another drug such as nortriptyline.

6. *Consider drug effects on the efficacy of other analgesics.* For example, although benzodiazepines are known to be excellent drugs for calming acute anxiety states associated with pain, they may interfere with opioid analgesia or complicate management of depressive disorders.

7. *Consider behavioral effects when prescribing.* What are the effects of a drug on critical neuropsychological functions, such as learning, memory, and psychomotor performance, that are critical to outcome in rehabilitation yet often not considered when prescribing? Benzodiazepines interfere with memory and learning and disinhibit negatively conditioned behavior. These effects are particularly problematic in pain rehabilitation, which relies on the premise that patients will learn new coping skills. What is the abuse liability of a drug? Diazepam's rapid onset of action makes abuse more likely than clonazepam. What are a drug's behavioral consequences? To avoid unpleasant withdrawal a patient dependent on regular doses of a short-acting sedative such as alprazolam or butalbital (in Fiorinal and Fioricet) may develop secondary drug-seeking pain behavior, sometimes manifest as pain symptoms.

8. *Select combinations of medications from different classes.* Consider appropriate combinations of medication to influence the various nociceptor and neurotransmitter systems of pain perception: *nociception, transmission of nociception, pain perception, suffering, pain modulation* and *pain behavior,* as outlined in Fig. 19.1, and their neurophysiological substrates. The tra-

ditional strategy of staying with one or two familiar drugs in each class is often ineffective in chronic pain, no matter what its cause. One must be willing to try drugs of different classes in combination and also different drugs within the same class.

The clinical problem of herniated lumbar disc suggests the importance of this principle. Thus, for a patient with an acute disc and radicular leg pain without surgical indications, the following medication combinations might be useful to consider:

- To reduce the inflammatory response and related nociception at the site of the herniation: ibuprofen 400 to 800 mg t.i.d.-qid. If ineffective in 5 to 7 days, change to another NSAID. In high-risk patients, choose a COX-2 inhibitor. Also, consider epidural steroids.

- To reduce pain perception, related CNS arousal and secondary noradrenaline release at nociceptive sites leading to "sensitization" of nociceptors: For short-term use, Tylenol with codeine 30 mg, 1 to 2 tabs every 4 hours PRN to control moderate to severe pain. If ineffective, successively try hydrocodone or oxycodone combination products as increasing opioid analgesic potency is required. Increase the potency of opioid rather than the number of pills to avoid acetaminophen toxicity. If longer-term opioid use is required, use sustained-action opioids such as OxyContin, methadone, MS Contin, or transdermal fentanyl patches until adequate analgesia is achieved (or until limited by side effects). Treat episodic anxiety with a short-acting benzodiazepine, such as lorazepam 0.25 to 0.5 mg, and train the patient in behavioral and relaxation techniques.

- To reduce neuropathic pain and to restore disturbed sleep: Doxepin, amitriptyline, or nortriptyline, titrating upward from 10 mg HS every 3 to 5 days until sleep improves or adequate analgesia is reached. In patients with concurrent depression, use higher doses. Maintain for at least a 3-week trial. If idiosyncratic effects occur, switch to another HCA. If side effects are intolerable, consider an SSRI (citalopram, sertraline, paroxetine, or fluoxetine) or anticonvulsant. If any one of these agents is ineffective or creates intolerable or bothersome side effects, systematically substitute another agent. Try to change only one drug at a time to be able to assess which drug and what dose are effective. Institute behavioral pain management techniques simultaneously.

9. *Establish a reliable method of monitoring pain and activity levels.* Pain diaries should be used to establish baseline pain levels prior to treatment and to monitor the patient's response to treatment. Instructions are provided during the first visit, and charts are reviewed at subsequent clinic visits to reinforce diary keeping and the patient's responsibility for outcome. Diaries provide

detailed information about factors that worsen or alleviate pain, about patient behavior, and about the effects of medication and other interventions. Daily diaries help identify critical points at which utilization of short-acting medication, physical methods (e.g., icing and stretching), or behavioral methods (e.g., pacing and relaxation) might change the pain pattern and course of treatment.

10. *Avoid irrational polypharmacy.* When patients report unrelieved or increased pain, in their eagerness to alleviate suffering physicians may prescribe higher doses or a new drug without considering other factors that might impact outcome. Physicians should consider the possibility of untoward drug interactions, side effects, toxicity, and behavioral effects and also investigate the possibility that either disease progression or nondisease factors, such as a change in activity or stress, may be responsible for nonresponse or an increase in pain. The reinforcement paradigm of Figure 19-1 helps explain this tendency. Well-established, unconscious operant pain behaviors powerfully induce medication prescription. Our social role as physicians creates enormous pressure to relieve pain and suffering with prescriptions, a behavior that is positively reinforced by grateful and approving patients. Not prescribing elicits punishing disapproval from the patient, providing another incentive to prescribe. *Keep in mind that almost any new intervention, including a new medication, may have an initial placebo effect: The patient will actually feel better despite there being no specific pharmacological advantage to the medication prescribed.*

What are some useful clinical strategies to minimize the tendency to polypharmacy? First, medication trials should be carefully planned after adequate data gathering. The database prior to starting drugs should include:

- A complete medical and pain history
- A selective physical and mental status examination
- A comprehensive formulation of the clinical problem including an assessment of the various types of pain (e.g., nociceptive, neuropathic); hypotheses about mechanisms perpetuating pain (e.g., deconditioning, sleep disturbance, depressive illness, poor adherence to indicated treatment); medical problems (including comorbid psychiatric disorders); and psychosocial factors that might influence treatment
- A diagnostic list, including pain diagnoses, hypothesized mechanisms (e.g., neuropathic, nociceptive, mixed, psychogenic), and associated other medical problems including psychiatric disorders
- A baseline record of pain levels and fluctuations by using the pain diaries, usually for at least a week

Second, do not assume that every pain requires a pharmacological response or that flareups necessarily require new or more medication. Often, other interventions, including physical (e.g., icing, TENS, and stretching), behavioral (e.g., relaxation training with and without biofeedback, pacing, cognitive restructuring, and stress management), and trigger point therapies (e.g., spray and stretch with fluoromethane or ethyl chloride) can be quite effective in controlling pain. If psychological symptoms occur, do not assume a psychiatric disorder (e.g., major depression, panic disorder) is present requiring a full therapeutic trial of psychotropic medication. Often reassurance, brief support, and cognitive behavioral techniques will suffice.

Third, select medication based upon careful formulation of the type of pain, the mechanisms perpetuating pain, and the presence of comorbid or secondary psychiatric disorder. Figure 19-2 proposes a general algorithm for drug selection.

Fourth, close monitoring, every 1 to 2 weeks but occasionally several times weekly, may be necessary to establish optimum dosing for a medication and to minimize noncompliance. Thus, medication will be given a full therapeutic trial. A common problem is inadequate dosing and noncompliance. For example, heterocyclic antidepressants, commonly used and effective in neuropathic pain, are often stopped before effective doses are reached. Instead of appropriately titrating the dose upward, the tendency is to add another medication.

MEDICATIONS USED FOR CHRONIC PAIN

Peripherally Acting Medications

The first category of medications to be discussed is that useful with pain related to inflammation. Thermal and chemical nociceptors involve prostaglandin receptors on nerve endings. The nociceptive process can be generated from a multitude of sources. In most pathophysiological conditions, however, the presence of inflammation causes thermal stimulation, edema causes pressure, and the presence of such autocoids as serotonin, bradykinin, histamine, and other substances released from injured tissues initiates the nociceptive process.

Antiinflammatory Agents

Aspirin and Acetaminophen   Despite the proliferation of NSAIDs on the market, aspirin continues to be widely used as a drug of choice for early treatment of chronic pain because of its low cost and efficacy (17–19). The appropriate dosage for nonarthritic pain is related to aspirin's ceiling effect at approximately 1000 mg. Halpern notes that the optimal dose may be less than the 600-mg oral dose commonly used and that at higher doses aspirin's therapeutic effects do not increase, although at oral doses of more than 1000 mg toxicity increases dramatically (20). In the treatment of mild to moderate pain, aspirin is generally given every 3 to 4 hours. To avoid toxicity, the interval between doses should be increased as the dose itself is increased. As the dose increases, so does the half-life (from 3 or more hours with 300 mg to 9 hours with 2 gm), while urinary excretion decreases (21). Toxicity from aspirin may carry its own warning signal—tinnitus—although this is not always present. Difficulties with aspirin are that excessive doses over a long time can produce central nervous system damage and salicylate poisoning. Furthermore, aspirin must be taken cautiously with such gastrointestinal problems as gastritis, peptic ulcer disease, and other ulcerative conditions of the stomach. Angioedema, rhinitis, nasal polyposis, and bronchial asthma are also contraindications and complications. Less common toxic effects include abdominal pain, nausea, shock, tinnitus, acid-base disturbances, and respiratory alkalosis.

Fortunately, the preceding side effects are relatively rare, and even the more common complications afflict fewer than 5% of the overall population. However, approximately 10% of adverse drug reactions in U.S. hospitals are aspirin related. It may well be that this high percentage reflects the high usage of aspirin compounds.

Aspirin does not generally cause liver damage in healthy adults, but it may exacerbate preexisting liver disease. It may also exacerbate already diminished kidney function, especially among the elderly, by causing further renal impairment, such as diminished glomerular filtration and decreased renal tubular tissue secretion, leading to the retention of toxic levels of salicylate. The toxicity appears to be related to serum rather than blood levels. The margin of safety for aspirin is said to be relatively high when compared with other nonsteroidal antiinflammatory drugs (NSAIDs). Aspirin also increases prothrombin time and inhibits the second phase of platelet aggregation (19).

Salicylates can cause pathological cochlear changes and deafness, but this ototoxicity is generally reversible. Tinnitus is not always a reliable indicator of toxicity. Serum levels may also monitor salicylate dosages. When aspirin is used in high doses for rheumatoid arthritis, supplementation with vitamin C should be considered. Aspirin occasionally causes an iron-deficiency anemia and may precipitate aplastic anemia in the elderly (22).

Some people cannot tolerate aspirin for a variety of reasons. For them, acetaminophen is often a substitute. This drug is rapidly absorbed from the gastrointestinal (GI) tract, reaches a peak plasma concentration within 30 minutes to 2 hours after ingestion, and is primarily metabolized by the liver. Liver damage has been described with the ingestion of more than 10 to 15 gm; 25 gm or more is said to be a potentially fatal dose for adults (22). Whereas aspirin is antipyretic and antiinflammatory, acetaminophen does not have antiinflammatory properties. This reduces its usefulness in certain conditions, although its analgesic and antipyretic capabilities are equal to those of aspirin, and the ceiling dosage is the same. As with aspirin,

acetaminophen should be used cautiously by people taking anticoagulants. In addition, taking tricyclic antidepressants or benzodiazepines along with acetaminophen may lead to hypersensitivity, hepatitis, or cholestasis. There are also interactions when acetaminophen is taken with antibiotics or indomethacin (22,23).

Other Antiinflammatory Agents A number of drugs in addition to aspirin fall within the class of medications for which the primary actions seem to be caused by the inhibition of prostaglandin synthesis. The ability of these drugs to induce analgesia and to relieve the pain associated with inflammatory processes is now well established. Indeed, studies have shown that, in some circumstances, these agents have a potency comparable to that of the opioids (24). Their usefulness in such conditions as rheumatoid arthritis and osteoarthritis is equally well established (25). In general, they may provide symptomatic improvement for ankylosing spondylitis, but they do not generally alter the natural course of the disease (26).

Contraindications to the use of NSAIDs are the same as those generally noted for aspirin. They may cause gastritis, gastric bleeding, and peptic ulcer in some patients, especially those with a history of peptic ulcer disease. Alcoholism, smoking, and concurrent steroid use may pose additional risk factors. With NSAIDs the incidence of GI irritation is similar to that of aspirin, approximately 2% to 10% with occasional use and 30% to 50% with high-dosage regular use. A recent study shows that the prophylactic use of famotidine at 40 mg b.i.d. reduced the incidence of duodenal ulcers from 13% to 2%, gastric ulcers from 20% to 8% (27). Lower doses (20 mg b.i.d.) reduced duodenal, but not gastric, ulcers. Mild changes of liver-function test results may occur in about 15% of patients taking NSAIDs. These elevations may stabilize, progress, or be transient despite continued therapy. Allergic reactions may occur with any of these agents. As with aspirin, the other NSAIDs may induce asthmatic attacks in susceptible individuals. It is estimated that, in the United States, approximately 10% of the population are aspirin intolerant. Symptoms include nasal polyposis, bronchial asthma, and skin reactions (21). In an individual known to be intolerant to aspirin or another NSAID, there is increased risk to subsequent NSAID trials.

Conservative estimates indicate that more than 100 000 patients are hospitalized each year for NSAID-related gastrointestinal (GI) complications and that at least 16 500 NSAID-related deaths occur each year among arthritis patients alone (28). A prospective study (29) reviews patient status and outcomes, drug side effects, and the economic impact of illness for more than 11 000 patients at participating institutions in the United States and Canada and indicates: "1. Osteoarthritis (OA) and rheumatoid arthritis (RA) patients are 2.5 to 5.5 times more likely than the general population to be hospitalized for NSAID-related GI events; 2. The absolute risk for serious NSAID-related GI toxicity remains constant and the cumulative risk increases over time; 3. There are no reliable warning signals—more than 80% of patients with serious GI complications had no prior GI symptoms; 4. Independent risk factors for serious GI events were age, prednisone use, NSAID dose, disability level, and previous NSAID-induced GI symptoms; and 5. Antacids and H2 antagonists do not prevent NSAID-induced gastric ulcers, and high-risk NSAID users who take gastro-protective drugs are more likely to have serious GI complications than patients not taking such medications." It was concluded that limiting NSAID use is the only way to decrease the risk of NSAID-related GI events.

Special advice must be given to certain patients for whom NSAIDs are prescribed. In children, for example, toxic reactions may occur at lower dosages than those that would produce similar toxicity in an adult. Because these agents alter platelet aggregation, patients with coagulation disorders (e.g., hemophilia and some forms of malignancy with bleeding diathesis) must be carefully monitored when these drugs are administered. Patients requiring coumadin-type anticoagulants, heparin, sulfonamides, sulfonylurea, or hydantoins should be observed for signs of toxicity when concurrently taking NSAIDs. When prescribing these drugs for the elderly, lower dosages may have to be considered because of the greater possibility of inducing hepatic and renal toxicity (21). NSAIDs can reduce the antihypertensive effect of propranolol and other β-blockers, inhibit the naturetic effect of furosemide, and inhibit renal lithium clearance.

Acute interstitial nephritis and renal failure, associated with prostaglandin depletion, are well-known complications of NSAIDs. In the presence of preexisting renal insufficiency, renal function should be carefully monitored, and smaller doses should be used because the reduced excretion will increase the half-life of these drugs, may exacerbate already diminished renal functioning, and precipitate overt renal decompensation (21). Peripheral edema has been observed in some patients. Therefore, NSAIDs (especially those with higher sodium content) should be used cautiously in patients with hypertension, fluid retention, or heart failure (21).

Diflunisal: One of the major advantages of this salicylic acid derivative is that it has a plasma half-life of from 8 to 12 hours, and therefore the frequency of administration need be only two to three times a day. It has antiinflammatory and general analgesic actions but is not recommended as an antipyretic.

Indomethacin: This drug is said to be more effective than aspirin for conditions such as ankylosing spondylitis, osteoarthritis, acute gout, pleurisy, pericarditis, and pericardial effusion and is useful as an antipyretic in Hodgkin's disease. Complications and toxicity with this drug are common, affecting up to 50% of those receiving therapeutic dosages. About 20% of these patients are forced to discontinue the medication. It is also a general analgesic, but its side effects often prevent its use for non-inflammation-related pain. Indomethacin's interactions include enhancement of the action of anticoagulants, as well as possible cardiac toxicity when used with thyroid medications (21).

Sulindac: An analog of indomethacin, sulindac was synthesized as a result of a search for a compound as effective as indomethacin but less toxic. It has a long duration of action of 16 hours and is often useful for a long-term antiinflammatory treatment because the dosing can be accomplished twice daily.

Naproxen and naproxen sodium: Naproxen and naproxen sodium are rapidly absorbed from the gastrointestinal tract with peak plasma levels attained at 1 to 2 hours. Mean plasma half-life is 13 hours, making it appropriate for twice-daily dosing. These are recommended for mild to moderate pain and for the treatment of primarily dysmenorrhea and for the treatment of rheumatoid arthritis, osteoarthritis, ankylosing spondylitis, tendonitis, bursitis, and acute gout. Multiple studies (22,30,31) suggest a favorable long-term gastrointestinal profile. This is related to rapid dispersion, reducing exposure of the gastric mucosa to the concentrated drug and lactose-free naproxen, eliminating the risk of gastrointestinal side effects associated with lactose intolerance.

Diclofenac sodium: Diclofenac sodium is a phenylacetic acid with established antiinflammatory and analgesic effects. Its indications include the treatment of rheumatoid arthritis, osteoarthritis, and ankylosing spondylitis. It is rapidly absorbed from the GI tract with peak plasma levels reached in 2 to 3 hours. Despite its relatively short half-life, diclofenac sodium diffuses into and persists in synovial fluid from 4 to 24 hours (although it has not been established that diffusion into the joint plays a role in the drug's effectiveness). As with other NSAIDs, the most frequent side effects are GI related. When compared to other NSAIDs, diclofenac sodium was found to have a high therapeutic index based on analgesic and antiinflammatory effects (32).

Phenylbutazone and oxyphenbutazone: The butazones are effective antiinflammatory drugs for the treatment of ankylosing spondylitis, acute gout, bursitis, capsulitis, peritendonitis, and other arthropathies. However, because of the potentially severe adverse effects (agranulocytosis and aplastic anemia) their use should be limited to short-term intervention with close monitoring for evidence of bone marrow failure (33). The pyrazoles are also contraindicated in patients with peptic ulcer disease, congestive heart failure, hypertension, and reduction in granulocytes (20).

Azapropazone: This is a pyrazole derivative with a spectrum of activity similar to phenylbutazone but without its severe toxicity. In contrast to many of the NSAIDs, 62% of azapropazone is excreted unchanged in the urine. In patients with renal impairment, the dosage should be reduced and the patients monitored carefully (33).

The Propionic Derivatives   Most widely used NSAIDs in U.S. clinical practice are the propionic derivatives represented by ibuprofen, naproxen, fenoprofen, keto-profen, and flurbiprofen. In addition to their effect on prostaglandin synthesis, they are thought to affect the histamine and kinin systems of inflammation mediation. Side effects include nonspecific edema and GI irritation. These drugs have a wider margin of safety than indo-methacin. In addition to their application for inflammatory conditions, the Food and Drug Administration (FDA) now approves them for noninflammatory painful conditions, although their mechanism of action is not clear. These drugs are also used for menstrual cramps with the proposed mechanism involving reduction of prostaglandin levels in menstrual fluid (34). Long-acting preparations of these medications (e.g., naproxen) potentially improve patient compliance through a more convenient dosing schedule of once or twice daily.

Pyranocarboxylic acid: Etodolac is an NSAID that exhibits analgesic, antiinflammatory, and antipyretic properties. Its indications include the management of pain as well as acute and long-term use in the management of osteoarthritis. Unlike other NSAIDs, which significantly suppress gastric and duodenal prostaglandins, contribut-ing to undesirable gastric side effects, etodolac appears to selectively spare cytoprotective prostaglandins in the gas-tric mucosa. This has been suggested as a possible mecha-nism for the gastric safety of etodolac (35,36).

COX-2 inhibitors: The newest class of nonnarcotic analgesics is the COX-2 inhibitors, which include celecoxib (Celebrex) and rofecoxib (Vioxx). They have been shown to have analgesic efficacy in osteoarthritis, rheumatoid arthritis, dysmenorrhea, and dental pain (37–39). Payne (40) suggests that further research is necessary prior to concluding that COX-2 drugs are efficacious in chronic medical illnesses other than arthritis. Aspirin and the tra-ditional NSAIDs block both COX-1 and COX-2 enzymes. Because pain and inflammation are caused primarily by COX-2 inhibition, and many of the GI side effects are relieved primarily by COX-1 inhibition, this new class of medication offers significant advantages in terms of pro-viding analgesia with fewer adverse GI problems. The newer COX-2 drugs have a longer half-life and are lipid soluble. In a recent article, Sunshine (41) suggests that because of different mechanisms of action, consideration may be given to combining traditional NSAIDs and COX-2 drugs in a select patient population who get some, but inadequate, analgesia with one class if used alone.

As with traditional NSAIDs, the COX-2 drugs are also limited as analgesics for severe pain by their ceiling effect.

Trials of glucosamine and chondroitin preparations for osteoarthritis symptoms demonstrate moderate to large effects, but quality issues and likely publication bias suggest that these effects are exaggerated. Because of their safety, these remedies would have great utility in the treatment of osteoarthritis even if they were only modestly effective (42).

Capsaicinoids are molecules derived from chili peppers. In 1997, a gene that encoded for a receptor specific for cap-saicinoids was identified. Called VR1, this fatty acid recep-tor is present only on C fibers and when activated produces desensitization or degeneration of the sensory afferent. Today, capsaicinoids are being studied as effective treatments for a number of sensory nerve fiber disorders, including pain associated with arthritis, cystitis, human immunodeficiency virus, and diabetic neuropathy (43).

Opioid Analgesics

With severe acute pain, cancer pain, and postoperative pain, the use of opioid analgesics is usually appropriate. In these situations, physicians' reluctance to use narcotics because of fear of causing physical dependence and toler-ance is generally inappropriate. Twycross has emphasized that, in a cancer pain population, increasing requirements for opioid analgesia generally do not represent tolerance but rather progression of the disease (44). It should also be noted that the dosage of opioid frequently can be decreased through balanced analgesia utilizing adjuvants and peripherally acting nonnarcotic analgesics. Judicious use of these drug combinations not only can enhance anal-gesia but also can diminish adverse side effects and treat symptoms other than pain (14,17). Nonpharmacological pain management techniques of proven efficacy (45) should also be employed to reduce suffering and improve analgesic efficacy (16,46–48). Unfortunately, training in these techniques is often considered as a last resort when frequent practice and long use lead to better efficacy (45).

Although there is no doubt that opiates are often the drugs of choice for severe acute pain and chronic cancer pain, in the authors' opinion their use in chronic nonma-lignant pain must be selective (14–16,48). As recently as 10 years ago, one of the outcome measures for a success-ful multidisciplinary pain center was the percentage of patients "successfully" weaned and maintained off of opioids during followup. In retrospect, we can say that many of these patients had not done well prior to their admission when they were on opioids, and, therefore, jus-tification of the medication taper was not difficult. How-ever, with 2001 knowledge and hindsight, many pain medicine practitioners believe that a disservice has been done to a group of patients who would have benefited from long-term opioid treatment but for whom we might have dogmatically refused to prescribe opioids (49). This issue now needs revisiting.

Much has been learned, especially from clinical studies and treatment of cancer pain. We now know that in appro-priately selected patients, opioids have a low morbidity (often less than NSAIDs) and a low addiction potential. Although tolerance may occur in some cases, generally patients become tolerant to bothersome side effects (other than constipation) more so than to analgesic effects. Evi-dence from cancer studies suggests that when patients who are clinically stable on a certain opioid dose request a dose escalation, it may be more related to progression in their disease than to tolerance. When principles from the WHO analgesic ladder paradigm (50) are followed appropriately, combining NSAIDs, adjuvants, and opioids, we can manage the vast majority of patients with severe chronic pain.

There is a subgroup of the nonmalignant pain population who can be treated effectively with long-term opioids (51,52–56) (Table 19-1). These individuals, who have a well-documented medical condition as the cause of their pain, have attempted alternative techniques of pain management and are being carefully monitored by a physician. In general these patients may not have responded either to treatment with nonnarcotic analgesics, adjuvants, or alternative techniques of pain management (e.g., physical therapy, psychotherapy, relaxation therapy, and pain center therapy) or may receive added benefit from the selective use of opioids in combination with these other medications and treatment. In addition, it should be demonstrated that these patients remain functional while receiving narcotic analgesics, but attempts to taper the medications result in diminished function, impairment in overall activities of daily living, and increased suffering.

TABLE 19-1. *Guidelines for maintenance: opioid use in chronic nonmalignant pain*

1. Documented medical condition as the cause of the pain.
2. Prior systemic therapeutic trials of alternative pain-control regimens (analgesics, adjuvants, psychosocial interventions, appropriate medical treatments, and behavioral approaches) have been unsuccessful.
3. Documentation that nonopioid treatments have resulted in (a) inadequate analgesia impairing functional activities of daily living (ADL) and (b) continued suffering.
4. Prior to initiating opioid maintenance, nonalgologists should (a) obtain consultation with an algologist or (b) consult with a specialist in management of the specific problem being treated. Consultation report should document occurrence with opioid treatment.
5. Document detailed discussion of short- and long-term effects and risks. Signed informed consent is suggested.
6. One physician should be responsible for writing prescriptions (which should be on a time-contingent rather than pain-contingent basis) and monitoring clinical progress. Recommended initial frequency of appointments is at least monthly. Patients must be seen and records must show reason for continuing opioids.
7. Documentation that maintenance opioids improve analgesia and functional ADL and diminish suffering.
8. Use lowest clinically effective opioid dose. Peripherally acting nonnarcotics and adjuvants used concurrently may allow lower-dose opioid usage.
9. A history of substance dependence or abuse is a relative contraindication.
10. Any evidence of drug-seeking behavior, obtaining opioids from multiple sources, or frequent requests for dose escalation without documentation of significant worsening of the clinical condition should be a cause for careful review and reconsideration of opioid use.

Supported by a research grant from Purdue Pharma L.P.

With balanced analgesics, they can remain active and productive with diminished pain and suffering. When this occurs, they do not exhibit significant pain behaviors. When it does not occur, some will find alternative ways to obtain the medication they need for pain control. It has been suggested that this behavioral pattern should not be viewed as addiction but rather as pseudoaddiction related to inadequate treatment (56). There is little evidence that exposure to opioids in patients with painful conditions leads to true addiction unless predisposing factors, such as prior substance abuse, are present (57,58). Patients with a history of substance abuse or addiction, significant psychopathology, high risk factors, or environmental stressors contributing to escalating pain and suffering in general should only cautiously, if at all, be maintained on opioids for nonmalignant pain. It needs to be emphasized that most chronic pain syndrome patients can be effectively managed without the regular daily use of narcotic analgesics. Yet, in patients carefully selected for opioid maintenance, addiction is rarely a clinical problem.

Opioid Agonists

Opioids can be classified as agonists, agonist-antagonists, and antagonists. In this section only the agonist and agonist-antagonist groups will be discussed because the antagonist drugs are not analgesics.

The opioid agonists have generally similar clinical effects when given at equianalgesic doses. The differences among the individual drugs are important because a patient may have an adverse reaction to one of the opioids but not to others. Usually, the reason for choosing one agonist rather than another is that one confers some advantage—for instance, in route of administration or in the time action of the agent. It should be emphasized, however, that at equianalgesic dosages the reasons for choosing one agonist over another are the specific adverse effects of a particular opioid for an individual patient and the differences in oral absorption or time action of analgesic effect (59).

The use of opioids in pregnancy may result in neonatal withdrawal symptoms. This may be a special problem with such longer-acting opioids, such as methadone, because the abstinence syndrome may be delayed until after the infant leaves the hospital. Also, the physician must be cognizant of the possibility that long-term exposure to systemic opioids may have some adverse effect on the CNS development and weigh that possibility against the adverse effects in the infant of poorly controlled pain in the mother.

The agonists are useful in relieving anxiety, which is normally associated with severe pain. At usual clinical dosages the emotional reaction to the pain is changed, and it is believed that this may be due largely to the action of the agonists on the limbic system. Other central nervous system effects include analgesia, drowsiness, mood changes, mental clouding, and, on occasion, respiratory depression.

The major toxic effects of the agonist opioids include vomiting and respiratory depression. In the supine patient, therapeutic doses of agonists do not generally have significant effects on blood pressure or cardiac rate and rhythm. However, these substances do cause vasodilation, therefore one must watch for the development of orthostatic hypotension and syncope in susceptible individuals. Opioids also cause a marked decrease in contractility in the small and large intestine, often resulting in constipation.

Morphine is the standard to which other opioid agonists are often compared.

Studies have found that, with postoperative pain, 10 mg of [cf6] D-amphetamine combined with morphine is twice as potent as morphine alone and that a combination of 5 mg is 1½ times as potent as morphine (60). It has also been found that, in proportion to its dose, [cf6] D-amphetamine generally improves performance that has been diminished by morphine. Researchers have discovered that a potent, common, nonsedating analgesic can be produced by a combination of the well-absorbed oral opioid anileridine in combination with amphetamine. A dose of 25 mg of anileridine plus 5 mg of [cf6] D-amphetamine taken orally leads to an analgesic equivalent to approximately 12 to 15 mg of injectable morphine (61).

Agonist-Antagonist Opioids

The agonist-antagonist group consists of pentazocine, butorphanol, nalbuphine, and buprenorphine. The raison d'etre for this class of drugs is not that they provide better analgesia than the agonist opioids, but rather that they were thought to have a much lower incidence of physiological dependence (61). Despite having said this, the authors do note that, although somewhat diminished compared to the agonist drugs, there is a definite abuse potential, and the possibility of a withdrawal syndrome should be recognized after chronic use (17).

One of the more worrisome side effects of pentazocine has been the incidence of psychotomimetic effects, which seems to be reduced (although still present) with the newer members of this class, and in clinical trials this is described as approximately 1%. Caution must be exercised with these medications. Patients should not have taken opioids for a period of time depending on the half-life of the narcotic because the agonist-antagonist drug will precipitate an abstinence syndrome.

The authors generally do not recommend this class of opioids for use with chronic nonmalignant pain.

Sustained-action Opioids

When the physician now considers the use of opioids in a chronic pain patient, the advent of long-acting opioid preparations has improved the likelihood of getting good analgesia with a lower incidence of adverse side effects.

Long-acting oxycodone, morphine, and fentanyl enable the patient to reach a steady state while avoiding the fluctuations in blood levels, often either contributing to inadequate analgesia (with low blood levels) or adverse side effects (with high blood levels). The side-effect profile of these medications appears to be lower as well. Methadone, used for decades as a heroin substitute for drug addicts being maintained on narcotics, has also been useful for chronic pain; however, its use carries the burden of its pharmacokinetics—its analgesic effects last 4–8 hours, but its pharmacological half-life is far longer, with the result that toxic levels can accumulate as a patient and physician attempt to reach an analgesic "steady state." There are times, however, when cost considerations make methadone the opioid analgesic drug of choice. It must be emphasized that although all patients maintained on chronic opioids must be monitored carefully for adverse side effects, those on methadone should be monitored even more carefully to avoid toxicity.

Generally, in chronic pain patients, physicians should avoid using meperidine (Demerol) because of the toxicity of its principal metabolite, normeperidine, and pentazocine because of its psychotomimetic effects and its lower efficacy when compared with pure agonists.

In the context of a rehabilitation focus for patients with chronic pain, a concern about the use of opioids while driving or using other potentially dangerous machinery has been expressed. The effects of opioids on performance have been exaggerated. In fact, there is good evidence that patients acclimate to the sedative and psychomotor effects of opioids (57), whereas they do not acclimate to the negative effects of pain on task performance (62). It appears that pain is more deleterious than opioids on functional performance!

Occupational Issues

Pain center experience has demonstrated that the dysfunctional process known as the chronic pain syndrome (associated with dysfunctional pain behaviors and self-limitations of activity level with associated pain deconditioning, poor coping skills, and significant life disruption) is often modifiable with appropriate treatment (63). In selected patients this may involve the use of long-term opioids, and many individuals who were receiving or applying for disability prior to opioid treatment were able to return to work and resume useful, productive lives as a result of getting adequate analgesia from opioids. Prior to releasing patients to return to work, they must be carefully evaluated regarding mental acuity in cognitive functioning, they must be alert and have no difficulty with concentration or attention span, and essentially they must be found to not have any drug effect that would interfere with job performance or endanger themselves or coworkers. In our clinical experience, this is most likely to occur with regular use of sustained-action opioids rather than with short-acting opioids.

Driving and the Use of Opioids

Many physicians are hesitant to recommend that patients drive while on opioids. Our clinical experience is consistent with an emerging research (64–74) suggesting that this hesitancy is unfounded with patients having a normal mental status who are on stable doses of sustained-action opioids. It is important to emphasize several points, however.

Frequently, patients are being prescribed other centrally acting medications such as antidepressants and benzodiazepines, and these may interact with opioids, adversely influencing mental acuity. It is also essential that the physician take a careful history of all prescribed over-the-counter medications. The senior author (GMA) monitors reaction time as well as mental status and has developed a test called the Aronoff test of reaction time (75). With a patient not anticipating the event, a soft rubber ball is thrown across the desk, and the patient's reaction observed. A normal response is for the patient to react appropriately and catch the ball. A patient sedated, with decreased mental acuity or impaired reflexes, will generally not be able to pass this test and will be struck by the ball or be unable to catch it. Although this has not been tested for scientific validity, I have found that this test, combined with a detailed mental status examination, gives a good estimate of whether a patient has adequate reaction time to function in a number of situations, including driving. As the dosage of opioid is increased, caution patients not to drive or put themselves in at-risk situations until they find that they are at full mental acuity.

In summary, we have learned that (a) nociceptive pain is most opioid responsive, (b) neuropathic and central pain are less but variably responsive, and (c) psychologically maintained pain is generally nonresponsive and inappropriate for chronic opioid treatment. As always, optimal management of the patient with chronic pain depends on comprehensive assessment, and we still have much to learn about identifying which patients are most appropriate for opioids.

Antidepressants and Anticonvulsants

Centrally active drugs such as antidepressants and anticonvulsants are commonly used medications in chronic pain and are considered first-line drugs in the treatment of neuropathic pain and psychiatric comorbidity. These medications affect pain experience through four distinct, but often complementary, clinical actions (14). First, these drugs are known to be effective *adjuvants to opiate analgesia,* and they constitute an integral part of the three-step analgesic ladder recognized by the World Health Organization in 1990 (50). Second, certain of these drugs possess *independent analgesic efficacy* for specific pain disorders within the present classification of chronic pain, particularly neuropathic pain. Third, these drugs have *psychotropic effects on psychiatric syndromes,*

such as depression, anxiety, and sleep disorders that frequently cooccur with pain disorders and exacerbate pain-related disability. Fourth, these drugs may be used to treat *troublesome physiological symptoms,* such as sleep disturbance or muscle spasm, that often accompany pain and may importantly contribute to the disability associated with chronic pain states.

Antidepressants in Chronic Pain

Antidepressants are probably the most commonly prescribed psychotropic drugs for chronic pain. A metaanalysis of 39 placebo-controlled, double-blind studies of the effectiveness of antidepressants in chronic pain indicated that antidepressants are significantly more effective than placebo in reducing pain in chronic pain patients (76). In this study, the average chronic pain patient receiving an antidepressant experienced less pain than 74% of the patients who received placebo. This effect appears to be consistent with a direct analgesic activity of the medication that is independent of antidepressant activity. However, because of the relatively uneven methodologies of the studies, the generalizability of these findings in chronic pain in general is questioned (16,77). The multiple physical and psychosocial factors that may confound or interact with antidepressant response must be controlled for, either through sampling strategies or analyses, to establish these effects (78,79).

Antidepressants may be clinically effective in chronic pain through one or more of several mechanisms:

1. *Direct analgesic effect:* These medications are thought to modulate pain perception through activity on noradrenergic and serotonergic neurophysiological systems that descend from the midbrain to the dorsal horn (80). Like certain anticonvulsants, inhibition of sodium channel activity in the neuronal membrane may contribute to their analgesic properties in neuropathic pain.
2. *Amelioration of comorbid psychiatric disorder:* Depressive illnesses may worsen pain perception, interfere with coping, and contribute additional morbidity (81). In this category, effects on pain could be through either of two mechanisms: first, by the treatment of masked depression that is causing the pain symptom (82); and second, by the treatment of manifest depression, which enables the patient to better tolerate the pain (83). Panic disorder also specifically responds to antidepressants.
3. *Reduction of pain-related symptoms:* These might include changes in appetite and sleep that contribute to morbidity and disability (16).
4. *Potentiation or enhancement of opioid analgesia* (84,85): This probably results from a combination of the first three mechanisms.

Pain defined by region, mechanism, or description may respond to specific medication. However, controlled, standardized trials comparing antidepressants with other medications, and with each other, in specific conditions are lacking.

Heterocyclic Antidepressants

First-generation heterocyclic antidepressants (HCAs) (e.g., amitriptyline, imipramine, and doxepin) have been the most widely used for the management of chronic pain, alone or comorbid with depression. In studies of neuropathic pain, HCAs have demonstrated an analgesic effect even when depression is controlled for or patients with depressive illness are excluded from the study (86,87). HCAs have been reported to relieve lancinating pain as well as constant pain (88,89). The hypothesis that myofascial pain may indeed be an expression of deafferentation neuralgia (84) suggests that these medications may be used successfully in diverse myofascial disorders.

Most studies of HCAs report on older drugs, such as amitriptyline, imipramine, and doxepin, which consistently show an analgesic effect. However, the problematic side-effect burden of amitriptyline related to its anticholinergic and antihistaminergic activity has led to comparative studies of other tricyclics. Desipramine, which has far fewer side effects, may approach the efficacy of amitriptyline for relief of neuropathic pain. Both amitriptyline and desipramine block norepinephrine reuptake; their effectiveness compared to selective serotonin reuptake inhibitors (SSRIs) such as fluoxetine, suggested to investigators that norepinephrine reuptake blockade contributes to the analgesic effect of antidepressants. Nortriptyline, with activity in both NA and 5-HT systems, and like desipramine with a lower side-effect profile than amitriptyline, also seems effective, and blood levels can be reliably obtained.

In summary, the clinical pharmacology literature and clinical experience suggest that the HCAs constitute useful treatment for central deafferentation and neuropathic pain, particularly when predominantly dysesthetic or burning. A trial of antidepressants may be useful in any patient with primary neuropathic pain and certainly should be considered when pain has responded inadequately to standard pharmacological management with NSAIDs and/or opiates. Unlike HCA's antidepressant effect, which may require several weeks, these drugs may relieve pain within a few days. However, pain relief may not occur for 1 to 3 weeks and may require titration to higher doses, often at the same level for depression, for some patients (14,80).

Side effects of HCAs: The usefulness of HCAs in chronic pain patients is limited somewhat by troublesome side effects, by problematic interaction with other medications, and by their potential deleterious effects on medical problems other than chronic pain. These effects reflect each drug's profile of receptor affinities such as anticholinergic, antihistaminic H-1 and H-2, adrenergic, and serotonergic (14). HCAs commonly produce a benign elevation in heart rate, particularly desipramine due to its stronger norepinephrine reuptake blockade effect, and dry mouth and constipation. Orthostatic hypotension can be dangerous, particularly in cardiac patients or elderly patients because of the risk of fractures from falls. Urinary retention can be problematic in the elderly.

Drug-drug interactions of HCAs: Dangerous interactions occur particularly with MAOIs (MAOI crisis) and SSRIs (serotonin toxicity). Other HCA interactions include cimetidine, methylphenidate, acetaminophen, oral contraceptives, chloramphenicol, isoniazid, monoamine oxidase inhibitors, and disulfiram—inhibition of metabolism increasing blood levels and toxicity of HCAs. Disulfiram—induction of psychosis and a confusional state. Guanethidine, propranolol, clonidine—blockage of neuronal reuptake. Methyldopa—agitation, tremor, tachycardia. Thiazides, acetozolamide—decreased HCA effect, hypotension augmentation. Cardizem, quinidine, procainamide—decreased cardiac conduction and prolongation of QT interval. Coumadin—increased bleeding. Neuroleptics—increased HCA effect, ventricular arrhythmias, and sedation. Psychostimulants—blocked HCA metabolism, increased cardiotoxicity. Cyclobenzaprine (Flexeril)—synergistic effect. Halothane anesthetics—tachycardia, synergistic anticholinergic effect. Testosterone—psychosis. Opiates—potentiate analgesia, synergistic anticholinergic effects. Benzodiazepines, alcohol—sedation, confusion, increased suicide risk, impaired motor function. Propranolol—agitation, tremor, tachycardia. Anticholinergic drugs—increased anticholinergic toxicity. Anticonvulsants—induction of hepatic metabolism decreasing HCA levels. Valproate—increased HCA levels. HCAs increase Dilantin levels, decrease Tegretol levels.

Drug-disease interactions of HCAs: It is important to note that HCAs are contraindicated with post-A–V node conduction disturbance, that they may lower the seizure threshold, and that they may have a hypoglycemic effect. Rarely do they precipitate narrow-angle glaucoma.

Selective Serotonin Reuptake Inhibitors (SSRIs)

SSRIs specifically inhibit the neuronal reuptake of serotonin with little other receptor activity. Because these drugs lack anticholinergic and antihistamine activity compared with the HCAs, their side-effect profile and risk of problematic interactions with other drugs and medical illnesses are minimal. Despite the purported role of serotonin in pain modulation, a clear-cut analgesic role for the SSRIs has not been empirically established. Even so, fluoxetine showed analgesic activity in experimental animal pain models (90) and chronic pelvic pain (79), and case reports suggest its utility in the management of headache (91), fibrositis (92), diabetic neuropathy (93), and phantom limb pain (84). However, these studies did not control for depression. Paroxetine (Paxil) is effective in the treatment of neuropathic pain (93). Both fluvoxamine and mianserin were more effective than placebo in chronic tension-type headache; however, fluvoxamine, the SSRI, was more effective than mianserin in the nondepressed patients, suggesting that the therapeutic activity of fluvoxamine was unrelated to a direct effect on depression (94).

The most common side effects of SSRIs include agitation, anxiety, sleep disturbance, tremor, sexual dysfunction, and headache. Citalopram (Celexa) has been reported to have a lesser rate of sexual side effects than other SSRIs. Rarely, SSRIs have been associated with EPS-like symptoms, arthralgias, lymphadenopathy, inappropriate antidiuretic syndrome, agranulocytosis, and hypoglycemia. SSRIs interact with MAOIs causing the life-threatening central serotonin syndrome manifested by abdominal pain, diarrhea, sweating, fever, tachycardia, elevated mood, hypertension, altered mental state, delirium, myoclonus, increased motor activity, irritability, and hostility. Severe manifestation of this syndrome can include hyperemia, cardiovascular shock, and death. SSRIs are essentially devoid of Type 1A antiarrhythmic effects of tricyclics, nor do SSRIs have any (alpha) adrenergic antagonistic effect; therefore, they rarely are associated with orthostatic hypotension. Sertraline, fluoxetine, and paroxetine are relatively free of interactions with CNS depressants such as benzodiazepines, alcohol, barbiturates, or lithium. Combining paroxetine or fluvoxamine with anticoagulants such as warfarin increases bleeding time; therefore, anticoagulants must be adjusted. Fluvoxamine potentiates the effects of diazepam, terfenadine, astemizole, theophylline, and warfarin. SSRIs in combination with HCAs generally increase HCA levels.

The relatively benign side-effect and toxicity profiles of SSRIs, when compared to HCAs, favor their use in clinical situations in which there is no therapeutic advantage to using the HCAs, or the HCAs are relatively contraindicated because of risk (e.g., cardiac conduction defects, suicidality, seizures).

Atypical Antidepressants

Bupropion (Wellbutrin), *trazodone* (Desyrel), *nefazadone* (Serzone), and *venlafaxine* (Effexor) are so-called atypical antidepressants that may be useful in chronic pain (60). Trazodone has little intrinsic analgesic activity but has been used to treat comorbid depression and to induce sleep. It has the disadvantage of association with priapism, even though rare, which makes its use unacceptable to many men. Bupropion, nefazadone, and venlafaxine have not been studied in pain. Bupropion has the advantages of low side-effect profile, including low sexual impairment, unique mechanism of action (good for treatment-resistant depressions), and short half-life, which avoids buildup in geriatric patients. Significantly increased seizure risk in at-risk patients and slightly increased risk in normal patients merit attention to avoiding peak plasma levels by prescribing multiple divided doses.

Venlafaxine and nefazadone are two newer antidepressants that have not been studied for their analgesic proper-

ties. Venlafaxine, like HCAs, affects NE and 5HT systems and so may have analgesic properties as well; it has fewer side effects and minimal drug interaction risk and does not build up in geriatric patients. Its major problems include increased diastolic blood pressure (usually at doses over 300 mg/day), nausea (tolerance develops in 2 to 6 weeks), twice-daily dosing requirement, and variable final dosing. It is the drug of choice for severe melancholic or geriatric depression (22). Nefazadone, a phenylpiperazine similar to trazodone, has fewer anticholinergic side effects than the HCAs and is less likely to impair sexual functioning than either HCAs or SSRIs. It has a potentially lethal interaction with the commonly used antihistamines terfenadine (Seldane) and temizole (Histamil) because it inhibits their hepatic metabolism.

Choosing an Antidepressant

The SSRIs have largely replaced the HCAs as first-line drugs for most patients with depression. However, the unproven efficacy of SSRIs for pain makes selection of an antidepressant more complicated in pain patients. Figure 19-2 (95) outlines one of the authors' (RMG) simple algorithms for choosing antidepressants in populations of chronic pain patients with and without comorbid depression. For any one patient, the choice of the most appropriate antidepressant trial may be confounded by the complex interaction of factors that determine efficacy. Positive effects must be weighed against the potential for negative effects. Optimal judgment requires a specific knowledge of the pharmacology, efficacy, and side-effect profile of the medications themselves and the clinical evaluation of the patient, including a detailed knowledge of the following factors: *the characteristics of the medication, the phenomenology of the pain syndrome, the presence of other medical problems, the use of other medications, the presence of comorbid psychiatric disorder, and the psychological characteristics of the patient.*

Pain medicine lacks clinical algorithms based upon controlled clinical trials comparing the efficacy of one antidepressant to another in specific pain syndromes. However, the evidence for efficacy of HCAs is better established than for SSRIs. Therefore, if there are no medical contraindications, HCAs and atypical antidepressants are preferable in a clinical trial. Choice of medication requires knowledge of side effects and drug and disease interactions.

Neuropathic pain (e.g., radiculopathy, causalgia, diabetic neuropathy) alone may respond to HCAs. The favorable side-effect profile of nortriptyline and desipramine increases patient acceptance of titration to higher doses. Desipramine is much less expensive than nortriptyline but not as cheap as amitriptyline. Start with low doses, such as nortriptyline 10 mg, desipramine 25 mg, or amitriptyline 25 mg and titrate weekly up to antidepressant doses if necessary until relief or side effects intervene. If *myofascial pain* or *inflammatory pain* exist as part of a more systemic clinical syndrome such as fibromyalgia, which is often associated with evidence of CNS disorder such as sleep disturbance and depression, a trial of HCAs may be warranted. *Migraine headache* prophylaxis with tricyclics or SSRIs may be effective (96); however, newer abortive approaches, such as self-administered sumatriptan or DHE, which have strong serotonin agonist activity, often successfully prevent progression of headache to a full-blown incapacitating migraine (97) while avoiding the attendant risks and side effects associated with taking regular HCAs. Combining injected abortive approaches such as sumatriptan or DHE with SSRIs and HCAs must be done cautiously for fear of precipitating serotonin toxicity.

Other medical problems such as cardiac conduction disturbance, post-A–V node blocks particularly, are a relative contraindication to HCAs. In patients with heart disease or risk factors or the elderly, if a trial of HCAs is warranted, obtain an EKG prior to starting these and monitor EKG as doses are titrated. Start with SSRIs such as paroxetine, fluoxetine, and sertraline, which are reasonable choices for a trial. Use HCAs cautiously in the context of medical problems that may worsen, such as orthostatic hypotension and urinary retention. Antidepressants may lower the insulin needs of diabetics. HCAs, particularly maprotiline, may lower seizure threshold.

Comorbid psychiatric disorder often complicates pain disorder (98,99) and influences treatment outcome. Because a pain medicine evaluation often overlooks psychiatric disorder, such as depressive illness, even when present, the clinician must actively screen for its presence repeatedly during the course of treatment (99). Depression appears to lower pain threshold and tolerance (100), to increase analgesic requirements, and generally to add to the debilitating effects of pain. Patients in pain often suffer insomnia and fatigue, which are also extremely common vegetative symptoms of depression. Patients usually attribute insomnia to pain rather than depression because pain is the more socially acceptable malady (21). It is difficult to distinguish cause and effect within the pain-depression-insomnia cycle, but after the cycle is established, it becomes self-perpetuating and requires active intervention. If comorbid *major depression (MDD)* exists, antidepressants should be titrated to therapeutic levels for depression over 2 to 3 weeks. SSRIs (fluoxetine 20 mg, paroxetine 20 mg, sertraline 50 mg) should be given for 2 weeks to assess response and then titrated appropriately. HCAs usually start with nortriptyline 25 mg HS or desipramine 50 mg HS and increase to 75 mg and 150 mg, respectively, over about 10 days, monitoring side effects. (Lower doses are used for geriatric populations.) Give the dose about 3 weeks to work and monitor serum levels for therapeutic range.

Clinical depression is often overlooked in medical practice (101,102) and, when diagnosed, often inadequately treated (103). In pain populations the diagnosis of depression can be difficult and unreliable because of denial or response bias (patients not reporting symptoms when asked because of fears of stigma) and confounding of the physical symptoms of MDD, such as sleep disturbance and fatigue, by pain, medical problems, or medications (59). Several common errors may lead to inadequate treatment of comorbid MDD (14,103): (a) choosing a medication not effective for MDD (e.g., diazepam); (b) underdosing with an effective medication; (c) ineffectively managing side effects causing noncompliance; (d) stopping medication too soon. If MDD occurs with neuropathic pain, HCAs are the drug of choice but must be titrated to antidepressant doses, usually higher than needed for neuropathic pain alone. For MDD in the absence of neuropathic pain, SSRIs are the drug of choice because their low side-effect profile, fewer interaction problems, and better acceptance make adequate dosing more likely. Often, we will use a tricyclic antidepressant in low doses for insomnia and for neuropathic pain (e.g., nortriptyline or doxepin 10 to 50 mg) and an SSRI in the usual antidepressant dosage for a clinically depressed patient. When physicians are uncomfortable treating MDD, they should have a low threshold for psychiatric consultation or referral because of the physical, psychological, and social morbidity associated with untreated depression (104).

The timing of depression, relative to onset of pain, and the type of depression, whether or not there is a personal or family history of depression, may influence treatment choice. In a recent study of depression in chronic myofascial facial pain patients and their families and in controls and their families, Dohrenwend and colleagues (105) showed that pain patients with late onset depressive illness have rates of prepain depression and rates of depression in first-degree relatives that are equivalent to those of pain patients without depression and controls without depression; in other words, it appears that depression in these myofascial pain patients is not familial and that other, nonfamilial, mechanisms, such as learned helplessness (106), must be considered. What are treatment implications of this finding for pain patients? In some chronic pain patients who first present with major depression after the onset of pain-related disability, depressive symptoms respond well to effective control of pain without using antidepressants (14,16). Particularly if the depressive symptoms are relatively mild, if there is no family history, and if medical cautions exist, we may delay using antidepressants for 2 weeks to evaluate response to effective pain treatment. However, the risks associated with this procedure (e.g., untreated depression leading to poor pain treatment outcome and higher risk for chronic disability and suicide) are sufficiently high so that the general clinician without considerable experience should treat with an appropriate SSRI agent and seriously consider appropriate psychiatric consultation.

Suicide is always a risk in patients with depression, a risk heightened by the suffering and chronicity of intractable pain. The salience of this issue is heightened by our contemporary heated debate on physician-assisted suicide. The risks of antidepressant medications differ. If taken in overdose, HCAs have far greater potential for successful suicide than do SSRIs. *Yet the key to preventing suicide is identification of depression early in its course and rapid and effective treatment combined with effective pain management.* Consultation with a psychiatric colleague is essential, and hospitalization must be considered.

In all cases of depression, appropriate psychotherapies (e.g., cognitive behavioral and interpersonal) should be added to medications for even greater benefit, perhaps in conjunction with behavioral pain management training. When medical problems or a patient's beliefs preclude medication, the clinician must rely on psychotherapeutic treatments; but in the latter instance, the clinician should continue trying to help patients overcome the cognitive distortions and negative emotions that prevent them from using medication.

In patients with comorbid *panic disorder,* antidepressants can very effectively block panic attacks, often at doses lower than in major depression. Benzodiazepines can *temporarily* provide control of symptomatic anxiety but should be replaced by anxiety control training (45,47) to avoid other problems (see the section on antianxiety medications).

Patients' reluctance to accept antidepressant treatment—for example, because of religious beliefs—can impede successful outcome. The clinician should explore their ideas and beliefs to identify misunderstanding about the nature of pain and depression and to educate about the mecha-

nism of action of these drugs. When a physician prescribes antidepressants for neuropathic pain, even in the absence of depression, patients may believe that the physician is suggesting that depression is causing pain; they may become defensive and even overtly hostile because of negative past experience, such as an insurer's efforts to discredit the patients by attempting to establish psychological causation to avoid financial responsibility. In fact, among disabled LBP patients with equal spinal pathology, those with more psychological distress (elevated depression score on the MMPI) are more likely to be judged as less severely impaired even when they are not (107). Thus, physicians must explain, when antidepressants are being used as analgesics for comorbid depression, why and how common depression is as a complication of chronic disabling pain. Also, they must explain that depression does not invalidate nociceptive or neuropathic pathology or suffering, nor does it mean that the pain is "all in their head" or caused by depression or that depression is caused by personal weakness.

Figure 19-2 presents simplistic, but rational, clinical guidelines for treating depression, pain, and insomnia in persons with chronic pain (14). To regulate sleep, low doses of sedating HCAs (e.g., doxepin or amitriptyline) are preferable to benzodiazepines; zolpidem (Ambien) is our choice for episodic stress-related, sleep-onset insomnia. We do not generally use HCAs for regional myofascial low back pain unless seeking antidepressant effects. Antidepressant trials should be considered in any patient whose pain has

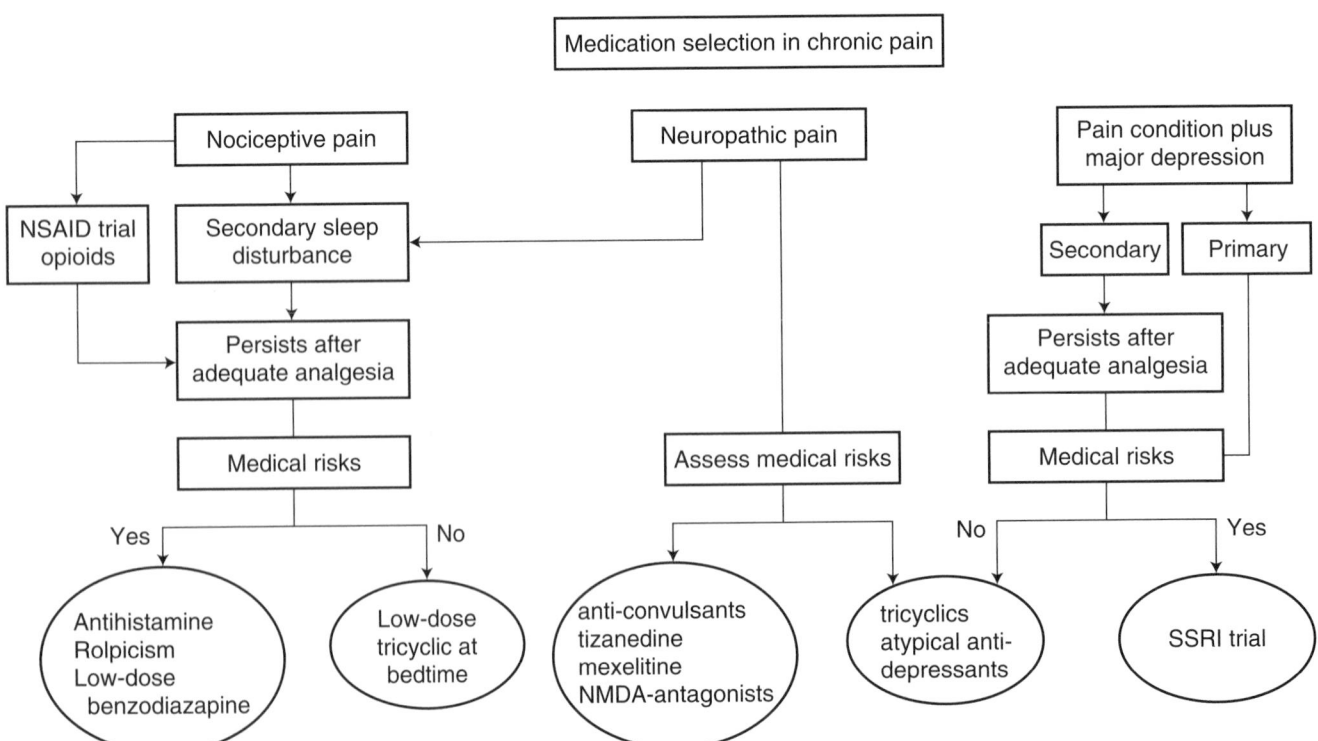

FIG. 19-2. Algorithm for antidepressant selection (Gallagher and Pasol, 1997, with permission, *Current Therapies*).

responded inadequately to standard pharmacological management with opiates, particularly malignant pain. We advise titrating from low doses, to which some will respond, to the higher doses customarily used for depression. Analgesic benefits may not occur for 1 to 3 weeks.

Anticonvulsants in Chronic Pain

Anticonvulsants, widely accepted in the management of chronic neuropathic pain, particularly when lancinating, burning, and dysesthetic, are postulated to cause their analgesic effect primarily by suppressing ectopic neuronal discharges. Spontaneous aberrant electrical activity has been recorded from different levels of the neuroaxis in experimental models of nerve injury, also found in patients with chronic neuropathic pain (108–111). Phenytoin (Dilantin), carbamazepine (Tegretol), valproic acid (Depakote), and clonazepam (Klonopin) suppress spontaneous neuronal firing (112), and phenytoin reduces cortical responses to paired stimuli and decreases posttetanic potentiation (113). The anticonvulsant effect of carbamazepine may be mediated by the so-called peripheral benzodiazepine receptors located in the brain and possibly also by the potentiation of adeno receptors and stabilization of sodium channel ion neurons; this latter effect may also mediate its analgesic effects in chronic pain. Anticonvulsants have been used in chronic neuralgias, sometimes in combination with tricyclic antidepressants (114). Multiple clinical studies suggest that carbamazepine (115–117), phenytoin (118–120), clonazepam (121), and valproic acid (88,122) are useful in pain management. Several studies have documented the successful use of anticonvulsants for cancer-related neuropathic pain caused by neural invasion by tumor, radiation fibrosis, and surgical scarring (123); these drugs have also been used successfully in postherpetic and deafferentation neuralgias (124). The clearest indications for anticonvulsants are lancinating neuropathic pain and chronic dysesthetic pain. With the exception of gabapentin, their potentially toxic interactions with other medications and their toxic and side-effect burden (18,114,125) restrict their general use to patients not responding to other medications, except in the case of trigeminal neuralgia where carbamazepine is the drug of first choice.

Gabapentin, a drug initially developed as an adjunctive to anticonvulsant therapies (77,126), is now being widely used in various pain conditions, particularly in neuropathic pain. Its immediate and widespread acceptance is based upon clinician reports of efficacy for RSD (127) and neuropathic pain disorders (128) and its relative safety and low side-effect profile (77,129,130). Gabapentin has demonstrated efficacy in reducing pain from moderate to mild in patients with diabetic neuropathy and postherpetic neuralgia. It also exhibits positive effects on mood and quality of life and improves sleep (131,132).

Unlike other anticonvulsants, gabapentin has no documented long-term toxicity, active metabolites, hepatic enzyme induction, or major drug interactions (124). Side effects are minimal, dose dependent, and similar in description to those of other anticonvulsants (e.g., sedation, disequilibrium, ataxia, and nausea). Gabapentin is recommended as a first-choice drug for neuropathic pain, particularly when there is a potential for HCA-related side effects or toxic drug-disease or drug-drug interactions (14). Dosing regimens are not established empirically. Clinical experience suggests a regimen of starting at 100 mg b.i.d. and titrating by 100-mg increments every 5 days, switching to a 300-mg capsule when appropriate. Some practitioners have reported success at doses above 3600 mg.

Carbamazepine has well-established efficacy in the management of trigeminal neuralgia as well as a reported case of successful treatment of painful traumatic mononeuropathy. However, its side-effect burden and potential toxicity make it a second-line anticonvulsant for neuropathic pain treatment (133).

Two carbamazepine analogs, dihydroketo and dihydromohydroxy, require higher doses than carbamazepine to achieve a symptom-free state, but unwanted side effects in the form of dizziness and ataxia occur much less frequently than with carbamazepine (134).

Oxacarbazepine has potent antineuropathic properties in the absence of significant side effects and is useful in the management of intractable trigeminal neuralgia (135,136). With oxacarbazepine, a high rate of control of pain can be achieved in those who do not respond fully to carbamazepine. It should be used as a monotherapy. Carbamazepine can be immediately exchanged for equivalent dosages of oxacarbazepine, thus reducing the dropout rate due to side effect and, presumably, also reducing the time to onset response (137).

Patients with multiple sclerosis have a higher incidence of trigeminal neuralgia than the general population. Treatment with carbamazepine has been reported to relieve symptoms of trigeminal neuralgia in 75% of patients, with complete relief in 50% of patients in one study. Phenytoin, baclofen, and clonazepam can be used as alternative medical therapy (138). It has been reported that the long-acting PGE1 analog misoprostol produced pain relief in six of seven patients with TN and MS who failed to respond to conventional pharmacological therapy (139).

Recent clinical experience and anecdotal evidence suggest that lamotrigine, which is active at glutaminergic excitatory synapses, is effective in neuropathic pain. However, more double-blind, placebo-controlled studies are needed to substantiate these findings (140,141). In a double-blind, placebo-controlled crossover trial in 14 patients with refractory trigeminal neuralgia, a maintenance dose of 400 mg lamotrigine was superior to placebo (P = 0.011) based on analysis of a composite efficacy index, which compared the numbers of patients assigned greater efficacy on lamotrigine with those assigned greater efficacy on placebo (142,143). However, in 100 patients with neuropathic pain, a randomized, double-blind, placebo-controlled trial of lamotrigine in doses up to 200 mg did not show beneficial effects on either pain, component pain symptoms, or quality of life variables (144). In a clinical case series of 20 patients with neuropathic pain, lamotrigine was reported to show additive effects to morphine (145), and in a case series of four patients it was effective in long-standing central pain (146).

Topiramate is well tolerated at a low therapeutic level and has few interactions with other drugs. Although there are no placebo-controlled studies to report as of yet, clinical experience and case series indicate that it may be a reasonable alternative for neuropathic pain in patients failing to respond to other neuropathic analgesics and anticonvulsants (147,148).

Valproic acid's starting dose is 250 mg once or twice daily, titrating by increments of up to 250 mg per week while monitoring blood levels. Therapeutic doses range from 250 mg to 1000 mg per day, divided in three doses with a therapeutic level between 50 and 100 mcg/mL. Valproic acid can be used as an adjunct to other anticonvulsants, such as phenytoin, benzodiazepines, as well as with antidepressants; however, these combinations require careful monitoring of serum levels and PT and PTT, particularly with coumadin and NSAIDs. Prior to initiating a trial with valproic acid, baseline hepatic function should be tested, and serum levels must be monitored throughout treatment. Abrupt withdrawal in epileptic patients is contraindicated. Valproate may potentiate the CNS effects of alcohol and MAOIs and increase blood levels and toxicity of phenobarbital, primidone, and phenytoin. Valproic acid has been associated with exfoliative dermatitis such as Steven Johnson's syndrome, hypotension, cardiovascular collapse, arrhythmias, depression, confusion, tremors, headaches, peripheral neuropathy, hepatic dysfunction, and GI symptoms of nausea, vomiting, constipation, and abdominal cramps. Hematological effects include thrombocytopenia and leukopenia.

Phenytoin is used for neuropathic pain at a dose range of 100 to 250 mg two to four times daily while monitoring for therapeutic blood levels between 10 to 20 mcg/mL, with therapeutic effects occurring 3 to 5 days after initial treatment. Serum levels increase with the use of benzodiazepines, chloramphenicol, dicumarol, disulfiram, tolbutamide, salicylates, halothane, cimetidine, and alcohol. Reserpine, carbamazepine, and calcium-containing antacids impede absorption. Phenytoin diminishes the effects of corticosteroids, coumadin, anticoagulants, quinidine, digoxin, and furosemide.

Clonazepam, a long-acting benzodiazepine often used as an anticonvulsant and for anxiety, may be an effective adjuvant in chronic pain management, particularly for chronic neuropathic pain. Its analgesic activity is probably related to a combination of its effect on the GABA A receptor and secondary effects on autonomic arousal and pain perception, as well as additional analgesic properties possibly related to its anticonvulsant properties. It is used primarily combined with other analgesics such as opiates, nonsteroidal antiinflammatories, and antidepressants (14), with the usual dose of 0.5 to 2 mg and a range between 0.25 mg and 10 mg daily. Peak plasma levels occur 1 to 2 hours after a single dose without active metabolites. Abrupt discontinuation will precipitate withdrawal symptoms, although they are not as severe as with other benzodiazepines without active metabolites, but with shorter half-lives, such as alprazolam and lorazepam. Symptoms of withdrawal include anxiety, nervousness, diaphoresis, restlessness, irritability, fatigue, lightheadedness, tremors, insomnia, and weakness. Liver function tests should be checked periodically. If a trial of clonazepam is not successful within 2 to 4 weeks, a discontinuation by progressive dose reduction of approximately 25% per week is recommended. Clonazepam should be used cautiously with other sedatives, particularly in combination with opiates, due to the risk of respiratory suppression; its effects are antagonized by flumazenil. Clonazepam and lithium together may be neurotoxic.

Elmiron (pentosan polysulfate sodium) appears to be an efficacious long-term treatment for a constellation of debilitating symptoms associated with interstitial cystitis in some patients. Patients with a positive response to Elmiron appear to maintain this response over time (149). Elmiron is specifically approved for the treatment of IC in the United States in 1996.

Chronic pain can be maintained by a state of sensitization within the central nervous system that is mediated in part by the excitatory amino acids glutamate and aspartate binding to the N-methyl D-aspartate (NMDA) receptor. Activation of NMDA receptors causes the spinal cord neuron to become more responsive to all of its inputs, resulting in central sensitization. NMDA-receptor antagonists can suppress central sensitization in experimental animals. Commercially available NMDA-receptor antagonists include ketamine, dextromethorphan, memantine, and amantadine. NMDA-receptor activation not only increases the cell's response to pain stimuli, but also decreases neuronal sensitivity to opioid receptor agonists. In addition to preventing central sensitization, coadministration of NMDA-receptor antagonists with an opioid may prevent tolerance to opioid analgesia (150, 151).

Two randomized, double-blind crossover trials compared 6 weeks of oral dextromethorphan to placebo in two groups, made up of 14 patients with painful distal symmetrical diabetic neuropathy and 18 with postherpetic neuralgia. Thirteen patients with each diagnosis completed the comparison. Dosage was titrated in each patient to the highest level reached without disrupting normal activities; mean doses were 381 mg/day in diabetics and 439 mg/day in postherpetic neuralgia patients. In diabetic neuropathy, dextromethorphan decreased pain by a mean of 24% (95% CI: 6% to 42%, p = 0.01), relative to placebo. In postherpetic neuralgia, dextromethorphan did not reduce pain (95% CI: 10% decrease in pain to 14% increase in pain, p = 0.72). It was concluded that dextromethorphan or other low-affinity NMDA channel blockers might have promise in the treatment of painful diabetic neuropathy (152).

Ketamine has shown to be analgesic in both controlled trials and case reports of various neuropathic pains (153,154). Current application as a topical gel stems from the theory that ketamine has peripheral action at both opioid and Na+-K+ channels. A systematic case study of five patients with CRPS using topical ketamine gel reported alteration in temperature sensation, feeling of relaxation, decreased tension in the area of application, and significant pain relief at initial application. No significant side effects were reported (155).

Neuroleptics in Chronic Pain

Neuroleptic medications, often referred to as antipsychotics, have four potential uses in chronic pain patients (14). They are the drugs of choice when pain is part of a *delusional system*. In major depression with psychosis, neuroleptics may be used initially to treat psychosis while antidepressant treatment such as with HCAs and/or SSRIs or with ECT progresses. If pain is a delusional symptom of a schizophrenic disorder, neuroleptics may be maintained long term. Because the disturbance is primarily psychiatric, these patients are best treated by a psychiatric team, similar to an internist treating diabetes with neuropathy in consultation with pain specialists. Neuroleptics are useful when patients with chronic pain lose control of *anger*. Patients with chronic pain are often caught in irrational bureaucracies that are not responsive to their real needs for financial support and timely, effective treatment. These patients can become angry and threatening. Neuroleptics, including the phenothiazines and butyrophenones, and the newer agents with less toxicity, such as olanzapine (Zyprexa) and risperidone (Risperdal), may be helpful as *adjunctive medications* in a variety of chronic or episodic pain syndromes. The regular use of these agents is restricted by their side-effect profile and significant risk for toxicity such as tardive dyskinesia. Low-potency neuroleptics such as the phenothiazines are more prone to cause sedation, orthostatic hypotension, and anticholinergic side effects. High-potency neuroleptics such as haloperidol and fluphenazine are more prone to causing extrapyramidal symptoms, such as dystonia and parkinsonism, best managed with benztropine (cogentin) and antihistamines such as diphenhydramine (Benadryl). Some intractable akathisias have been treated with beta-blockers. Rarely, neuroleptic use is complicated by *neuroleptic malignant syndrome*, a dangerous condition manifested by rigidity, fever, and autonomic instability. Management consists of physiological supportive therapy, discontinuation of neuroleptics, and, in some cases, bromocriptine and dantrolene. Long exposure to neuroleptics may induce tardive dyskinesia. Neuroleptics lower the seizure threshold. Phenothiazines should be avoided in

patients who take MAOIs and should be used cautiously with antihypertensives, opiates, barbiturates, antihistamines, atropinic medications, and anticholinergic drugs such as TCAs.

Because of design problems in many studies showing efficacy and the problem of toxicity with regular use, neuroleptics are secondary adjuvant analgesic drugs, most useful for managing acute agitation or psychotic symptoms and for controlling nausea and vomiting. Their use as adjuvant analgesics has been limited to intractable neuropathic pain, which has failed to respond to the use of antidepressants, anticonvulsants, and antianxiety agents in combination with opiates. Neuroleptics are the mainstay for managing agitated delirium in hospitalized patients. The selection of a neuroleptic as an adjuvant will be based upon the therapeutic needs of the individual patient. If a low-potency neuroleptic has been chosen, an EKG should be run and liver function tests obtained because of the potential for low-potency neuroleptics to cause cholestatic jaundice. Start with the lowest dose possible, titrating slowly while evaluating clinical response and side effects: For example, start Zyprexa 2.5 mg b.i.d.-t.i.d. or haloperidol (Haldol) at 0.5 mg b.i.d.-t.i.d., or chlorpromazine, at 10–25 mg b.i.d.-t.i.d. In all cases, review potential medication interactions, particularly when used in combination with anticonvulsants and antidepressants. After acute agitation is controlled, refer for psychiatric consultation before committing to longer-term use.

Parenteral lidocaine reduces the symptoms of nerve injury pain, but its regular use is likely to be limited by tachyphylaxis and dose-related toxicity. Orally administered lidocaine-like antiarrhythmics, such as mexiletine, may be an alternative to parenteral lidocaine and have been shown to reduce nerve injury pain in several controlled clinical trials (156–158). Side-effect burden, such as dizziness and nausea, can limit the effectiveness of mexiletine.

Physicians are using transdermal lidocaine for several types of neuropathic pain with variable effects but avoiding the side-effect and toxicity burden of parenteral lidocaine. Topical applications of lidocaine relieve pain from postherpetic neuralgia by direct local anesthetic effect (159). Recently, 5% lidocaine patch was approved for the treatment of postherpetic neuralgia. We often use this patch to help relieve allodynia associated with CRPS.

Psychostimulants in Chronic Pain

Stimulants increase central release of norepinephrine, dopamine, and serotonin and may be serotonin agonists. They increase arousal and decrease fatigue in normal adults and are used to treat apathy in disorders such as geriatric depression, dementia, and narcolepsy. Amphetamines increase analgesia and decrease sedation both in animals and humans (14). In postsurgical patients, they potentiate morphine analgesia with a single dose (60). Side effects caused by alpha and beta adrenergic activity include increased systolic and diastolic blood pressure and reflexive slowing of heart rate. Large doses may cause cardiac arrhythmias. Side effects include gastrointestinal disturbance, urinary hesitancy, anorexia, dryness of mouth, hypertension, tachycardia, insomnia and restlessness, agitation, confusion, dysphoria, and delirium. Amphetamines inhibit the cytochrome P450 enzyme system, raising blood levels of TCAs, neuroleptics, and other medications metabolized by P450. Interaction with other medications such as phenylpropanolamine, used as a decongestant, may produce hypertension. Psychostimulants may increase the hypotensive effect of guanethidine, decrease metabolism of anticoagulants, anticonvulsants, and heterocyclic antidepressants, cause hypertensive crisis with MAOIs, and lower the seizure threshold. Because of potential for abuse and addiction, careful drug monitoring is mandatory.

Caffeine increases the analgesic effect of aspirin and acetaminophen by 40% in postpartum pain (160) and is typically used in over-the-counter preparations. Caffeine, amphetamine, and cocaine induce an increased sense of well-being, energy, alertness, concentration, self-confidence, motivation for work, a desire to talk to people, and reduced sleepiness. Caffeine is safe and effective when used in recommended dosage of 100 to 200 mg not more than every 3 to 4 hours (14). Tolerance to caffeine develops after abrupt cessation; symptoms of withdrawal include headache, drowsiness and yawning, decreased energy and alertness, difficulty concentrating, a diminished sense of well-being and contentment, decreased sociability and talkativeness, flulike symptoms, blurring of vision, and impaired psychomotor performance. Acute and chronic caffeine intoxication (caffeinism) causes anxiety, insomnia, and cardiovascular and gastrointestinal symptoms. Caffeine should be eliminated in patients with anxiety disorder, insomnia, palpitations, tachycardia, arrhythmia, hernia, ulcers, and pregnancy.

Cocaine potentiates morphine analgesia by blocking the reuptake of serotonin (59) and is used in combination with opiates for cancer pain, primarily as a local and regional anesthetic in the oral and nasal cavity (46). Cocaine's cardiovascular toxicity, high abuse liability, and very short half-life of approximately 40 minutes regardless of the route of administration limit its use in pain management (59).

Clinical use of psychostimulants: Psychostimulants are most commonly prescribed to alleviate the sedative effect due to narcotic administration for pain in advanced malignancy. Amphetamines have been useful in combination with morphine for severe postoperative pain and spasmodic torticollis. Occasionally they are used to promote energy, initiative, and mood in depressed patients when conventional antidepressants are not helpful. In these cases, methylphenidate treatment is usually started at a dose of 2.5 mg at 8 AM and at noon. The dosage gradually increases for several days until therapeutic objectives are achieved or side effects such as overstimulation, anxiety,

insomnia, paranoia, or confusion intervene. Typically, effective doses are less than 30 mg per day, although some patients may require up to 60 mg. Methylphenidate doses are maintained for 1 to 2 months, after which many patients are successfully withdrawn (14). The recommended dose range for dextroamphetamine is from 5 to 20 mg a day. Chronic use of high doses can lead to personality changes, paranoid psychosis, psychological and physical dependency and withdrawal symptoms, mild fatigue, and depression. Contraindications to stimulants include anxiety disorders, paranoid disorders and schizophrenia, hyperthyroidism, seizures, arrhythmias, uncontrolled hypertension, and angina. The daily oral dose range for methylphenidate is from 10 to 40 mg a day.

Antianxiety Agents in Chronic Pain

Anxiety, a psychological state associated with stress and ubiquitous in acute pain and anxiety disorders, is frequently comorbid with chronic pain. Stress and anxiety play an important role in precipitating and perpetuating pain. Several related mechanisms may explain the efficacy of anxiolytic medications (14): (a) *Pain causes anxiety and the stress response;* reducing anxiety in pain states may prevent the negative psychophysiological sequelae of these states described later. (b) *Anxiety causes autonomic nervous system (ANS) arousal, leading to skeletal muscle tension;* this mechanism is thought to be at least partially responsible for the precipitation and perpetuation of episodic muscle spasm postinjury and in muscle contraction (tension) headaches associated with psychological and/or biomechanical stress. Symptoms of myofascial pain syndromes may worsen with anxiety. (c) Ectopic firing of injured nerves causes neuropathic pain, precipitating muscle tightening and vulnerability to spasm, particularly when anxiety activates muscle tension. (d) ANS arousal activates vasomotor changes that liberate nociceptive algogens at the site of injury. (e) ANS arousal liberates noradrenaline at the site of injury, which, by increasing the sensitivity of nociceptors, lowers the threshold for pain perception. (f) Pain-related anxiety activates psychophysiological and functional disorders such as irritable bowel syndrome, chest pain, and headache. (g) Anxiety interferes with effective cognitive and behavioral coping.

Benzodiazepines

Benzodiazepines (BZDs) are commonly prescribed in both acute and chronic pain states, often incorrectly. Their reputation for inducing dependency and abuse overshadows the more clinically important problem of behavioral toxicity. Understanding this latter problem, which is generally overlooked by physicians, is key to their successful use in chronic pain states (14,16). These drugs depress presynaptic release of serotonin and excite GABA (161). Their analgesic effects in acute pain are attributed to reductions in anxiety, tension, and insomnia. Diazepam and midazolam reduce pain in the postoperative patient (162, 119). BZDs can be useful for short-term management of acute musculoskeletal pain.

The efficacy of BZDs in cancer-related pain and chronic nonmalignant pain appears to be limited (161). Clonazepam and alprazolam may be beneficial for certain chronic pain conditions, most notably neuropathic pain (161,163). The authors have used clonazepam, a benzodiazepine often used as an anticonvulsant, successfully in treating trigeminal neuralgia, paroxysmal postlaminectomy pain, and posttraumatic neuralgias. Physicians often prescribe BZDs for sleep problems that frequently accompany chronic pain. They are not recommended for regular and frequent use in sleep disorders because of tolerance, dependency, and cognitive effects. BZDs may also be useful for the management of comorbid anxiety disorder, such as generalized anxiety disorder. Alprazolam and clonazepam have been most thoroughly studied for use in panic disorder, and the former may have some antidepressant properties. Outside of clonazepam, BZDs play a limited role in chronic pain management. Their long-term use has not become fully accepted because of the potential development of dependence and because they may interfere with opioid analgesia.

The *neurobehavioral toxicity* of BZDs is clinically salient. They impair memory and psychomotor performance and are associated with increased incidence of falls, a particular problem for those with musculoskeletal disorders. A more insidious effect, inhibiting new learning, may prove to be particularly deleterious during pain rehabilitation because the ability to learn the new cognitive and motor coping skills is prerequisite to functional recovery and return to work (16,164,165).

The longer the half-life of a BZD and its active metabolites, the greater the risk for cumulative side effects such as sedation, amnesia, psychomotor impairment, and ataxia with risk for falls. The 3-hydroxy compounds with short half-lives and a lack of active metabolites, such as oxazepam (Serax), lorazepam (Ativan), alprazolam (Xanax), triazolam (Halcion), and temazepam (Restoril), have less potential for accumulation. Those with longer elimination half-lives, such as diazepam (Valium), chlordiazepoxide (Librium), clorazepate (Tranxene), prazepam (Centrax), and flurazepam (Dalmane), are more likely to cause cumulative toxic effects—a particular problem in the medically compromised patient and elderly. A single dose of BZDs with a very short half-life, such as triazolam and midazolam, may produce confusion and amnesia, particularly in patients with organic brain disease. Patients taking regular doses of short-acting BZDs are subject to withdrawal symptoms that may be accompanied by seizures and other symptoms such as tinnitus, amnesia, psychosis, delirium, rebound anxiety, panic, headache, dizziness, diaphoresis, myalgias, tremors, and muscle twitching. BZDs potentiate other sedatives, such as alcohol, narcotics, barbiturates,

phenothiazines, MAO inhibitors, and volatile anesthetics, in causing sedation, confusion, and psychomotor impairment; they also potentiate opiate-caused respiratory depression. Doses should be adjusted down for elderly patients and those with renal, liver, CNS, and pulmonary disease. Cimetidine increases BZD levels. Anticonvulsants and adrenal steroids decrease BZD levels. BZDs are contraindicated in sleep apnea. Toxicity from BZDs may be antagonized with the use of flumazenil 0.2 to 1 mg.

Antihistamines, such as hydroxyzine and diphenhydramine, are commonly used to sedate patients in acute pain; they may also be used for anxiety or sleeplessness, often to avoid benzodiazepines, at doses ranging of 25 to 50 mg I.M. or 25 to 100 mg P.O. These drugs do not produce physical dependence.

We avoid using barbiturate preparations such as Fiorinal and Fioricet because their short-acting barbiturate, butalbital, is addictive and may cause transformational headaches. Also, other more effective interventions are available. Carisoprodol (Soma), a sedative marketed for its muscle-relaxing properties, may be useful in patients with recurrent muscle spasm; doses are usually 350 mg b.i.d.– qid, but it is also addicting.

Buspirone, an antianxiety agent unrelated to the BZDs, does not interact with the GABA receptor system, has a strong affinity for serotonin (5HT1A) receptors in vitro, and a moderate affinity for dopamine receptors in the brain. However, its anxiolytic mechanism is not well known. Buspirone's principal use is for chronic anxiety, particularly generalized anxiety disorder. Buspirone is ineffective in single doses, taking about 2 weeks for full therapeutic effects to occur. In contrast to the benzodiazepines, buspirone does not sedate, impair motor function, interact with other sedative-hypnotics, develop tolerance, produce drug dependency, potentiate alcohol, or suppress sedative withdrawal (125). There is no "drug rebound," as found with short-acting BZDs, and little, if any, abuse liability exists.

Choosing an Anxiolytic or Sedative Consider clonazepam (Klonopin) for patients with *neuropathic pain* if they cannot tolerate, or do not respond to, HCAs. Starting doses might be 0.25 to 0.5 mg HS or b.i.d., titrating up carefully while watching for sedation. For patients with *acute anxiety* due to breakthrough pain we tend to use hydroxyzine 25 to 50 mg or lorazepam because of its short half-life, 0.25 mg to 0.5 mg, and reliable IV, I.M. and P.O. absorption. Buspirone, starting at 5 mg b.i.d. and titrating to 10 mg t.i.d. to 15 mg qid, may be helpful for *chronic anxiety.* Behavioral methods of anxiety control (47) are preferable to regular long-term use of BZDs, which can be used as a "backup" system for breakthrough anxiety. When regular BZD use is warranted, we use clonazepam starting at 0.25 to 0.5 mg HS; higher doses may produce sedation and mental changes. We avoid regular use of high-potency, short-acting BZDs such as alprazolam, which are associated with potentially dangerous withdrawal and are often not clinically effective when used several times daily for long periods. Because of the short duration of these drugs, patients cannot go for more than a few hours without having breakthrough anxiety and/or withdrawal symptoms, a pattern that induces multiple daily dosing and psychological dependency.

Capsaicin, a topical analgesic cream, has been used for the treatment of postherpetic neuralgia, arthritis, diabetic neuropathy, causalgia, and reflex sympathetic dystrophy syndrome (18,20). Studies suggest that capsaicin renders the skin insensitive to pain by depleting and preventing a reaccumulation of substance P in peripheral sensory neurons (20). There are no known systemic side effects or drug interactions with topically applied capsaicin cream, making it potentially helpful for older patients who may have coexisting diseases and often take concomitant systemic medications. The initial enthusiasm for capsaicin, as for most new pain treatments that are often considered a panacea when introduced, has been tempered by its failure to cure pain. But it has its place alongside the many other pharmacological and nonpharmacological techniques in the armamentarium of the physician treating pain disorders.

A recent report has suggested that calcitonin is useful in the treatment of phantom limb pain (115,166). Patients receiving a 100 IE s-calcitonin IV injection over 5 minutes experienced immediate pain relief. This is encouraging, considering the difficulty in treating phantom limb pain (167).

The antiarrhythmic drugs lidocaine and tocainamide have been shown to be useful in the treatment of the pain of diabetic peripheral neuropathy, trigeminal neuralgia, and Dercum's disease (adiposis dolorosa) (168). With lidocaine, a 5-mg/kg dose was administered by IV infusion over 30 minutes. Significant benefit was obtained, which lasted from 3 to 21 days.

Antispastic Medication

Many patients with chronic pain syndromes are maintained on centrally acting antispastic medication. These include drugs of the mephenesin class, benzodiazepines, baclofen, and dantrolene. The mephenesin class is perhaps the most widely prescribed of the muscle relaxants currently available. There are no well-controlled studies in which the relative safety and efficacy of these compounds are compared. The mechanism of action of this class is poorly understood. The most prominent action is to depress polysynaptic reflexes preferentially over monosynaptic reflexes. The degree of muscle relaxation appears to be achieved only with considerable sedation. It is difficult to determine whether these are true relaxants or sedative drugs. Their use should be discouraged in view of newer and more effective agents (14,18).

The mechanism of action of quinine is by increasing the refractory time of the muscle so that the response to multiple stimulations is reduced. This particular property seems to make it useful for special types of muscle cramps, such as nocturnal leg cramps, which is the most frequent usage. The dose is 200 to 300 mg before retiring. With some patients, only a brief trial of quinine therapy is required to provide relief from muscle cramps. In other individuals, even large dosages may fail to give relief.

The three most effective antispastic medications are baclofen, dantrolene, and diazepam. From a clinical viewpoint, baclofen appears to act on presynaptic mechanisms rather than postsynaptic γ-aminobutyric acid (GABA) receptors, as does diazepam. Furthermore, baclofen may act preferentially in part to reduce the release of excitatory transmitters (possibly including substance P) from nociceptive afferent nerve endings—those coming from the skin and elsewhere, which tend to produce flexor reflexes when activated. It has also been demonstrated that baclofen produces a dose-dependent, stereospecific, antinociceptive effect in the intact animal, suggesting that baclofen may be useful in pain syndromes unrelated to flexor spasms (162).

A number of studies comparing baclofen and diazepam report that their overall antispastic effects are comparable. However, baclofen is usually preferred, at least initially, because it is much less likely to produce sedation or to reduce residual voluntary power. Similarly, baclofen does not produce generalized muscle weakness, as does dantrolene. It also differs from dantrolene in that it appears to produce essentially no abnormalities of other organ systems, such as the liver. Therapy begins with one-half of a 10-mg tablet twice a day, to be increased by one-half of a tablet every 3 days to a usual maximum of two tablets four times a day. Occasionally, 100 to 150 mg per day is useful. In many patients, 5 or 10 mg four times a day is sufficient. Abrupt withdrawal of baclofen should be avoided because it often produces a temporary rebound in the number and severity of flexor spasms and, in a few patients, may precipitate temporary hallucinations.

Therapeutic blood levels of baclofen are considered to be 80 to 400 ng/mL. A 40-mg dose in healthy subjects produces levels remaining above 200 ng/mL for 8 hours. The serum half-life of baclofen is 3 to 4 hours. The use of baclofen may be limited by its adverse effects, which include drowsiness, insomnia, dizziness, weakness, and mental confusion.

Although dantrolene does reach the central nervous system, its primary action is peripheral. It appears to reduce muscle tension through a direct effect on the contractile mechanism. It is said to produce pronounced skeletal muscle relaxation without affecting coordination or neuromuscular transmission. A number of placebo-controlled clinical trials have demonstrated its efficacy in relieving spasticity due to cerebrovascular damage, spinal cord lesions, multiple sclerosis, or cerebral palsy. In the few studies in which dantrolene has been compared with diazepam, the drugs have been said to be of approximately equal efficacy. Theoretically, if the two agents are of equal efficacy in patients with certain types of spasticity, dantrolene may be useful for those in whom the sedative side effects of diazepam are more of a problem, such as the elderly and persons with central nervous system lesions or other disorders of cerebral function. Simultaneous use of dantrolene and diazepam (and perhaps also baclofen) might control the troublesome symptoms of spasticity better than either drug alone, with smaller doses and fewer side effects (162).

Dantrolene may be hepatotoxic; therefore therapy with this agent should be continued only if it can be shown clearly that dantrolene itself is of considerable benefit. Its major drawback is provoking generalized weakness because it acts peripherally on skeletal muscle. Patients begin therapy with one 25-mg tablet daily; dosage can initially be increased by one tablet twice a day, but this is rarely indicated. If no definite benefit is demonstrable within 6 weeks—or within 2 weeks of reaching the maximum tolerated dosage if adjustments in dosage have taken longer than 6 weeks—therapy should be discontinued (162).

Benzodiazepines directly potentiate the action of GABA. Some studies show that diazepam is useful alone or as adjunct therapy for spasticity, especially in patients with lesions affecting the spinal cord and occasionally in patients with cerebral palsy. There is no convincing evidence that diazepam is better than either baclofen or dantrolene. Diazepam is probably not as effective as baclofen in patients who primarily have intermittent, painful flexor spasms. Studies show few demonstrable differences between diazepam and baclofen with various types of spasticity, except that the incidence of such unwanted side effects as somnolence, dizziness, and increased muscular weakness is markedly higher with diazepam (169).

Many clinicians treating intractable chronic pain are dismayed by the frequency with which the benzodiazepine drugs are prescribed for chronic pain patients with concurrent depression (170). Lipman has noted that benzodiazepines cause an increase in anger and hostility when given over an 8-week period (171). This can be an adverse response for this already difficult population of chronic pain sufferers. It has been suggested that one of the mechanisms by which the benzodiazepines and the barbiturates adversely affect pain is by action on the neurotransmitters. It is suggested that benzodiazepines deplete serotonin, often adding to depression, paradoxical rage, habituation, disrupted sleep, and hangovers due to alterations of stage 3 and 4 sleep and rapid eye movement (REM) sleep. It has also been suggested that the benzodiazepines inhibit serotonin release and that theoretically they may increase pain perception as well (162). These theories, combined with the authors' clinical experience, suggest that this class of medication should not be used for long-term treatment of chronic pain.

Diazepam is said to be useful in the treatment of various nonspastic types of involuntary muscle activity, such as those seen in tetanus, the stiff man syndrome, or local muscle spasms of various traumatic causes. For elderly patients or patients with major symptoms of higher central nervous system dysfunction, the initial dose should not exceed 2 mg per day, and increments must be made extremely cautiously. In the treatment of spasticity, intramuscular or intravenous diazepam may occasionally be useful in the treatment of acute low back muscle spasm. Because its common side effects include drowsiness, lightheadedness, weakness, fatigue, dizziness, vertigo, and ataxia, diazepam must be used cautiously in patients who are receiving other central nervous system active medications or alcohol, the side effects of which tend to be problems in individuals with risk factors for addiction.

There is considerable anecdotal evidence of an analgesic effect of the muscle relaxant tizanidine, an alpha 2 agonist. Although double-blind clinical trials have not been reported, tizanidine has shown promising effect in several pain conditions. For example, there is a report of its effectiveness in chronic cluster headache resistant to traditional pharmacological management (172). We use it routinely as one of the medications of choice for pain conditions associated with muscle spasm, particularly when related to nerve injury and neuropathic pain conditions. Because of its sedating effects, we often start with 1 to 2 mg at bedtime and then try small doses of 1 mg two or three times daily, cautioning the patient about sedation. We then increase it gradually as tolerated, giving higher doses (4–8 mg) at bedtime when the sedating effect can also help sleep. At higher doses, liver enzyme changes, reversible by lowering or eliminating the drug, have been reported, so LFTs should be followed, and the drug should be used with caution in those with known liver disease.

Botulinum toxin type A (BTX-A) is a neurotoxin that has proved safe and effective in the treatment of strabismus, blepharospasm, and VII nerve disorders (173). Intramuscular injection of BTX-A produces highly specific cholinergic neuromuscular blockade that is useful in treating abnormal muscle movement and spasticity, as well as pain due to involuntary or excessive muscle contraction. In a recent review, Raj (174) discussed BTX-A in the treatment of various focal dystonias, including cervical dystonia or torticollis, and in writer's cramp (occupational dystonias). BTX-A is also noted to be effective in treating pain associated with upper motor neuron disorders, including stroke, traumatic brain injury, cerebral palsy, multiple sclerosis, and Parkinson's disease. Raj notes that use of BTX-A in many clinical settings where pain is associated with muscle contraction represents an important new treatment modality that may be more cost-effective than invasive and irreversible surgeries, better tolerated than systemic pharmacotherapy for pain, and highly valuable as an aid in achieving the overall objectives of physical therapy.

SUMMARY

Some of the more common medications considered useful in the treatment of chronic pain have been discussed. The practitioner should begin medication trials with the least potent medication capable of alleviating the patient's symptoms with an eye to minimizing side effects and avoiding toxicity. After successful control is achieved, self-control techniques should be added to eventually help lower dose requirements (12,14,16,45,47). Patients should be periodically reassessed for their need to maintain dose, and reliance on daily pharmacotherapy should be reduced or discontinued when feasible if the patient can maintain functioning. No medication is entirely benign, and patients should not be given prescriptions for indefinite periods of time without monitoring. In all instances the physician should ask the same fundamental question as when administering any treatment—namely, do the potential benefits of treatment outweigh the risks? Any significant morbidity associated with treatment should be discussed with the patient, who should decide, ultimately, whether or not to use a specific medication.

REFERENCES

1. Muller J. Handbuch der Physiologie des Menschen, Vol. 2, English translation by W. Baly Taylor and Walton, London, 1840.
2. Latze, Dallenbach KM. Pain: history and present status. *Am J Psychol* 1939;52:331–347.
3. Von Frey M. Bertrage zur physiologie des schmerzsennes, *Ber Verhandl Koneg Sachs Ges Wess Leipzeg* 1984;46:185-196, 288–296.
4. Erb, Luckey GWA. Some recent studies of pain. *Am J Psychol* 1985;7:109.
5. Goldscheider A. Du spezifesche energre der gefiihlsnerven der haut, *Monatsschr Prakt Dermatol* 1984;3:282.
6. Hardy JD, Wolff, HG, Goodell H. Studies on pain; a new method for measuring pain threshold; observation on spatial summation of pain. *J. Clin Investigation* 1940;19:649.
7. Beecher HK. Pain in men wounded in battle. *Ann Surg* 1946;123:96.
8. Wall PD, Melzack R. *Textbook of pain.* Churchill: Livingstone, 1984.
9. Bonica JJ. Introduction. In: Bonica JJ ed. *Pain: research publications—association for research in nervous and mental disorders, Vol. 58.* New York, Raven Press, 1980:1–17.
10. Todd EM. Pain: historical perspectives. In: Crue BL ed. *Chronic pain.* New York: SP Medical & Scientific Books, 1979:39–56.
11. Bennett GJ. Chronic pain due to peripheral nerve damage: an overview. In: Fields HL, Leibeskind JC, eds. *Progress in pain research and management, Vol. 1.* Seattle: IASP Press, 1994:51–59.
12. Price D, Mao J, Mayer DJ. Central mechanisms of normal and abnormal pain states. In:.Fields HL, Leibeskind JC, eds. *Progress in pain research and management, Vol. 1.* Seattle: IASP Press, 1994, 61–84 .
13. Aronoff GM, Evans WO. Chronic pain: a pharmacological approach. In: Aronoff GM, ed. *Mediguide to pain, Vol. 3.* Lawrence New York: DellaCorte Publications, 1983:1–4.
14. Gallagher RM, Pasol E. Psychopharmacologic drugs in the chronic pain syndromes. *Current Review of Pain* 1997;1(2):138–152.
15. American Pain Society and the American Academy of Pain Medicine. *Joint statement on the use of opioids in intractable pain.* 1997.
16. Gallagher RM, Woznicki M. Low back pain rehabilitation. In: Stoudemire A, Fogel BS, eds. *Medical psychiatric practice, Vol 2.* APA Press, 1993.
17. *American Medical Association Drug Evaluations,* ed. 5, Chicago: The Association, 1983.
18. Amoi S. *The pain handbook.* Mosby, 1995.
19. Baskin SI, Smith L, Hoey LA, et al. Age-associated changes of responses to acetylsalicyclic acid. *Pain* 1981;2:1–8.
20. Halpern IM. Analgesic and anti-inflammatory medications. In: Tollison CD, ed. *Handbook of chronic pain management.* Baltimore: Williams & Wilkins, 1989:57.
21. Aronoff GM, Evans WO. *Handbook on the rational use of medication for pain.* New York: DellaCorte Publications, 1987.
22. Martin FW. *Hazards of medications.* Philadelphia: J.B. Lippincott Co., 1971.
23. Canalese J, Gimson AES, Davis M, Williams R. Factors contributing to mortality paracetamol-induced hepatic failure. *Br Med J* 1981;282:199–201.
24. Beaver WT. Nonsteroidal anti-inflammatory analgesics and their combinations with opioids. In: Aronoff GM ed. *Evaluation and treatment of chronic pain,* 3rd ed. Lippincott Williams & Wilkins, 1999:465.
25. IBID #24:455-473.
26. Maier R, Menasse R, Riesterer L. The pharmacology of diclofenac sodium (Voltarol). *Rheumatol Rehabil* 1979;(Suppl 2):1121.
27. Taha AS, Hudson N, Hawkey CJ, et al. Famotidine for the prevention of gastric and duodenal ulcers caused by steroidal anti-inflammatory drugs. *N Eng J Med* 1996;334,1434–1439.
28. Singh G. Recent considerations in nonsteroidal anti-inflammatory drug gastropathy. *Amer J Med* 1998;105:31S–38S.
29. Singh G, Ramey DR, Morfeld D, et al. Gastrointestinal tract complications of non-steroidal anti-inflammatory drug treatment in rheumatoid arthritis—a prospective observational cohort study. *Arch Intern Med* 1996;156:1530–1536.
30. Luggen ME, Gartside PS, Ness V. Nonsteroidal antiinflammatory drugs in rheumatoid arthritis: duration of use as a measure of relative value. *J Rheumatol* 1989;18(12):1565–1569.
31. Van Den Ouweland FA, Corstens FNM, Van DePutte LBA. Gastrointestinal blood loss during treatment with maproxen for rheumatoid arthritis. *Scand J Rheumatol* 1987;18:365–370.
32. Maier R, Menasse R, Riesterer L. The pharmacology of diclofenac sodium (Voltarol). *Rheumatol Rehabil* 1979;(Suppl 2):11–21.
33. Dewson DD, Mather IE. Non-steroidal anti-inflammatory agents. In: Raj PP ed. *Practical management of pain.* Chicago:Year Book Medical Publishers Inc., 1986:523–524.
34. Alvin PE, Lett IF. Current status of the etiology and management of dysmenorrhea in adolescence. *Pediatrics* 1982;70(14):516–525.
35. Dvorwik D, Lee DKN. Possible mechanisms for the gastric safety of etodolac. *J Musculoskel Med* 1991;8(Suppl 4):S47–S53.
36. Russell RI, Sturrock RD, Tana AS. Endoscopic studies of patients treated with etodolac. *J Musculoskel Med* 1991;8(Suppl 4): S60–S64.
37. Cannon GW, Caldwell JR, Holt P, et al. Rofecoxib, a specific inhibitor of cycloogenase 2, with clinical efficacy comparable with that of diclofenac sodium: results of a one-year, randomized clinical trial in patients with osteoarthritis of the knee and hip. *Arthritis Rheum* 2000;43: 978–987.
38. Schnitzer T, Truitt K, Fleishmann R, et al. The safety profile, tolerability, and effective dose range of rofecoxib in the treatment of rheumatoid arthritis. *Clin Thera* 1999;21:1653–1665.
39. Malmstrom K, Daniels S, Kotey P, et al. Comparison of rofecoxib and celecoxib, two cyclooxygenase-2 inhibitors, in postoperative dental pain: a randomized, placebo- and active comparitor controlled clinical trial. *Clin Thera* 1999;21:1653–1665.
40. Payne R. Limitations of NSAIDS for pain management: toxicity or lack of efficacy. *J Pain.* 2000;3(Suppl 1):14–18.
41. Sunshine A. A comparison of the newer COX-2 drugs and older oral analgesics. *J Pain* 2000;3(Suppl 1):10–13.
42. McAlindon TE. LaValley MP. Gulin JP. Felson DT. Glucosamine and chondroitin for treatment of osteoarthritis: a systematic quality assessment and meta-analysis. *JAMA* Mar 15 2000;283(11): 1469–1475.
43. Robbins W. Clinical applications of capsaicinoids. *Clin J Pain* June 2000;16(2 Suppl):S86–9.
44. Twycross RG. Morphine and diamorphine in the terminally ill patient. *Acta Anesthesiol Scand* 1982;(Suppl) 74(26):128–134.
45. Gallagher RM. Behavioral and biobehavioral treatment in chronic pain: perspectives on the evidence of effectiveness. *Mind-Body Medicine* 1997;2(4)(in press).

46. Jacox A, Carr DB, Payne R, et al. Management of cancer pain. Clinical Practice Guideline No.9. AHCPR Publication No. 94-0592. Rockville, MD. Agency for Health Care Policy and Research, U.S. Department of Health and Human Services, Public Health Service, March 1994.

47. Gallagher RM, McCann W, Hughes J, et al. The behavioral medicine service: an administrative model for biopsychosocial teaching, research and clinical care. *General Hospital Psychiatry* 1990;12(5),283–295.

48. Sanders SH, Rucker KS, Anderson KO, et al. Clinical practice guidelines for chronic non-malignant pain syndrome patients. *J Back Musculoskelatal Rehabilitation* 1995;5:115–120.

49. Aronoff GM. Southern Pain Society News, p. 10, Summer 1997.

50. World Health Organization. Cancer pain relief and palliative care. Report of a WHO expert committee [World Health Organization Technical Report Series, 804] Geneva, Switzerland: World Health Organization, 1990:1–75.

51. Mayne GE, Brown M, Arnold P, Moya F. Pain of herpes zoster and postherpetic neuralgia. In: Raj RP ed. *Practical management of pain.* Chicago: Year Book Medical Publishers, Inc., 1986:345–361.

52. Portenoy RK. Chronic opioid therapy in nonmalignant pain. *J Pain and Sympt Manag* 1990:5(Suppl):S46–S62.

53. Portenoy RK. Chronic opioid therapy in nonmalignant pain. *J Pain Sympt Manag* 1990;5(Suppl):46–61.

54. Portenoy RK. Chronic opioid therapy for persistent noncancer pain: can we get past the bias? APS Bull 1(2):1, 4-5, 1991.

55. Portenoy RK, Foley KM. Chronic use of opioid analgesics in non-malignant pain: report of 38 cases. *Pain* 1986;25:17–186.

56. Savage SR. Long-term opioid therapy: assessment of consequences and risks. *J. Pain and Symptom Management* 1996;11(5):274–286.

57. Zacny JP. A review of the effects of opiates on psychomotor and cognitive functioning in humans. *Experimental and Clinical Psychopharmacology* 1995;3 :432–466.

58. Zacny JP. Should people taking opioids for medical reasons be allowed to work and drive? *Addiction* 1996;91, 1581–1584.

59. Jaffe J, Martin WRP. Opioid analgesics and antagonists. In: Gillman AG, Goodman LS, Gilman A, eds. *The pharmacological basis of therapeutics.* 6th ed. New York: MacMillan Publishing Co., 1980.

60. Forrest WH, et al. Dextroamphetamine with morphine for the treatment of postoperative pain. *N Engl J Med* 1977;296:712–715.

61. Webb SS, Smith GMP, Evans WO, Webb NC. Toward the development of a potent nonsedating oral analgesic. *Psychopharmacol* 1978;60:25–28.

62. Crombez G, Eccleston C, Baeyens F, Eelen P. Habituation and the interference of pain with task performance. *Pain* 1997;70(2,3): 149–154.

63. Aronoff GM. Pain centers treatment for intractable suffering and disability resulting from chronic pain. In: Aronoff GM, ed. *Evaluation and treatment of chronic pain,* 3rd ed. Baltimore: Lippincott Williams and Wilkins, 1999:591–602.

64. Zacny JP. Opioids and chronic pain. Letter to the editor. *Clin J Pain* 1998;14:89–91.

65. Zacny JP. A review of the effects of opioids on psychomotor and cognitive functioning in humans. *Exp Clin Psychopharmacol* 1995; 3:432–466.

66. Starmer GA. A review of the effects of analgesics on driving performance. In: O'Hanlon JF, deGier JJ, eds. Drugs and driving. London: Taylor & Francis, 1986:251–269.

67. Chesher GB. Understanding the opioid analgesics and their effects on skills performance. *Alcohol Drugs Driving* 1989;5:111–138.

68. Hanks GW, O'Neill WM, Simpson P, et al. The cognitive and psychomotor effects of opioid analgesics. II. A randomized controlled trial of single doses of morphine, lorazepam and placebo in healthy subjects. *Eur J Clin Pharmacol* 1995;48:455–460.

69. Vainio A, Ollila J, Matikainen E, et al. Driving ability in cancer patients receiving long-term morphine analgesia. *Lancet* 1995;346: 667–670.

70. Hanks GW. Morphine sans morpheus. *Lancet* 1995;346:652–653.

71. Smith AM. Patients taking stable doses of morphine may drive [letter]. *Br Med J* 1996;312:56–57.

72. Kappes S, Laux G. Driving performance of opiate addicts under methadone supported rehabilitation. *Pharmacopsychiatry* 1995;28:191.

73. Lodemann E, Leifer K, Kluwig J, et al. Methadone maintenance and driving ability. *Pharmacopsychiatry* 1995;28:199.

74. O'Neill WM, Hanks GW, McIntyre E, et al. An investigation of the cognitive effects of repeated doses of opioid analgesics in volunteers. *Eur J Clin Invest* 1995, 25:379.

75. Aronoff GM. Opioids in chronic pain management: is there a significant risk of addiction? *Current RevPain* 2000;4:112–121.

76. Onghena P, Van Houdenhove B. Antidepressant-induced analgesia in chronic non-malignant pain: a meta-analysis of 39 placebo-controlled studies. *Pain* 1991;49:205–219.

77. Goa KL, Sorkin EM. Gabapentin: A review of its pharmacological properties and clinical potential in epilepsy. *Drugs* 1993;3:46.

78. Goodkin K, Guillian CM. Antidepressants for the relief of chronic pain: Do they work? *Annals of Behavioral Medicine* 1989;11:83–101.

79. Walker EA, Sullivan MD, Stenchever MA. Use of antidepressants in the management of women with chronic pelvic pain. *Obst Gyne Clin N Am* 1993;20(4):743–751.

80. Max M. Antidepressants as analgesics. *Progress in pain research and management, vol 1.* Seattle: IASP Press, 1994.

81. France RD. The future of antidepressants; treatment of pain. *Psychopathology* 1987;20 (Suppl 1);99–113.

82. Blumer D, Heilbron M. Chronic pain as a variant of depressive disease: the pain-prone disorder. *J Ner Men Dis* 1982;170(7): 381–406.

83. Aronoff GM, Evans WO. Doxepin as an adjunct in the treatment of chronic pain. *J Clin Psychiatry* 1982;43(8/Sec 2):42–45.

84. Ventafridda V, Bonezzi C, Caraceni A, et al. Antidepressants for cancer pain and other painful syndromes with deafferentiation component; comparison of amitriptyline and trazodone. Ital. *J Neuro Sci* 1987;8:579–587.

85. Botney M, Fields HL. Amitriptyline potentiates morphine analgesia by direct action on the central nervous system. *Ann Neurology* 1983;13(2):160–164.

86. Matthew NT. Prophylaxis of migraine and mixed headache: a randomized controlled study, *Headache* 1981;21:105–109.

87. Max MB, Culnane M, Schafer SC, et al. Amitriptyline relieves diabetic neuropathic pain in patients with normal and depressed mood. *Neurology* 1987;37(4):589–596.

88. Raftery H. The management of postherptic pain using sodium valporate and amitriptyline. *J Irish Med. Association* 1959;72:399–407.

89. Watson CPN, Chipman M, Reed K, et al. Amitriptylene versus maprotilene in post-herpetic neuralgia: a randomized, double-blind, crossover trial. *Pain* 1992;48:29–36.

90. Hynes MD, Lochner MD, Bemisk, et al. Fluoxetine, a selective inhibitor of serotonin uptake. Potentiates morphine analgesia without altering its discriminative stimulant properties or affinity for opioid receptors. *Life Science* 1985;36:2317–2323.

91. Diamond S, Frietag FG. The use of fluoxetine in the treatment of headache. *Clin J Pain* 1989;5:200–201.

92. Geller SA. Treatment of fibrositis with fluoxetine. *Am. J. Med* 1989; 87:594–595.

93. Theesen KA, Marsh WR. Relief of diabetes neuropathy with fluoxetine. *DILP* 1989;23:572–574.

94. Sindrup SH, Gram LF, Brosen K, et al. The selective serotonin reuptake inhibitor paroxetine is effective in the treatment of diabetic neuropathy symptoms. *Pain* 1990;42:135–144.

95. Manna V, Bolino F, DiCicco L. Chronic tension type headache, depression and serotonin: therapeutic effects of fluvoxamine and mianserine. *Headache* 1994;44–49.

96. Bank J. A comparison study of amitriptylene and fluvoxamine in migraine prophylaxis. *Headache* 1994;476–478.

97. Pramond R, Saxena, Felt-Hansen PT. *Sumatriptan-migraine; the headache.* New York: Raven Press, 1993:329–341.

98. Atkinson JH. Psychopharmacologic agents in the treatment of pain syndromes. In: Tollison CD ed. *Handbook of chronic pain management.* Baltimore: Williams & Wilkins, 1989:69–99.

99. Gallagher R M, Moore P, Chernoff I. The reliability of depression diagnosis in chronic low back pain: a pilot study. *General Hospital Psychiatry* 1995;17:399–413.

100. Krass S, Gallagher RM, Myers P, Friedman R. Pain threshold and sensitivity in depressed and non-depressed patients with chronic pain. *Proceedings, Annual Meeting of the American Pain Society.* Nov. 1996.

101. Wells KB, Golding JM, Burnham MA. Psychiatric disorder in a sample of the general medical population with and without chronic medical conditions. *Am J Psychiat* 1988;145:976–981.

102. Depression Guideline Panel. Depression in Primary Care: Vol 1. Detection and Diagnosis. Clinical Practice Guideline, Number 5. Rockville, MD, US Department of Health and Human Services, Public Health Service, Agency for Health Care Policy and Research, AHCPR Publication No. 93-0551. April 1993.

103. Depression Guideline Panel. Depression in Primary Care: Vol 2. Treatment of Major Depression. Clinical Practice Guideline, Number 5. Rockville, MD, US Department of Health and Human Services, Public Health Service, Agency for Health Care Policy and Research, AHCPR Publication No. 93-0551. April 1993.

104. Wells KB, Golding JM, Burnham MA. The functioning and well-being of depressed patients: results from the Medical Outcomes Study. *JAMA*, 1989;262(7):914–919.

105. Dohrenwend B, Marbach J, Raphael, Gallagher RM. Why is depression co-morbid with chronic facial pain? A family study test of alternatives hypotheses. *Proceedings, Annual Meeting American Pain Society* 1995;APS169.

106. Seligman MEP. *Helplessness: on depression, development, and death.* San Francisco: WH Freeman, 1975.

107. Gallagher, RM, Williams B, Skelly J, et al. Worker's compensation and return-to-work in low back pain. *Pain* 1995;61(2):299–307.

108. Loeser JD, Ward AA, White LE. Chronic deafferentation of human spinal cord neurons. *J Neurosurg* 1968;29:48–50.

109. Nashold BE, Wilson WE. Central Pain and irritable midbrain. In: Crue B, ed. *Pain and suffering.* Springfield: Charles C. Thomas: 1970:95.

110. Nysfrom B, Hagbarth KE. Miloelectrode recording from transmiter nerves in amputes with phantom limb pain. *Neurosciences Letter* 1981;27:211–216.

111. Tasker RR, Dostrovsky JO. Deaferentation and central pain. In: Wall PD, Melzack R, eds. *Textbook of pain.* New York: Churchill and Livingstone 1989:154–180.

112. Maciewicz R, Bouckoms A, Martin JB. Drug therapy of neuropathic pain. *Clin J Pain* 1985;1:39–49.

113. Englander RN, Johnson RSN, Brickley JJ, Nanna GR. Effects of antiepileptic drugs on thalamocortical excitability. *Neurology* 1977;27:1134–1139.

114. Swerdlow M. Anticonvulsant drugs and chronic pain. (CW Book). Management of cancer pain. *Clinical Neuropharmacology* 1984;7(1):51–82.

115. Dunsker SB, Mayfield FN. Carbamazepine in the treatment of flashing pain syndrome. *Journal of Neurosurgery* 1976;45:49–51.

116. Nicol CF. A four year double blind trial of carbamazepine in facial pain. *Headache* 1969;9:54–57.

117. Elliot F, Little A, Mebrandt W. Carbamazepine for phantom limb phenomena. *N Eng J Med* 1956;295:678.

118. Canton FK. Phenytoin treatment of thalamic pain. *Br Med Journal* 1972;2:590.

119. Chadda VS, Mathur MS. Double blind study of the effect of diphenylhydantoin sodium in neuropathy. *J Assoc Physicians India* 1978;26:403–406.

120. Ellenberg M. Treatment of diabetic neuropathy with diphenylhydantoin. *N.Y. State J Med* 1976;68:295:6J8.

121. Caccia MR. Clonazepam in facial neuralgia and cluster Ha. Clinical and electrophysiological study. *Eur Neurology* 1975;13:560–563.

122. Peiris JB, Perera GLS, Devendra SV, Lionel NOW. Sodium valproate in trigeminal neuralgia. *Med J Aust* 1980;2:278.

123. Bruera E, Nauigante A, Barugel M, et al. Treatment of pain and other symptoms in cancer patients: patterns in a North American and South American hospital. *J Pain Sympt* Manag 1990;5:78.

124. Monks R. Psychotropic drugs. In: Bonica JJ, ed. *The management of pain.* Philadelphia: Lea & Febiger, 1990:1677.

125. Maxmen JS, Ward NG. *Psychotropic drugs: fast facts.* New York: Norton, 1995.

126. Chadwick D. Gabapentin. *Lancet* 1994;343:89–91.

127. Mellick GA, Mellicy LB, Mellick LB: Gabapentinn in the management of reflex sympathetic dystrophy. *J Pain Symptom Management* 1995;10 :265–266.

128. Rosner H, Rubin L, Kestenbaum H. Gabapentin adjunctive therapy in neuropathic pain staes. *Clin J Pain* 1996;12:56–58.

129. Andrew J, Chadwick D, Bates D: Gabapentin in partial epilepsy. *Lancet* 335 :1114–1115, 1990.

130. Melick GA, Seng ML. The use of gabapentin in the treatment of reflex sympathetic dystrophy and a phobic disorder. *Am J Pain Management* 1995;5:7–9.

131. Backonja M, Beydoun A, Edward KR, et at. Gabapentin for the symptomatic treatment of painful neuropathy in patients with diabetes mellitus: a randomized controlled trial. *JAMA* 1998; 280:1831–1836.

132. Rowbotham M, Harden N, Stacy B, et al. Gabapentin for the treatment of postherpetic neuralgia: a randomized controlled trial. *JAMA* 1998;280:1837–1842.

133. Rizzo MA. Successful treatment of painful traumatic mononeuropathy with carbamazipine: insights into a possible molecular pain mechanism. *J Neurol Sci* 1997;152:102–106.

134. Farago F. Trigeminal neuralgia: its treatment with two new carbamazepine analogues. [Clinical Trial.] *European Neurology.* 1987;26(2): 73–83.

135. Zakrzews JM, Patsalos PN. Oxacarbazepine: a new drug in the management of intractable trigeminal neuralgia. *J Neurology, Neurosurgery Psychiatry* 1989;52;472–476.

136. Lindstrom P, Lindstrom U. The analgesic effect of tocainide in trigeminal neuralgia. [Clinical Trial] *Pain* 1987;28(1):45–50.

137. Remillard G. Oxacarbazepine and intractable trigeminal neuralgia. *Epilepsia* 1994; 35(Suppl,3):S28-S29.

138. Hooge JP, Redekop WK. Trigeminal neuralgia in multiple sclerosis. [Journal Article] *Neurology* July 1995;45(7):1294–1296.

139. Reder AT, Arnason BG. Trigeminal neuralgia in multiple sclerosis relieved by a prostaglandin E analogue. [Journal Article] *Neurology* Jun 1995;45(6): 1097–1100.

140. di Vadi PP, Hamann W. The use of lamotrigine in neuropathic pain. [Journal Article] *Anaesthesia* Aug. 1998;53(8):808–809.

141. Carrieri PB, Bonuso S, Bruno R, et al. Efficacy of lamotrigine on sensory symptoms and pain in peripheral neuropathies [letter]. [Letter] *J Pain Symp Manag* Sept. 1999;18(3):154–156.

142. McCleane G. Lamotrigine can reduce neurogenic pain associated with multiple sclerosis [letter]. [Letter] *Clin J Pain* Sep. 1998;14(3):269–270.

143. Zakrzewska JM, Chaudhry Z, Nurmikko TJ, et al. Lamotrigine (lamictal) in refractory trigeminal neuralgia: results from a double-blind placebo controlled crossover trial [see comments]. [Clinical Trial. Journal Article. Randomized Controlled Trial] *Pain* Nov. 1997;73(2):223–230.

144. McCleane G. 200 mg daily of lamotrigine has no analgesic effect in neuropathic pain: a randomised, double-blind, placebo controlled trial [see comments]. [Clinical Trial. Journal Article. Randomized Controlled Trial] *Pain* Oct. 1999;83(1):105–107.

145. Devulder J, De Laat M. Lamotrigine in the treatment of chronic refractory neuropathic pain. *J Pain Sympt Manag* May 2000;19(5): 398–403.

146. Canavero S, Bonicalzi V. Lamotrigine control of central pain. *Pain* 1996;68(1):179–181.

147. Rosenfeld WE. Topiramate: a review of preclinical, pharmacokinetic, and clinical data. *Clinical Therapeutics* Nov-Dec 1997;19(6): 1294–1308; discussion 1523–1524.

148. Bajwa ZH, Sami N, Warfield CA, Wootton J. Topiramate relieves refractory intercostal neuralgia. *Neurology* June 10 1999;52(9):1917.

149. Hanno PM. Analysis of long-term Elmiron therapy for interstitial cystitis. [Clinical Trial. Journal Article] *Urology* May 1997;49(5A Suppl):93–99.

150. Bennett GJ. Update on the neurophysiology of pain transmission and modulation: focus on the NMDA-receptor. *J Pain Symptoms Management* 2000;19:S2–S6.

151. Hewitt DJ. The use of NMDA-receptor antagonists in the treatment of chronic pain. *Clin J Pain* June 2000;16(2 Suppl):S73–79.

152. Nelson KA. Park KM. Robinovitz E. Tsigos C. Max MB. High-dose oral dextromethorphan versus placebo in painful diabetic neuropathy and post herpetic neuralgia. [Clinical Trial. Journal Article. Randomized Controlled Trial] *Neurology.* May 1997;48(5):1212–1218.

153. Mathisen LC, Skjelbred P, Skoglund LA, Oye I. Effect of ketamine, an NMDA receptor inhibitor, in acute and chronic or facial pain. *Pain* 1995;61:215–220.

154. Persson J, Axelsson G, Hallin RG, Gustafsson LL. Beneficial effects of ketamine in a chronic pain state with allodynia, possibly due to central sensitization. *Pain* 1995;0:217–222.

155. Gammaitoni A, Gallagher RM, Welz MP, Topical ketamin gel: possible role in treating neuropathic pain. *Pain Medicine* 2000;1:97–100.

156. Chabal C, Jacobson L, Mariano A, et al. The use of oral mexiletine for the treatment of pain after peripheral nerve injury. *Anesthesiology* 1992;76:513–517.

157. Deugard A, Petersen P, Kastrup J. Mexiletine for treatment of chronic painful diabetic neuropathy. *Lancet* 1988;1:9–11.

158. Galer BS, Harle J, Rowbotham MC. Response to intravenous lidocaine infusion predicts subsequent response to oral mexiletine: A prospective study. *J Pain Symptom Manage* 1996;12:161–167.

159. Rowbotham MC, Davis PS, Fields HL. Topical lidocaine get relieves post-herpetic neuralgia. *Ann Neurol* 1995;37:246–253.

160. Laska EM, Sunshine A, Zighelboim I, et al. Effect of caffeine on acetaminophen analgesia. *Clin Pharmacol Toxicol* 1983;33:4,498–509.

161. King SA, Strain JJ. Benzodiazepine use by chronic pain patients. *Clin J Pain* 1990;6:143–147.

162. Singh PN, Sharma P, Gupta PK, Pandey K. Clinical evaluation of diazepam for relief of post operative pain. *Bri J Anesthesia* 1981;53:831–836.

163. Fernandez F, Adams F, Holmes VF. Analgesic effect of alprazolam in patients with chronic, organic pain. *J Clin Psychopharmacology* 1987;7:167–169.

164. Mayer TG, Gatchel RJ, Mayer H, et al. A prospective two-year study of functional restoration in industrial low back pain. *JAMA* 1987;258:1763–1768.

165. Hazard RG, Genwich JW, Kalish SM, et al. Functional restoration with behavioral support: a one year prospective study of patients with chronic low back pain. *Spine* 1989;14:157–161.

166. Martens RA, Martens S. *The milk sugar filemma: living with lactose intolerance.* East Lansing, MI: Meoi-Ed Press, 1987.

167. Zrbanec D, Spaventi S. Effect of calcitonin on the skeleton and bone pain in patients with osteolytic metastases. *Acta Med Iugoslavia* 1987;41:33–42.

168. Kastrup J, Peterson P, Dejgard A, et al. Intravenous lidocaine infusion. A new treatment of pain in diabetic neuropathy. *Pain* 1987;28:69–75.

169. Young RR, Delwaide PM. Spasticity. I and II. *N Engl J Med* 1981;304:28–33,96–99.

170. Aronoff GM, Adams JR. Spasticity and spasmolytic agents. *Int Med Special* 10(1):89, 122–129.

171. Lipman RS. Pharmacotherapy of anxiety and depression. *Psychopharmacol Bull* 1981;17:3,91–103.

172. D'Aalessandro, R, Granella, F. Tizanidine for chronic cluster headache. *Archieves of Neurology* Nov. 1996:53(11);1093.

173. Tsui JKC, Botulinum toxin as a therapeutic agent. *Pharmacol Ther* 1996;72;13–24.

174. Raj P. Prithvi. Toxin in the treatment of pain associated with musculoskeletal hyperactivity. *Current Review of Pain* 1997;1:403–416.

CHAPTER **20**

Anticonvulsants and Muscle Relaxants

R. Michael Gallagher

The management of chronic pain presents a difficult problem for the clinician. The patient with chronic pain suffers either continuously or frequently and often is subjected to severe limitations in daily life. Fear that the pain is caused by unrecognized pathology, and the illogical, sometimes causes patients to see many physicians and engage in an endless search for explanation and relief. Compassion and competent professional assistance, along with the development of patient coping skills, can mean the difference between productive and unproductive lives.

The perception of pain is an individual experience that differs from person to person. Similar injuries may not always produce similar pain in a variety of people. The situation, individual, state of mind, and expectation of pain can influence exactly how the pain is perceived (e.g., an athlete in the heat of competition who experiences serious injuries goes on, or the mother who experiences serious injuries but is still able to save her child). Similarly, analgesia can be influenced by expectation and suggestion of pain relief. These differences may be the result of pain modulation activity of the brain, which can increase or decrease pain perception (1).

The differences among individuals, and neurobiologic variations, probably account for the variability of the effectiveness of medications. Pharmacologic pain management with anticonvulsants or muscle relaxants may require trials with more than one medication or combinations of medications. It is important to allow an adequate trial at a maximum dose before medications are changed.

Unlike acute pain, which lessens or resolves with altered nociceptive input, chronic pain continues, and seeking relief can become the sufferer's most consistent activity. Frequently narcotic and nonnarcotic analgesics are the first line of defense, but the potential for addiction or habituation makes them impractical for the majority of patients. In addition, many patients with chronic pain syn-

dromes do not respond to the opioid and nonopioid analgesics. This may be in part due to changes in opioidal receptor expression (2). Safe and tolerable medications that interfere with chronic pain mechanisms are preferable as a part of a pain management program. Various medications, including antiinflammatory drugs, tricyclic antidepressants, anticonvulsants, and muscle relaxants, have been utilized with success in many patients.

Chronic benign pain, which limits patient activity, but doesn't threaten an early demise, often involves not only complex neurophysiologic mechanisms, but also extremely complex psychosocial issues. The psychosocial aspects of the sufferer's "whole being" are a critical part of treatment. In many patients, combinations of medications can be helpful in dealing with anxiety, depression, and muscle tension, all of which may be contributing to the pain paradigm. The anticonvulsants or muscle relaxants can be utilized individually or in combinations with each other or other agents to maximum benefit. When pain control is achieved, some patients can undergo a weaning process that may allow maintenance with a single agent.

When prescribing these medications, it is important to review the appropriate prescribing information details of precautions, side effects, contraindications, and interactions.

ANTICONVULSANTS

Anticonvulsant medications have been utilized in the treatment of chronic pain for many years with varying degrees of success. Initially used for neuropathic and lancinating pain, treatment options have expanded and a wide array of pain syndromes/conditions have been studied. It has been suggested that, since common inhibitory and excitatory amino acids or voltage dependent channels are involved in the neurophysiology of both pain and epilepsy, antiepileptic drugs are a reasonable treatment option (3).

Anticonvulsants are infrequently used in the treatment of acute pain. Few studies have been conducted and those that have been done to date have not been promising (4).

In numerous studies, anticonvulsants have demonstrated effectiveness for patients suffering with varying types of chronic pain. Their effectiveness, and use in combination with other anticonvulsants for seizure disorders, has led to combinations being used in difficult cases. The anticonvulsants also are used in combination with antidepressants, muscle relaxants, NSAIDs, and tranquilizers for greater effectiveness, or when the maximum dosage cannot be used because of adverse effects (5).

The precise mechanism of action of anticonvulsant drugs is uncertain. Various mechanisms have been proposed involving gamma-aminobutyric acid inhibition, stabilizing effects on neuronal membranes, changes in N-methyl-D-aspartate receptor sites, and changes in action potential (3,5,6). Table 20-1 lists some anticonvulsants along with their brand names.

Carbamazepine

Carbamazepine is structurally related to imipramine and is utilized with fairly good success in the treatment of trigeminal neuralgia. Approximately 70 percent of patients will respond, and those patients who do not or who have partial responses may benefit from the addition of phenytoin or chlorphenesin (7,8).

Carbamazepine has been shown to depress synaptic transmission in the trigeminal system (1,9). It probably has analgesic efficacy in lancinating pain regardless of the pathology that induces it. In addition, it has muscle relaxant, sedative, and analgesic effects (10). The dosage of carbamazepine generally is 200 to 600 mg/day with individual titration to the severity of pain. In some patients suffering with trigeminal neuralgia, higher doses may be necessary. Its half-life is variable, from 20 to 50 hours, which may account for a wide therapeutic dosage range. Major side effects include drowsiness, ataxia, confusion, and rash. There is a possibility of serious blood dyscrasias, and for this reason, laboratory monitoring is recommended.

TABLE 20-1. *Anticonvulsants*

Medication	Brand name
Carbamazepine	Tegretol
Clonazepam	Klonopin
Felbamate	Felbatol
Divalproex sodium	Depakote, Depakote ER
Gabapentin	Neurontin
Lamotrigine	Lamictil
Phenytoin	Dilantin
Topiramate	Topamax
Valproate sodium	Depacon

Because of the increased incidence of epilepsy in migraine sufferers and a possible association, carbamazepine has been used in the prophylaxis of migraine headache (11). Few studies have been done that have demonstrated its efficacy in migraine (12).

Other conditions in which carbamazepine is utilized with varying success are cluster headache, posttraumatic headache, myofascial pain syndrome, facial pain, post-stroke syndrome, diffuse pain syndrome, postherpetic neuralgia, and glossopharyngeal neuralgia (13–17) Although not dramatic, carbamazepine is more effective than placebo in treating diabetic neuropathy pain (18).

Clonazepam

Clonazepam is a benzodiazepine anticonvulsant that is used as an adjuvant in pain management. It demonstrates enhancing effects on gamma-aminobutyric acid (GABA) inhibition and has secondary effects on autonomic arousal and pain perception. Clonazepam has significant muscle relaxation effects.

Clonazepam is administered 4 to 12 mg/day in divided doses. Side effects are similar to other benzodiazepines with the more common being drowsiness, confusion, depression, muscle weakness, slurred speech, and transient liver enzyme elevations. Habituation can occur and caution should be exercised in prescribing clonazepam.

Clonazepam is not commonly used in pain management, but has been shown to be of benefit in trigeminal neuralgia, myofascial pain, and migraine prophylaxis (1,19).

Felbamate

Felbamate is a newer anticonvulsant that was originally investigated as an analgesic and has been shown to induce analgesia in animal models (20,21). Because of a high incidence of blood dyscrasias and hepatic effects, it does not appear to be practical for chronic pain management in its present form (3).

There have been anecdotal reports of benefit in hemifacial spasm and other forms of pain (22).

Divalproex Sodium and Valproate Sodium

Divalproex sodium is an anticonvulsant that has been used in various chronic pain syndromes with efficacy in many patients. However, there is little evidence to suggest that divalproex sodium is useful in acute pain, although limited studies have been completed (23). It has GABA-ergic enhancement mechanisms within the central nervous system (CNS), which have been linked to the opioid system and is thought to alter or stabilize neurotransmission (24,25). Divalproex sodium is often preferred over carbamazepine or phenytoin for adjuvant pain therapy because of increased tolerability.

Divalproex sodium dissociates in the gastrointestinal tract to the valproate ion. Pharmacologic action and drug profiles are similar.

Divalproex sodium is administered orally for chronic pain or headache in divided doses or in an extended-release form. Effective dosage varies from patient to patient and may be due to poor correlation between plasma concentrations and efficacy in the treatment of epilepsy (26). An average daily range varies from 250 mg to 1500 mg. Initial gastric upset frequently occurs and lower starting dosage with gradual upward titration is recommended. The more commonly reported side effects include nausea, dyspepsia, diarrhea, asthenia, somnolence, dizziness, tremors, weight gain, and alopecia. Hepatic dysfunction and coagulation abnormalities can occur.

Although widely used, limited clinical trials have been reported on varied chronic pain syndromes. In a study of 70 patients treated with sodium valproate (600 mg) or phenytoin (150 mg) for "shooting" pain, a 67 percent success rate was reported (27). Some of the patients were taking concomitant antidepressant medications and the success rates of valproate or phenytoin were not individually reported. Partial to marked improvement was reported in the treatment of herpetic neuralgia in 23 patients taking sodium valproate and amitriptyline in combination. The valproate daily dosage was 200 to 600 mg and 10 to 25 mg with amitriptyline (28).

A retrospective study of neuropathic pain among 65 advanced cancer patients showed a 67 percent efficacy in pain improvement with valproate sodium. Patients were on concomitant medications, which included antidepressants, corticosteroids, or opiates. However, the improvement was attributed to the addition of/or increase in dosage of the valproate sodium. Daily dosage ranged from 200 mg to 2000 mg (29).

Divalproex sodium is approved for migraine headache prophylaxis by the Food and Drug Administration (FDA), and it is frequently used as a preventative (30,31). In general, a 50 percent reduction in frequency and a decrease in pain intensity and/or duration are expected, although many responsive patients show greater improvement for migraine headache. The dosage varies from 250 to 750 mg/day in most patients. In a double-blind, placebo-controlled, crossover study of 29 patients treated with valproate sodium, there was a decrease in attacks from an average 15 to 8 per month in 25 patients, and a decrease in duration and pain intensity. The dosage was 800 mg/daily and only one patient withdrew because of active drug side effects (32).

A multicenter retrospective study of 248 patients with migraine or cluster who were treated with 500 to 1500 mg/day divalproex sodium showed efficacy and patient toleration. Fifty-one migraine and 13 cluster patients were treated with divalproex sodium as monotherapy and 184 migraine and 36 cluster patients were treated with divalproex sodium in combination with a multitude of other medications (33). Of all treated patients, 14 percent discontinued divalproex sodium because of side effects.

In a large, retrospective study of 540 patients with chronic daily headache treated with antidepressants (SSRIs and tricyclics), beta blockers, or valproate sodium, 46 percent of patients treated with all medications achieved long-term relief. Valproate sodium and SSRIs were the most effective preventatives at 35% each (34). Divalproex sodium has been used with success in a variety of other headache conditions, including chronic cluster headache, intractable migraine, and pediatric migraine (35,36,37).

Divalproex sodium has been used in combination with baclofen with success in the treatment of spasticity-related chronic pain. A limited report of four patients demonstrated significant improvement over an extended period while taking 750 mg (38). Patients with other conditions such as polyneuropathy, facial pain and central pain, have been treated with divalproex sodium with varied effectiveness (39).

Gabapentin

Gabapentin is an antiepileptic drug available in the United States since 1994. It is structurally related to gamma-aminobutyric acid (GABA), a neurotransmitter involved in pain modulation and transmission. The mechanism is not completely understood, but gabapentin is thought to modulate spinal cord neuronal calcium channels and alters the synthesis and release of GABA in the brain (40). Other more complicated pharmacologic activities have been proposed and described (41).

Gabapentin has been widely used by pain specialists to treat neuropathic pain. It is considered to be a relatively safe medication with no hepatic metabolism and no known drug–drug interactions. The analgesic effects are generally dose dependent.

Treatment is initiated at 300 mg/day and increased gradually until pain relief, to as high as 3200 mg/day in divided doses. Gabapentin is well tolerated in most individuals. The more common side effects include somnolence, dizziness, ataxia, and edema.

There have been various studies evaluating the efficacy of gabapentin in the treatment of pain. It was shown to be more effective than placebo in a comparative trial of diabetic peripheral neuropathy patients with 1- to 5-year histories of chronic pain (42).

The more common nonepileptic use of gabapentin is in treating neuropathic pain. Gabapentin effectiveness in trigeminal neuralgia was reviewed in an open-label study of 13 patients. Eighty-three percent of patients who had never been treated with carbamazepine and 57% of patients who had minimal benefit with carbamazepine improved significantly (43).

Case reports have been documented in the successful use of gabapentin in HIV patients with reflex sympathetic axonopathy, and in patients with pain from radiation myelopathy (44–46). Nine patients treated with gabapentin 900 to 2400 mg/day for reflex sympathetic dystrophy experienced excellent or good pain relief and most showed early evidence of disease reversal. Eight patients who were treated with 2000 to 2400 mg/day for distal symmetric axonopathy showed a significant reduction in pain.

Gabapentin also is used in the prophylactic treatment of vascular headache. Seventy patients experiencing migraine with aura or migraine without aura were treated with 900 to1800 mg/day in an open-label study. Both migraine types showed significant reduction in frequency and severity of headaches (46,47). Gabapentin sometimes is added to the prophylactic regimen of migraine and cluster headache for enhanced results.

Lamotrigine

Lamotrigine is a newer adult anticonvulsant with less sedating and psychomotor performance effects than the traditional medications. It is postulated that its mode of action in pain involves its effect on voltage gated cation channels and inhibition of glutamate release (48,49). It has demonstrated effectiveness in decreasing pain in animal models, anecdotally in various types of pain, and in a limited number of studies or controlled clinical trials (50).

Lamotrigine is administered orally in a wide range from 100 to 400 mg/day in divided doses. In patients who are taking valproic acid or other enzyme-inducing anticonvulsants simultaneously, the lamotrigine dose is reduced and steadily increased based on toleration, from 25 mg every other day. The more frequently encountered side effects include dizziness, headache, visual changes, nausea, rhinitis, and rash. Serious, potentially life-threatening rashes have been reported with lamotrigine and the risk may be increased with concomitant valproic acid.

In a study of 20 patients with chronic neuropathic pain refractory to previous treatment, four patients experienced temporary relief and six had sustained relief (50). Patients included suffered with neuralgias, surgical deafferentation, failed back surgery syndrome, myelopathy, neurolytic nerve destructions, spinal cord tumor, and postsurgical limb pain. Dosage ranged from 150 to 400 mg, and of the responders morphine was continued in four patients.

Lamotrigine dosage of 100 mg/day was studied in an open label pilot trial of 24 migraine with aura patients. The patients had suffered with frequent attacks and there was a substantial decrease in attacks over a 3-month period (51). A double-blind, placebo-controlled study of 53 patients with migraine with and without aura showed no difference between placebo and lamotrigine (52).

A study of 20 patients suffering with trigeminal neuralgia treated with lamotrigine showed significant improvement in most. Fifteen patients with trigeminal neuralgia and five patients with trigeminal neuralgia with concomitant multiple sclerosis taking 100 to 400 mg/day of lamotrigine were studied (53). All five of the trigeminal neuralgia

with multiple sclerosis patients showed complete remission of pain and 11 of the 15 trigeminal neuralgia patients experienced remission.

Lamotrigine is also used as adjunctive therapy in various pain conditions, including pain from multiple sclerosis. An open label study of 21 multiple sclerosis patients showed improvement of 17 patients with a dosage to 400 mg/day (54).

Phenytoin

Phenytoin is structurally related to the barbiturates and has been available for use since 1938. It is believed to reduce cortical responses to stimuli and reduces posttetanic potentiation (55). It is used with varying degrees of success in the treatment of neuropathic pain, cancer pain, trigeminal neuralgia, rheumatoid arthritis, irritable bowel pain, diabetic neuropathy, postherpetic neuralgia, Fabry's disease, glossopharyngeal neuralgia, and posttraumatic neuralgia (56). The half-life of phenytoin is quite unpredictable, varying from 7 to 42 hours, but steady plasma concentrations are achieved in 7 to 10 days. Concomitant medications, such as the antidepressants, can displace this highly protein-bound drug and result in toxicity (57).

Dosage is variable, depending on the individual patient and must be carefully titrated starting with 3 mg/kg/day. Side effects include ataxia, slurred speech, variable CNS effects, rash, gastrointestinal disorders, hematologic disorders, osteomalacia, and hypersensitivity.

Topiramate

Topiramate is a sulfonamate-substituted monosaccharide with antiseizure effects. It is thought to exact its effects by blocking action on sodium channels and it potentiates the activity of GABA. Topiramate has been used in the treatment of various pain disorders although few have been documented.

Topiramate is administered orally in divided doses. Treatment is initiated with 15 to 25 mg/day and gradually increased with an average range of 25 to 400 mg/day. In seizure disorders, plasma concentrations do not necessarily correlate with therapeutic effectiveness. Topiramate is generally well tolerated with the more common side effects being dizziness, somnolence, speech difficulties, psychomotor slowing, nervousness, visual changes, and memory difficulties.

There have been encouraging results with topiramate in the treatment of headache. Four migraine headache prophylactic studies were recently reported that showed significant patient improvement in frequency of attacks (58–61). One study documented a dramatic remission in 14 of 18 patients with cluster headache with topiramate (62). Topiramate was well tolerated in all studies.

A limited case report documented the positive response of one patient with refractory intercostal neuralgia to topiramate 75 mg (63).

MUSCLE RELAXANTS

Introduction

Complex neurologic mechanisms combine to maintain muscle tone. Any malfunction within this system can mean sustained abnormal muscle contraction, producing marked stiffness and pain. Such insult can be precipitated by a variety of sources, including injury, inflammation, or anxiety.

Muscles are prone to spasm from a variety of causes. The muscles of the neck are particularly prone to spasm, which may result in headache, as well as pain in the neck, shoulders, and upper back. Usually, the cause is injury, often from a motor vehicle accident, fall, work mishap, athletic participation, or overstretching. Inflammatory diseases and prolonged anxiety or stress also may cause painful spasm.

Persistent pain, for any length of time, can frustrate both the patient and the clinician. The problem is compounded by the potential muscle-spasm–pain–anxiety cycle that is self-perpetuating (Fig. 20-1).

The comprehensive approach is usually used to treat patients suffering with chronic musculoskeletal disorders such as strains or sprains. Such an approach would include muscle relaxants as adjunctive therapy, as an alternative to NSAIDs or opioids. Though this approach is accepted by most clinicians, there are few well-controlled efficacy studies.

A group of pharmacologic agents frequently used to treat acute musculoskeletal pain are the central-acting muscle relaxants (Table 20-2). These agents do not produce a direct effect on muscle, the myoneural junction, or motor nerves. Instead, muscle relaxation is produced through a depression of the central nerve pathway and possibly through the effect on higher centers.

Since the central-acting muscle relaxants have effects on higher brain centers, this group is sometimes used as anxiolytics and analgesics. Muscular pain is decreased by mod-

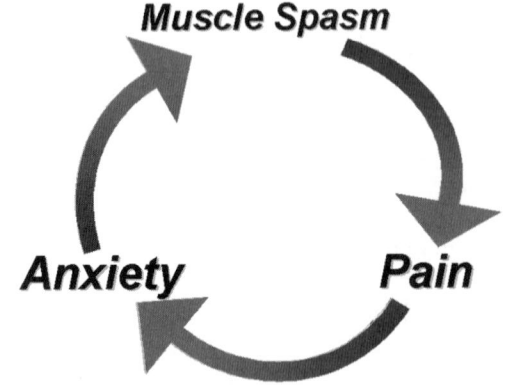

FIG. 20-1. Muscle-Spasm–Pain–Anxiety Cycle

TABLE 20-2. *Muscle relaxants*

Medication	Brand name
Baclofen	Lioresal
Carisoprodol	Soma
Chlorphenesin carbamate	Maolate
Chlorzoxazone	Parafon Forte DSC, Paraflex
Cyclobenzeprine HCl	Flexeril
Diazepam	Valium
Metaxalone	Skelaxin
Methocarbamol	Robaxin
Orphenadrine citrate	Norflex, Norgesic, Orphengesic
Tizanidine	Zanaflex

ifying central perception, without interrupting normal peripheral pain reflexes or motor activity. This group of medications is well tolerated and has a low toxicity profile.

Baclofen

Baclofen is a muscle relaxant with agonist properties at the gamma-aminobutyric acid β receptor (GABA$_B$). It is not clear if its clinical effects are related to GABA activity. Its effects may be related to its inhibition of monosynaptic and polysynaptic reflexes at the spinal level. In addition, baclofen may depress the response to maxillary nerve stimulation of mechanoreceptive neurons in the spinal trigeminal nucleus oralis (64).

Baclofen has shown efficacy in neuropathic pain of the episodic lancinating or paroxysmal type and especially in those patients resistant to carbamazepine (65). It has been used as an adjuvant and as monotherapy in various types of chronic pain, including trigeminal neuralgia, glossopharyngeal neuralgia, and chronic peripheral nerve disease (66–68).

For chronic pain, baclofen is administered orally starting with 5 mg two to three times daily and titrating the dose upward as tolerated. Average dosage is 30 to 90 mg/day. Abrupt cessation of baclofen can result in withdrawal syndrome, including seizures and delirium. For this reason, a gradual weaning of the medication is recommended. The more common side effects include drowsiness, dizziness, weakness, fatigue, nausea, and confusion.

In a double-blind, crossover study of ten patients taking 60 to 80 mg/day, seven experienced a significant reduction of paroxysms of typical trigeminal neuralgia (65). In another open label study by the same researchers, 37 of 50 typical trigeminal neuralgia patients experienced significant relief while taking 40 to 60 mg/day (65). Baclofen does not appear to be effective in atypical trigeminal neuralgia.

Carisoprodol

Carisoprodol is a central nervous system depressant with a structure similar to meprobamate. It is reported to have analgesic properties and to reduce local muscle spasm without significantly interfering with muscular or neuromuscular function (69). The exact mechanism of action is not well understood, but it is believed that it depresses the polysynaptic transmission in interneuronal pools at the supraspinal level in the brainstem reticular formation. Its sedative qualities may also play a role in the muscle relaxation effect.

Carisoprodol is a relatively short-acting drug with minimal cumulative effect. It is generally well tolerated and its potential for organic toxicity is extremely low. Drug interactions are an additive sedative effect when taken with central nervous system depressants such as alcohol or antihistamines.

The adult oral dose for carisoprodol is 350 mg three to four times daily. It is most often recommended for use in adults; however, its use in pediatric patients is not uncommon. The suggested dosage for children above 5 years of age is 25 mg/kg four times daily (70). Carisoprodol should be used cautiously in children.

Carisoprodol (200 mg) is sometimes combined with aspirin (325 mg) or aspirin and codeine (16 mg) for patients suffering significant pain, adding antiinflammatory properties and analgesia. These preparations are given in a dose of one or two tablets four times daily. The usual aspirin and codeine prescribing information should be followed.

Side effects are usually transient and occur within the initial several days of use. Side effects may include drowsiness, dizziness, vertigo, ataxia, tremor, agitation, irritability, headache, depression, syncope, and insomnia.

In one study of 65 patients, 42 patients were treated with 350 mg of carisoprodol or placebo, four times daily for 10 days (71). Carisoprodol was significantly more effective than placebo in relieving muscle spasm, pain, and stiffness of the cervical, thoracic, lumbar, and iliac regions.

Various other studies have compared carisoprodol to other muscle relaxants, analgesics, and sedatives. Carisoprodol demonstrated more effectiveness in a comparative study with butalbital or placebo, a comparative study with propoxyphene or placebo, and a comparative study with diazepam (72–74).

Chlorphenesin Carbamate

Chlorphenesin is a central-acting skeletal muscle relaxant that is structurally and pharmacologically similar to methocarbamol. Its exact mechanism of action is unknown and its direct muscle relaxation effects are minimal. Its benefits probably are derived from its sedative effects. Chlorphenesin sometimes is used as an adjuvant in pain related to musculoskeletal pain.

The usual adult daily dosage is 1600 mg in divided doses. In more severe cases, 2400 mg in divided doses can be administered and reduced with improvement. Treatment with chlorphenesin should be limited to no more than 8 weeks. It should be used with caution in patients with hepatic dysfunction. It is not recommended for children under 12.

Side effects include drowsiness and dizziness. Less common side effects include confusion, insomnia, headache, and nausea. Rash, fever, or anaphylaxis are rare. Chlorphenesin should not be given to patients with liver dysfunction.

Chlorzoxazone

Chlorzoxazone is a central-acting skeletal muscle relaxant with sedative qualities. Its mode of action has not been clearly identified. It acts at the spinal cord level and subcortical areas of the brain, inhibiting reflex arcs that play a role in muscle spasm.

In chronic pain chlorzoxazone is administered orally. The usual initial adult dosage is 750 to 2000 mg daily in three to four divided doses. The dosage can be increased to 3000 mg in unresponsive patients and lowered with improvement. Chlorzoxazone can be used in children, at 375 to 1000 mg in three to four divided doses, taking into account the age and weight of the child. As with numerous other medications, chlorzoxazone should be given to children only when clearly necessary.

Chlorzoxazone is usually well tolerated and undesirable side effects are not common. Side effects include gastrointestinal disturbances, drowsiness, dizziness, lightheadedness, overstimulation, and allergic skin rash. Serious reactions are extremely rare.

In a study, 59 patients were treated with chlorzoxazone or placebo for musculoskeletal back conditions over 6 to 8 days (75). By day two, patients receiving 750 mg of chlorzoxazone four times daily reported reduced spasm, pain, and tenderness and had regained some of their restricted range of motion. At the end of the study, 97 percent of the chlorzoxazone group had complete remission of symptoms, contrasted with 39 percent of the placebo group.

In a controlled, double-blind study of 53 patients treated with chlorzoxazone 300 mg or diazepam 20 mg for muscular spasm, chlorzoxazone was shown to be significantly more effective and have fewer side effects than diazepam (76).

Cyclobenzaprine

Cyclobenzaprine is a central-acting muscle relaxant similar to the tricyclic antidepressants. It is believed to relieve skeletal muscle spasm with the central nervous system at the brainstem level, although it may have an effect at the spinal cord level (77). Cyclobenzaprine initially was studied for psychotherapeutic use with limited benefit and is more widely used for the relief of muscle spasm (78). Cyclobenzaprine can be sedating, but does not appear to interfere with muscle function (79).

Cyclobenzaprine is administered orally in divided doses of 20 to 40 mg/day. It is a relatively long-acting drug, like the tricyclic antidepressants, as compared to other muscle relaxants. Because of an elimination half-life of 1 to 3 days and its sedating effects, it can be taken in a single bedtime dose.

Drowsiness is the most common side effect, occurring as often as 40%, but lessens with time in most individuals. Other more frequently encountered side effects include dry mouth, dizziness, nausea, constipation, dyspepsia, tachycardia, and urinary retention.

In a study of 78 patients with thoracolumbar strain and sprain taking cyclobenzaprine or carisoprodol, both drugs equally relieved muscle spasm and pain (80). Another study of 55 patients treated with cyclobenaprine 30 to 50 mg/day or placebo with chronic neck spasm and pain showed a significant reduction of spasm and pain in the active drug group (81).

Diazepam

Diazepam is a benzodiazepine, which is commonly used as a sedative. The benzodiazepines act on the central nervous system, resulting in sedation, hypnosis, decreased anxiety, anticonvulsant activity, and muscle relaxation. The effects are believed to be from a potentiation of GABA on neurons at all levels (81). Other benzodiazepines are sometimes prescribed, including clonazepam, chlordiazepoxide, meprobamate, or alprazolam.

Diazepam is rapidly absorbed, reaching peak blood levels in one hour in adults and as soon as 15 minutes in children. Secondary peak blood levels can occur at 6 to 12 hours. Tolerance and dependency can occur. Benzodiazepines should only be prescribed when absolutely necessary.

Diazepam is administered orally and sometimes by injection in the most severe cases of muscle spasm. The usual adult daily dosage is 6 to 40 mg in three to four divided doses. The daily dosage for children is 1 to 2.5 mg in three to four divided doses.

Ataxia is the most common side effect of diazepam. Dizziness, confusion, headache, gastrointestinal disturbances, rash, and chills are infrequent side effects.

A study of 40 patients treated with diazepam, phenobarbital, or placebo over four days, showed that patients treated with diazepam experienced a significant improvement over the phenobarbital or placebo groups (82). The patients included had muscle spasm and pain due to trauma, nervous tension, cold weather, degenerative joint disease, overexertion, and unknown causes.

A study comparing diazepam to carisoprodol showed diazepam to be of benefit in skeletal muscle spasm (74).

Metaxalone

Metaxalone is a central-acting skeletal muscle relaxant that is chemically similar to the mild tranquilizer, mephenoxalone. Its mode of action is unclear, but it is believed to cause muscle relaxation through depressing the central nervous system, and it has been used as adjunctive therapy for many years in acute musculoskeletal conditions. It is absorbed rapidly, with an onset of action about one hour after it is given. Metaxalone is administered orally. The adult daily dosage is 2400 to 3200 mg in divided doses. It should be prescribed with caution in patients with diminished liver function.

Metaxalone is usually well tolerated. Side effects include nausea, vomiting, drowsiness, headache, nervousness, irritability, rash, and pruritus. Leukopenia, jaundice, and hemolytic anemia are extremely rare.

In a multicenter study of 228 patients, those treated with metaxalone for spasm and pain showed a significant improvement over the placebo group when given 1600 to 3200 mg of metaxalone over 7 to 9 days (83).

A study of 100 patients suffering with low back muscular pain treated with metaxalone or placebo showed a 97 percent medically significant improvement (84). The same study was repeated and corroborated previous results demonstrating a 75 percent improvement with metaxalone.

Methocarbamol

Methocarbamol is a central-acting skeletal muscle relaxant with a structure similar to mephenesin. It has been used in the United States for more than 40 years with success in treating acute musculoskeletal conditions. Its method of action is not clear, and it does not have a direct effect on striated muscle or the myoneural junction. In animals, it inhibits nerve signals in the internuncial neurons of the spinal cord and blocks polysynaptic reflexes.

Methocarbamol can be given orally or by injection. The average starting daily oral dosage is 6 g in four divided doses, then decreasing to 4.0 to 4.5 g for maintenance therapy. Methocarbamol can be combined with aspirin and is given two tablets three to four times daily in most cases.

The injectable form of the drug can be given intramuscularly, via intravenous push, or by slow intravenous drip. Intramuscularly, 200 to 500 mg can be injected into each gluteal region, repeated at 8-hour intervals until there is sufficient improvement to place the patient on the oral form. As much as 3000 mg of methocarbamol can be administered intravenously in divided doses daily for up to 3 days. Patients receiving the drug intravenously may have immediate side effects and should remain in the recumbent position while methocarbamol is administered and for 15 minutes after it is given.

Methocarbamol is generally well tolerated. Side effects usually improve with time and include light-headedness, vertigo, headache, blurred vision, rash, flushing, gastrointestinal upset, nasal congestion, and with the injectable form a metallic taste in the mouth.

In a double-blind parallel study of 180 patients taking either methocarbamol or placebo for acute musculoskeletal disorders caused by trauma or inflammation, methocarbamol was significantly more effective (80%) than placebo (45%) after 2 days (85). After 9 days, methocarbamol remained more effective, but to a far less degree. This difference may be a result of the self-limiting nature of many musculoskeletal conditions.

Few controlled comparison studies using methocarbamol have been done. A comparative placebo controlled study of 227 patients treated with methocarbamol or cyclobenzaprine demonstrated a slight advantage to methocarbamol and significantly more effectiveness than placebo (86). Another study comparing methocarbamol, chlorphenesin, carisoprodal, and placebo did not demonstrate more effectiveness than the other two active medications (87).

Orphenadrine Citrate

Orphenadrine is a central-acting skeletal muscle relaxant with anticholinergic properties. It is thought to work by relaxing skeletal muscles through blocking neuronal circuits where hyperactivity may play a role in hypertonia and spasm.

Orphenadrine can be given in oral form or in injectable form for hospitalized patients. The drug is available in 100-mg sustained-release tablet, 25 mg in combination with caffeine and aspirin, and 50 mg in combination with caffeine and aspirin. The 100-mg sustained-release tablet is given twice daily. Combination tablets are administered three to four times daily.

Many of the side effects for orphenadrine are related to its anticholinergic effects and are related to dosage. Potential side effects include tachycardia, palpitations, urinary retention, dry mouth, blurred vision, increased intraocular pressure, weakness, nausea, vomiting, headache, and drowsiness.

In one 40-patient placebo-controlled study, those treated with orphenadrine intravenously showed statistically significant improvement in overall effectiveness in patients with painful muscle spasm (88). Another study of 38 tension-type headaches treated with orphenadrine, diazepam, or placebo showed equal effectiveness of the active drugs (89).

Tizanidine

Tizanidine is a central alpha 2 adrenoreceptor agonist that is used in the management of spasticity and the palliation of pain. It is structurally related to clonidine with multiple effects that are not completely understood. Its myospasmolytic effects are the result of presynaptic action at the spinal cord level and a resultant decrease in the effectiveness of excitatory transmitters (90). It also

exerts inhibitory action on alpha motor neurons, which may be related to its efficacy in pain and spasm (91).

Tizanidine is administered orally in divided doses of 4 to 16 mg/day. It is helpful to begin with a low starting dose and gradually increase as tolerated. Abrupt cessation can cause transient signs of withdrawal, and for this reason weaning from the tizanidine is recommended. Side effects include somnolence/sedation, asthenia, dizziness, and dry mouth, and hallucinosis has been reported. Elevations in liver enzymes can occur, which are usually reversible on drug withdrawal.

Tizanidine has been shown to be effective in neck and back pain in clinical trials and appears to be as effective as diazepam or chlorzoxazone (90–92). In a 78-patient tension headache study, 68% showed improvement while taking 3 mg/day for 4 weeks (93). Tizanidine also has been shown to be effective in myofascial pain, chronic daily headache, tension-type headache, and neuropathic pain (94–97).

CONCLUSION

Chronic pain presents a difficult challenge for clinicians attempting to bring relief to suffering patients. Patients may describe their pain as sharp, dull, burning, or stabbing and give a myriad of other explanations. Their pain may be frequent or it may be constant. Many times, there are numerous variables that have an impact on patients' chronic pain, including disease state, environment, mental and emotional status, and more. Almost always, chronic pain is difficult to endure.

Frequently, traditional pain medications do not afford adequate relief or are ineffective. Narcotic and non-narcotic medications have helped, but present problems. The clinician must always be on guard against addiction and habituation. Nonsteroidal antiinflammatory drugs (NSAIDs) have proved to be of help against pain and inflammation, but are not without difficult side effects. Used in high doses, over lengthy periods, NSAIDs can cause significant gastrointestinal disturbances and sometimes bleeding.

While the comprehensive approach to treating patients suffering with chronic pain continues to be critical to breaking the cycle of pain and anxiety, the addition of nontraditional medications can be of great benefit. It is important for the clinician not to overlook these therapies.

Two such critical drug groups are the anticonvulsants and the muscle relaxants. Medications in each of these groups have demonstrated their efficacy in numerous clinical studies and in modern patient practice, when given alone or in combination with other drugs. Anticonvulsants and muscle relaxants have earned a place in a comprehensive treatment plan for many patients suffering with chronic pain. This approach has proved to be helpful and likely to enable patients to move more freely and function better in their daily lives.

REFERENCES

1. Naidu MU, Ramesh K, Anuradha RT, et al. Evaluation of phenytoin in rheumatoid arthritis: an open study. *Drugs Exp Clin Res* 1991; 17:71–275.
2. Maekawa K, Minami M, Masuda T, et al. Expression of mu- and kappa-, but not delta-, opioid receptor mRNAs is enhanced in the spinal dorsal horn of the arthritic rats. *Pain* 1996;64:365–371.
3. Hansen HC. Treatment of chronic pain with antiepileptic drugs: a new era. *So Med J* 1999;92 (7):642–649.
4. Martin C, Martin A, Rud C, et al. Comparative study of sodium valproate and ketoprofen in the treatment of postoperative pain. *Ann Fr Anesth Reanim* 1988;7:387–392.
5. McQuay H, Tramer M, Nye B, et al. A systemic review of antidepressants in neuropathic pain. *Pain* 1996;68:217–227.
6. Wiffen P, McQuay H, Carroll D, et al. Anticonvulsant drugs for acute and chronic pain. In: *The Cochrane Library* 2000;Issue 2.
7. Loeser JD. Tic douloureux and atypical facial pain. In: Wall PD, Melzack R, eds. *Textbook of pain*, 3rd ed. London: Churchill Livingstone 1994:699–710.
8. Campbell FG, Graham JG, Zilkha KJ. Clinical trial of carbamazepine in trigeminal neuralgia. *J of Neuro Neurosurg and Psychiatry* 1966;29:265–267.
9. Fromm GH, Landgren S. Effect of diphenylhydantoin on single cells in the spinal trigeminal nucleus. *Neurology* 1963;13 (1):34–37.
10. Dalessio DJ, ed. *Wolff's headache and other head pain*, 5th ed. New York: Oxford University Press, 1987.
11. Ziegler DK. The treatment of migraine. In: D'Alessio DJ, ed. *Wolff's headache and other head pain*, 5th ed. New York: Oxford University Press, 1987:87–111.
12. Rompel H, Bauermeister PW. Aetiology of migraine and prevention with carbamazepine (Tegretol): results of a double-blind, cross-over study. *S Afr Med J* 1970;44 (4):75–80.
13. Gonakowska M. Treatment of Horton's headache with small doses of pilocripine and carbamazepine. *Wiad Lek* 1984;37:1093–1095.
14. Kienast HW, Boshes LD. Clinical trials of carbamazepine in suppressing pain. *Headache* 1968;8:1–5.
15. Westerholm N. Treatment of facial pain with g32883 (Tegretol). *Scan J Dent Res* 1970;78:144–148.
16. Leijon G, Boirre J. Central post-stroke pain—a controlled trial of amitriptyline and carbamazepine. *Pain* 1989;36:27–36.
17. Killian JM, Fromm GH. Carbamazepine in the treatment of neuralgia. Use and side effects. *Archives of Neurology* 1968;19:129–136.
18. Rall TW, Schleifer LS. Drugs effective in the therapy of the epilepsies. In: Goodman LS, Gilman A, Rall TW, Nies AS, Taylor P, eds. *The Pharmacological basis of therapeutics*, 8th Edition. Toronto: McGraw-Hill, 1990:436–462.
19. Stensrud P, Sjaastad O. Clonazepam in migraine prophylaxis. *Headache* 1979;19: 333–334.
20. Hunter JC, Gagas KR, Hedley LR, et al. The effect of novel antiepileptic drugs in rat experimental models of acute and chronic pain. *European Journal of Pharm* 1997; 324:153-160.
21. Imamura Y, Bennett GJ. Falbamate relieves several abnormal pain sensations in rats with an experimental peripheral neuropathy. *Journal of Pharmacol Exp* 1995;275:177.
22. Portenoy RK. Adjuvant analgesics in pain management. In: Doyle D, Hangs GW, MacDonald N, eds. *Oxford textbook of palliative medicine*. Oxford: Oxford University Press, 1998;361–390.
23. McQuay H, Carroll D, Jadad AR, et al. Anticonvulsant drugs for management of pain: a systemic review. *BMJ* 1995;311(7012):1047–1052.
24. Gram L. Experimental studies with controlled clinical testing of valproate and vigabatrin. *Acta Neurol Scand* 1988;78:241–270.
25. Thomas JR. Long term safety of divalproex Na prophylactic treatment of patients with migraine. *Cephalalgia* 1995;(suppl 14):266(Ab).
26. Abulan FS, Shariwal MA, Al-Bekairi AM, et al. Antinociceptive activity of sodium valproate in mice after chronic treatment. *Gen Pharmac* 1977;29(3):463–467.
27. Swerdlow M. The treatment of "shooting" pain. *Postgrad Med J* 1980;56(653):159–161.
28. Rafferty H. The management of post herpetic pain using sodium valproate and amitriptyline. *J IR Med Assoc* 1979;72(9):399–401.
29. Snare AJ, Tett SE, Kaye K, et al. Sodium valproate: retrospective analysis of neuropathic pain control in patients with advanced cancer. *J Pharm Tech* 1993;9:114–117.
30. Rothrock, JF. Clinical studies of valproate for migraine prophylaxis. *Cephalalgia* 1997;17(2)000:81–83.
31. Cutrer FM, Limmroth J, Moskowitz MA. Possible mechanisms of valproate in migraine prophylaxis. *Cephalalgia* 1997;17:83–100.
32. Herring R, Kuritsky A. Sodium valproate in the prophylactic treatment of migraine: a double-blind study vs. placebo. *Cephalalgia* 1992;12:81–84.
33. Gallagher RM, Mueller L, Freitag F. Divalproex Na in the treatment of migraine and cluster headache. *JAOA* 2001. In Press.
34. Robbins L, Maides JF. Efficacy of preventive medications for chronic daily headache. *Am J of Pain Mgmt* 1999;9(4):139–142.
35. Freitag F, Diamond S, Diamond ML, et al. Preventative treatment of chronic cluster headache with divalproex sodium *Cepalalgia* 2000;20:403(Ab).
36. Kapisyzi M, Kruja J. Use of valproic acid in chronic daily headache. *Cephalalgia* 2000;20:337(Ab).
37. Pakalnis A, Greenberg G, Drake ME, et al. Paediatric migraine prophylaxis with divalproex. *Cephalalgia* 2000;20:388(Ab).
38. Zachariah SB, Borges EF, Varghese R, et al. Positive response to oral divalproex sodium in patients with spacity and pain. *Am J Sci* 1994;72(9):399–401.
39. Skelton WP, Skelton NR. Nutritional depletion polyneuropathy with valproic acid. *Arch Intern Med* 1993;153:902–903.
40. Ronibotham M, Harden N, Stacey B, et al. Gabapentin for the treatment of post-herptic neuralgia. *JAMA* 1998;280:1837–1842.
41. Taylor CP, Gee NS, Su TZ, et al. A summary of mechanistic hypothesis of gabapentin pharmacology. *Epilepsy Res* 1998;29:233–249.
42. Backonja M, Beydoun A, Edwards KR, et al. Gabapentin for the symptomatic treatment of painful neuropathy in patients with diabetes mellitus: a randomized controlled trial. *JAMA* 1998;280(21):1831–1836.
43. Valcania F, Strafella AP, Naserti A, Tassinari CA. Gabapentin in idiopathic trigeminal neuralgia. *Neurology* 1998;50:A379(Ab).
44. Mellick LB, Mellick GA. Successful treatment of reflex sympathetic dystrophy with gabapentin. *Am J Emerg Med* 1995;13:96.
45. Gatti A, Jana S, Sandro B, Manuela B. Gabapentin for treatment of distal symmetric axonopathy in HIV-infected patients. *Neurology* 1998;50:A216(Ab).
46. Cheville A, Narcessian E, Elliot K. Neuropathic pain in radiation myelopathy: a case report. *Proc 14th Ann Sci Mtg Am Pain Soc* 1995; A115(Ab).
47. Mathew NT, Tucker C. Gabapentin in migraine prophylaxis, a preliminary open label study. *Neurology* 1996;46:A169(Ab).
48. Lees G, Leach MJ. Studies on the mechanism of action of the novel anticonvulsant lamotrigine using primary neurological cultures from rat cortex. *Brain Res* 1993;612:190–199.
49. Teoh H, Fowler U, Bowery NG. Effect of lamotrigine on the electrically-evoked release of endogenous amino acids from slices of dorsal horn of the rat spinal cord. *Neuropharmacology* 1995;34:2173–1278.
50. Devulder J, DeLaat M. Lamotrigine in the treatment of chronic refractory neuropathic pain. *J Pain and Symt Mgmt* 2000;19(5):398–403.
51. D'Andrea G, Granella F, Caldaldini M, et al. Effectiveness of lamotrigine in the prophylaxis of migraine with aura: an open label study. *Cephalalgia* 1999;19:64–66.
52. Steiner TJ, Findley LJ, Yuen AWC. Lamotrigine versus placebo in the prophylaxis of migraine with and without aura. *Cephalalgia* 1997;17: 109–112.
53. Lunaradi G, Leandri M, Albano C, et al. Clinical effectiveness of lamotrigine and plasma levels in essential and symptomatic trigeminal neuralgia. *Neurology* 1997;48:1714–1717.
54. Cianchetti C, Zuddas A, Randazzo AP, et al. Lamotrigine adjunctive therapy in painful phenomena in MS: Preliminary observations. *Neurology* 1999;53(2):433.
55. Englander RN, Johnson RSN, Brickley JJ et al. Effects of antiepileptic drugs on thalamocortical excitability. *Neurology* 1977;27:1134–1139.
56. Symptom management. In: Doyle D, Hanks GWC, MacDonald N, eds. *Oxford textbook of palliative medicine*, 2nd ed. New York: Oxford University Press Inc, 1998:247–774.

57. Atcheson R, Rowbotham DJ. Pharmacology of acute and chronic pain. In: Rawal N, ed. *Management of acute and chronic pain.* London: BMJ Books, 1998:23–50.
58. Wilson MC. Efficacy of topiramate in the prophylactic treatment of intractable chronic migraine: a retrospective chart analysis. *Cephalalgia* 2000;20(4):301(Ab).
59. Edwards KR, Glantz MJ, Norton JA, et al. Prophylactic treatment of migraine with topiramate: a double blind, placebo controlled trial in 30 patients. *Cephalalgia* 2000;20 (4):316(Ab).
60. Trapani G, Mei D, Marra C, et al. Use of topiramate as a prophylactic treatment in migraine: results of a pilot study. *Cephalalgia* 2000;20(4):426(Ab).
61. Drake ME, Greathouse NI, Pakalnis A. An open label study of topiramate for migraine prevention. *Cepalalgia* 2000;20(4):421(Ab).
62. Wheeler SDE, Carrazana EJ. Topiramate-responsive cluster headache. *Cepalalgia* 2000;20(4):330(Ab).
63. Bajwa ZH, Sami N, Warfield CA, et al. Topiramate relieves refractory intercostals neuralgia. *Neurology* 1999;52:1917.
64. Fromm GH, Chattha AS, Terrance CF, et al. Role of inhibitory mechanisms in trigeminal neuralgia. *Neurology* 1981;31:683–687.
65. Fromm GH, Terrence CF, Chattha AS. Baclofen in the treatment of trigeminal neuralgia: double-blind study and long-term follow-up. *Annals of Neurology* 1984;15:240–244.
66. Fromm GH. Baclofen as an adjuvant analgesic. *J Pain and Symp Mgmt* 1994;9:500–509.
67. Ringel RA, Roy EP. Glossopharyngeal neuralgia: successful tratment with baclofen. *Annals of Neurology* 1987;21:14–15.
68. Terrence CF, Fromm GH, Tenicela R. Baclofen as an analgesic in chronic peripheral nerve disease. *European Neurology* 1985;24:380–385.
69. Bergen FM, Kletzstein M, Ludwig BJ, Margolin S. History, chemistry and pharmacology of carisoprodol. *Ann NY Acad Sci* 1960;86:90–107.
70. McEvoy GK. Autonomic drugs. *Drugs Info 85.* Bethesda, MD: American Society of Hospital Pharmacists 1985:417–548.
71. Cullen AP. Carisoprodol (Soma) in acute back conditions. *Curr Ther Res* 1976;20:556–562.
72. Hindle TH. Comparison of carisprodol, butalbital and placebo in treatment of low back syndrome. *Calif Med* 1972;117:7–11.
73. Baratta RR. A double-blind comparative study of carisprodol, propoxephine and placebo in the management of low back syndrome. *Curr Ther Res* 1976;20:233–239.
74. Boyles WF, Glassman JM, Soyka MD. Management of acute musculoskeletal condition. *Today Ther Trend* 1983;1:1–16.
75. Vernon WG. A double-blind evaluation of Parafon Forte in the treatment of mesculo-skeletal back conditions. *Curr Ther Res* 1972;14(12):801–806.
76. Scheiner JJ. Muscle relaxants: chlorzoxazone compared with diazepam (a double-blind study). *Curr Ther Res* 1976;19(1):51–57.
77. Share NN, McFarlane CS. Cyclobenzeprine: a novel centrally acting skeletal muscle relaxant. *Neuropharmacology* 1975;14(9):675–684.
78. Basmajian JV. Cyclobenzeprine HC effect on skeletal muscle spasm in the lumar region and neck: two double-blind controlled clinical and laboratory studies. *Arch Phys Med Rehabil* 1978;59:58–63.
79. Nibbelink DW. Flexeril (cyclobenzeprine HCL/MSD). Review of clinical double-blind evaluations of efficacy and tolerability. *Postgrad Med Commun May* 1978;19–24.
80. Rollings HE, Glassman JM, Soyka JP. Management of acute musculoskeletal pain conditions—thoracolumbar strain and sprain; a double blind evaluation comparing the efficacy and safety of carisoprodol and cyclobenzeprine. *Cuer Ther Res* 1983;34(6):917–928.
81. Harvey CH. Hypnotics and sedatives. In: Gilman AG, Goodman LS, Rall TW, Murad S, eds. *Pharmacological basis of therapeutics.* New York: MacMillan, 1985:345.
82. Basmajian JV. Reflex cervical muscle spasm: treatment by diazepam, phenobarbital or placebo. *Arch Phys Med Rehabil* 1983;64:121–124.
83. Dent RW, Ervin MS. Study of metaxalon (Skelaxin) vs placebo in acute musculoskeletal disorders: a comparative study. *Curr Ther Res* 1975;18(3):433–440.
84. Fathie K. Second look at a skeletal muscle relaxant: a double-blind study of metaxalone. *Curr Ther Res* 1964;6(1):677–683.
85. Tisdale SA, Ervin DK. A controlled study of methocarbamol (Robaxin) in acute painful musculoskeletal conditions. *Curr Ther Res* 1975;17:524–530.
86. Preston EJ, Miller CB, Herbertson RK. A double-blind, multicenter trial of methocarbamol (Roboxin) and cyclobenzeprine (Flexeril) in acute musculoskeletal conditions. *Today Ther Trends* 1984;1(4):1–11.
87. Stern TH. A controlled comparison of three muscle relaxant agents. *Clin Med* 1961;Feb:367–372.
88. Gold RH. Orphenadrine citrate in low back pain. *Clin Trial J* 1978;15(5):145–149.
89. Bakris GL, Mulopulos GP, Subhash T, Franklin C. Orphenadrine citrate: an effective alternative for muscle contraction headaches. *Ill Med J* 1982;161(2):106–108.
90. Milanov I, Georgiev D. Mechanism of tizanidine in spasicity. *Acta Neurol Scanda* 1994;89:274–279.
91. Wisendanger M, Coboz M, Palmeri A, et al. Noradrenergic mechanisms involved in muscle relaxation: significance for the treatment of spacicity. *Schweiz Acta Neurol Psychiatr* 1991;142:132–134.
92. Fryda-Kaurimsky Z, Muller-Fassbender H. Tizanidine (DS 103-282) in the treatment of acute paravertebral muscle spasm: a controlled trial comparing tizanidine and diazepam. *J Intl Med Res* 1981;9(6):501–505.
93. Shimomura T, Awaki E, Kowa H, et al. Treatment of tension-type headache with tizanidine: Its efficacy and relationship to the plasma MHPG concentration. *Headache* 1991;10:601–604.
94. Longmire DR. Bimodal dose-response to adjunctive use of tizanidine HCL in the control of myofascial pain. 18th Annual Scientific Meeting Proceedings, American Pain Society 1999:Poster #869.
95. Krusz JC, Belanger J. Tizanidine: an effective novel agent for treatment of chronic headaches. 18th Annual Scientific Meeting Proceedings, American Pain Society 1999: Poster #657.
96. Diamond S, Freitag F, Diamond ML, et al. Tizanidine in the preventative treatment of chronic tension-type headache. *Cephalalgia* 2000;20(4):335.
97. Semenchuk MR, Sherman S. Efficacy of tizanidine in neuropathic pain. 18th Annual Scientific Meeting Proceedings, American Pain Society 1999:Poster #716.

CHAPTER **21**

Pediatric and Geriatric Medication Considerations

Brenda C. McClain and Carmen R. Green

Medical advances have led to significant gains in life expectancy of Americans between the present and last century. The survival of low birth weight and extremely low birth weight infants (i.e.,1,000 g born at 23 weeks gestation) is 67 percent or better when managed at a tertiary center (1,2). The average life expectancy of Americans at birth is 77 years. The likelihood of one experiencing pain that is related to a procedure or to disease will be more probable for those at each end of the age spectrum. In addition, physiological perturbations due to age require an adapted approach to pain management. Both age groups have concerns with pharmacokinetics and pharmacodynamics. Renal clearance and hepatic metabolism of various agents will vary. Many agents have not been formally studied in children, thus the pediatric population has been described as "therapeutic orphans" (3). Recent studies on drug bioavailability, stereospecificity, and metabolism reveal that children may have metabolic pathways that are undetectable in adults. Biotransformation of theophylline into caffeine occurs in infants via N7 methylation, a metabolic process that is not found in adults (4). The volume of distribution is higher in infants for select agents and lower in the elderly; adjustments in the dose and schedule of administration are required and can vary from standard tables. Gastric motility and reflux are problems for the young and the old. Each age group is susceptible to unique alimentary dysfunctions; intestinal pneumotosis and necrotizing enterocolitis in the young and diverticulitis and colon cancer in the elderly can cause prolonged bouts of pain and/or the need for surgical intervention.

The psychosocial facet of these populations finds a significant proportion of each group dependent on others for care. Therefore, the beliefs of caregivers with regards to pain management will directly affect the patient's compliance with prescribed care regimens. Many who care for children echo fear of dispensing an overdose or that regular administration will lead to the development of addiction (5). Adult caretakers of the elderly also voice such concerns. These facts, coupled with the misconceptions that neither the very young nor the very old are reliable in conveying their pain complaint, places these populations at risk of inadequate pain control. Thus, the extremes of age present unique challenges to the pain management practitioner.

PEDIATRIC PAIN MANAGEMENT

There remains insufficient representation of pediatric pain management issues in the daily care of children with acute and chronic pain. The complexity of the pediatric pain experience is vast and is an area that is often avoided by many adult pain specialists. Neonatal, toddler, school age, and adolescent age groups each have unique concerns. Acute, persistent, and recurrent pain and chronic pain are other delineating perspectives from which pain in infants, children, and adolescents can be addressed.

The impact of the pediatric pain experience on subsequent pain and illness issues is underestimated, if not ignored. The pediatric pain experience is often discounted as being a predominantly emotional response to fear, anxiety, separation, anger, and sadness. All too often, the outcries are dismissed as something they will soon get over or not remember. Longitudinal research on early childhood pain experiences suggests long-lasting behavioral and physiological effects as a result of permanent structural and functional changes due, in part, to central sensitization (6–8). Therefore, good pain management may have far-reaching effects in a child's development of pain tolerance and coping skills.

Executing pediatric pain management services requires creativity and foresight. The daily function of a pediatric pain service relies heavily on communication among physicians, nurses, child life specialists, and other support services (9–10). The pediatric services must be distinctive for the institution and should be tailored to serve the community's needs (11). Consistency in care, administrative support, and institutional commitment are keys to success.

Pain Assessment

Because of general skepticism of self-reports of pain from children, health care professionals tend to depreciate the validity of a child's pain complaint. Further muddying of the water results from the persistence of myths regarding the presence and severity of pain in children. As a result, regular and consistent assessment of pain is not a pervasive practice. At Yale New Haven Children's Hospital, age-appropriate scales are incorporated into the biophysical profile flow sheets and pain scores are regularly recorded along with the vital signs.

The neonatal infant pain scale (NIPS) is used in the newborn special care and toddler units. The NIPS was adapted from the Children's Hospital of Ontario Pain Scale (CHEOPS). The NIPS is scored at one-minute intervals prior to, during, and after procedures. Its validity has been established and a high interrater reliability of .92 to .97 has been observed with independent observers (12). The Objective Pain Scale (OPS) is used at Yale New Haven Children's Hospital for preverbal and nonverbal children. It consists of five domains, each assessed by a 3-point scale (0–2). Concurrent validity established with the CHEOPS revealed a correlation value of .88 to .98 for postoperative pain assessment (12). Since children first learn to quantify in a vertical direction, our preferred self-report tool for young children is the Oucher scale (Fig. 21-1). The Oucher has good reliability and sensitivity and is utilized by children as young as 3 years of age. Ethnic versions of the Oucher scale are also available (Fig. 21-2). Verbal analogue scales (VAS) with anchoring descriptors of "0 equals no pain and 10 equals the worst pain you could imagine" are used for older children.

ACUTE PEDIATRIC PAIN

The first description of an anesthesiology based acute pain service was by Ready et al in 1988. This service was designed to treat severe postoperative pain in adults (13). The development of pediatric pain management programs soon followed suit; however, they did not flourish as did the upgrowth of adult pain services. There are multiple reasons for the lag in development of pediatric pain management services. Pediatric pain management, as it currently exists, is not a profitable entity for most hospitals, and therefore, it may not be given the attention or funding the issue deserves. Myths and fears about delivery of pain intervention techniques in infants, children, and adolescents persist today, despite the acknowledgment of

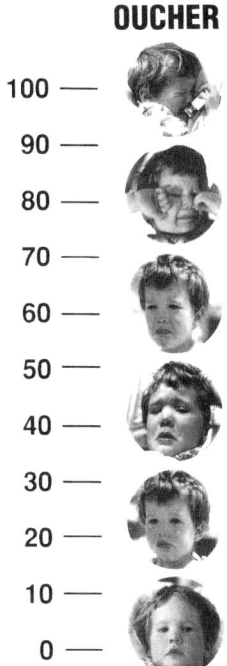

FIG. 21-1. The Caucasian version of the OUCHER score was developed and copyrighted by Judith Beyer, PhD, RN, 1983.

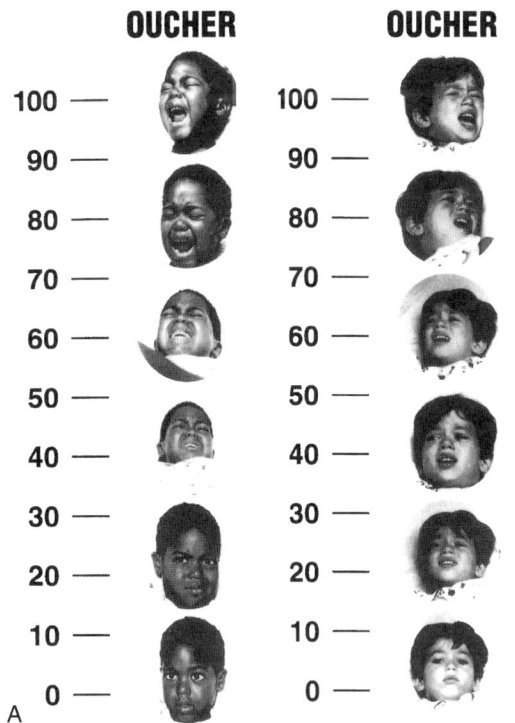

FIG. 21-2. A. The African-American version was developed and copyrighted by Mary J. Denyes, PhD, RN, Wayne State University and Antonia M Villaruel, PhD, RN, Children's Hospital of Michigan, 1990. Cornelia P. Porter, PhD, RN, and Charlotta Marshall, RN, MSN, contributed to the development of this scale. **B.** The Hispanic version was developed and copyrighted by Antonia M. Villaruel, PhD, RN, and Mary J. Denyes, PhD, RN, 1990.

necessity for pain management. These misconceptions hinder the acceptance of change in philosophies of pediatric pain management.

The evolving intricacies of pain pathophysiology and the psychosocial facets of the pain experience have resulted in the recognition of pain management as a distinct discipline. Pain can become a disease in its own right. Education is going to be key in changing the present medical culture's perspectives in pediatric pain management. Currently, educating health care professionals at the postgraduate level does not significantly change their behavior about treating pain (14). A growing number of institutions are introducing lectures on pain into their undergraduate curriculum. Changes in perspectives will take a massive and unrelenting educational effort to reshape the attitudes and behaviors of professionals toward pain management. Concerted efforts among pediatric subspecialists will be needed to make an impact on the care philosophies of children in pain.

Children encounter multiple types of acute pain due to organic or systemic disease. The pain experience is invariably impacted by the severity of the disease process, the patient's coping skills, family structure, and the timbre of the parent's rapport with the medical and nursing staff. Procedure-related pain and postoperative pain are predominant types of conditions cited in our pediatric pain service census.

PROCEDURE-RELATED PAIN

Procedural pain (e.g., bone marrow biopsies, lumbar punctures, or wound care) is usually brief and can be a daily occurrence. These encounters, despite their brevity, can be traumatic, if not brutal. There must be a well-thought-out plan of execution prior to undertaking procedures in children. Multiple modalities may be required. Current philosophy suggests the implementation of imagery and distraction since these techniques have been shown to be very effective in children. The use of topical analgesics has lessened the trauma of many procedures. A sedation unit now exists in many hospitals and affords safe completion of procedures with minimal duress for the child.

Preparation

An age-appropriate educational presentation of the potential postoperative, procedural, or disease-related pain should take place for each child. The family should be instructed with as real a description as possible of the type and potential intensity of pain that the youngster may experience. The child should be given the option of incorporating any desired support systems into the development of a pain intervention plan. This may involve bringing in a special stuffed animal, a doll, or any other toy, including electronic video games.

INTERVENTIONS

Parental Presence

Parents should be encouraged and, in most circumstances, expected to participate in the pain management of their child. Parents serve as the most fundamental source of comfort for every youngster. Parents can be quite helpful in determining the pain level experienced by the child. It is, therefore, common practice for parents to be present with the child during their entire hospital stay, including nights. In addition, it is beneficial for parents to participate in a variety of comforting measures for children during painful procedures. The analogies to the discussion of parental presence during the induction of anesthesia are obvious.

Distraction

Preschool and early school-age children are easily distracted. Techniques that have proved helpful in the management of painful procedures or painful conditions include the use of activity books, party blowers, puppet play, storytelling, and kaleidoscopes. Child-life therapists and social workers can be invaluable in designing programs of distraction to help children cope with painful situations. The pediatric anesthesiologist is well versed in a variety of distraction techniques. Many of the measures employed for induction of general anesthesia are examples of distraction.

Guided Imagery/ Hypnosis

It is critical not to underestimate the usefulness of various cognitive and behavioral techniques for pain management in children. These techniques can be applied in virtually any pain setting and can prove to be invaluable as aids for the completion of painful procedures in children. In addition, they can be exploited as an adjunct of acute pain management in postoperative, posttraumatic, or disease- and therapy-related pain crises. Hypnotic techniques require the involvement of a hypnotherapist. For the physician who is not trained in any of these techniques, it is desirable to find a nurse, social worker, child-life specialist, or psychologist who may possess these skills in addition to those of their primary profession and should be made an integral part of the pain management plan. Often the several minutes spent in teaching the young adolescent self-relaxation, guided imagery, or hypnotic techniques will prove invaluable in the course of their pain management.

A simpler technique that can be used is repeated deep breathing (15). Deep, rhythmic breathing can be accomplished by having the child blow onto a spinning pinwheel. Blowing bubbles also results in deep breathing and various types of bubble rings exist that convert this inexpensive toy into a powerful tool of relaxing distraction.

Conscious Sedation (Moderate sedation/analgesia)

The term *conscious sedation* has been revised and is now referred to as moderate sedation/analgesia and is defined as "a drug-induced depression of consciousness during which patients respond purposefully to verbal commands, either alone or accompanied by light tactile stimulation. No interventions are required to maintain a patent airway, and spontaneous ventilation is adequate. Cardiovascular function is usually maintained" (16). While criteria for credentialing in sedation are not standardized, it is clear that skills in airway management and a fund of knowledge of the sedation pharmacopoeia are crucial to safe execution of sedation. Proper monitoring and adherence to recognized guidelines are key to limiting adverse outcomes (17).

The following guidelines address pertinent issues in pediatric procedural pain (18–20).

The Children's Hospital at Yale Guidelines for Management of Painful Procedures

1. Procedures should never be completed in any of the safe havens for children (playrooms, patient rooms, waiting areas). Procedures should be conducted in a treatment room.
2. Parents should almost invariably be present for procedures, except when the parent feels that they are too uncomfortable and that their presence could heighten anxiety. Several minutes of preparation and role assignment for the parent will prove helpful for the child and the parent. Parents should not be asked to restrain children. If restraint is required, other professional caretakers should be called upon.
3. Preparation and behavioral interventions should be employed in an age- and procedure-specific way.
4. If pharmacological sedation will be employed, appropriate monitoring and personnel guidelines with adequate documentation are essential (see American Academy of Pediatrics Guidelines for Conscious Sedation, 1992, or ASA Practice Guidelines for Sedation and Analgesia by Non-Anesthesiologists, 1996).
5. Local anesthetics for skin preparation should be employed in almost every circumstance. Anticipatory use of EMLA cream (eutectic mixture of local anesthetics) or injectable 1% lidocaine should be used. If 1% lidocaine is diluted as nine parts lidocaine to one part of standard sodium bicarbonate solution, considerably less burning occurs with injection. Use a 27 to 30 g needle to inject. Numby stuff® is an iontophoretic approach that is quick and effective and should be readily available on most units. Ametop, although not yet obtainable in the United States, is applied like EMLA and is stated to have rapid onset and should be considered when it becomes available.
6. Inexperienced operators should not perform procedures on awake or minimally sedated children. The awake and frightened child should not serve as the practice subject.

The administration of sedatives, hypnotics, and analgesics for noxious procedures require adherence to the fasting guidelines as established by the American Academy of Pediatrics. At Yale New Haven Children's Hospital, 4-6-8 hour rule applies to ingestion of solids, including milk, for those children ≤4 months, ≤6 months, and >6 months, respectively. The fasting period for clear liquids is 2 hours for all age groups (19). The approved clear liquids are golden grape or apple juices, water, and Pedialyte®. There is only a modest difference in the digestibility of breast milk in comparison to cow's milk and therefore we make no distinction. The practice of sending infants for a procedure with a milk bottle to comfort them is not encouraged. If such practice is allowed and the child is unable to complete the procedure, then repeat tries of the procedure are delayed until proper Non per os (NPO) criteria are met. Children who have significant neurological, cardiac, or pulmonary histories that meet ASA III classification probably should be referred to an anesthesiologist for sedation management since the frequency of adverse events is higher for ASA classes III and IV when compared to ASA classes I and II (21).

Many mistakenly believe that orally administered agents are inherently safer because of presumed lesser potency than intravenous preparations. Only the onset of clinical effects is reliably slower. Recent studies show that the incidence of adverse events are related to drug overdose, inadequate monitoring, inadequate skills, or premature discharge (21).

The development of sedation units is controversial in part due to the confusion as to defining conscious sedation (i.e., sedation/analgesia) and which agents and doses are considered as sedative. The literature is replete with articles about ketamine and propofol in doses considered standard for the induction of general anesthesia but being described by nonanesthesiologists as sedation doses (22–24). In addition, the supervisory staff physician must be readily available to respond at a moments' notice. Remote coverage is not acceptable. Recent studies show that the frequency and severity of adverse outcomes is higher in non-hospital-based facilities. Death and permanent neurologic sequelae occurred more frequently in non-hospital-based facilities (92.8% versus 37.2%) (25). Poor outcome was due to lack of recognition of problems, inappropriate or lack of resuscitative equipment, and inadequate skills. Thus, vigilant monitoring, age-appropriate equipment, and certification in sedation and airway management are mandatory for safe execution of sedation.

SEDATIVE-HYPNOTICS

The selected agent should be based on the type of procedure. Will it be painful? Will the child need to remember or forget? What is the length of the procedure? Will the clinical effects of the selected agent outlast the procedure or is the agent short acting as to need repeated or continuous infusion? These queries are crucial to insuring the appropriate selection of agents for a given procedure.

Chloral Hydrate

Chloral hydrate is the only chloral derivative used in the United States. It is one of the most popular agents utilized in pediatric sedation. However, its margin of safety is too narrow to permit the drug to be used as a general anesthetic (23). Chloral hydrate is rapidly converted to the active metabolite trichloroethanol, which probably contributes a larger fraction to the witnessed sedative-hypnotic effects. In therapeutic doses, chloral hydrate has little effect on respiratory function or blood pressure in healthy patients. In large doses, hypotension occurs and with toxic doses untoward cardiac effects such as reentry phenomena, including torsade de pointes and severe respiratory depression, are probable (26,27). At-home administration of chloral hydrate prior to transit to a facility for a procedure has resulted in death (25). Ergo, premedication by parents without onsite professional supervision should be forbidden.

Chloral hydrate is irritating to skin and gastric mucosa, yet it should be given on an empty stomach in accordance with NPO guidelines. Vomiting may be prolonged and such patients should be observed until palliated. Excitement and delirium may occur if the patient experiences a painful stimulus. Prolonged sedation may occur since the $T_{1/2}$ is variable (4 to 12 hours). The drug should be avoided in patients with significant cardiac or hepatic disease. The combination of ethanol and chloral hydrate is known as a "Mickey Finn" (27). Chloral hydrate is available in liquid, capsule, and suppository formulations. The therapeutic oral dose is 50 to 75 mg/kg. The maximum oral pediatric dose is 2 gm. A procedural success rate of 89% has been cited for chloral hydrate. The frequencies of postdischarge side effects are sleepiness for > 4 hours in 28%, hyperactivity in 29%, unsteadiness in 68% and vomiting in 15%. Sleep deprivation does not improve the success rate (28).

Midazolam

Midazolam is a benzodiazepine with a fused imidazo ring. Like most benzodiazepines, midazolam produces prominent sedation, hypnosis, anxiolysis, muscle relaxation, and anterograde amnesia, and anticonvulsant activity. The $T_{1/2}$ is variable and is quoted as ranging from 4 to 20 hours. Potentiation of GABA-ergic pathways have been ascribed to the CNS effects (27). When used as the sole sedative, the drug has a good record of cardiopulmonary stability. However, when midazolam is administered as cotherapy with a narcotic, the results are unpredictable and a reduction in the dosing of each agent is suggested (29).

Oral doses of 0.5 to 0.75 mg/kg up to a maximum dose of 20 mg of midazolam will reliably produce anxiolysis. The unpleasant taste of midazolam can make patient acceptance difficult. The taste is disguised in cherry syrup. Intranasal administration results in stinging of the nasal mucosa, but no irritation or damage has been noted. An intranasal dose of 0.2 mg/kg produces anxiolysis in

approximately 5 minutes. This dose can be repeated once, for a maximum dose of 0.4 mg/kg (30). The 5.0 mg/ml concentration of midazolam is used for intranasal instillation. Because of possible emotional trauma, Yale New Haven Children's Hospital recommends the avoidance of rectal dosing of midazolam in children past the toddler stage. Intravenous administration has rapid onset and produces the most profound effect of the given routes of delivery. The suggested dose is 0.2 mg/kg up to 5.0 mg total. In small children, a maximum dose of 2.5 mg is usually sufficient to bring about the desired effects. If the patient is not cooperative despite administration of the maximum dose, one should reconsider the appropriateness of the drug choice. If cotherapy with a narcotic is subsequently pursued after the patient has received the maximum midazolam dose, then smaller doses of the opioid should be titrated to effect as one should proceed with caution in this situation.

Pentobarbital

Pentobarbital is a barbiturate with a $T_{1/2}$ of 15 to 48 hours. The clinical sedation may last for several hours after a hypnotic dose has been received. Oral pentobarbital was prospectively studied in infants up to 12 months with a mean age of 7 months. An oral dose of 4 to 6 mg/kg was well tolerated by the infants. Adverse effects were limited and the drug had better parental acceptance than chloral hydrate (31). Intravenous dosing ranges from 1 to 2 mg/kg, and the maximum dose is 6 mg/kg. Cardiovascular changes resemble those of natural sleep in healthy patients. However, rapid injection can cause cardiovascular collapse. Respiratory effects are minimal except in patients with pulmonary insufficiency. The barbiturates are absolutely contraindicated in patients with porphyria (i.e., acute intermittent and variegate forms), while a relative contraindication exists for patients receiving antihistamines, tricyclic antidepressants, and thyroxine (27).

Ketamine

Ketamine is a phencyclidine analog and is classified as a dissociative anesthetic due to what appears to be a disconnection between the limbic and thalamocortical areas of the brain that results in immobility, amnesia, analgesia, and a sense of being dissociated from one's surroundings (32). Nystagmus is often noted and the gaze is stuporous. Drooling can be severe and may compromise airway safety. Oral ketamine at 5 to 8 mg/kg has been effective for minimally invasive procedures, while intravenous ketamine at 1 to 2 mg/kg rapidly renders most patients anesthetized. Yet, current perspectives by nonanesthesiologists cite the aforementioned intravenous doses as the range for sedation. Generally, a much smaller dose, such as 0.25 to 0.5 mg/kg, will result in conscious sedation (33,34). Patients will appear to be awake with induction doses of 1 to 2 mg/kg; however, close examination reveals a patient who demonstrates criteria for general anesthesia. Daily dosing for repetitive procedures has shown good tolerance when the drug is administered with a benzodiazepine and antisialogogue (35). Intramuscular injection is usually withheld for combative or difficult patients. While there are no predictors for adverse outcome, intravenous access is always suggested regardless of the route of administration. Despite ketamine's safety profile, airway compromise due to laryngospasm, apnea, and emesis can occur unpredictably (36,37).

Clonidine

Clonidine is an α-2 agonist that can be administered by transdermal, epidural, intrathecal, intravenous, and oral routes. Clonidine decreases the sympathetic signs and symptoms of opioid abstinence syndrome. In children, oral clonidine has a good safety record and has been used in the treatment of attention deficit hyperactivity disorder, aggressive behavior, and self-injurious behavior (38,39). A single dose of 100 micrograms renders most patients in a cooperative state while a dose of 4 to 5 micrograms/kg often results in marked sedation with minimal cardiovascular changes when compared to a benzodiazepine premedicant (40). Administration should be at least 30 minutes prior to the procedure. The central sympatholytic effects cause sedation and a decrease in heart rate. Atropine is seldom required for bradycardia but should be readily available. Blood pressure is only mildly decreased in normal subjects, but profound hypotension can occur in patients who are dehydrated or have a history of hypertension.

PERIOPERATIVE PAIN

Postoperative pain management for children has greatly improved over the past decade. In 1984, Hawley described the misconceptions that perpetuated inadequate postoperative pain management in children, while Beyer, in 1989, documented inadequate treatment of postoperative pain for children in comparison to adults who had undergone similar operations (41,42). Since that time, the administration of analgesics to children has improved although the frequency and dosing still lags behind that of adults.

Neuraxial and Peripheral Analgesia

The use of epidural analgesia in children has waxed and waned and is again becoming popular as the field of pediatric anesthesia grows. Improvements in techniques and equipment have led to better applications of the entire spectrum of regional anesthesia in pediatric pain and anesthesia (43).

A marked difference between pediatric and adult implementation of regional anesthesia is that in children, regional techniques are often actualized after the induction of general anesthesia (44). Some may argue that the safety of inserting catheters into unaware patients is ques-

tionable since these patients are rendered unresponsive and cannot warn the physician of nerve root irritation. Thoracic epidural placement in children is more controversial and should be performed only by the most experienced physicians.

Safety in the placement of neuraxial catheters in children is paramount. Several philosophies are upheld to improve outcome. The Bromage grip with a saline-filled syringe for loss of resistance is our preferred technique for epidural insertion. The loss-of-resistance technique with an air-filled syringe has been cited in the literature as a cause of perioperative death (45). Therefore, this technique is forbidden by our pediatric pain management policies. Obtaining access into the thoracic epidural space of neonates is possible and has limited use. Because of the low anatomical placement of the neonatal spinal cord, we choose to perform epidurals in neonates at or below the L3–4 interspace. Below are suggested methods and agents for application of neuraxial analgesia.

Epidural Solutions for Continuous Infusions

The use of continuous neuraxial analgesia in children requires close monitoring and frequent and open communication among the pain service, the primary service, and the nursing staff. Some institutions have limited the use of regional techniques to a single ward or unit due to the required nursing experience and availability of monitoring. Our institution provides this service to all pediatric units. Regularly scheduled nursing in-services are required to insure education of new and rotating staff. Resuscitation equipment and parenteral agents for reversal or resuscitation must be available at all times. ECG and pulse oximetry are required for children less than one year of age, whereas only pulse oximetry is required for continuous monitoring in older children. Regular vital signs and pain scores are obtained.

Epidural solutions typically contain an opioid or clonidine plus a dilute local anesthetic. The opioids used in equal frequency by Yale Pediatric Pain Management Services are fentanyl and hydromorphone. Neonatal solutions contain either 1 microgram of fentanyl per ml of solution or 3 micrograms of hydromorphone per ml. Epidural opioid solutions for infants and older children contain either 3 micrograms of fentanyl or 10 micrograms of hydromorphone per ml.

Clonidine solutions are mixed at a concentration of 2.5 or 5.0 micrograms per ml with the maximum dose limited to 1.0 microgram/kg/hr. In our experience, bradycardia becomes most prominent at 4 to 6 hours after the start of the continuous infusion. Parameters for administration of atropine are automatically rendered in the order set as a precautionary measure. Epidural clonidine infusions are not used in our neonatal population.

The local anesthetic solutions most frequently chosen are bupivacaine at 0.031% or ropivacaine at 0.1% or 0.2%

concentrations. Regardless of the solution devised, the highest hourly dose of either amide anesthetic is 0.4 mg/kg/hr for infants and 0.2 mg/kg/hr for neonates as determined by previous clinical findings (46,47). The use of epidural lidocaine solution has the advantage of being readily assayed in any hospital. However, the occurrence of tachyphylaxis limits the use of this local anesthetic for perioperative pain management.

Caudal anesthesia and analgesia remain the cornerstones in pediatric conduction anesthesia and can be applied in a single shot or continuous fashion. Bupivacaine 0.125% to 0.5% is used for the single shot or loading dose not to exceed 2.5 mg/kg; alternatively, ropivacaine 0.1% to 0.2% is used in a similar fashion. The addition of a single dose of 5 µg/kg of caudal clonidine to the local anesthetic enhances both sensory and motor blockade, decreases intraoperative anesthetic requirements, and reduces early postoperative pain scores and analgesic requirements (48). A 2.0 microgram/kg dose of clonidine in combination with 0.1% ropivacaine provides excellent analgesia without loss of motor function (49). Typically, caudal clonidine is used if the patient has not received the drug by any other route in the preoperative period.

The use of caudal morphine mandates in-hospital observation and is reserved for planned admissions. These patients are monitored by the same protocol for continuous epidural analgesia. The duration of analgesia of caudal morphine ranges from 6 to 24 hours. Peak plasma levels of morphine after epidural injection in man occurs at 10 min-

utes (50). The dose range is 25 to 100 µg/kg; however, the lower dose has been found to have fewer complications and is as effective as the higher dose for pain control. Respiratory depression has been noted without concomitant administration of additional opiates by any other route (51,52). Therefore, it is imperative in the postoperative period that the patient be observed for a reasonable amount of time after the first administration of additional opiate, regardless of its potency. The length of observation should be based on the time of onset by route and the half-life of the given opioid. Nonsteroidal antiinflammatory agents (NSAIDs) may be tried at first complaint post-caudal morphine; however, if analgesia is inadequate from this drug class, then the pain must be appropriately treated with systemic opioids. The NSAIDs commonly used in pediatric pain management are listed in Table 21-1.

Intrathecal anesthetics are used predominantly in young and premature infants in an attempt to avoid CNS depression from general anesthesia. Positioning the patient for optimum exposure is key and care must be taken to avoid excessive head flexion and respiratory compromise. Intravenous access should be secured prior to attempting intrathecal anesthesia in the event of total spinal and respiratory embarrassment or cardiovascular collapse.

Peripheral nerve block techniques are often actualized under general anesthesia with the aid of a peripheral nerve stimulator. Insulated B-beveled regional block needles are preferred to avoid nerve trauma and to precisely locate the nerve with low frequency stimulation. Contin-

TABLE 21-1. *Nonopioid analgesic drug doses for children*

Drug	Dose(mg/kg)	Route/formulation	Comments
Acetaminophen	10–25 q 4h	PO/liquid, tablets	Limited antiinflammatory effect
Acetyl salicylic acid	10–25 q 4h	PO/tablets, chewable	Associated with Reye syndrome Antiplatelet effect, GI upset
Choline magnesium trisalicylate (Trilisate)	25 q 8–12h	PO/liquid, tablets	Less GI upset and antiplatelet effect than other NSAIDs
Ibuprofen	5–10 q 6h	PO/liquid, tablets	Antiplatelet effect, GI upset; interstitial nephritis and hepatic toxicity with chronic use
Indomethacin	1 q 8h	PO, IV, PR/liquid, tablet, suppository	Used in premature infants to close patent ductus arteriosus, suppository in postop pain
Ketorolac	0.5 (load) 0.5 q 6h 10 (total dose) q 6h	IV, IM/injectable IV, IM/injectable PO/tablets Not metabolized by cytochrome P 450	Limit to 72 hours Marked GI upset
Naproxen	5–10 q 6–8h	PO/liquid, tablets	See Ibuprofen
Tramadol	1–2 q 6h Maximum 100 mg total dose	PO/tablets	Some sedation, light-headedness Contraindicated for pts. taking systemic antifungals, tricyclic antidepressants, SSRIs

uous infusions of local anesthetics can be maintained by indwelling catheters; as a result, the postoperative pain management avoids the use of opioids and their related side effects.

Complications

The types of complications resulting from regional anesthesia are the same for children as for adults; however, because these techniques are typically initiated in an unaware, anesthetized patient, the complications may not manifest until arrival in the postanesthesia care unit (PACU) or later. Total doses and times of administration of local anesthetics and opioids and adjuvants should be documented to alert the PACU staff of propensities for changes in alertness, irritability, seizure, cardiac arrhythmias, or respiratory depression.

Post-dural puncture headaches do occur in children. Obtaining a clear history of symptoms in a younger child may be difficult, but upon examination, discomfort will increase with assumption of the upright posture. A Finnish study of children ages 6 months to 10 years revealed that approximately 5.0% of children undergoing spinal anesthesia developed position-dependent headaches (53). Treatment is supportive and includes hydration, antiemetics for nausea, and analgesics for pain. Epidural blood patch has been performed; however, the total volume of blood used can only be reported in an anecdotal fashion.

Patient-Controlled Analgesia (PCA)

PCA is a valuable tool, but the problems with its application in children are aligned with the adult experience. Some children have mastered the use of PCA as early as 4 years of age, but this is an exception, and consistent, appropriate use is not seen before 7 years of age. This cutoff correlates to the expansion of abstract thought. Generally, the guideline for a lower age limit is that at which a child can demonstrate appropriate understanding after a suitable explanation of the concept of PCA. A standardized educational program for children has been shown to alleviate concerns about addiction and overdose and empowers the child with the proper use of the technique (54). PCA has been successfully employed in the management of perioperative pain, burn care, sickle cell-related pain, mucositis pain from chemotherapy, and in at-home care of cancer pain (55–59).

Morphine remains the gold standard and is the first choice for PCA and continuous infusions. Unless it is contraindicated, a loading dose is given prior to the start of PCA. Protracted inadequacy of pain relief heightens anxiety and the likelihood of improper PCA utilization. The aim is to have the pain controlled within one hour of initiation of the intervention. Meperidine is limited to 24 hours of use due to the CNS effects of its metabolite,

normeperidine. Agents for PCA use in children do not differ from the adult experience.

Techniques of delivery vary from PCA with low-dose or high-dose continuous infusion opioid to PCA alone. There is evidence that the use of continuous background infusions are not advantageous in perioperative pain control (60). Parent-controlled and nurse-controlled analgesia (NCA) are techniques that are used in special circumstances. In a study of nurses' pain beliefs it was found that nurses appeared to judge the suitability of PCA for pediatric and geriatric patients by different criteria (61). The assumption was that children would use too much and that the elderly would use too little. Additionally, the likelihood of nurse implementation of PCA depends on their past experiences and comfort level (61). Thus, NCA should be used only with proper clinical support from the pain service.

Continuous infusions of morphine are appropriate for infants greater than 3 months of age and for children who are too young or who cannot physically use the PCA apparatus. In all cases, care must be taken to avoid oversedation, and hypoxemia has been noted, especially at nighttime. It is important to recognize that one cannot treat all pain by a single modality (62). Thus the addition of opioid-sparing agents such as NSAIDs should be added when possible.

Methadone Sliding Scale

The methadone sliding scale or "reverse PRN" is a technique that is useful in patients who are not appropriate for the use of PCA. In this regimen, the patient is assessed every 4 hours for pain intensity for 24 hours and every 6 hours thereafter. The drug is administered at the time of assessment. The dose of methadone is titrated according to the pain intensity at the time of assessment. The drug is given around the clock and is held only if significant side effects occur. The ventilatory effects of methadone in children are significantly different in comparison to morphine and meperidine. End tidal CO_2 rises to a maximum mean at 8 minutes after intravenous administration of methadone and remains elevated for 81 minutes after a single dose (63). Therefore, concomitant administration of other potentially sedating agents is withheld for one hour prior to or after the scheduled methadone dose.

Pain score	Methadone dose
Zero–Mild	25 mcg/kg
Mild–Moderate	50 mcg/kg
Moderate–Severe	75 mcg/ kg

Accumulation occurs after several days of methadone administration, and therefore, the dosing frequency is less with prolonged administration. A reduction in methadone dose may also be required. If the patient is opioid tolerant, then a 25 microgram/kg incremental increase in the sliding scale dose may be needed. Should breakthrough pain occur, it is first treated with nonsteroidal analgesics. If pain persists, then intravenous or immediate-release oral morphine is administered on a q 1 to 2 hourly Pro re nata (PRN) schedule. the next scheduled dose, then the timing of the methadone dose is adjusted and no morphine is given. Long-term use of methadone in children has been employed and the oral formulation should be utilized when appropriate.

Methadone may prove to have added benefits. There is a wealth of evidence that the d-isomer of methadone has N-methyl-D-aspartate (NMDA) receptor antagonist activity. The l-isomer may have some NMDA receptor activity as well. Methadone has also been found to lessen the development of morphine tolerance and NMDA-induced hyperalgesia thus, this agent could have a wider application than first imagined (64,65). While pain management physicians are often comfortable with the use of methadone for chronic pain, this drug still carries the stigma of being used for treatment of drug addiction.

PEDIATRIC CHRONIC PAIN

Pediatric pain management does not always mirror its adult pain counterparts in treatment philosophies. Neuroablative and implantable techniques have limited application in children and are often introduced late, being turned to as a last resort. Thus, treatment philosophies that are utilized in adults may not be widely embraced in pediatric practice. Parental perspectives on the execution of procedures and the administration of analgesics must be appreciated and can affect treatment. Most parents find the administration of rectal medications unpleasant while approximately 20% find intramuscular injections acceptable (66). This is contrary to the current pediatric pain management philosophy where we attempt to avoid intramuscular injections when possible.

Secondary gain is an issue for children as well. Release from chores, garnered attention, and school absences can cause tension among family units. The disruption of daily routines can have far-reaching effects. School absenteeism and return to the classroom environment can become a major problem if the child is allowed to remain at home for a protracted period. At-home tutoring is often instituted but does not replace the socialization provided by in-school interactions (67).

The approaches to chronic pain in children require a candid review since standard adult practices do not readily transfer to the pediatric practice. As a result of the uniqueness of pediatric chronic pain, special training in established pediatric pain centers is needed.

Types of Pediatric Chronic Pain

The true incidence of chronic pain in children is unknown but appears to be significantly less than that of the adult population. The major types of recognized pain disorders in children are as follows.

Headaches are the most common reason for a consultation with a neurologist. Over 75% of children experience headaches by age 15. The main task facing the physician evaluating childhood headache is to determine whether the headache is due to underlying systemic disease, head and neck pathology, or a benign condition. The most common organic causes of headache in children include infection, tumor, hypertension, pseudotumor cerebri, and ocular disorders (68). The presentation of children's headaches may be quite different from the adult counterparts. For example, nausea, vomiting, and abdominal pain are more pronounced in children with migraine, especially in the younger patient.

Treatment response to ibuprofen and acetaminophen is high. In those with persistent, or poorly controlled pain, sumatriptan at 0.06 mg/kg has proved effective in 91% of males; however, females experience only 68 percent resolution (69). Also, there are some children in whom the headache plays a minor role in the clinical presentation of the syndrome.

Recurrent abdominal pain syndrome (RAP) affects one in seven school-age children in the United States. Extensive testing to prove absence of disease may only heighten anxiety. Invasive examination, such as laparoscopy, is unwarranted in most cases since the percentage of patients with identifiable organic pathology is less than 10%. On the other hand, endoscopy and gastric biopsy may be worthwhile. In a small study, Helicobacter pylori had been found in half of the patients with microscopic gastritis and RAP. Eighty-four percent of all the patients with RAP had marked improvement after triple antibiotic therapy (70).

Chest pain is more common in healthy children than in children with heart disease. Episodes of Tietze's syndrome (i.e., localized swelling and pain of the costochondral joints) or Texidor's twinge (i.e., precordial postexertional pain), while benign, can be frightening and debilitating. Thus, the absence of pathology does not discount the magnitude of the problem. Reassurance is key since children may limit their activities because of unfounded fear of morbidity and contrived anticipation of death (71,72).

Fifteen percent of all school-age children experience musculoskeletal pain and approximately one-third of these children have an interruption of normal activities for longer than 3 months (73). Increasing numbers of cases of nonmalignant low back pain and sports-related injuries are requiring pediatric physical therapists, nurses, and pediatricians to be more knowledgeable of these disorders.

Fibromyalgia (FM) in children often does not strictly adhere to the 1990 criteria for fibromyalgia as set forth by the American College of Rheumatology. Preadolescent cases of FM are usually limited. Outcome studies show resolution of symptoms within one year in 75% of patients (74,75). Juvenile rheumatoid arthritis has an annual incidence of 13.9 cases per 100,000 children, resulting in persistent and recurrent pain of childhood. Pauciarticular and polyarticular forms are found.

Sickle cell disease affects 7% of African Americans. The disease is heralded by a life punctuated by acute painful episodes due to vaso-occlusion, vascular sludging, and microinfarction of bone, muscle, and viscera. Some patients endure chronic pain due to avascular necrosis of the hip or shoulder, chronic or recurrent leg ulcers, or unrelated, coexisting pain disorders. Sickle cell pain has been likened to cancer pain and similar treatment for the two diseases has been offered. However, there are frank differences. Cancer pain is mostly chronic and focal, whereas sickle cell–related pain is acute and may vary in the site and number of locations affected at each presentation (76).

Other emerging syndromes that present special problems include cystic fibrosis pain, HIV-related pain, and protracted neonatal pain. Pain due to disease is often thought of as inevitable and inadequate pain relief is mistakenly accepted as normal. However, the growing body of literature suggests lasting, untoward physiological problems may result from the undertreatment of pain.

The philosophies of treatment in pediatric chronic pain syndromes are also unique. The drug residence times for many agents differ between the child and adult. The age related pharmacodynamics and pharmacokinetics are dissimilar and dosing schedules may vary. The halflife of nortriptyline is shorter in children than in adolescents and a divided dosing schedule is sometimes recommended (77).

One must be cautious in extrapolating adult conditions and their management to the pediatric experience. Complex regional pain syndrome, Type I (CRPS I) is more common in the lower extremity in children, whereas adults experience the disorder primarily in the upper extremity. The mainstay of treatment is physical therapy for both adult and pediatric onset of CRPS I; regional blockade has not shown to have great advantage over the use of tricyclic antidepressants in children. Many believe that invasive measures to treat CRPS I may yield little benefit in children (78). The pathophysiology of CRPS I in children may differ in the prevalence of the sympathetically maintained component. Lumbar sympathetic blockade and even dense spinal blockade may not provide relief in some children. In addition, some fear that repeated invasive measures will reinforce the sick role for the child. More than one mechanism can operate in a single patient and these mechanisms may change over time (79). Psychosocial issues should be addressed in most children with chronic pain in order to foster healthy coping skills and outlooks. Thus a multidisciplinary approach involving a pain medicine physician, psychologist, physical therapist, and child-life specialist is necessary in the management of these complex presentations.

CANCER-RELATED PAIN

Malignancy is the leading cause of death due to disease in children. Trauma is the number-one cause of death in children. Approximately 10% of deaths during childhood in

the United States is related to cancer (80). Cancer pain can be divided into three major types. These are pain from direct tumor invasion, pain resulting from cancer therapy, and pain unrelated to cancer or its therapy (81). Fortunately, most pediatric neoplastic disorders do not initially present with pain. However, most children with cancer will experience pain due to procedures or therapeutic interventions. For example, the diagnostic workup may include bone marrow biopsies, repeated spinal taps, or tumor debulking and/or biopsy. Therapeutic interventions may require central venous catheter placement. Radiation therapy or chemotherapy may induce neuropathies or mucositis. Limb salvage procedures can result in direct nerve trauma. A study of 75 children who had undergone amputation secondary to trauma or cancer without chemotherapy showed similar rates of phantom limb pain (12%); however, once chemotherapy was introduced, the rate of phantom limb pain increased to 74% (82). Thus patients may experience multiple pains and discomforts throughout all phases of cancer management.

The World Health Organization ladder for cancer pain management is employed in children as well as adults. However, the use of adjuvants may be minimized or alleviated during the course of cancer therapy because of the propensity to cause blood dyscrasias. Secondly, patients may be intolerant of oral intake at a time when rectal administration is forbidden secondary to immunosuppression. Thus, exploration of alternate routes of delivery such as transdermal, intranasal, and buccal administration may be required. Epidural implantation, subarachnoid infusions, and neurolytic blocks are performed more commonly during the terminal phases of a malignancy in children (83,84). These invasive techniques are attempted later in children in comparison to the adult philosophy of cancer pain management.

The challenges of end-of-life care are many. In the pediatric experience, acceptance of the terminal illness may be late. Anxiety and anticipatory grief regarding termination of therapy, orders of "do not resuscitate," and a sense of helplessness can lead to despair. This parity compounded by inadequate pain relief for the child with cancer can lead to hopelessness and despondency for the patient and family. The use of sedative-hypnotics for intentional sedation can provide relief for the patient and will likely empower the family. Treatment is given with the intent to provide relief, but it may hasten death. Caregivers may be uncertain about whether their actions will be viewed as killing or caring because of the double effect (85,86). Educating the family that euthanasia is not the intent is mandatory prior to starting a continuous infusion of hypnotics.

Hospice care for children represents a comprehensive approach to delivering quality care to families confronting terminal illness. This specialized care is delivered in both hospital and at-home settings. The benefits of home include more freedom, less disruption of family life and assurance of privacy. Successful at-home care depends on adequate support from hospital-based teams. This will help lessen the family's fears about symptomatic care (87,88).

PHARMACOTHERAPEUTICS IN PEDIATRIC PAIN

The use of pharmaceuticals is key to pain intervention during many aspects of pain management in children. In cancer pain management, opioids are the cornerstone of care. The management of nonmalignant pain in children usually does not require chronic opioid administration. However, the use of opioids should not be withheld when indicated. The risk of addiction is low in children where opioids are given appropriately for pain.

Opioids

Codeine is the most frequently prescribed narcotic for children. Its safety and efficacy have been overrated. Respiratory depression and obtundation have been documented at doses greater than 5 mg/kg/d. The antitussive claims of codeine have not been proven (89). Codeine is not less addictive than other opioids and prescribing with such intent is the misconception of many (90). The published dose recommendation for codeine is 1 mg/kg/day in four divided doses (89); however, higher doses of 0.5 to 1.0 mg/kg/dose are common in perioperative pain management. A greater frequency than every 6 hours may be needed for control of moderately severe pain.

Tramadol is available in the United States only in an oral formulation. The potency is similar to that of meperidine. The respiratory depressant effects are less than the latter. Tramadol is a μ-receptor agonist and serotonin reuptake inhibitor and has the potential of precipitating a hypertensive event when given to patients chronically receiving tricyclic antidepressants. The serotonin syndrome characterized by acute autonomic instability, neuromuscular changes, and cognitive-behavioral changes has been described for tramadol when given in co-administration with fluoxetine, paroxetine, or sertraline (91–93).

To date, there have been two pediatric prospective studies examining the efficacy and appropriateness of transdermal fentanyl analgesic delivery in children (94,95). Children with cancer pain and sickle cell disease have displayed limited adverse response and good tolerance of this technique. In these studies it appears that transdermal fentanyl is more appropriate for cancer pain than for recurrent pain. Prior opioid exposure and demonstration of well-established opioid requirements are mandatory for safe use. Patients must be receiving at least 45 mg of oral morphine equivalents to use the 25 microgram/hr patch. The pharmacokinetics in children reveal a slightly higher rate of clearance, but this difference does not alter the prescribing regimen (95). The patch is changed every 72 hours. A stable analgesic requirement is preferred, but this mode of opioid delivery can be employed in patients with

breakthrough or escalating pain where co-administration of immediate-release opioid preparations is needed. A 12.5 microgram/hr patch is being developed and will be marketed in the near future.

Subcutaneous infusion of opioids is an alternative mode of delivery when intravenous access is not possible. Effective analgesia can also be obtained via a secured butterfly needle or via a 22- or 24-gauge intravenous catheter placed subcutaneously. The site must be rotated weekly to avoid irritation. Morphine or hydromorphone can be used for this mode of delivery, but the latter has a higher solubility and is preferred (96). Most patients will experience some discomfort during bolus administration, but in general, patients tolerate this technique well. The dosing used is similar to intravenous PCA (Table 21-2).

Sustained-release preparations of morphine and oxycodone are available with a recommended scheduling of 12- or 24-hour intervals. Bioequivalence of these preparations shows marked differences in plasma levels with the least fluctuations noted with once daily (eg., Kapanol®) formulations. MS Contin tablets can be administered rectally and results in a slower rate but greater extent of adsorption. Controlled-release suppositories designed for rectal administration have less variability (97).

Nonsteroidal Antiinflammatory Drugs (NSAIDs)

NSAIDs are used in a wide spectrum of pediatric indications. Uses for NSAIDs in pediatrics include treatment of juvenile rheumatoid arthritis, musculoskeletal pain, dysmenorrhea, patent ductus arteriosus closure, opioid sparing, and perioperative pain (98). NSAIDs are the first step in the World Health Organization's cancer pain ladder and are used in chronic nonmalignant pain in children. The risks of renal failure, gastritis, and NSAIDs toxicity must always be kept in mind with chronic administration (Table 21-1)

COX-2 selective inhibitors such as celecoxib and rofecoxib are sulfonamides that are selective cyclooxygenase-2 isoform inhibitors. Platelet function is not affected by COX-2 inhibitors (99). Less gastric irritation has been noted when compared to nonselective NSAIDs and rofecoxib has fewer effects on the GI tract than does celecoxib. Guidelines for the use of COX-2 inhibitors in children are not established; however, these agents may prove beneficial in pediatric pain management. NSAIDs and COX-2 inhibitors should not be given to patients with a history of asthma, nasal polyps, rhinitis, or renal dysfunction.

Adjuvants

The use of adjuvant therapy in the management of neuropathic pain is a long-accepted practice. The utility of antidepressants in the management of neuropathic pain is better established than antiepileptics (100). Tricyclic antidepressants have been found to consistently improve pain

TABLE 21-2. *Opioid analgesic drugs—pediatric dosing*

Drug	Dose (mg/kg)	Dosing interval	Comments
Codeine	0.25–1.0 PO	Q 4 h	Dose limited by side effects of constipation, nausea, vomiting, combined with fix amount of acetaminophen
Fentanyl	0.001 L.D. (IV)	Q 1–2 h	For acute perioperative or procedure pain
	0.002–0.004 (CI)	Hourly infusion rate	Continuous infusion ± PCA for moderate to severe pain
	0.010–0.015 (Oral)	X 1 transmucosal solid formulation	For procedures, pt. self-titrates to sedative effect
Hydromorphone	0.015–0.020 (IV)	Q 3–4 h	
	0.004–0.006 (IV)	Hourly rate	Continuous infusion ± PCA for moderate to severe pain
Meperidine	0.5–1.0 (IV)	Q 2–4 h	Do not exceed 600 mg/day, active metabolite lowers seizure threshold
Methadone	0.05–0.10 (IV)	Q 4 h x 24h then q 6–8 h	Long acting after 4th dose, observe closely
	0.10–0.30 (PO)	Q 8–12 h	For established patients receiving opioid
Morphine	0.10 (IV)	Q 2–3 h	Histamine release, pruritus
	0.015–0.03 (IV)	Hourly rate	Continuous infusion ± PCA
	0.3 (PO)	Q 3–4 h	
PCA	0.05–0.1	Loading dose	For postoperative pain; higher doses may be needed in sickle cell or cancer-related pain
	0.01–0.02	Bolus wth 6–10 min L.O.	
	0.01–0.02	Hourly background infusion rate	
Oxycodone	0.15 (PO)	Q 4h	Commonly used for postoperative pain when oral meds are appropriate

as opposed to the selective serotonin reuptake inhibitors (SSRIs). Antidepressants are used to aid sleep, improve opioid analgesia, and provide inherent analgesia when used alone. Because of the propensity of the tricyclics to cause rhythm disturbances, all patients should undergo baseline electrocardiogram, liver function testing, and complete blood count before starting chronic administration (Table 21-3).

Anticonvulsants that are commonly used in pediatric pain include carbamazepine and phenytoin. Gabapentin is a second-generation antiepileptic. This γ amino acid drug crosses the blood–brain barrier. There is no interaction with other antiepileptics. Starting doses of 5 to 10 mg/kg/d have been used with minimal side effects. New onset behavioral changes may be seen at doses of 15 mg/kg/d, but these improve with dose reduction or cessation of the drug (100). Gabapentin, with its low incidence of adverse effects, may prove to be a better first-line choice in the management of neuropathic pain in children.

CONCLUSION

There is a desire to establish better pain management protocols for children, but myths and unfounded fears impede progress. It is imperative that the pain clinician commit to addressing all the facets of the pediatric pain experience. The psychological and psychosocial risk factors for the onset and development of chronic pediatric pain may be significant. Since there is some evidence of a continuum of the pain experience, it is requisite that the treatment of acute pain be addressed with the vigilance that is used in adult chronic pain intervention.

PAIN MANAGEMENT IN THE ELDERLY

Medical advances and interventions have yielded significant gains in the life expectancy of Americans between the present and last century. Americans who are now 65 years of age can expect to live an additional 18 years (age 83), while those 75 years of age can be expected to live an average of 11 years more (86 years) (101). Increased longevity has not necessarily yielded improvements in quality of life. By the year 2030, an estimated 20% of the nation's population will be over 65 years of age. At the same time every other patient seen by a family doctor will be elderly. Thus, physicians will be challenged to evaluate and treat an older population with multiple medical problems and end-of-life issues in unprecedented numbers.

TABLE 21-3. *Adjuvants in pediatric pain management*

Drug	Drug and oral dosage	Uses	Comments
Tricyclic antidepressants	Amitriptyline 0.2–2.0 mg/kg q HS Starting dose is 10 mg	TCAs	Anticholinergic effects (somnolence, dry mouth, tachycardia) Start low and increase slowly
		Decrease pain by altering central processing Aid sleep	Obtain baseline ECG and LFTs for TCAs
	Nortiptyline: same as above Desipramine: same as above	Augment opioid analgesia	Less sedating than amitriptyline
	Doxepin: same as above		Most sedating
	Trazodone 0.2–2.0mg/kg		Avoid in males due to risk of priapism
Anticonvulsants	Phenytoin 5mg/kg/day ÷ BID Carbamazepine 10–20 mg/kg/day ÷ BID	Neuropathic pain Same as above	Obtain baseline CBC for anticonvulsants SI. Sedation with all anticonvulsants listed
	Clonazepam 0.5–1.0 mg/dose	Same as above + restless leg syndrome, TMJ	
	Gabapentin 10–30 mg/kg/day ÷ TID		Dizziness; occas.mild, reversible behavioral changes
Benzodiazepines	Midazolam: 0.1–0.2	For postoperative muscle spasm and associated pain	Maximum oral dose is 20 mg regardless of weight
	Midazolam: 0.4–0.7	Anxiolysis, premedicant	
	Diazepam: 0.02–0.1 q 6–8 h	Anxiolysis, muscle spasm	
	Lorazepam 0.02–0.05	Sedation	

Health and well-being is a broader concept than that typically applied in clinical medicine, transcending both physical disease and emotional distress (102–104). Healthy days (a health-related quality-of-life measure) are limited by chronic conditions such as pain. The contribution of spiritual and psychological factors to health must also be evaluated. Chronic pain affects more than 75 million Americans and is associated with greater than 60 billion dollars in health care expenditures in the United States annually (105–108). Contributing to the age-related differences in chronic pain is an increased incidence of chronic conditions in the elderly (e.g., osteoarthritis, back pain, leg pain, and neuropathic pain) (109). However, the increased prevalence of chronic pain in older people is not well characterized nor has it been well studied. Psychological functioning, quality of life, level of disability, and pain perception in the elderly patient with chronic pain are important factors to consider in an aging population. Most studies of pain in this population have suffered from a significant selection bias: using predominantly Caucasian and nursing-home populations (110). Very little information is available about older Americans with chronic pain living independently in the community and receiving care in a tertiary care (e.g., pain clinic) or primary care setting. A confounding variable of most epidemiologic studies of pain in the elderly is that pain was not the primary symptom evaluated.

Improvements in life expectancy and health status have not been uniform for all Americans (111–124). Pain is one of the most frequent complaints of older Americans. Clearly, inadequate pain control has a significant impact on patient well-being and quality of life. The potential impact of the racial, ethnic, and gender variables on chronic pain has also not been well studied (125,126). Many chronic conditions such as osteoporosis put women at an increased risk for chronic pain and disability (106,127–131). In our aging society, women comprise nearly 60% of the population greater than 60 years of age (132). If this trend continues, women will account for nearly 75% of persons over 85 years of age. The impact of chronic pain in elderly women cannot be minimized (133,134). Despite an increased life expectancy, the quality of life of older women may be worse than their male counterpart (135,136). Minority elderly currently account for 16% of the elderly population and are expected to grow to 22% in the next 20 years. Studies in racial and ethnic minority elders show an increased number of comorbidities (e.g., cardiac disease, diabetes), as well as increased severity of these chronic diseases (111,126,137,138). Overall racial minority elders rate their health status lower (i.e., fair or poor) than Caucasian elders (139). These findings support the reported health disparities and a reduction in life expectancy, quality of life, and healthy years for minority elders while putting them at increased risk for the disabling effects of chronic pain (135,136).

PAIN PERCEPTION

The interactions between aging and pain perception have significant relevance to chronic pain management. Many studies have attempted to evaluate the effect of aging on pain perception and pain thresholds with variable results (139,140). A number of studies have pointed to decreased pain sensitivity in the elderly. However, these aging effects in the laboratory have not been able to be extrapolated or correlated with clinical pain. Age seems to have a variable influence on the experience of pain. What is clear is that advanced age appears to increase the risk of silent myocardial ischemia, afebrile pneumonia, and postherpetic neuralgia. When treating elderly patients, physicians should have a high index of suspicion since the pain experience may differ from younger patients.

PAIN ASSESSMENT

The measurement of pain is an exquisitely personal experience, which is poorly quantified in the elderly. Overall the basic tools utilized to assess for the presence of chronic pain in a general adult population can be used in the elderly population as well (141–145). Initial assessment of pain requires a thorough history and physical. The gold standard of pain assessment remains self-report. All attempts to identify the etiology of the pain complaint in the elderly should be identified. Most pain scales have been shown to be reliable in the elderly even in the presence of mild to moderate cognitive impairment (146). However, elderly patients may minimize the impact of pain on their lives and use descriptors other than "pain" to describe their condition. This may be due in part that older patients frequently believe that pain is a normal part of aging.

Pain in the aging patient does not occur in isolation and has a significant impact on the caregiver (147,148). Thus the adequate assessment and treatment of chronic pain in the elderly requires evaluation of multiple and often competing psychosocial, financial, cultural, social, and spiritual factors. Many tools have been modified or developed specifically for the elderly in order to provide a comprehensive assessment of the intensity of pain and to identify the impact of pain in this population (Fig. 21-3).

   I. On initial presentation of any older person to any health care service, a health care professional

should assess the patient for evidence of chronic pain.

  II. Any persistent or recurrent pain that has a significant impact on function or quality of life should be recognized as a significant problem.

 III. A variety of terms synonymous with pain should be used to screen older patients (e.g., burning, discomfort, aching, soreness, heaviness, tightness).

 IV. For those with cognitive or language impairments, nonverbal pain behavior, recent changes in function, and vocalizations suggest pain as a potential cause (e.g., changes in gait, withdrawn or agitated behavior, moaning, groaning, or crying).

  V. For those with cognitive or language impairments, reports from a caregiver should be sought.

 VI. Conditions that require specific interventions should be identified and treated definitively if possible.
    A. Underlying disease should be managed optimally.
    B. Patients who need specialized services or skilled procedures should be referred for consultation to a health care specialist who has expertise in such services and procedures.
      1. Patients identified as having debilitating psychiatric complications should be referred for psychiatric consultation.
      2. Patients identified as abusing or as being addicted to any legal or illicit substance should be referred for consultation with an expert who has experience in pain and addiction management.
      3. Patients with life-altering intractable pain should be referred to a multidisciplinary pain management center.

 VII. All patients with chronic pain should undergo comprehensive pain assessment. (Figure 21-3 provides an example of a medical record form that can be used to summarize the initial pain assessment.)
    A. Comprehensive pain assessment should include a medical history and physical examination, as well as a review of the results of the pertinent laboratory and other diagnostic tests, with the goals of recording a temporal sequence of events that led to the present pain complaint and establishing a definitive diagnosis, plan for care, and likely prognosis.
    B. Initial evaluation of the present pain complaint should include characteristics such as intensity, character, frequency (or pattern, or both), location, duration, and precipitating and relieving factors.
    C. Initial evaluation should include a thorough analgesic medication history, including current and previously used prescription medications, over-the-counter medications, and "natural"

GERIATRIC PAIN ASSESSMENT

Date:_____   Medical Record_____

Patient's Name _____

Problem List: Medications:

_____   _____

_____   _____

_____   _____

_____   _____

_____

Pain Description

Pattern:	Constant	Intermittent	Pain Intensity
			0 1 2
Duration:_____			None
Location:_____			
Character:			Worst Pain
Lancination	Burning	Stinging	0 1 2
Radiating	Shooting	Tingling	None

Other Descriptors:

FIG. 21-3. Example of a medical record form that can be usesd to summarize pain assessment in older persons (From anonymous: *J Am Geriatr Soc* 1998;46(5):635–651.)

remedies. The effectiveness and any side effects of current and previously used medications should be recorded.

D. Initial evaluation should include a comprehensive physical examination with particular focus on the neuromuscular system (e.g., search for neurologic impairments, weakness, hyperalgesia, hyperpathia, allodynia, numbness, paresthesia) and the musculoskeletal system (e.g., palpation for tenderness, inflammation, deformity, trigger points).

E. Initial evaluation should include evaluation of physical function.

   1. Evaluation of physical function should include a focus on pain-associated disabilities, including activities of daily living (e.g., Katz ADLs, Lawton IADLs, FIMS, Barthel Index).

   2. Evaluation of physical function should include performance measures of function (e.g., range of motion, Up-and-Go Test, Tinetti Gait and Balance Test).

F. Initial evaluation should include evaluation of psychosocial function.

   1. Evaluation of psychosocial function should include assessment of the patient's mood, especially for depression (e.g., a Geriatric Depression Scale, Brief Symptom Inventory, Beck Depression Inventory, CES-D scale).

   2. Evaluation of psychosocial function should include assessment of the patient's

social networks, including any dysfunctional relationships.

G. A quantitative assessment of pain should be recorded by the use of a standard pain scale (e.g., visual analogue scale, word descriptor scale, numerical scale).

   1. Patients with cognitive or language barriers should be presented with scales that are tailored for their needs and disabilities (e.g., scales adapted for speakers of a foreign language, scales in large print, or scales for the visually impaired that do not require visual-spatial skills).

   2. Quantitative estimates of pain based on clinical impressions or surrogate reports should not be used unless the patient is unable to reliably make his or her needs known.

VIII. Patients with chronic pain and their caregivers should be instructed to use a pain log or pain diary with regular entries for pain intensity, medication use, response to treatment, and associated activities.

IX. Patients with chronic pain should be reassessed regularly for improvement, deterioration, or complications attributable to treatment. The frequency of follow-up should be a function of the severity of the pain syndrome and the potential for adverse effects of treatment.

A. Reassessment should include evaluation of significant issues identified in the initial evaluation.

B. The same quantitative assessment scales should be used for follow-up assessments.

C. Reassessment should include an evaluation of analgesic medication use, side effects, and adherence problems.

D. Reassessment should include an evaluation of the positive and negative effects of any non-pharmacologic treatments (149).

COMORBIDITIES IN ELDERLY PATIENTS WITH PAIN

Depression and Sleep Disorder

Older patients are more likely to suffer from more than one chronic condition or disease at any time. Sleep perturbations and depression are quite common in older patients and are not merely a function of aging (150–162). Unfortunately, in the elderly, symptoms of clinical depression are subtle and easily dismissed as part of the aging process, thereby contributing to further disability. It is estimated that nearly 2 million of the 34 million Americans greater than 65 years of age suffer from some form of depression. There is also data to suggest that physicians often miss mental health problems or misdiagnose depression in older adults, leading to their undertreatment (154, 156,159).

Elderly patients often do not discuss their symptoms of sadness due to the potential stigma associated with depression and fears that these revelations may lead to their loss of independence. New data suggests that the elderly may benefit more from a multidisciplinary approach to the management of depression.

Depression and concomitant sleep disturbance are very prevalent in patients with chronic pain. It is difficult to have a worthwhile reduction in pain intensity without improving depression and enhancing the quality of sleep (104). In the geriatric chronic pain patient, it is important for physicians to have a high index of suspicion for confounding problems of depression and sleep disturbance (163). Physicians treating elderly patients with pain must also recognize that (1) they often do not present with classic symptoms, (2) problems with sleep and symptoms consistent with depression are not a normal function of aging, (3) psychotherapy and supportive counseling are often helpful, and (4) in order to obtain the best clinical pain outcomes these problems must be recognized and treated. Small doses of antidepressants in the elderly can yield modest improvements in sleep and depression. Improvements in sleep and depression can in turn lead to significant reductions in pain resulting in a dramatic impact on quality of life.

PHARMACOKINETICS OF MEDICATIONS USED FOR PAIN CONTROL

Pharmacokinetics depicts the absorption, distribution, metabolism, and elimination of drugs, which are of significant importance in the elderly. Age-related changes in pharmacokinetics are often manifested as a prolongation of elimination half times, making the elderly particularly vulnerable to cumulative drug effects and adverse drug reactions. Absorption is reduced with aging due to reduction in gastric emptying and cardiac output. Both renal and hepatic changes occur due to decreased vascularity and perfusion as well as loss of tissue mass leading to functional changes in the liver and kidney. Reductions in the metabolic capacity of the liver with liver disease lead to decreases in hepatic blood flow, hepatocellular mass, and plasma protein binding. Aging is associated with a progressive decline in renal blood flow, which may put elderly patients at an increased risk of fluid overload and the nephrotoxic effects of drugs (e.g., NSAIDs) (Table 21-4). The increase in total body water and the resulting edema can lead to alterations in the distribution characteristics of a drug. Three major alterations in the elderly body components occur: (1) an increase in lipid content from 14% to 30% by age 70, (2) a 25% to 30% decrease in soft tissue and muscle, and (3) an 18% decline in intracellular water. The net result is decreased drug clearance and an inability to withstand salts or water loads. With aging, there is a progressive reduction in CNS activity and peripheral nerve conduction. Increased permeability of the blood–brain barrier may occur with aging, which may result in increased sensitivity to pharmacologic agents. Elderly patients are particularly vulnerable to cumulative drug effects with repeated dosing due to decreased clearance and an increased volume of distribution (Table 21.5).

Beyond pharmacokinetic changes, pharmacodynamic changes in the elderly play a major role and account for the primary differences seen in drug effects in the elderly. Overall, the elderly are more sensitive to a given concentration of a drug and may require a decreased dose of most drugs. This is important to consider since multiple diagnoses may lead to the concomitant administration of multiple medications, which require the same pathway for metabolism, clearance, and elimination (Figures 21-4 and 21-5).

THERAPEUTIC APPROACHES TO THE MANAGEMENT OF PAIN IN THE ELDERLY

General Principles

Major efforts in health care policy and education have been directed at the prevention of medical errors and adverse events. The past few years have revealed excessive prescribing of inappropriate and unnecessary drug therapies in the elderly. Concerns about excess drug prescribing in this population are reasonable, but underprescribing to improve quality of care may be seriously misdirected. A number of studies have illustrated the adverse consequences associated with underprescribing of beneficial therapies in the elderly. Adverse effects in the elderly may be a function of the number of drugs and not merely a function of age (164,165).

The major goal of chronic pain management is to provide effective analgesia with minimal side effects. First, it is necessary to determine the source of the pain. Management begins with the use of nonpharmacologic techniques, NSAIDs, antidepressants, anticonvulsants, and opioids in an attempt to control pain and to reduce nerve firing that relay painful impulses. Although designed for the management of cancer pain, the World Health Organization (WHO) stepwise progression from weak to strong opioid ladder provides a sound framework for the management of all types of pain regardless of the age of the patient. Supportive care and psychological counseling are not mentioned in the WHO ladder but are important therapies to utilize to enhance pain management in the elderly (166). Of particular importance is the use of a multidisciplinary team, which allows the elderly patient with pain to receive total care.

Alternative/Complementary and Nonpharmacologic Approaches

It is estimated that greater than 10% of Americans utilize some form of alternative or complementary medication in the pursuit of natural regimens to treat disease or to maintain health (167). Alternative and complementary

TABLE 21-4. *Nonsteroidal antiinflammatory drugs for the elderly*

Drug	Maximum dosage	Pharmacologic changes	Precautions and recommendations
Acetaminophen	4000 mg/24 h (q 4–6 h dosing)	Hepatotoxic above maximum dose	Mild pain, avoid exceeding maximum recommended dose
Aspirin	4000 mg/24 h (q 4–6 h dosing)	Gastric bleeding, dyspepsia, abnormal platelet function, hypersensitive	Mild pain, avoid high doses for prolonged periods of time, may enhance effects of oral hypoglycemics
Ibuprofen	2400 mg/24 h (q 4–6 h dosing)	Gastric bleeding, dyspepsia, renal, and abnormal platelet function, hyper-sensitive, side effects may be more common in older patients	Mild pain, joint pain, avoid high doses for prolonged periods, caution in renal insufficiency
Naproxen	1000 mg/24 h (q 8–12 h dosing)	Similar toxicity to ibuprofen	Mild pain, joint pain, avoid high doses for prolonged periods, caution in renal insufficiency
Rofecoxib	25 mg/24 h (q 12–24 h dosing)	Not metabolized by cytochrome P 450	Mild pain, joint pain, avoid high doses for prolonged periods, caution in renal insufficiency Drug interactions can occur with rifampin, methotrexate, and warfarin Similar to rofecoxib
Celecoxib	400 mg/24 h (q 12–24 h dosing)	Contraindicated in patients with a sulfa allergy • Borderline elevations of LFTs can occur • Avoid in aspirin-sensitive patients • Can cause fluid retention and edema if there are no contraindications Metabolized by cytochrome P 450	Mild pain, joint pain, avoid high doses for prolonged periods, caution in renal insufficiency May be used for acute pain at higher doses of up to 50 mg/24 h for 5 days • Use lowest dose possible to prevent GI bleeding • Caution in renal insufficiency • Caution in patients with history of perforated ulcer or bleeding • Avoid in patients with uncontrolled hypertension, peripheral edema, CHF • May need to reduce dose in the elderly • Avoid in aspirin-sensitive patients

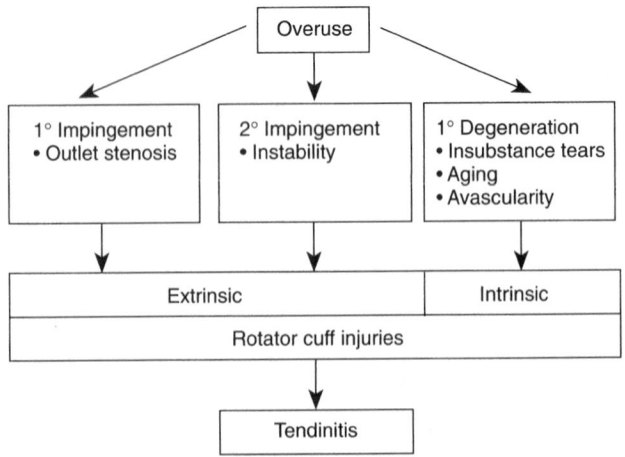

FIG. 21-4. Etiology of rotator cuff tendinitis. Tendinitis is multifactorial and not just due to primary impingement. Extrinsic causes are from outside the rotator cuff. Intrinsic causes are a primary breakdown of the cuff. Extrinsic and intrinsic injuries to the rotator cuff are exacerbated by overuse syndromes. Primary and secondary causes of impingment lead to an indistinguishable tendinitis pattern.

techniques have gained great popularity for the management of pain (168). The problem with these techniques is that complementary pharmacologic agents are not without risks. Often the mechanisms of action and side effect profiles of these agents are not well described. Elderly patients may be at an increased risk of adverse events due to unforeseen drug interactions (169). It is critical during the assessment and history phase of the interview that patients are specifically asked about their use of complementary and alternative therapies.

Nonpharmacologic strategies are rarely sufficient for the management of mild or severe pain but can be utilized as adjuncts to pharmacologic care (Table 21-5). Cognitive and behavioral techniques (e.g., relaxation training, guided imagery, biofeedback, counseling), as well as physical interventions (e.g., ice, heat, massage), are extremely helpful for patients with pain. Studies have also documented that utilization of the TENS unit, acupressure, and acupuncture can enhance the activity of traditional opioid analgesics to help modulate the pain response.

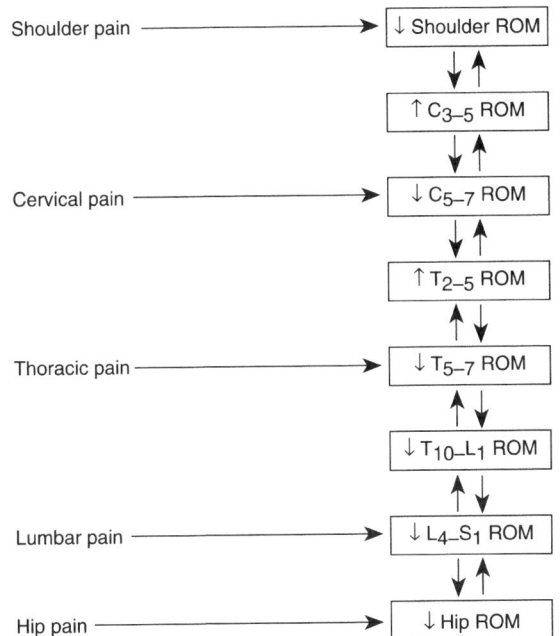

FIG. 21-5. The motion cascade. C = cervical, T = thoracic, L = lumbar, S = sacral, ROM = range of motion. Downward arrows indicate a decrease, upward arrows an increase. (Courtesy of Aquatecnics Consulting Group, Aptos, CA.)

TABLE 21-5. *Opioid analgesic drugs— geriatric dosing*

Drug	Oral equivalent	Starting dosage
Mild		
Tramadol		50 mg q 6–12 h
Propoxyphene		
Moderate		
Codeine	120 mg	30–60 mg q 4–6 h
Hydrocodone	30 mg	5–10 mg q 3–4 h
Oxycodone	20–30 mg	5–10 mg q 3–4 h
Sustained-release* oxycodone	20–30 mg	10–20 mg q 12 h or 24 h
Severe		
Morphine sulfate	30 mg	15–30 mg q 4 h
Sustained-release* morphine	30 mg	15–30 mg q 12 h or 24 h
Hydromorphone	7.5 mg	1.5 mg q 3–4 h
Methadone	2.5–5 mg	2.5-5 mg q 8–12 h
Transdermal fentanyl	12.5 mg	25 mg/h q 3 days
*Activity may last longer in the elderly		

*Sustained-release formulas are not to be broken, crushed, or dissolved in order to provide continuous activity.

Nonopioid Analgesics

A variety of agents other than opioids are useful analgesics for pain management (170). The most prominent of these are the nonsteroidal antiinflammatory drugs (NSAIDs). Many studies have supported a reduction in analgesic requirements with this class of agents. Acetaminophen has been shown to have significant analgesic and opioid-sparing effects. A maximum daily dose of 4000 mg of acetaminophen limits its use alone and as a combination product. Aspirin is useful due to its significant antiinflammatory properties but has minimal analgesic effects.

NSAIDs have the ability to provide prostaglandin analgesia both peripherally and centrally via inhibition of cyclooxygenase-1(COX-1). Side effects associated with NSAIDs (e.g., ibuprofen, indomethacin) include impairment of platelet aggregation and other nonspecific complaints (171,172). Reductions in gastric emptying in the elderly can lead to nausea and gastrointestinal irritation. Unlike the opioids, NSAIDs provide analgesia with less nausea, vomiting, sedation, and constipation. A number of studies have shown the efficacy of these drugs with a reduction in pain scores. The introduction of agents that inhibit cyclooxygenase-2 (COX-2) (e.g., rofecoxib, celecoxib), has provided an alternative for those patients who have not been able to tolerate the gastrointestinal (GI) side effects or are at risk for gastrointestinal bleeding associated with NSAID. However, the outcome data for the use of the new COX-2 agents in the elderly is limited. Caution should be used when using these agents (especially rofecoxib) in the elderly patient with a history of gastrointestinal bleeding,

peripheral edema, and congestive heart failure since it may worsen these problems (173). Celecoxib is contraindicated in the patient who is allergic to sulfa compounds. The use of NSAID alone for the management of moderate to severe pain remains controversial and probably depends on the underlying etiology of the pain (174).

Antidepressants and Anticonvulsants

Use of antidepressants in the elderly population is very common (175). Important considerations when treating the elderly patient with antidepressants include evaluation of the efficacy and safety profile. The elderly are more prone to the side effects of the antidepressants (especially the older tricyclic antidepressants), which are often used for the management of pain and sleep disturbance. Although tricyclic antidepressants (TCA) remain a mainstay for the management of neuropathic pain, their anticholinergic side effects can be problematic in elderly patients. Patients at risk for serious anticholinergic toxicity include those with benign prostatic hypertrophy (BPH), dementia of organic basis, and narrow angle glaucoma. In the elderly patient who frequently gets up during the night, TCA administered at nighttime can put them at risk for falls due to sedation and orthostatic hypotension. The incidence of orthostatic hypotension increases in patients with congestive heart failure, peripheral neuropathy, and those patients utilizing antihypertensives (Table 21-6).

TABLE 21-6. *Adjuvants for analgesia in the elderly*

Drug	Starting dose (PO)	Indications	Major side effects	Precautions and recommendations
Anticonvulsants				
Clonazepam	0.25–0.5 mg	Neuropathic pain	Sedation	
Carbamazepine	100 mg	Only for lancinating pain (e.g., trigeminal neuralgia, postherpetic neuralgia)	Common sedation, anxiety, ataxia, dizziness, leukopenia, thrombocytopenia, and rarely aplastic anemia	Start at 100 mg qd, increase slowly bid, 200 mg qd, then bid; check LFTs, CBC, RF at baseline; CBC at 2 then 8 weeks
Valproate	125 mg	Neuropathic pain	Gastrointestinal, tremor	Similar to carbamazepine
Gabapentin	100 mg	Neuropathic pain	Less serious side effects but nausea, confusion, and dizziness may occur more frequently in the elderly	Start with low dose (100 mg) and titrate up slowly to effect; neuropathic doses not yet established; titrate to tid dosing; monitor for idiosyncratic side effects (e.g., ankle swelling, ataxia), dose range for efficacy anecdotally reported 100–800 mg tid
Lamotrigine	25 mg	Neuropathic pain		
Antiarrhythmics				
Mexiletine (Mexitil)	150 mg	Neuropathic pain	Side effects such as tremor, dizziness, unsteadiness, paresthesias are common; rarely hepatic damage and blood dyscrasias occur	Avoid use in patients with preexisting heart disease; start with low dose and titrate slowly; recommend initial and follow-up ECGs; titrate to tid-qid dosing
Lidoderm	Patch size 4 × 5½ cm (may be cut)	Postherpetic neuralgia		Maximum time frame is 12 hours with a maximum of 3 patches at a time. Avoid in patients on Class I antiarrhythmic.
Other agents				
Baclofen	5 mg	Neuropathic pain, muscle spasms	Probable increased sensitivity and decreased clearance	Monitor for weakness, urinary dysfunction; avoid abrupt discontinuation due to CNS irritability

CBC = complete blood cell count
CNS = central nervous system
ECG = electrocardiogram
LFT = liver function tests
RF = renal function
HS = hour of sleep or at bedtime

Newer nontricyclic antidepressants (e.g., selective serotonin reuptake inhibitors (SSRIs) have fewer side effects and are generally safer than the TCA. Although fluoxetine, citalopram, and paroxetine are in the SSRI class, studies have demonstrated successful treatment in patients with neuropathic pain. However, downward dosage adjustments of SSRIs are often required to prevent side effects, and they should be avoided in patients with Parkinson's disease. Trazodone is well tolerated and its safety profile has made it particularly attractive for the management of sleep in the elderly (Table 21-7).

Fear of side effects should not be a reason for delaying the introduction of antidepressant therapy in the elderly. To avoid adverse events associated with antidepressants in the dosing regimen in the elderly, one should always take into account the possibility of side effects. Judicious use of

antidepressants entails knowledge of their common side effects, conservative dosing schemes (e.g., start at the lowest dose possible, which may be half of the smallest available tablet), and consideration of physiologic alterations in pharmacokinetics and pharmacodynamics. For instance, amitriptyline and desipramine have similar efficacy but amitriptyline has more side effects. In general, antidepressant medications in elderly patients should be slowly titrated to effect and the patient should be carefully monitored to prevent untoward side effects.

Anticonvulsants have been extremely helpful in the management of neuropathic and radicular pain. Their proposed mechanism of action is the slowing of nerve conduction. The older anticonvulsants (e.g., carbamazepine, valproate, phenytoin) were commonly associated with sedation, lethargy, ataxia, as well as potential hema-

TABLE 21-7. *Antidepressant medications for analgesia*

Drug	Starting dose (PO) mg	Half-life hours	Indications and precautions	Major side effects			Uptake blocking activity	
				Anticholinergic	Sedation	Orthostatic hypotension	Norepinephrine	Serotonin
Antidepressants								
Tricyclics								
Amitriptyline	10	31–46	Pain, neuropathy, sleep	++++	++++	++	++	++++
Desipramine	10	12–24	Pain, neuropathy,sleep	+	+	+	++++	++
Doxepin	10	8–24	Pain, neuropathy, sleep	++	+++	++	+	++
Imipramine	10	11–25	Pain, neuropathy, sleep	++	++	+++	++	++++
Nortriptyline	10	18–44	Pain, neuropathy, sleep	++	++	+	++	+++
Triazolopyridine								
trazodone	25	4–9	Pain, neuropathy, sleep May be too sedating	+	++	++	++	+++
Selective SSRI								
Citalopram	10 (scored)	35	Depression, anxiety, PTSD. May exacerbate insomnia. Often combined with SSRI					
Fluoxetine	10	2–9 days	Depression, anxiety, PTSD	0+	0+	0+	0+	4+
Fluvoxamine	50	15.6	Depression, anxiety, PTSD	0+	0+	0+	0+	4+
Sertraline	12.5 (scored)	1–4	Depression, anxiety, PTSD	0	0+	0	0+	4+
Paroxetine	10	10–24	Depression, anxiety, PTSD	0	0+	0	0+	4+

Key: 0 = None + = Slight ++ = Moderate +++ = High ++++ = Very High

Start dose as low as possible and increase by 10 mg every 3–5 days as tolerated.

tologic abnormalities (Table 21-6). Gabapentin has virtually replaced these agents due to a significant reduction in side effects and the fact that it is well tolerated. Lamotrigine is helpful and often used for patients who cannot tolerate gabapentin. Nonetheless, despite an enhanced profile of the newer anticonvulsants, it is important to start with a low dose and increase gradually in the elderly population.

Opioid Analgesics

At therapeutic doses, opioid analgesics provide analgesia and may improve quality of life by reducing pain (165). Medical professionals may constitute a barrier to the provision of adequate pain management with opioid analgesics (166). Their inaccurate knowledge as well as regulatory issues may contribute to physician's reluctance to provide opioid analgesics for the management of chronic pain (176–179). Opioids have many undesirable side effects: sedation, nausea, vomiting, respiratory depression, dysphoria, tolerance, and constipation (180–182). Physicians also may fear addiction and diversion of opioids. The underprescribing of opioids for all types of pain may lead to inadequate pain control and suffering (164,165,183). Overall, there appears to be a general reluctance to prescribe opioid analgesics for the elderly patient (184). Often when opioid analgesics are prescribed for elderly patients with pain, the dose may be inadequate because of a fear of increased side effects in this population. It is important to note that the use of opioids in the elderly or in the chronic pain population rarely leads to addiction (185). When opioid-related side effects occur, they can be easily managed by changing the opioid, patient education, and treatment with other medications. It is important to anticipate and prevent side effects and anticipate and begin a bowel regimen early in elderly patients.

Many studies show a small but significant decrease in opioid clearance in the elderly (186). The metabolites of morphine (morphine-6-glucuronide) and meperidine (normeperidine) may increase, causing prolonged effects in the elderly. In general, the liver is the major site of biotransformation for most opioids. Morphine is the most widely used opioid analgesic worldwide. It is metabolized by conjugation in the liver primarily, and secondarily in the kidney, and is eliminated renally as two metabolites (morphine-6-glucuronide and morphine-3-glucuronide). Morphine-6-glucuronide has a more potent analgesic effect than its parent drug and the half-life of both glucuronides is considerably longer than that of their parent compound. Thus, with repeated administration these metabolites can accumulate in the cerebral spinal fluid (CSF) and plasma, resulting in sedation and potentially life-threatening respiratory depression. The dose of morphine should also be reduced in the elderly patient who has renal or hepatic insufficiency and the patient should be carefully monitored.

The use of fentanyl in patients with kidney failure is less marked but can yield a decrease in plasma protein binding. Renal failure may potentially alter the free fraction of the fentanyl metabolites and lead to accumulation of the inactive metabolites. The disposition of fentanyl is affected more by changes in hepatic blood flow than by changes in hepatocellular function. It is important to suspect an increase in sensitivity in patients with end stage renal disease or those with chronic liver disease, and a reduction in dose is suggested. The transdermal fentanyl patch also is particularly useful for those patients with compliance issues. Methadone is particularly attractive for chronic neuropathic pain because of its action on the NMDA receptor and its lack of mental status changes. Differences in bioavailability and its renal elimination can lead to sedation and prolonged effects. Thus, it should be started at low doses and the elderly patient should be monitored closely.

Codeine and dihydrocodeine are metabolized to morphine and dihydromorphine. Tramadol has an active metabolite, 0-demethyltramadol, the exact analgesic significance of which is unclear. When combined with nortriptyline, it has been associated with seizures by lowering the seizure threshold, and this combination should be avoided. Oxycodone use has increased due to an increase in availability; however, it tends to be more expensive than the older opioid analgesics. Hydromorphone is metabolized in the liver and has a shorter half-life than morphine. The metabolites of hydromorphone are inactive and are not affected by renal factors. Due to increased sensitivity in the elderly, the dose of hydromorphone may need to be decreased. The metabolic product of meperidine (normeperidine) is renally excreted and is associated with seizures. As such, meperidine is not recommended for use in the elderly population.

Technology

Simple techniques such as the application of topical anesthetic agents can alleviate the need for additional analgesics and can be used as adjuncts to pharmacologic therapies for the management of pain in the elderly. Nerve blocks have been successfully utilized during the perioperative period to provide anesthesia and analgesia (187). The same procedures can be safely utilized in the elderly to provide improved quality of life and to decrease pain associated with acute, chronic, or cancer pain (188). Outcome studies or cost-benefit analysis for the use of the more expensive technology (e.g., intrathecal pumps, spinal cord stimulators) for the management of chronic pain in the elderly population are rare (189,190). In general, when considering nerve blocks for the elderly patient, care must be taken to consider other potential comorbidities. The administration of steroids in the diabetic elderly patient can lead to poor wound healing, alterations in glucose control, and inability to respond to stress (191). Patients in this age group should also be monitored and evaluated for the concomitant use of anticoagulants and medications that interfere with platelet activity (192).

Specific Recommendations

I. All older patients with diminished quality of life as a result of chronic pain are candidates for pharmacologic therapy.
II. The least invasive route of administration should be used (this is usually the oral route).
III. Fast-onset, short-acting analgesic drugs should be used for episodic (i.e., chronic recurrent or noncontinuous) pain.
IV. Acetaminophen is the drug of choice for relieving mild to moderate musculoskeletal pain. The maximum dosage of acetaminophen should not exceed 4000 mg per day.
V. NSAIDs should be used with caution.
   A. High-dose, long-term NSAIDs use should be avoided.
   B. When used chronically, NSAIDs should be used as needed, rather than daily or around the clock.
   C. Short-acting NSAIDs may be preferable to avoid dose accumulation.
   D. NSAIDs should be avoided in patients with abnormal renal function.
   E. NSAIDs should be avoided in patients with a history of peptic ulcer disease.
   F. NSAIDs should be avoided in patients with a bleeding diathesis.
   G. The use of more than one NSAID at a time should be avoided.
   H. Ceiling dose limitations should be anticipated (i.e., maximum dose may be unattainable because of toxicity or may be accompanied by lack of efficacy).
VI. Opioid analgesic drugs may be helpful for relieving moderate to severe pain, especially nociceptive pain.
   A. Opioids for episodic (i.e., chronic recurrent or noncontinuous) pain should be prescribed as needed, rather than around the clock.
   B. Long-acting or sustained-release analgesic preparations should be used only for continuous pain.
     1. Breakthrough pain should be identified and treated by the use of fast-onset, short-acting preparations. Breakthrough pain includes the following three types:
       a. End-of-dose failure is the result of decreased blood levels of analgesic with concomitant increase in pain before the next scheduled dose.
       b. Incident pain is usually caused by activity that can be anticipated and pretreated.
       c. Spontaneous pain, common with neuropathic pain, is often fleeting and difficult to predict.

     2. Titration should be conducted carefully.
       a. Titration should be based on the persistent need for and use of medications for breakthrough pain.
       b. Titration should be based on the pharmacokinetics and pharmacodynamics of specific drugs in the older person and the propensity for drug accumulation.
       c. The potential adverse effects of opioid analgesic medication should be anticipated and prevented or treated promptly.
     3. Constipation should be prevented.
       a. A prophylactic bowel regimen should be initiated with commencement of analgesic therapy.
       b. Bulking agents should be avoided.
       c. Adequate fluid intake should be encouraged.
       d. Exercise, ambulation, and physical activities should be encouraged.
       e. Bowel function should be evaluated with every follow-up visit.
       f. Rectal examination and disimpaction should occur before use of motility agents.
       g. An osmotic, stimulant, or motility agent should be prescribed, if necessary, to provide regular bowel evacuation.
       h. Motility agents should not be used if signs or symptoms of obstruction are present.
       i. If fecal impaction is present, it should be relieved by enema or manual removal.
     4. Mild sedation and impaired cognitive performance should be anticipated when opioid analgesic drugs are initiated. Until tolerance for these effects has developed:
       a. Patients should be instructed not to drive.
       b. Patients and caregivers should be cautioned about the potential for falls and accidents.
       c. Monitoring for profound sedation, unconsciousness, or respiratory depression (defined as a respiratory rate of <8 per minute or oxygen saturation of <90%) should occur during rapid, high-dose escalations. Naloxone should be used carefully to avoid abrupt reversal of pain and autonomic crisis.
     5. Severe nausea may need to be treated with antiemetic medications, as needed.
       a. Mild nausea usually resolves spontaneously in a few days.
       b. If nausea persists, a trial of an alternative opioid may be appropriate.
       c. Anti-emetic drugs should be chosen from those with the lowest side-effect profiles in older persons (149).

CONCLUSIONS

Chronic pain in the elderly is a significant health concern. Despite tremendous improvements in knowledge and addition to the armamentarium of currently available analgesic techniques, all types of pain in the elderly remain undertreated (193–195). The presence of chronic pain in the elderly can be managed appropriately and safely. New literature suggests that elderly patients with chronic pain may be better served by management in specialty pain centers. Multidisciplinary teams can be utilized to optimize the management of pain and improve the quality of life in the elderly (109). Effective January 2001, the standards set by the Joint Commission on the Accreditation of Hospital Organizations (JCAHO) required the assessment for pain in all patients (141,196). As such, the management of pain will become a priority for all patients, including the elderly patients. Thus, understanding the subtleties of managing pain (e.g., communication challenges, the impact on the caregiver) in elderly patients with pain will be of critical importance. There is a need for further research to evaluate not only the efficacy and side effects of treatment but also the quality-of-life implications in an aging population in order to reduce suffering due to the undertreatment of pain.

REFERENCES

1. Finnstrom O, Olausson PO, Sedin G, et al. The Swedish national prospective study on extremely low birthweight (ELBW) infants. Incidence, mortality, morbidity and survival in relation to level of care. *Acta Paediatr* 1997;86(5):503–511.
2. Donovan EF, Ehrenkranz RA, Shankaran S, et al. Outcomes of very low birth weight twins cared for in the National Institute of Child Health and Human Development Neonatal Research Network's intensive care units. *Am J Obstet Gynecol* 1998;179(3):742–749.
3. Berde C, Cairns B. Developmental pharmacology across species: promise and problems. *Anesth Analg* 2000;91(1):1–5.
4. Pons G, Rey E. Stable isotopes labeling of drugs in pediatric clinical pharmacology. *Pediatrics* 1999;104(3):633–639. Supplement part 2 of 3.
5. Anderson BJ, Ellis JE. Common errors of drug administration in infants: causes and avoidance. *Paediatr Drugs* 1999;1(2):93–107.
6. Porter FL, Grunau RE, Anand KJ. Long-term effects of pain in infants. *Paediatr Drugs* 1999;20(4):253–261.
7. Grunau RE, Whitfield MF, Petrie J. Children's judgement about pain at age 8–10 years: do extremely low birthweight (< or = 1000 g) children differ from full birthweight peers? *J Child Psychol Psychiatry* 1998;39(4):587–594.
8. Taddio A, Katz J, Ilersich AL, Koren G. Effect of neonatal circumcision on pain response during subsequent routine vaccination. *Lancet* 1997;349(9052):599–603.
9. Saucier BL. Play therapy: a nursing intervention. *Adv Clin Care* 1989; 45(5):22–23.
10. Committee on Hospital Care. American Academy of Pediatrics. Child Life Programs. *Pediatrics* 1993; 91(3):671–673.
11. McClain BC. Organization of pain management services for children. In: Raj PP, ed. 3rd ed. *Practical management of pain.* St. Louis: Mosby. 2000:59–67.
12. Stevens B. Composite Measures of Pain. In: Finley GA, McGrath PJ, eds. *Measurement of pain in infants and children. Progress in pain research and management.* Seattle: IASP Press 1997(10)161-178.
13. Rawal N. 10 years of acute pain services—achievements and challenges. *Reg Anesth Pain Med* 1999;24(1):68–73.
14. Hill CS, Jr. When will adequate pain treatment be the norm? *JAMA* 1995;274(23):1881–1882.
15. Peretz B, Gluck GM. Assessing and active distracting technique for local anesthetic injection in pediatric dental patients: repeated deep breathing and blowing out air. *J Clin Pediatr Dent* 1999;24(1):5–8.
16. Revisions to Anesthesia Care Standards for Comprehensive Accreditation Manual for Hospitals. Available at: http://www.jcaho.org/standard/aneshap.html.
17. Kraft M, Arellano RS, Mueller PR. Conscious sedation for the non-anesthesiologist: a primer. *Seminars in Intervent Radiol* 1999;16(2):89–98.
18. Anonymous. American Academy of Pediatrics Committee on Drugs: Guidelines for monitoring and management of pediatric patients during and after sedation for diagnostic and therapeutic procedures. *Pediatrics* 1992;89(6, pt 1):1110–1115.
19. American Society of Anesthesiologists Task Force on Sedation and Analgesia by Non-Anesthesiologists. Practice Guidelines for Sedation and Analgesia by Non-Anesthesiologists. *Anesthesiology* 1996; 84(2):459–471.
20. McClain BC. Chronic pain in children: current issues in recognition and management. *Pain Digest* 1996;6:71–76.
21. Malviya S, Voepel-Lewis T, Tait AR. Adverse events and risk factors associated with the sedation of children by nonanesthesiologists. *Anesth Analg* 1997;85:1207–1213.
22. Parker RI, Mahan RA, Giugliano D, Parker MM. Efficacy and safety of intravenous midazolam and ketamine as sedation for therapeutic and diagnostic procedures. *Pediatrics* 1992;89:1110–1114.
23. Lowrie L, Weiss AH, Lacombe C. The pediatric sedation unit: a mechanism for pediatric sedation. *Pediatrics* 1998;102(3).
24. McCarty EC, Mencio GA, Walker LA, Green NE. Ketamine sedation for the reduction of children's fractures in the emergency department. *J Bone & Joint Surg* 2000;82–A(7):912–918.
25. Cote CJ, Notterman DA, Karl HW, Weinberg JA, McCloskey C. Adverse sedation events in pediatrics: a critical incident analysis of contributing factors. *Pediatrics* 2000;105(4):805–814.
26. Nazziola E, Sharma AN, Hoffman RS. Sedation and analgesia for procedures in children. *NEJM* 2000;343(4):302–303
27. Rall TW. Hypnotics and sedatives: ethanol. In: Goodman GA, ed. *The pharmacological basis of therapeutics,* 8th ed. New York: Pergamon Press. 1990:345–382
28. Kao SC, Adamson SD, Tatman LH, Berbaum KS. A survey of post-discharge side effects of conscious sedation using chloral hydrate in pediatric CT and MR. *Pediatric Radiol* 1999;29(4):287–290.
29. Kraft M, Arellano RS, Mueller PR. Conscious sedation for the non-anesthesiologist: a primer. Seminars in *Interventional Radiology* 1999; 16(2):89–99.
30. Ljungman G, Kreuger A, Andreasson S, et al. Midazolam nasal spray reduces procedural anxiety in children. *Pediatrics* 2000;105(1 Pt 1):73–78.
31. Chung T, Hoffer FA, Connor L, et al. The use of oral pentobarbital sodium (Nembutal) versus oral chloral hydrate in infants undergoing CT and MR imaging—a pilot study. *Pediatr Radiol* 2000;30(5):332–335.
32. Reich DL, Silvay G. Ketamine: an update on the first twenty-five years of clinical experience. *Can J Anaesth* 1989;36:186–197.
33. Dachs RJ, Innes GM. Intravenous ketamine sedation of pediatric patients in the emergency department. *Ann Emerg Med* 1997;29(1):146–150
34. Rockoff M, Cote C, Kaplan R. Sedation for procedures. *Pediatrics* 1997;100(6):1045–1046.
35. Rauch DA. Use of ketamine in a pain management protocol for repetitive procedures. *Pediatrics* 1998;102(2):404–405.
36. Green SM, Kupperman N, Rothrock SG, et al. Predictors of adverse events with intramuscular ketamine sedation in children. *Ann Emerg Med* 2000;35(1):35–42.
37. Pena BMG, Krauss B. Adverse events of procedural sedation and analgesia in a pediatric emergency department. *Ann Emerg Med* 1999;34(4, Pt 1):483–491.
38. Scahill L, Barloon L, Farkas L. Alpha-2 agonists in the treatment of attention deficit hyperactivity disorder. *J Child Adolesc Psychiatr Nurs* 1999;12(4):168–173.
39. Blew P, Luiselli JK, Thibadeau S. Beneficial effects of clonidine on severe self-injurious behavior in a 9-year-old girl with pervasive developmental disorder. *J Child Adolesc Psychopharmacol* 1999;9(4):285–291.
40. Fujii Y, Saitoh Y, Tanaka H, Toyooka H. Pretreatment with oral clonidine attenuates cardiovascular responses to tracheal extubation in children. *Paediatr Anaesth* 2000;10(1):65–67.

41. Hawley DD. Postoperative pain in children: misconceptions, descriptions and interventions. *Pediatr Nurs* 1984;10(1):20–23.
42. Beyer JE, Bournaki MC. Assessment and management of postoperative pain in children. *Pediatrician* 1989;16(1-2);30–38.
43. Sethna NF, Berde CB. Pediatric regional anesthesia equipment. *Int Anesthesiol Clin* 1992;30(3):163–176.
44. Krane EJ, Dalens B, Murat I, Murrell D. The safety of epidurals placed during general anesthesia [editorial]. *Reg Anesth Pain Med* 1998;23(5):433–438.
45. Sethna NF, Berde CB. Venous air embolism during identification of the epidural space in children [editorial;comment]. *Anesth Analg* 1993; 76(5):925–927.
46. Larsson BA, Lonnqvist PA, Olsson GL. Plasma concentrations of bupivacaine in neonates after continuous epidural infusion. *Anesth Analg* 1997;84:501–505.
47. Berde CB. Toxicity of local anesthetics in infants and children. *J Pediatr* 1993;122(5 pt 2):S14–20.
48. Eisenach JC, DeKock M, Klimscha W. α_2-Adrenergic agonists for regional anesthesia. A clinical review of clonidine (1984-1995). *Anesthesiology* 1996;85(3):655–674.
49. Ivani G, DeNegri P, Conio A, et al. Ropivacaine-clonidine combination for caudal blockade in children. *Acta Anaesthesiol Scand* 2000; 44(4):446–449.
50. Drost RH, Ionescu TI, vanRossum JM, Maes RA. Pharmacokinetics of morphine after epidural administration in man. *Arzneimittel-Forschung* 1986;36(7):1096–1100.
51. Krane EJ, Tyler DC, Jacobson LE. The dose response of caudal morphine in children. *Anesthesiology* 1989;71(1):48–52.
52. Leong CK, Ng AS, Chew SL. Caudal morphine in paediatric patients: a comparison of two different doses in children after major urogenital surgery. *Ann Acad Med, Singapore* 1998;27(3):371–375.
53. Kokki H, Heikkinen M, Ahonen R. Recovery after paediatric daycase herniotomy performed under spinal anaesthesia. *Paediatr Anaesth* 2000;10(4):413–417.
54. Kotzer AM, Coy J, LeClaire AD. The effectiveness of a standardized educational program for children using patient-controlled analgesia. *J Soc Pediatr Nurs* 1998;3(3):117–26.
55. Gaukroger PB, Chapman MJ, Davey RB. Pain control in paediatric burns—the use of patient controlled analgesia. *Burns* 1991;17(5): 396–399.
56. Collins JJ, Geake J, Frier HE, et al. Patient controlled analgesia for mucositis pain in children: a three period crossover study comparing morphine and hydromorphone. *J Pediatr* 1996;129(5):722–728.
57. Shapiro BS, Cohen DE, Howe CJ. Patient controlled analgesia for sickle cell-related pain. *J Pain Symptom Manage* 1993;8(1):22–28.
58. Trentadue NO, Kachoyeanos MK, Lea G. A comparison of two regimens of patient controlled analgesia for children with sickle cell disease. *J Pediatr Nurs* 1998;13(1):15–19.
59. Beaulieu P, Cyrenne L, Mathews S, et al. Patient-controlled analgesia after spinal fusion for idiopathic scoliosis. *Int Orthop* 1996;20(4):295–299.
60. McNeely JK, Trentadue NC. Comparision of patient-controlled analgesia with/without nighttime morphine infusion following lower extremity surgery in children. *J Pain Symptom Manage* 1997;13(5): 268–273.
61. Fulton TR. Nurses' adoption of a patient-controlled analgesia approach. *West J Nurs Res* 1996; 18(4):383–396.
62. Rowlingson JC. Just when we thought we understood patient-controlled analgesia. *Anesth Analg* 1999;89:3–6.
63. Hamunen K. Ventilatory effects of morphine, pethidine and methadone in children. *Br J Anaesth* 1993;70:414–418.
64. Davis AM, Inturrisi CE. D-Methadone blocks morphine tolerance and N-methyl-D-Aspartate-induced hyperalgesia. *JPET* 1999;289: 1048–1053.
65. Ebert B, Thorkildsen C, Andersen S, et al. Opioid analgesics as non-competitive N-Methyl-D-aspartate (NMDA) antagonists. *Biochem Pharmacol* 1998;56:553–559.
66. Seth N, Llewellyn NE, Howard RE. Parental opinions regarding the route of administration of analgesic medication in children. *Paediatr Anaesth* 2000;10(5):537–544.
67. Dutta S, Mehta M, Veima IC. Recurrent abdominal pain in Indian children and its relation with school and family environment. *Indian Pediatr* 1999;36(9):S17–20.
68. Gladstein J. Headaches: the pediatrician's perspective. *Semin Pediatr Neurol* 1995;2(2):119–126.
69. Linder SL. Subcutaneous sumatriptan in the clinical setting: the first 50 consecutive patients with acute migraine in a pediatric neurology office practice. *Headache* 1996;36(7):419–422.
70. Kimia A, Zahavi I, Shapiro R, et al. The role of Helicobacter Pylori and gastritis in children with recurrent abdominal pain. *IMAJ* 2000;2(2):126–128.
71. McGrath PJ, Unruh AM. Other medical pain. In: McGrath PJ, ed. *Pain in children and adolescents.* Amsterdam: Elsevier 1987:255–273.
72. Kocis KC. Chest pain in pediatrics. *Pediatr Clin of North Am* 1999; 46(2):189–203.
73. Walco GA, Oberlander TF. Musculoskeletal pain syndromes in children. In: Schecter NL, Berde CB, Yaster M, eds. *Pain in infants, children and adolescents.* Baltimore: Williams & Wilkins, 1993:459–471.
74. Breau LM, McGrath PJ, Ju LH. Review of juvenile primary fibromyalgia and chronic fatigue syndrome. *J Dev Behav Pediatr* 1999; 20(4):278–288.
75. Mikklesen M. One year outcome of preadolescents with fibromyalgia. *J Rheum* 1999;26(3)674–282.
76. Ballas SK. Sickle cell pain. *Progress in pain research and management.* Seattle: IASP Press 1998(11)3-18.
77. McClain BC. Chronic pain in children: current issues in recognition and management. *Pain Digest* 1996;6:71–76.
78. Wilder RT, Berde CB, Wolohan M et al. Reflex sympathetic dystrophy in children: clinical characteristics and follow-up of seventy patients. *J Bone Joint Surg Am* 1992;74:910–919.
79. Woolf CJ, Mannion RJ. Neuropathic pain: aetiology, symptoms, mechanisms and management. *Lancet* 1999;353:1959–1964.
80. Robison LL. General principles of the epidemiology of childhood cancer. In: *Principles and practice of pediatric oncology,* 3rd ed. Lippencott-Raven, 1997:1–10.
81. Foley KM. Pain syndromes in patients with cancer. *Med Clin of North Am* 1987;71(2):169–184.
82. Smith J, Thompson JM. Phantom limb pain and chemotherapy in pediatric amputees. *Mayo Clin Proc* 1995;70(4):357–364.
83. Collins JJ, Grier HE, Sethna NF, et al. Regional anesthesia for pain associated with terminal pediatric malignancy. *Pain* 1996;65(1): 63–69.
84. Queinnec MC, Esteve M, Vedrenne J. Positive effect of regional analgesia (RA) in terminal stage paediatric chondrosarcoma: a case report and the review of the literature. *Pain* 1999;83(2):383–385.
85. Truog RD, Berde CB, Mitchell C, Grier HE. Barbiturates in the care of the terminally ill. *N Engl J Med* 1992;327(23):1678–1682.
86. Kenny NP, Frager G. Refractory symptoms and terminal sedation of children: ethical issues and practical management. *J Palliat Care* 1996;12(3):40–45.
87. Collins JJ, Stevens MM, Cousens P. Home care for the dying child. A parent's perception. *Aust Fam Physician* 1998;27(7):610–614.
88. Sagara M, Pickett M. Sociocultural influences and care of dying children in Japan and the United States. *Cancer Nurs* 1998;21(4):274–281.
89. Anonymous. Use of codeine-and dextromethorphan-containing cough remedies in children. *Pediatrics* 1997;99(6):918–920.
90. Agble, YM. Management of sickle cell disease: non-addictive analgesics can be as effective as morphine and pethidine. *BMJ* 1998; 316(7135):935.
91. Kesavan S, Sobala GM. Serotonin syndrome with fluoxetine plus tramadol. *J R Soc Med* 1999;92(9):474–5.
92. Egberts AC, terBorgh J, Brodie-Meijer CC. Serotonin syndrome attributed to tramadol addition to paroxetine therapy. *Int Clin Psychophamacol* 1997;12(3):181–182.
93. Mason BJ, Blackburn KH. Possible serotonin syndrome associated with tramadol and sertraline coadministration. *Ann Pharmacother* 1997;31(2):175–177.
94. Christensen ML, Wang WC, Harris S, et al. Transdermal fentanyl administration in children and adolescents with sickle cell pain crisis. *J Pediatr Hematol Oncol* 1996;18(4):372–376.
95. Collins JJ, Dunkel IJ, Gupta SK, Inturrisi CE, Lapin J, Palmer LN, Weinstein SM, Portenoy RK. Transdermal fentanyl in children with cancer pain: feasibility, tolerability and pharamcokinetic correlates. *J Pediatr* 1999;134(3):319–323.
96. Bruera E, MACEachern T, Macmillan K, et al. Local tolerance to subcutaneous infusions of high concentrationsn of hydromorphone: a prospective study. *J Pain Symptom Manage* 1993;8:201–204.
97. Gourlay GK. Sustained relief of chronic pain. Pharmacokinetics of sustained release morphine. *Clin Pharmacokinet* 1998;35(3):173–90.

98. Lindsley CB. Uses of nonsteroidal anti-inflammatory drugs in pediatrics. *Am J Dis Child* 1993;147(2):229–236.

99. Malmstrom K, Daniels S, Kotey P, et al. Comparison of rofecoxib and celecoxib, two cyclooxygenase –2 inhibitors, in postoperative dental pain: a randomized, placebo-and active-comparator-controlled clinical trial. *Clin Ther* 1999; 21(10):1653–1663.

100. McClain BC, Ennevor S. The use of gabapentin in pediatric patients with neuropathic pain. *Semin Anesth Perioperat Med Pain* 2000;19(2):83–87.

101. Services U.S.D.o.H.a.H., Healthy People 2010: *Understanding and Improving Health.* Department of Health and Human Services, Government Printing Office: Washington DC.2000.

102. Breslow L. A quantitative approach to the World Health Organization definition of health: physical, mental and social well-being. *Int J Epidemiol* 1972;1(4):347–355.

103. Kelly MP. The World Health Organisation's definition of health promotion: three problems. *Health Bull* (Edinb) 1990;48(4):176–180.

104. Skevington S.M. Investigating the relationship between pain and discomfort and quality of life, using the WHOQOL. *Pain* 1998; 76(3):395–406.

105. *Study show 1.2 million michigan adults suffer from chronic pain; many say treatment ineffective.* Lansing MI: EPIC, MRA 1997.

106. Becker N, Hojsted J, Sjogren P, et al. Sociodemographic predictors of treatment outcome in chronic non-malignant pain patients. Do patients receiving or applying for disability pension benefit from multidisciplinary pain treatment? *Pain* 1998;77(3):279–287.

107. Crombie IK, Davies HT, Macrae WA, The epidemiology of chronic pain: time for new directions [editorial]. *Pain* 1994;57(1):1–3.

108. Crook J, Rideout E, Browne G. The prevalence of pain complaints in a general population. *Pain* 1984;18(3):299–314.

109. Gibson SJ, Littlejohn GO, Gorman MM, et al. Pain in older persons. *Disabil Rehabil* 1994;16(3):127–139.

110. Werner P, Cohen-Mansfield J, Watson V, Pasis S. Pain in participants of adult day care centers: assessment by different raters. *J Pain Symptom Manage* 1998;15(1):8–17.

111. Allison JJ, Kiefe CI, Centor RM, et al. Racial differences in the medical treatment of elderly Medicare patients with acute myocardial infarction. *J Gen Intern Med* 1996;11(12):736–743.

112. Ayanian JZ, Epstein AM. Differences in the use of procedures between women and men hospitalized for coronary heart disease [see comments]. *N Engl J Med* 1991;325(4):221–225.

113. Ayanian JZ, Kohler BA, Abe T, Epstein AM. The relation between health insurance coverage and clinical outcomes among women with breast cancer [see comments]. *N Engl J Med*1993;329(5):326–331.

114. Dawkins FW, Laing AE, Smoot DT, et al. The impact of health insurance on an African-American population with colorectal cancer. *J Natl Med Assoc* 1995;87(4):301–303.

115. Eley JW, Hill HA, Chen VW, et al. Racial differences in survival from breast cancer. Results of the National Cancer Institute Black/White Cancer Survival Study [see comments]. *JAMA* 1994;272(12):947–954.

116. Elixhauser A, Ball J. Black/White Differences in Colorectal Tumor Location in a National Sample of Hospitals. *J Natl Med Assoc* 1993;86(6):449–458.

117. Hicks ML, Kim W, Abrams J, et al. Racial differences in surgically staged patients with endometrial cancer. *J Natl Med Assoc* 1997; 89(2):134–140.

118. Johnson PA, Lee TH, Cook EF, et al. Effect of race on the presentation and management of patients with acute chest pain [see comments]. *Ann Intern Med* 1993;118(8):593–601.

119. Kales HC, Blow FC, Bingham CR, et al. Race and inpatient psychiatric diagnoses among elderly veterans [In Process Citation]. *Psychiatr Serv* 2000;51(6):795–800.

120. Lauver D. Care-seeking behavior with breast cancer symptoms in Caucasian and African-American women. *Res Nurs Health* 1994;17 (6):421–431.

121. Lieu TA, Newacheck PW, McManus MA, Race, ethnicity, and access to ambulatory care among US adolescents [see comments]. *Am J Public Health* 1993;83(7):960–965.

122. Mouton CP. Special health considerations in African-American elders. *Am Fam Physician* 1997;55(4):1243–1253.

123. Williams, DR, Lavizzo-Mourey R, Warren RC. The concept of race and health status in America. *Public Health Rep* 1994;109(1):26–41.

124. Schulman KA, Berlin JA, Harless W, et al. The effect of race and sex on physicians' recommendations for cardiac catheterization [see comments] [published erratum appears in *N Engl J Med* Apr 8, 1999;340(14):1130]. *N Engl J Med* 1999;340(8):618–626.

125. McCulloch BJ. Gender and race: an interaction affecting the replicability of well-being across groups. *Women Health*, 1992;19(4):65–89.

126. Ortega R, Youdelman B, Havel R. Ethnic variability in the treatment of pain. *The Am J Anesthesiology* 1999;26(9):429–432.

127. Mudrick NR. Predictors of disability among midlife men and women: differences by severity of impairment. *J Community Health* 1988;13(2):70–84.

128. Unruh AM. Gender variations in clinical pain experience. *Pain* 1996;65(2-3):123–167.

129. LeResche L. Gender Differences in Pain: Epidemiologic Perspectives. *Pain Forum* 1995. 4;(4):228–230.

130. Fillingim R, Maixner W. Gender differences in the responses to noxious stimuli. *Pain Forum* 1995;4(4):209–221.

131. Taenzer AH, Clark C, Curry CS. Gender affects report of pain and function after arthroscopic anterior cruciate ligament reconstruction. *Anesthesiology* 2000;93(3):670–675.

132. Manton KG. Demographic trends for the aging female population. *J Am Med Womens Assoc* 1997;52(3):99–105.

133. Butler RN, Collins KS, Meier DS, et al. Older women's health: clinical care in the postmenopausal years. A roundtable discussion part 2 [clinical conference]. *Geriatrics* 1995;50(6):33–6,39–41.

134. Roberto KA. Chronic pain in the lives of older women. *J Am Med Womens Assoc* 1997;52(3):127–131.

135. Butler RN, Collins KS, Meier DS, et al. Older women's health: 'taking the pulse' reveals gender gap in medical care [see comments]. *Geriatrics* 1995;50(5):39–40,43–6,49.

136. Hopper SV. The influence of ethnicity on the health of older women. *Clin Geriatr Med* 1993;9(1):231–259.

137. Nelson DV, Novy DM, Averill PM, Berry LA. Ethnic comparability of the MMPI in pain patients. *J Clin Psychol* 1996;52(5):485–497.

138. Bates M, Edwards W. Ethnic Variations in the chronic pain experience. *Ethnicity & Disease* 1992;2:63–83.

139. Collins K, Hall A, Neuhaus C. *U.S. minority health: a chartbook.* New York: The Commonwealth Fund 1999:161.

140. Islam AK, Cooper ML, Bodnar RJ. Interactions among aging, gender, and gonadectomy effects upon morphine antinociception in rats. *Physiol Behav* 1993;54(1):45–53.

141. Standards, Intents, Examples, and Scoring Questions for Pain Assessment and Management -Comprehensive Accreditation Manual for Hospitals. *JCAHO* Department of Standards. 1999:1–11.

142. Quality improvement guidelines for the treatment of acute pain and cancer pain. American Pain Society Quality of Care Committee [see comments]. *JAMA*, 1995;274(23):1874–1880.

143. Miaskowski C, Donovan M. Implementation of the American Pain Society quality assurance standards for relief of acute pain and cancer pain in oncology nursing practice. *Oncol Nurs Forum* 1992; 19(3):411–415.

144. Cancer pain assessment and treatment curriculum guidelines. Ad Hoc committee on cancer pain of the American Society of Clinical Oncology. *Support Care Cancer*, 1993;1(2):67–73.

145. Fishman B, Pasternak S, Wallenstein SL, et al. The Memorial Pain Assessment Card. A valid instrument for the evaluation of cancer pain. *Cancer* 1987;60(5):1151–1158.

146. Sriwatanakul K, Weis OF, Alloza JL, et al. Studies with different types of visual analog scales for measurement of pain. *Clinical Pharmacol Ther* 1982;34(2):234–269.

147. Flor H, Turk DC, Scholz OB. Impact of chronic pain on the spouse: marital, emotional and physical consequences. *J Psychosom Res* 1987;31(1):63–71.

148. Rapp SE, Wild LM, Egan KJ, Ready LB. Acute pain management of the chronic pain patient on opiates: a survey of caregivers at University of Washington Medical Center. *Clin J Pain* 1994;10(2):133–138.

149. The management of chronic pain in older persons: AGS Panel on Chronic Pain in Older Persons. American Geriatrics Society [published erratum appears in *J Am Gerriatr Soc* Jul 1998;46(7):913] [see comments]. *J Am Geriatr Soc* 1998;46(5):635–651.

150. Late-life depression: Usually treatable, usually ignored, in Consumer Reports on Health. 1998:6–8.
151. Averill PM, Novy DM, Nelson DV, Berry LA. Correlates of depression in chronic pain patients: a comprehensive examination. *Pain* 1996;65(1):93–100.
152. Cleeland CS. The impact of pain on the patient with cancer. *Cancer*, 1984;54(11 Suppl):2635–2641.
153. Doan BD, Wadden NP. Relationships between depressive symptoms and descriptions of chronic pain. *Pain* 1989;36(1):75-84.
154. Dworkin SF, Von Korff M, LeResche L. Multiple pains and psychiatric disturbance. An epidemiologic investigation. *Arch Gen Psychiatry* 1990;47(3):239–244.
155. Fields H. Depression and pain; a neurobiological model. *Neuropsychiatry, neuropsychology, and behavioral neurology* 1991;4(1):83–92.
156. Fishbain DA, Culter R, Rosomoff HL, Rosomoff RS. Chronic pain-associated depression: antecedent or consequence of chronic pain? A review. *Clin J Pain* 1997;13(2):116–137.
157. Fishbain DA, Goldberg M, Meagher BR, et al. Male and female chronic pain patients categorized by DSM-III psychiatric diagnostic criteria. *Pain* 1986;26(2):181–197.
158. Geisser ME, Roth RS, Theisen ME, et al. Negative affect, self-report of depressive symptoms, and clinical depression: relation to the experience of chronic pain [In Process Citation]. *Clin J Pain* 2000;16(2):110–120.
159. Geisser ME, Roth RS, Robinson ME, Assessing depression among persons with chronic pain using the Center for Epidemiological Studies-Depression Scale and the Beck Depression Inventory: a comparative analysis. *Clin J Pain* 1997;13(2):163–170.
160. Lancee WJ, Vachon ML, Ghadirian P, et al. The impact of pain and impaired role performance on distress in persons with cancer. *Can J Psychiatry* 1994;39(10):617–622.
161. McCracken LM. Learning to live with the pain: acceptance of pain predicts adjustment in persons with chronic pain. *Pain* 1998;74(1):21–27.
162. Von Korff M, Le Resche L, Dworkin SF. First onset of common pain symptoms: a prospective study of depression as a risk factor. *Pain* 1993;55(2):251–258.
163. Kelsen DP, Portenoy RK, Thaler HT, Niedzwiecki D, et al. Pain and depression in patients with newly diagnosed pancreas cancer. *J Clin Oncol* 1995;13(3):748–755.
164. Gurwitz JH, Avorn J. The ambiguous relation between aging and adverse drug reactions. *Ann Intern Med* 1991;114:956–966.
165. Rochon PA, Gurwitz JH. Prescribing for seniors: neither too much nor too little. *JAMA* 1999;282(2):113–115.
166. Bernabei R, Gambassi G, Lapane K, et al. Management of pain in elderly patients with cancer. SAGE Study Group. Systematic Assessment of Geriatric Drug Use via Epidemiology *[see comments] [published erratum appears in JAMA 1999 Jan 13;281(2):136]*. *JAMA* 1998;279(23):1877–1882.
167. Eisenberg D.M. Advising patients who seek alternative medical therapies [see comments]. *Ann Intern Med* 1997;127(1):6–19.
168. Cleeland CS. Nonpharmacological management of cancer pain. *J Pain Symptom Manage* 1987;2(2):S23–28.
169. Shimp LA. Safety issues in the pharmacologic management of chronic pain in the elderly. *Pharmacotherapy* 1998;18(6):1313–1322.
170. O'Hara DA. Non-opioid. *Analgesics.* 1–5.
171. Conaway DC. Using NSAIDs safely in the elderly. *Hospital Medicine* 1995.
172. Fries JF. NSAID gastropathy: the second most deadly rheumatic disease? Epidemiology and risk appraisal. *J Rheumatol Suppl* 1991;28:6–10.
173. Page J, Henry D. Consumption of NSAIDs and the development of congestive heart failure in elderly patients: an underrecognized public health problem. *Arch Intern Med*, 2000;160(6):777–784.
174. Green CR, Pandit SK, Levy L, et al. Intraoperative ketorolac has an opioid-sparing effect in women after diagnostic laparoscopy but not after laparoscopic tubal ligation. *Anesth Analg* 1996;82(4):732–737.
175. Sullivan MJ, Reesor K, Mikail S, Fisher R. The treatment of depression in chronic low back pain: review and recommendations [see comments]. *Pain* 1992;50(1):5–13.
176. Morrison RS, Wallenstein S, Natale DK, et al. "We don't carry that"—failure of pharmacies in predominantly nonwhite neighborhoods to stock opioid analgesics [see comments]. *N Engl J Med* 2000;342(14):1023–1026.
177. Turk DC. Clinicians' attitudes about prolonged use of opioids and the issue of patient heterogeneity. *J Pain Symptom Manage* 1996;11(4):218–230.
178. Turk DC, Brody MC, Okifuji EA. Physicians' attitudes and practices regarding the long-term prescribing of opioids for non-cancer pain. *Pain* 1994;59(2):201–208.
179. Max MB. Improving outcomes of analgesic treatment: is education enough? [see comments]. *Ann Intern Med* 1990;113(11):885–889.
180. Society, T.A.A.o.P.M.a.t.A.P. The Use of Opioids for the Treatment of Chronic Pain (Consensus Statement). *J Pharmaceutical Care in Pain and Symptom Control* 1998;6(1):97–102.
181. Greenwald BD, Narcessian EJ, Pomeranz BA. Assessment of physiatrists' knowledge and perspectives on the use of opioids: review of basic concepts for managing chronic pain. *Am J Phys Med Rehabil* 1999;78(5):408–415.
182. The use of opioids for the treatment of chronic pain. *American Academy of Pain Medicine and the American Pain Society.* 1997.
183. Friedrich MJ. Experts describe optimal symptom management for hospice patients [news]. *JAMA* 1999;282(13):1213–1214.
184. Von Roenn JH, Cleeland CS, Gonin R, et al. Physician attitudes and practice in cancer pain management: a survey from the Eastern Cooperative Oncology Group. *Ann Intern Med* 1993;119(2):121–126.
185. Gomez-Lechon MJ, Ponsoda X, Jover R, et al. Hepatotoxicity of the opioids morphine, heroin, meperidine, and methadone to cultured human hepatocytes. *Mol Toxicol* 1987;1(4):453–463.
186. Jacox A, Carr DB, Payne R. New clinical-practice guidelines for the management of pain in patients with cancer. *N Engl J Med* 1994;330(9):651–655.
187. Yeager MP, Glass DD, Neff RK, Brinck-Johnson T. Epidural anesthesia and analgesia in high-risk surgical patients. *Anesthesiology* 1987;66(6):729–736.
188. Yeager MP, Cronenwett JL. Effect of anesthetic technique on outcome after abdominal aortic surgery. *J Vasc Surg* 1992;15(5):875–878.
189. Whedon M, Ferrell BR. Professional and ethical considerations in the use of high-tech pain management. *Oncol Nurs Forum* 1991;18(7):1135–1143.
190. Ferrell BR, Griffith H. Cost issues related to pain management: report from the Cancer Pain Panel of the Agency for Health Care Policy and Research. *J Pain Symptom Manage* 1994;9(4):221–234.
191. Kay J, Findling JW, Raff H. Epidural triamcinolone suppresses the pituitary-adrenal axis in human subjects. *Anesth Analg* 1994;79(3):501–505.
192. Horlocker TT, Wedel DJ, Schlichting JL. Postoperative epidural analgesia and oral anticoagulant therapy. *Anesth Analg* 1994;79(1):89–93.
193. Cleeland CS. Undertreatment of cancer pain in elderly patients [editorial; comment]. *JAMA* 1998;279(23):1914–1915.
194. Cleeland CS, Gonin R, Hatfield AK, et al. Pain and its treatment in outpatients with metastatic cancer [see comments]. *N Engl J Med* 1994;330(9):592–596.
195. Cleeland CS, Gonin R, Baez L, et al. Pain and treatment of pain in minority patients with cancer. The Eastern Cooperative Oncology Group Minority Outpatient Pain Study. *Ann Intern Med* 1997;127(9):813–816.
196. *New standards: a pain in the assessment.* Briefings on JCAHO, 1999:6–7.

CHAPTER **22**

Opiate, Hypnosedative, Alcohol, and Nicotine Detoxification Protocols

David A. Fishbain

OPIATE DETOXIFICATION

Following long-term use of opiates, physical dependence and tolerance can develop. It is estimated that of those who use opiates sporadically (nondaily), 25% will become dependent (1). Physical dependence is a function of the dosage schedule of the opiate, but can be produced by very little opiate exposure, can persist for a long period after drug cessation, and will develop in every patient so exposed. In general, of those who advance to twice-daily use, the majority will become physically dependent within 6 to 8 weeks (1). Each opiate apparently has its own capacity for inducing physical dependence (2).

In a patient who is opiate physically dependent, abrupt opiate discontinuation leads to the development of the opiate withdrawal syndrome (*distressing physical reaction*) (3). The signs and symptoms of this syndrome are well described (3–6) and will not be delineated here. Some of these signs and symptoms have been incorporated into the *DSM-IV-TR* Criteria for Opiate Withdrawal (7). The elimination half-life of the opiate drug will determine when withdrawal will begin, because this syndrome usually begins two to three half-lives after the last opiate dose (3). Thus, for short–half-life opiates such as morphine, withdrawal begins in 6 to 12 hours, whereas for long–half-life opiates such as methadone, withdrawal begins in 36 to 48 hours. Opiate plasma half-lives are well documented in most reference works (2). In terms of time, the opiate withdrawal syndrome will begin within 6 to 8 hours after the last opiate dose, peak in 48 to 72 hours, and last for 7 to 14 days. However, lingering physical effects of opiate withdrawal can appear for up to 6 months after resolution of acute symptoms (3). The severity of the withdrawal is a function of which opiate was being taken, at what dose, and for how long (3). Generally the severity of opiate withdrawal will reflect the degree of physical dependence.

Significant confusion exists over the use of such terms as *drug/alcohol abuse, physical dependence,* and *addiction* (8). As a result, data on the percentages of chronic pain patients who abuse opiates or are dependent or addicted to this group of drugs, appear to be limited (8). For chronic pain patients, opiate abuse, dependence, or addiction, in most cases, may not be an adequate reason for opiate detoxification. There are, however, other reasons for detoxifying chronic pain patients from opiates, which have been reported (8).

Until quite recently, opiate detoxification had been a relatively standard procedure whose primary purpose was to *minimize* or *eliminate* the signs and symptoms associated with opiate withdrawal via a slow taper. However, because of the development of new medications such as clonidine for opiate withdrawal, there has been an explosion in the variety of opiate detoxification protocols used. This part of the chapter presents a review of some of the opiate detoxification protocols advocated in the literature.

Principles

A number of major principles have been outlined for the management of opiate withdrawal (2–4, 9, 10):

1. Opiate withdrawal can be associated with major patient discomfort, both psychological and physiological, but has no serious medical consequence, such as death, if untreated. Thus opiate physical dependence should not impede rapid tapering. This is not the case for sedative/hypnotic withdrawal.
2. Opiate withdrawal can be treated with any opiate, but if a long-acting opiate is used (long half-life), withdrawal symptoms are milder and there is less patient distress.
3. Opiate dosage equivalencies can be utilized to withdraw patients from methadone or any opiate. Generally, in all

314

detoxification procedures the total amount of opiate that the patient takes over 24 hours is translated via dosage equivalencies into the equivalent amount of opiate with which detoxification will proceed. This is why dosage equivalencies are so important to detoxification protocols. Dosage equivalencies are well documented in most reference works (2) and will not be presented here. However, for detoxification to proceed in a correct fashion, the treating physician should have a dosage equivalencies chart. He or she should be prepared to use such a chart especially when a patient is found to use more than one opiate.

4. Titration of methadone, or any opiate, for control of opiate withdrawal should be based on objective withdrawal signs (e.g., dilation of pupils, stuffy nose, gooseflesh). However, there appears to be little correlation among patients' subjective ratings, objective nurse ratings, and physical parameters of severity of withdrawal (9). Thus, clinicians should not base their decision as to the severity of opiate withdrawal syndrome solely on physical parameters. There are opiate withdrawal symptoms rating scales available (10). These should be used if the amount of opiate that the patient will receive is to be determined by the presence or absence of withdrawal symptoms and signs.

5. Some patient discomfort is inevitable; the signs and symptoms of withdrawal can rarely be entirely abolished, unless the detoxification process is much prolonged.

6. Detoxification can be blind (cocktail) or open (pills), depending on patient and physician preference.

7. Usual daily dose *required to prevent withdrawal is equal to 25% of the previous daily dose.* Therefore, daily tapers can be from 75% to 5%, depending on preference. However, the usual figure is 50%.

8. At higher dose levels, the daily dose reduction can be greater because it represents a smaller percentage of the total. As daily dose falls, reduction should be more gradual.

PROTOCOLS

All opiate detoxification protocols generally adhere to the principles outlined above. These protocols can be characterized by the type of opiate that is used in the detoxification process and the time required to complete detoxification. Time is an important element because it is thought that short–half-life opiates require 5 to 7 days to complete detoxification and that intermediate–half-life and long–half-life opiates require 10 to 14 days and 14 to 21 days, respectively (2). Many protocols are designed to decrease the time required for detoxification even further. This is because drug treatment programs usually wish to taper opiates as quickly as possible. To date, the protocols that have appeared in the literature can be classified as follows: methadone substitution/detoxification, codeine or other opiate substitution/detoxification, opiate of choice

detoxification, buprenorphine substitution/detoxification, opiate antagonist precipitated withdrawal/detoxification, and clonidine-assisted detoxification.

Methadone is an opiate with an extremely long half-life (2). It has some euphoria, it plateaus in 2 hours, and its onset of action is in 0.5 hour. It cannot be used to detoxify patients dependent on mixed agonist/antagonist opiates. Additionally, it may accumulate between the 24th and 48th hours, and therefore patients on this drug must be assessed for toxicity (4). Because of its long half-life, methadone has been used in a number of opiate detoxification protocols. The best example of this is a protocol presented by Halpern (Table 22-1) (11). This protocol is notable for the following: There is an initial 48-hour time span during which the patient is on an opiate Pro-Re-Nata (PRN) (as medically necessary) demand schedule; a pain cocktail is used, adjunct medications are used in the cocktail, and the time required to complete this protocol from 50 mg of methadone at 20% reduction is 17 days. Two alternatives to this protocol are presented in Table 22-2. Alternative *A* takes 20 days, whereas alternative *B* requires 11 days to complete from 50 mg of methadone.

An example of a nonmethadone opiate substitution/ detoxification protocol is presented in Table 22-3. This protocol will take 8 to 9 days to complete from an equivalent dose of 50 mg of methadone. There are two reasons for considering this protocol over a methadone substitution/detoxification protocol. First, the longer the half-life of the opiate, the longer the detoxification protocol required. It does not make any sense to transfer patients taking short– and intermediate–half-life drugs to long–half-life drugs and then, by necessity, prolonging detoxification if the goal is rapid detoxification. Second, many drug addicts believe, although there

TABLE 22-1. *Methadone opiate substitution/ detoxification protocol*

1. Patients given any and as much medication as they need for 24 to 48 hours.
2. From the amount of drug taken in no. 1 (above), calculate equivalent daily dose of methadone (Table 22.11) required.
3. If unable to determine above, give methadone 15 mg q4h until respiratory rate decreases to 16 breaths/min.
4. The total daily substitution dose of methadone is the total dose given to reduce the respiratory rate to 16 breaths/min.
5. This dose is given in four divided doses for 24 hours.
6. Methadone dose is reduced daily by 15 to 20 percent in a "pain cocktail" (drug plus masking vehicle to blind patient to detoxification).
7. Doxepin 50 to 100 mg is added to cocktail if sleep is a problem.
8. Hydroxyzine 50 mg t.i.d. added to cocktail if patient is anxious.

Compiled from Halpern L. Substitution-detoxification and its role in the management of chronic benign pain. *J Clin Psychiatry* 1982;43:10–14.

TABLE 22-2. *Alternative methadone substitution/detoxification protocol*

A. As in Table 22-5, except decrease methadone at 7 mg/day over 20 days.
B. As in Table 22-5, but as follows:
　1. If taking greater than 30 mg/day, drop at 10 mg/day to 30 mg/day, then
　2. Drop at 5 mg/day to 20 mg/day; then
　3. Drop at 2.5 mg/day to zero.
　4. If taking less than 30 mg/day, start at step 2.

From Frances RJ, Franklin JE. Alcohol and other psychoactive substance use disorders. In: Talbott JA, Hales RE, Yudofsky SC, eds. *American Psychiatric Press textbook of psychiatry.* Washington, D.C.: American Psychiatry Press, 1988:67–75.

is little evidence for this, that methadone may be more difficult to detoxify from than other opiates. In support of this, methadone detoxification protocol with true opiate addicts can be extremely prolonged.

Another example of a nonmethadone detoxification protocol is presented in Table 22-4. This protocol has a number of advantages over others: it is simple; it does not use methadone; it does not use cocktails; it can be very rapid, with most patients being detoxified in 10 days; the patient is detoxified with the opiate of his or her choice and preference (i.e., the one he or she is most familiar with); and for patients taking one opiate only, there is no need for conversions to other opiates. The major disadvantage to this protocol is that, in most cases, detoxification proceeds with an opiate that has a short or intermediate half-life, thereby potentially permitting more patient discomfort than with methadone. However, this is minimized by *dose* detoxification first, followed by *time* detoxification. This distinction between time and dose detoxification is very important because patients using short–half-life opiates will be taking these at frequent intervals. There is one (12,13) literature report of the successful use of this protocol (14). At the University of Miami Pain Center, we have used this protocol for about 10 years without major problems.

TABLE 22-3. *Codeine or other opiate substitution/detoxification protocol*

1. Patient given as much opiate of choice as he or she requires for 24 to 48 hours.
2. Total intake of opiate over the 48 hours is calculated and translated into opiate of doctor's choice (e.g., codeine).
3. This total dose of codeine is divided into four doses and given over 24 hours (q6h).
4. This dose is given for 2 days.
5. Then this dose is decreased by 50 percent every 2 days.
6. When a dose equivalent to 10 mg methadone is reached, that dose is given for 2 days.

From Inturrisi CE. Role of opioid analgesics. *Am J Med* 1984;10:27–36.

TABLE 22-4. *Opiate of choice detoxification protocol*

1. Patient given as much opiate of choice as he or she requires for 3 days (i.e., a PRN demand schedule).
2. No intramuscular or intravenous opiates are allowed, and these routes are immediately switched to p.o.
3. At the end of 3 days, total dose of opiate is calculated and is translated into a daily opiate dose.
4. If the patient is taking two or three opiates, as is often the case, the opiates taken less frequently are translated into the opiate taken most frequently, and the daily opiate dose is calculated.
5. Detoxification will proceed with the opiate taken most frequently.
6. The daily opiate dose is split over the day according to the original demand schedule of the patient. For example, if the patient was taking Percodan at q2h intervals, the daily opiate dose will be split at q2h intervals.
7. Patient will be maintained on the q2h schedule for 2 days. This is not a demand schedule, and the patient is brought his or her medications.
8. Detoxification then proceeds by decreasing the dosage by 25% to 50% per day. For example, if patient is taking three Percodans every 2 hours, he or she would be detoxified to two every 2 hours, then one every 2 hours.
9. Once dosage detoxification is complete (i.e., patient is taking *one* pill at the time interval), then *time detoxification* begins. An example of this would be:
　a. one tab q4h × 1 day, then
　b. one tab q6h × 1 day, then
　c. one tab q8h × 1 day, then
　d. one tab q12h × 1 day, then
　e. one tab q.h.s. × 1 day, then
　f. D/C
10. No adjunct medications (doxepin, hydroxyzine) are given unless indicated (i.e., reasons other than detoxification problems).
11. Clonidine is given only if the patient has major withdrawal difficulties.
12. This protocol requires the cooperation of the patient. He or she is therefore advised of the following:
　a. During the first 3 days, he or she should take as much medication as he or she requires; if he or she takes less, detoxification may be more difficult than necessary.
　b. Total minimization of discomfort is not possible.
　c. Once the detoxification schedule is written, it will not be changed, no matter how much discomfort the patient experiences.
　d. During the detoxification, no PRN opiates will be administered.
　e. The patient is advised not to worry about his or her schedule during detoxification, because it is now the nurse's responsibility to bring the medications to the patient.
　f. The patient may refuse a dosage; however, this is not advisable and he or she will not be able to have any medication until the next scheduled dosage.
　g. If a patient is asleep during the time that he or she should receive an opiate dose, he or she will not be awakened.

Buprenorphine is an opiate with mixed agonist/antagonist properties and has a long duration of action, which may be a function of slow disassociation from opioid receptors and not a long half-life, as for methadone (12,13). Buprenorphine can also block the effects of exogenously used opiates and therefore reduce heroin self-administration (12). The drug is also associated with a very mild withdrawal syndrome which, however, can be prolonged. These properties suggested that this drug could be used in an opiate detoxification protocol. Buprenorphine was demonstrated to be as effective as methadone using such a protocol (12). This protocol is presented in Table 22-5. In addition, buprenorphine treatment has been shown to be superior to clonidine (discussed below) in controlling subjective and psychological withdrawal symptomatology (15). In the future, buprenorphine may be substituted for methadone in opiate detoxification protocols.

When working with opiate addicts, it is important to determine whether the addict in alleged opiate withdrawal is indeed physically opiate-dependent. To make this determination, a test using naloxone, an opiate antagonist, has been developed. This test is presented in Table 22-6. The naloxone challenge test appears to predict treatment outcome in opiate addicts (16). High naloxone challenge test scores at intake (high levels of opiate dependence) predict poor program retention (16).

In addition to determining whether the patient is physically opiate-dependent, opiate antagonists such as naloxone can be used to reduce the time required for opiate detoxification (17). This is called *opiate antagonist precipitated withdrawal*. The opiate withdrawal is compressed into as short a time as possible, with the hope that a short period of severe symptoms may be easier to cope with than a prolonged period of milder symptoms. This technique is demonstrated in the next section for opiate detoxification with clonidine (Tables 22-10 and 22-11), rapid detoxification (to be discussed below; Table 22-16), and ultra rapid detoxification (to be discussed below; Table 22-7)

Naltrexone (Trexan) is a nonaddicting, long-acting opioid antagonist. It has been approved for the treatment of opioid addiction in detoxified opioid addicts. This drug blocks the usual euphoric effects of opioids and thereby may pre-

vent the redevelopment of opioid dependence (17) and the drug-seeking behavior. Naltrexone does not cause physical or psychological dependence nor is there development of tolerance to this drug (18). Thus, naltrexone does not produce a "high" and thereby has no potential for abuse. Patients may discontinue this drug at any time without experiencing withdrawal symptoms (18). Naltrexone can be utilized after the completion of an opioid detoxification regimen (as in Table 22-16) for the purpose of preventing the redevelopment of opioid dependence/addiction. A general suggested procedure is as follows: (1) 7 days after completion of opioid taper, get urine toxicology; (2) if urine is negative for opioids, give patient a Narcan challenge test; (3) if test is negative and patient does not develop any withdrawal symptoms, begin

TABLE 22-5. *Buprenorphine substitution/ detoxification protocol*

1. Two mg of buprenorphine equivalent to 30 mg methadone.
2. Determine the patient's opiate stabilization dose in milligrams of methadone.
3. Buprenorphine is prepared in 20% aqueous alcohol and given once daily sublingually.
4. Buprenorphine detoxification is to proceed for 4 weeks with cuts of 25% in the first week and of 50% thereafter.

From Bickel WK, Stitzer ML, Bigelow GE, Liebson IA, Jasinski DR, Johnson RE. A clinical trial of buprenorphine: comparison with methadone in the detoxification of heroin addicts. *Clin Pharmacol Ther* 1988;43:72–78.

TABLE 22-6. *Naloxone opiate physical dependence test*

1. Administer naloxone 0.4 to 0.6 mg IM.
2. Watch for signs of opiate withdrawal syndrome.
3. If no effect, subject is not physically dependent.
4. To relieve withdrawal syndrome, give morphine 15 to 30 mg.

From Kosten TR, Krystal JH, Charney DS, et al. Rapid detoxification from opioid dependence. *Am J Psychiatry* 1989;146:1349.

TABLE 22-7. *Ultra rapid opioid detoxification protocol (operative protocol)*

Premedication i.v:	0.1 mg kg^{-1} diazepam 0.01. mg kg^{-1} atropine 150 mg clonidine
Induction of anesthesia	0.4 mg kg^{-1} midazolam 1.5 mg kg^{-1} propofol 0.6 mg kg^{-1} atracurium
Orotracheal intubation and mechanical ventilation (FiO$_2$=0.4).	
Insertion of naso-gastric tube and bladder catheter.	
Maintenance of anesthesia for 6 h:	0.15 mg kg^{-1}h^{-1} midazolam 1 mg kg^{-1}h^{-1} propofol 0.4 mg kg^{-1}h^{-1} atracurium
Monitoring:	ECG, non-invasive arterial BP pulse oximetry, capnography blood gas analysis
Infusion of hydosaline solutions	
Receptorial wash-out:	0.8 mg h^{-1} naloxone (infusion for 5h)
Evaluation of withdrawal symptoms (modified Wang Score).	
Awakening:	decurarization
Observation in intensive care for 24 h	
The day after:	naloxone test (0.8 mg IV) naltrexone induction

Adapted from Lorenzi P, Marsili M, Boncinelli S, Fabbri LP, Fontanaari P, Zorn AM, Mannaionit PF, Masini E. Searching for a general anaesthesia protocol for rapid detoxification from opioids. *Euro J Anaesth* 1999;16:719–727.

naltrexone 12.5 mg daily; (4) titrate dose up to 50 mg daily or to patient tolerance; (5) continue treatment for 1 to 2 years. Naltrexone is usually administered three times per week (19). Data indicates that opiate addicts who receive naltrexone are more likely to complete detoxification and less likely to relapse (19).

Levo-alpha-acetylmethadone (LAMM) (Orlaam) is a μ-opioid agonist approved for the maintenance treatment of opioid dependence. It is similar to methadone but has a longer half-life (48 to 72 hours), requiring a dosing frequency of three times per week (20). LAMM is also as safe and as effective as methadone but may have lower patient retention as it has a slower onset of action than methadone (20). As such, it is less likely to be abused as it does not produce an immediate high when ingested (21). Opioid detoxification protocols utilizing LAMM have yet to be developed. Patients on LAMM requiring detoxification should probably be detoxified with this drug utilizing a reduction schedule of 25% every week.

In recent years, *rapid and ultra rapid* opioid detoxification protocols have been developed. These are designed to dramatically shorten detoxification time by *precipitating* withdrawal through the administration of opioid antagonists such as naloxone or naltrexone. This approach is thought to have the advantage of getting patients through detoxification more rapidly and thus to minimize risk of relapse. In addition, such an approach allows a more rapid placement into follow-up treatment such as naltrexone maintenance and/or suitable psychosocial therapies. An example of such a rapid opioid detoxification protocol is presented in Table 22-16. Opioid antagonists such as naltrexone have also been utilized with buprenorphine (agonist-antagonist) in order to shorten detoxification. This method has also proved safe and effective (22). Ultra rapid opioid detoxification (UROD) represents a variant of the rapid opioid detoxification technique. Here patients undergo opioid antagonist-precipitated withdrawal such as in rapid opioid detoxification, but now under general anesthesia or heavy sedation (23,24). Advantages of this technique are alleged to be the potential cost saving and for the patient, a fear-free, comfortable withdrawal (24). At the present time there are no standardized protocols for ultra rapid opioid detoxification (24). One example of this type of protocol, which is claimed to stabilize vital signs and check withdrawal symptoms, is presented in Table 22-7. Rapid opioid detoxification studies have recently been reviewed (23). It was concluded that this literature was limited in terms of numbers of subjects evaluated, variations in protocols studied, lack of randomized design and use of control groups, and the short-term nature of the outcomes reported (23). In addition, the ultra rapid detoxification protocol literature indicates that this technique does not necessarily ameliorate all withdrawal symptoms (25). Finally, it appears that this approach, like other approaches, is associated with high relapse rates (25,26).

Clonidine Opiate Protocols

Opiate withdrawal is a state of adrenergic hyperactivity in which neurons of the locus caeruleus become markedly activated. Clonidine is an alpha-2 adrenergic agonist, which suppresses the acute dysphoric state associated with opiate withdrawal and appears to act by inhibiting the firing of the locus caeruleus via opening potassium channels (27). The ability of clonidine to suppress the symptoms and signs of opiate withdrawal has made the use of this drug popular for this purpose (28). Clonidine has some opiate-like properties, but does not bind to the opiate receptor and does not produce euphoria. Most signs and symptoms of withdrawal are reversed or prevented by 5 to 30 μg/kg oral clonidine (28). Clonidine is not the ideal agent for opiate withdrawal. It cannot be precisely titrated and higher doses may be limited by side effects such as hypertension. As a result, clonidine has limitations in its ability to suppress withdrawal manifestations as compared with methadone (29), and opiate addicts being detoxified with clonidine are more likely to fail at detoxification (30).

As an adjunct to methadone opiate detoxification, clonidine has many assets. With the addition of clonidine, the percentage of narcotic addicts who achieve a symptom-free state in inpatient studies is greater than with methadone alone, and the same in outpatients (28). It is also claimed that clonidine can decrease the time required for opiate detoxification to 3 to 5 days for short-acting opiates, 5 to 7 days for intermediate-acting opiates, and 7 to 10 days for long-acting ones (4). Clonidine can be used to detoxify from mixed agonist-antagonist opiates, which is a major plus. Clonidine, therefore, appears to offer additional options in the amelioration of the opiate withdrawal syndrome. Physicians must remember that abrupt discontinuation of clonidine can result in a withdrawal syndrome, however. Therefore, patients placed on clonidine detoxification protocols should then be tapered off this drug (4).

Clonidine opiate detoxification protocols can be classified as follows: clonidine alone, clonidine plus opiate antag-

TABLE 22-8. *Clonidine alone detoxification protocol*

1. At the first sign of withdrawal, 0.3 to 0.4 mg p.o. (5 μg/kg body wt.) stat clonidine.
2. Then 0.1 to 0.25 mg q4h for a total of 0.9 to 1.6 mg (or 15–20 μg/kg) on the first day.
3. Vital signs are taken hourly the first day, every 2 hours on the second, and every 4 hours thereafter.
4. Hold clonidine if blood pressure is less than 90/50 combined with a bradycardia of 50 beats or less per min. Hold until vital signs acceptable.
5. When vital signs are acceptable, reinstate clonidine q4h.
6. On the second day, and each day thereafter, reduce clonidine dosage by 50 percent.

From Cuthill JD, Beroniade V, Salvatori VA, Viguie F. Evaluation of clonidine suppression of opiate withdrawal reactions: a multidisciplinary approach. *Can J Psychiatry* 1989;35:377–382.

onist (naloxone or naltrexone), methadone followed by clonidine, clonidine alone–transdermal patch, and adjunct clonidine. These detoxification protocols are presented in Tables 22-8 through 22-14. The following observations apply to these protocols:

1. There is major variability on how much clonidine is given initially. The doses vary from 0.1 to 1.6 mg per day.
2. With the clonidine-antagonist protocol, one can detoxify a patient in 3 days.
3. The methadone-clonidine protocol does not contain a clonidine detoxification step. I believe this is necessary.

4. Transdermal clonidine offers the advantage of weekly application and stable blood levels of clonidine (31). This protocol requires 2 days of oral clonidine and continues for 21 days, however.
5. The adjunct clonidine protocol is only used if there are difficulties in detoxification and is the protocol used by our pain center. The patient is placed on clonidine until the opiate detoxification is complete, at which point he or she is detoxified from clonidine.

TABLE 22-9. *Variant of clonidine alone detoxification protocol*

1. Calculate the amount of daily opiate required from the history or observe intake.
2. Translate into methadone equivalents.
3. If the required equivalent is 25 mg methadone or less, begin at 0.05 mg clonidine b.i.d.
4. If the required equivalent is greater than 25 mg methadone, use 0.1 mg clonidine b.i.d.
5. Maintain on this dose for 3 days.
6. Then decrease clonidine by 25% per day.

From Ghodse H. *Drugs and addictive behavior: a guide to treatment.* Oxford: Blackwell Scientific Publications, 1990.

TABLE 22-10. *Clonidine plus opiate antagonist (naloxone) detoxification*

1. Clonidine 0.1 mg t.i.d. first day.
2. Clonidine 0.2 to 0.3 mg t.i.d. (monitor blood pressure) and naloxone 0.2 mg IM, then 0.4 mg IM q2h for four doses on the second day.
3. Clonidine (same dose as on day 2), naloxone 0.8 mg IM, five doses at 2-hour intervals on third day.
4. Demonstrate completeness of detoxification by a naloxone challenge: 0.4 mg IM should cause no withdrawal; then follow with 0.8 mg IM 1 hour later (no withdrawal should be noted); this is day 4.

From Ghodse H. *Drugs and addictive behavior: a guide to treatment.* Oxford: Blackwell Scientific Publications, 1990.

TABLE 22-11. *Clonidine, naloxone, and naltrexone detoxification protocol*

Day 1	Naloxone 0.8 mg IM; total clonidine 0.3–0.9 mg; naltrexone 12.5 mg.
Day 2	Total clonidine 0.3 to 0.9 mg; naltrexone 12.5 mg.
Day 3	Total clonidine 0.3 to 0.6 mg; naltrexone 25 mg.
Day 4	Total clonidine 0.3 to 0.6 mg; naltrexone 50 mg.
Day 5 and thereafter	Naltrexone 100 mg.

Compiled from Rawson RA, Washton AM, Resnick RB, Tennant FS Jr. Clonidine hydrochloride detoxification from methadone treatment—the value of naltrexone aftercare. *Adv Alcohol Subst Abuse* 1984;3:41–49.

TABLE 22-12. *Methadone followed by clonidine detoxification protocol*

1. Stabilize the patient on methadone.
2. Taper methadone to 20 mg/day.
3. Then switch to clonidine 0.1 to 0.3 mg t.i.d. for 2 days.
4. Then clonidine 0.2 to 0.7 mg t.i.d. for 8 to 14 days.
5. Then none.

From Frances RJ, Franklin JE. Alcohol and other psychoactive substance use disorders. In: Talbott JA, Hales RE, Yudofsky SC, eds. *American Psychiatric Press textbook of psychiatry.* Washington, D.C: American Psychiatry Press, 1988:67–75.

TABLE 22-13. *Clonidine alone–transdermal patch detoxification protocol*

1. Test dose oral clonidine 0.1 mg administered and blood pressure measured 1 hour later. If blood pressure systolic less than 90, patient is not to get patch.
2. Place two no. 2 transdermal clonidine patches or three patches (if patient weighs more than 150 lbs.) on a hairless area of the upper body.
3. For first 24 hours after patch application, give oral clonidine 0.2 mg q6h.
4. For the next 24 hours, give oral clonidine 0.1 mg q6h.
5. Change patches weekly.
6. After 2 weeks of two patches, switch to one no. 2 patch (or two no. 2 patches if the patient weighs more than 150 lbs.).
7. After 1 week of no. 6 (above), D/C patches.

From Spencer L, Gregory M. Clonidine transdermal patches for use in outpatient opiate withdrawal. *J Subst Abuse Treatment* 1989;6:113–117.

TABLE 22-14. *Adjunct clonidine detoxification protocol*

1. Only start clonidine if the patient demonstrates signs of withdrawal syndrome and/or exhibits major behavioral problems with detoxification.
2. Clonidine 0.1 to 0.4 mg per day in divided doses to start.
3. Increase gradually to a maximum of 1.2 mg/per day (divided into three doses) according to symptoms.
4. Blood pressure taken lying and standing q.i.d. If less than 90 systolic, clonidine is held for the next dose.
5. Stop increases as soon as symptoms decrease.
6. Maintain on this dose until completion of opiate detoxification.
7. Then begin clonidine detoxification at 25% to 50% decrease per day.
8. Space clonidine detoxification over 1 week.

In using clonidine for opiate detoxification, the physician will need to monitor blood pressure and should try to use the lowest possible dose of clonidine necessary. I believe that patients should be carefully selected for adjunct clonidine opiate detoxification using two criteria: difficulties in the detoxification process and presence of addictive behaviors. This selection is necessary because clonidine use will prolong detoxification, because clonidine itself requires a taper.

LOFEXIDINE

Lofexidine is an alpha-2 adrenergic agonist with similar properties to clonidine (32). As presented above, the usefulness of clonidine for opioid detoxification has been significantly restricted by its marked hypotensive effects (32). Lofexidine in contrast to clonidine was not found to have strong antihypertensive properties and as such its production was abandoned in the United States. However, in the United Kingdom lofexidine has been utilized for opioid detoxification since 1992 (32).

There have been a number of studies performed with this drug (32). Three reports compared lofexidine with clonidine. These three studies found this drug to be similar to clonidine at moderating the effects of withdrawal but without the problem of hypotension (32). Two studies compared lofexidine with methadone for opioid detoxification. Interestingly methadone demonstrated a more rapid resolution of withdrawal symptoms with lofexidine, especially so in a rapid opioid detoxification protocol. It is likely that when this drug becomes available in the United States, it will be substituted for clonidine in all clonidine opioid detoxification protocols.

PROTOCOLS USING OTHER MEDICATION

Detoxification protocols using medications other than opiates and clonidine are presented in Table 22-15. These protocols will ameliorate opiate withdrawal syndrome, but less successfully than opiates or clonidine will. The protocols mainly affect anxiety generated by the syndrome.

The medications used in these protocols are used as *adjuncts* in the detoxification process. Propranolol is one such medication. Often, in opiate withdrawal syndrome, the patients complain of restlessness that presents like anxiety. Propranolol, at doses of 20 to 40 mg/day, has been used successfully for this problem during detoxification (33).

Doxepin is another adjunct medication used successfully during opiate detoxification. Doxepin appears to augment methadone opiate withdrawal (34). It is administered in doses of 50 to 100 mg by mouth at bedtime during detoxification and is maintained for 6 weeks. It is not clear by what mechanism doxepin augments opiate withdrawal. Doxepin may act by simply increasing the levels of methadone or by combating anxiety and/or depression.

TABLE 22-15. *Detoxification protocols using other medications*

I. *Neuroleptics*
  1. Thioridazine 25 mg p.o., b.i.d. and 75 mg h.s. for 2 weeks
  2. Then tapered for 1 week

II. *Diphenoxylate (Lomotil)*
  1. Two tabs q.i.d. for 4 days
  2. Then slowly tapered
  3. Can be combined with thioridazine

III. *Beta-Adrenoreceptor Blocking Drugs*
  1. Reduces craving after heroin withdrawal
  2. May be helpful in high somatic anxiety, as indicated by raised pulse rate and high blood pressure
  3. Propranolol, 80 to 160 mg in divided doses for 2 to 3 weeks
  4. Then slowly tapered

IV. *Sedative Protocol for Opiate Detoxification*
  1. Does not relieve opiate withdrawal syndrome, only the anxiety
  2. Not the treatment of choice
  3. Use diazepam as follows:
     a. 10 mg q.i.d. × 3 days; then
     b. 10 mg t.i.d. × 1 day; then
     c. 10 mg b.i.d. × 1 day; then
     d. 5 mg b.i.d. × 1 day; then
     e. 5 mg h.s. × 1 day; then
     f. D/C

Compiled from Ghodse H. *Drugs and addictive behavior: a guide to treatment.* Oxford: Blackwell Scientific Publications, 1990.

Doxepin may therefore be the ideal adjunct for opiate detoxification.

Naloxone-precipitated opiate detoxification is often uncomfortable. Therefore, researchers have concentrated on adjunct medications to make this process more tolerable. Methohexitone, a barbiturate (35), and midazolam, a short-acting benzodiazepine (36), appear to be such agents. Both of these agents appear to block objective signs of withdrawal precipitated by naloxone. The use of midazolam for this purpose is presented in Table 22-16.

Although there have been a number of reports (33) on the usefulness of acupuncture in easing opioid detoxification, there has only been one controlled study (37) on this issue. This study (37) found that for some outcome variable acupuncture did demonstrate some efficacy. A recent review (38) has also concluded that acupuncture was effective in the treatment of drug withdrawal (i.e., detoxification). Thus, acupuncture can be considered as an adjunct to existing opioid detoxification protocols.

Conclusions

At issue is whether there is good evidence for the superiority of one opiate detoxification protocol over another. The answer to this question is that at the present time there is

TABLE 22-16. *Midazolam, naloxone, flumazenil, and naltrexone detoxification protocol*

1. Twenty-four hours after last oral dose of methadone, give bolus of 30 mg midazolam IV.
2. Dilute 4 mg of naloxone in 200 ml of 0.9% saline and inject IV via infusion pump. This step is performed 10 min after step 1 above.
3. Maintain sedation with repeated midazolam injections of 50 to 75 mg.
4. After completion of naloxone infusion, give repeated doses of flumazenil 2 to 6 mg until fully awake.
5. Then continue with oral naltrexone treatment at 50 mg/day.
6. During the procedure, record heart rate continuously by EKG and blood pressure by automatic cuff manometer.

Compiled from Rawson RA, Washton AM, Resnick RB, Tennant FS Jr. Clonidine hydrochloride detoxification from methadone treatment—the value of naltrexone aftercare. *Adv Alcohol Subst Abuse* 1984;3:41–49.

TABLE 22-17. *Advantages and disadvantages of different opiate detoxification protocols*

	Addictive potential	Dangers	Time required to complete	Detoxification with opiate of preference	Severity of withdrawal (methadone as reference compound)	Failure of detoxification (methadone as reference compound)	Ability to detoxify from mixed agonist antagonists
Methadone substitution/ detoxification	High	May accumulate	17+ days	No	Same	Same	No
Codeine or other opiate substitution/ detoxification	Lower for codeine	None	8–9+ days	No	More severe	?	No
Opiate of choice detoxification	Same as drug utilized	As for drug utilized	10+ days	Yes	Usually more as detoxifying with drug utilized	Less	Yes, if utilizing an agonist– antagonist
Buprenorphine substitution detoxification	Low	None	28 days	No	Less severe and more severe	Less	Yes
Clonidine alone	None	Decreased BP	6+ days	No	Severe	More	Yes
Clonidine plus opiate antagonist (naloxone)	None	Decreased BP	4 days	No	Very severe	More	Yes
Clonidine, naloxone, and naltrexone	None	Decreased BP	5 days	No	Very severe	Less	Yes
Methadone followed by clonidine	High	Accumulation and decreased BP	33 days	No	Less severe	Should be less than for methadone alone	No
Adjunct clonidine	Low	Decreased BP	Variable	Yes	More	Should be less than for methadone alone	No
Rapid and ultra rapid opioid detoxification	None	Cardiac arrest	Hrs. to one day	No	Can be severe	Less	Yes

no reliable scientific evidence that would lead this author to recommend one opioid detoxification protocol over another. The choice of a particular protocol should then be dictated by such clinical factors as the need for rapid detoxification, safety concerns, patient and clinician comfort with severity of detoxification symptoms, and the patient population dealt with. However, to compare the various opioid detoxification protocols and to help the clinician choose a protocol appropriate to his or her needs, a comparison table (Table 22-17) was developed.

HYPNOSEDATIVE DETOXIFICATION

Of the hypnosedatives, the barbiturates and nonbarbiturates are rarely administered. The benzodiazepines are now the most important hypnosedative group to the pain physician. This group is widely used for the treatment of anxiety and insomnia within the general population (39) and with chronic pain patients (40). There is much controversy over abuse/dependence/addiction to benzodiazepines in the chronic pain population (41). This issue and the reasons for benzodiazepine detoxification in chronic pain patients have been reviewed in detail (41).

Benzodiazepines differ in abuse liability (i.e., attractiveness as drugs of abuse). This abuse liability is rated as follows (highest to lowest): diazepam, lorazepam, alprazolam, oxazepam, and chlordiazepoxide (42). Abuse potential does not appear to depend on the half-life of the drug.

Physical dependence to the benzodiazepines can occur even with doses in the clinical range, but requires 6 to 8 months to develop (43). The short-acting benzodiazepines may have a stronger potential for physical dependence (34). Interestingly, tolerance to the therapeutic effect *does not* develop (39). Three types of benzodiazepine dependence syndromes have been described (44). The patient takes several times the normal therapeutic dose: primary high-dose dependency. The patient takes therapeutic doses: primary low-dose dependency. The patient takes benzodiazepines to treat alcohol or opiate withdrawal: secondary dependency. Patients who manifest primary high-dose dependence are most likely to display addictive behaviors.

Although the hypnosedatives generally cause the same type of withdrawal syndrome, the different classes of hypnosedatives can vary in some signs and symptoms of withdrawal. Barbiturate withdrawal can result in a classic severe withdrawal syndrome that is much like that of alcohol. The signs and symptoms of this withdrawal syndrome are described in most reference texts (45). In general, the hypnosedative withdrawal syndrome will occur from the 2nd to the 14th day after drug cessation (46), and the withdrawal reaction can last 5 to 20 days (43). It is claimed that unless a hypnosedative has been administered daily for more than 1 month in amounts equivalent to 400 to 600 mg of a short-acting barbiturate, a severe withdrawal syndrome will not develop (46). To determine whether the patient may or may not develop a severe hypnosedative withdrawal syndrome,

the treating physician should add the total amount of the hypnosedative taken by the patient per day and translate that total amount into a short-acting barbiturate dosage. This conversion can be made with a hypnosedative dosage equivalence chart (47).

Hypnosedative withdrawal has been divided into two types: with delirium and uncomplicated withdrawal. The *DSM-IIV-TR* has developed diagnostic criteria for uncomplicated withdrawal (7). Barbiturates and alcohol use are more likely to be associated with withdrawal delirium, whereas benzodiazepine withdrawal is more likely to be of the uncomplicated type (48).

Benzodiazepine withdrawal has also been divided into major and minor types. Owen (43) has described the signs and symptoms of these two types of withdrawal. These signs and symptoms will also differ between abrupt withdrawal and gradual benzodiazepine discontinuation (48,49). Even a gradual discontinuation, however, appears not to suppress all the signs and symptoms of benzodiazepine withdrawal. Thus, a benzodiazepine withdrawal syndrome will develop even when a gradual taper of *25% per week* is undertaken (47). It is not clear whether these symptoms are withdrawal, rebound, or simply the return of anxiety in a patient being treated for anxiety (43). It is now clear that some form of withdrawal syndrome can be observed in about half the patients discontinuing benzodiazepines (46).

The tendency to experience the benzodiazepine withdrawal syndrome is a function of dosage and duration of treatment and occurs more rapidly in patients taking short–half-life benzodiazepines (43). In addition, the more rapid the fall in benzodiazepine blood level the more likely a withdrawal will occur (43). Severity of withdrawal may be related to benzodiazepine potency, with high-potency drugs such as lorazepam producing more severe withdrawal than medium-potency drugs such as diazepam and low-potency drugs such as chlordiazepoxide (44). In addition, individuals with a psychobiologic predisposition to addiction (often with a past history or family history of alcoholism) may manifest severe benzodiazepine withdrawal symptoms on abrupt benzodiazepine cessation.

Rebound is the return of a symptom for which the drug was originally prescribed, to a degree that is worse than before the drug (44). The benzodiazepine drugs are associated with rebound, especially the short-acting hypnotic benzodiazepine triazolam, which produces prompt and severe rebound. Because of rebound and reemerging anxiety symptoms even in a gradual benzodiazepine taper (25% per week), a large percentage (approximately 36%) of patients treated for anxiety syndromes will not complete detoxification. Patients on long–half-life benzodiazepines may achieve detoxification in greater numbers, however (49).

In summary, after benzodiazepine drug reduction or cessation, the patient could experience the following syndromes: none, return of preexisting disorder, rebound, major withdrawal symptoms, minor withdrawal symptoms, combination of rebound and withdrawal, disturbed social/behavioral problems, mood disturbance (major depression), and new anxiety symptoms not before exhibited, such as panic and emotional reaction to anticipated drug withdrawal (50). It is difficult to make a distinction among these syndromes. The pain physician detoxifying a patient from benzodiazepines should be aware of the possibility of the development of these syndromes, however.

Chronic pain patients taking benzodiazepines for anxiety present a special problem. These patients should have a psychiatric examination to determine the type of anxiety syndrome, and whether this syndrome existed before the onset of chronic pain. If the syndrome existed before the pain condition, that patient is less likely to be successfully detoxified and may not be a candidate for detoxification. Efforts should be made, however, according to the anxiety syndrome diagnosed, to place the patient on other agents that may control his or her anxiety syndrome (e.g., buspirone, MAO inhibitors, tricyclics, beta-blockers). Patients who do not have preexisting anxiety syndromes but who have current anxiety problems may also have difficulties during detoxification for reasons described above. These difficulties may complicate pain treatment and may occur no matter how slow the taper.

Benzodiazepine Detoxification Protocols

Drugs within the hypnosedative group are mutually cross-tolerant. Thus, as long as dosage equivalencies are calculated correctly (47), any drug within this group can be detoxified by using any other drug within the group (3). There are three major types of benzodiazepine detoxification protocols: graded reduction of the benzodiazepine of dependence, substitution of long-acting benzodiazepine, and phenobarbital substitution. All three, together with their indications, are presented in Table 22-18. Selection of the technique depends on a variety of factors, including severity of dependency, interaction with other drugs, setting for detoxification, and physician expertise (51).

There is disagreement regarding the speed of detoxification for graded reduction. Some authors advocate a 25%

reduction every 3 days, which should be titrated according to the severity of withdrawal symptoms (51). Other authors advocate a detoxification schedule of 6 to 12 weeks in which dose reduction is no greater than 5 mg of diazepam per week (52). The manufacturer of alprazolam has recommended that for this drug, dosage should be reduced *weekly*. If taking over 3 mg/day of alprazolam, the dosage reduction should be 0.5 mg/week, whereas for patients taking less than 3 mg the reduction should be 0.25 mg/week. Some authors, however, allege that alprazolam can be detoxified much faster, and they advocate a reduction of 1 mg every 3 days, or 0.5 mg every 3 days, with a gradual reduction over 3 to 12 weeks (53). Again, the pain physician will need to decide between a slow taper and an expeditious taper on clinical grounds.

According to my experience if problems or difficulties appear during benzodiazepine detoxification, they can be attributed to one or more of the factors listed in Table 22-19. Difficulties in the detoxification process are best avoided by a high index of suspicion for the presence of these factors and by a patient education approach (52). Because of the great likelihood for the development of detoxification problems, patients characterized by the following problems should have a slow taper: preexistent anxiety syndromes (prepain), intense anxiety, trouble coping with current anxiety, increased anxiety with increased pain, and dependent personality features (52).

Substitution of a long-acting benzodiazepine as a detoxification protocol has been advocated for withdrawal from short-acting benzodiazepines. This is because short-acting benzodiazepines, such as alprazolam, may be associated with more withdrawal symptoms than the longer-acting agents, such as clonazepam (54). Thus, to make detoxification more tolerable, four long-acting agents have been used in substitution detoxification: chlordiazepoxide, diazepam, clonazepam, and phenobarbital. Examples of long-acting benzodiazepine substitution protocols are presented in Table 22-20. An example of phenobarbital substitution protocol is presented in Table 22-21. For some patients, substitution to long-acting benzodiazepines for alprazolam withdrawal has not been effective, but phenobarbital has been (51).

TABLE 22-18. *Acute benzodiazepine detoxification methods*

Detoxification method	Indications	Drugs used
Graded reduction of the benzodiazepine of dependence	Primarily used in medical setting for therapeutic range dependency	Drug used
Substitution of long-acting benzodiazepine	Primarily used for alcohol and/or alcohol-benzodiazepine combination dependency Also now used for therapeutic range dependency	Chlordiazepoxide, diazepam, clonazepam
Phenobarbital substitution	Primarily used for benzodiazepine-poly drug use Also useful for high-dose benzodiazepine dependency This method has the broadest utility for all sedative-hypnotics	Phenobarbital

Adapted from Smith DE, Wesson DR. Phenobarbital technique for the treatment of barbiturate dependence. *Arch Gen Psychiatry* 1971;24:56–60, and Smith DE, Landry MJ. Benzodiazepine dependence discontinuation: focus on the chemical dependency detoxification setting and benzodiazepine-poly-drug abuse. *J Psychiatr Res* 1990;24(Suppl 2):145–156.

TABLE 22-19. *Factors involved in benzodiazepine detoxification problems*

1. Taper too rapid
2. Dosage decrease too large
3. Fear of tapering, patient was not sufficiently prepared
4. Caffeine use
5. Alcohol use
6. Illicit drug use
7. Menstrual syndrome (PMS) symptoms
8. Medical condition problem (e.g., increased pain)
9. Life stressors
10. Difficulties in handling tapering problems in a flexible manner
11. Return of preexisting disorder
12. Rebound
13. Major and minor withdrawal symptoms
14. Mood disorder
15. New anxiety symptoms

Adapted from Dupont RL. A practical approach to benzodiazepine discontinuation. *J Psychiatr Res* 1990;24(Suppl 2): 81–90.

Adjunct Medications

To assist hypnosedative detoxification, adjunct medications have been used. Research for opiate and alcohol withdrawal syndrome has recommended clonidine for benzodiazepine withdrawal. Unfortunately, it is only partially effective at a dose of 0.1 to 1.2 mg/day (55). Propranolol in doses of 20 mg four times per day is also only partially effective, but should be used for rebound and symptom reemergence (51,55). Because carbamazepine demonstrated efficacy in alcohol withdrawal, it was used in benzodiazepine with-

TABLE 22-20. *Benzodiazepine detoxification protocol using substitution of long-acting benzodiazepine*

A. Using Diazepam[a]
The dosage of diazepam equivalent to the patient's total benzodiazepine daily dose is calculated (38) for high-dose benzodiazepine abuse, and a loading dose of diazepam of 40% of the patient's total benzodiazepine daily dose is given. Diazepam is then reduced 10% per day for a probable 14-day taper. A slower variant of this technique is to estimate total daily dose by history. Divide this dose into four equivalent doses and administer for 2 days. Then, decrease by 10% per day. If required, give 5 mg Valium PRN for signs of withdrawal syndrome. When remaining diazepam dose reaches 10%, reduce over 4 days. Although slower, the authors recommend this latter method.

B. Using Clonazepam to Substitute for Alprazolam[b]
1. First day, transfer to clonazepam at a milligram-to-milligram equivalency.
2. Divide clonazepam into b.i.d. dosage.
3. Taper clonazepam at 1 to 1.5 mg every 2 days.
4. Taper completed in 7 to 10 days.

[a]From Harrison M, Busto U, Navanjo CA, Kaplan HL, Sellers EM. Diazepam tapering in detoxification for high-dose benzodiazepine abuse. *Clin Pharmacol Ther* 1984;36:527–533.
[b]Patterson JF. Withdrawal from alprazolam dependency using clonazepam: clinical observations. *J Clin Psychiatry* 1990;51(Suppl 5):47–49.

TABLE 22-21. *Benzodiazepine detoxification protocol using phenobarbital substitution*

1. To calculate the amount of hypnosedative that the patient requires per day, he or she is given the phenobarbital challenge test (43).
2. The amount of pentobarbital (in milligrams) required for 24 hours is calculated from the test.
3. This dose is translated into phenobarbital equivalency (38).
4. Phenobarbital is divided in q8h doses.
5. Detoxification proceeds at one-tenth the starting dose per day.

From Shader RI, Caine ED, Meyer RE. Treatment of dependence on barbiturates and sedative-hypnotics. In: Shader RI, ed. *Manual of psychiatric therapeutics.* Boston, Little Brown, 1989; and from Smith DE, Wesson DR. Phenobarbital technique for the treatment of barbiturate dependence. *Arch Gen Psychiatry* 1971;24:56–60.

drawal. Carbamazepine was initiated at 200 mg by mouth twice a day at the onset of detoxification, and increased to 800 mg per day, depending on symptoms. It was then discontinued in 3 to 14 days after completion of benzodiazepine detoxification (56). Of these three agents, carbamazepine may have the greatest effectiveness as an adjunct medication for benzodiazepine withdrawal.

Recently, a new nonbenzodiazepine anxiolytic has been developed: buspirone. This drug was used in one study of alprazolam detoxification and has demonstrated that it can decrease the manifestations of withdrawal (57). Buspirone was initiated 2 weeks before beginning the taper at a dosage of 5 mg three times per day. Because buspirone appears not to have any abuse liability, it could be very useful. A final approach could be the addition of an antipanic agent, such as imipramine Tri-Cyclic Antidepressants (TCA) or phenelzine Mono-Amine Oxidase Inhibitors (MAO), before beginning detoxification. Such an approach could minimize rebound and symptom reemergence problems.

Alcohol Abuse/Dependence/Withdrawal and Psychiatric Dual Diagnosis

Alcohol or ethanol is a depressant drug and is classified under the hypnosedative group. Current alcohol abuse/ dependence has been reported to be present in 4.3% of a large sample of chronic pain patients (58). Alcohol abuse/dependence in remission has been reported to be present in 7.4% of chronic pain patients (58). Thus, approximately 12% of chronic pain patients appear to have had a problem with alcohol at one point. As with other drugs of abuse, patients who abuse and/or are dependent on alcohol suffer from other psychiatric disorders (dual diagnosis) (56). The pain physician should therefore maintain a high index of suspicion for potential dual diagnosis in alcoholic patients, because the dual diagnosis problem can interfere with alcohol detoxification and the concomitant treatment of chronic pain.

Alcohol withdrawal signs and symptoms have been well described and subdivided into mild, moderate, and severe forms (59). The *DSM-IV-TR* divides alcohol withdrawal syndrome into *uncomplicated alcohol withdrawal* and *alcohol withdrawal delirium* (7). This classification is simpler and therefore less confusing. In the mild, moderate, and severe classification, both the moderate and severe forms contain some signs and symptoms of delirium, and this is confusing. The mild, moderate, and severe classification, however, lends itself more to the alcohol withdrawal detoxification protocol to be described below. The most effective treatment of alcohol withdrawal, however, is a preventive approach. The pain physician should be alert to the development of alcohol withdrawal in any patient he or she suspects of alcohol abuse/dependence. These patients should be closely monitored; if they demonstrate symptoms of withdrawal, prophylactic aggressive treatment to prevent delirium should be initiated.

ALCOHOL WITHDRAWAL DETOXIFICATION PROTOCOLS

Benzodiazepines are clearly the drugs of choice for the treatment of alcohol withdrawal. This group has consistently demonstrated superiority to placebo in controlled trials for the treatment of alcohol withdrawal (47). Of the benzodiazepines, two drugs—chlordiazepoxide and diazepam—have emerged as the drugs of choice. Chlordiazepoxide may be preferable over diazepam because of its lower abuse potential (42). The use of these benzodiazepines for the treatment of various types of alcohol withdrawal is demonstrated in Table 22-22. This alcohol withdrawal detoxification protocol demonstrates the treatment of alcohol withdrawal according to the type of syndrome. In addition it advises on the use of other benzodiazepines (e.g., lorazepam) in other specific situations. This protocol also lists adjunct treatments such as magnesium. According to my experience, this protocol can be extremely effective. Often, however, the mistake is made of placing the patient on a PRN chlordiazepoxide schedule after the initial dosage. This is not correct, because generally the nursing staff withholds the PRN benzodiazepine and the patient continues in withdrawal, especially if the routine dosage has not been calculated correctly. Thus, if a PRN order is written, it should specify the symptom for which the medication should be given (e.g., agitation, tremor). A better way to give the benzodiazepine is as in numbers 4 and 5 of Table 22-22, but at the interval specified *unless the patient is asleep.* This type of order will ensure that the patient will get enough benzodiazepine over a short period to terminate the alcohol withdrawal syndrome and prevent delirium. The prevention of delirium in an alcohol withdrawal syndrome should be of primary concern.

Other Alcohol Withdrawal and Alcohol Addiction Treatments

In addition to the benzodiazepines, other drugs also appear to control the autonomic dysfunction in alcohol withdrawal. Clonidine is claimed to be as useful as the benzodiazepines, but will not prevent seizures or delirium (60). Atenolol (a beta-blocker) appears to decrease the symptoms of tremor, rapid heart rate, and hypertension in this syndrome (60). In

TABLE 22-22. *Alcohol withdrawal detoxification protocol*

1. Because of severe medical consequences of alcohol abuse and potential for dehydration/seizure/death, all patients should have adequate medical evaluation for concomitant medical/surgical/psychiatric conditions, including full-range laboratory work-up.
2. *Minimal syndrome*—Drug-free, reassurance given, adequate but appropriate stimulation, milieu support (social setting detoxification).
3. *Mild syndrome*—Chlordiazepoxide 10 to 25 mg p.o. q.i.d. for 2 to 5 days, regular contact with clinician, titrate dosage as needed.
4. *Moderate syndrome*—Chlordiazepoxide 50 to 100 mg p.o. initially, then 25 mg. q. 3 to 4 h. for first 24 hours, then taper total dose by 25% to 33%/day.
5. *Severe syndrome*—Chlordiazepoxide 50 to 100 mg p.o. initially, then 50–100 mg q1 to 2h until adequately sedated, then D/C and observe for at least 48 hours.
6. *Emergency management*—If very severe, diazepam 5 to 10 mg IV slow push (2 to 5 mg/min), may be repeated PRN or lorazepam 2 to 5 mg IM or IV may be given and repeated. When stable, use p.o. regimen as above.
7. Thiamine 100 mg orally four times daily.
8. Folic acid 1 mg orally four times daily.
9. Multivitamin, one per day.
10. Magnesium sulfate 1 g IM every 6 hours for 2 days (if status following withdrawal involves seizures).
11. Use lorazepam or oxazepam in debilitated patients and those with chronic obstructive pulmonary disease (COPD) or severe liver disease.
12. If benzodiazepine must be taken IM, do not administer chlordiazepoxide or diazepam, because they are poorly absorbed by IM route; use lorazepam.
13. Patients must be carefully monitored. Signs of oversedation should lead to withholding doses and decreasing subsequent doses. Continued withdrawal should prompt increased dose or reevaluation of choice of drug, increased dosing interval, and/or route of administration, checking for presence of hypoglycemia or hypomagnesemia.
14. Phenytoin 100 mg p.o. q.i.d., if history of seizure disorder and/or previous withdrawal seizures.

Adapted from Wartenberg AA. Detoxification of the chemically dependent patient. *Rhode Island Med J,* 1989;72:451–456.

addition, the anticonvulsants carbamazepine and valproic acid have been tried (61,62). These drugs retard the development of kindling foci in the limbic system, thereby controlling seizure development (60). Carbamazepine in doses of 800 mg per day has been found to be as efficacious as oxazepam (60) and may have some efficacy in the treatment of alcohol dependence/addiction (63). Thus, these drugs may have some utility for these two indications. Detoxification protocols utilizing these two drugs have not yet been developed. These drugs could, however, be added to a benzodiazepine alcohol withdrawal detoxification protocol to further ease the symptoms of withdrawal.

Many studies have shown that alcoholics often suffer from comorbid psychiatric disorders such as depression and anxiety (64). These disorders are thought to increase the risk of relapse (64). As such, the detection of these disorders in an alcoholic completing an alcohol detoxification regimen should lead the pain physician into considering utilizing buspirone for anxiety and/or the tricyclic antidepressants for depression. These drugs have proven efficacy in some alcoholics (64). In addition, there are some studies that suggest that the serotonin reuptake inhibitors (citalopram, fluoxetine) reduce alcohol consumption (65,66).

Naltrexone properties have been described above. Recently this drug, trade name Revia, was approved for the adjunct treatment of alcoholism. Naltrexone seems to interfere with the craving for alcohol that abstinent alcoholics feel (67). Patients on naltrexone drink less, take longer to relapse, and have longer times between relapses (68). Thus, alcoholics completing alcohol withdrawal detoxification protocols can be considered for naltrexone maintenance. In this case, placement would begin immediately after completion of the detoxification protocol. Thus, the clinician may consider utilizing the above drugs (anticonvulsants, antidepressants, naltrexone) either during or after completion of an alcohol detoxification protocol.

There are two other drugs that have recently been reported to have some efficacy in alcoholism. The first, ondansetron (Zofran), a serotonin 5-HT3 receptor antagonist approved as an antiemetic, has been shown to decrease drinking among some alcoholics (21). The 5-HT3 receptor has been associated with regulating dopamine release in the nucleus accumbens. This blockade may underlie the effectiveness of ondansetron. Ondansetron is currently available in IM form only. The second drug is isradipine (DynaCirc). This is a calcium channel blocker currently approved for hypertension that may prevent relapse in alcohol addiction. In a double-blind controlled study, isradipine was compared to naltrexone for prevention of alcohol relapse. The isradipine group remained abstinent significantly longer (69).

Finally, there are two other drugs that are currently not available but appear to have significant efficacy for alcohol relapse prevention. These drugs are nalmefene and acamprosate. Nalmefene is an opioid antagonist similar to naltrexone but has a longer duration of antagonist action and less tendency toward liver toxicity (70). It has been shown

to be effective in reducing heavy drinking episodes (70). Acamprosate (calcium acetyl homotaurinate) appears to act by restoring normal N-metyl D-aspartate (NMDA) receptor tone in the glutamate system (71), thus relieving the discomfort of not having alcohol. Several studies have demonstrated the efficacy of this drug for maintaining abstinence with long-term benefits (72). This medication has also been reported to lower the rates of consumption during periods of relapse (71). It is expected that these two drugs will become available soon. As such, in appropriate patients, they can be added to the end of alcohol detoxification protocols. Finally, a recent review (73) has concluded that acupuncture may also help alcoholics become abstinent. Thus, this modality can also be added to alcohol detoxification protocols.

NICOTINE DETOXIFICATION

There are 50 million smokers in the USA (74). Of these, 27%, 32%, and 26% are white, black, and Hispanic males, respectively. For females, 23%, 22%, and 14% are white, black, and Hispanic, respectively (74). There is some evidence that a large percentage of chronic pain patients (CPPs) smoke (75) and that these percentages may even be higher than that of the general U.S. population. This is because nicotine dependence is frequently associated with two types of comorbid psychiatric conditions: other substance abuse disorders (76,77) and affective disorders (78). The presence of these comorbidities often means that the patient is more highly dependent on nicotine and thereby has greater difficulty quitting (77,78). The increased prevalence of nicotine dependence within CPPs may, therefore be partially related to the frequent presence of these two comorbidities within CPPs (79). Thus, the pain physician may frequently come into contact with a CPP who may wish to be detoxified from nicotine or the pain physician may deem that such treatment may help the CPP eliminate some other drug dependencies such as alcohol or opioids.

Nicotine dependence can be visualized as being determined by two types of reinforcers: positive and negative (Table 22-23). Positive reinforcers are associated with the positive aspects of using nicotine, whereas the negative reinforcers are associated with the negative consequences of not utilizing nicotine (i.e., withdrawal symptoms). Nicotine replacement has now become the cornerstone of nicotine detoxification and appears to work by decreasing withdrawal symptoms and intense craving (80). It is then to be noted here that the object of nicotine replacement *is not to* provide the positive reinforcers to smoking (Table 22-23), which smokers crave. Nicotine dependent smokers wishing to quit, then, have to be advised of the objectives of the nicotine replacement regimen in helping them to detoxify from nicotine (i.e., prevention withdrawal symptoms only). Smokers wishing to quit using the nicotine replacement regimen will have to deal with the lack of positive reinforcers behaviorally.

TABLE 22-23. *Reinforcers in nicotine dependence*

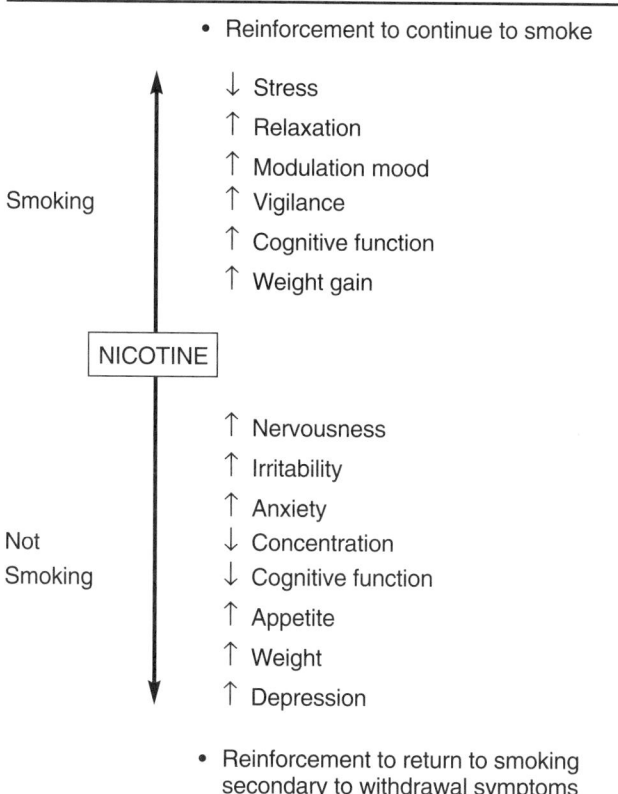

- Reinforcement to continue to smoke

Smoking
- ↓ Stress
- ↑ Relaxation
- ↑ Modulation mood
- ↑ Vigilance
- ↑ Cognitive function
- ↑ Weight gain

NICOTINE

Not Smoking
- ↑ Nervousness
- ↑ Irritability
- ↑ Anxiety
- ↓ Concentration
- ↓ Cognitive function
- ↑ Appetite
- ↑ Weight
- ↑ Depression

- Reinforcement to return to smoking secondary to withdrawal symptoms

The various available nicotine replacement methods, along with their advantages and disadvantages, are presented in Table 22-24. The most important aspect of Table 22-24 is the nicotine blood levels generated by the use of these various systems. To understand this statement one needs to realize that the frequency of utilizing nicotine in the form of cigarettes is determined by the positive and negative reinforcers in Table 22-23. These come into play when nicotine blood levels approach a certain blood level for positive reinforcement and drop to a certain blood level for negative reinforcement. Thus, nicotine blood levels gener-

ated by smoking are most closely approximated within the nasal spray system. However, for a patient to successfully complete nicotine detoxification to zero, that patient has to be willing to tolerate the withdrawal of positive reinforcement or the rush associated with high nicotine blood levels. As such, the patch system provides less nicotine than the nasal system, but the steady nicotine blood levels prevent the negative reinforcement (withdrawal symptoms). Withdrawal symptoms can be associated with all the other nicotine replacement systems because of the rise and fall in nicotine blood levels. As one would expect, the patch systems appear to be more effective for lower than higher dependence smokers. In contrast, the nasal spray system appears to have a greater relative benefit for highly dependent smokers (78). All of these replacement systems reduce the tar, carbon monoxide, or other chemicals associated with cigarette smoking. As such, if the patient can reduce the number of cigarettes smoked per day, utilizing any replacement system can be considered a partial success (78).

A nicotine detoxification protocol has been published by the American Psychiatric Association (81). This protocol is presented in Table 22-25 and is divided into first-line treatment and second-line treatment. Second-line treatments are to be initiated if the first-line treatments fail (81). Bupropion and the nicotine inhaler have been added to this protocol. At the time this protocol was published, these methods were not yet FDA approved for the treatment of nicotine dependence.

Bupropion has dopaminergic and noradrenergic activity that seems to reduce nicotine's withdrawal symptoms (78). Bupropion should be started before actual smoking cessation in order to attain effective blood levels. This drug is started at 150 mg per day and raised to a maximum dose of 300 mg per day. Other drugs that have also been shown to be effective in assisting nicotine abstinence are the following: the antidepressants nortriptyline (Pamelor), doxepin (Sinequan), fluoxetine (Prozac); the alpha-adrenergic agonist clonidine (Catapres); and the nicotine antagonists mecamylamine (Inversine) and gamma-vinyl-GABA

TABLE 22-24. *Nicotine replacement methods (NRM)*

NRM	Trade name(s)	Available doses	Advantages	Disadvantages	Nicotine blood levels
Gum	Nicorette[a]	2,4 mg	PRN use	Sore jaw	Less than smoking Rise and fall
Patch	Habitrol Nicoderm[a] Nicotrol[a] ProStep	7,14,21 mg	Continuous delivery enhanced compliance	Skin rash Less likely to substitute for oral craving	Less than smoking Steady
Spray (nasal)	Nicotrol NS	1 mg	Rapid peak	Nasal irritation	Same as smoking Rise and fall
Inhaler	Nicotrol	10 mg	PRN use Mimics hand to mouth ritual of smoking	Throat irritation	Less than smoking Rise and fall

[a]Available over the counter

TABLE 22-25. *Nicotine replacement protocol*

First line
- Brief advice
- Group behavior therapy
- Nicotine patch or gum
- Bupropion (Zyban, Wellbutrin)

Second line
- Nicotine patch plus gum
- Nicotine inhaler
- Nicotine nasal spray
- Clonidine

From Hughes JR, Fiester S, Goldstein MG, Resnick MP, Rock N, Ziedonis D. American Psychiatric Association practice guideline for the treatment of nicotine dependence. *Am J Psych* 1996;153:S1–3.

(Vigabatrin) (available in Europe) (78). The rationale for using the nicotine antagonists would be to block any positive reinforcers for nicotine use (Table 22-23).

DETOXIFICATION DRUGS OTHER THAN OPIATES, HYPNOSEDATIVES, AND NICOTINE

The psychomimetic drugs do not require a detoxification protocol. The stimulants, alpha-adrenergic blocking agents, antidepressants, beta-adrenergic blocking agents, and muscle relaxants may or may not be associated with a withdrawal syndrome, however. Thus, in some situations this last group may require a detoxification protocol. For some of these (e.g., stimulants) protocols have been developed. For details of these protocols, the reader is referred to a recent review (41).

REFERENCES

1. Newman RG. The need to redefine "addiction," *N Engl J Med* 1983; 18:1096–1098.
2. Inturrisi CE. Role of opioid analgesics. *Am J Med* 1984;10:27–36.
3. Ludwig AM. *Principles of clinical psychiatry.* New York: Free Press, 1980.
4. Ghodse H. *Drugs and addictive behavior, a guide to treatment.* Oxford: Blackwell Scientific Publications, 1990.
5. Madden C, Ong B, Singer G. Mood state of heroin-dependent persons undergoing methadone detoxification. *Int J Addict* 1989;22: 93–102.
6. Haertzen CA, Hooks NT. Changes in personality and subjective experience associated with chronic administration and withdrawal of opiates. *J Nervous Mental Dis* 1969;148:606–614.
7. *American Psychiatric Association Diagnostic and Statistical Manual of Mental Disorders,* ed IV-TR Washington, D.C., 2000.
8. Fishbain DA, Rosomoff HL, Steele-Rosomoff R. Chronic pain patients opiate and other drug dependence/addiction. A review of the evidence. *Clin J Pain* 1992;8:77–85.
9. Turkington D, Drummon DC. How should opiate withdrawal be measured? *Drug-Alcohol Depend* 1989;24:151–153.
10. Cuthill JD, Beroniade V, Salvatori VA, Viguie F. Evaluation of clonidine suppression of opiate withdrawal reactions: a multidisciplinary approach. *Can J Psychiatry* 1989;35:377–382.
11. Halpern L. Substitution-detoxification and its role in the management of chronic benign pain. *J Clin Psychiatry* 1982;43:10–14.
12. Bickel WK, Stitzer ML, Bigelow GE, et al. A clinical trial of buprenorphine: comparison with methadone in the detoxification of heroin addicts. *Clin Pharmacol Ther* 41988;3:72–78.
13. Kosten TR, Krystal JH, Charney DS, et al. Rapid *detoxification* from opioid dependence. *Am J Psychiatry* 1989;146:1349.
14. Goldstein E, Pollack R, Weiner B, Lazoritz R. Rapid treatment of percodan addiction: a case report. *Int J Addiction* 1978;13:1003–1007.
15. Janiri L, Mannelli P, Persico AM, et al. Opiate detoxification of methadone maintenance patients using lefetamine, clonidine and buprenorphine. *Drug Alcohol Dep* 1994;36:139–145.
16. Jacobsen LK, Kosten TR. Naloxone challenge as biological predictor of treatment outcome in opiate addicts. *Am J Drug Alcohol Abuse* 1989;15:355–366.
17. Martin WR, Jasinski D, Mansky P. Naltrexone, an antagonist for the treatment of heroin dependence. *Arch Gen Psych* 1973;23: 784–789.
18. Callahan EJ, Rawson RA, McCleave B, et al. The treatment of heroin addiction: naltrexone alone with behavior therapy. *Am J Drug Alcohol Abuse* 1980;7:795–807.
19. Rawson RA, Washton AM, Resnick RB, Tennant FS Jr. Clonidine hydrochloride detoxification from methadone treatment—the value of naltrexone aftercare. *Adv Alcohol Subst Abuse* 1984;3:41–49.
20. Jones HE, Strain EC, Bigelow GE, et al. Induction with levomethadyl acetate. *Arch Gen Psych* 1998;55:729–736.
21. Childs ND. Long-acting heroin substitute slow to catch on. *Clin Psych News,* Nov: 20 1971.
22. Umbtricht A, Montoya ID, Hoover DR, et al. Naltrexone shortened opioid detoxification with buprenorphine. *Drug & Alcohol Dependence* 1999;56(3):181–190.
23. O'Connor PG, Kossten TR. Rapid and ultrarapid opioid detoxification techniques. *JAMA* 1998;279(3):229–234.
24. Lorenzi P, Marsili M, Boncinelli S et al. Searching for a general anaesthesia protocol for rapid detoxification from opioids. *Euro J Anaesth* 1999;16:719–727.
25. Gold CG, Cullen DJ, Gonzales S, et al. Rapid opioid detoxification during general anesthesia: a review of 20 patients. *Anesthesiology* 1999;91(6):1639–1647.
26. Rabinowitz J, Cohen H, Tarrasch R, Kotler M. Compliance to naltrexone treatment after ultra-rapid opiate detoxification: an open label naturalistic study. *Drug & Alcohol Dep* 1997;47(2):77–86.
27. Aghajanian GK, Vander Mallen CP. Alpha-2-adreno-receptor-induced hyperpolarization of locus ceruleus neurons: intracellular studies in vivo. *Science* 1982;215:1394–1396.
28. Kleber HD, Riordqan CE, Rounsaville B, et al. Clonidine in outpatient detoxification from methadone maintenance. *Arch Gen Psychiatry* 42:391–394.
29. San L, Cami J, Peri JM, et al. Efficacy of clonidine quanfacine and methadone in the rapid detoxification of heroin addicts: a controlled clinical trial. *Br J Addict* 1990;85:141–147.
30. Kosten TR, Rounsaville BJ, Kleber HD. Comparison of clinician ratings to self reports of withdrawal during clonidine detoxification of opiate addicts. *Am J Drug Alcohol Abuse* 1985;11:1–10.
31. Fertig JB, Pomerleau OF, Sanders B. I Nicotine-produced antinociception in minimally deprived smokers and ex-smokers. *Addict Behav* 1986;11:239–248.
32. Strang J, Bearn J, Gossop M. Lofexidine for opiate detoxification: review of recent randomised and open controlled trials. *Amer J Addictions* 1999;8:337–348.
33. Roehrich HJ, Gold MS. Propranolol as adjunct to clonidine in opiate detoxification. *Am J Psychiatry* 1987;144:1099–1100.
34. Dufficy RG. Use of psychotherapeutic drugs in the acute detoxification of heroin addicts. *Milit Med* 1973;138:748.
35. Loimer N, Schmid R, Lencz K, et al. Acute blocking of naloxone precipitated opiate withdrawal symptoms by methohextone. *Br J Psychiatry* 1990;157:748–752.
36. Loimer N, Lencz K, Schmid R, Presslich O. Technique for greatly shortening the transition from methadone to naltrexone maintenance of patients addicted to opiates. *Am J Psychiatry* 1991;148:933–935.
37. Washburn AM, Fullilove RE, Fullilove MT et al. Acupuncture heroin detoxification: a single-blind clinical trial. *J Substance Abuse Treatment* 1993;10(4):345–351.
38. Ceniceros S, Brown GR. Acupuncture: a review of its history, theories, and indications. *S Med J* 1998;91(12):1121–1125.
39. Uhlenhuth E, DeWit H, Balter MB. Risks and benefits of long-term benzodiazepine use. *J Clin Psychopharmacol* 1988:161–167.
40. King SA, Strain JJ. Benzodiazepine use by chronic pain patients. *Clin J Pain* 1990;6:143–147.

41. Fishbain DA, Rosomoff HL, Steele-Rosomoff R. The detoxification of non opiate drugs in the chronic pain setting and clonidine opiate detoxification: a review. *Clin J Pain* 1992;8:191–203.
42. Griffiths RR, Wolf B. Relative abuse liability of different benzodiazepines in drug abusers. *J Clin Psychopharmacol* 1990;10:237–243.
43. Owen RT, Tyrel P. Benzodiazepine. A review of the evidence. *Drugs* 1983;25:385–398.
44. Lader M. Long-term anxiolytic therapy: the issue of drug withdrawal. *J Clin Psychiatry* 1987;48(Suppl 12):12–16.
45. Shader RI, Caine ED, Meyer RE. Treatment of dependence on barbiturates and sedative-hypnotics. In: Shader RI, ed. *Manual of psychiatric therapeutics.* Boston: Little Brown, 1989.
46. Noyes R, Garvey MN, Cook BL, et al. Benzodiazepine withdrawal: a review of the evidence. *J Clin Psychiatry* 1988;49:382–389.
47. Wartenberg AA. Detoxification of the chemically dependent patient. *Rhode Island Med J* 1989;72:451–456.
48. Rickels K, Schwerzer E, Case WG, Greenblatt DJ. Long-term therapeutic use of benzodiazepines. I: Effects of abrupt discontinuation. *Arch Gen Psychiatry* 1990;47:899–907.
49. Schwerzer E, Rickels K, Case WG, Greenblatt DJ. Long-term therapeutic use of benzodiazepines. II: Effects of gradual taper. *Arch Gen Psychiatry* 1990;47:908–915.
50. Burrows GD, Norman TR, Judd FK, et al. Short-acting versus long-acting benzodiazepines: discontinuation effects in panic disorders. *J Psychiatric Res* 1990;24(Suppl 2):65–72.
51. Smith DE, Landry MJ. Benzodiazepine dependence discontinuation: focus on the chemical dependency detoxification setting and benzodiazepine-poly-drug abuse. *J Psychiatric Res* 1990;24(Suppl 2):145–156.
52. DuPont RL. A practical approach to benzodiazepine discontinuation. *J Psychiatric Res* 1990;24(Suppl 2):81–90.
53. Burrows GD. Managing long-term therapy for panic disorder. *J Clin Psychiatry* 1990;51(Suppl 11):9–12.
54. Herman JB, Rosenbaum JF, Brotman AW. The alprazolam to clonazepam switch for the treatment of panic disorder. *J Clin Psychopharmacol* 1987;7:175–178.
55. Lader M. Long-term anxiolytic therapy: the issue of drug withdrawal. *J Clin Psychiatry* 1987;48(Suppl 12):12–16.
56. Ries RK, Roy-Byrne PP, Warang, et al. Carbamazepine treatment for benzodiazepine withdrawal. *Am J Psychiatry* 1989;146:536–537.
57. Udelman HD, Udelman DL. Concurrent use of buspirone in anxious patients during withdrawal from alprazolam therapy. *J Clin Psychiatry* 1990;51(Suppl 9):46–54.
58. Fishbain DA, Goldberg M, Meagher BR, et al. Male and female chronic pain patients categorized by DSM-III psychiatric diagnostic criteria. *Pain* 1986;26:181–197.
59. Miller GW Jr. Principles of alcohol detoxification. *Am Fam Physician* 1984;30:145–148.
60. Castaneda R, Cushman P. Alcohol withdrawal: a review of clinical management. *J Clin Psychiatry* 1989;50:278–284.
61. Rosenthal RN, Perkel C, Singh P, Anand O, Miner CR. A pilot open randomized trial of valproate and phenobarbital in the treatment of acute alcohol withdrawal. *Amer J Addictions* 1998;7(3):189–197.
62. Pages KP, Ries RK. Use of anticonvulsants in benzodiazepine withdrawal. *Am J Addictions* 1998;7(3):198–204.
63. Mueller TI, Stout RL, Rudden S, et al. A double-blind, placebo-controlled study of carbamazepine for the treatment of alcohol dependence. *Alcoholism: Clin & Experimental Research* 1997;21(1):86–92.
64. Sherman C. Isradipine may prevent relapse of alcohol dependence. *Clin Psych News* 2000 Feb 9:
65. Miller NS. Pharmacotherapy in alcoholism. *J Addictive Dis* 1995; 14(1):23–46.
66. Litten RZ, Allen JP. Advances in development of medications for alcoholism treatment. *Psychopharmacology* 1998;139: 20–23.
67. O'Malley SS, Jaffe AJ, Chang G et al. Six month follow-up of naltrexone and psychotherapy for alcohol dependence. *Arch Gen Psych* 1996;53(3):217–224.
68. Anton RF, Moak DH, Waid R et al. Naltrexone and cognitive behavioral therapy for the treatment of outpatient alcoholics: results of a placebo-controlled trail. *Am J Psych* 1999;156(11):1758–1764.
69. Sherman C. Isradipine may prevent relapse of alcohol dependence. *Clinical Psychiatric News.* 2000 Feb 9.
70. Mason BJ, Salvato FR, Williams LD et al. A double-blind, placebo-controlled study of oral nalmefene for alcohol dependence. *Arch Gen Psychiatry* 1999;56:719–724.
71. Mason BJ, Ownby RL. Acamprosate for the treatment of alcohol dependence: a review of double-blind, placebo-controlled trials. *CNS Spectrums* 2000;5(2):58–59.
72. Spanagel R, Zieglgansberger W. Anti-craving compounds for ethanol: new pharmacological tools to study addictive processes. *Trends Pharmacol Sci* 1997;18(2):54–59.
73. Brewington V, Smith M, Lipton D. Acupuncture as a detoxification treatment: an analysis of controlled research. *J Substance Abuse Treatment* 1994;11(4):289–307.
74. Moon MN. Traditional smoking programs don't help women. *Clinical Psychiatric News* 2000 May:24–25.
75. Leboeuf-Yde C. Smoking and low back pain. A systematic literature review of 41 journal articles reporting 47 epidemiologic studies. *Spine* 1999;24(14):1463–1470.
76. Hughes JR. Treatment of smoking cessation in smokers with past alcohol/drug problems. *J Substance Abuse Treatment* 1993;10(2): 181–187.
77. Burling TA, Ramsey TG, Seidner AL, Kondo CS. Issues related to smoking cessation among substance abusers. *J Substance Abuse* 1997;9:27–40.
78. Knowlton L. Nicotine and psychiatric disorders. *Psych Times* 2000 Nov:12–14.
79. Fishbain DA. Comorbidity between psychiatric disorders and chronic pain. *Curr Rev Pain* 1998;2(1):1–10.
80. Zarin DA, Pincus HA, Hughes JR. Treating nicotine dependence in mental health settings. *J Prac Psych Behav Hlth* 1997;250–254.
81. Hughes JR, Fiester S, Goldstein MG, et al. American psychiatric association practice guideline for the treatment of nicotine dependence. *Am J Psych* 1996;153:S1–31.

CHAPTER **23**

Pharmacological Management of Pain in the Terminally Ill

Perry G. Fine

ETHICAL FOUNDATIONS AND BASIC PRECEPTS

The duty to relieve suffering is an ethical imperative of the medical profession (1,2). This admonition is most weighty in the care of those who are dying, since comfort care in terminally ill patients wholly fulfills the obligation to "do good" (beneficence) while concurrently "doing no harm" (nonmaleficence). This is in keeping with the view that the greatest harm to be done to persons with limited life expectancy is to abandon them in their need for comfort, of which relief from pain is paramount. As reflected in a report by Singer et al. (3), patients expect that their physicians will honor this need, by being both available and clinically capable of treating pain. Although the age-old principle of double effect—an unintended "bad" outcome (e.g., hastened death) from a likely beneficial and therapeutic intervention (e.g., opioid analgesic therapy) is both morally and legally defensible—has been invoked frequently in the recent past (even in legislative language) to assure physicians of the ethical nature of aggressive pain control, there is no scientific evidence to support any claim that appropriately titrated analgesics hasten death. In fact, there is far more anecdotal evidence to the contrary, and burgeoning literature that suggests unabated pain increases morbidity and mortality (4,5).

Mindful of these ethical duties, it is tragic, and no less ironic, that at a time in our medical history when we have greater technological capability of effectively relieving pain than ever before, it seems that we have lost sight of the need to attend to this obligation, as evidenced by the high percentages of patients who die without adequate pain control (6). This sad truth has been repeatedly corroborated over the last decade in a variety of health care settings, including hospitals (7) and long-term care facilities (8) where the majority of people die. However, most people, when given the opportunity, voice their preference to conclude their lives at home (9,10). Hospice focuses on caring for terminally ill people in their places of residence if at all possible and strongly emphasizes symptom management; hospice is greatly underutilized even though there is a specific Medicare benefit for this type of care. The reasons for this disturbing data have also been well described, and hopefully, corrective actions in medical education and public policy, including appropriate incentives for palliative care, will lead to improvements in the near future (6).

Notwithstanding the many systems barriers and poorly aligned incentives that preclude appropriate and timely referral to comprehensive end-of-life care services (11), conscientious practicing physicians need readily available resource materials so that, as individuals with independent moral agency, we can attempt to do our best to practice in an ethically and clinically acceptable fashion. It is my contention that when it is recognized that a patient has limited life expectancy, measured in months, hospice is the optimal care path. Patients who are in the last phase of life have complex and intertwined medical, psychosocial, and spiritual needs that no single practitioner can hope to fully support, manage, or contend with 24 hours a day. Hospice becomes the fully featured extension of the compassionate physician. And, in addition to the provision of human clinical services, under the Medicare Hospice Benefit (as well as most proprietary insurance plans and Medicaid), durable medical equipment, supplies, and very importantly, pharmaceuticals are fully covered. Lastly, bereavement support is provided to family well after the death of the patient.

Why are these thoughts pertinent to a section describing pharmacological management of pain in terminally ill patients? Unlinking pain from other non-nociceptive/visceral/neuropathic etiologies of suffering can be a daunting task in patients with far-advanced disease. This becomes even more challenging in individuals who are aware and capable of confronting the imminence of their mortality. Therefore, expertise in the pharmacological management of pain, per se, is an absolutely necessary starting point but insufficient destination in the care of terminally ill patients. A full discussion of nonpharmacological approaches to the management of pain and suffering is beyond the scope of this chapter, but those who embark upon care of these patients should be well aware of the breadth and depth of competencies required for proficiency in this type of practice (12).

CLINICAL CONTEXT

Continuous and/or intermittent pain that interferes with basic functions, activities, sleep, social interaction, or otherwise erodes quality of life to an appreciable extent affects the majority of patients with late-stage cancer and is common in most other chronic, progressive, life-limiting disease states (13–15). Along with severe anxiety/agitation and dyspnea, pain that is out of control represents one of the urgent-emergent symptom complexes encountered by patients with far-advanced disease. Because of the high incidence and prevalence of pain, frequent assessment (including an understanding of realizable patient goals) and plans for intervention should be put into place as a high priority. The ability to respond to calls for help when pain is out of control, and the capacity to assess and intervene effectively in a timely manner (without having to transfer the patient to an inpatient facility unless absolutely necessary) are key and fundamental measures of quality pain management. This is why an interdisciplinary team approach that focuses on anticipated needs and continuity of care, such as that modeled by hospice, is so crucial.

CAUSES OF PAIN IN THE TERMINALLY ILL

From the biomedical perspective, the basic pain assessment and management principle of identifying the cause of pain and treating it with the most etiologically specific intervention applies equally to patients who are in the terminal stage of disease (16). However, an important difference is that patients who are no longer candidates for curative therapies or who otherwise have limited life expectancy may not elect to undergo even minimally invasive diagnostic procedures. In this clinical context, "work-ups" may add greater burden than benefit due to short life expectancy. In these circumstances it is especially important not to defer pain therapies, treating what is the most likely etiology of pain, and monitoring the results of therapy closely to ascertain the correctness of one's hypothesis (17).

Cancer accounts for about 20% of deaths in the United States, and much of what has been learned about chronic disease-related severe pain comes from investigations and longitudinal studies of cancer patients. Pain associated with direct or metastatic tumor involvement of bone, nerves, viscera, or soft tissues affects 60% to 80% of all cancer patients. Treatment-related pain, resulting from surgery, radiation therapy, or chemotherapy affects 20% to 25% of cancer patients (18). Painful disorders experienced by both cancer and noncancer patients in the advanced stages of life-limiting diseases include (14):

1. Myofascial pain (muscle trigger point pain with radiating and referred pain)
2. Arthropathies (joint pains most commonly due to osteoarthritis, degenerative joint disease, or rheumatoid arthritis)
3. Neuropathies (e.g., diabetes, peripheral vascular disease, herpes zoster, neurodegenerative disorders such as multiple sclerosis, Parkinson's disease, or amyotrophic lateral sclerosis)
4. Headache (tension pattern, migraine, mixed, other)
5. Skin and mucosal ulceration
6. Constipation
7. Back pain (e.g., spinal stenosis, facet disease, spondylosis/disc disease)

ASSESSMENT IN PATIENTS WHO CANNOT SELF-REPORT

The gold standard for pain assessment is the patient's self-report (refer to Chapter 4). These standard principles and approaches to pain assessment apply to all self-reporting patients, regardless of life expectancy (Figs. 23-1 and 23-2). Since it has been shown that observers (both professional and nonprofessional caregivers) are not very accurate at approximating patients' intensity of pain (19), and memory for pain is also not reliable, it is helpful to use a written recording device such as a pain diary, especially during periods when a new intervention or a dose change is being prescribed (Fig. 23-3).

Patients who cannot self-report represent a great challenge for the conscientious practitioner. It has been well documented that patients with dementia who lack the cognitive capacity to describe or rate their pain receive significantly less opioid analgesic for similar clinical conditions (20). The same problem applies to patients with far-advanced disease who may be too obtunded, due to their clinical condition, to self-report. In these cases, proxy measures must be taken into account, and documented, to ensure that suffering is minimized without overconcern that analgesics or other pain-reducing therapies are being applied purely to hasten death. These include (21,22):

- Facial expressions or body posturing suggestive of pain (e.g., grimacing, guarding)
- Vocalizations suggestive of pain
- Tachycardia, tachypnea, hypertension, diaphoresis (Note: Absence of these autonomic findings do not rule out pain, but the presence of these findings in a

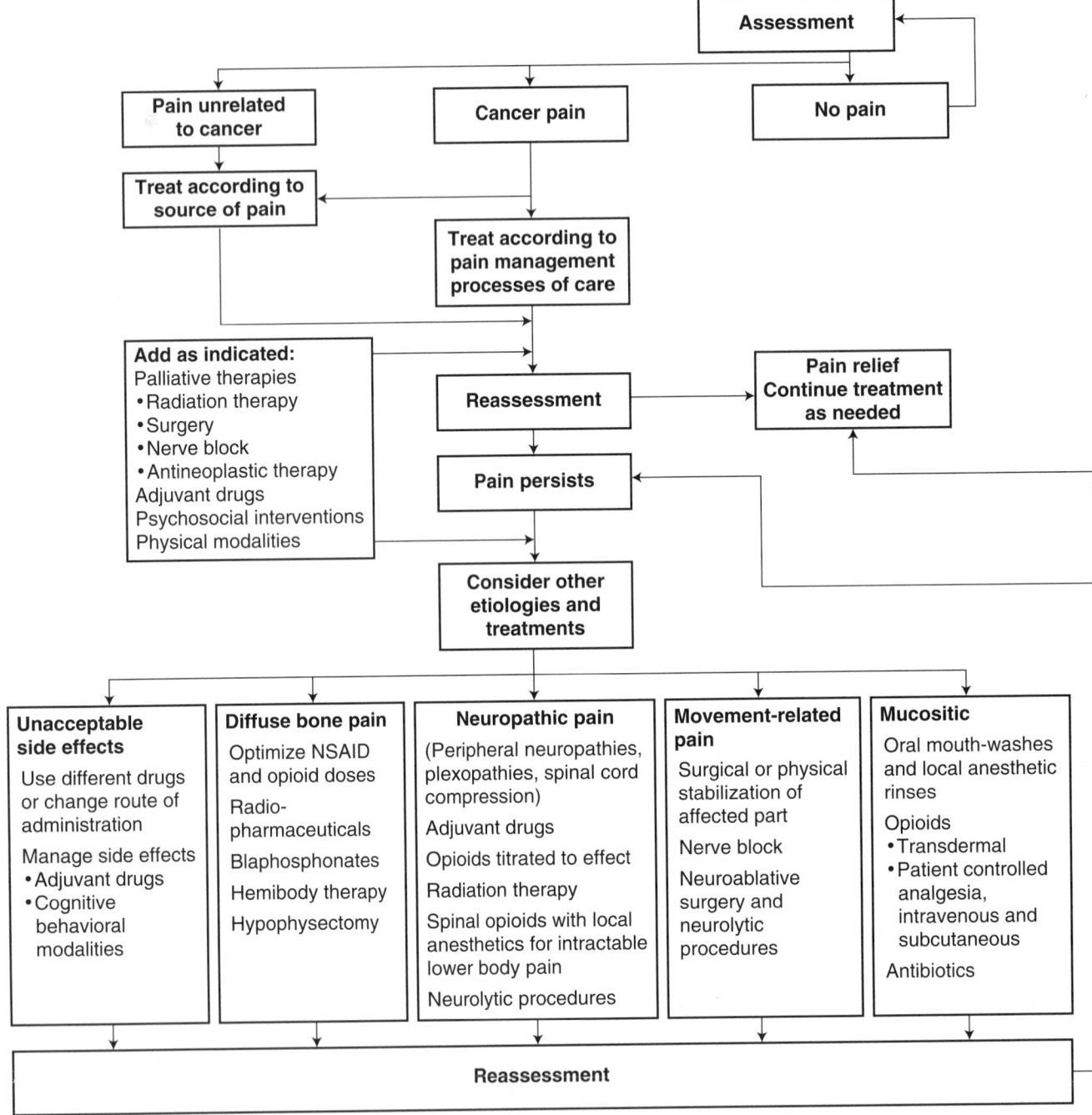

FIG. 23-1. Flow chart for continuing evaluation and treatment of pain (Adapted from AHCPR Clinical Guideline No. 9)

noncommunicating patient are highly suggestive of pain, especially during repositioning of the patient.)

Absent other apparent causes, findings that suggest pain in a patient who cannot self-report are

- poor sleep or change in sleep patterns;
- agitation/restlessness;
- withdrawal from social interaction or other behavioral change;
- decreased interest in previous enjoyments (e.g., music,

feeding, personal care, massage, bathing);
- other signs and symptoms of depression or anxiety.

PHARMACOLOGICAL INTERVENTION FOR PAIN CONTROL IN TERMINALLY ILL PATIENTS

Basic Priniciples

Practical and humanistic issues should take high priority in care decisions around dying patients. It is important to remember that time is limited. Potential barriers to ready

Pain Rating Scales for Adults [all of these scales can be "transcribed" into a 0-10 numeric rating for purposes of recording data]

A. 0 - 10 numeric scale:

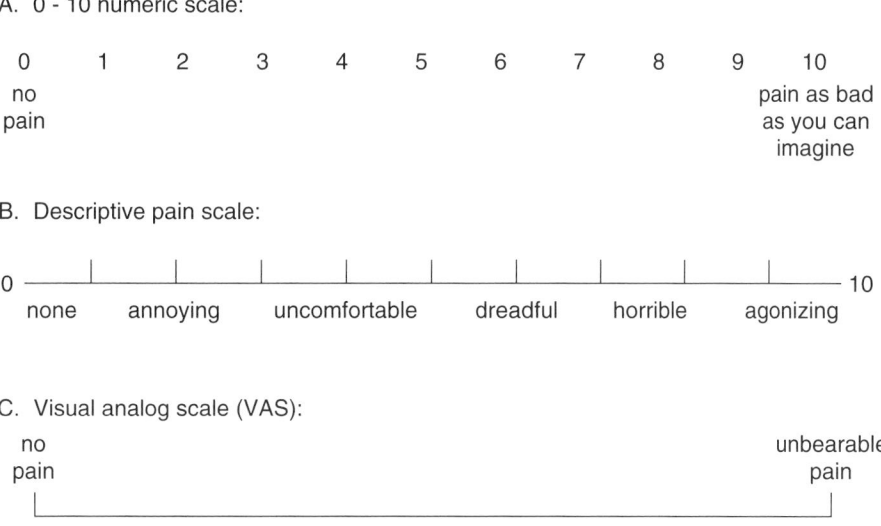

B. Descriptive pain scale:

C. Visual analog scale (VAS):

Pain Rating Scale for Children

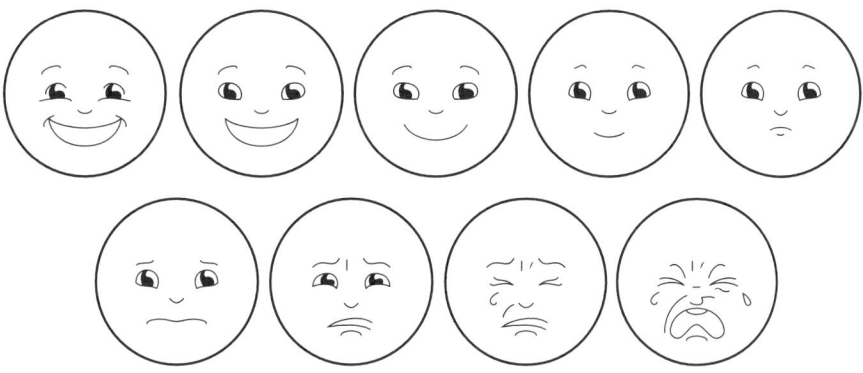

FIG. 23-2. Pain rating scales for adults (Adapted from AHCPR Clinical Guildline No. 9)

access to pharmaceuticals for noninpatients (e.g., supply availability) should be anticipated. Dignity counts enormously, and the *perceptions* of the circumstances surrounding the death of the patient by his or her family and loved ones will be revisited for the rest of their lives. These concerns apply to choices of pharmacological therapies, even though these are not pharmacological issues, per se. Some practical guidelines include:

• Use the least invasive and most readily available and acceptable (to the patient/caregiver) agent/route of administration possible. This is usually the oral route, but anticipatory planning around the inability to ingest or absorb drugs by the enteral route should precede this event so that pain crises can be averted.

• Administer analgesics on a regularly scheduled basis—around-the-clock (ATC) rather than prn (as needed) for continuous pain problems. Sustained or continuous-release formulations make this easier.

• Prescribe for and educate patients/caregivers about breakthrough pains.

Pharmacotherapeutic Options

Acetaminophen and Nonsteroidal Antiinflammatory Drugs (NSAIDs) (23,24)

Indications/Advantages

• Mild to moderate pain
• Inflammatory pain syndromes, including bone pain

Twenty-four Hour Pain Diary

Patient Name: _____ Date: _____

TIME	Maximal Pain 0-10 scale	Minimal Pain 0-10 scale	Medication: name, dose, route of administration	Activities: lying, sitting, walking, eating, toilet, etc.
12 Midnight				
1 am				
2				
3				
4				
5				
6				
7				
8				
9				
10				
11				
12 Noon				
1 pm				
2				
3				
4				
5				
6				
7				
8				
9				
10				
11				

FIG. 23-3. Pain diary and pain scales

- Minimal effect on mental functioning
- Supplement with opioid analgesics for moderate to severe pain
- Available over the counter in a variety of forms
- Cyclooxygenase 2 (COX-2) selective antagonists with less GI bleeding risk
- Nonselective NSAIDs available in liquid and nonoral (rectal suppository/parenteral) dosage forms for patients unable to swallow capsules/pills

Contraindications/Disadvantages (Table 23-1)

- GI distress and ulceration (nonselective NSAIDs)
- Platelet dysfunction/bleeding (nonselective NSAIDs)

- Hypersensitivity reactions (all NSAIDs)
- Hepatic/renal impairment (all NSAIDs and acetaminophen)
- COX-2 selective NSAIDs only available in oral dosage form (paracoxib, a parenteral COX-2 selective NSAID is under review by the FDA at the time of this writing)

Acetaminophen has been determined to be one of the safest analgesics for long-term use in the management of mild to moderate pain, or as a supplement in the management of moderate and more severe pain syndromes (14,25,26). It is especially useful in the management of nonspecific musculoskeletal pains or pain associated with osteoarthritis, and it should be considered as an adjunct to

TABLE 23-1. *Acetaminophen and a selection of OTC and prescription NSAIDs*

Drug	>50 kg dose	<50 kg dose
Acetaminophen[a,b]	4000 mg/24 h (q4–6 h dosing)	10–15 mg/kg/q4 h (oral) 15–20 mg/hg q4 h (rectal)
Aspirin[a,b]	4000 mg/24 h (q4– h dosing)	10–15 mg/kg q4 h (oral) 15–20 mg/kg q4 h (rectal)
Ibuprofen[a,b]	2400 mg/24 h (q6–8 h dosing)	10 mg/kg q6–8 h (oral)
Naproxen[a,b]	1000 mg/24 h (q8–12 h dosing)	5 mg/kg q8 h (oral/rectal)
Choline magnesium trisalicylate[a,d]	3000 mg/24 h (q8–12 h dosing)	15 mg/kg q8 h (oral)
Indomethacin[c]	75–150 mg/24h (q8–12 h dosing)	0.5–1 mg/kg q 8–12 h (oral/rectal)
Celecoxib[d,e]	200 mg/24 h (q12–24 h dosing)	3 mg/kg/24 h (max 200 mg)
Rofecoxib[d,e]	25–50 mg/24 h (q24 h dosing)	0.75 mg/kg/24 h (max 50 mg)
Ketorolac	30–60 mg IM/IV initially, then 15–30 mg q6 h bolus IV/IM or continuous IV/SQ infusion; SHORT-TERM USE ONLY	

[a]commercially available in a liquid form
[b]commercially available in a suppository form
[c]potent antiinflammatory (short-term use only due to GI side effects)
[d]minimal platelet dysfunction
[e]minimal GI adverse effects

any chronic pain regimen. It is often overlooked when severe pain is being treated, or in terminal conditions, but its availability in liquid and suppository form make it especially useful as a "co-analgesic" under these circumstances. Concerns about dose accumulation in the face of renal insufficiency or liver toxicity become mute in the face of pain control during the last few days of life.

Nonsteroidal antiinflammatory drugs affect analgesia by reducing the biosynthesis of prostaglandins, thereby inhibiting the cascade of inflammatory events that cause, amplify, or maintain nociception. Other peripheral or central mechanisms of analgesia that do not necessarily involve mediators of inflammation may also contribute to the analgesic properties of the NSAIDs (27). The traditional (nonselective) NSAIDs, exemplified by aspirin, are nonselective in their inhibitory effects on the enzymes that convert arachidonic acid to prostaglandins (28). The new class of cyclooxygenase-2 (COX-2) selective NSAIDs mostly inhibits the inducible form of the enzyme, caused by tissue injury or other inflammatory conditions. For this reason, there is less risk of gastrointestinal bleeding with the chronic use of these newer compounds (29,30).

As a drug class, the NSAIDs are very useful in the treatment of many pain-producing conditions, especially those mediated by inflammation and including those caused by cancer (31,32). There is insufficient data to determine whether the newly available COX-2 selective agents (celecoxib and rofecoxib) have any specific advantages, or more or less efficacy, compared to the relatively nonselective NSAIDs in the management of conditions that lead to severe pain (e.g., bone metastases) in patients with far-advanced, life-limiting disease. All of the NSAIDs do offer the potential advantage of being opioid sparing in patients with moderate to severe pain where opioids are indicated. This opioid sparing effect may lead to less nausea and constipation, as well as decreased sedation or other effects on mental functioning (33). Although there is some risk of short-term memory impairment induced by NSAIDs in older patients (34), this is probably inconsequential in the care of terminally ill patients compared to the benefits of pain reduction. As in the choice of any pharmacotherapy, a balance must be struck between potential therapeutic benefits and all associated burdens, including cost. The COX-2 selective NSAIDs are much more expensive than generic

NSAIDs, and this may be of considerable importance for patients with limited income and for fixed per diem payment programs such as the Medicare (and Medicaid) Hospice Benefit. On the other hand, in the care of patients with far-advanced disease who have significant pain and a high risk of bleeding, the COX-2 selective drugs may offer meaningful advantages.

Opioid Analgesics (Table 23-2)

As a pharmacological class, the opioid analgesics offer great efficacy and flexibility in the treatment of a wide range of pain-producing conditions, especially in patients with limited life expectancy where a focus on comfort care, pain relief, and maximizing quality of life are the goals. It is very important for clinicians who are involved in the care of these patients to know that careful titration of opioid analgesics to effect pain relief is rarely associated with induced respiratory depression and iatrogenic death (35). This is critical, because fears of hastening death (and, as a result, leaving patients with intolerable pain) have been greatly exaggerated compared to any evidence base for this concern. Indeed, the obverse seems to be supported by exigent data, suggesting that insufficient pain relief hastens death by increasing physiological stress, possibly decreasing immunological resistance, decreasing mobility with consequences of increasing risk for pneumonia and thrombosis, increasing work of breathing and myocardial oxygen requirements (36–39). Since there is great inter- and intraindividual variation in clinical responses to the various opioids, methodical dose titration should be used to optimize therapy and minimize adverse effects. This implies close follow-up to determine whether clinical endpoints have been reached. Also, idiosyncratic responses often require trials of more than one agent to determine the most effective drug and route of delivery for a given patient and as patients' conditions change (40). A description of the essentials for use of opioid analgesics in the care of terminally ill patients is provided below.

Indications, Contraindications, and Precautions   Opioid analgesics are indicated for moderate to server pain; they are absolutely contrandicated when allergy or specific sensitivity is present.

Use of agonist-antagonist drugs is contraindicated (pentazocine, butorphanol, nalbuphine) due to limited efficacy, psychotomimetic effects, and potential for inducing an acute abstinence syndrome in patients using opioid agonists (41). Meperidine use discouraged due to toxic metabolite (normeperidine) (42–45). Intramuscular use is highly discouraged except in "pain emergency" states while other routes are being established or transdermal drugs are being titrated. The oral transmucosal route for rapid delivery of fentanyl may obviate the necessity to ever use the intramuscular route for pain control in cooperative patients (46).

Dose Conversions (47)   Changing from one opioid to another, or one route to another, is often necessary, and facility with this process is an absolute necessity. Triple check all dose calculations and ask a colleague to check your conclusions if there is any question. Remember the following points:

- Incomplete cross-tolerance occurs, leading to decreased requirements of a newly prescribed agent.
- Use morphine parenteral equivalents as a "common denominator" for all dose conversions to avoid errors.

Opioid Analgesics: Specific Features, Caveats, Cautions, and Quirks

Morphine (48)

- Morphine is most often considered the "gold standard" of opioid analgesics.
- Some patients cannot tolerate morphine due to itching, headache, dysphoria, or other adverse effects.
- The metabolites of morphine (morphine-3-glucuronide and morphine-6-glucuronide) are active and may contribute to sedation, myoclonus, and psychotomimetic effects, especially in the face of renal insufficiency, dehydration, and hepatic dysfunction, commonly occurring findings in dying patients (49).
- Usual and predictable effects such as sedation and nausea often resolve within a few days, but may require adjunctive medications while habituation occurs. Adap-

TABLE 23-2. *Approximate equianalgesic doses of most commonly used opioid analgesics (47)[a,b]*

Drug	Parenteral dose	Enteral dose
Morphine[c]	10 mg	30 mg
Codeine	130 mg	200 mg
Fentanyl[d]	50–100 mcg	
Hydrocodone		30 mg
Hydromorphone[e]	1.5 mg	7.5 mg
Levorphanol[f]	2 mg	4 mg
Methadone[f]	10 mg	20 mg
Oxycodone[g]		20–30 mg

[a]Dose conversion should be closely monitored since incomplete cross tolerance may occur.

[b]Meperidine (Demerol, pethidine) is not included since it is a contraindicated opioid analgesic due to its toxic metabolite, normeperidine.

[c]Available in continuous- and sustained-release formulations lasting 8 to 24 hours.

[d]Also available in both transdermal and oral transmucosal forms.

[e]May be available soon as a continuous-release formulation lasting 12 to 24 hours.

[f]These drugs have long half-lives so accumulation can occur; close monitoring during the first few days of therapy is very important.

[g]Available in several continuous-release doses formulated to last 12 hours.

tation to constipation does not usually occur, so a chronic preventative approach to maintenance of bowel function is required (see section below on treating and preventing adverse effects).

- Convert to an equianalgesic dose of a different opioid if adverse effects exceed benefit.
- Oral morphine solution can be swallowed, or small volumes (1/2 to 1 ml) of a concentrated solution (e.g., 20 mg/ml) can be placed under the tongue for partial mucosal absorption into the bloodstream, although most of the effect is obtained by enteral absorption after swallowing.
- Morphine's bitter taste may be prohibitive in unflavored forms, especially if immediate release tablets are left in the mouth to dissolve.

Fentanyl (50)

- Transdermal fentanyl (fentanyl patch) (51). Opioid naive patients should start with a 25 mcg per hour patch and be very closely observed for the first 24 to 48 hours of therapy until steady-state blood levels are attained. Use 12-hour oral morphine equivalent dose to convert to microgram per hour dose size of patch (e.g., for a patient using 100 mg oral morphine every 12 hours, use a 100 mcg per hour fentanyl patch). Time to peak and steady-state blood levels for patients starting the patch is usually 18 to 24 hours. Make sure other rapid-onset dosage forms of an opioid analgesic are available during this time period and for breakthrough pains later on. Although the currently available fentanyl patch is formulated for 72-hour use, end-of-dose failure occasionally occurs as early as 48 hours. Close monitoring of efficacy, duration of effect, breakthrough pain episodes and medication use, and adverse effects is important during the first several days of use and during periods of advancing disease with increasing pain, until a stable pattern of effectiveness is reached. Patients with massive ascites, those with unstable body temperature, very low or very high body fat levels, and those who have decreased peripheral circulation (as often occurs during the phase of so-called active dying) have variable and unpredictable uptake of transdermal drugs. This may require use of a different delivery system under these clinical circumstances.

Instructions to Patient or Caregiver

1. *Place patch on the upper body in a clean, dry, hairless area.*
2. *Choose a different site when placing a new patch, then remove the old patch.*
3. *Remove the old patch or patches and fold sticky surfaces together, then flush down the toilet.*
4. *Wash hands after handling patches.*
5. *All unused patches (patient discontinued use or deceased) should be removed from wrappers, folded in half with sticky surfaces together, and flushed down the toilet.*

- Oral transmucosal fentanyl citrate (OTFC) (46,52). For adults, start with the 200 mcg dose for breakthrough pain, and monitor efficacy, advancing to higher dose units as needed. Onset of pain relief can usually be expected in about 5 minutes after beginning use. Any remaining partial units should be disposed of safely by placing under hot water or clipping the unused medication off of the stick and flushing down the toilet.

Hydromorphone (47,53,54)

- Hydromorphone is 5 to 8 times more potent than morphine, permitting analgesic equivalence at lower doses and smaller volumes.
- Hydromorphone can be administered through oral, parenteral (subcutaneous, intramuscular, and intravenous), rectal, or intraspinal (epidural and intrathecal) routes.
- Hydromorphone's relatively short half-life of elimination (2 to 3 hours) facilitates dose titration. Onset of action occurs within 15 minutes after parenteral administration and within 30 minutes after oral or rectal administration.
- Since hydromorphone is highly soluble in water (about 300 mg/ml), it is particularly suitable for subcutaneous administration, including continuous subcutaneous infusion (CSCI) and patient-controlled analgesia (PCA).
- Hydromorphone is hydrophilic and extensively distributes in the cerebral spinal fluid (CSF) upon epidural administration.
- A high-potency preparation (10 mg/ml) is commercially available for opioid-tolerant patients. This preparation is particularly useful for CSCI in patients where small volumes are necessary.
- Side effects associated with hydromorphone are qualitatively similar to those associated with opioids in general and most often include constipation, nausea, and sedation. Hydromorphone may be preferred for patients with decreased renal clearance in order to prevent toxic metabolite accumulation associated with other opioid analgesics.

Levorphanol and Methadone (55,56)

- These drugs are useful in selected patients as time-contingent analgesics due to their long biological half-lives, making dosing intervals (q6–8 h) relatively convenient. The potential for drug accumulation prior to achievement of steady-state blood levels (4 to 6 doses) puts patients at risk for oversedation and respiratory depression. Close monitoring for these potentially adverse effects is required by an observant caregiver. Methadone offers the advantage of relatively low cost compared to other long-acting opioid formulations, which may be critically important for patients with limited financial resources and no or limited insurance.

Sustained or Continuous-Release Enteral Formulations
Several opioids are now available in sustained or continuous-release form, facilitating compliance and maintaining blood levels between dosing intervals for improved overall control of continuous types of pain.

- Morphine: commercially available continuous-release pill formulations of morphine last 8 to 12 hours. The continuous-release formulations have similar effects when administered rectally, applied with a small amount of water-based lubricant to ease insertion (no encapsulation is necessary). A sustained-release morphine formulation of pellets in a capsule is available that lasts up to 24 hours but cannot be used per rectum. The capsules can be opened and the contents sprinkled on to a palatable food (e.g., apple sauce) as an alternative to swallowing them whole.
- Oxycodone: continuous-release oxycodone lasts 8 to 12 hours and is available in several dose sizes.
- Hydromorphone: at the time of this writing continuous-release hydromorphone is under review by the FDA and it may be available soon in several dose sizes, formulated to last 12 to 24 hours.

Note: Chewing or crushing continuous-release formulations causes them to be *immediate release*, potentially subjecting the patient to overdosage.

Preventing and Treating Opioid Adverse Effects

Constipation (57)

Always begin a prophylactic bowel regimen when commencing opioid analgesic therapy.

- Avoid bulking agents (e.g., psyllium) since these tend to cause a larger, bulkier stool, increasing defecation time in the large bowel.
- Encourage fluid (fruit juice) intake.
- Encourage dietary regimens (use of senna tea and fruits).
- Prescribe bowel motility and softening agents, as needed (e.g., senna derivatives, bisacodyl, docusate, lactulose).

Excessive Sedation (58)   After dose titration for appropriate pain control, and other correctable causes have been identified and treated if possible, use of psychostimulants may be beneficial.

- Dextroamphetamine 2.5 to 5 mg PO q am and midday.
- Methylphenidate 5 to 10 mg PO q am and 2.5 to 5 mg midday.
- Adjust both dose and timing to prevent nocturnal insomnia.
- Monitor for undesirable psychotomimetic effects (agitation, hallucinations, irritability).

Respiratory Depression (36,59)   This is rarely a clinically significant problem for opioid-tolerant patients in pain.

When undesired depressed consciousness occurs along with a respiratory rate < 8/min or hypoxemia (O_2 saturation <90 percent) associated with opioid use, cautious and slow titration of naloxone can be instituted, if the circumstances warrant. Excessive administration may cause abrupt opioid reversal with pain and autonomic crisis. Dilute 1 ampule of naloxone (0.4 mg/ml) 1:10 in injectable saline (final concentration 40 mcg/ml) and inject 1 ml every 2 to 3 minutes while closely monitoring level of consciousness and respiratory rate.

Nausea/Vomiting (60,61)   Common with opioids, but habituation occurs in most cases within several days. Assess for other treatable causes. Doses of antiemetics below are initial doses, which can be increased as required.

- Phenothiazine dopamine antagonists
  - prochlorperazine 25 to 50 mg PO/PR q 6h
  - promethazine 25 to 50 mg PO/PR q 6h
- Butyrophenone dopamine antagonists
  - haloperidol 0.5 mg IV q 6h or 2 mg PO q 6h
  - droperidol 1/4 to 1/2 cc IV q 6h
- Other dopamine antagonists
  - metoclopramide 10 mg PO/IV q 6h
- 5-HT$_3$ antagonists
  - ondansetron 4 mg PO/IV q 8h
  - granisetron 500 mg IV q 12h
- H$_1$ antihistamines
  - diphenhydramine 25 mg PO/IV q 6h
  - dimenhydrinate 25 mg PO/IV q 6h
  - hydroxyzine 25 mg PO/IV q 6h
- Benzodiazepines
  - lorazepam 0.5 to 1 mg SL/PO/IV q 4 to 6h
- Anticholinergics
  - transdermal scopolamine patch (0.5 mg q 3 days)
- Cannabinoids
  - dronabinol 7.5 mg PO q 4h
  - nabilone 1 mg PO q 4h
- Corticosteroids
  - dexamethasone 4 mg PO/IV q 8h

Myoclonus (62-64)   Myoclonus occurs more commonly with high-dose opioid therapy. Use of an alternate drug is recommended, especially if using morphine, due to metabolite accumulation. A lower dose of the substitute drug may be possible due to incomplete cross tolerance. First-line pharmacotherapy is use of low-dose benzodiazepines:

- Clonazepam 0.5 mg PO q 6 to 8h may be useful in treating myoclonus in patients who are still alert and able to communicate and take oral preparations. Increase as needed and tolerated.
- Diazepam 2 to 5 mg IV as needed to control myoclonus in imminently dying patients with intravenous access may be helpful.

Pruritus (65)   Pruritus is most common with morphine and is thought to be due to histamine release, but it can occur with most opioids. Treatment-induced sedation must be viewed by the patient as an acceptable trade-off. First-line approaches include antihistamines and/or sedatives:

- Antihistamines
  - diphenhydramine 25 to 50 mg PO/IV q 6h
  - hydroxyzine 25 mg PO q 6h
- Benzodiazepines
  - lorazepam 1 mg SL/PO/IV q 6 h

Pain-Modulating Drugs (Table 23-3)

An increasing number of drugs from various pharmacological classes seem to modulate or attenuate different kinds of pain, especially when used in combination with analgesics. A basic principle of pain management is to consider the addition of pain-modulating agents when there is a specific pathophysiologic indication (e.g., bone pain, neuropathic pain), when there is inadequate pain control with primary analgesic therapy alone, when there is sleep disturbance, or when opioid adverse effects predominate.

Pain Crises

Table 23-4 outlines a basic approach to immediate analgesic treatment for patients taking around-the-clock opioid analgesics.

The first approach to treating pain that has increased beyond the patient's level of comfort is to methodically evaluate the cause to determine the most therapeutically specific means to treat it, while ensuring comfort as quickly and effectively as possible (76). Most somatic and visceral pain is controllable with appropriately administered analgesic therapy. Some neuropathic pains (e.g., invasive and compressive neuropathies, plexopathies, and myelopathies) may be poorly responsive to analgesic therapies, short of inducing a nearly comatose state. Widespread bone metastases or end-stage pathologic fractures may present similar challenges.

- Differentiate terminal agitation or anxiety from physically based pain, if possible. Terminal restlessness/agitation symptoms unresponsive to rapid upward titration of opioid may respond to benzodiazapines, phenothiazines or barbiturates if not controlled by "milieu" therapy, and symptoms appear distressing to the patient or those in attendance.
- Make sure drugs are getting absorbed. The only *guaranteed* route is the intravenous route. Although this is to be avoided unless necessary, if there is any question about absorption of analgesics, parenteral access should be established.
- Preterminal pain crises that are poorly responsive to basic approaches to analgesic therapy merit consultation

TABLE 23-3. *Pain-modulating drugs*

Drug	Daily adult starting dose range	Route(s) of administration	Indications
Corticosteroids (66)			cerebral edema, spinal cord compression, bone pain, neuropathic pain
dexamethasone	2–4 mg tid-qid	PO/IV/SQ	
prednisone	15–30 mg tid-qid	PO	
Tricyclic antidepressants (67)	10–25 mg hs	PO	neuropathic pain, sleep disturbance
amitriptyline desipramine imipramine nortriptyline doxepin			
Anticonvulsants (68–70)			neuropathic pain
clonazepam	0.5–1 mg hs-bid-tid	PO	
carbamazepine	100 mg qd-tid	PO	
gabapentin	100 mg qd-tid	PO	
Local Anesthetics (71–73)			neuropathic pain
mexiletine	150 mg qd-tid	PO	
lidocaine	10–25 mg/hr	IV or SQ infusion	
Bisphosphonates (74)			
pamidronate	30 mg over 8–12 hr	IV infusion	osteolytic bone pain
Calcitonin (75)	25 IU/day	Nasal	neuropathic and bone pain

TABLE 23-4. *Example of analgesic protocol for escalating pain in opioid-tolerant patients (recommended for inpatient use or in-home or residential environments only where registered nurse care is available)*

Time (hours)	Treatment
0	Definition of pain out of control: Continuous pain > 4–5/10 not responsive to current analgesic Rx and distressing to patient. 1. Bolus dose (PO, SL, PR, IV, SQ) 50% of equivalent hourly dose with immediate-release dose of opioid analgesic and 2. Increase ATC doses 50% (notify physician as soon as time allows).
1	3. If pain still out of control after 1 hour, rebolus as per number 1.
2	4. If no appreciable change, notify physician for further orders.
3–4	5. If recommendations by physician(s) do not lead to adequate pain control (pain continues > 4–5/10 and distressing to patient): *Recommend:* (a) opioid rotation (i.e., equivalent dose of alternative opioid analgesic), (b) parenteral opioid administration (if not already route of administration) with dose titration at bedside.
6–8	6. If pain continues out of control, contact pain management consultant. 7. If not an inpatient, consider transfer of patient to inpatient facility with pain management consultation service unless specifically countermanded by patient's advance directives. 8. Review indications for other approaches to pain control.

with a pain management consultant as quickly as possible. Radiotherapy, anesthetic, or neuroablative procedures may be indicated. Consider spinal/epidural opioid/local anesthetic approaches, neurolytic celiac plexus block, or spinothalamic tractotomy. Expertise in these techniques is required. Epidural/intrathecal catheters can be placed in a home or residential care setting under terminal care circumstances that warrant the risks, when proper informed consent has been obtained. From a case-management standpoint, these interventions can add greatly to quality of life and decrease costs if a patient's pain is inadequately controlled by appropriate dose titration of opioid analgesics and adjuvants.

- For truly intractable end-stage pain, parenteral administration of ketamine will provide relief for the patient and ease the great distress that witnessing such agony can cause family and other caregivers who need or want to remain in attendance. One published technique (77) is:
  - *Bolus*: ketamine 0.1 mg/kg IV. Repeat as often as indicated by the patient's response. Double the dose if no

clinical improvement in 5 minutes. Follow the bolus with an infusion. Decrease opioid dose by 50%.
- *Infusion*: Start ketamine at 0.015 mg/kg/minute IV (about 1 mg/min for a 70 kg individual). Subcutaneous infusion is possible if IV access is not attainable. In this case, use an initial IM bolus dose of 0.3 to 0.5 mg/kg. Decrease opioid dose by 50%.
- It is advisable to administer a benzodiazepine (e.g., diazepam or lorazepam) concurrently to mitigate against the possibility of hallucinations or frightful dreams, since patients under these circumstances may never be able to communicate such experiences.

Another published technique (78) is:

- *Infusion*: ketamine (2 mg/ml) plus fentanyl (5 mcg/ml) plus midazolam (0.1 mg/ml) titrated upward from 2 ml/hr.
- Observe for problematic increases in secretions; treat with glycopyrrolate, scopolamine, or atropine.

Breakthrough Pain

Breakthrough pain is variously defined, but generally is thought of as intermittent episodes of moderate to more severe pains that occur in spite of control of baseline continuous pains (79). Most of the studies evaluating breakthrough pain have been done with cancer patients (80,81) although there is evidence that patients with other pain-producing, life-limiting diseases experience breakthrough pains a few times a day, lasting moments to many minutes (19). The risk of increasing the ATC analgesic dose is increasing adverse effects, especially sedation, once the more short-lived, episodic breakthrough pain has remitted.

Subtypes and Treatment

Incident Pains   Incident pain is predictably elicited by specific activities. Use a rapid-onset, short-duration analgesic formulation in anticipation of pain-eliciting activities or events. Adjust dose to severity of anticipated pain or the intensity/duration of the pain-producing event. Past experience will serve as the best guide.

Spontaneous Pains   Unpredictable pain, not temporally associated with any activity or event, is referred to as spontaneous pain. These pains are more challenging to control. Use of adjuvants for neuropathic pains may help diminish frequency and severity of these types of pains (Table 23-3). Otherwise, immediate treatment with a potent, rapid-onset opioid analgesic is indicated.

- Conventionally, oral morphine solution or other immediate-release oral formulations of opioid analgesics have been used most commonly to avoid parenteral administration, but relatively long and inconstant/unpredictable onset times coupled with duration of effect exceeding the typical breakthrough pain episode limits the utility of this traditional approach.

- Oral transmucosal fentanyl (46) is a reliable, predictable, and noninvasive means of treating these symptoms in cooperative patients.

- Intravenous bolus dosing for patients with intravenous access may be necessary in those circumstances where oral or transmucosal drugs are not able to be used (PCA devices may be helpful).

End-of-dose failure   End-of-dose failure is the phrase used to describe pain that occurs toward the end of the usual dosing interval of a regularly scheduled analgesic. This results from declining blood levels of the ATC analgesic prior to administration or uptake of the next scheduled dose. Appropriate questioning will ensure rapid diagnosis of end-of-dose failure. Shortening the dose interval to match the onset of this type of breakthrough pain should remedy this problem. For instance, a patient who is taking continuous-release morphine every 12 hours whose pain "breaks through" after about 8 to 10 hours is experiencing end-of-dose failure. If increasing the dose of drug by 25% to 50% leads to too much sedation, the dosing interval should be increased to every 8 hours.

SUMMARY AND GOALS OF THERAPY

Pain is a common manifestation of far-advanced disease. Death is an inevitability, but a painful death is not. When attention is focused on relief of pain, backed by a solid grounding in the available means to relieve pain, both simple and more technically demanding, a promise of a comfortable dying can be a promise kept. Some basic standards that can be adopted by most health care systems can define pain management goals, which, when implemented, can be measured and made part of routine continuous quality improvement processes. For instance:

- Pain out of control (patient self-report of > 3/10 pain, or pain greater than patient's acceptable level) is brought under control within 24 hours of admission to *XYZ Care Setting* (e.g., hospital, hospice, skilled nursing facility, etc.).

- Pain out of control is responded to with effective interventions so that no patient dies in *XYZ Care Setting* with pain out of control.

- Analgesic adverse effects and side effects are anticipated, prevented, or attempts at effective management are documented in all patients.

REFERENCES

1. Hippocrates. The Art. Reprinted in: Reiser SJ, Dyck AJ, Curran WJ, eds. *Ethics in Medicine.* Cambridge (MA), MIT Press, 1977.
2. American Medical Association. *Code of Medical Ethics.* Chicago: American Medical Asssociation, 1997: 2.20.
3. Singer PA, Martin DK, Kelner M. Quality end-of-life care: patients' perspectives. *JAMA* 1999;281:163–168.
4. Scull T, Motamed C, Carli F. The stress response and pre-emptive analgesia. In: Ashburn MA, Rice LJ, eds. *The management of pain.* New York: Churchill-Livingstone, 1998:557–576.
5. Liebeskind JC. Pain can kill. *Pain* 1991;44:3–4.
6. Institute of Medicine. *Approaching death: improving care at the end of life.* Washington, D.C.: National Academy Press, 1997.
7. The SUPPORT Principal Investigators. A controlled trial to improve care for seriously ill hospitalized patients. *JAMA* 1995;274:1591–1598.
8. Bernabei R, Gambassi G, Lapane K, et al. Management of pain in elderly patients with cancer. *JAMA* 1998;279:1877–1882.
9. The Gallup International Institute. Spiritual beliefs and the dying process: a report on a national survey. Funded by the Nathan Cummings Foundation, 1997
10. Townsend JA, Frank O, Fermont D, et al. Terminal cancer care and patients' preferences for place of death: a prospective study. *BMJ* 1990;301:415–417.
11. Rich BA. An ethical analysis of the barriers to effective pain management. *Cambridge Quarterly of Healthcare Ethics* 2000;9:54–70.
12. Doyle D, Hanks GWC, MacDonald N. *Oxford textbook of palliative medicine,* 2nd ed. New York: Oxford University Press, 1998.
13. Conner E, Amorosi S. *The study of pain and older Americans.* New York: Louis Harris and Associates, 1997.
14. American Geriatrics Society Panel on Chronic Pain in Older Persons. The management of chronic pain in older persons. *JAGS* 1998;46: 635–651.
15. Jacox A, Carr DB, Payne R, et al. Management of Cancer Pain: Clinical Practice Guideline Number 9. AHCPR Publication No. 94-0592. Rockville, MD: Agency for Healthcare Policy and Research. U.S. Department of Health and Human Services, Public Health Service, 1994.
16. Foley KM. Pain management in the elderly. In: Hazzard WR, Bierman EL, Blass JP, Ettinger WH, Halter JB, eds. *Principles of geriatric medicine and gerontology,* 3rd ed. New York: McGraw Hill, 1994:317–331.
17. Ferrell BR, Ferrell BA, Ahn C, Tran K. Pain management for elderly patients with cancer at home. *Cancer* 1994;74:2139–2146.
18. Bonica JJ. Cancer pain. In: Bonica JJ, ed. *The management of pain,* 2nd ed, vol. I. Philadelphia: Lee and Febiger, 1990.
19. Fine PG, Busch MA. Characterization of breakthrough pain by hospice patients and their caregivers. *J Pain Symptom Manage* 1998;16:179–183.
20. Fox P, Raina P, Jadad A. Prevalence and treatment of pain in older adults in nursing homes and other long-term care institutions. A systematic review. *CMAJ* 1999;160:329–333.
21. Herr KA, Mobily PR, Kohout FJ, Wagenaar D. Evaluation of the faces pain scale for use with the elderly. *Clin J Pain* 1998;14:29–38.
22. Gagliese L, Katz J, Melzack R. Pain in the elderly. In: Wall PD, Melzack R, eds. *Textbook of pain.* Toronto: Churchill-Livingstone, 1999:991–1006.
23. Rawlins, MD. Non-opioid analgesics. In: Doyle D, Hanks GWC, MacDonald N, eds. *Oxford textbook of palliative medicine,* 2nd ed. New York: Oxford University Press, 1998:355–361.
24. Stambaugh JE. Role of nonsteroidal anti-inflammatory drugs in the management of cancer pain. In: Patt RB, ed. *Cancer pain.* Philadelphia: Lippincott Company, 1993:105–117.
25. Bradley JD, Brandt KD, Katz BP, et al. Comparison of an antiinflammatory dose of ibuprofen, an analgesic dose of ibuprofen and acetaminophen in the treatment of patients with osteoarthritis of the knee. *N Engl J Med* 1991;325:87–91.
26. Avorn J, Gurwitz JH. Drug use in nursing homes. *Ann Int Med* 1995;123:87–91.
27. Vane JR, Botting RM. Mechanism of action of aspirin-like drugs. *Semin Arthritis Rheum* 1997;26(suppl):2–10.
28. Cryer B, Feldman M. Cyclooxygenase-1 and cyclooxygenase-2 selectivity of widely used nonsteroidal anti-inflammatory drugs. *Am J Med* 1998;104:413–421.
29. Garcia Rodriguez LA. Nonsteroidal antiinflammatory drugs, ulcers and risk: a collaborative meta-analysis. *Semin Arthritis Rheum* 1997; 26(suppl):16–20.
30. Cryer B, Dubois A. The advent of highly selective inhibitors of cyclooxygenase—A review. *Prostaglandins* 1998;56:341–61.
31. Lipsky PE, Isakson PC. Outcome of specific COX-2 inhibition in rheumatoid arthritis. *J Rheum* 1997;24(suppl):9–14.
32. Foley KM. Treatment of cancer pain. *N Engl J Med* 1985;313:84–95.
33. Grond S, Zeck D, Schug SA, Lynch J. Validation of the World Health Organization guidelines for cancer pain relief during the last days and hours of life. *J Pain Symptom Manage* 1991;6:411–22.

34. Goodwin JS, Regan M. Cognitive dysfunction associated with naproxen and ibuprofen in the elderly. *Arthritis Rheum* 1982;25: 1013–1016.
35. Dahl JL. Effective pain management in terminal care. *Clinics in Geriatric Medicine* 1996;12:279–300.
36. Twycross RJ. Misunderstandings about morphine. In: Twycross RJ, ed. *Pain relief in advanced cancer.* New York: Churchill Livingstone, 1994:333–347.
37. Page GG, Ben-Eliyahu S, Yirmiya R, Liebeskind JC. Opioids attenuate surgery-induced enhancement of metastatic colonization in rats. *Pain* 1993;54:21–8.
38. Cousins MJ. Prevention of postoperative pain. In: Bond MR, Charlton JE, Woolf CJ, eds. *Pain research and clinical management, vol 4.* Amsterdam: Elsevier, 1991.
39. Sklar LS, Anisman H. Stress and coping factors influence tumor growth. *Science* 1979;205:513–515.
40. Watanabe S. Intraindividual variability in opioid response: a role for sequential opioid trials in patient care. In: Portenoy R, Bruera E, eds. *Topics in palliative care, vol I.* New York: Oxford University Press, 1997:195-203.
41. Hoskin PJ, Hanks GW. Opioid agonist antagonist drugs in acute and chronic pain states. *Drugs* 1991;326–344.
42. Kaiko RF, Foley KM, Grabinski PY, et al. Central nervous system excitatory effects of meperidine in cancer patients. *Annals of Neurology* 1983;13:180–185.
43. Goetting MG, Thirman MJ. Neurotoxicity of meperidine. *Ann Int Med* 1985;14:1007–1009.
44. Hagmeyer KO Mauro LS, Mauro VF. Meperidine-related seizures associated with patient-controlled analgesia pumps. *Ann Pharmacotherapy* 1993;27:29–31.
45. Krstenansky P. Adverse Drug Reaction Report, Drug Information Service Newsletter. Department of Pharmacy, Stanford University Hospital. 1995;15(2).
46. Fine PG. Clinical experience with Actiq® (oral transmucosal fentanyl citrate) for the treatment of cancer pain. *J New Developments in Clinical Medicine* 1999;17:1–11.
47. American Pain Society. *Principles of analgesic use in the treatment of acute pain and cancer pain,* 4th ed. Glenview, IL: American Pain Society, 1999.
48. Twycross RJ. Oral morphine. In: Twycross RJ, ed. *Pain relief in advanced cancer.* New York: Churchill Livingstone, 1994:307–332.
49. Sjøgren P. Clinical implications of morphine metabolites. In: Portenoy RK, Bruera E, eds. *Topics in palliative care, vol I.* New York: Oxford University Press, 1997:163–176.
50. Gauthier ME, Fine PG. The emerging role of the fentanyl series in the treatment of chronic cancer pain. In: Portenoy RK, Bruera E, eds. *Topics in palliative care, vol I.* New York: Oxford University Press, 1997:177–194.
51. Simmonds MA. Transdermal fentanyl: long-term analgesic studies. *J Pain Symptom Manage* 1992;7(suppl):S36–9.
52. Fine PG, Streisand JB. A review of oral transmucosal fentanyl citrate: Potent, rapid and noninvasive opioid analgesia. *J Palliative Med* 1998;1:55–63.
53. Hill CS. Oral opioid analgesics. In: Patt RB, ed. *Cancer pain.* Philadelphia: J.B. Lippincott Company, 1993:129-142.
54. Lipman AG, Gauthier ME. Pharmacology of opioid drugs: basic principles. In: Portenoy RK, Bruera E, eds. *Topics in palliative care, vol I.* New York: Oxford University Press, 1997:137–162.
55. Wallenstein SL, Rogers AG, Kaiko RF, Houde RW. Clinical analgesic studies of levorphanol in acute and chronic cancer pain. In: Foley KM, Inturrisi CE, eds. *Advances in pain research and therapy, vol 8.* New York: Raven Press, 1986:211–215.
56. Fainsinger R, Schoeller T, Bruera E. Methadone in the management of cancer pain: a review. *Pain* 1993;52:137–147.
57. Curtis E, Krech R, Walsh T. Common symptoms in patients with advanced cancer. *J Palliative Care* 1991;7:25.
58. Bruera E, Brenneis C, Paterson AH, MacDonald N. Use of methylphenidate as an adjuvant to narcotic analgesics in patients with advanced cancer. *J Pain Symptom Manage* 1989;4:3–6.
59. Hanks G, Cherny N. Opioid analgesic therapy. In: Doyle D, Hanks GWC, MacDonald N, eds. *Oxford textbook of palliative medicine,* 2nd ed. New York: Oxford University Press, 1998:331–355.
60. Campora E, Merlini L, Pace M, et al. The incidence of narcotic-induced emesis. *J Pain Symptom Manage* 1991;6:428–434.
61. Lichter I. Results of anti-emetic management in terminal illness. *J Palliative Care* 1993;9:19–25.
62. Tiseo PJ, Thaler HT, Lapin J, et al. Morphine-6-glucuronide concentrations and opioid-related side effects: a survey of cancer patients. *Pain* 1995;61:47–54.
63. Eisele JH. Clonazapam treatment of myoclonic contractions associated with high dose opioids: a case report. *Pain* 1992;49:231–232.
64. Mercadante S. Dantrolene treatment of opioid-induced myclonus. *Anesth Analg* 1995;81:1307–1308.
65. Bernard JD. *Mechanisms and management of pruritus.* New York: McGraw Hill, 1994.
66. Ettinger AB, Portenoy RK. The use of corticosteroids in the treatment of symptoms associated with cancer. *J Pain Symptom Manage* 1988; 3:99–103.
67. Onghena P, Van Houdenhove B. Antidepressant induced analgesia in chronic nonmalignant pain. A meta-analysis of 39 placebo-controlled studies. *Pain* 1992;49:205–219.
68. McQuay H, Carroll D, Jadad A, Wiffeh P, Moore A. Anticonvulsant drugs for management of pain: a systematic review. *Br Med J* 1995;311:1047–1052.
69. Merren MD. Gabapentin for treatment of pain and tremor: a large case series. *South Med J* 1998;91:739–44.
70. Tecoma ES. Oxcarbazepine. *Epilepsia* 1999;40(suppl):S37-S46.
71. Dejgard A, Petersen P, Kastrup J. Mexiletine for treatment of chronic painful diabetic neuropathy. *Lancet* 1988;I:9–11.
72. Brose WG, Cousins MJ. Subcutaneous lidocaine for treatment of neuropathic cancer pain. *Pain* 1991;45:145–148.
73. Mao J, Chen LL. Systemic lidocaine for neuropathic pain relief. *Pain* 2000;87:7–17.
74. Koeberle D, Bacchus L, Thuerlimann, Senn H-J. Pamidronate treatment in patients with malignant osteolytic bone disease and pain. *Support Care Cancer* 1999;7:21–27.
75. Lyritis G, Paspati, I, Karachalios T, et al. Pain relief from nasal calcitonin in osteoporotic vertebral crush fractures: a double blind, placebo-controlled clinical study. *Acta Orthop Scand* 1997(Suppl);68:112–114.
76. Hagen NA, Elwood T, Ernst S. Cancer pain emergencies: a protocol for management. *J Pain Symptom Manage* 1997;14:45–50.
77. Fine PG. Low dose ketamine in the management of opioid nonresponsive terminal cancer pain. *J Pain Symptom Manage* 1999;17: 296–300.
78. Berger JM, Ryan A, Vadievelu N, et al. Ketamine-fentanyl-midazolam infusion for the control of symptoms in terminal care. *American J Hospice Palliative Care* 2000;17:127–136.
79. Portenoy RK, Hagen NA. Breakthrough pain: Definition, prevalence, and characteristics. *Pain* 1990;41:273–281.
80. Portenoy RK, Payne D, Jacobsen P. Breakthrough pain: characteristics and impact in patients with cancer pain. *Pain* 1999;81:129–34.
81. Fine PG. Breakthrough cancer pain: epidemiology, characteristics and management. *CNS Drugs* 2000;13:313–319.

CHAPTER 24

Migraine and the Primary Headaches

Steve D. Wheeler

Migraine and the other primary headache disorders affect not only the individual sufferers, but often have a major impact on the lives of their family and friends. The poor quality of life, comorbidity, and frequent medical contacts at the office, pharmacy, emergency department, or hospital all plague the migraineur. The societal economic burden is great, amounting to over $13 billion annually in America (1). The good news is that there has been an explosion in our understanding of migraine and, to a lesser extent, some of the other primary headache disorders. The fallout has produced new therapeutic options that, with time, will translate to headache sufferers and eventually improve their physical and emotional well-being.

However, there exists a certain paradox wherein recent developments may not fully benefit or extend to all headache sufferers. Amazingly, 52% of migraineurs have never even been correctly diagnosed, and of those who are diagnosed, 38% have suffered 3 years or more before being diagnosed. Additionally, 60% of migraineurs exclusively use over-the-counter preparations for acute headache attacks, 80% say their headaches are severe or extremely severe, 39% seek bed rest, and 24% have sought emergency room care. In many ways, there seems to be a disconnection between what is known about headache and what happens in patient care (2).

The purpose of this chapter is to teach you something about headache. Hopefully, at least in part, you will learn to recognize and modify attitudes in yourself and others that impair validation of the primary headaches as genuine disorders associated with considerable suffering.

The primary headache disorders, and to a small extent, how differential diagnosis has an impact on the secondary or symptomatic headache will be discussed. However, it must be recognized from the start that chronic recurrent headache presenting to the physician's office is typically represented by one of the benign primary headaches. The secondary or symptomatic headaches, on the contrary, often present with an interesting constellation of historical features and physical findings that begin to hint and define their malicious nature.

Since migraine is the best understood headache, it serves as a model for the primary headaches. Here we will first review migraine, then the disorders associated with autonomic dysfunction, the trigeminal autonomic cephalalgias, including cluster headache, the paroxysmal hemicranias, hemicrania continua, and SUNCT (short-lasting unilateral neuralgiform headache with conjunctival injection and tearing) (3). Second, idiopathic stabbing headache and tension-type headache will complete the discussion of the primary headaches. Third, the significant issues of analgesic rebound headache and medication induced headache will be discussed. Finally, we will consider comorbidity, then review acute and preventative pharmacotherapy.

EPIDEMIOLOGY OR VITAL STATISTICS

The best population-based epidemiological studies relate to migraine and some of that information will be reported here.

Data from the American Migraine Study II, recently presented by Lipton, shows no major changes since the original report in 1992 (2,4). The overall well-being, disability, diagnosis, and treatment of migraine sufferers has not changed in any significant fashion in the last decade. Currently, there are nearly 28 million migraine sufferers in America and growing. Today more people know they have migraine, but unhappily 52% of migraine sufferers remain undiagnosed. There exists a situation where neither the sufferers nor their physicians know they have migraine. Unfortunately, without proper diagnosis, appropriate treatment will never be possible. Some argue that undiagnosed migraine represents a milder, less-disabling disorder. However, in Lipton's study the data are clear—the diagnosed and undiagnosed migraine sufferers have nearly equivalent disability, albeit diagnosed migraineurs have more frequent severe attacks.

The likelihood of misdiagnosing migraine as sinus or tension-type headaches is greater than the chance of diagnosing migraine correctly. Although episodic tension-type headaches occur most frequently, they rarely result in office visits. Additionally, tension-type headaches are not severe; they are, by definition, of mild to moderate intensity. When tension-type headache sufferers present to the office, it is most often because they have undiagnosed migraine or are in a transformational phase evolving toward chronic daily headache. Migraine, idiopathic stabbing headache, cluster headache, and hemicrania continua typically present to primary and neurologic physicians. Unfortunately, the characteristic headache features are not defined and the specific diagnosis remains unrecognized.

PATHOGENESIS

Migraine and many of the other primary headaches are neurovascular disorders. Much is known about the pathogenesis of migraine; however, it is fair to say that more is unknown. Moreover, it is likely that some of the present notions, in time, will be found incorrect. Nevertheless, these ideas serve as thought-provoking hypotheses. Additionally, although many of the current suppositions segregate headache from aura, a unified hypothesis is needed.

In any migraine postulation, the contribution of genetics cannot be ignored. In some hemiplegic migraine families there is evidence of a missense mutation in the α_1-subunit of the P/Q-type, voltage-gated calcium channel on chromosome 19 (5–7). Thus, whether migraine is a channelopathy, a disorder of dopamine receptors, or a disorder of other neuromodulary systems remains to be determined (8). Population-based genetic analysis suggests that migraine is a multifactorial, polygenic disorder (9). Yet, clinical experience suggests autosomal dominant inheritance since probands have an affected first-degree relative 70% to 90% of the time. Perhaps, like other autosomal dominant neurologic conditions, it may well be that variable expression and incomplete penetrance are involved. Additionally, it must be considered that different genes express the headache and aura of migraine.

We now know that migraine sufferers have a region in the midbrain near the dorsal raphe nucleus, ipsilateral to unilateral headache, that has come to be known as the migraine generator (10). However, whether the migraine generator truly resides in the brainstem or the occipital cortex is not clear. Presumably the generator is genetically determined and predisposes to migraine attacks. Apparently, once the generator becomes active there is subsequent activation of trigeminal nucleus caudalis and thalamic and cortical areas. The occipital cortex appears to be the seat of spreading cortical depression, which, in humans, represents spreading hypoperfusion. Spreading hypoperfusion occurs in waves and travels at a rate of 3 to 6 mm/minute as it advances anteriorly through the occipital cortex. However, spreading hypoperfusion is not characterized by vasoconstriction; it is associated with vasodilatation.

Soon after migraine initiation, there is activation of trigeminal nucleus caudalis and subsequently the trigeminal sensory nerve via pseudo-bipolar fibers. Stimulation of the trigeminal system is associated with the release of potent vasoactive substances like calcitonin gene-related peptide (CGRP), vasoactive intestinal peptide (VIP), and substance P. These vasoactive substances contribute to the neurogenic inflammation that is released at the level of the pain-sensitive meningeal vessels. There is dilation of meningeal vessels and, consequently, pain. It has been suggested that nitric oxide release occurs early, produces vasodilatation and a cascade of events, eventuating in neurogenic inflammation, vasodilatation, and pain.

The aura is associated with cortical hyperexcitability and spreading hypoperfusion. Aurora (11) has demonstrated cortical hyperexcitability in the transcranial magnetic stimulation model in humans where phosphenes are produced at a threshold considerably lower in migraineurs than in nonmigraineurs. Moreover, some migraineurs have had migraine triggered by this technique.

Recent studies by Burstein (12) suggest that peripheral and central nervous system sensitization occurs during migraine. Sensitization, manifested by cutaneous allodynia, has been noted during migraine attacks. Allodynia initially affects the head ipsilateral to the headache. However, as the attack proceeds, the contralateral head and subsequently the ipsilateral forearm develop allodynia. Recurrent, frequent central nervous system sensitization may eventuate in a chronic allodynic state represented by chronic daily or intractable headaches. This pathological sensitization suggests that the elimination of attacks is tantamount and, failing this, attacks must resolve rapidly.

Some of the primary headaches, particularly those associated with autonomic dysfunction, involve the trigeminal autonomic reflex. In this reflex, trigeminal system stimulation results in stimulation of the parasympathetic system. Stimulation of the parasympathetic system is associated with orbital-nasal autonomic dysfunction like that typically seen in cluster headache.

Studies have shown that CGRP is the single most important vasoactive substance in migraine. In a series of unilateral migraineurs, when ipsilateral jugular blood was sampled for CGRP and VIP, there was a marked elevation in CGRP, but no significant change in VIP (13). In cluster headache where the trigeminal autonomic reflex is active, there is marked elevation not only in CGRP, but also in VIP (14). Additionally, studies have shown that in some migraineurs with evidence of ipsilateral orbital-nasal autonomic dysfunction, the jugular venous neuropeptide pattern is similar to that of cluster patients. Thus, suggesting that the trigeminal autonomic reflex is active in these migraineurs.

DIAGNOSIS AND IHS DIAGNOSTIC CRITERIA

The primary headache disorders are represented by benign, recurrent head pain. Benign suggests that neurological examination and neuroradiological studies, if performed, are normal or have no clinical relevance to the headache condition. Recurrent typically means that individual sufferers have experienced at least five headache attacks in their lifetime. Head pain location is not specific to the diagnosis. However, the duration of the individual attacks is rather specific. Likewise, the severity of the headache attacks and the quality of the pain often yield useful diagnostic information. For example, migraine is often pulsating or throbbing. Cluster headaches frequently produce hot poker or sharp, ice-pick pain, whereas tension-type headaches generally are described as tight, pressure, or dull in nature.

In addition to some of the more specific diagnostic features as formalized in the International Headache Society (IHS) classification and diagnostic criteria (15), there are other properties that provide clues to the headache type. Behavioral characteristics during acute attacks often suggest a more specific diagnosis. Migraine sufferers tend to be somewhat withdrawn during an attack and seek a dark, quiet room, resting or sleeping, and assume their special position. Many times the migraineur weeps quietly, as more vigorous crying tends to exacerbate headache. Some cultures, particularly those of African and Hispanic descent, often tie socks, belts, or towels around their head.

Contrast the quiet, resolved behavior of a migraineur during an attack with a cluster headache sufferer. The cluster sufferer is usually restless. They walk and pace. If they do seek a dark, quiet room, they rarely lie flat. They may reduce head pain by traumatizing their heads.

Chronobiological or biological clock disturbances often hint or indicate the diagnosis of cluster headache. Cluster headache has a propensity to occur with a certain periodicity such that certain seasons, months, or times of the day serve as points of peak cluster attacks.

The IHS criteria were formulated to allow a commonality of diagnoses across countries, cultures, languages, and specialties. Originally intended for clinical trials, the usefulness of these criteria allows applicability to clinical practice. Despite this, there remains considerable hesitance by physicians to utilize these criteria in daily practice.

Migraine and the IHS

Migraine is a benign, recurrent, moderate to severe, disabling headache that is often unilateral and pulsatile and associated with certain environmental sensitivities or nausea. The criteria discussed in this section are in reference to the two most common types of migraine, migraine without aura and migraine with aura (Tables 24-1 and 24-2). Previously, these were known as common and classical migraine, respectively. Migraine without aura is the most common of the migraines and repre-

sents 80% to 85% of all cases. Migraine with aura occurs in the minority and represents approximately 15% to 20% of all migraineurs.

Twelve% of Americans have migraine, and women suffer migraine three times as often as men do. This represents 18% of American women and 6% of American men. The prevalence of migraine in childhood is similar in boys and girls until puberty when the prevalence takes off in women. Prevalence peaks between the ages of 25 and 44. However, with advancing age, prevalence begins to wane, particularly after menopause in women. After age 70 prevalence is similar in men and women. The changes in migraine prevalence appear to be effected by hormonal issues in women,

TABLE 24-1. *IHS migraine without aura diagnostic criteria*

A. At least five attacks fulfilling B–D
B. Headache attacks lasting 4 to 72 hours
C. Headache has at least two of the following:
   1. Unilateral
   2. Pulsating quality
   3. Moderate or severe intensity
   4. Aggravation by walking stairs or similar routine physical activity
D. During headache at least one of the following:
   1. Nausea and/or vomiting
   2. Photophobia and phonophobia
E. At least one of the following:
   1. History, physical, and neurological examinations do not suggest one of the symptomatic disorders
   2. History, physical, and neurological examinations do suggest one of the symptomatic disorders, but it is ruled out by appropriate investigations
   3. Such disorder is present, but migraine attacks do not occur for the first time in close temporal relation to the symptomatic disorder

(From Headache Classification Committee of the International Headache Society. Classification and diagnostic criteria for headache disorders, cranial neuralgias and facial pain. *Cephalalgia* 1988;(Suppl 7):1–96, with permission.)

TABLE 24-2. *IHS migraine with aura diagnostic criteria*

A. At least two attacks fulfilling B
B. At least three of the following four characteristics:
   1. One or more fully reversible aura symptoms indicating focal cerebral cortical and/or brainstem dysfunction
   2. At least one aura symptom develops gradually over 4 minutes or two or more symptoms occur in succession
   3. No aura symptom lasts more than 60 minutes. If more than one aura symptom is present, accepted duration is proportionally increased.
   4. Headache follows aura with a free interval of less than 60 minutes. (It may also begin before or simultaneously with the aura.)
C. The benign clause (see Table 24.1, section E)

(From Headache Classification Committee of the International Headache Society. Classification and diagnostic criteria for headache disorders, cranial neuralgias and facial pain. *Cephalalgia* 1988;(Suppl 7):1–96, with permission.)

particularly menarche and menopause. However, stress seems to play a role in triggering the migraine genetic predisposition, particularly after menarche where dating and marriage issues are relevant.

According to IHS criteria, migraine is a benign, recurrent disorder with head pain attacks that last 4 to 72 hours, untreated or unsatisfactorily treated. The headaches are associated with at least two features of a four-part criterion. Headache is frequently *unilateral*. Often, too much is made of unilaterality when, in fact, 33% to 40% of sufferers have bilateral headache. The headache is *moderate or severe* in intensity. However, it must be recognized that severity and the other features described here represent only one part of a four-part criterion. Thus, it is possible for individuals to experience mild migraine. In our experience, many patients believe they have mild migraine when, in fact, they do not. Often they are satisfied with poor headache control. They do not recognize that current treatments allow improved pain control and diminished disability.

> A young woman experienced menstrual migraine since adolescence. She claimed her migraine was mild, as only one attack occurred monthly. Attacks start two days premenstrually and last three days. On each day she takes eight butalbitals for headache control (i.e., 24 butalbital per migraine attack). Fifty percent of the time she misses work because of the headaches, and when she goes to work she functions at 60% to 70% of full capacity.

Migraine pain is often *pulsatile*. Unfortunately, many migraineurs, as well as other headache sufferers, share a certain difficulty describing the nature of their pain. Their inability to describe pain quality offers several opportunities. First, it allows patients to recognize that their headache insight ("I know my body!") may not be as good as they thought, and better methods of headache identification or quantification (e.g., a diary) would be appropriate. Second, lack of insight into the quality of the pain often suggests that important behavioral opportunities will be available. Third, if the examining physician offers a series of adjectives that describe headache quality, patients begin to realize that there really is no "normal" or "regular" headache (Table 24-3).

Migraine headache is *aggravated by routine physical activity,* which, according to the IHS, is defined as climbing stairs. However, in Florida stairs are rare. Thus, we ask whether jumping up and down or shaking the head worsens the pain. Usually, the awful facial expression in response to this question is sufficient. Finally, the last two criteria define whether *photophobia and phonophobia* or *nausea or vomiting* are present.

Migraine with aura represents migraine associated with a focal neurological syndrome. However, one of the major weak points in the IHS classification concerns the lack of specific features for the headache of migraine with aura. Essentially any headache associated with aura meets criteria for migraine with aura; however, we prefer that the headache meet criteria for migraine without aura.

The most common aura is characterized by a visual disturbance. Visual aura can be variable, but in the individual it is usually stereotyped. It can represent the classical fortification spectra or it may be experienced as bright lights, halos, flashes, kaleidoscopic images, or other visual phenomena. It may be colorful, lively, or frightening, and it is often pulsatile. Bizarre peduncular hallucinations may occur, particularly in children, and can be characterized by active images like stars or cowboys. Positive phenomenon with brightness, shininess, glares, scintillation, and heat wave characteristics are typical presentations of visual aura.

Next most commonly, sensory aura occurs. The best-defined sensory syndrome is represented by cheilo-oral paresthesias. Paresthesias involve the hand and ipsilateral face, lips, tongue, or mouth and may start in either the hand or the head or both simultaneously.

The third most common aura is characterized by a language disturbance. Many migraineurs who experience language aura do not recognize that it occurs, mostly because they limit communication during headache. On other occasions, there are no witnesses to their disturbed speech. Lastly, disordered language may go unrecognized because migraine-associated cognitive dysfunction may be present (16).

> A 40-year-old woman with migraine claimed that people could not hear her during a migraine. Therefore, she shouted loudly so they could hear. When asked whether people could understand her, she was puzzled, but during the next migraine she paid particular attention. It was clear that people could not understand her and she could not understand them. In an attempt to understand she shouted and demanded that they speak louder, but the louder they got, the more phonophobic she got.

Migraine aura typically is time locked or linked to the headache. It often occurs before the headache, usually resolving at headache onset. However, it may occur at headache onset or during the headache. The aura to headache interval should last no more than 60 minutes (Table 24-2). The rule of thumb, however, is that aura should not occur independent of the headache.

Uncomplicated migraine aura typically lasts 10 to 15 minutes, but never, by definition, lasts more than 60 minutes. It usually evolves slowly over 4 minutes and rarely starts suddenly. Aura can have a repetitive quality in that it may recur several times during the headache. However, most fail to report this phenomena, as they suffer so severely from the headache, besides they believe it to be a

TABLE 24-3. *A headache by any name is still a pain*

Sharp	Biting	Hammering
Dull	Beating	Heavy
Pulling	Banging	Pressure
Grabbing	Jabbing	Stiff
Tight	Jolting	Burning
Stabbing	Throbbing	Tingling
Aching	Pulsating	Electrical
Twisting	Bursting	Lancinating
Gnawing	Exploding	Empty

common experience. Some undergo multiple auras. Each aura lasts the usual time, but can last as long as 60 minutes. The most common order in which multiple auras occur is similar to aura frequency in that visual, sensory, and language disturbances are encountered.

Some migraineurs experience aura-like phenomena that are rather short lived. They usually last seconds, frequently occurring as the headache peaks, and are most often described as flashes, dots, or zigzags. These symptoms most likely represent clinical evidence of cortical hyperexcitability (11).

Many migraineurs endure symptoms that tend to predict the coming migraine. These represent premonitory or prodromal symptoms. Fatigue, yawning, cravings, euphoria, depression, anger, and irritability occur. Many women encounter premenstrual cravings that likely represent a combination of migraine and menstrual cravings. After the migraine has passed, many experience postdromal fatigue, irritability, and diminished cognitive awareness and efficiency, although euphoria occurs occasionally.

Migrainous disorder is an IHS diagnosis, wherein all but one criterion for IHS migraine is met. Many times this is called migrainous headache or migraine minus one because of a single missing criterion. From a clinical and therapeutic standpoint, migrainous disorder represents migraine. However, these individuals cannot be entered into migraine clinical trials since they do not meet IHS migraine criteria.

Migraine status, by definition, describes a circumstance where migraine is experienced continuously or near-continuously for more than 72 hours, with headache-free periods of no more than 4 hours. Migraine status can be an isolated event or it can represent deterioration in episodic migraine or a chronic daily headache syndrome. It is serious, however, as it can be associated with dehydration and needs to be treated aggressively.

Recent studies have attempted to define the different types of headaches that occur in headache sufferers with migraine, migrainous disorder, and tension-type headache. It is clear that these headache sufferers experience a spectrum of headaches. In the migraineur, tension-type and migrainous headaches respond well to sumatriptan (17); however, there is no reason to expect that the other triptans (e.g., zolmitriptan, naratriptan, rizatriptan) will not be effective. In the tension-type headache sufferer, some have "pure" tension-type headaches and never have migraine, whereas others also have migraine or migrainous disorder. Thus, those with migraine most likely represent migraineurs who predominately have tension-type headaches.

Complicated Migraine

Migraine can be complicated by or associated with significant neurologic features that often suggest a symptomatic process. The presence of cortical, brainstem, prolonged, or isolated neurologic symptoms and signs typify the complicated migraines (Table 24-4).

TABLE 24-4. *The complicated migraines*

Hemiplegic migraine, familial or nonfamilial
Basilar migraine
Migraine with prolonged aura
Migraine aura without headache
Migraine with acute onset aura
Ophthalmoplegic migraine
Migrainous infarction

Hemiplegic migraine is characterized by the presence of unilateral weakness. This can be subtle and minimal or mild, but at times it is severe and produces complete hemiplegia. The use of the term *hemiplegic* in this circumstance does not necessarily indicate a true hemiplegia since hemiparesis is often present. Many physicians consider the presence of a hemisensory disturbance to be a manifestation of complicated migraine. Fortunately, this is not the case, as sensory aura is the second most common migraine aura. Nevertheless, if there is evidence of a subtle hemiparesis associated with a sensory disturbance, then this represents hemiplegic migraine rather than migraine with sensory aura.

Brainstem symptoms or signs imitating vertebrobasilar transient ischemic attack (TIA) or stroke define basilar migraine. Individuals can experience diplopia, dysarthria, hemiparesis, quadriparesis, or diagonal paresis. Sensory features may be crossed and limb or gait ataxia may be present.

Migraine with prolonged aura is manifested by aura, most often visual then next most commonly sensory, that persists for more than 60 minutes but less than 7 days. It is unassociated with routine neuroimaging abnormalities.

Migraine with acute onset aura is unlike typical migraine with aura in that the headache is specifically defined as migraine headache. However, the aura is sudden in onset, typically developing in less than 4 minutes. The paroxysmal nature of the aura may suggest a symptomatic etiology.

Migraine aura without headache is defined by the unique situation wherein typical neurologic features compatible with migraine aura are experienced separate and distinct from the headache. To make this diagnosis, migraine with aura must be experienced. Once this initial criterion is met, attacks of migraine without aura, migraine with aura, and migraine aura without headache occur. This is not unlike the situation where migraine with aura or migraine without aura can be experienced at different times. Additionally, there is the peculiar circumstance where migraine aura is never associated with headache. Often there is a family or remote personal history of migraine headache in these cases. However, when aura occurs independent of headache, particularly when it occurs for the first time, TIA, stroke, and other neurologic disorders must be considered. Although uncommon, typical migraine aura, usually visual aura, can be triggered by ischemia. Rarely, occipital lobe lesions (e.g., meningioma and arteriovenous malformations) have been associated with visual disturbances imitating migraine aura.

A 50-year-old hypertensive, diabetic woman had migraine with and without aura and began to experience visual aura without headache. She was found to have critical stenosis of the ipsilateral internal carotid artery and endarterectomy resulted in complete resolution of the migraine aura without headache.

Complicated migraine *cannot* be diagnosed at the time of first presentation. Additionally, IHS criteria require that at least two stereotypical episodes must be experienced before this diagnosis should ever be made. Thus, complicated migraine remains a diagnosis of exclusion, otherwise symptomatic disorders will be missed.

In migraineurs it has been suggested that the risk of persistent neurologic dysfunction, that is stroke, occurs at a rate higher than normally anticipated. An estimated stroke risk of 5% is thought to occur in hemiplegic and basilar migraine, but this seems to be an overestimate. The use of the triptans (sumatriptan, zolmitriptan, naratriptan, and rizatriptan) and ergot derivatives (dihydroergotamine, ergotamine, methysergide, or methylergonovine) is, in general, contraindicated in complicated migraine. The Food and Drug Administration (FDA) has deemed triptans to be contraindicated in basilar and hemiplegic migraine, although there is no strong evidence for this conclusion. Complicated migraineurs historically have been excluded from triptan trials. Thus, there are no controlled studies in this patient population and therefore no evidence supporting safety, tolerability, or efficacy. However, we have seen individuals with previously undiagnosed hemiplegic and basilar migraine who were treated with triptans and had no untoward reactions. Klapper and Mathew recently reported several complicated migraineurs who demonstrated safety, tolerability, and efficacy with triptan use (18). However, until convincing evidence is available, manifested by ample clinical experience by headache experts or randomized controlled trials, we generally suggest compliance with FDA recommendations.

Migraine and Stroke

Stroke can occur in migraine sufferers. Migraine stroke or migrainous infarction (Table 24-5) represents migraine associated with a neurological deficit that persists in excess of 7

TABLE 24-5. *IHS migrainous infarction diagnostic criteria*

A. Patient has previously fulfilled criteria for migraine with aura
B. The present attack is typical of previous attacks, but neurological deficits are not completely reversible within 7 days and/or neuroimaging demonstrates ischemic infarction in relevant area
C. Other causes of infarction ruled out by appropriate investigations

(From Headache Classification Committee of the International Headache Society. Classification and diagnostic criteria for headache disorders, cranial neuralgias and facial pain. *Cephalalgia* 1988;(Suppl 7):1–96, with permission.)

days, with or without neuroradiographic correlation (15). Some migraineurs with antiphospholipid or anticardiolipin syndrome may have a slightly greater risk for stroke, but these disorders are often heralded by recurrent deep vein thrombosis or miscarriages (19). The presence of mitral valve prolapse in a high percentage of migraineurs (20% of women and 6% of men) does not seem to dramatically increase the stroke risk (20). Recent studies suggest that patent foramen ovale occurs more often in young women with migraine with aura. Thus, it is more likely that stroke can occur with patent foramen ovale than with mitral valve prolapse (21).

Some evidence suggests that migraine with aura in young woman less than 45 years old has a slightly greater risk for stroke than age-matched controls without aura. There are concerns about oral contraceptives increasing the stroke risk in this population, particularly high-dose estrogen contraceptives. Additionally, there is interplay with other vascular disease risk factors, especially smoking.

Headache occurs in approximately one-third of patients presenting with new stroke. Certainly, in our clinical experience, many stroke sufferers often have a preexisting history of active or remote migraine, no matter what their age.

Cluster Headache

Severe pain and ipsilateral orbital-nasal autonomic dysfunction characterize cluster headache. However, it is often accompanied by chronobiological and behavioral disturbances. Cluster is associated with severe to excruciating, unilateral temporal-orbital pain that is often described as piercing, boring, knife, ice-pick, stake, dagger, or swordlike (Table 24-6). Cluster attacks, by definition, last 15 to 180 minutes untreated (not unsatisfactorily treated) and are associated with at least one symptom or sign of ipsilateral orbital-nasal autonomic dysfunction (lacrimation, con-

TABLE 24-6. *IHS cluster diagnostic criteria*

A. At least 5 attacks fulfilling B–D
B. Severe unilateral orbital and/or temporal pain lasting 15 to 180 minutes (untreated)
C. Headache is associated with at least one of the following on pain side:
  1. Conjunctival injection
  2. Lacrimation
  3. Nasal congestion
  4. Rhinorrhea
  5. Forehead and facial sweating
  6. Miosis
  7. Ptosis
  8. Eyelid edema
D. Attack frequency: 1 every other day to 8/day
E. The benign clause (see Table 24.1, section E)

(From Headache Classification Committee of the International Headache Society. Classification and diagnostic criteria for headache disorders, cranial neuralgias and facial pain. *Cephalalgia* 1988;(Suppl 7):1–96, with permission.)

junctival injection, eyelid edema, ptosis, periorbital sweating, miosis, nasal congestion, and rhinorrhea).

The chronobiological disturbance of cluster suggests a hypothalamic locus for cluster generation (22). Hypothalamic dysfunction results in a certain predilection for headache attacks to occur with circannual or circadian rhythmicity. Attacks tend to occur at particular times during the year, most often January and July, but generally occur at higher frequency during certain times of the season, month, week, or day. Frequent cluster attacks are noted to occur around 2:00 A.M., awakening people from sleep, typically at the onset of the first REM cycle, but they also occur with high frequency at 3:00 P.M. and 9:00 P.M. These latter times are associated with a predisposition for cluster attacks to occur after school or work.

Agitation, restlessness, and hyperactivity best characterize cluster behavioral features. Sufferers commonly walk or pace. Typically they are unable to lie flat, preferring a 30- to 45-degree angle. When flat, they become increasingly restless, tossing and turning, finally arising to walk and pace. They often stand in open windows or doors seeking the relief of a cool breeze. These features can be associated with banging or rubbing the head on the floor, wall, or bed. Sometimes the trauma is so vigorous that abrasions and contusions occur. These efforts briefly relieve cluster pain, replacing it with the milder discomfort of traumatic counterirritation until the cluster headache returns.

Cluster headache is not particularly common. It occurs with a prevalence of 0.1% to 0.4% and affects men more often than women. In the past, the male-to-female ratio was reported as high as 6–10:1. However, more recently the ratio has fallen to 2.1–2.5:1 (23,24). The increase in women is thought to be associated with lifestyle changes more typical of those traditionally found in men, particularly cigarette smoking. Cluster affects all ethnic populations; however, women, particularly African American women, are less likely to be diagnosed early.

Paroxysmal Hemicranias

Chronic and episodic paroxysmal hemicrania represent indomethacin or nonsteroidal antiinflammatory drug (NSAID) responsive primary headache disorders (3). Typically, they are associated with attacks of severe unilateral temporal orbital pain lasting on average 2 to 4 minutes. By definition, however, attacks last 2 to 45 minutes, occur more than eight times daily, and are associated with ipsilateral orbital-nasal autonomic dysfunction. The major difference between episodic and chronic paroxysmal hemicrania is that the latter occurs daily or nearly daily, whereas in episodic paroxysmal hemicrania there may be long periods of headache remission.

Chronic paroxysmal hemicrania can be distinguished from hemicrania continua by recognizing that daily unilateral background headache is only present in hemicrania continua. Interval headache is not present in the paroxysmal hemicranias. There should be complete headache freedom between attacks. Making this history-dependent differential diagnosis is often difficult since many patients report only the severe headaches, resigned to live with the mild or moderate daily headache.

Hemicrania Continua

Hemicrania continua is said to be a rare headache disorder, but Nahmias et al. (25) have noted that it is not all that rare. In our experience it occurs considerably more frequently than cluster headache (26). Hemicrania continua represents an indomethacin or NSAID-responsive trigeminal autonomic cephalalgia. It is characterized by a daily unilateral background headache that varies in severity from minimal to mild to moderate, but it is present for at least one month. Superimposed on the daily unilateral background headache, severe headache attacks occur (Table 24-7). Indomethacin or NSAID-responsiveness for the entire headache syndrome and/or ipsilateral orbital-nasal autonomic dysfunction characterize the severe headache attacks. Women predominate in this population at a ratio of approximately 7:1. Analgesic rebound headaches often accompany this disorder. In the original description, Sjaastad and Spierings (27) reported patients who experienced moderately severe headaches. However, there appears to be a clinical spectrum of hemicrania continua. Severe headache attacks vary in frequency and duration, last anywhere from seconds to one week but, on average, last 40 hours and occur two to three times weekly. Often the severe headaches are associated with idiopathic stabbing headache.

It is extremely important to make the diagnosis of hemicrania continua, as treatment is highly effective with an appropriate NSAID. When hemicrania continua is

TABLE 24-7. *Proposed diagnostic criteria for hemicrania continua (modified)*

A. Continuous but fluctuating daily headache, present for one month
B. Moderate severity
C. Lack of precipitating mechanisms
D. Headache must have either one of these features:
  1. Complete response to indomethacin or NSAID
  2. Autonomic features in association with severe pain attacks:
    a. Conjunctival injection
    b. Lacrimation
    c. Nasal congestion
    d. Rhinorrhea
    e. Ptosis
    f. Eyelid edema
E. The benign clause (see Table 24.1, section E)

(From Goadsby PJ, Lipton RB. A review of paroxysmal hemicranias, SUNCT syndrome and other short-lasting headaches with autonomic features, including new cases. *Brain* 1997;120:193–209, with permission.)

NSAID-unresponsive, it is typically highly refractory to pharmacotherapeutic interventions, although some respond well to long-acting opioids. In this syndrome, diagnosis is facilitated by a diagnostic/therapeutic trial with an NSAID (e.g., naproxen sodium or rofecoxib) (28). If a less potent and less toxic NSAID fails, a trial with indomethacin is appropriate.

SUNCT

SUNCT (short-lasting unilateral neuralgiform headache with conjunctival injection and tearing) syndrome is extremely rare. Hundreds of attacks occur daily with duration of 5 to 250 seconds. The acronym describes this syndrome well, and most of the cases reported in the literature have been men. No therapies have been found to be consistently useful for this disorder; it is highly refractory to treatment.

Idiopathic Stabbing Headaches

Idiopathic stabbing headache represents a common headache in clinical practice. It is a paroxysmal disorder of a sharp, stabbing, jabbing, or jolting nature typically lasting less than one second. However, it can trigger a migraine or tension-type headache and it is often associated with hemicrania continua. In isolation it is not associated with autonomic dysfunction. Fairly typical clinical features often suggest the diagnosis. Patients are usually frightened by this headache, as they fear an impending vascular catastrophe. It typically stops them in their tracks, they wince and grab the painful area. However, by the time the hand gets to the head, the pain is usually gone. These headaches are "head grabbers." They represent an indomethacin/NSAID-responsive disorder. However, as long as they are infrequent, pharmacotherapy is not necessary; education is sufficient. Yet, if they occur many times an hour or produce a true status, then treatment is usually required.

Tension-Type Headache

Episodic tension-type headaches are the most common headaches of all (Table 24-8). They are characterized by bilateral mild to moderate pain, typically of a pressing, dull, tight, or achy quality. Nausea and vomiting are absent, but photophobia or phonophobia can be present. Chronic tension-type headaches are represented by 180 days per year of headache with similar qualities as noted with episodic tension-type headaches. In our experience, we rarely see episodic tension-type headaches in our clinic. Instead, we see individuals with frequent migraine and chronic tension-type headaches. Tension-type headaches can be associated with myofascial involvement of pericranial musculature. One of the major pitfalls in the diagnosis of tension-type headache has to do with headache severity. Many physicians believe that tension-type headaches can be severe.

TABLE 24-8. *IHS tension-type headache diagnostic criteria*

A. At least 10 previous headache episodes fulfilling criteria B–D listed below. Number of days with such headache < 180/year (<15/month).
B. Headache lasting from 30 minutes to 7 days
C. At least two of the following pain characteristics:
   1. Pressing/tightening (nonpulsating) quality
   2. Mild or moderate intensity (may inhibit, but does not prohibit activities)
   3. Bilateral location
   4. No aggravation by walking stairs or similar routine physical activity
D. Both of the following:
   1. No nausea or vomiting (anorexia may occur)
   2. Photophobia and phonophobia are absent, or one but not the other is present
E. The benign clause (see Table 24.1, section E)

(From Headache Classification Committee of the International Headache Society. Classification and diagnostic criteria for headache disorders, cranial neuralgias and facial pain. *Cephalalgia* 1988;(Suppl 7):1–96, with permission.)

However, this feature strongly suggests the presence of migraine or another primary headache disorder.

ANALGESIC REBOUND HEADACHES

Many of the medications we use for primary headache treatment can cause headaches. Analgesic rebound headache represents the most insidious and malicious process that can occur in headache sufferers. This is a state wherein analgesics actually cause more headaches. Typically, there is an increase in headache frequency, duration, and severity. Transformation into a chronic daily headache process develops over many years, 1 to 2 years when caused by triptans or ergotamine, and 4 years for analgesics (29). Patients report that the offending analgesic is effective for control of any given headache, however, they rarely recognize the deceptive nature of this process wherein there is an increasing headache burden. Fearful of being withdrawn from the offending analgesics, many patients argue to continue the status quo, thus dooming themselves to more headaches in the future. Many times, these patients have never been placed on a preventative headache medication. Unfortunately by the time analgesic rebound is present, acute and preventative headache treatments have lost considerable efficacy and often fail. Typically, acute medications are increasingly ineffective, patients require larger doses to get increasingly faltering efficacy. Similarly, preventative regimens lose efficacy. The patient's paradox is such that acute and preventative efficacy rarely returns until the analgesics that initiated the process have been eliminated and replaced with low-risk agents.

Analgesic rebound headache issues are difficult and complex. Patients report how well the offending medicines work based on maintained job function but, at the same time, home life deteriorates. There is considerable disability, and family lifestyle adjustments are made because of the headaches. Often, it is useful to discuss these issues with the spouse and family members, since patients usually argue medication efficacy based on their continued ability to work. Additionally, we believe that these agents need to be called headache poisons (Table 24-9) simply because such terminology clearly indicates how good these agents are at initiating the rebound process wherein a certain toxicity or intoxication takes place in their bodies, allowing generation of more headaches. Patients need to know that continued use of these headache poisons will result in less effect on the severe headaches with time, require increased analgesic quantities, and at the same time, condemn them to more headaches. Asking patients if they want to have more headaches in the future often will help enlist their full support. Additionally, the term *headache poison* has a negative connotation that enforces the idea that patients should not continue to take these medications at the risk of personal medical harm.

> Headache poisons are medications that are at high risk of causing analgesic rebound headaches. Such a wonderfully negative connotation guarantees that patients will think about what medications they take. Use this term liberally!

The treatment of analgesic rebound headache requires withdrawal of the offending substance. Unfortunately, simply withdrawing the rebounding medication usually does not result in complete resolution of this process. Initially, there will be an increase in headache for the first 1 to 2 weeks in those who acutely withdraw rebounding medication. Thereafter, in the next 1 to 3 months, there will be a decrease in frequency, duration, and severity with the baseline nonrebound headache frequency finally returning. This time course is typical of the simple analgesics. However, with the combination agents, particularly those containing caffeine, aspirin, acetaminophen, and/or butalbital, it may take as long as 6 to 12 months to return to a nonrebounding baseline. Patients need to know that this will not be a rapid process, but that it will take a lot of time and hard work.

To break the analgesic rebound headache process, acute treatments, usually administered as short-term preventatives to bridge the gap between acute and preventative medications, can be effective. These treatments are combined with appropriate long-term preventatives. In general, the antiepileptic drugs seem best at breaking up the rebound process and then, secondly, the tricyclic antidepressants.

Short-term prevention involves the use of an acute agent on a daily basis for a limited period of time, usually 3 to 14 days. We have found sumatriptan, modifying Ducker and

Tepper's (30) protocol, at a dose of 25 mg t.i.d. for 3 to 5 days to be particularly useful for short-term prevention. The other triptans can be used similarly (e.g., rizatriptan 5 mg t.i.d., zolmitriptan 1.25 mg t.i.d., or naratriptan 1.25 mg b.i.d). Usually, adding an NSAID to short-term prophylaxis for a slightly longer period of time, typically 5 to 14 days, augments the triptans. Naproxen sodium 550 mg b.i.d. for 14 days, rofecoxib 50 mg q.d. for 5 days, and diclofenac 50 mg t.i.d. for 7 to 14 days are the agents we use most frequently. Additionally, some have found indomethacin and chlorpromazine suppositories useful for bridging therapy.

Dihydroergotamine administered subcutaneously or intramuscularly on an outpatient basis can be used to interrupt the analgesic rebound headache process. If this and other treatments fail, then hospitalization for repetitive intravenous dihydroergotamine is indicated.

MEDCATION INDUCED HEADACHES

Many medications can induce headache; unfortunately physicians rarely recognize the nature of this problem. When medications induce headache, improvement typically occurs shortly after exposure to the offending substance ceases. This is unlike analgesic rebound headache where headache persists independently, once initiated, for months to years after headache poisons are stopped. Many recognize that estrogen (e.g., oral contraceptives and menopausal hormone replacement therapy) can initiate or induce migraine, particularly in the genetic predisposed.

In 1989 Askmark et al. (31) reviewed data regarding medications associated with headaches reported to the World Health Organization and the FDA (Table 24-10). However, more than 10 years later these associations remain poorly recognized.

COMORBIDITY

The primary headache disorders, in particular migraine, are commonly associated with other medical conditions. These associated disorders occur at a rate considerably greater than that anticipated by chance occurrence and are said to be comorbid. Comorbidity implies genetic, neurochemical, and

TABLE 24-9. *Medications prone to produce analgesic rebound headaches*

Butalbital derivatives
Aspirin, acetaminophen, caffeine combinations
Acetaminophen

TABLE 24-10. *Medications that induce headaches*

Indomethacin	Isotretinoin
Nifedipine	Captopril
Cimetidine	Piroxicam
Atenolol	Metoprolol
Trimethoprim-sulfamethoxazole	Diclofenac
Zimelidine	Methyldopa
Glyceryl trinitrate	Terfenadine
Isosorbide dinitrate	Propranolol
Zomepirac	Benoxaprofen
Ranitidine	Metronidazole

(From Askmark H, Lindberg PO, Oisson S. Drug-related headache. *Headache* 1989;29:441–444, with permission.)

neuroanatomical shared pathophysiology. The three most common clusters of comorbid disorders are exemplified by psychological, gastrointestinal, and cardiac problems.

Psychological conditions that commonly occur in migraine include depression, anxiety disorders, panic attacks, and bipolar disorder. Depression, in fact, is more comorbid than any other disorder. The risk of a migraine sufferer being depressed is essentially the same as the risk of a depressed person having migraine. They are equally comorbid. Because of the frequency of the comorbid psychological states, many physicians incorrectly assume that these disorders, or stress, cause migraine, when, in fact, migraine is highly comorbid with these psychological conditions and will be worsened by these disorders, as well as by stress.

Other psychological conditions may occur in migraineurs; however, phobias stand out prominently. The phobia we see most often in migraineurs is represented by fear of migraine or migraine phobia. These individuals are frightened that stroke, "vascular explosion," death, or some other bizarre neurologic catastrophe will be produced by their headache. They are inordinately concerned that each headache will never end, even though they have had hundreds. They are scared, often anxious, or experience full-blown panic attacks. In some circumstances neuroimaging can be therapeutic as it can help allay some of the unfounded fears. Behavioral interventions are necessary in this population.

Gastrointestinal comorbid disorders include gastritis, gastroesophageal reflux disorder, irritable bowel syndrome, and H. pylori infection. These disorders, when associated with gastrointestinal hemorrhage, often secondary to NSAID overuse, can be fatal. Some of the agents that are used to treat these disorders, particularly cimetidine and ranitidine, are at high risk of inducing headache.

> A 60-year-old man with peptic ulcer disease had a remote history of migraine and was placed on ranitidine. Subsequently, he experienced frequent visual disturbances lasting 10 to 15 minutes that were thought to represent TIA. Scintillating fortification spectra with a pulsatile characteristic occurred and was unassociated with headache. He stopped the ranitidine, concerned that migraine headaches would return, and had immediate and complete resolution of the migraine aura without headache.

Cardiac comorbidity is typically represented by mitral valve prolapse and, less commonly, patent foramen ovale. These are commented on in the Migraine and Stroke section of this chapter.

Several chronic pain syndromes are comorbid with migraine. There is some suggestion that chronic low back pain sufferers have an increased risk of developing migraine (32). Some migraineurs have multiple tender points in a pattern consistent with fibromyalgia. Typically the tender points are most prominent in the pericranial musculature where knotting, tightness, and spasm are noted. Many times tenderness over the occipital nerves is so severe that true trigger points occur. Tinel's sign is evident and an interesting collection of painful reactions occurs where patients jump and scream during palpation. These responses make up the so-called jump and scream signs, which are reminiscent of the chandelier sign. Some patients actually meet criteria for the clinical diagnosis of fibromyalgia.

Individuals with epilepsy appear to have a significantly increased migraine risk, whereas migraineurs have a slightly greater risk of seizures compared to nonmigraineurs. In our experience, many of the migraineurs who develop seizures typically develop them in isolation, often associated with the use of anticholinergic medications (e.g., tricyclic antidepressants, antihistamines, antiemetics, or antipsychotic major tranquilizers). Eliminating the anticholinergic agent may result in seizure resolution.

Vertigo, particularly benign positional vertigo and motion sickness occur commonly. Children often experience car sickness. Some adults get carsick too, particularly when they are not driving. Sometimes, driving in the mountains may trigger this phenomenon even though not present at other times.

COEXISTING MEDICAL ILLNESSES

Migraine and other primary headache sufferers are not resistant to other medical conditions. Although, generally speaking, migraine sufferers experience fewer significant medical problems than nonmigraineurs, migraine may be a risk factor for cardiovascular and cerebrovascular disease (33,34). In our experience, coronary artery disease, diabetes mellitus, and peripheral arterial vascular disease occur less frequently in migraine clinic populations. However, African Americans with hemicrania continua have considerably more significant or potentially life-threatening coexisting medical illnesses.

It is important to recognize that the coexisting and comorbid disorders often allow insight into appropriate treatment selection and, when treated successfully, better migraine control occurs.

ACUTE AND SYMPTOMATIC TREATMENT

Primary headache disorders, particularly migraine, require treatment aimed at rapid amelioration of pain and, in many circumstances, the associated symptoms. The most common disabling symptoms associated with the acute headache attack are represented by gastrointestinal disorders. Vomiting is most common, quite disabling, and particularly likely to produce dehydration. Dehydration typically makes the headache less likely to respond to acute therapies and in many cases worsens it. Additionally, the medical complications of dehydration, including hypotension, worsen the overall condition. Some individuals experience diarrhea, but if not questioned specifically, will not volunteer its presence. Diarrhea, like vomiting, can lead or add to a dehydrated state. However, it is clear that effective, rapid treatment of migraine results in marked reduction in vomiting. Likewise, in our experience, diarrhea improves with acute headache treatment, albeit clinical trials have not assessed response of this particular associated symptom.

When vomiting or diarrhea does not respond well to acute treatment, dehydration and its medical complications occur and require intravenous hydration and treatment with additional agents. Metoclopramide orally or intravenously or prochlorperazine orally, rectally, intramuscularly, or intravenously are extremely useful, as are other antiemetic agents. However, metoclopramide and prochlorperazine when administered intravenously have considerable efficacy in the management of acute headache (35,36).

Adequate hydration must be maintained. This particularly applies to the care of pregnant women where ketosis may indicate a high risk for fetal injury. Without adequate hydration, escalation to migraine status may occur.

In terms of acute pain management, basically, there are two approaches to pain control. Historically, a step care approach for acute headache therapy has been taken. In step care, analgesics are selected in a stepwise fashion, typically starting with agents of low efficacy and advancing toward agents of high efficacy (e.g., the triptans). This approach has been criticized, since it is slow, poorly efficacious, and deludes patients into thinking that effective therapy is not available for their headache. It typically takes 3 years and cycling through five different headache preparations before adequate headache control is obtained. The step care approach requires that migraineurs hang in there long enough to be successful, but many cannot. Managed care formularies typically recommend that physicians provide step care headache management simply because the medications are less expensive. These near-sighted formulary decisions rarely take the overall cost of care into consideration, opting to pay for an emergency department visit to treat the headache out of control. Clearly, with these features in mind the evidence is overwhelming that step care is inappropriate in most circumstances.

The alternative to stepped care is stratified care. The concept of stratified care is that each headache sufferer is treated as an individual and treatment decisions are based on the severity of the headache, associated features, frequency, disability, and coexisting medical illnesses. In this model, headache education and nonpharmacotherapeutic options (e.g., biofeedback with stress management, relaxation, conflict resolution, and physical therapy modalities) are utilized early.

In mild headache sufferers, a simple analgesic may be sufficient as long as there are no significant analgesic rebound issues. The goal is to get treatment right the first time and to use an effective agent early for good headache control rather than dooming patients to years of inadequate therapy. If headaches are too frequent (generally, two or more headaches weekly), disabling, or if paroxysmal vomiting or complicated neurologic features are present, an appropriate preventative regimen is required.

Acute headache treatment should be aimed toward complete and rapid pain control. The triptans are the best acute headache therapies currently available. Sumatriptan was the first triptan introduced to the American market. Subsequently, zolmitriptan, naratriptan, and rizatriptan have become available. Eletriptan, frovatriptan, and almotriptan are on the horizon. No single triptan will be ideal for all patients, particularly since some patients appear to respond well to one and perhaps not at all to another triptan. Additionally, there is evidence that sumatriptan nonresponders may respond, at least sometimes to naratriptan—41% headache relief at 4 hours with naratriptan versus placebo (37)—which, in clinical trials, has a 4-hour efficacy that is inferior to sumatriptan. Moreover, zolmitriptan and rizatriptan have been shown in open label studies to be effective in sumatriptan nonresponders; headache response of 73% and 81%, respectively at 2 hours (38). This kind of evidence suggests that triptan response may have more to do with patient idiosyncrasies, rather than to pharmacokinetic or pharmacodynamic properties.

Physicians need to be familiar with the currently available triptans and recognize certain contraindications such as coronary artery disease, cerebrovascular disease, peripheral arterial disease, uncontrolled hypertension, and hemiplegic and basilar migraine. As well, package inserts suggest that two different triptans should not be used within a 24-hour period of one another, and triptans should not be used with ergot derivatives. Safety issues are tantamount. There is considerable concern that myocardial infarction or other untoward vascular events may occur in situations where triptans are mixed or used with ergot derivatives.

In some patient populations there remains a role for some of the nonspecific analgesics, particularly NSAIDS, and short-acting opioids. These needs are most evident in diabetes and coronary artery disease, where the vascular risk is great.

RESCUE THERAPY

Migraine status and intractable chronic daily headache syndromes, particularly when analgesic rebound headache is present, require intravenous therapies. Over the years, dihydroergotamine has been the agent of choice (39). We prefer to mix 1 mg of dihydroergotamine in 50 ml of normal saline and run it over 15 to 60 minutes every 8 hours for up to 9 doses or so, depending on the severity of the headache under treatment. If dihydroergotamine produces nausea or vomiting, then a subnauseating dose can be reached by decreasing the dose by 0.25 mg to 0.75 mg every 8 hours. Further dose adjustments can be made in a similar fashion. Typically, we premedicate with metoclopramide or prochlorperazine 10 mg intravenously given 15 to 30 minutes before dihydroergotamine. Recently, valproate sodium administered intravenously, 300 to 500 mg run in over 5 to 7 minutes, has shown some efficacy (40). Steroids may also be useful in some situations; however, we limit their use because of long-term safety issues.

PREVENTATIVE TREATMENT

The goals of preventative treatment in migraine and other primary headaches are to decrease headache frequency, duration, or severity and improve acute treatment efficacy. Preventative medications are indicated when either the patient or the migraine is out of control. For example, if two or more migraines are experienced weekly, headaches last more than 3 days, neurological symptoms and signs occur particularly if prolonged or complicated, poor acute medication tolerability or contraindications or failure, paroxysmal vomiting, frequent bed rest, or analgesic rebound issues are noted.

Currently there are only four FDA-approved migraine preventative agents available. These include methysergide, divalproex, propranolol, and timolol. On the other hand, there are three major migraine/headache preventative groups and most of the agents are used off label. These agents consist of antidepressants, anticonvulsants, antihypertensives, and a miscellaneous group. Headache preventatives provide a wide range of pharmacotherapeutic options and allow tailoring of drug selection to the patient. Recognizing therapeutic opportunities often depends on comorbid and coexisting disorders. In the setting where hypertension and coronary artery disease are present, beta or calcium channel blockers would be appropriate choices. In the situation where epilepsy or bipolar disorder is present, divalproex, topiramate, or gabapentin would be good choices. When depression is present, an antidepressant is appropriate. Many preventative agents cause weight gain, thus topiramate, an agent associated with weight loss, may be a useful adjunct. Additionally, recent studies suggest that lamotrigine may be efficacious for aura and migraine with aura (41, 42).

Because many preventative agents cause drowsiness or fatigue, when initiating therapy adopt the rule of starting at a low dose and slowly titrating upward to an appropriate dose. Adequate therapy for migraine prevention requires 2 to 8 weeks of continued use at an appropriate dose. Many times, finding the appropriate dose requires several dose adjustments. During this titration phase, the patient has to be reminded that preventative agents usually manifest their effects slowly. and they will need to continue to take the medication as prescribed. If tolerability issues arise, usually titrating downward to the previous dose, maintaining that dose for 3 to 7 days, and then titrating upward half as fast as before often allows dose increments with good tolerability

SUMMARY

We now have considerable understanding of migraine and the primary headaches. Yet, migraine remains a huge burden manifested by high societal cost and horrendous suffering. Despite present knowledge, there remains a major gap in how new advances are translated to headache sufferers. The present situation is such that migraine remains undiagnosed, too often mistaken for stress, sinus, or tension-type headaches. A step care approach to treatment is usually selected and, unfortunately, typically dooms migraineurs to years of inadequate treatment eventuating in a lapse from headache care. In many circumstances, the best medications (e.g., the triptans) have never ever been prescribed and preventatives are rarely utilized. It is a paradox that so many effective treatments are available, yet many migraine sufferers never benefit.

It is hoped that by pointing out these major discrepancies, attitudes toward headache sufferers will improve and primary headaches will be validated as real disorders with disabling consequences.

REFERENCES

1. Hu XH, Markson LE, Lipton RB, et al. Burden of migraine in the United States: disability and economic costs. *Arch Intern Med* 1999;159: 813–818.
2. Lipton RB. Update on Prevalence—The American Migraine Study: Ten years later. 13th Annual practicing physicians approach to the difficult headache patient. 2000.
3. Goadsby PJ, Lipton RB. A review of paroxysmal hemicranias, SUNCT syndrome and other short-lasting headaches with autonomic features, including new cases. *Brain* 1997;120:193–209.
4. Stewart WF, Lipton RB, Celentano DD, et al. Prevalence of migraine headaches in the United States. *JAMA* 1992;267:64–69.
5. Ophoff RA,Terwindt GM, Vergouwe GM, et al. Familial hemiplegic migraine and episodic ataxia type-2 are caused by mutations in the Ca2+ channel gene CACNLA4. *Cell* 1996;87:543–552.
6. May A, Ophoff RA,Terwindt GM, et al. Familial hemiplegic migraine locus on chromosome 19p13 is involved in common forms of migraine with and without aura. *Hum Genet* 1995;96:604–608.
7. Nyholt DR, Lea RA, Goadsby PJ, et al. Familial typical migraine: linkage to chromosome 19p13 and evidence for genetic heterogeneity. *Neurol* 1998;50:1428–1432.
8. Peroutka SJ, Wilhoit T, Jones K. Clinical susceptibility to migraine with aura is modified by dopamine D2 receptor (DRD2) Nco1 alleles. *Neurol* 1997;49:201–206.
9. Russell MB. Genetic epidemiology of migraine and cluster headache. *Cephalalgia* 1997;17:683–701.
10. Weiller C, May A, Limmroth V, et al. Brain stem activation in spontaneous human migraine attacks. *Nature Med* 1995;1:658–660.
11. Aurora SK, CaoY, Bowyer SM, et al. The occipital cortex is hyperexcitable in migraine experimental evidence. *Headache* 1999;39:469–476.
12. Burstein R, Cutrer MF, Yarnitsky D. The development of cutaneous allodynia during a migraine attack: clinical evidence for the sequential recruitment of spinal and supraspinal nociceptive neurons in migraine. *Brain* 2000;123:1703–1709.
13. Goadsby PJ, Edvinsson L, Ekman R. Vasoactive peptide release in the extracerebral circulation of humans during migraine headache. *Ann Neurol* 1990;28:183–187.
14. Goadsby PJ, Edvinsson L. Human in vivo evidence for trigeminovascular activation in cluster headache. Neuropeptide changes and effects of acute attacks therapies. *Brain* 1994; 117:427–434.
15. Headache Classification Committee of the International Headache Society. Classification and diagnostic criteria for headache disorders, cranial neuralgias and facial pain. *Cephalalgia* 1988;(suppl) 7:1–96.
16. Farmer K, Cady R, Bleiberg J, et al. A pilot study to measure cognitive efficiency during migraine. *Headache* 2000;40:657–661.
17. Lipton RB, Stewartt WF, Cady R, et al. Sumatriptan for the range of headaches in migraine sufferers: results of the spectrum study. *Headache* 2000;40: (*in press*).

18. Klapper J, Mathew N, Nett R. Basilar migraine and familial hemiplegic migraine treated with triptans. *Cephalalgia* 2000;20:340.
19. Tietjen GE. The relationship of migraine and stroke. *Neuroepidemiology* 2000;19:13–19.
20. Rothrock J, North J, Madden K, et al. Migraine and migrainous stroke: risk factors and prognosis. *Neurol* 1993; 43:2473–2476.
21. Anzola GP, Magoni M, Guindani M, et al. Potential source of cerebral embolism in migraine with aura: a transcranial doppler study. *Neurol* 1999;52:1622–1625.
22. May A, Bahra A, Buchel C, et al. Hypothalamic activation in cluster headache attacks. *Lancet* 1998;352:275–278.
23. Manzoni GC. Male preponderance of cluster headache is progressively decreasing over the years. *Headache* 1997;37:588–589.
24. Manzoni GC. Gender ratio of cluster headache over the years: a possible role of changes in lifestyle. *Cephalalgia* 1998;18:138–142.
25. Nahmias S, Silberstein SD, Rozen T, et al. Hemicrania continua is not that rare: 26 new cases. *Headache* 2000;54(Suppl 3):A21.
26. Wheeler SD. Clinical spectrum of hemicrania continua. *Neurol* 2000; 54 (Suppl 3): A42.
27. Sjaastad O, Spierings ELH. "Hemicrania continua": another headache absolutely responsive to indomethacin. *Cephalalgia* 1984;4:65–70.
28. Wheeler SD. Rofecoxib-responsive hemicrania continua. *Headache* 2000;40:436–437.
29. Katsarava Z, Fritsche G, Diener HC, et al. Drug-induced headache (DIH): following the use of different triptans. *Cephalalgia* 2000;20:293.
30. Ducker P, Tepper S. Daily sumatriptan for detoxification from rebound. *Headache* 1998;38:687–690.
31. Askmark H, Lundberg PO, OIsson S. Drug-related headache. *Headache* 1989;29:441–444.
32. Duckro PN, Schultz KT, Chibnall JT. Migraine as a sequela to chronic low back pain. *Headache* 1994;34:279–281.
33. Mitchell P, Wang JJ, Currie J, et al. Prevalence and vascular associations with migraine in older Australians. *Aust N Z J Med* 1998;28: 627–632.
34. Haapaniemi H, Hillbom M, Juvela S. Lifestyle-associated risk factors for acute brain infarction among persons of working age. *Stroke* 1997; 28:26–30.
35. Tek DS, McClellan DS, Olshaker JS, et al. A prospective, double-blind study of metoclopramide hydrochloride for the control of migraine in the emergency department. *Ann Emerg Med* 1990;9:1083–1087.
36. Jones J, Sklar D, Dougherty J, et al. Randomized double-blind trial of intravenous prochlorperazine for the treatment of acute headache. *JAMA* 1989;261:1174–1176.
37. Stark S, Spierings ELH, McNeal S, et al. Naratriptan efficacy in migraineurs who respond poorly to oral sumatriptan. *Headache* 2000;40:513–520.
38. Matew NT, Kailasam J, Gentry P, et al. Treatment of nonresponders to oral sumatriptan with zolmitriptan and rizatriptan: a comparative open trial. *Headache* 2000; 40: 464–465.
39. Raskin NH. Repetitive intravenous dihydroergotamine as therapy for intractable migraine. *Neurol* 1986;36:995–997.
40. Kailasam J, Mathew NT, Meadors L, et al. Intravenous valproate sodium (Depakon™) aborts migraine rapidly: a preliminary report. *Headache* 1999;39:361.
41. Lampl C, Buzath A, Klinger D, et al. Lamotrigine in the prophylactic treatment of migraine aura—a pilot study. *Cephalalgia* 1999;19:58–63.
42. D'Andrea G, Granella F, Cadaldini M, et al. Effectiveness of lamotrigine in the prophylaxis of migraine with aura: an open pilot study. *Cephalalgia* 1999;19:64–66.

The Treatment of Selected Pain Disorders

CHAPTER 25

Orofacial Pain: Differential Diagnosis and Treatment

Frank P. K. Hsu, Zvi H. Israel, Jeffrey A. Burgess and Kim J. Burchiel

It is our goal to provide a framework with which we deal with patients with orofacial pain problems. In this chapter we present a survey of the differential diagnosis of orofacial pain syndromes. No attempt has been made to produce an encyclopedic litany of exceptionally rare syndromes. Rather we discuss here the acute and chronic pain states that are encountered with any frequency in a busy practice specializing in the treatment of orofacial pain problems. Emphasis is on diagnosis, although where appropriate, brief mention of relevant medical and surgical therapy is made.

In most cases, the patient's history is the most important aspect of the diagnostic evaluation. Therefore, symptoms are of paramount importance. In fact, the critical determinants in sorting out facial pain syndromes are the temporal quality of the pain and the adjectives used to describe it. The diagnosis is usually apparent from the history and physical examinations. Recent utilization of high-resolution magnetic resonance imaging enables us to visualize any etiologic vascular compression on the posterior fossa cranial nerves. We hope to objectify and confirm the diagnosis of some facial pain syndromes based on diagnostic imaging studies.

NEURALGIAS OF THE TRIGEMINAL NERVE

Trigeminal Neuralgia I (TN1)

Classically known as tic douloureux, trigeminal neuralgia (type 1) is typically described as a fleeting, lancinating pain occurring in the sensory distribution of the trigeminal nerve. This story is strikingly reproducible and unmistakable. The pain characteristically lasts seconds to minutes and is almost always unilateral. Curiously, the disease course is not static and is notable for pain-free intervals that may last months to years. The pain is described as parox-

ysmal and electric in nature. Although attacks may be spontaneous, they are usually brought on by such triggering stimuli as talking, eating, oral hygiene, or even cool temperatures or wind on the face. Light tactile stimulation is often all that is needed to provoke such profound pain that sufferers will neglect grooming on the affected side because of it. The prevalence of TN1 is relatively rare; the incidence per annum is 3.4/100 000 for men and 5.9/100 000 for women (1). Age of onset is usually after the fourth decade, with peak onset during the fifth and sixth decades. Onset of pain before age 40 is uncommon and should at least suggest the possibility of multiple sclerosis.

Although not proven scientifically, the current belief that vascular compression near the root entry zone of the trigeminal nerve is the etiology for TN1 is increasingly accepted (2–9). Recently high-resolution magnetic resonance imaging (MRI) has been used to visualize the compression of the trigeminal nerve by vascular structures (10–16). Specific sequences employing the magnetic resonance angiography (MRA) and intravenous contrast administration enable us to visualize the trigeminal nerve and vascular structures near the nerve concurrently. This diagnostic methodology objectifies the diagnosis of TN1-based imaging evidence of vascular compressions.

Trigeminal Neuralgia 2 (TN2)

We propose that trigeminal neuralgia type 2 be used in place of atypical trigeminal neuralgia since it can be confused with "atypical facial pain," which is a different entity. TN2 differs from TN1 in that, in addition to the episodic lancinating pain, there exists a more persistent aching or burning pain (17–21). The constant painful component should be present for greater than 50% of the time. In this setting, careful consideration should be given to the presence of structural pathology in the nerve, or to an extrinsic compressive lesion such as a tumor or vascular malformation. This is particularly true if sensory loss is detected on the face. Patients with atypical features should undergo computed tomography or magnetic resonance imaging to rule out other pathology. In the absence of easily demonstrable pathology, we have theorized that TN2 may be a progression of TN1 if vascular compression of the trigeminal nerve is left untreated surgically (18). High resolution MRI/MRA should be performed to carefully examine the nerve for vascular compression as well.

Medical Treatment for Trigeminal Neuralgia

Approximately 70% of trigeminal neuralgia patients are well controlled nonoperatively. Perhaps the quintessential drug used is carbamazepine (Tegretol) (22–26) started at 100 mg PO b.i.d. then increased by 200 mg a day every 2 to 3 days to a final effective dose in the range of up to 800 to 1000 mg. Most patients respond to this regimen, and it is also a powerful and reliable modality in the diagnosis of trigeminal neuralgia. That is, if a patient with facial pain responds to carbamazepine, the diagnosis of trigeminal neuralgia is ensured. Unfortunately, use of the drug is limited by development of hypersensitivity reactions or side effects such as drowsiness, decreased mental acuity, subjective dizziness and ataxia (particularly in older patients), dose-related mild leukopenia, or a very rare non-dose-dependent idiosyncratic bone marrow suppression (aplastic anemia), which can occur early in treatment. For these reasons, a baseline white blood count (WBC) is obtained and repeat studies are done at 3 to 4 week intervals. In patients who cannot tolerate carbamazepine, other options include baclofen (Lioresal) or phenytoin (Dilantin). Baclofen can be a good choice in patients who get effective relief from carbamazepine but cannot tolerate its side effects, and it is usually started at 5 mg t.i.d. and increased by 5 to 10 mg every 2 to 3 days to a maximum dose of 80 mg per day (27–31). It is usually not effective in patients who do not derive benefit from carbamazepine. Phenytoin is rarely of use when carbamazepine or baclofen have failed, but may be helpful in combination with one of the other medications (32). Gabapentin (Neurontin) can be used alone or in conjunction with the above-mentioned drugs to treat patients with trigeminal neuralgia (33–37). Relatively few side effects such as sedation can be caused by gabapentin at high dose. Otherwise most patients tolerate this drug fairly well. Doses should start low, at 300 mg per day, and should be increased slowly to reach as high as 2700 mg per day in t.i.d. dosing.

Although most patients are well controlled initially by medical management, many of these will become nonresponders in time; drug therapy becomes ineffective and breakthrough pain begins. In fact, in the author's opinion, the majority of patients will eventually fail medical man-

agement if followed up carefully over a period of years. Fortunately, most of these patients subsequently derive excellent relief from surgical modalities.

Surgical Treatment for Trigeminal Neuralgia

Once it becomes apparent that a patient has failed or become refractory to maximal medical management, a surgical decision point is reached. Particularly in patients with trigeminal neuralgia, numerous surgical options are available, and patients must make an informed decision on surgery based on factors such as age, general medical condition, and patient preferences.

Minor Procedures

Percutaneous injection of alcohol into the peripheral trigeminal nerve or its ganglion (ethanol block) and peri/intraganglionic injection of alcohol (gangliolysis) are procedures that are rarely performed and will not be discussed further (38–40). Peripheral neurectomy is no longer a state-of-the-art procedure, but it can be employed to provide simple effective pain relief for very sick elderly patients who would not tolerate surgery and in whom pain will almost certainly return within a few years requiring relesioning (41–46). It also will not be discussed further.

There are three main minor procedures: percutaneous retrogasserian glycerol rhizolysis (PRGR), percutaneous radiofrequency trigeminal gangliolysis (PRTG), and percutaneous trigeminal ganglion compression (PTGC) (47–50). The choice of procedure depends on the experience and preference of the surgeon. All are effective with relative advantages and disadvantages to each. PTGC is technically simple, causes only mild sensory loss, and has an acceptable recurrence rate (50–58). However, it is impossible to restrict the lesion to a single division. PRGR causes mild to no sensory loss, but is technically more difficult to perform (59–66). The failure rate also seems to be higher in most operators' hands, as is the relapse rate over 5 years. PRTG affords immediate pain relief in a very high percentage of patients with a low recurrence rate but produces a considerable sensory loss. It is also effective for trigeminal neuralgia associated with multiple sclerosis or tumor. It is easier to perform for V3 than V2 because of the potential overlap with V1. In general, the more minor denervation associated with PTGC and PRGR is preferable for V1 pain to avoid the complication of corneal keratitis, whereas in V2/V3 pain PRTG is preferred.

One of the primary criticisms of the minor procedures is that they do not address the underlying pathology and remove the cause of the pain. On the other hand, they are effective procedures with relatively minimal morbidity and almost nonexistent mortality, an important consideration for a nonlethal condition such as trigeminal neuralgia.

These procedures offer the substantial benefits of outpatient surgery with minimal anesthetic risk and morbidity/

mortality, and they utilize local or brief general anesthetics rather than general endotracheal anesthesia. In addition to effective short-acting general anesthesia, methohexital (Brevital) and propofol (Diprivan) also provide an amnestic effect. It is important to note that these agents provide no analgesia, however, and their use requires supplementation with analgesic agents. The surgical indication for these procedures is medically intractable trigeminal neuralgia. These techniques are particularly well suited for elderly or ill patients who do not desire or would be poor candidates for major operative procedures. However, the lesions seldom last more than a few years, necessitating repeat procedures (54,62,65,67–69).

Major Procedures

The primary major procedures are microvascular decompression (MVD) (70–74) and partial sensory rhizotomy (PSR) (70). In practice these two procedures are used in tandem. If a patient shows no trigeminal root compression on microsurgical exploration, or if a patient has recurrent pain after MVD, a PSR is performed. PSR may be performed in a patient with multiple sclerosis and symptomatic trigeminal neuralgia, who has failed to gain lasting relief from percutaneous denervation.

Although microvascular decompression is the only surgical modality directly addressing the presumed etiology of trigeminal neuralgia and probably provides the longest lasting pain relief, it has several significant drawbacks; it is a major surgical procedure with a reported mortality of 1%, nonnegligible postoperative complications, and transient or permanent cranial nerve deficits (50,75). Several authors have questioned the use of a procedure with defined morbidity and mortality for benign disease, and propose the use of the percutaneous procedures for most surgical management of trigeminal neuralgia (76).

The ultimate choice between major and minor procedures in patients refractory to medical management should be made between the patient and physician. Older patients are often biased toward minor procedures because of considerations such as life expectancy, other health concerns, longer hospital stay, increased recovery time, and avoidance of a craniotomy. On the other hand, in a young healthy patient the longer duration of effective pain relief offered by microvascular decompression may offset these considerations.

Symptomatic Trigeminal Neuralgia (STN)

Patients with multiple sclerosis (MS) can also develop trigeminal neuralgia (71,77–79). The description of the pain is similar to that of TN1, though atypical features of a constant pain component and sensory loss are more common. Patients with multiple sclerosis and trigeminal neuralgia are usually younger and more likely to have bilateral facial pain than those with TN alone (77). The pathology of these cases

appears to be demyelination either in the nerve or in the brainstem within the descending tracts of the trigeminal system. In patients less than 40 years of age with trigeminal neuralgia, not previously known to have MS, this diagnosis should at least be entertained, particularly if there is evidence of trigeminal sensorimotor dysfunction.

Trigeminal Neuropathic Pain (TNP)

Between 5% and 10% of patients will develop some degree of facial pain following facial fracture, or after reconstructive orthognathic surgery, and a further 1% to 5% of patients after removal of impacted teeth (18,19,80,81). The quality of the pain is sharp, with episodic triggered paroxysms and dull throbbing or burning background pain. Signs of this condition include tender palpable nodules over peripheral nerves or neurotropic effects. The course of the disorder is characterized by progression over a period of 6 months or so, then stabilization of the pain until treatment. The pathology is often vague, but may include neuromata or trigeminal deafferentation (82,83). This type of pain may also be termed *trigeminal neuropathic pain,* to indicate that it is a pain probably related to peripheral nerve injury. Peripheral neuropathic pains are well known in noncranial neuropathies (e.g., diabetic or posttraumatic neuropathic pain), and these posttraumatic trigeminal neuralgias often are quite similar in description and resistance to treatment. An hypothesis has been put forward proposing that the major difference between more typical trigeminal neuralgias and the trigeminal neuropathic pains is the *location* and *severity* of the nerve injury. That is, minimal injury of the trigeminal nerve at the root entry zone results in trigeminal neuralgia, whereas more distal injuries result in neuropathic pains. Trigeminal neuralgia 2, an overlap syndrome, possibly results from more severe compression or injury of the trigeminal nerve, which extends distal to the root entry zone.

Medical Treatment for TNP

There is no satisfactory medical treatment for neuropathic pain in the trigeminal distribution. Anticonvulsants such as carbamazepine or gabapentin can alleviate the lancinating component of the pain, if any. Antidepressants can be tried, but are rarely effective.

Surgical Treatment for TNP

Minor Procedures

Trigeminal neuropathic pain is similar in origin and clinical presentation to other peripheral neuropathic pains. Damage to the distal trigeminal nerve is the common feature of these related neuralgias. Although controversial, some patients that respond favorably to local anesthetic blockade of the involved branch may improve after peripheral neurectomy (19). There has also been some evidence that trigeminal electrical stimulation (84) may also produce analgesia, although implantable systems designed for this indication are currently not available in the United States.

Major Procedures

Caudalis dorsal root entry zone (DREZ) may be used in the most difficult cases (85–87), as can deep brain stimulation (DBS) (88) and motor cortex stimulation (89).

Trigeminal Deafferentation Pain (TDP)

Patients with prior trigeminal deafferentation surgery may develop trigeminal deafferentation pain (90). Pain that is felt in an insensate region of the face is termed *anesthesia dolorosa*. The pains are variously described as burning, crawling, itching, or even tearing; they are thought to be "central" in origin and thus not dependent on peripheral stimuli. Tricyclic antidepressants can be tried for anesthesia dolorosa, but as with other deafferentation pains, the outlook for improvement is bleak.

Postherpetic Neuralgia

Pain associated with an acute outbreak of herpetic lesions in the distribution of a branch or branches of the trigeminal nerve does not usually present a diagnostic dilemma. The etiologic agent is herpes zoster, or varicella virus, and affects middle-aged to elderly individuals; males and females about equally. Pain is described as burning or tingling with occasional lancinating components felt in the skin. The pain usually precedes the onset of herpetic eruption by one or two days, or may develop coincident with the eruption. The pain is severe and usually lasts one to several weeks (91).

Associated symptoms include malaise, low fever, and headaches. Clusters of small vesicles, almost invariably located in the distribution of the ophthalmic division of the trigeminal nerve, appear. Herpetic eruptions are often seen in patients undergoing treatment for systemic lymphoma, carcinomatous metastasis, or any other condition that predisposes to or creates immunosuppression. Elevated protein and pleocytosis of the spinal fluid are also observed. Corneal ulceration due to vesicles has been reported. The pathology of the lesions is small cell infiltrates in the affected skin and bullous cutaneous changes. Similar infiltrates in the trigeminal ganglion and root entry zone are also seen.

In the usual case, spontaneous and permanent remission is the rule. However, in the older age group, progression to chronic (postherpetic) neuralgia is more the rule.

Acute herpetic neuralgia can be managed symptomatically with oral or parenteral narcotic pain medication. Due to the limited duration of the syndrome, tricyclic and anticonvulsant medications are probably not appropriate. Some evidence indicates that repeated sympathetic blockade (i.e.,

stellate block) may reduce the acute pain as well as the incidence of postherpetic neuralgia. Other agents, which have been reported to be effective in the prevention of postherpetic neuralgia, when given in the acute phase include corticosteroids, amantadine, levodopa and benserazide, vidarabine, and interferon-alpha (91).

Chronic neuralgia that occurs in the distribution of one or more divisions of the fifth cranial nerve subsequent to an acute herpes zoster outbreak is described as postherpetic neuralgia. Pain of this type is usually associated with chronic skin trophic changes or scarring and most commonly occurs in the first (ophthalmic) division. It is a relatively infrequent disorder, predominantly seen in patients in their fifties or older, and is more common in males. The quality of the pain is described as burning, tearing, crawling, or itching dysesthesia in the affected area, and is exacerbated by mechanical contact with the skin. The pain is moderate, but present constantly and may last for years, although spontaneous remission can occur. Due to the chronic and unremitting nature of the pain, depression and irritability are common associated symptoms.

On examination, the skin of the painful region may show scarring, loss of normal pigmentation, hypesthesia or hyperesthesia, or hypalgesia or hyperpathia (allodynia). In the early phase of the disorder, pathologically there are chronic inflammatory changes in the trigeminal ganglion and demyelination in the root entry zone. Later on, Wallerian degeneration of the peripheral nerve fiber with fibrosis, and a relative depletion of the large more than small myelinated and unmyelinated axons, is seen (91).

Treatment of established postherpetic neuralgia is difficult. Fortunately, there is a tendency for the pain to diminish with time. Medications that are effective for trigeminal neuralgia are of little benefit in this disorder, although carbamazepine or clonazepam may be useful in the treatment of any component of postherpetic neuralgia that is described as being paroxysmal and lancinating. For the more typical constant burning dysesthetic pain, tricyclic antidepressant medications are probably the most effective choices for pharmacologic treatment. Amitriptyline 75 mg given at bedtime with fluphenazine 1 mg three times a day is a commonly utilized regimen (91,92).

In the light of the natural history of postherpetic neuralgia, surgical therapy should be reserved for those patients with severe, unremitting pain that is refractory to medical management. Currently, stereotaxic trigeminal tractotomy and open radiofrequency tractotomy/nucleotomy are probably the only surgical procedures that have been shown, albeit in only a few cases, to be effective for the management of postherpetic trigeminal neuralgia (87,92).

Destruction of the descending spinal tract of the trigeminal nerve in the dorsal medulla, or trigeminal tractotomy, produces analgesia and thermoanalgesia in the distribution of the ipsilateral nerve with preservation of tactile sensation. This can be performed as either an open

(93) or percutaneous stereotaxic (94) procedure and can be done bilaterally. The open medullary tractotomy is generally ineffective in cases of deafferentation pain, although the literature presents mixed success in treating postherpetic neuralgia. Stereotactic trigeminal nucleotomy of the second-order neurons at the oral pole of nucleus caudalis has been found to be quite effective in such patients with deafferentation pain (95). Unlike essential trigeminal neuralgia, the dysesthetic pain in deafferentation is directly proportional to the extent of sensory deficit.

The theoretical basis for performing caudalis DREZ lesions is the belief that central pain is localized to the secondary neurons (95). These are thought to be "hyperirritable" and become destabilized after deafferentation, firing erratically and resulting in severe pain. Although technically not the trigeminal DREZ, the nucleus caudalis of the trigeminal nerve is the first relay station for central transmission of facial pain. The nucleus caudalis of the trigeminal system is effectively the anatomic equivalent of the spinal dorsal horn. The caudalis DREZ lesion is aimed at destroying the second-order neurons theoretically responsible for maintaining the ongoing pain sensation, and in this respect the operation differs from trigeminal tractotomy. In general, DREZ lesions are thought to be most efficacious for deafferentation pain and should probably be limited to patients failing the first-line procedures.

Deep brain stimulation (DBS) directed at Ventro Posterior Medial (VPM) (VCi) may benefit some patients with this disorder. It is probably somewhat less morbid than caudalis DREZ, but the efficacy is difficult to gauge from the literature.

Secondary Trigeminal Neuralgia

This entity constitutes a clinical syndrome of trigeminal neuralgia, which is thought to be due to a definable structural pathologic lesion, such as tumor, aneurysm, or other vascular abnormality. These lesions are thought to produce a trigeminal neuropathy or neuritis by destruction, irritation, or demyelination of the nerve, and this in turn is responsible for the production of pain. It is much less common than primary trigeminal neuralgia, representing only about 2% of trigeminal neuralgia. The age of onset corresponds to the appearance of the tumor or vascular abnormality and may be somewhat younger than the TN1 and TN2 cases. Cases are equally distributed between males and females. The description of the pain is identical to that seen in TN1, with the exception that nonparoxysmal pain of a dull or more constant type may occur, which is similar to features in TN2. The timing and progression of the pains mimic primary trigeminal neuralgia, and the severity is equal.

Structural lesions that may produce this syndrome include tumors in Meckel's cave or in the cerebellopontine angle, which account for about 50% of cases. A partial list of associated conditions is given in Table 25-1. The

TABLE 25-1. *Conditions associated with secondary trigeminal neuralgia*

Tumors
  Meningioma
  Epidermoid tumor
  Acoustic neurinoma
  Nasopharyngeal carcinoma
  Metastatic tumors
  Brainstem glioma
Vascular lesions
  Basilar artery or cavernous sinus aneurysm
  Arteriovenous malformation
  Tortuous basilar artery
Sarcoidosis
Connective tissue disease
  Scleroderma
Syringobulbia
Pseudotumor cerebri
Paget's disease or acromegaly
Amyloidosis
Toxins
Syphilis
Dejerine-Sottas disease
Arnold-Chiari malformation

likelihood of detecting one of these abnormalities is increased by documentation of hypesthesia in the trigeminal distribution or depression of the corneal reflex (96). In these instances, a CT or MRI scan is mandatory.

Atypical Facial Pain (AFP)

Unfortunately, the diagnosis of trigeminal neuropathic pain overlaps to some extent with the term *atypical facial pain*, a catch-all diagnosis that is not useful from a taxonomic, diagnostic, or therapeutic standpoint (see below, Pain of Psychological Origin in the Head and Face). The differential diagnosis of this type of pain is difficult since it lacks many of the characteristic attributes that signify primary or secondary (nontraumatic) trigeminal neuralgia. The differential diagnostic possibilities include idiopathic trigeminal neuralgia, secondary trigeminal neuralgia from intracranial lesions, postherpetic neuralgia, odontalgia, and musculoskeletal pain.

In general, the more these pains resemble typical trigeminal neuralgia, the more likely patients will respond to the anticonvulsant medications such as carbamazepine or diphenylhydantoin. If the pain has a constant or burning character, a tricyclic antidepressant such as amitriptyline, in doses of 100 to 150 mg at bedtime, in combination with fluphenazine 1 to 2.5 mg PO b.i.d., represents a reasonable option. More recently, clonazepam 2 to 3 mg/day in divided doses can also provide some relief.

If a discrete area of nerve injury (neuroma) can be demonstrated, and the pain responds completely to local anesthetic block, surgical excision can be recommended. However, these problems are very complex. Detailed evaluation including psychologic screening is essential, since the standard caveat in these cases is that further trigeminal deafferentation by neurectomy, gangliolysis, or rhizotomy is frequently unsuccessful in the management of this condition, and often worsens the pain state.

NEURALGIAS OF CRANIAL NERVES (OTHER THAN TRIGEMINAL)

Geniculate Neuralgia (VIIth Cranial Nerve)

The nervus intermedius is a component of the seventh (facial) cranial nerve, which contains primary sensory afferent fibers whose somata are located in the geniculate ganglion. These fibers innervate part of the external canal and tympanic membrane, the skin of the angle between ear and mastoid process, the tonsillar region, and some other deep structures of the head and neck. Severe lancinating pain felt within the territory of the nervus intermedius (i.e., deeply within the external auditory canal, auditory meatus, concha, or retroauricular region) constitutes geniculate neuralgia.

The clinical syndrome of geniculate neuralgia, or intermedius neuralgia, occurs in young or middle-aged adults, predominantly in women. The pain can be described as sharp, shocklike, lancinating, and located in the external auditory meatus with retroauricular radiation. Local tenderness in the pinna or external auditory canal may be present, and manifestations such as excessive salivation or nasal secretion, tinnitus, vertigo, or a bitter taste may accompany the pains.

This is an extremely rare entity, with only a few cases reported in the world's literature. Nevertheless, the syndrome is instructive since it demonstrates a pain syndrome due to involvement of the sensory component of the seventh cranial nerve, the nervus intermedius. Pain of this type must be differentiated from otic varieties of trigeminal and glossopharyngeal neuralgias (97,98).

Geniculate neuralgia is not usually responsive to medical management, and a surgical procedure is therefore required. The most efficacious technique has been surgical division of the nervus intermedius, glossopharyngeal, and upper two strands of the vagus nerve in the posterior fossa. Ideally, this procedure should be performed under local anesthesia such that electrical stimulation of the cranial nerves VII, VIII, IX, and X can be achieved. If, under these circumstances, pain can be reproduced by stimulation only of VII, IX, and the upper fibers of X, then rhizotomy of these nerves should be carried out. Otherwise, a medullary tractotomy is the procedure of choice (97).

Glossopharyngeal Neuralgia (IXth Cranial Nerve)

Glossopharyngeal, or more appropriately vagoglossopharyngeal, neuralgia is a rare syndrome that denotes episodic bursts of pain in the sensory distribution of the ninth and tenth cranial nerves (99). The vagal and glossopharyngeal nerves are concerned with touch, pain, and temperature sensation in the posterior third of the tongue, tonsillar pillars, and fossa, naso-, oro-, and laryngeal pharynx, including pyriform recess, larynx, eustachian tube, middle ear, external auditory canal, part of the pinna, and a small cutaneous area anterior and posterior to the pinna. Pains in these regions can be mild to severe, may be described as being sharp, stabbing, shocklike, hot, or burning. Other uncomfortable sensations, not frankly painful, may occur in isolation or simply precede painful paroxysms. A dull aching or burning sensation may persist after an attack.

Swallowing, particularly of cold or acid fluids, often triggers the pain, and less commonly chewing, eating, talking, or other movements that involve the oropharyngeal musculature may also precipitate attacks. A discrete trigger point is commonly localizable on the fauces or tonsil, although this may be absent. Individual pains may last from seconds to minutes, and may occur from a few per year to dozens per day. Episodes may last for weeks to months and subside spontaneously, although commonly there is recurrence of the pain.

Bradycardia, tachycardia, syncope, hypotension, or seizures may accompany the painful paroxysms. The cardiovascular effects are thought to be mediated by the carotid sinus nerve or its central connections via the glossopharyngeal or vagus nerves.

The pathophysiology of glossopharyngeal neuralgia is unknown. However, vascular cross-compression by ectatic vessels in the region of the entry zones of the ninth and tenth cranial nerves, akin to what has been observed in the fifth nerve in trigeminal neuralgia, has been suggested as a possible etiology. A possible variant of this syndrome is neuralgia of the superior laryngeal nerve (vagus nerve neuralgia). In these cases paroxysms of unilateral lancinating pain radiate from the side of the thyroid cartilage or pyriform sinus to the angle of the jaw and occasionally to the ear. All other aspects of this syndrome are similar to glossopharyngeal neuralgia. The differential diagnosis for pains in this area includes carotidynia, Eagle's syndrome, or local lesions such as carcinoma.

Like trigeminal neuralgia, glossopharyngeal neuralgia typically does respond to anticonvulsant agents such as carbamazepine (100). If medical management fails to satisfactorily control the pain, the most promising approach has recently been to surgically explore the region of cranial nerves IX and X in the posterior fossa. Frequently, vascular loops impinging on the nerve can be identified and repositioned. This results in pain remission in the majority of cases (99). If no vascular cross-compression is identified, the ninth and upper one-half of the tenth nerve are divided. Again, this rhizotomy is effective in relieving pain in most cases. If the syndrome is attributed to the superior laryngeal nerve, then temporary relief may be obtained from analgesic nerve block, alcohol nerve block, or nerve section.

Occipital Neuralgia

In contradistinction to other cranial neuralgias, occipital neuralgia is quite common. Paresthesias may occur in the occipital nerve distributions. Pain is usually deep, aching, or stabbing in the distribution of the second (greater occipital nerve) or third (lesser occipital nerve) cervical dorsal root [i.e., unilaterally from the suboccipital area to the vertex (C2), or to the retromastoid and supraauricular areas (C3)]. Temporal pattern of the pain is irregular, but usually worse later in the day, and may range from moderate to severe in intensity. A history of chronic recurring episodes is typical, although spontaneous cessation of the pain may also occur. Pains of this kind often occur after acceleration-deceleration injuries and are more common in the third to fifth decades of life. Hyperesthesia of the scalp is a common complaint, and hypesthesia to pin prick in the C2-3 region of the scalp or tenderness or Tinel's sign of the greater occipital nerve may be found, and local anesthetic/corticosteroid block of the occipital nerve may produce effective temporary relief.

The pathophysiology of occipital neuralgia is unknown, although it may be secondary to trauma, including flexion-extension (whiplash) injuries. The mechanism may be related to increased muscle activity in the cervical region or entrapment of the C-2 root or dorsal root ganglion by paravertebral ligamentous structures (101,102). The differential diagnosis of occipital neuralgia includes cluster headaches, posterior fossa, high cervical, or foramen magnum tumors, herniated cervical intervertebral disc, uncomplicated flexion-extension injury, and metastatic neoplasm at the base of the skull.

Since occipital neuralgia is merely a symptom of radicular or peripheral nerve pathology, treatment varies with the actual, or supposed, etiology. Treatment ranges from therapy directed at specific lesions of the C1-2 region such as Arnold-Chiari malformation, gout, or neoplasm to generalized disorders such as diabetes. Often a specific etiology can only be postulated, and in these cases a wide variety of treatments have been advocated such as rhizotomy, collar placement, massage, infrared heat, procaine and alcohol infiltrations, avulsion of the greater occipital nerve, traction, steroid injections, and excision or alcohol injection of all of the nerves in the back of the head (101). Another mechanism has been proposed, that being entrapment of the second or third cervical root and dorsal root ganglion either by ligamentous or fascial structures in their respective neural foramina or by osteoarthritis and spondylosis in these areas (101,102). Surgical exploration of the C-2 or C-3 foramen may demonstrate neural compression, which when relieved may result in pain remission without the necessity for a neurodestructive procedure.

Other Facial Neuralgias

These syndromes are unusual and are mentioned here only to complete the differential diagnostic possibilities in patients with paroxysmal facial pain secondary to presumed neuralgia.

Sphenopalatine neuralgia

Sphenopalatine neuralgia (Sluder's syndrome or lower-half headache) consists of paroxysmal pains that begin on the medial side of the nose or medial canthus of the eye and radiate to the roof of the mouth, retroorbitally, or rarely to the ipsilateral neck, shoulder, and upper extremity (103). Attacks occur many times a day and are often precipitated by sneezing or preceded by a sensation of nasal congestion. Unilateral lacrimation and conjunctival injection may accompany the attacks. Cocaine injection into sphenopalatine ganglion affords temporary relief. Vidian neuralgia, or Vail's syndrome, is a variant of sphenopalatine neuralgia. It is paroxysmal unilateral facial pain attributed to "irritation" of the vidian nerve, an afferent branch of the sphenopalatine ganglion. Pain may radiate backward into the ear, nape of the neck, and shoulder, and is occasionally associated with tinnitus and vertigo (103).

Raeder's Paratrigeminal Neuralgia

Raeder's syndrome, or "paratrigeminal" neuralgia, is characterized by frontotemporal pain and oculosympathetic paresis (incomplete Horner's syndrome). The syndrome may be due to the proximity of the ophthalmic division of the fifth nerve to the ocular sympathetic fibers, which travel with the carotid artery in the region of the cavernous sinus (104,105). Two types of pain result: a migrainous variant with episodic and recurrent pains lasting hours or days, and a symptomatic, more persistent type, often secondary to an aneurysm or tumor in the region of the middle fossa or cavernous sinus.

Craniofacial Pain of Musculoskeletal Origin

Craniofacial pain of musculoskeletal origin may arise from the muscles of mastication or the temporomandibular joint (TMJ), depending on the sites of pathology, or be referred from the neck musculature (106). In this section we discuss chronic orofacial pain thought to originate specifically from the muscles of mastication or the TMJ. Information regarding head pain originating from the scalp muscles can be found in Chapters 20 thorugh 22 and the neck musculature in Chapters 27 through 31 of Handbook of Pain Management, 2nd edition.

Chronic orofacial pain of musculoskeletal origin can be divided into four major subcategories: temporomandibular pain and dysfunction syndrome (107) (also called myofascial pain and dysfunction syndrome) (108); specific myofascial disorders; osteoarthritis of the temporomandibular joint; and bone infections and tumors. Diagnosis in some cases may be confounded by the overlapping of conditions, pain referral from nonmasticatory muscles, lack of clear pathology, and psychosocial and behavioral factors contributing to symptom expression.

Temporomandibular Pain and Dysfunction Syndromes

Temporomandibular pain and dysfunction syndrome has been equated by the IASP (109) with myofascial pain and dysfunction syndrome (MPDS). In contrast, some workers consider these conditions to be distinctly different entities, with temporomandibular pain and dysfunction syndrome (TMPDS), by definition, associated with altered TMJ physiology, and myofascial pain and dysfunction syndrome primarily identified with sustained muscle activity (110). Practically, however, both conditions are characterized by the same triad of signs and symptoms: pain and tenderness of the masticatory muscles, joint sounds with jaw opening, and limited mandibular movement (111). While the International Association for the Study of Pain (IASP) has chosen to utilize the terms *TMPDS* and *MPDS*, the reader should be aware that the American Dental Association has recommended use of the term *temporomandibular disorder* (TMD) to define all conditions involving the temporomandibular joint and muscles of mastication. A number of recently proposed classification schemes present standardized terminology and diagnostic criteria for TMD (112,113).

Diagnosis is based on the patient's history and clinical findings. In general, extensive radiographic evaluation is not necessary. However, radiographic analysis with panography or tomography may be required to rule out degenerative joint disease or other forms of joint pathology (114), and in some complex cases, special procedures such as arthrography and CT scanning may be needed to define the nature of joint dysfunction or to rule out other forms of muscular disease such as myofibrositis. Unless the history or clinical findings are suggestive of systemic muscle pathology, rheumatoid arthritis, or lupus erythematosus, laboratory blood studies are not generally useful. Additional laboratory tests, such as surface or needle electromyography or thermography, have been recommended to assess TMPDS, but the significance of the data gathered from such testing is not presently understood. Since psychosocial stressors may be easily assessed by detailed psychosocial interview, the use of more extensive psychometric testing is not generally necessary, unless to confirm or underscore a clinical impression.

Pain may be perceived on one or both sides of the face around the ear, in the cheek, jaw, or temple. Generally characterized as a dull, continuous, poorly localized ache of moderate intensity with a boring or gnawing quality, it may vary in degree of discomfort through the course of the day. Yawning, chewing, or moving the mandible will often result in stabs of severe pain and precipitate cramping or jaw locking. Long-term pain may also include cyclical periods of remission.

In addition to pain, patients frequently report symptoms such as jaw muscle fatigue with chewing, episodic jaw locking in either an open or closed position, and deviation with opening. Many patients note the presence of soft or hard clicking or popping joint sounds. If questioned, they may also relate grinding their teeth at night (bruxism), keeping their teeth together during the day (clenching), or other parafunctional habits (gum chewing or fingernail biting). There may be a history of trauma to the face or jaws (115),

and onset may often be associated with recent psychosocial stress. Other signs and symptoms that have been irregularly associated with TMPDS include ear pain (116), headache (117), tinnitus and dizziness (118), malocclusion (119), and psychogenic pain.

TMPDS patients with chronic pain will display many of the psychological characteristics that have been observed for other chronic pain states, including anxiety, stress, depression, anger, and frustration. They may also demonstrate assorted illness behaviors, including increased treatment seeking and medication usage.

Examination will often reveal a limited mouth opening; while normal jaw opening is highly variable between individuals, an opening of less than 40 mm (or three finger widths) is generally considered restricted (120). Reduced jaw opening may be the result of muscle dysfunction, such as spasm or splinting (121); the result of meniscal displacement, such as failure of the condylar head to capture the meniscus (reduce) during opening; or a combination of both conditions. Audible soft clicking or popping sounds resulting from meniscal reduction may occur at any point during jaw opening or closing and are not generally considered to be of significance. However, hard clicking consistently occurring late in opening (greater than 25 mm) coupled with periodic closed locking may indicate pathologic change in the meniscus or joint. In these rare cases arthrography may be useful in defining the nature of meniscus function and potential pathology. Palpation of the jaw opening muscles, particularly the masseter, temporalis, and internal (lateral) pterygoid, will frequently elicit tenderness, but the pathophysiologic significance of such pain is presently unclear. Intraoral examination will sometimes demonstrate marked tooth attrition, cheek biting, or tongue indentations, findings associated with bruxism or clenching. In cases of dislocation of the meniscus, there may be marked alteration in occlusion.

The prevalence of TMPDS has been estimated to be between 10% to 15% of the population (122). It is a disease of the young (e.g., ages 15–45) with a three to five times greater incidence in females. Although TMPDS is generally acknowledged to be a psychophysiologic disease, its etiology remains unsettled. Fortunately, for approximately 80% of patients, the condition is self-limiting. Conditions that must be considered in the differential diagnosis of TMPDS are presented in Table 25-2.

The American Dental Association has recommended that, until differences concerning the etiology, pathophysiology, and diagnosis of TMPDS are resolved, treatment strategies should be conservative and noninvasive (123). Interventions that address the muscular component of the problem include psychophysiologic (habit control, hypnotherapy, relaxation therapy, and biofeedback), psychologic (counseling/stress management, communication/cognitive therapy, and behavioral modification), and pharmacologic (antidepressants, antianxiety agents, or muscle relaxants) modalities as well as massage, physical exercises,

TABLE 25-2. *Conditions associated with TMPDS*

Tumors
    Synovial chondromatosis
    Coronoid hyperplasia
    Sarcoma
Arthritis
    Infectious arthritis
    Traumatic arthritis
    Rheumatoid arthritis
    Osteoarthritis (degenerative joint disease)
    Psoriatic arthritis
    Juvenile rheumatoid arthritis
Connective tissue disease
    Systemic lupus erythematosus
    Dermatomyositis
Condylar agenesis
Myofascial disorders (myositis, fibrositis)
Myositis ossificans
Odontogenic or nonodontogenic infection
Otitis media
Parotitis
Reflex sympathetic dystrophy of the face
Elongated styloid process (Eagle's syndrome)
Pain of psychological origin in the face (psychogenic pain
    disorder)

physiotherapy, splints, transcutaneous electric nerve stimulation (TENS), or myofunctional therapy. Relatively noninvasive strategies such as acupuncture and trigger point injections may also be useful. Aggressive intervention with orthodontics or dental reconstruction is very rarely necessary. In cases of severe TMJ dysfunction involving meniscus pathology, surgical therapy (e.g., disc repositioning and plication of the distal ligament, disc removal, or artificial meniscus implantation) may be indicated. The efficacy of the latter strategy, however, is increasingly being questioned because of premature breakdown and rejection. For greater detail about treatment methodologies, the reader is referred to in Chapter 24 of Handbook of Pain Management, 2nd edition.

Specific or Diffuse Myofascial Pain Syndromes The cardinal feature of what the IASP has described as myofascial pain syndromes, upon which diagnosis is based, is the presence of latent or active myofascial trigger points (109). These are discrete nodular areas of hyperirritable muscle or fascial tissue that, when compressed, predictably produce what has been termed a "jump sign" and a reproducible pain referral pattern (124). Satellite tender points may be found within the area of pain reference of the initial trigger point. The presence of multiple trigger points distinguishes this pain disorder from pain of other muscle conditions (e.g., TMPDS).

Pain, described as deep, aching, or pressure-like, may be induced by passive stretch, functional movements, strong voluntary contraction of the shortened muscle, or cold, damp weather, trauma, hyperactivity or inactivity, fatigue, and emotional distress. Activation of an initial trigger point

may excite satellite points within the zone of reference and trigger points within synergistic muscles (125). If myospasm becomes a feature of trigger point activation, associated orofacial symptoms may include limited opening or joint clicking. Evidence associating trigger points with specific or nonspecific pathologic features is limited (126), and there is virtually no experimental evidence supporting the presence of such discrete areas of pathophysiologic change within the muscles of mastication. Nonetheless, distinctive regions of tenderness described as trigger points have been reliably measured with a pressure algometer in the masseter and temporalis muscles (127). Laboratory procedures such as electromyography and thermography have not been thoroughly investigated in relation to masticatory trigger points and at present offer limited diagnostic utility. Blood studies are negative and not necessary, unless there is suspicion that the condition is secondary to systemic disease. Radiography with soft tissue imaging has not demonstrated abnormalities and is not recommended.

While myofascial pain associated with the masticatory musculature appears to be quite common, its epidemiologic characteristics are unknown. In a recent study of 296 patients with complaints of head and neck pain, 55.4% were found to have a primary diagnosis of myofascial pain syndrome based on the presence of multiple trigger points (128).

Myofascial pain syndromes may occur within an individual muscle (e.g., "specific" type) or involve several muscles (e.g., "diffuse" type). Synonyms for this condition include fibrositis (syndrome), myalgia, tenomyositis, muscular rheumatism, and nonarticular rheumatism. Conditions from which myofascial pain syndromes should be differentiated are listed in Table 25-3.

Specific myofascial pain syndromes involving the masticatory muscles respond well to stretch and spray techniques, trigger point compression, massage, injection, or acupuncture. Low dose amitriptyline, 50 to 75 mg, may be helpful. The elimination of perpetuating postural or behavioral factors should be part of the management strategy. Additional information concerning management of myofascial pain syndromes is found in Chapters 24 and 43 of Handbook of Pain Management, 2nd edition.

TABLE 25-3. *Conditions associated with myofascial pain syndromes*

Temporomandibular pain and dysfunction syndrome
Myofascial pain and dysfunction syndrome
Connective tissue disease
    Systemic lupus erythematosis
    Dermatomyositis
Myositis ossificans
Odontogenic or nonodontogenic infection
The arthritides
Reflex sympathetic dystrophy of the face
Elongated styloid process
Pain of psychological origin in the face

Osteoarthritis and the Temporomandibular Joint   Pain is a frequent, but not consistent, finding in patients presenting with osteoarthritis of the TMJ. When present, it is often described as a deep ache within the ear or preauricular area of the face (with minimal radiation to surrounding regions) that increases in intensity from morning to evening and is exacerbated with use or cold weather. It may persist for months or years with cyclical periods of remission. Crepitus is the symptom most consistently related to osteoarthritis of the TMJ (129), but limitation of mandibular movement, presumably associated with muscle splinting, has also been reported (130). The sound of crepitus is distinctly different from clicking and has been described as a gristle, crackle, or soft-hard grating. It is assumed that damage to the soft tissue articulating components contributes to the noise, but the degree to which joint morphology, as opposed to degenerative change, contributes to the quality of sound is presently unknown. There is often a history of trauma. Patients with chronic osteoarthritis will appear to be less psychologically disturbed than those with myofascial conditions.

Diagnosis is based on history, the presence of crepitus revealed through stethoscopic evaluation, TMJ palpation pain (lateral and intrameatal), and radiographic interpretation. Changes in occlusion may also be noted if joint degeneration has been rapid. Laboratory tests (e.g., blood or synovial fluid analysis) are not generally necessary, unless there is suspicion of infectious arthritis (bacterial, fungal, tubercular), connective tissue diseases (rheumatoid arthritis, systemic lupus erythematosus, dermatomyositis), or the rheumatoid variants (psoriatic arthritis, Reiter's syndrome, juvenile rheumatoid arthritis). Gross radiographic bone changes can be observed in panoramic and transcranial radiographs, but tomograms are currently considered the most accurate means of assessing the full extent of pathology. Osseous changes include flattening of the condyle or eminence, osteophytes, marginal lipping of the anterior portion of the condyle, subarticular cystic changes or erosions in the lateral or superior portion of the condyle, sclerosis of marginal bone, and medullary distortions (131). Severe erosion of the TMJ is more indicative of connective tissue disease rather than osteoarthritis. Joint space narrowing has also been suggested as a sign of pathology, but this view remains controversial and unsupported. Other radiographic diagnostic techniques [e.g., magnetic resonance imaging (MRI) and single photon emission computed tomography (SPECT)] show promise for improving diagnostic capability.

Osteoarthritis of the TMJ is most likely to be observed in women after the age of 40 (132). It has, however, been reported in young females (130). Epidemiologic studies suggest that between 4% and 14% of the population may have TMJ degenerative disease based on the presence of crepitus (133). Far fewer have pain or seek treatment. The histopathology of TMJ osteoarthritis is well documented, consisting of primary articular erosion and secondary joint space dystrophic calcification in the absence of inflammation (134). Histopathologic studies suggest that degenerative change may be correlated with articular disc perforations or deformations (135).

The etiology of TMJ osteoarthritis is unknown. The literature identifies a plethora of causes that include age, various forms of trauma (136), and functional or dysfunctional loading. The effects of genetic predisposition, systemic disease, metabolic-endocrine processes, and inflammation have not been thoroughly investigated. Recent evidence suggests that osteoarthritis may be related to condylar dysfunction, particularly chronic anterior meniscus displacement (135). However, the hypothesis that osteoarthritis may result from intermittent joint clicking remains speculative. Conditions that should be considered in the differential diagnosis are listed in Table 25-4.

In general, osteoarthritis of the temporomandibular joint follows a pattern similar to skeletal joints with symptoms lasting 1 to 3 years and including bone remodeling. The condition may be conservatively managed with therapeutic strategies outlined under the Temporomandibular Pain and Dysfunction Syndrome section. In addition, anti-inflammatory medications and anesthetic injection into the joint may be helpful. Severe cases may require surgical management but recurrence is likely.

Bone Infections and Tumors   Orofacial pain resulting from infection and neoplasia is described as a constant, deep, aching sensation, sometimes localized to the teeth, but more often of a diffuse quality. Diagnosis is based on the patient's history and laboratory, radiographic, and clinical findings. In cases of nonpurulent infection (osteitis), radiography may reveal demineralization or remineralization of the bone. Signs and symptoms associated with chronic osteomyelitis include paresthesia (if the condition involves the mandibular nerve canal), low-grade fever, elevated WBC and increased Erythrocyte Sedimentation Rate (ESR) values, sinus tract formation, limitation of opening, and occasionally, exposed bone. Bone death and necrosis results in a distinctive radiographic presentation, with islands of bone, termed *sequestra*, surrounded by demineralization.

TABLE 25-4. *Conditions associated with osteoarthritis and TMJ*

Temporomandibular pain and dysfunction syndrome
Myofascial pain and dysfunction syndrome
Infectious arthritis (bacterial, fungal, tubercular)
Connective tissue diseases
    Rheumatoid arthritis
    Systemic lupus erythematosis
    Dermatomyositis
Rheumatoid variants
    Psoriatic arthritis
    Reiter's syndrome
    Juvenile rheumatoid arthritis
Traumatic arthritis

The condition may result from periapical tooth abscess, fracture, or surgical contamination. Osteoradionecrosis, one form of osteomyelitis, may result from radiation treatment to the jaws or from radiation treatment that is followed by trauma (e.g., tooth extraction).

When neoplastic activity in the mandible (osteogenic sarcoma) is the source of the pain, there may be concurrent altered skin sensation (e.g., hypesthesia, dysesthesia, or paresthesia over the chin or lower face). Chondrosarcoma, a relatively rare but exquisitely painful tumor, is most commonly found in the anterior maxilla. Diagnosis of neoplasm is straightforward and based on history, and clinical, laboratory, and radiographic findings.

LESIONS OF THE EAR, NOSE, AND ORAL CAVITY

Orofacial pain resulting from acute sinus infection can be mild to severe and is often described as aching, throbbing, or as headache. Frontal or ethmoidal sinus involvement generates bilateral forehead pain or pain felt between the eyes, whereas pain originating from the maxillary sinus is often experienced on one or both sides of the face in the upper cheek (zygoma) or the entire side of the face. Pain arising from chronic (as opposed to acute) maxillary sinusitis may be described as mild and continuous with a burning quality. Other associated symptoms may include a feeling of fullness in the face or, in cases of maxillary sinus involvement, tenderness of the maxillary premolar or molar teeth.

The diagnosis of chronic sinusitis is based on history and clinical and radiographic findings. Forward bending or pressure applied over the affected sinus may intensify or exacerbate the pain in some cases. Examination may reveal hypertrophy or atrophy of the nasal mucosa and/or polyp formation. With maxillary involvement, the upper teeth on the affected side will frequently be percussion sensitive. Cultures of the nose or nasal discharge, however, are often negative (137). In these cases the examiner should be alert to the possibility of allergy or a reaction to irritating dusts or toxic chemicals. Standard radiography may demonstrate a fluid level but may not be helpful in assessing mucosal changes. CT may be necessary to rule out neoplasm.

Acute sinusitis is quite prevalent in adults, with chronic sinusitis being less common. Males and females are equally affected. Inflammation of the sinus mucosal lining is considered to be the pathophysiological mechanism responsible for facial pain genesis and inflammation of elements of the superior alveolar nerve plexus, the cause of tooth pain. Orofacial conditions that should be considered in the differential diagnosis include odontogenic infection and malignant disease.

Relief may be gained from antibiotics, decongestants, analgesics, moist heat, or lying down on the opposite side to promote drainage. Surgical lavage or drainage is necessary for intractable cases.

Orofacial Pain of Odotogenic Origin

Odontogenic pain or toothache, also termed *odontalgia*, is the commonest source of orofacial discomfort. Highly variable in presentation, odontogenic pain may be intermittent or continuous, spontaneous or induced, and will often simulate other pain syndromes. It is most often described as a mild to unbearable aching or sometimes throbbing sensation with a dull or depressing quality. The IASP has chosen to differentiate five varieties of odontalgia: pain due to dentinoenamel defects; pain arising from the pulp, such as pulpitis; pain arising from the periodontal structures, such as periapical periodontitis and abscess; pain not associated with lesions, such as atypical odontalgia; and cracked tooth syndrome. With the exception of pain due to dentinoenamel defects, all of these conditions can be chronic in nature. Since atypical odontalgia is not associated with a known pathophysiological mechanism, we have elected to describe this condition under the section Pain of Psychological Origin in the Head and Face below. A complete discussion of therapeutic considerations related to pain conditions of odontogenic origin is presented in Chapter 25 of Handbook of Pain Management, 2nd edition.

Odontalgia: Toothache-Pulpitis

The term *pulpitis* implies that the etiology of this pain is due only to pulpal inflammation and not periapical infection. In these cases pain is very often poorly localized within the teeth, jaws, face, or head. It may occur spontaneously, or be activated (in severe cases exacerbated) by hot or cold stimuli. Pulpal pain is often perceived as a sharp or dull ache of moderate or severe intensity.

Diagnosis is based on clinical signs and radiologic findings. Examination and radiography will often reveal deep dental caries, sometimes with erosion into the pulp chamber or root canal. Application of stimulants such as cold, heat, electric stimulation, and probing will induce pain. If inflammation progresses to infection and periodontal involvement, pain will be aggravated by percussion.

Differential diagnosis includes other forms of dental disease, trigeminal neuralgia, sinusitis, and migrainous headache syndromes.

Odontalgia: Toothache-Periapical Periodontitis and Abscess

Pain related to periodontal structures is similar in quality, occurrence, intensity, and duration to pain of pulpal origin. However, in contrast to pulpal pain, it is easily localized by the patient and diagnosis generally does not present difficulty. Pressure applied to the offending tooth will initiate or exacerbate tenderness. Associated symptoms may include localized redness, cellulitis, lymphadenitis, and drainage through the formation of a sinus tract. More severe complications can involve diffuse cellulitis and spread of the infection to parapharyngeal spaces with airway compromise, CNS with cerebral abscess, or endocardium (138). Radiographic data is useful for initial diagnosis and for defining extensive fascial plane involvement. In cases involving diffuse cellulitis, hematological, histopathologic, and microbiological laboratory tests may be necessary to augment diagnosis or to provide baseline information should the infection not respond to initial treatment. Differential diagnosis includes other dental disease, nonodontogenic infections, and neoplasia.

Cracked Tooth Syndrome

Pain originating from a tooth with a fine crack can be acute or chronic and is described as sharp or shocklike and of brief duration, often produced by biting or chewing. Upon examination, percussion directed laterally toward the affected tooth cusp will usually exacerbate the pain. A visible crack may sometimes be apparent or the cusp may move with manipulation. Radiography is not beneficial. The differential diagnosis includes other forms of toothache associated with the dentine or pulp.

Orofacial Pain of Mucosal Origin

Mucosal diseases produce pain that is intermittent in nature, although the patient may experience chronic discomfort. There are, however, a number of conditions that may produce persistent facial pain of an aching quality, including chronic periodontitis, benign mucous membrane pemphigoid (BMMP), ulcerative lichen planus, major recurrent aphthous, Wegener's granulomatosis, and oral cancer with superimposed infection. Diagnosis in these cases is generally confirmed by history, examination, or laboratory findings (139).

One type of orofacial mucosal pain that may be encountered has been termed *burning mouth syndrome* (glossodynia). The typical patient is a postmenopausal woman. The onset of the disorder is often associated with a prior dental procedure. In these cases, pain, described as a persistent, severe, burning sensation, may occur in the tongue or other mucosal tissues within the mouth, often in association with other altered sensations, such as taste or dryness (140). It may fluctuate during the day. The etiology and pathophysiology of this disorder remain unknown. The condition has been associated with local irritation (ill-fitting dentures), xerostomia, systemic disease, and nutritional deficiencies (especially B_{12}, but also B_1, B_2, and B_6). Burning tongue has also been reported following the development of adenoid cystic carcinoma in the floor of the mouth. In addition, many workers consider burning mouth a psychogenic pain problem since symptoms are often associated with emotional upset in the absence of organic findings (see below).

PAIN OF PSYCHOLOGICAL ORIGIN IN THE HEAD AND FACE

The IASP has chosen to describe two general categories of pain of psychological origin in the head and face: delusional or hallucinatory pain and hysterical or hypochondriacal pain (109). Classification of a pain condition as such requires that there be no known physical cause or pathophysiological mechanism and, in addition, there must be proof of the presence of contributing psychological factors. As a result, these categories are roughly equivalent to what the American Psychiatric Association has described as *psychogenic pain disorder* (141).

Historically, atypical facial pain, or prosopalgia, has been the term most commonly used to describe diffuse, nonanatomic orofacial pain of unknown pathophysiology. In the authors' opinion, the diagnosis of atypical facial pain should be made only on the following basis: (1) When other etiologies for facial pain have been considered and evaluated where appropriate; (2) when objective evidence for most of the facial pain syndromes is lacking; and (3) when specific antecedent psychologic or behavioral factors can be identified.

The predominant characteristic of psychologically induced pain is that it mimics pain of known pain syndromes. It is usually constant, often bilateral, and is not confined to the trigeminal distribution. The description of the pain quality is often vague and variable, as is the location and precipitating factors. A constant aching or burning sensation is the dominant feature, paroxysmal pain being uncommon. Psychological features, such as delusions, hallucinations, multiple physical complaints with classical conversion or pseudoneurological symptoms, exaggerated symptom reporting, excessive concern or fear of the symptoms, depression, illness behaviors, and excessive treatment seeking or medication usage are common. The patient often appears morose with evident suffering. Neurologic exam is usually normal except for some poorly localized tenderness and vague sensory loss in the painful region. Anticonvulsant medication is distinctly not helpful in these patients; psychiatric evaluation with psychotherapy and antidepressant medication is perhaps the only reasonable course (98).

CONCLUSION

Orofascial pain is a wide area in clinical medicine. It presents the clinician many challenges in diagnosis and treatment since the presentation may be diverse and syndromes can be overlapping. In this chapter we present a rational algorithm in dealing with patients with the more common facial pain syndrome to patients with less prevalent syndromes. It is our hope that this chapter can provide a framework for practicing clinicians to methodically examine the patients with facial pain syndromes that they may face in their clinic.

REFERENCES

1. Katusic S, et al. Incidence and clinical features of trigeminal neuralgia, Rochester, Minnesota, 1945–1984. *Ann Neurol* 1990;27(1):89–95.
2. Childs AM, et al. Neurovascular compression of the trigeminal and glossopharyngeal nerve: three case reports. *Arch Dis Child* 2000;82(4):311–315.
3. Haines SJ, Jannetta PJ, Zorub DS. Microvascular relations of the trigeminal nerve. An anatomical study with clinical correlation. *J Neurosurg* 1980;52(3):381–386.
4. Jannetta, PJ, Arterial compression of the trigeminal nerve at the pons in patients with trigeminal neuralgia. *J Neurosurg* 1967;26(1): p. Suppl:159–162.
5. Jannetta PJ. Trigeminal neuralgia and hemifacial spasm—etiology and definitive treatment. *Trans Am Neurol Assoc* 1975;100:89–91.
6. Jannetta, PJ. Observations on the etiology of trigeminal neuralgia, hemifacial spasm, acoustic nerve dysfunction and glossopharyngeal neuralgia. Definitive microsurgical treatment and results in 117 patients. *Neurochirurgia (Stuttg)* 1977;20(5):145–154.
7. Petty, PG, Southby PG, Siu K. Vascular compression: cause of trigeminal neuralgia. *Med J Aust* 1980;1(4):166–167.
8. Wepsic JG. Tic douloureux: etiology, refined treatment. *N Engl J Med* 1973;288(13):680–681.
9. Wilkins RH. Neurovascular compression syndromes. *Neurol Clin* 1985;3(2):359–372.
10. Furuya Y, et al. MRI of intracranial neurovascular compression. *J Comput Assist Tomogr* 1992;16(4):503–505.
11. Hutchins LG, et al. Trigeminal neuralgia (tic douloureux): MR imaging assessment. *Radiology* 1990;175(3):837–841.
12. Masur H, et al. The significance of three-dimensional MR-defined neurovascular compression for the pathogenesis of trigeminal neuralgia. *J Neurol* 1995;242(2):93–98.
13. Meaney JF, et al. Vascular contact with the fifth cranial nerve at the pons in patients with trigeminal neuralgia: detection with 3D FISP imaging. *AJR Am J Roentgenol* 1994;163(6):447–452.
14. Meaney JF, et al. Demonstration of neurovascular compression in trigeminal neuralgia with magnetic resonance imaging. Comparison with surgical findings in 52 consecutive operative cases. *J Neurosurg* 1995;83(5):799–805.
15. Papke K, et al. Three-dimensional MR imaging of neurovascular compression in trigeminal neuralgia [letter; comment]. *Radiology* 1998;208(2):550–552.
16. Sens MA, Hige HP. MRI of trigeminal neuralgia: initial clinical results in patients with vascular compression of the trigeminal nerve. *Neurosurg Rev* 1991;14(1):69–73.
17. Brown CR, Shankland W. Atypical trigeminal neuralgia. *Pract Periodontics Aesthet Dent* 1996;8(3):285.
18. Burchiel KJ, Slavin KV. On the natural history of trigeminal neuralgia. *Neurosurgery* 2000;46(1):152–154; discussion 154–155.
19. Burchiel KJ. Trigeminal neuropathic pain. *Acta Neurochir Suppl (Wien)* 1993;58:145–149.
20. Cusick JF. Atypical trigeminal neuralgia. *JAMA* 1981;245(22):2328–2329.
21. Shankland WED. Trigeminal neuralgia: typical or atypical? *Cranio* 1993;11(2):108–112.
22. Keuter EJ. Treatment of trigeminal neuralgia with tegretol. *Psychiatr Neurol Neurochir* 1966;69(6):439–451.
23. Murphy JP. Tegretol (carbamazepine): a new and effective medical treatment of trigeminal neuralgia, with a note concerning its use in the syndrome of thalamic hyperpathia. *Med Ann Dist Columbia* 1966;35(12):658–663.
24. Nicol CF. A four year double-blind study of tegretol in facial pain. *Headache* 1969;9(1):54–57.
25. Rasmussen P, Riishede J. Facial pain treated with carbamazepin (Tegretol). *Acta Neurol Scand* 1970;46(4):385–408.
26. Walsh TJ, Smith JL. Tegretol—a new treatment for tic douloureux. *Headache* 1968;8(2):62–64.
27. Baker KA, Taylor JW, Lilly GE. Treatment of trigeminal neuralgia: use of baclofen in combination with carbamazepine. *Clin Pharm* 1985;4(1):93–96.
28. Fromm GH, et al. Baclofen in trigeminal neuralgia: its effect on the spinal trigeminal nucleus: a pilot study. *Arch Neurol* 1980;37(12):768–771.
29. Fromm GH, Terrence CF, Chattha AS. Baclofen in the treatment of trigeminal neuralgia: double-blind study and long-term follow-up. *Ann Neurol* 1984;15(3):240–244.
30. Hershey LA. Baclofen in the treatment of neuralgia. *Ann Intern Med* 1984;100(6):905–906.
31. Zakrzewska JM, Patsalos PN. Drugs used in the management of trigeminal neuralgia. Oral *Surg Oral Med Oral Pathol* 1992;74(4):439–450.
32. Zakrzewska JM. Medical management of trigeminal neuralgia. *Br Dent J* 1990;168(10):399–401.
33. Carrazana EJ, Schachter SC. Alternative uses of lamotrigine and gabapentin in the treatment of trigeminal neuralgia [letter; comment]. *Neurology* 1998;50(4):1192.
34. Khan OA. Gabapentin relieves trigeminal neuralgia in multiple sclerosis patients. *Neurology* 1998;51(2):611–614.
35. Magnus L. Nonepileptic uses of gabapentin. *Epilepsia* 1999;40(Suppl 6):S66–72; discussion S73–74.
36. Sist T, et al. Gabapentin for idiopathic trigeminal neuralgia: report of two cases. *Neurology* 1997;48(5):1467.
37. Solaro C, et al. An open-label trial of gabapentin treatment of paroxysmal symptoms in multiple sclerosis patients. *Neurology* 1998;51(2):609–611.
38. Crimeni R. Clinical experience with mepivacaine and alcohol in neuralgia of the trigeminal nerve. *Acta Anaesthesiol Scand Suppl* 1966;24:173–176.
39. Ecker A, Perl T. Alcoholic injection of the gasserian ganglion for tic douloureux. *N Y State Dent J* 1967;33(3):149–158.
40. Ecker A. Tic douloureux; eight years after alcoholic gasserian injection. *N Y State J Med* 1974;74(9):1586–1592.
41. Braun TW, Sotereanos GC. Transantral maxillary neurectomy for intractable neuralgia. *J Oral Surg* 1977;35(7):583–584.
42. Freemont AJ, Millac P. The place of peripheral neurectomy in the management of trigeminal neuralgia. *Postgrad Med J* 1981;57(664):75–76.
43. Mason DA. Peripheral neurectomy in the treatment of trigeminal neuralgia of the second and third divisions. *J Oral Surg* 1972;30(2):113–120.
44. Murali R, Rovit RL. Are peripheral neurectomies of value in the treatment of trigeminal neuralgia? An analysis of new cases and cases involving previous radiofrequency gasserian thermocoagulation. *J Neurosurg* 1996; 85(3):435–437.
45. Oturai AB, et al. Neurosurgery for trigeminal neuralgia: comparison of alcohol block, neurectomy, and radiofrequency coagulation [see comments]. *Clin J Pain* 1996;12(4):311–315.
46. Quinn JH, Weil T. Trigeminal neuralgia: treatment by repetitive peripheral neurectomy. Supplemental report. *J Oral Surg* 1975;33(8):591–595.
47. Brown JA, McDaniel MD, Weaver MT. Percutaneous trigeminal nerve compression for treatment of trigeminal neuralgia: results in 50 patients. *Neurosurgery* 1993;32(4):570–573.
48. Brown JA, Preul MC. Percutaneous trigeminal ganglion compression for trigeminal neuralgia. Experience in 22 patients and review of the literature. *J Neurosurg* 1989;70(6):900–904.
49. Abdennebi B, et al. Percutaneous balloon compression of the Gasserian ganglion in trigeminal neuralgia. Long-term results in 150 cases. *Acta Neurochir (Wien)* 1995;136(1-2):72–74.
50. Fraioli B, et al. Treatment of trigeminal neuralgia by thermocoagulation, glycerolization, and percutaneous compression of the gasserian ganglion and/or retrogasserian rootlets: long-term results and therapeutic protocol. *Neurosurgery* 1989;24(2):239–245.
51. Arias MJ. Percutaneous retrogasserian glycerol rhizotomy for trigeminal neuralgia. A prospective study of 100 cases. *J Neurosurg* 1986;65(1):32–36.
52. Beck DW, Olson JJ, Urig E. Percutaneous retrogasserian glycerol rhizotomy for treatment of trigeminal neuralgia. *J Neurosurg* 1986;65(1):28–31.
53. Bergenheim AT, Hariz MI, Laitinen LV. Selectivity of retrogasserian glycerol rhizotomy in the treatment of trigeminal neuralgia. *Stereotact Funct Neurosurg* 1991;56(3):159–165.
54. Burchiel KJ. Percutaneous retrogasserian glycerol rhizolysis in the management of trigeminal neuralgia. *J Neurosurg* 1988;69(3):361–366.
55. Fujimaki T, Fukushima T, Miyazaki S. Percutaneous retrogasserian glycerol injection in the management of trigeminal neuralgia: long-term follow-up results. *J Neurosurg* 1990;73(2):212–216.

56. North RB, et al. Percutaneous retrogasserian glycerol rhizotomy. Predictors of success and failure in treatment of trigeminal neuralgia. *J Neurosurg* 1990;72(6):851–856.

57. Sweet WH, Poletti CE, Macon JB. Treatment of trigeminal neuralgia and other facial pains by retrogasserian injection of glycerol. *Neurosurgery* 1981;9(6):647–653.

58. Sweet WH, Poletti CE. Problems with retrogasserian glycerol in the treatment of trigeminal neuralgia. *Appl Neurophysiol* 1985;48(1-6):252–257.

59. Apfelbaum RI. A comparision of percutaneous radiofrequency trigeminal neurolysis and microvascular decompression of the trigeminal nerve for the treatment of tic douloureux. *Neurosurgery* 1977;1(1):16–21.

60. Burchiel KJ, et al. Comparison of percutaneous radiofrequency gangliolysis and microvascular decompression for the surgical management of tic douloureux. *Neurosurgery* 1981;9(2):111–119.

61. Hakanson S. Comparison of surgical treatments for trigeminal neuralgia: reevaluation of radiofrequency rhizotomy [letter; comment]. *Neurosurgery* 1997;40(5):1106–1107.

62. Kanpolat Y, et al. Percutaneous controlled radiofrequency rhizotomy in the management of patients with trigeminal neuralgia due to multiple sclerosis [In Process Citation]. *Acta Neurochir (Wien)* 2000;142(6):685–689; discussion 689–690.

63. McKenzie S. Stereotaxic radiofrequency coagulation: a treatment for trigeminal neuralgia. *J Neurosurg Nurs* 1972;4(1):75–81.

64. Nugent GR. Technique and results of 800 percutaneous radiofrequency thermocoagulations for trigeminal neuralgia. *Appl Neurophysiol* 1982;45(4-5):504–507.

65. Taha JM, Tew JM Jr. Treatment of trigeminal neuralgia by percutaneous radiofrequency rhizotomy. *Neurosurg Clin N Am* 1997;8(1):31–39.

66. Tew JM, Jr., Keller JT. The treatment of trigeminal neuralgia by percutaneous radiofrequency technique. *Clin Neurosurg* 1977;24:557–578.

67. Abdennebi B, Mahfouf L, Nedjahi T. Long-term results of percutaneous compression of the gasserian ganglion in trigeminal neuralgia (series of 200 patients). *Stereotact Funct Neurosurg* 1997;68(1-4 Pt 1):190–195.

68. Taha JM, Tew, JM, Jr. Comparison of surgical treatments for trigeminal neuralgia: reevaluation of radiofrequency rhizotomy [see comments]. *Neurosurgery* 1996;38(5):865–871.

69. van Loveren, H., et al. A 10-year experience in the treatment of trigeminal neuralgia. Comparison of percutaneous stereotaxic rhizotomy and posterior fossa exploration. *J Neurosurg* 1982;57(6):757–764.

70. Bederson JB, Wilson CB. Evaluation of microvascular decompression and partial sensory rhizotomy in 252 cases of trigeminal neuralgia. *J Neurosurg* 1989;71(3):359–367.

71. Broggi G, et al. Role of microvascular decompression in trigeminal neuralgia and multiple sclerosis [letter] [see comments] [published erratum appears in *Lancet* 2000 Apr 29;355(9214):1560]. *Lancet* 1999;354(9193):1878–1879.

72. Burchiel KJ, et al. Long-term efficacy of microvascular decompression in trigeminal neuralgia. *J Neurosurg* 1988;69(1):35–38.

73. Jannetta PJ. Outcome after microvascular decompression for typical trigeminal neuralgia, hemifacial spasm, tinnitus, disabling positional vertigo, and glossopharyngeal neuralgia (honored guest lecture). *Clin Neurosurg* 1997;44:331–383.

74. Lovely TJ, Jannetta PJ. Microvascular decompression for trigeminal neuralgia. Surgical technique and long-term results. *Neurosurg Clin N Am* 1997;8(1):11–29.

75. McLaughlin MR, et al. Microvascular decompression of cranial nerves: lessons learned after 4400 operations [see comments]. *J Neurosurg* 1999;90(1):1–8.

76. Morley TP. Case against microvascular decompression in the treatment of trigeminal neuralgia. *Arch Neurol* 1985;42(8):801–802.

77. Brisman R. Trigeminal neuralgia and multiple sclerosis. *Arch Neurol* 1987;44(4):379–381.

78. Friedlander AH, Zeff S. Atypical trigeminal neuralgia in patients with multiple sclerosis. *J Oral Surg* 1974;32(4): 301–303.

79. Friedman CE. Trigeminal neuralgia in a patient with multiple sclerosis. *J Endod* 1989;15(8):379–380.

80. Delcanho RE. Neuropathic implications of prosthodontic treatment. *J Prosthet Dent* 1995;73(2):146–152.

81. Eide, PK, Rabben T. Trigeminal neuropathic pain: pathophysiological mechanisms examined by quantitative assessment of abnormal pain and sensory perception. *Neurosurgery* 1998;43(5):1103–1110.

82. Goldstein NP. Gibilisco JA, Rushton JG. Trigeminal neuropathy and neuritis: a study of etiology with emphasis on dental causes. *JAMA* 1963;184:458–462.

83. Thrush DC, Small M. How benign a symptom is face numbness? *Lancet* 1970;2:851–853.

84. Lazorthes Y, Armengaud JP, Da Motta M. Chronic stimulation of the Gasserian ganglion for treatment of atypical facial neuralgia. *Pacing Clin Electrophysiol* 1987;10(1 Pt 2):257–265.

85. Bullard DE, Nashold, BS, Jr. The caudalis DREZ for facial pain. *Stereotact Funct Neurosurg* 1997;68(1-4 Pt 1):168–174.

86. Gorecki JP, Nashold BS. The Duke experience with the nucleus caudalis DREZ operation. *Acta Neurochir Suppl (Wien)* 1995;64:128–131.

87. Nashold BS, et al. Trigeminal DREZ for craniofacial pain. In: Samii M, ed. *Surgery in and around the brain stem and third ventricle.* Berlin: Springer-Verlag, 1986:54–59.

88. Roldan P, Broseta J, Barcia-Salorio JL. Chronic VPM stimulation for anesthesia dolorosa following trigeminal surgery. *Appl Neurophysiol* 1982;45(1-2):112–113.

89. Ebel H, et al. Chronic precentral stimulation in trigeminal neuropathic pain. *Acta Neurochir (Wien)* 1996;138(11):1300–1306.

90. Sweet WH. Deafferentation pain after posterior rhizotomy, trauma to a limb, and herpes zoster. *Neurosurgery* 1984;15(6):928–932.

91. Loeser JD. Herpes zoster and postherpetic neuralgia. *Pain* 1986;25:149–164.

92. Watson PN, Evans RJ. Postherpetic neuralgia: A review. *Arch Neurol* 1986;43:836–840.

93. Hosobuchi Y, Rutkin B. Descending trigeminal tractotomy. Neurophysiological approach. *Arch Neurol* 1971;25(2):115–125.

94. Schvarcz JR. Craniofacial postherpetic neuralgia managed by stereotactic spinal trigeminal nucleotomy. *Acta Neurochir Suppl (Wien)* 1989;6:62–64.

95. Sampson J, Nashold BS, Jr. Facial pain due to vascular lesions of the brain stem relieved by dorsal root entry zone lesions in the nucleus caudalis. *J Neurosurg* 1992;77:473.

96. Bullitt E, Tew JM, Boyd J. Intracranial tumors in patients with facial pain. *J Neurosurg* 1986;64(6):865–871.

97. White JC, Sweet WH. *Pain and the neurosurgeon.* Springfield: Thomas, 1969:264-265.

98. Hart RG, Easton JD. Trigeminal neuralgia and other facial pains. *Mo Med* 1981;78(11):683–693.

99. Laha RK, Jannetta PJ. Glossopharyngeal neuralgia. *J Neurosurgery* 1977;47:316–320.

100. Ekbom KA, Westerberg CE. Carbamazepine in glossopharyngeal neuralgia. *Arch Neurol* 1966;14(6):595–596.

101. Ehni G, Benner B. Occipital neuralgia and the C1-2 arthrosis syndrome. *J Neurosurg* 1984;61(5):961–965.

102. Poletti CE. Proposed operation for occipital neuralgia: C-2 and C-3 root decompression. Case report. *Neurosurgery* 1983;12(2):221–224.

103. Aubry M, Pialoux P. Sluder's syndrome. In: Vinken PJ, Nruyn GW, eds. *Handbook of clinical neurology.* Elsevier North Holland: Amsterdan, 1968:350–361.

104. Appen RE, and Sturm RJ. Raeder's paratrigeminal syndrome. *Ann Ophthalmol* 1978;10(9):1181–1187.

105. Toussaint D. Raeder's syndrome. In: Vinken PJ, Nruyn GW, eds. *Handbook of clinical neurology.* Elsevier North Holland: Amsterdan, 1968:333–336.

106. Travell J. Temporomandibular joint pain referred from head and neck. *J Prosthet Dent* 1960;10:745–763.

107. Schwartz L. *Disorders of the temporomandibular joint.* Philadelphia: W. B. Saunders, 1969.

108. Laskin DM. Etiology of the pain-dysfunction syndrome. *J Am Dent Assoc* 1969;79(1):147–153.

109. Classification of chronic pain: description of chronic pain syndromes and definitions of chronic pain terms. *Pain* 1986;(Suppl.) 3:S1–S225.

110. Moss RA, Garrett J. Temporomandibular joint dysfunction syndrome and myofascial pain dysfunction syndrome: a critical review. *J Oral Rehabil* 1984;11(1):3–28.

111. Rugh JD, Solberg WK. Psychological implications in temporomandibular pain and dysfunction. *Oral Sci Rev* 1976;7:3–30.

112. Truelove EL, et al. Clinical diagnostic criteria for TMD. New classification permits multiple diagnoses [see comments]. *J Am Dent Assoc* 1992;123(4):47–54.

113. Craniomandibular disorders: guidelines for evaluation, diagnosis and management. McNeill C, ed. Chicago: Quintessence Publishing, 1990.

114. Laskin DM, Block S. Diagnosis and treatment of myofacial pain-dysfunction (MPD) syndrome. *J Prosthet Dent* 1986;56(1): 75–84.

115. Burgess J. Symptom characteristics in TMD patients reporting blunt trauma and/or whiplash injury. *J of Craniomandibular Disorders: Fascial and Oral Pain* 1991;5(4):251–257.

116. Dolowitz DA, et al.The role of muscular incoordination in the pathogenesis of the temporomandibular joint syndrome. *Laryngoscope* 1964;74:790–801.

117. Magnusson T, Carlsson GE. A 21/2-year follow-up of changes in headache and mandibular dysfunction after stomatognathic treatment. *J Prosthet Dent* 1983;49(3):398–402.

118. Sharov Y, et al. Muscle pain index in relatio to pain dysfunction and dizziness associated with the myofascial pain dysfunction syndrome. *Oral Surg* 1978;46:742–747.

119. Agerberg G, Carlsson GE. Symptoms of functional disturbances of the masticatory system. A comparison of frequencies in a population sample and in a group of patients. *Acta Odontol Scand* 1975;33(4):183–190.

120. Bell W. *Clinical management of temporomandibular disorders.* Chicago: Year Book. 1982.

121. Griffin CJ, Munro RR. Electromyography of the masseter and anterior temporalis muscles in patients with temporomandibular dysfunction. *Arch Oral Biol* 1971;16(8):929–949.

122. Solberg WK, Woo MW, Houston JB. Prevalence of mandibular dysfunction in young adults. *J Am Dent Assoc* 1979;98(1):25–34.

123. Griffiths RH. Report of the president's conference on the examination, diagnosis, and management of temporomandibular disorders. *JADA* 1983;106:75–77.

124. Travell J, Rinzler SH. The myofascial genesis of pain. *Postgrad Med* 1952;11:425–434.

125. Travell J, Simon DJ. *Myofascial pain and dysfunction. The trigger point manual.* Baltimore: Williams and Wilkins, 1983.

126. Awad EA. Interstitial myofibrisitis: hypothesis of the mechanism. *Arch Phys Med Rehabil* 1973;54:449.

127. Reeves JL, Jaeger B, Graff-Radford SB. Reliability of the pressure algometer as a measure of myofascial trigger point sensitivity. *Pain* 1986;24(3):313–321.

128. Friction JR, et al. Myofascial pain syndrome of the head and neck: a review of clinical characteristics of 164 patients. *J Oral Surg Oral Pathol Oral Medicine* 1985;60:615–623.

129. Shira R.B. Temporomandibular degenerative joint disease. *Oral Surg* 197;40(2):1651–1682.

130. Ogus H. Degenerative disease of the temporomandibular joint in young persons. *Br J Oral Surg* 1979;17(1):17–26.

131. Wilkes C.H. Structural and functional alterations of the temporomandibular joint. *Northwest Dent* 1978;57(5):287–294.

132. Toller PA. Osteoarthrosis of the mandibular condyle. *Br Dent J* 1973;134(6):223–231.

133. Gross A, Gale EN. A prevalence study of the clinical signs associated with mandibular dysfunction. *J Am Dent Assoc* 1983;107(6):932–936.

134. Moffett GC, Johnson LC, McCabe JB. Articular remodeling in the adult human temporomandibular joint. *Amer J Anatomy* 1964;115: 119–142.

135. Wesstesson PL, Rohlin M. Internal derangement of the temporomandibular joint: morphologic description with correlation to joint function. *Oral Surg Oral Med Oral Pathol* 1985;59: 323–331.

136. Truelove EL, et al. Incidence of trauma associated with temporomandibular disorders. *J Dent Res* 1985;64:339.

137. Weinstein L. Disease of the upper respiratory tract. In: Wilson J, ed. *Harrison's principle of internal medicine.* McGraw-Hill: New York. 1983:1570–1571.

138. Hohl T, et al. *Diagnosis and treatment of odontogenic infections.* Seattle: Stoma Press 1983.

139. Wood NK, Goaz P. *Differential diagnosis of oral lesions.* St. Louis: Mosby Co 1980.

140. Basker RM, Sturdee DW, Davenport JC. Patients with burning mouths. A clinical investigation of causative factors, including the climacteric and diabetes. *Br Dent J* 1978;145(1):9–16.

141. *American Psychiatric Association: Quick diagnostic and statistical manual (DSM-III).* Washington, DC: American Psychiatric Association, 1980.

CHAPTER **26**

Differential Diagnosis and Management of Cervical Spine Pain

John Aryanpur and Thomas B. Ducker

"Pain in the neck" is such a common complaint and is so universally understood that the expression alone is used to describe certain people, situations, and experiences. Within any given month approximately 10% of the population will experience pain in the neck, with or without radicular pain into the arms (1). More than one-third of the population can recall a significant episode of severe neck pain, often with radicular components (1). In epidemiologic studies, a history of significant stiff neck with or without arm pain has been found in one-half to three-quarters of all individuals (2–4). Often these people will see their physician with this complaint. The scope of this problem is therefore tremendous.

Fortunately, 70% of people with the complaint of new-onset neck pain who visit a doctor are well or improving within 1 month (2), and a majority of the remaining 30% obtain symptomatic relief with time and appropriate therapeutic interventions. Thus, only a small proportion of patients with acute neck pain goes on to develop more chronic pain problems.

The human neck is evolutionarily an extremely complex structure with multiple bony, ligamentous, muscular, vascular, and neural components, all of which are capable of generating "neck pain." As such a structure, the neck can be affected by such processes as degenerative osteoarthritis, inflammatory diseases of muscle and ligament, vascular insufficiency, and neural compression syndromes, to mention only a few. Dermatomal, myotomal, and sclerotomal pain patterns may be distinguished.

More importantly, in a social sense the neck acts as a fulcrum from which our eyes, ears, nose, and mouth function to interact with our environment. Neck mobility is essential for the full appreciation of the world around us. More than we realize, the neck is active in common activi-

ties—nodding, turning, smiling, and shaking hands. Any disruption of its normal function may quickly be appreciated as uncomfortable, and even painful.

To complicate the situation, pathologic processes in other areas, such as the shoulder, the diaphragm, the heart, or the jaw, may cause pain that is referred to the neck—thus the complaint of "neck pain" in patients with acromioclavicular joint disease, diaphragmatic irritation, hypertension and myocardial infraction, or temporomandibular joint syndromes. Disease of the apical lung and pleura also may impinge on the brachial plexus to give pain in a C-8 or T-1 distribution.

Finally, even the most minor discomfort in the neck may be colored by certain psychosocial and psychoneurotic factors, in which case the complaint of "pain in the neck" is in reality but a physical outlet for a variety of personal and psychological problems.

The differential diagnosis of cervical spine pain is therefore quite large, and it is often only with repeated office visits and multiple investigations and therapies that the proper diagnosis is made.

In the next few pages we review some basic aspects of cervical anatomy and biomechanics as well as bony and neurologic pathology and specific referred pain syndromes. Following that, diagnostic studies are outlined. From a synthesis of the above, a list of differential diagnoses can in most cases be made, with the ultimate goals of focusing on the most appropriate diagnosis and treatment for each patient.

ANATOMY AND BIOMECHANICS

The neck is the most mobile region of the spine. Over 50% of all neck motion occurs at the atlanto-occipital and atlantoaxial joints; and the remaining 50% of neck motion is equally distributed through the C3-7 segments. In quadruped animals the motion allowed at the atlanto-occipital and atlantoaxial joints is even greater than it is in humans.

Mechanically there are many places where the system may cause pain. In the 7 cervical vertebrae there are 14 zygoapophyseal joints (usually referred to as facet joints) as well as 5 Luschka's joints (referred to as uncinate processes), and a muscular and ligamentous apparatus that is innervated not only by the 11th cranial nerve but also by all of the 8 cranial nerves on both sides. Muscle and ligamentous tears and sprains are by far the most common causes for neck pain, but other pathologies may exist as well. The facet joints and joints of Luschka are lined with synovial membrane and are subject to the same inflammatory pain-producing pathologies as synovial joints elsewhere. The normal intervertebral disc absorbs axial loading pressures on the spine, serving as a "shock absorber." Disc rupture or degeneration or annulus tear can produce severe focal pain that may be difficult to diagnose and treat. Bony structures themselves may degenerate secondary to osteoporosis or metabolic or infiltrative processes, leading to pathologic fractures and pain. Finally, the neural tissues themselves may be a source of pain when compressed or irritated. These pathologic mechanisms are discussed in more detail below.

Cervical Spine

The anatomy and relevant biomechanics of the cervical spine are most pertinent to clinical disorders if considered segmentally. Thus, the occiput–C-1 region (comprising the occiput and C-1 vertebrae, the joints between them, the muscles and ligaments affecting movement at these joints, and the spinal cord and nerve roots exiting at that level) may be considered an independent segment, and so on for the C1-2, C2-3, and remaining regions down C-7–T-1.

The seven small cervical vertebrae balance the 15-pound weight of the head and its contents. The center of weight of the skull is slightly anterior to the midaxis of the spine, and naturally causes the head to fall forward. For this reason, there is constant tension on the posterior cervical musculature to hold the head in the upright position. Relaxation and contraction of this posterior musculature, aided by the upper one-third of the trapezius, allows cervical flexion and extension. The vast majority of this flexion and extension occurs at the atlanto-occipital joint, and this joint is commonly referred to as the "yes" joint. Conversion of the emotion of "yes" into the "yes" motion of the head is mediated by branches of the 11th cranial nerve supplying the trapezius and sternocleidomastoid muscles, as well as by all eight cervical roots, including the C-1 motor root, which exists at this level. There is no C-1 sensory root.

Beneath this atlanto-occipital joint the neural anatomy is terribly complex. Within the spinal cord at that level there is the decussation of the long motor tracts as well as the descending spinal tract of the fifth cranial nerve, which is responsible for pain and temperature sensation over the face. The lower cranial nerve nuclei are also vulnerable at this location. Compression of the cord at this level can cause a variety of signs and symptoms (neck pain, limitation of flexion and extension, headaches, "onionskin" facial numbness, lower cranial nerve palsies, upper extremity weakness, and lower extremity spasticity) that may be diffuse enough to confuse even the best-trained clinician. Suffice it to say that a patient presenting with complaints and physical findings as listed above should be suspected of having pathology at the occiput–C-1 level.

Movement at the C1-2 level is greatly influenced by the dens, which acts as a stable pin about which rotation may occur. The rotary movement of the atlantoaxial joint has led to its being referred to as the "no" joint. Again, motion through a cervical joint is controlled by one's emotions! Extremes of rotation, up to 80% to 100°, are possible at this joint.

The actual turning of the neck to produce a "no" movement is primarily a function of the sternocleidomastoid muscle. This muscle, with its attachments on the mastoid process at the base of the skull, clearly provides the major fulcrum for turning of the atlantoaxial joint. Posteriorly, the smaller capitis musculature, with attachments onto the spinous process of C-2 extending up to the skull, acts primarily as a stabilizer and servomechanism balance system to maintain the head in proper alignment with the motions initiated by the stronger sternocleidomastoid muscle. Other posterior muscle groups, including the trapezius, complement this stabilizing action. Motor innervation for the sternocleidomastoid occurs primarily through the 11th cranial nerve, supplemented by small fibers from C-2 and C-3 to the lower half of the muscle. At the C1-2 segment, a sensory nerve component is present in the form of large C-2 sensory nerve roots. These divide peripherally into several branches, the largest of which on each side is the greater occipital nerve. This nerve provides sensory innervation of the superior aspect of the neck and the entire posterior half of the hemicranium, including the occiput and superior parietal areas of the skull and scalp. The greater occipital nerve may be trapped peripherally as it passes through the thick fascial attachments of the posterior neck musculature over the occipital region. This can be a source of pain and tenderness on the posterior aspect of the head. Prolonged contraction of the posterior cervical musculature, due to stress or fatigue, can cause compression of both greater occipital nerves, contributing to the tension headache syndrome.

The C2-3 segment is in a sense a transitional segment between the hypermobile occiput–C-2 area and the remaining cervical segments. The C2-3 joint has multiple components: the intervertebral disc, the vertebral joints, and the zygoapophyseal joints. These limit the degrees of freedom at the segment, but also provide a degree of stability not present at higher levels. This joint will allow approximately 10° of motion in flexion and extension and 5° to 8° in rotation or lateral flexion. It is rarely involved in the degenerative arthritic changes that are so common at lower cervical levels.

The C-3 vertebra has the C-3 nerve root above and the C-4 nerve root below. The motor innervation of the diaphragm, and of the accessory muscles of respiration in the neck, basically comes from these two nerve roots. (Occasionally the C-5 roots make several smaller contributions to this innervation.) These motor roots also contribute to the innervation of the intrinsic neck muscles, as do all motor roots in the cervical region. The sensory component of the C-3 root supplies the superior half of the neck anteriorly and can extend up to the angle of the jaw and ear. Below, the C-4 dermatome covers the lower half of the neck and will extend over the clavicles. C-5 through C-8 dermatomal patterns are carried primarily out through the brachial plexus into the upper extremities.

From the C3-4 segment caudally the motion of each vertebra on its adjacent vertebra is basically the same. All are associated with approximately 10° of rotation and/or lateral flexion. All have intervertebral discs and uncovertebral and zygoapophyseal joints. Although disease within any of these vertebrae, adjacent ligaments, or joint structures can cause focal pain, more commonly the pathologic process is associated with a prominent component of local nerve root irritation, and a strong radicular element is apparent. Pathology in the C-4–T-1 segments, therefore, commonly produces varying degrees of upper extremity pain and neurologic deficit. For this reason, the discussion of the caudal cervical segments simplifies to a neuroanatomic discussion of each of the individual cervical nerve roots that lead to the brachial plexus, although the specific organization of the brachial plexus complex's individual nerve root patterns are well recognized and easy to distinguish.

The C-5 nerve root, which exits between the fourth and fifth cervical vertebrae, supplies the major innervation of the deltoid muscle. It also contributes to the biceps, the supra- and infraspinatus, serratus anterior, and levator scapulae. All are muscles involved in stabilizing the shoulder and in abduction of the arm. The biceps reflex can be associated with the C-5 nerve root, although in fact the C-6 root may make a significant contribution. The sensory innervation of the C-5 root is fairly specific, covering the shoulder and down the radial aspect of the arm to the mid-distal forearm.

The motor component of the C-6 nerve root, which exits between the C-5 and C-6 vertebrae, is responsible for the innervation of the brachioradialis and biceps muscles, as well as the extensors of the wrist. Clinically, the brachioradialis reflex is linked with the C-6 root—in truth the C-5 root is also involved. The C-6 dermatomal pattern is very specific and definitely involves the dorsal radial aspect of the dorsal surface of the index finger.

The C-7 nerve root makes an important contribution to the posterior aspect of the brachial plexus, which leads directly into the radial nerve. For that reason C-7 strongly influences the triceps musculature, as well as the extensors of the wrist and the intrinsic muscles of the hand. Its sensory dermatomal pattern always involves the middle finger, but can involve the index finger as well. The triceps reflex is subserved by this nerve root.

The C-8 nerve root, which comes off beneath the seventh cervical vertebra just above the first thoracic vertebra and the first rib, contributes heavily to the inferior cord of the brachial plexus and the medial cord. Its primary myotome includes the flexors of the hand—it is responsible for grip. The sensory innervation of this root covers the ulnar aspects of the forearm and the dorsal and palmar ulnar aspects extending up over the fourth and fifth fingers. This differs from the sensory distribution of the ulnar nerve in that the latter covers only the ulnar half of the fourth finger and does not extend proximally beyond the palmar crease.

Although it exits outside the cervical spine at the T1-2 region, the T-1 nerve root obviously contributes to the brachial plexus and the intrinsic muscles of the hand. Its sensory contributions are into the axilla and down the medial aspect of the upper arm. There is no specific reflex associated with this nerve root.

Spinal Cord

The relationship between the spinal cord and nerve roots at the C-3–T-1 levels is clinically important and is constant in the mid and lower cervical spine. The spinal cord lies within the vertebral canal, with nerve roots exiting via foramina at each level. The neural foramen at each level is bounded dorsolaterally by the facet joint capsule, anteromedially by the disc space and uncovertebral joints, and superiorly and inferiorly by the arches of the vertebra above and below. Each foramen can therefore be impinged on in many ways. Degenerative changes leading to hypertrophy of the facet joint and/or the uncovertebral joints can often cause foraminal stenosis. The nucleus pulposus of the intervertebral disc is usually held in place by strong posterior longitudinal ligaments. Under certain extremes of pressure and stress, however, the disc material can herniate posteriorly or posterolaterally to impinge on the spinal cord or nerve root. The neural foramina are slightly large at C2-3 and become progressively smaller down to C6-7. Generally speaking, the foramina have an average vertical diameter of 10 mm and a transverse diameter of 5 mm. The nerve roots lie near the upper vertebral pedicle, and as they exit further they descend slightly toward the intervertebral joint space itself. Because the nerve roots themselves occupy only one-third of the cross-sectional area of the foraminal space, the actual shape of the foramen may be the most important consideration in determining its adequacy. A decrease in foraminal height is not as critical as a decrease in foraminal width. Consequently foraminal stenosis may be fairly advanced before the patient becomes symptomatic.

Cross-sectionally, the normal spinal cord has a diameter in the lateral dimension of 12 to 13 mm throughout most of the cervical regions. In the anteroposterior (AP) dimension, this diameter is generally less, from 8 to 9 mm. The spinal canal is largest in the high cervical region, and tapers progressively from there down. Assuming a normal AP diameter of 8 to 9 mm and allowing for the 1-mm thickness of cerebrospinal fluid and 1-mm thickness of dural coverings surrounding the cord anteriorly and posteriorly, a minimal spinal canal diameter of 12 to 13 mm is required to allow for a healthy, noncompressed spinal cord. Clinically, the AP diameter of the spinal canal is easily obtainable from plain films or computed tomography (CT), thus allowing quick estimates of the adequacy of the spinal canal. In practice, an AP diameter of 14 mm is considered normal, and anything less than that indicates a degree of central spinal stenosis with narrowing of the canal that could adversely effect the spinal cord.

Vascular Supply

The vertebral artery travels through the transverse foramina of the C8-1 vertebrae, making a tight arch over the atlas as it pierces the dura between the atlas and occiput. The spinal cord and nerve roots derive their blood supply bilaterally from myeloradicular arteries that branch from each vertebral artery and accompany specific nerve roots toward the cord substance itself. In the neck there are often three or four of these arteries, the largest of which usually accompanies the C-6 or C-7 root and is usually larger on the left than the right. This is commonly termed the artery of the cervical enlargement. This supply feeds into bilateral contributions from the intracranial vertebral artery, which joins at the midline to form the anterior spinal artery. A system of parallel posterior spinal arteries also exists. Although anastomoses between anterior and posterior spinal arteries are numerous, in general the anterior spinal artery supplies blood to the anterior two-thirds of the cord (including the anterior and lateral funiculi and gray matter of the cord). The posterior spinal artery system supplies the posterior columns exclusively. In rare individuals, the anterior spinal artery may be vestigial, and a single large myeloradicular artery may supply most of the cervical spinal cord. Embolic or thrombotic events, or occlusion of major spinal arteries or veins during surgical interventions or by trauma, can lead to spinal cord ischemia, and ultimately spinal infarction.

PATHOLOGY

Pathology within the cervical spine can involve the central nervous system and its adjacent nerve roots, the vertebral joints, or the bones themselves. When initially attempting to ascertain where the pathology lies, the first major division is between involvement of bony and soft tissue struc-

tures. In many cases both go hand in hand, and consequently may be difficult to tease apart. For discussion's sake, we will begin centrally with problems of the spinal cord itself, and then proceed peripherally to quickly review pathology of the bones, joints, and muscles.

Clinically, the prototypical intrinsic spinal pathology is an expansile mass of the cord, and the simplest of central spinal masses is the syrinx. These can develop idiopathically or as a long-term sequela of spinal trauma, and may be initially associated with arm and facial pain and discomfort, especially at night. This latter is thought to be secondary to changes in differential pressure between syrinx and subarachnoid space that occur during recumbency. The pain then becomes less prominent as the neurologic deficit becomes more pronounced. There can be focal sensory loss on the face as well as over the trunk and limbs as a consequence of compression of the anterior white commissure and lateral spinothalamic tracts. Clumsy, wasted hands and a stiff gait reflect a combination of upper and lower motor neuron deficits in the upper extremities and pure upper motor neuron deficits in the lower extremities. Bowel and bladder problems may occur as well.

On occasion, a spinal cord cyst is associated with a tumor, such as an ependymoma. More frequently the tumor itself can develop cystic degeneration, as in astrocytomas of the cord.

Other degenerative processes besides intrinsic compressive cord lesions may lead to neurologic deficit and pain. Anterior motor horn cell loss, as in amyotrophic lateral sclerosis and polio, or ischemic processes of the cord may result in clinical syndromes that are difficult to distinguish from those of the more common spinal cord compressive syndromes.

Rather than being in the spinal cord itself, the mass may be centered along the meninges or adjacent nerve roots. These are locations at which meningiomas and neurofibromas are commonly found. Even though these tumors may initially develop on one root alone, they progress so slowly that the true pathology may not be fully appreciated. Again, the common initial symptom is pain, but it is often only when spinal cord compression has reached the point of upper extremity weakness, myelopathy, or gait disturbance that the clinical syndrome is recognized.

Extradural processes as well may cause a syndrome identical to the one described above. By far the most common source of extradural compression is degenerative joint disease of the intervertebral joints. Normal degenerative joint changes lead, over time, to reactive pannus and bony spur formation that when severe can cause spinal cord or nerve root compression. These degenerative processes can be accelerated by coexistent disease, such as rheumatoid arthritis, which characteristically attacks predominantly the atlanto-occipital and atlantoaxial regions of the spine, leading to ligamentous laxity and spinal column instability as well as cord and nerve root compression. In contrast, ankylosing spondylitis causes calcification of joints and longitudinal spinal ligaments, leading to spinal fusion and abnormal bone formation that once again may compress neural tissues.

Other epidural masses such as metastatic tumors (usually from the breast or lung) and benign and malignant primary bone tumors may cause cord or root compression as above and can therefore be included in this category of extradural compressive masses.

Intervertebral disc herniation typically affects only a single nerve root. The herniation may be directly posterior into the canal to cause acute spinal cord compression and symptoms similar to those of other extradural lesions, however. In addition, joint and ligamentous pathology may cause pain independent of a compressive effect on neural tissue. Joints that are inflamed or unstable may produce focal, mechanical pain quite different from that of neural compression. Thus, a common clinical presentation is that of the patient with severe degenerative changes of the cervical spine who has both mechanical (joint and ligamentous) and radicular (neural compressive) pain components.

Intrinsic pathology of the bone, such as with osteoporotic fractures, bony tumors, or Paget's disease of the spine, may produce focal pain. This pain may be exacerbated by neck movement, as is pain originating from the joints, but more commonly is not. Palpation of the involved vertebra, however, almost invariably reproduces the pain. The pain from bony lesions is characteristically described as dull or aching.

Finally, all the above pathologies may contribute to the development of cervical muscle spasm and irritation, making this a nearly universal accompaniment of all complaints of neck pain. Pain on movement and superficial palpation, and muscle tightness, are characteristic.

MEDICAL HISTORY

In evaluating a patient with cervical pain, as with any patient, the physician has the responsibility of directing the interview process. If this is skillfully done, in 70% to 80% of patients a reasonable initial diagnosis can be made even without a physical examination or further diagnostic studies. As always, open-ended questions yield the greatest information.

The interview begins as the patient enters the room, and his or her habitus, posture, and gait should be observed. Age, sex, and occupation are all readily ascertained. Next, a description of the pain is needed.

Pain always has at least three characteristics—onset, course, and severity. These need to be described in terms of location, exacerbating and relieving factors, quality, and severity. It is essential to have the patient begin by pointing to the painful area of the neck or arm. One must literally have the patient stand up and show the examiner where he or she hurts. This will allow the examiner to sidestep any confusion the patient may have with anatomic description or terms.

Leading questions about particular activities (e.g., twisting the neck, running, doing sports, working) are useful. If the patient does not spontaneously provide descriptions of the type and severity of the pain, then questions such as how sharp or dull, aching or burning, throbbing or cramping the pain is may be employed. Although it is important not to put words in the patient's mouth, certain general types of pain may indicate certain pathologies. For example, pain deep within the bone is usually described as dull and nagging, whereas fracture pain is sharp, severe, and immediately associated with muscle spasm. Pain that is worse at night can suggest a spinal cord tumor or mass. Pain that radiates sharply is usually radicular in origin.

Finally, patients may have initiated treatments on their own or sought advice elsewhere prior to being seen. Responses to over-the-counter drugs such as aspirin, Motrin, Tylenol, and the like are important. Some patients have seen physical therapists or chiropractors, and knowledge of the response to such manipulations is always beneficial. As always, how the patient reacts to his or her disease psychologically is of paramount importance. If there is obvious secondary gain or malingering involved, the examiner may do better to direct treatment toward these psychological factors.

It is also important to be cognizant of the many patterns of referred pain. As discussed earlier, numerous noncervical pathologies may cause various types of neck pain. Consequently, in difficult cases where no conspicuous cervical pathology can be held accountable for the patient's pain, consultation with colleagues in other specialties should be the rule rather than the exception.

CLINICAL EXAMINATION

In dealing with patients with neck pain, the physical examination must have two basic components. The first component must involve an examination of the anatomy and mechanics of the neck itself. The second component must include an accurate assessment of the patient's neurologic status.

Anatomy and Mechanics of the Neck

In evaluating the mechanics of the neck, it must be appreciated that, as described above, 50% of cervical motion occurs at the occipital C-1 and C-2 joints alone. Thus the "yes" and "no" motions may be intact in the face of many a severe cervical disorder. The first three cervical vertebrae are anatomically located behind the face and are covered by the jaw at the base of the skull. C-4 through C-7 are centrally placed, as are the vertebrae that make up the neck as we view it from the surface.

Grossly the neck should have a gentle lordotic curve, as in the lumbar region. Most patients should be able to easily extend their neck to look at the ceiling and to flex their neck to look at the floor. A neck that is fixed and lacks motion has either mechanical or pain-evoked limitations to a full range of motion. The head compression, or Spurling's, test is a valuable aid in localizing the level of the pathology (5). This maneuver causes compression of the vertebral bodies on one another and narrows the neural foramina. If this maneuver produces radicular pain, a nerve root pathology is probable. If only local neck pain is elicited, however, joint or ligamentous disease is more likely. The reverse of compression (i.e., distraction) is often helpful as well. The radicular pain of a soft disc herniation or foraminal stenosis may be relieved by the opening of the foramina caused by cervical distraction. If pain is from joint disease, distraction will simply accentuate the pain as much as compression will. In cervical nerve root disorders due to either soft disk disease or osteophytes, extending the neck and turning the head to the side of the pain commonly reproduces the radicular pain symptoms. Patients will often volunteer that they will not turn or extend their neck because of this discomfort.

In addition to testing the range of motion of the neck, the range of motion of the shoulder and upper extremity must be evaluated as well. In many cases, it is very difficult to distinguish between shoulder joint disorders and certain nerve root compression syndromes. Furthermore, with certain neck disorders weakness within the deltoid or biceps leads to shoulder stiffness and tightness, so the patient may in actuality have both problems. Nonetheless, if the patient has pain in the neck that radiates down the arm, it is useful for the patient and examiner to demonstrate that passive movement of the wrist, elbow, or shoulder will not reproduce the pain, thereby confirming that the upper extremity pain is not caused by pathology in the limb itself. If this is followed by measures that do reproduce the upper extremity pain (i.e., compression, extension, and rotation of the neck), ordering radiographs and other diagnostic studies of the neck will seem logical to the patient as well as reassuring to the physician.

Neurologic Status

The neurologic examination should be performed in a systematic way. The patient can be sitting on an examining table, although it may be helpful to have the patient sitting in a chair. This way the examiner can walk around the patient to observe at many angles. A motor, sensory, and reflex examination can be done in a matter of a few minutes. The examiner begins by walking behind the patient and observing as he or she raises the arms above the head and lowers them back down. By looking at how the neck is held and at the mechanics of the neck and shoulders throughout this movement, one has already learned a good deal of information. Palpation of neck muscles and individual spinous processes may also yield valuable information regarding the origin of neck pain.

Next, the patient is instructed to flex the arms at the elbows and abduct at the shoulder, and to maintain this position. By exerting counterpressure the strength of the deltoid muscles may be tested simultaneously. This is essen-

tial because, although absolute strength is important, it is more crucial to detect an asymmetry in strength from side to side. The patient now lowers the arms to his or her side, keeping them flexed at the elbow. In this position, biceps strength can be assessed. Again, one is looking above all for symmetry. Moving behind the patient, the patient's fist is then placed inside the examiner's hands with instructions to extend the arms, thus utilizing the triceps muscle. If the arm is only minimally flexed to begin with, the mechanical advantage will be with the examiner, and no patient will be able to overcome the examiner. A false impression of weakness might thus be given. It is therefore always crucial to examine individual muscles in positions that allow the patient maximal mechanical advantage. The triceps musculature has widespread innervation (C5-8), so that asymmetry of the strength of this muscle is often a very sensitive indicator in patients with neurologic dysfunction. Finally the examiner faces the patient and has him or her extend the wrist, spread the fingers, and squeeze down tightly, all as a measure of the strength of the wrist extensors and intrinsic hand musculature. Although more-sophisticated motor examinations are possible, these simple maneuvers can be rapidly performed and will pick up the majority of upper extremity dysfunctions. The lower extremities can be tested in a similar fashion.

The sensory examination is best done with a safety pin. This will not cause bleeding, can be used to test the patient's ability to distinguish between sharp and dull, and can be discarded after each examination. Comparing dermatomal patterns from side to side is usually the best way to appreciate a subtle hypoalgesia. As discussed above, a simple way to remember dermatomal patterns is to think of C-5 as covering the shoulder, C-6 covering the thumb, C-7 involving the index and middle fingers, and C-8 the ring and little fingers. Often testing down onto the chest wall is helpful, and it is important to remember that the C-4 dermatomal pattern is on the anterior chest wall. Thus, a change in the sensation just below the clavicle may reflect a C-4 sensory level deficit. Often, assessment of lower extremity proprioception is useful.

When cervical problems are suspected, the reflex examination should include the upper and lower extremities as well as a comparison between the two. The biceps, triceps, and brachioradial reflexes are the significant deep tendon reflexes in the upper extremities. Inversion of the upper extremity reflexes or a positive Hoffmann's sign are evidence of hyperreflexia. Subsequent to this, lower extremity reflexes should be evaluated, especially at the knees. If the reflexes are perfectly normal in the upper extremities and at the knees, assessment of ankle and Babinski's reflexes are unlikely to yield much new information and may be omitted in the interest of time. However, if any pathologic reflexes are noted, then full lower extremity reflex assessment, including Babinski's reflex, is mandatory. The examination may be concluded by watching the patient walk from the examining room.

DIAGNOSTIC STUDIES

The investigation of any complaint of neck pain must first begin with plain films of the cervical spine. Any acute post-traumatic surgical pain, or persistent nontraumatic surgical pain, should be evaluated first using plain cervical spine x-rays. Often, plain films alone will show pathology such as bony erosion or degenerative osteoarthritis with osteophyte formation, which will guide further investigations and diagnostic decisions. If indicated, flexion and extension views of the cervical spine are indispensable in evaluating spinal stability radiographically. Oblique views allow visualization of the neural foramina. Other views such as the swimmer's view or the odontoid view may be tailored to the specific area being investigated.

With the plain film information in hand, further radiologic, electrophysiologic, or laboratory investigations may be ordered.

Any patient with a complaint or history suggestive of a radicular pattern who fails conservative therapy should be evaluated further. In the past, this evaluation has consisted of myelography, with or without CT scanning. Recently, magnetic resonance imaging (MRI) techniques have, to a large degree, supplanted this cervical myelogram. In general, following the plain x-ray evaluation of the patient with neck pain, the next radiologic study of choice should be an MRI scan. MRI studies, with the their ability to combine sagittal, axial, and coronal views of the cervical spine, allow for exquisite visualization of the spinal cord and nerve roots. Intraspinal lesions such as herniated disks, osteophytes, and tumors are easily visualized using MRI techniques. Intrinsic diseases of the cervical spinal cord such as intramedullary tumors, syringes, or the Chiari malformations are, in fact, best visualized by MRI techniques (Fig. 26-1).

However, if visualization of fine bony detail or bony destruction is desired, supplementation of MRI with CT scanning will be essential. Particularly in the area of osseous destructive lesions of the spinal column and bony osteophytes, MRI fails to provide enough bony detail to guide surgical intervention. In these circumstances, a high-resolution plain CT scan through the area of pathology is often an indispensable supplement to the MRI scan.

Although MRI has, to a large degree, supplanted myelography as an imaging modality, in certain patients the cervical myelogram is still indicated. Examples include patients with severe degenerative or postsurgical kyphosis in whom distortion of the normal anatomy prevents easy recognition of abnormalities using multiple plain or MRI formats. Another example is the patient who is suspected of having a cervical spinal arteriovenous malformation. In this case, MRI may miss the lesion altogether, and the diagnosis can oftentimes only be made by detecting the classic serpiginous defect on the cervical myelogram.

Nuclear medicine studies, such as gallium- and leukocyte-tagged scans, are not capable of providing detailed anatomic information. They are useful, however, when

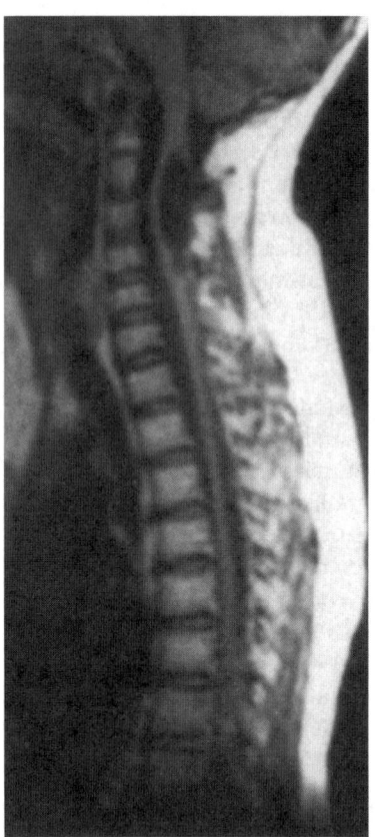

FIG. 26-1. MRI scan reveals a high cervical spinal cord syrinx with associated Chiari I malformation.

infectious etiologies are suspected as a cause of neck pain. It is always necessary to remember that these are fairly nonspecific tests and that they may be positive for several months after surgery or other interventions.

Electrophysiologic testing utilizing electromyography (EMG) and nerve conduction velocity (NCV) testing techniques is indicated when evidence exists of damage to neural tissue. Decrease in motor potential and muscle groups and/or slowing of conduction velocities along nerves are among the many pathologic responses detected by these tests. In particular, EMG/NCV tests are useful in delineating the level and extent of neurologic injury. Nerve conduction velocities may be decreased relatively quickly after injury to the involved nerve, whereas electromyographic changes may take weeks to become apparent. For this reason, the nerve conduction velocity is a more sensitive test early in the disease course.

Laboratory investigations will supplement all the above tests. Determination of the complete blood count and differential, serum protein electrophoresis, the erythrocyte sedimentation rate, rheumatoid factor, or the serum calcium may be crucial to arriving at the final diagnosis.

Occasionally, a patient will be encountered in whom all investigations, including radiographic, electrophysiologic, and serologic, will be negative, despite the complaint of persistent neck pain. In such difficult diagnosis, the use of discography has gained some recent popularity. The percutaneous injection of the small amounts of radiographic contrast material into the cervical disc spaces may demonstrate annular tears or frank extrusion of contrast material, which could help localize the pathological level. Reproduction of the patient's pain with injection of a small amount of contrast material is also thought to be diagnostic of pathology at the injected level. It is possible to control for the effects of injection at one level by subsequently injecting a small amount of local anesthetic. Relief of the patient's typical neck pain following the intradiscal injection of local anesthetic is reported to be a highly specific test of discogenic disease, and is reported to correlate well with relief of pain following subsequent surgery at that level. This technique has not yet been evaluated in a controlled fashion, and it remains to be seen whether such techniques find a wider applicability in the management of patients with intractable cervical pain.

Obviously, the individual tests described above will be ordered for each patient depending on the details of the history, physical examination, and radiographic studies. As a rule, however, the sequence of diagnostic evaluation should progress from plain spine films and simple serologic tests to more-extensive and -invasive evaluations only if the patient's neck pain persists. In over 90% of all patients with neck pain, a simple plain spine series is sufficient to rule out serious pathology and to reassure the patient that the episode of neck pain currently being experienced will most likely resolve with conservative therapy.

SPECIFIC CERVICAL PAIN SYNDROMES

Based on the history and physical examination, it should be possible to arrive at a tentative diagnosis. Diagnostic studies can bolster or refute these initial impressions. Certain disorders are common and should be familiar to every clinician. These are listed in Table 26-1 and are discussed individually. This table is in no way meant to be all-inclusive. Creating a huge differential diagnosis is not helpful in the day-to-day practice of treating cervical pain syndromes. Once again, the key differential here is to determine whether the disease syndrome is primarily neurologic or bony in nature. Deciding this will allow a narrowing of the differential diagnosis list into manageable subclasses and will direct further studies that will allow the final diagnosis to be reached. Obviously there are other esoteric diseases that may cause pain in the neck and upper extremities. A full discussion of these disorders is beyond the scope of this chapter. For this the reader is referred to a more comprehensive text (6).

Spinal Cord Compression

Compression of the spinal cord can occur from mass lesions either extrinsic or intrinsic to the cord itself. The most common intra-axial spinal mass lesions are syringes, and the

TABLE 26-1. *Common disorders of the cervical spinal area causing neck and upper extremity pain*

Spinal cord compression due to tumor or syrinx
Intrinsic motor and sensory disorders of the cord (including torticollis, toxins, and viral, vascular, and metabolic diseases)
Extrinsic spinal cord neoplasms
Osteoarthritis
Nerve root irritations (soft and hard disk protrusions)
Traumatic injury to the cervical spine
Rheumatoid arthritis
Ankylosing spondylitis and diffuse idiopathic skeletal hyperostosis
Infections

most common primary spinal tumors are spinal ependymomas and spinal gliomas, respectively, accounting for 60% and 30% of all primary spinal tumors (7).

The ependymoma literally starts from the central spinal canal, taking origin from vestigial ependymal cells lining this cavity. The tumor expands slowly to compress the spinal cord between it and the confines of the spinal canal.

Spinal gliomas arise from malignant transformation of astrocytes or other glial elements. These tumors are more infiltrative than ependymomas and are consequently much more difficult to deal with surgically.

The pain from such lesions is usually insidious in onset and is poorly localized. It is often worse at night or in the early morning, for reasons discussed above. It may occasionally be exacerbated by activity, leading to the speculation that increased blood supply to the tumor during exercise may aggravate any ongoing compression.

The key to arriving at the proper diagnosis is in recognizing that this pain is invariably associated with a defined but sometimes subtle neurologic deficit. There may be slight lower extremity hyperreflexia or subtle weakness of the upper extremities. Often, a capelike distribution of sensory deficit over the shoulders and upper arms is the first appreciable evidence of neurologic problems. These deficits rapidly progress, however, to become more readily apparent. Soon there is loss of motor function and coordination in the hands. Invariably at some point in the progression of the syndrome lower extremity hyperreflexia will develop, as will stiffness of gait and other signs of myelopathy.

There are often intradural tumors that may be associated, initially at least, predominantly with unilateral symptoms. These are tumors that usually lie within the dura but are extramedullary, the classic examples being neurofibromas and meningiomas. Here again, the history of night pain is common. These tumors may grow to totally envelop a single nerve root with no appreciable neurologic deficit on examination. Often, the patient presents with unilateral radicular pain and numbness only. Once again, as the mass grows and the spinal cord is compressed, signs and symptoms of myelopathy point the way to the correct diagnosis.

Once the tentative diagnosis of intrinsic spinal cord compression is reached, the diagnosis may be confirmed by radiologic studies. Intrathecally enhanced CT and MRI scans are most commonly available and should be the radiologic studies of choice following the plain x-ray. Treatment of these lesions is surgical and, in the case of tumors, is often supplemental by local radiation.

Intrinsic Motor and Sensory Disorders

Many primary neurologic disorders can disrupt spinal cord function. When the disorder primarily involves the motor system, it may disrupt spinal cord circuitry and cause a lack of balance between agonist and antagonist motor functions. This may cause constant paradoxical muscle spasms, or torticollis. This disorder can quickly be recognized by the patient's posturing. In severe torticollis, there is almost constant head jerking to one side or the other, and the patient soon develops osteoarthritic changes in the facet and uncinate joints that may be a source of additional pain. Unfortunately, there is no good treatment for spontaneous idiopathic torticollis. Cutting the various motor roots that innervate the involved muscles can indeed reduce the constant and abnormal motor movement; however, this comes at the price of muscle denervation and associated atrophy. Such treatment is justified only in extreme cases. Other experimental procedures are being tested that may have more promise.

Toxins can affect the nervous system and cause severe burning pain as well as neurologic deficit. In our highly industrialized society, the chance of significant exposure to potential neurotoxins is always present. The heavy metals lead and mercury, as well as more complex organic compounds, are in this group.

There are natural factors as well that have been implicated in neurologic disease. Recent reports of linkage between plants and amyotrophic lateral sclerosis (8) and the long-standing suspicions of a viral/infectious etiology for multiple sclerosis are prominent examples. Certain coral elements in the Caribbean, when eaten by fish and then by humans in the food cycle, may cause severe cervical pain. This is called *ciguatera*. Treatment of such conditions is directed toward ending exposure to the offending agent and providing supportive and curative care as needed.

On rare occasions, vascular insufficiency to the spinal cord can itself cause pain. This may occur as a result of surgery, trauma, or preexistent cardiovascular disease.

Characteristically the early stages of spinal cord ischemia will cause truncal pain that is poorly localized. Within a matter of hours, if not sooner, spinal infarction may occur, guaranteeing a devastating neurologic deficit and poor ultimate progress. Unfortunately, we do not know a great deal about how these various metabolic, toxic, or infectious disorders bring about disease on a cellular level. Further advances will be required for rapid and more effective treatment and diagnosis of such disorders.

Extrinsic Spinal Cord Neoplasms

Extra-axial neoplastic lesions of the cervical spine may cause mechanical symptoms and localized pain or may lead to neurologic deficit, depending on the site of origin of the process. Bony tumors may be divided into benign primary tumors of bone, malignant primary tumors of bone, and metastatic tumors to bone. Malignant tumor metastases to bone are far and away most common. A list of various tumor types is presented in Table 26-2.

Primary malignant bony tumors such as chordomas, osteosarcomas, and chondrosarcomas may occur in the cervical regions. Unfortunately, the bones of the cervical spine can also be involved by metastatic tumor processes. Hematologic malignancies such as multiple myeloma or lymphoma very commonly involve the axial skeleton, causing bony destruction and neurologic deficit.

It is obvious that with such an extensive list of pathologic processes it would be impossible to formulate a "typical" clinical presentation. However, some typical clinical features exist that would allow the clinician a hint.

Pain deep within the bone itself is the most common clinical presentation of all the above-listed processes. This complaint in any patient with previously diagnosed malignancy should trigger a full diagnostic workup aimed at detection of possible bony metastases. The pain is initially mechanical in nature and may be worse with motion. In addition, there is often an element of night pain. The

TABLE 26-2. *Tumors of the cervical spine*

Primary tumors
  Giant cell tumor
  Osteoblastoma
  Osteochondroma
  Eosinophilic granuloma
  Plasmacytoma
  Chondromyxoid fibroma
  Desmoid tumor
  Hemangioma
  Osteocartilaginous exostosis
  Rheumatoid pannus
Malignant tumors of the cervical spine
  Chordoma
  Chondrosarcoma
  Osteosarcoma
  Ewing's sarcoma
  Aggressive solitary plasmacytoma
  Hemangiopericytoma
Metastatic from solitary organs
  Breast
  Prostate
  Renal
  Gastrointestinal
  Thyroid
  Lung
  Nasopharyngeal
Hematogenous metastatic process
  Multiple myeloma
  Hodgkin's disease
  Lymphoma

patient typically falls asleep only to be awakened in the middle of the night with a deep underlying gnawing pain, possibly due to tumor expansion. As the pain increases in severity a radicular component usually develops. If the tumor irritates adjacent nerve roots, a radiculopathy with definite motor and sensory loss becomes apparent. As the tumor expands into the spinal canal a cervical myelopathy will readily occur. Usually, however, the neurologic symptoms occur well after the onset of pain.

Fortunately the radiologic appearance of these diseases is fairly specific. Cervical spine films with oblique views followed by CT scanning will reveal osteolytic lesions, pathologic fractures, and abnormal soft tissue masses in the majority of cases. Definitive diagnosis requires tissue biopsy, either from the cervical lesion itself or, as is sometimes possible in metastatic lesions, from the primary tumor site itself. Multiple myeloma produces "punched out" osteolytic lesions of the spine as well as a severe generalized osteoporosis, and pathologic fractures may ensue. Appropriate hematologic evaluations will usually clinch the diagnosis in these cases.

In all cases in which the cervical spine is involved by tumor there are two important treatment considerations. Ensuring the stability of the spine and maintaining neurologic functions are of paramount importance in planning treatment. Nonsurgical interventions such as radiation or chemotherapy and bracing are appropriate first-line treatments in many cases if a tissue diagnosis is already available. These may eliminate the need for surgical intervention. Close follow-up with radiologic studies and serial neurologic exams is necessary to detect progression of disease. If spinal stability or neurologic function is at risk, further consultation is required with specialists who are honestly interested in spinal surgical problems, be they neurologic or orthopedic surgeons. Many new techniques are now available to stabilize and decompress the spine, even in the most advanced of disease states. Patients with reasonable life expectancies (usually greater than 6 months) who are in medical condition to tolerate extensive operative procedures are candidates for these techniques. Unfortunately, for inpatients with a very limited prognosis as a result of extensive tumor spread or general poor health, simple bracing, supportive care, and radiation or chemotherapy are often all that is possible.

Osteoarthritis

In the vertebral column, osteoarthritic changes are usually associated with intervertebral disc degeneration. Disc degeneration, resulting from trauma or advanced age, reduces the shock absorber effect of a well-hydrated intervertebral disc and causes abnormal stresses to be applied to the vertebral body, the adjacent uncinate process (joint of Luschka), and the posterior facet areas. Over time, reactive osteophyte formation occurs along the joint interfaces. The buildup of these bony spurs may extend directly posteriorly

toward the spinal canal and cause cord compression and myelopathy. More commonly spur formation occurs at the uncinate process and facet joint, resulting thereby in neural foraminal stenosis. The most common sites of degenerative osteophytes are the C5-6 and C6-7 joint spaces.

Pure cervical osteoarthritis in itself (when not involving the nervous system) is not usually associated with a great number of symptoms. On occasion the patient may describe mechanical neck pain with radiation suggestive of but not corresponding to a radicular distribution. This may be associated with a variety of symptoms—headaches, shoulder pains, clicking sounds—that seem to be exacerbated by purely mechanical factors. For unclear reasons, high cervical disc degeneration with joint collapse and osteoarthritic changes is commonly associated with a headache that at times is impossible to separate from a tension headache. Periodically the patient may suffer acute attacks with increased neck discomfort and severe muscle pains resembling acute torticollis. These episodes are often triggered by activity and physical exertion, and peak after 2 to 3 days, with total recovery within 7 to 10 days.

When the cervical osteoarthritis has progressed to cause nerve root compression, radicular pain and symptoms are common. Lesions of this type are often referred to as "hard" discs (to be discussed below). When the cervical osteoarthritis extends posteriorly and causes central canal stenosis, cord compression and cervical spondylotic myelopathy occur. The common term for this myelopathy is *cervical spondylosis*, and the classic references describing this disorder were written in 1967 and 1971 (9,10). The combination of neck pain, increased lower extremity reflexes, stiff gait, and plain spine films showing osteophytic spurs is sufficient to make the presumptive diagnosis. The next diagnostic study of choice under these circumstances is the MRI scan. In some instances, bony anatomy may be insufficiently visualized, in which case a plain or intrathecally enhanced CT scan should be obtained. In all types of osteoarthritic disease, nonsteroidal antiinflammatory medications often speed recovery from mechanical symptoms (such as local pain and muscle spasm) and are helpful in keeping the patient active. Once the osteoarthritic changes have progressed to cause problems related to compression of neural tissue, remission of the symptoms is rare. Antiinflammatory medications and mechanical stabilization in bracing devices may prevent progression of symptoms for a long time; however, in the majority of cases well-planned operative decompressions will afford relief of symptoms and ensure that further neural tissue compression does not occur.

Nerve Root Irritations

The spinal cord is the conduit for carrying information to and from the brain. At the segmental level nerve roots gather information from the periphery and deliver motor messages to the trunk and limbs. Each of these nerve roots exits through a foramen and can be compressed by disc protrusion or osteophytes. Such compression will lead to pain in the distribution of the nerve root, and often locally as well. In explaining the problem to the patient it is often helpful to use the analogy of a telephone wire being rubbed on by a tree, which in turn produces static on the line.

Cervical radiculitis is a term applied when a nerve root is irritated and inflamed. The extension of this term, *cervical radiculopathy*, implies that damage to the root has produced a clinically appreciable motor or sensory neurologic deficit in the distribution of the root. Typically, patients with cervical root pain syndromes have neck pain made worse by extension and turning to the painful side. In addition, they will have pain that radiates either into the lower neck and shoulder (C4-5 roots) or well down into the upper extremity (C-8–T-1 roots). C-8 and C-7 root irritation in particular cause significant arm pain. These patterns are described above in the anatomic section of this chapter. Unfortunately, differentiation between these patterns can sometimes be difficult in a clinical setting. For example, differentiation between C-6 and C-7 root involvement may be difficult at times. In both of these syndromes biceps and triceps strength is affected and the patterns of sensation loss are similar: C-6 involvement causes sensation loss on the thumb and C-7 on the middle finger. Either of these syndromes can cause sensation loss on the index finger, although the C-7 syndrome does so more frequently.

The predominantly radicular nature of these patients' symptoms and complaints is the key element of the history and physical examination. Although the roots as they exit from the spinal canal can be compressed by numerous factors, by far the most common source of such irritation is either an acute disc herniation and/or a degenerative disc that in turn has caused focal osteoarthritic changes with foraminal stenosis. We commonly refer to these as "soft" and "hard" disc disease, respectively. The soft disc disorders tend to occur in patients under the age of 50. The hard disc/osteoarthritis spur formation tends to occur in the older population, although obviously there are no absolutes.

After obtaining a medical history and physical examination, diagnostic studies will often pinpoint which root is involved. Neurophysiologic studies such as EMG/NCV are helpful in pinpointing the level involved; however, diagnostic imaging is essential to making the correct diagnosis and in formulating treatment. In addition, in some patients (particularly those who have ill-defined neck and shoulder pain that is not clearly radicular in nature) plain shoulder films may be useful to rule out glenohumeral joint disease. The first and most basic diagnostic study, however, should be the plain cervical spine film with oblique views. In younger patients and in those who have normal-appearing plain x-rays, the next diagnostic study of choice is MRI, which will usually show the soft discs better than other diagnostic modalities will. In older patients and in those who have evidence of degenerative disc disease and spurs on plain films, the preferable next study is an intrathecally enhanced CT scan, which will allow better visualization of bony anatomy than MRI will.

Treatment of these lesions requires decompression of the affected root. In selected cases cervical bracing and traction or physical therapy may be of long-term benefit; however, in the vast majority this decompression is best accomplished surgically.

Gout, Multiple Sclerosis, Amyotrophic Lateral Sclerosis, Syringomyelia, Klippel-Feil Syndrome

Gouty arthritis is associated with elevation of uric acid levels and deposits within various joints. Although the disease commonly affects such joints as the big toe, it definitely can influence the spinal axis, including the cervical spine. Patients with known gouty arthritis have an increased incidence of degenerative changes in the cervical spine. The radiographic appearance is identical to that of osteoarthritis. The symptoms cannot be differentiated from those of the cervical myeloradiculopathies, and the treatment is basically the same. In the acute episode of the presentation, confirmation of the uric acid levels and use of uricosuric agents is appropriate as well.

Multiple sclerosis can occur in conjunction with osteoarthritic changes in the cervical spine. It is true that the two diseases together can accentuate an existing myelopathy. Decompressive procedures are only half as successful in this condition as they are in the routine setting, and the chance of symptomatic relief after surgery is less than 50%. Consequently, in these settings, only 50% of patients truly benefit from any type of decompressive laminectomy, foraminotomy, anterior cervical discectomy, or the like. It appears that when a fusion is done with an anterior discectomy, the spine is slightly more stabilized and there are better results in the relief of not only the pain but also the intrinsic neurologic problem. This probably is related to immobilization of the spinal cord, which is already diseased.

Amyotrophic lateral sclerosis can be present in patients with some pain caused by the associated arthritic changes that occur in the spine. The neurologic disease itself is painless. However, because of the imbalances along the spine caused by muscular weakness, arthritic changes can occur with some discomfort to the patients. Symptomatic treatment is all that is required. Rarely do any of these cases need operative surgery.

Syringomyelia was always thought to be a painless disease. In specific, patients experienced numbness in a cape-like distribution over the shoulders and arms, with muscle weakness primarily in the hands. Often they would have a myelopathy as well. As revealed by information obtained from MRI studies, however, syringomyelia usually presents initially as pain, often in a root fashion. This pain accompanies the initial development of the syrinx. As the syrinx enlarges, the pain fibers are destroyed and the patient has less pain. It is most beneficial to treat these patients early, with correction of the syrinx itself. This can be done by correcting the Arnold-Chiari malformation at the base of the skull if that exists and/or draining the syrinx into either the pleural or the peritoneal cavity. If the syrinx is adequately drained, patients will have less pain. Even with the most successful procedure, rarely is all the patient's discomfort obliterated.

When a patient has congenital blocked vertebrae, as in Klippel-Feil syndrome, there is an increased instance of osteoarthritic changes at an adjacent level, usually cephalad and rarely caudally. With an immobile joint in the cervical spine, the next superior joint often has accelerated degenerative changes with osteophyte formation. This can lead to a radiculitis and/or myelopathy. If the usual measures of physical therapy, proper exercises, and antiinflammatory medications fail, then the patients often do require decompressive procedures on the nerve roots. If there is marked compression anteriorly, an anterior operation can be done. Rarely do patients require more-extensive fusions posteriorly.

Cervical Trauma

Cervical spine trauma is almost invariably diagnosed on the historic facts alone. In taking a history, details of the traumatic event should be recorded succinctly and accurately, because this may prove germane to further events in our current litigious society. The trauma itself may be divided into its neurologic, bony and ligamentous, and muscular components, and each may give rise to significant pain. The most frequent cervical spine traumatic event that causes pain is muscle sprain or strain, more commonly referred to as whiplash injury. Under normal conditions of wear and tear, the cervical muscles modulate many of the forces being transmitted to the cervical spine via balanced contraction and relaxation. Rapid, large changes in motion or force, as occur in cervical spine injury, may exceed the capacity of the cervical musculature to compensate, leading to muscle strain and tears. Larger disruptive forces may cause bony and ligamentous damage in addition to the muscular injury. Classically the pain associated with muscle strain develops to a maximum after about 2 to 3 weeks. In the setting of trauma, local neck pain with spasm, and stiffness of cervical muscles, normal neurologic examination and normal diagnostic studies (if performed at all; usually plain films only) are the criteria that must be met before this diagnosis can be confidently made. If any one of these criteria is not met, then other cervical spine injury beyond muscle spasm must be suspected, and further diagnostic work-up is appropriate and necessary. Similarly, traumatic neck pain that persists for more than 3 weeks after injury should raise a red flag, and should be considered suspicious of bony or ligamentous origin until proven otherwise.

Mild cases of cervical sprain are usually best treated with mild nonnarcotic analgesics and application of heat packs. In more severe cases, decreasing cervical mobility with a bracing device such as a soft collar and the judicious use of antispasm medications such as cyclobenzaprine (Flexeril) or carisoprodol (Soma) may be required.

Trauma with bony or ligamentous disruption is caused by extreme abnormal movements or compressive forces in the neck. Although the head itself only weighs from 10 to 15 pounds, that weight alone is in extreme flexion and tension sufficient to damage bones. Furthermore, although protected from extremes of movement in flexion and extension by muscle and ligament, the cervical vertebrae are very vulnerable to axial compressive forces. These forces are commonly generated in diving and automobile accidents, thus accounting for the high percentage of cervical spine injury in such cases. The injury from such forces is variable, and may result in ligamentous tear, bony fracture, or dislocation and malalignment depending on the location and force vectors involved.

In general, bony and ligamentous cervical spine injuries can usually be classified into flexion, compression, or tension-type injuries. On rare occasions distraction injuries may occur, especially in the upper cervical and occipital areas. The pain associated with bony and ligamentous trauma is mechanical, sharp, and exacerbated by even the slightest cervical motion. In the absence of damage to neural structures, radicular or dysesthetic pain may not be present.

In the setting of trauma and neck pain, plain cervical spine films (particularly the lateral view) are essential. All seven cervical vertebrae must be visualized, as must be the occiput–C-1 and C-7–T-1 junctions. Additional views such as oblique views are often helpful. Cooperative patients may have flexion and extension films (with careful monitoring of neurologic function at each position, of course) to further document the degree of instability. Generally, the more abnormal the first lateral cervical spine radiograph, the lesser the need for further films. If the films initially appear normal and bony pathology is still suspected, then additional views such as oblique or flexion/extension should be attempted. If following adequate films any uncertainty remains regarding bony anatomy, CT scan becomes mandatory.

Trauma may leave the patient neurologically intact and with x-rays that are unimpressive. In these cases, ligamentous and/or joint capsular tearing is usually the source of pain. In most cases, the patients can localize the discomfort accurately to the level of the lesion. Local injection of damaged facets or ligaments with anesthetic agents is both diagnostic and therapeutic in this case.

In the neck with unstable bony disruption or significant malalignment secondary to trauma, skeletal tong traction must be initiated early to achieve stability. The only exceptions to this rule are disruption injuries causing distraction of the occiput from C-1 or C-2. In these cases, the application of traction can worsen the distraction and literally "pull the head off." In all other instances, however, bony alignment with judicious use of traction, multiple sequential lateral cervical spine films, and close monitoring of neurologic status is the appropriate course of action and should be carried out as rapidly as feasible.

Finally, cervical spine trauma may result in injury to the nervous tissue itself. Although this most commonly occurs in the setting of cervical spine fractures, damage to neural structures may also occur independently of this, as in traumatic anterior spinal artery or central cord syndromes. Focal pain at the site of injury and the presence of neurologic deficit are presumptive evidence of traumatic cord/root injury. The classic picture is of flaccid plegia or paresis during the spinal shock phase that eventually gives way to spasticity and upper extremity lower motor neuron deficits. Proximal motor function may be preserved, but the fine motor control needed for adequate hand function is invariably lost. Numbness, clumsiness, and even complete paralysis of the hands is the rule rather than the exception in these situations, and hand dysfunction may even exceed lower extremity dysfunction. This is particularly true with central cord syndromes, where upper extremity lower motor neuron lesions figure prominently.

When there is neurologic deficit in the presence of spinal trauma, adequate visualization of the spinal cord/thecal sac is essential for planning further treatment. Bony fragments, herniated discs, and epidural hematomas may all cause persistent cord compression independent of that caused by the initial traumatic blow itself. Intrathecally enhanced CT or MRI scanning is therefore required.

Treatment centers around the dual needs to stabilize the spinal column and to alleviate ongoing neural compression. The institution of skeletal traction is a valuable first step toward stabilizing the spinal column and may alleviate neural compression as well. Thus, judicious use of skeletal traction is the first treatment choice. Surgery, either to relieve ongoing neural compression or to internalize a stabilization construct, should be considered rapidly thereafter if the patient's clinical status will allow. This will be followed with 6 weeks to 3 months in a rigid cervical orthosis until the surgical fusion is stable.

RHEUMATOID ARTHRITIS

Rheumatoid arthritis is a chronic inflammatory disease of probable, although undefined, infectious etiology. Subsequent to the presumed infection, a broad immunologic response is generated that after prolonged periods of time leads to characteristic changes in many joints of the body. The prevalence of this disorder in the United States is roughly 1% of the population. Although juvenile forms exist, more frequently it is the elderly patient with rheumatoid arthritis who develops cervical spine pain and arthritic changes. The cervical spine is commonly involved, especially in the C-1–C-2 area. Inflammatory processes in this region cause exuberant pannus formation, bony destruction, and ligamentous laxity. Atlanto-occipital subluxation, basilar investigation, and atlantoaxial subluxation are frequent end results.

Mechanical neck pain is the initial presenting symptomatology. Occipital headache and muscle spasm can also

occur. Extremes of bony and ligamentous instability may allow cord compression, resulting in lower cranial nerve palsies, myelopathy, and facial numbness. Trivial trauma in the presence of this instability may cause acute, devastating neurologic deficit. More commonly, the patient presents with simple neck pain and as followed over time develops a gait disturbance with myelopathy and associated changes.

The diagnosis of rheumatoid arthritis is often made on physical examination alone because the findings in patients with rheumatoid arthritis are multiple and characteristic. Confirmatory laboratory evidence is obtained by elevated erythrocyte sedimentation rate and rheumatoid factor screen. Radiologic evidence of rheumatoid arthritis is best obtained on plain spine films. Tomograms will also disclose the loss of bony tissue with further appreciation of atlantoaxial subluxation. More recently, with MRI, the actual pannus buildup in and around the dens can be seen. Treatment of the mechanical pain of cervical spine rheumatoid arthritis relies on steroidal and nonsteroidal antiinflammatory agents. The development of significant (usually greater than 1 cm) subluxation at C-1–C-2, spinal instability, or neurologic deficit warrants serious consideration of surgical decompressive/stabilization procedures. Such a procedure is a major operation for many of the senior patients involved, and the morbidity of the postsurgical bracing devices (i.e., the halo brace) is not insignificant in this population. Nonetheless, such treatment is warranted since the natural history of this disease in a patient with symptomatic neural compression is indeed most bleak.

Ankylosing Spondylitis

Ankylosing spondylitis is an inflammatory joint disorder with a striking predilection for the cartilaginous joints of the axial skeleton. The main pathologic features involve abnormal deposition of calcium and spontaneous fusion of the ligamentous and facet structures. Although ankylosing spondylitis is commonly associated with the lumbosacral spine, it may also advance to involve the neck. It is initially associated with gradual onset of pain and aching in the lower back and buttocks. Morning stiffness is often present; this tends to improve with exercise during the day. There may be an associated mild peripheral arthritis. Mechanical spine pain and restriction of mobility go hand in hand. Compression of neural structures is rare, and radicular and myelopathic pain patterns are therefore rarely present. The abnormally fused spine becomes brittle and is therefore fractured easily even with minor trauma. This may cause acute onset of neurologic complaints.

Diagnosis may be made on the basis of plain spine films. The high association of this disease with BLA-B27 antigen type warrants this type of testing as well.

Often confused with ankylosing spondylitis is a hyperostotic disorder that primarily affects the anterior longitudinal ligament of the spine. This is referred to as the *diffuse idiopathic skeletal hyperostosis (DISH)* syndrome. It has also been termed *Forestier's disease* (11). Fortunately, this unusual form of ankylosing hyperostosis does not require specific therapy outside of occasional nonsteroidal antiinflammatory medications and continuous physical therapy modalities.

Infections

Although infections of the cervical spine are rare, the consequences of failure to make a proper diagnosis and initiate therapy in a timely fashion are so devastating that discussion is appropriate.

Whereas neoplastic processes usually begin in the bone and spare the disc space, infection is just the opposite; it usually begins in the disc space, with bony destruction occurring only later. The most common offending organisms are staphylococcal and streptococcal species, usually introduced into the area by iatrogenic means or by hematogenous spread from other foci. Other infectious organisms, such as tuberculosis, brucellosis, anaerobic bacteria, and fungi, are rare in this country except in specific host populations. Younger patients especially are susceptible to streptococcal infections, which may spread to the nasopharyngeal and tonsillar area and into the retropharyngeal space and on rare occasions become localized in a disc space. In the young adult the most common infection is usually staphylococcal. In the older person or in immunosuppressed individuals, tuberculosis and other more indolent infections may be seen. Finally, select patients with severe immunosuppression may develop fungal infections of the spine.

When the infections occur within the spine, there is relatively little systemic and/or immunologic response initially. Fever, sweats, and constitutional symptoms are common but not universal. Neck pain, with radiation to the shoulders and back of the head, is a predominant symptom of cervical spine infection. Invariably patients will have restricted range of motion of their neck and rather striking muscle spasms. These nonspecific complaints are often present for several weeks to months before the diagnosis is even entertained. If the infection tracks into the prevertebral space, dysphagia, dysphasia, and hoarseness may occur. Myelopathy is a late and ominous sign, indicative of epidural compression and possible epidural abscess.

Unfortunately, radiographic bony changes usually take 3 to 6 weeks to develop; thus the diagnosis of earlier, potentially more easily curable infection is difficult. Bone scanning with gallium or technetium or labeled white cells has become an important diagnostic adjuvant in these disorders. Elevated systemic white count as well as high erythrocyte sedimentation rate will point to possible infectious processes as well.

Making the proper microbiologic diagnosis may require aspiration or open biopsy and drainage. More recently more-aggressive care has been widely recommended. This protocol includes biopsy, drainage, curettage, and con-

comitant bony fusion occurring as the initial surgical procedure, and it has been very successful. The organism is identified, and appropriate antimicrobial coverage is continued for at least 6 weeks. After the cervical stabilization procedure, external immobilization with a rigid orthosis is commonly required.

CLINICAL CONCLUSIONS

The study of neck pain in cervical spine disorders is almost a specialty within itself, with rheumatologists, neurologists, orthopedic surgeons, and neurosurgeons all very interested in and committed to understanding these disorders. With a complaint so common as neck pain it is obvious that every patient cannot and should not see a specialist. Therefore some general guidelines should be outlined for the initiation of treatment of these patients.

Patients with pain in the neck with or without cord or root complaints will need to be seen on several occasions in order to make the proper diagnosis and assess treatment. The interval between these visits may vary, but in general should be proportionate to how ill the patient is. If the patient is suspected of harboring a serious neoplastic process or infection, or has suffered severe trauma with neurologic deficit, then hospitalization and more than two or three visits a day may be appropriate. The majority of patients with new-onset cervical pain will do well with an interval of 2 to 3 weeks between office visits. On the other hand, if the patient has a long-term complaint without impressive physical or radiographic findings, then the interval between visits can be 3 to 4 weeks, if not longer. The fundamental steps in managing the patient at each visit are basically the same and are outlined below.

Visit 1

Visit 1 includes the initial history and physical examination. Initial diagnostic testing, such as plain spine films, is often carried out at this time, although in most cases of simple neck pain from muscle sprain this is not indicated. It is wise at this time for the physician to give the patient an initial impression of what he or she believes the patient is suffering from. Treatment can be based on diagnostic impression, and oftentimes will be symptomatic only, such as with nonsteroidal antiinflammatory medications. The neck may be immobilized with some type of collar or brace, with instructions to evaluate response to immobilization. The majority of patients will not require more than a single office visit.

Visit 2

If the patient's neck pain has not improved after a sufficient period (usually 2 to 3 weeks) of initial treatment, several options exist. It is mandatory first, however, to reexamine the patient for evolution in signs and symptoms. If the patient is clinically stable at this point, medications could be changed to either another nonsteroidal antiinflammatory medication or to stronger pain medications. Utilization of such modalities as exercise and physical therapy also may be appropriate at this time. At this second visit complete cervical spine films with flexion, extension, and oblique views should be obtained regardless of diagnostic impressions. This study remains the single most important diagnostic study available to us. While the cervical spine x-rays are being done, screening hematologic evaluation, including complete blood count, rheumatoid factor, or erythrocyte sedimentation rate, could also be obtained.

Visit 3

If the patient has not responded to the second line of treatments after a reasonable time and all the studies obtained during the second office visit are normal, again repeat physical examination is warranted, and the differential diagnosis should be mentally reviewed. If the patient is clinically stable, medications should again be changed and additional studies ordered as below. In younger patients and those with normal cervical spine films, MRI is the next most important diagnostic study. This will point out soft tissue defects and herniated discs as well as visualize the neural elements. On the other hand, if there are significant arthritic changes, bony destruction, or malalignment on plain films, then the CT scan with or without intrathecal contrast is the study of choice.

Visit 4

In some patients an acceptable diagnosis will still not have been reached even after repeat physical examination, plain films, CT scan, and/or MRI. At this time looking for clinical oddities is warranted. Patients who have had MRI studies should have CT studies next, and vice versa. Other testing, such as EMG/NCV and bone scans, may be appropriate in specific situations. Additional blood work is also done.

Visit 5

If the patient is continuing to suffer from cervical spine pain at this point, now usually 2 to 3 months after initial presentation, then consultation and further diagnostic tests/procedures should be carried out. A more sophisticated mechanical examination of the neck by orthopedists or rheumatologists is warranted. A more detailed neuro-logic examination by neurologists or neurosurgeons is often appropriate as well. Further diagnostic studies also should be carried out, such as bone scanning, complete myelography, and lumbar puncture if indicated. Obviously, decisions need to be made on an individual basis. With each visit, if the patient is still failing to improve, medication changes should be considered. There are over a dozen nonsteroidal antiinflammatory medications, and it is important to try many, for patients may vary greatly in their response.

SUBSEQUENT PATIENT MANAGEMENT

Visits subsequent to the fifth one should be to either a competent rheumatologist or orthopedic surgeon or neurosurgeon, because the patient will probably not get well quickly, and further consultation and advice is needed. This is frequently the beginning of the chronic neck pain syndrome. It may be that nothing more can be done for the individual. It may also be that secondary gain or conversion disorders may be operative, especially in cases involving litigation and workers' compensation. In this case psychological evaluation should be seriously considered.

In any case, by following this guideline a logical and fairly complete evaluation of the patient with cervical spine pain will have been performed. In the vast majority of cases an appropriate diagnosis is obtained and appropriate treatments are started with excellent relief of symptoms.

REFERENCES

 1. Lawrence J. Disc degeneration, its frequency and relationship to symptoms. *Ann Rheum Dis* 1989;28:121.
 2. British Association of Physical Medicine. Pain in the neck and arm. *Br Med J* 1986;1:253.
 3. Hult L. Cervical, dorsal and lumbar spinal syndromes. *Acta Orthop Scand* 1954;(Suppl)17:1.
 4. Hult L. The Munkford Investigation. *Acta Orthop Scand* 1954;(Suppl)16:1.
 5. Spurling RG, Scoville WB. Lateral rupture of the cervical intervertebral discs. *Surg Gynecol Obstet* 1944;78:350.
 6. Bland J. *Disorders of the cervical spine.* Philadelphia: WB Saunders, 1987:40.
 7. Wilkins R. Regachary SP. *Neurosurgery.* New York: McGraw-Hill, 1985.
 8. Spencer P, Nunn P, Hugan J, et al. Guam amyotrophic lateral sclerosis-parkinsonism-dementia linked to a plant excitant neurotoxin. *Science* 1987;237:517–522.
 9. Brain W. *Cervical spondylosis.* Philadelphia: WB Saunders, 1967.
10. Wilkenson M. *Cervical spondylosis: its early diagnosis and treatment.* Philadelphia: WB Saunders, 1971.
11. Rosnick D, Niawayama G. Radiographic and pathological features of spinal involvement in diffuse idiopathic skeletal hyperostosis (DISH). *Radiology* 1978;119:558.

CHAPTER **27**

Differential Diagnosis of Low Back Pain

John A. McCulloch, Derek Snook and Bradley K. Weiner

The following question is frequently asked by doctors at various stages of training and practice experience: "How can I assess and treat a patient with back pain when the diagnosis is so elusive?" It is hard on the ego to assess a patient and fail to arrive at a concrete diagnosis on which to base a treatment program. All too often, a treatment program for low back pain is based more on hope than on science. This should not be so. In today's medical world, our clinical skills and our investigative tools are such that we should be able to arrive at the correct diagnosis for most patients with "lumbago or sciatica." This chapter outlines the simple steps needed to assess a patient who presents with a complaint of low back pain.

ASSESSMENT METHOD

Do not initiate your assessment with a long list of time-consuming differential diagnoses on your menu. In family practice, this presents an overwhelming burden to the multitude of chief complaints heard during a day. Instead, adopt a simple, methodical approach. Your goal is to sort those patients who have mechanical or structural problems in the low back from those who have not. In a family practice setting, perhaps 20% to 25% of patients presenting with low back pain will have a source outside of the back as the cause of their symptoms. This fact presents many pitfalls for the unwary. For this reason, accurate evaluation requires a logical, step-by-step method. The foundation of this method is the clinical assessment, the good old-fashioned history and physical examination. Investigations such as magnetic resonance imaging (MRI), computed tomography (CT) scanning, and myelography should play a secondary role to clinical assessment. Today, our investigative tools are so sophisticated that one can find pathology in almost every patient whether or not the patient is sick (1,2). Moreover, minor insignificant pathology can become

the red herring that causes you to miss the symptom-producing lesion.

CLINICAL APPROACH

In assessing a patient with a low back complaint, ask yourself five questions:

1. Is this a true physical disability, or are there a setting and a pattern on history and physical examination to suggest a nonphysical or nonorganic problem?
2. Is this clinical presentation a diagnostic trap?
3. Is this a mechanical low back pain condition, and if so, what is the syndrome?
4. Are there clues to an anatomical level on history and physical examination?
5. After reviewing the results of investigation, what is the structural lesion, and does it fit with the clinical syndrome?

Although these questions may not be answered sequentially during the history and physical examination, they ultimately must be answered sequentially before arriving at a diagnosis and prescribing a treatment program. That is to say, do not answer question 5 and plan a treatment program based on a radiographic diagnosis until you have satisfactory answers to each preceding question. Probably the biggest pitfall is to answer question 3 before you have satisfactorily answered questions 1 and 2. The answers to questions 1 and 2 should routinely be made outside the hospital and before CT, myelography, MRI, and other sophisticated investigative modalities are used. The classic trap is to ignore questions 1 and 2 and admit a patient with a complaint of low back pain to the hospital, order sophisticated tests, and then prescribe a treatment plan based on false-positive radiographic findings.

Each of the five questions listed here will be dealt with in its own section.

QUESTION 1

Is this a true physical disability, or are there a setting and a pattern on history and physical examination to suggest a non-physical or nonorganic problem?

That medicine should concern itself with the whole person is often stated but frequently ignored. The hallmark of a good clinician is the ability not only to diagnose disease but also to assess the "whole patient." No test of the art of medicine is more demanding than the identification of the patient with a nonorganic or emotional component to a back disability.

To start, recognize the disability equation:

$$\text{Disability} = A + B + C$$

where

A = the physical component (disease)

B = the patient's emotional reaction

C = the situation the patient is in at the time of disability (e.g., compensation claim, motor vehicle accident)

Each patient presenting with a back disability may have some component of each of these entities entwined in the disability. For example, a patient presenting a collection of symptoms, with no physical disability evident on examination, should lead one to think of the other aspects of the equation and look for emotional disability or situational reactions.

A classification of nonorganic spinal pain is outlined in Table 27-1. The term *nonorganic* has been chosen over other terms such as *nonphysical, functional, emotional,* and *psychogenic.* The following definitions are used for the classification in Table 27-1.

1. *Psychosomatic spinal pain.* Psychosomatic spinal pain is defined as symptomatic physical change in tissues of the spine that has as its cause anxiety. The expression of anxiety is mediated as a prolonged and exaggerated state that eventually leads to structural change (spasm) in the muscles of the neck or low back.

2a. *Psychogenic spinal pain.* Psychogenic spinal pain is defined as the conversion or somatization of anxiety into pain located in the neck or back, unaccompanied by physical change in the tissues of these regions. The pain is variously known in the literature as conversion hysteria, psychogenic regional pain, traumatic or accident neurosis, and hypochondriasis.

TABLE 27-1. *Nonorganic spinal pain*

1. Psychosomatic spinal pain
   a. Tension syndrome (fibrositis)
2. Psychogenic spinal pain
   a. Psychogenic spinal pain
   b. Psychogenic modification of organic spinal pain
3. Situational spinal pain
   a. Litigation reaction
   b. Exaggeration reaction

The emotional upset brings pains to the back just as it may bring tears to the eyes. The reason for the conversion is found in complex psychodynamic mechanisms beyond the scope of this chapter. The reaction represents a sincere unconscious emotional illness that offers the patient the primary gain of solving inner conflicts, fears, and anxieties. Inherent in the conversion reaction is the concept of suggestion and hypnosis, the importance of which will become apparent later in this chapter.

2b. *Psychogenic modification of organic spinal pain.* Psychogenic modification of spinal pain is a sincere emotional reaction that modifies the appreciation of an organic pain. Usually, the organic pain by itself would not be disabling, but with the psychogenic modification a significant disability ensues. No associated physical change occurs as a result of anxiety, and a conversion reaction may or may not coexist (3).

An example is the patient burdened with life-situational pressures (mortgage payments, car payments) who, because of his physical illness, believes he cannot sustain the effort necessary to meet these demands. A resulting depression may occur, and the symptoms of fatigue, loss of appetite, insomnia, impotence, constipation, and the like so dominate the history that the underlying physical condition is missed. Other examples are patients with passive-dependent personality, drug or alcohol dependence, or psychosis who, in the face of a minor physical problem, use their illness to step out of the demands of the real world.

Some obsessive-compulsive patients cannot adjust to a minor physical problem, and this personality trait leads them to believe they have a significant disability.

3. *Situational spinal pain.* Situational spinal pain is a reaction whereby a patient, through a collection of symptoms, maintains a situation (with potential secondary gain) through overconcern (3a) or conscious effort (3b).

3a. *Litigation reaction.* The litigation or compensation reaction is defined as overconcern by the patient for present and future health, arising out of a litigious or compensable event that initially affected health. The reaction manifests itself in patient's complaint of continuing neck or back pain coupled with a concern that, upon formal severance from her claim to compensation, deterioration in health may occur. The patient with this reaction is neither physically nor emotionally ill.

This reaction is not to be confused with the ambiguous terms *litigation neurosis* or *compensation neurosis.* Like "whiplash," these terms have no medical or legal value and should be dropped from our vocabulary. If a patient has a true neurosis arising out of a litigious or compensable event (accident), then those terms listed under *Psychogenic spinal pain (2a)* should be used for diagnostic purposes (e.g., traumatic neurosis or accident neurosis). If the patient's disability appears to be based more on his awareness of the commercial value of his symptoms, his reaction should not be legitimized by the use of the term *neurosis* in conjunction with the words *litigation* or *compensation* (thus *litigation reaction*).

3b. Exaggeration reaction. Exaggeration reactions are attempts by the patient to appear ill or to magnify an existent illness. *Malingering* is a term frequently applied to the reaction and is defined as "the conscious alteration of health for gain."

As is described later, it is possible for the physician to detect efforts to magnify pain, but it is not proper for him to assign motives (gain) to the patient. The lawyer involved is in a reversed role. He may raise doubts about the plaintiff's motives (gain), but he is in no position to clinically detect the effort to magnify or exaggerate. The choice of the word *malingering* implies proficiency in two professions, an uncommon occurrence. For this reason, the terms *malingering* and *conscious effort* are best not used by the physician when discussing nonorganic spinal pain.

Alteration of health in order to deceive, to evade responsibility, or to derive gain does occur. Those who would deny its occurrence deny the existence of human nature. The patient who tries to alter or reproduce symptoms or signs of a spinal problem may do so in a number of ways:

1. *Pretension:* No physical illness exists, and the patient willfully fabricates symptoms and signs. Occurring infrequently in the military during wartime, it is a rare civilian event.
2. *Exaggeration:* Symptoms and signs of a spinal disability are magnified to represent more than they really do.
3. *Perseveration:* As a manifestation of back disability, perseveration is a continuing complaint by the patient after the physical cause of the disability has ceased to exist.
4. *Allegation:* Genuine disability is present, but the patient fraudulently ascribes these to some cause, associated with gain, knowing that, in fact, his condition is of different origin (e.g., a fall at home instead of at work).

Civilian nonorganic situational spinal pain is usually of the exaggeration or perseveration type. Pretension and allegation are uncommon forms of gainful alteration of health in civilian practice. Like the patient with the litigation reaction, these patients are neither emotionally nor physically ill. They differ from patients with the litigation reaction, however, in that they are attempting to demonstrate physical illness through the effort of exaggeration or perseveration. The reason for this effort is usually, but not always, found in secondary financial gain.

Clinical Description

Before describing each of these entities, it is important to emphasize a few points. First, the preceding classification is a simplistic one that is useful only to the family practitioner or the spinal surgeon. It does not allow for the more complex assessments done by psychologists, psychiatrists,

and the like, but it does allow for a foundation on which to build clinical recognition of these entities so that the patient can be referred to others more skilled in the field. Second, one cannot rigidly define disability because there are gray areas. There is a tendency for a nonorganic disability to fall largely into one category, however. Third, it is most important to determine if one of the following settings exists for nonorganic disabilities:

1. A patient who has had previous emotional problems is prone to have an emotional component to a disability. Symptoms such as fatigue, sleeplessness, agitation, gastrointestinal upset, and excessive sweating should signal that an emotional component is likely present.
2. A patient who is in a secondary gain situation such as a motor vehicle accident claim has the potential for these nonorganic reactions. It is important to establish the presence of such circumstances early in the patient encounter. If a patient states that low back pain started suddenly with an incident, it is important to document whether or not the incident is a claim type of accident and whether or not insurance and legal factors are involved. Conversely, if there is no secondary gain detected on history, it is unusual to arrive at a secondary gain diagnosis such as litigation reaction or exaggeration reaction.
3. A vague and confusing history, a baffling physical examination, and an elusive diagnosis signal a possible nonorganic diagnosis. Reflect on this before taking the expensive step of hospital admission and sophisticated testing.
4. A patient who quickly establishes an abnormal doctor-patient relationship has a potential nonorganic component to his disability. These abnormal doctor-patient relationships include a hostile or effusively complimentary patient, a patient who has had many other doctors involved in care prior to your assessment, a patient who fails to respond to standard conservative treatment measures, and a patient who is critical of other doctors.

Psychosomatic Spinal Pain

The psychosomatic phenomenon of muscle spasm arising out of tension states usually affects the neck but may affect the low back. It should be known as the *orthopedic ulcer* but more often is given the label of *fibrositis.* Patients with this problem are overtly strained and tense, as evidenced by facial expression. They are fidgety and restless and may sit on the edge of the chair while they wring their hands. Some of these patients will place their hands on their neck or back during the history and literally wring the area while describing the pain. They have a general feeling of restlessness and a specific feeling of a tightness in their neck with associated sensations of cracking and a constant feeling of the need to stretch out the neck and shoulder muscles. The pain is not specifically mechanical but does tend to accumulate with the day's activity, especially when that activity is carried out in the tension-producing environment (e.g., work).

The pain typically responds to chiropractic or physiotherapeutic intervention, but relief is usually temporary, a fact that makes the patient tend to seek prolonged care.

Physical examination reveals a good range of movement in the back, with a complaint of pain only if movement is done too quickly or carried to extremes. The significant physical finding is the presence of firm, tender muscles when the affected part is examined in a position of rest—the so-called "trigger point." The patient may be able to demonstrate the "cracking" to the touch or hearing of the examiner.

No evidence of nerve root involvement exists in the lower extremities. Skin tenderness, the significance of which is explained later, is not a usual finding.

Psychogenic Spinal Pain

Patients with psychogenic spinal pain are emotionally ill. These patients often have a history of past illnesses replete with emotional problems. It follows that the history of the present illness contains a preponderance of emotional symptoms, and the description of the pain will not be typical of any organic condition. The patient is convinced that she is ill, and that conviction extends to the frequent demand for consultations with numerous doctors. Considerable financial hardship and aggravation will occur in some cases when these consultations take the patient great distances to and from major clinics or spas throughout the world. Throughout their constant demand for care, such patients notice times when their symptoms do improve. This is due to the institution of some new form of treatment that affects the patients through suggestion or hypnosis, a fact that makes placebo trial of little value in the evaluation of these problems.

It follows that because these patients are emotionally ill, no causative organic problem will be found on physical examination. The conversion reaction is associated with an upset body image appreciation such that a topographic unit (the back and leg), indifferent to matters of innervation or anatomical relationship, will contain physical findings of skin tenderness and dulled sensory appreciation (3). The somatization infrequently reaches the stage of weakness with wasting and depression of all the reflexes in the contiguous part (e.g., an arm or leg).

The important observation on physical examination of such patients is the paucity of physical findings, which separates these patients from the magnifier and exaggerator, who by definition has many "physical" findings.

Psychogenic Modification of Organic Spinal Pain

Of all the patients with nonorganic causes of spinal pain, the patient who psychogenically modifies organic pain presents the most difficult diagnostic and therapeutic challenge. Sometimes, but not always, the organic problem by itself would not be disabling. Thus, the historic and physical component of the disability related to the organicity is not significant. Those findings indicative of a physical illness will be appropriate and a quantitative guide to the extent of physical illness. The life-situational pressures or the personality of the patient modify the disability to a significant point, however. Also, the psychogenic reaction interferes with response to treatment and leads to persistence of the disability. In a surgical practice, this failure to respond to conservative treatment is the classic indication for operative intervention. If the surgeon fails to recognize that the failure to respond to treatment is due in this instance to a psychogenic disability, he will gradually build a practice containing a number of spinal surgery failures. Psychogenic modifications are commonly seen in the patient with an inadequate personality. By definition, the patient's personality may limit advancement up the social, educational, and occupational ladders and confine him to the unskilled worker classification. Some of these patients can be found in the worker's compensation board population and may be one of the reasons for poorer results of treatment sometimes obtained in the "comp" patient.

These patients are seen with a minor physical problem (e.g., back strain) yet have a total disability. All attempts at treatment fail to return patients to the workforce. Frequent office visits reinforce the disability for the patients. If the doctor fails to recognize this maladaptive reaction and reinforcement, he may add a scar to or stick a needle into the back, which will not help the patients in any way.

Other psychogenic modifications come about through drug addiction and alcohol dependence. Occasionally, psychotic behavior will convert a minor physical problem into a prolonged disability. Physical examination will reveal the nature and extent of the physical impairment. Usually the physical impairment by itself would not be significantly disabling. The loss of movement in the back is minor, the limitation of straight leg-raising is minimal, and the neurological changes are of questionable significance. In the face of repeated assessments and a continuing statement of disability, the patient's minor physical problem may become magnified in the mind of the clinician who does not assess personality and life-situational factors.

Situational Spinal Pain—Litigation Reaction

The litigation reaction patient is neither physically nor emotionally ill. Thus, few emotional symptoms will be present on historic examination. The patient is in the process of litigation or under the care of the worker's compensation board. Such patients often state that they do not care about the litigious or compensation issue, yet they also state that they are afraid to settle or return to work for fear that further illness will develop. Their continuing complaints are rather vague and would not normally be incapacitating. If they are on treatment, they are not improving. Physically, there may be an increased awareness of the part as manifested by skin tenderness in the affected area, but no organic illness is detectable, and there is no attempt to exaggerate or magnify a disability.

Situational Spinal Pain—Exaggeration Reaction

Some or most of the following historic characteristics will be obtained from the exaggeration reaction patient. The most obvious historic point is the secondary gain situation, which usually involves the fault of someone else and/or payment of financial compensation. Other secondary gain situations can occur. The initiating event is usually a trivial or minor incident. There may be a latent period of hours or days between the incident and the onset of symptoms, during which time the patient speaks to friends and relatives and learns the commercial value of the injury.

The patient describes the pain with some degree of indifference as evidenced by a smile or a laugh when describing his severe disability. He is vague in describing and localizing the pain, giving the examiner the impression of someone struggling to remember a dream. Specificity and elaboration require memory for repetition, a quality not present to a significant degree in this type of patient. The individual wishes you to believe that this pain is unique and severe. This attempt to have you believe in the pain is often accompanied by a salesman-like attitude with many examples of the disability spontaneously listed. Inability to engage in sex is frequently mentioned.

In spite of the trivial initiating event, the disability may have been present for a long time. Three types of treatment patterns occur:

1. The patient follows a "straight line" course of treatment; he does not respond to the standard treatment, nor to the suggestion of treatment (i.e., he does not improve, or he gets worse).
2. The patient is not on treatment because he is "allergic" to all medications prescribed, he "suffocates" in the neck or back braces, or he becomes ill in a physiotherapy setting.
3. The patient is not on treatment because he has not sought treatment.

Certain behavioral patterns become apparent after seeing a number of these patients. Some never appear for appointments in spite of weeks of notification. Others appear late for the appointment and do not apologize or state indifferently that the traffic was heavy. There may be an attempt to manipulate your feelings with a compliment about your reputation or your office. There may be an effort to play one doctor against another by making false statements about the other doctor. Finally, hostility may appear during the assessment. A patient truly ill will not be aware or afraid of exposure and will not be hostile unless provoked. A patient exaggerating a disability is suspicious. He may start out hostile, but the usual pattern is one of developing hostility as discrepancies in the history and physical examination are exposed. Examiners are advised, for obvious reasons, not to precipitate this final behavioral pattern.

The patient who is magnifying or exaggerating a disability can be exposed only through an adequate physical examination. Those physicians who do not physically examine patients will not recognize this reaction, which may explain the reluctance of the psychiatric community to accept this clinical entity.

The physical findings of exaggeration reaction are classified into those that demonstrate acting behavior, those that indicate anticipatory behavior, and those that fail to support the patient's claim to illness.

Acting Behavior

Exaggerating a disability requires acting by the patient. This acting may be general in nature, such as the Academy Award performances put on by some patients as they moan and groan through the examination, walk around the examining room with their eyes closed, and either reach for objects to support themselves or reach for their painful areas. The incongruity of this acting behavior may be evident when the patient mounts the examining table with considerable ease and/or dresses within minutes of the examination and smiles and waves goodbye as he leaves the office.

Specific examples of acting behavior are the rigid back, a condition that disappears on the examining table, the reduction of straight leg-raising (SLR) in the supine position (Fig. 27-1A) that disappears in the sitting position (Fig. 27-1B), tender skin, and the paralyzed insensitive extremity. That these findings are a result of acting can be demonstrated through the use of distraction testing (Table 27-2). Using nonpainful, nonemotional, and nonsurprising examination techniques, it is possible not only to change the acting behavior but also to demonstrate normal physical function. It is my opinion that proper distraction testing that abolishes an acted physical finding and demonstrates normal physical function is a method of demonstrating exaggeration behavior. The best distraction test is simple observation of the patient as he gets undressed and moves about the examining room.

Varying degrees of acting behavior occur in different patients. In general, the more sophisticated the patient, the more sophisticated the acting behavior, and the more sophisticated the examiner must be.

Anticipatory Behavior

The second group of physical findings in this reaction represent anticipation on the part of the patient to the test situations. This anticipatory behavior leads to an appropriate response by the patient in an attempt to indicate illness. An example of this test is illustrated in Fig. 27-2.

Contradictory Clinical Evidence

Statements by the patient to the effect that he is unable to work may not be supported by clinical observations. Some patients will say they are unable to drive yet will have driven by themselves great distances to get to the examination. Some patients will say that they require frequent medication

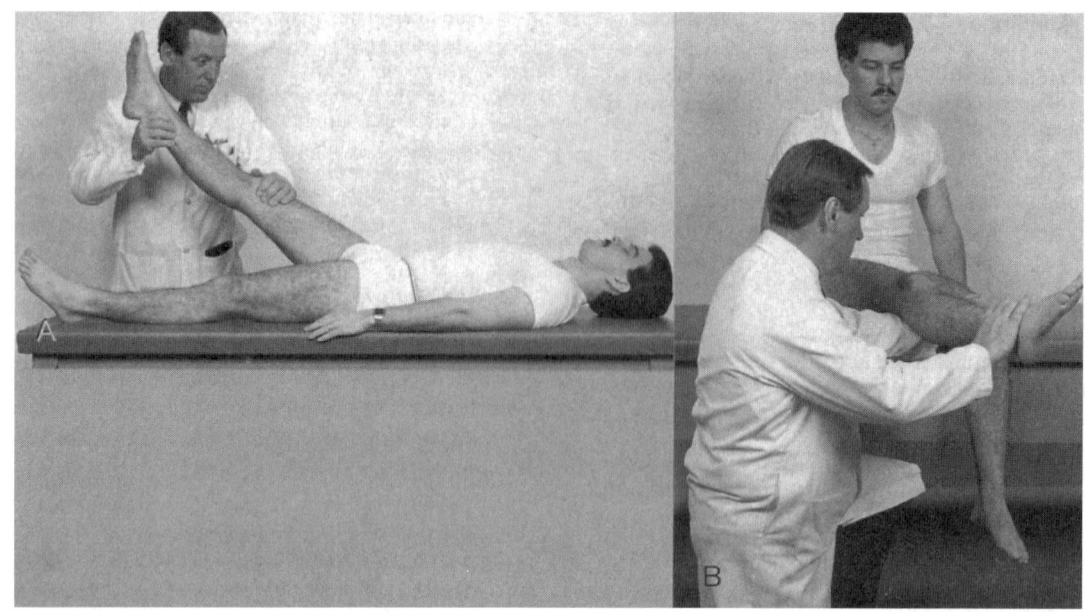

FIG. 27-1. A. Patient demonstrating significant SLR reduction in supine position. **B.** SLR ability in sitting position is 90°—a difference from **(A)** that cannot be explained by root involvement but rather represents magnification/exaggeration effort by the patient.

TABLE 27-2. *Demonstration of acting behavior*

Condition	Response
Physical finding (acting behavior)	Reduction in straight-leg raising
Distraction test (e.g., flip test): nonpainful, nonemotional, nonsurprising	Normal straight-leg raising (normal physical function)— sitting

yet will arrive from great distances without their medication. The patient who claims to be continuously wearing a collar or a brace should show signs of this wear on his body and the appliance. Patients with calluses on their hands and knees contradict their story of a prolonged inability to work. Other evidence of work may be in the form of paint stains or a particular distribution to their sunburn. Patients with nicotine stains on a grossly paralyzed limb should start to demonstrate similar stains on the opposite hand. Finally, those patients who demonstrate a prolonged and profound weakness in an extremity will not have associated wasting of that extremity.

It is important to stress that one swallow does not make a spring! The fact that a patient has one of these findings does not mean the patient should be classified as an exaggerator or litigant reactor. It is important to stress that a collection of symptoms and signs should be present with the appropriate clinical setting to make the diagnosis of exaggeration behavior. Waddell et al. (3) have documented the significant symptoms and signs that, when collected, suggest that a nonorganic component to a disability is pres-

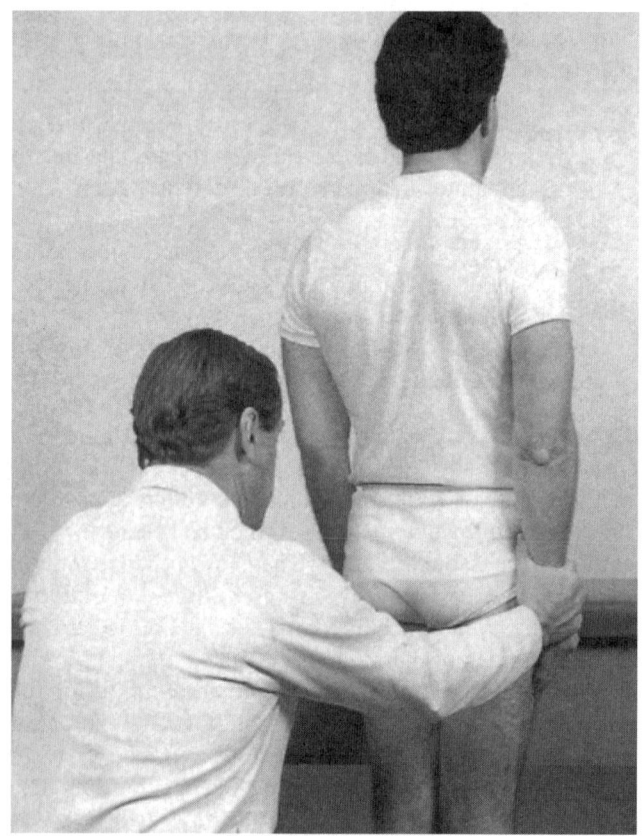

FIG. 27-2. Simulated movement testing. Holding the patient's arms fixed to the pelvis allows for rotation through the hip joints without moving the back. If the patient complains of back pain, this is considered anticipatory behavior, one of the many indications of nonorganic pain.

ent. These symptoms and signs have been scientifically documented as valid and reproducible. As a screening mechanism they are an excellent substitute for pain drawings and psychological testing (Table 27-3).

Conclusions

Every human attends the school of survival. Sometimes the lessons lead patients to modify or magnify a physical disability at a conscious or unconscious level. One word of caution—the presence of one of these nonorganic reactions does not preclude an organic condition such as a herniated nucleus pulposus. The art of medicine is truly tested by a patient with a physical low back pain who modifies the disability with a nonorganic reaction of tension, hysteria, depression, or emotional factors.

QUESTION 2

Is this clinical presentation a diagnostic trap?

It is too easy, when trying to arrive at a mechanical diagnosis, to fall into the many traps in the differential diagnosis of low back pain. An example is the young man in the early stages of ankylosing spondylitis who presents with vague sacroiliac joint pain and mild buttock and thigh discomfort who is thought to have a disc herniation. The patient with a retroperitoneal tumor invading the sacrum or sacral plexus may present with classic sciatica and also be misdiagnosed as having a disc herniation. It is not uncommon that patients with pathology within the peritoneal cavity will refer pain to the back.

To avoid missing these various diagnostic pitfalls, always ask yourself the second question: Is this clinical presentation a trap?

TABLE 27-3. *Symptoms and signs suggesting a nonorganic component to disability*

Symptoms
1. Pain is multifocal in distribution and nonmechanical (present at rest)
2. Entire extremity is painful, numb, and/or weak
3. Extremity gives way (as a result the patient carries a cane)
4. Treatment response:
   a. No response
   b. "Allergic" to treatment
   c. Not on treatment
5. Multiple crises, multiple hospital admissions/investigations, multiple doctors

Signs
1. Tenderness is superficial (skin) or nonanatomical (e.g., over body of sacrum)
2. Simulated movement tests positive
3. Distraction tests positive
4. Whole leg weak or numb
5. "Academy Award" performance

Two broad categories of disease are included in this question:

1. Back pain referred from outside the spine may come from within the peritoneal cavity (e.g., gastrointestinal tumors or ulcers) or from the retroperitoneal space (genitourinary conditions, abdominal aortic conditions, or primary or secondary tumors of the retroperitoneal space). These patients can be recognized clinically on the basis of two historic points. First, the pain is often nonmechanical in nature and troubles the patient just as much at rest as it does with activity. Second, the pain in the back often has the characteristics of the pain associated with the primary pathology.
2. Painful conditions arising from within the spinal column, including its neurological content. This group is subdivided into the differential diagnosis of low back pain or lumbago (Table 27-4) and the differential diagnosis of radicular pain or sciatica (Table 27-5).

These patients have nonmechanical back pain or a pain more characteristic for the primary pathology. Radiating extremity pain is not common unless neurological territory has been invaded by the disease process, which usually occurs late in the disease. Unfortunately, many of these conditions are not obvious on history and physical examination and are often missed on reviewing plain radiographs. The following diagnostic tests are useful as a screening mechanism:

1. Hemoglobin, hematocrit, white blood count, differential, and erythrocyte sedimentation rate
2. Serum chemistries, especially a fasting blood sugar, calcium, acid, and alkaline phosphatase, and serum protein electrophoresis
3. Bone scan

These three screening tests can be completed outside of the hospital and almost routinely identify these conditions. MRI now plays a significant role in the diagnosis of these various nonmechanical conditions.

Although the most common cause of leg pain in a radicular distribution is a structural lesion in the lumbosacral region, there are many other causes of radiating leg discomfort that must be considered. Missing these conditions

TABLE 27-4. *Differential diagnosis of nonmechanical low back pain*

1. Referred pain (e.g., from the abdomen or retroperitoneal space)
2. Infection—bone, disc, epidural space
3. Neoplasm
   a. Primary (e.g., multiple myeloma, osteoid osteoma)
   b. Secondary
4. Inflammation
5. Miscellaneous metabolic and vascular disorders such as osteopenias and Paget's disease

TABLE 27-5. *Differential diagnosis of sciatica*

1. Intraspinal causes
   a. Proximal to disc—conus and cauda equina lesions (e.g., neurofibroma, ependymoma)
   b. Disc level
      Herniated nucleus pulposus
      Stenosis (canal or recess)
      Infection—osteomyelitis or discitis (with nerve root pressure)
      Inflammation–arachnoiditis
      Neoplasm—benign or malignant with nerve root pressure
2. Extraspinal causes
   a. Pelvis
      Cardiovascular conditions (e.g., peripheral vascular disease)
      Gynecological conditions
      Orthopedic conditions (e.g., osteoarthritis of hip)
      Sacroiliac joint disease
      Neoplasms
   b. Peripheral nerve lesions
      Neuropathy (diabetic, tumor, alcohol)
      Local sciatic nerve conditions (trauma, tumor)
      Inflammation (herpes zoster)

TABLE 27-6. *Differential diagnosis of claudicant leg pain[a]*

Findings	Vascular claudication	Neurogenic claudication
Pain		
Type	Sharp, cramping	Vague and variously described as radicular, heaviness, cramping
Location	Exercised muscles (usually excludes buttock)	Either typical radicular or extremely diffuse (including buttock)
Radiation	Rare after onset	Common after onset, usually proximal to distal
Aggravation	Walking	Aggravated not only by walking, but also by standing
Relief	Stopping muscular activity even in the standing position	Walking in the forward flexed position more comfortably; once pain occurs, relief comes only with lying or sitting down
Time to relief	Quick (seconds to minutes)	Slow (many minutes)
Neurological symptoms (paresthesia)	Not present	Commonly present
Straight-leg raising tests	Negative	Mildly positive or negative
Neurological examination	Negative	Mildly positive or negative
Vascular examination	Absent pulses	Pulses present

[a]Be wary of the patient when both conditions coexist.

is probably the most common error made in a spine surgical practice. For example, the high sensitivity of today's investigative modalities is capable of showing a minor and insignificant herniated nucleus pulposus when in fact the patient has a conus tumor higher in the spinal canal. This situation is being abetted by the tendency to do a CT scan and skip myelography in an attempt to arrive at a structural diagnosis for mechanical low back pain. This may seem like a good idea to avoid the complications of myelography, but it will present problems unless you adhere to the following rule: An equivocal CT scan requires completion of myelography. Fortunately, the issue is being resolved by the use of MRI. All patients with low back pain who do not respond to usual conservative treatment measures will automatically have an outpatient hematologic and serum screen, a bone scan, and MRI. (Is it far down the road when robots will deal with the structural lesion?)

Etiology of Radiating Leg Pain

Space does not permit discussion of all the differential diagnoses of radiating leg pain, but three common conditions must be recognized: (a) cardiovascular conditions (peripheral vascular disease), (b) hip pathology, and (c) neuropathies.

Cardiovascular Conditions

Cardiovascular disorders in the form of peripheral vascular disease can cause leg discomfort that is easily confused with nerve root compression. Because these conditions tend to occur in the older patient population, they may coexist. Table 27-6 is an attempt to separate vascular claudication from neurogenic claudication.

Hip Pathology

Usually it is easy to diagnose conditions of the hip because they so commonly cause pain around the hip and specifically pain in the groin. In addition, walking causes a limp, and physical examination reveals a loss of internal rotation early in the disease. Occasionally, however, a patient with hip pathology will have no pain around the hip and will have only referred pain in the distal thigh. In these patients, it is easy to miss hip pathology unless one specifically examines the hip for loss of internal rotation. If there is any doubt, a radiograph of the pelvis must be taken.

Neuropathies

The most easily missed diagnosis is diabetic mononeuropathy. Although it more commonly occurs in poorly controlled diabetes mellitus, it may occur in an undiagnosed late-onset diabetic. It is thought to be due to an ischemic episode affecting the peripheral nerve and is characteristically manifested by acute onset with pain in a typical radicular distribution easily mimicking a disc herniation. If the peripheral neuropathy of diabetes is a mononeuropathy multiplex, a symmetrical polyneuropathy, or an autonomical neuropathy, the diagnosis is more readily apparent. The distinguishing features of diabetic mononeuropathy are as follows:

1. It occurs in the older patient with or without known diabetes.
2. There will be a history of the sudden onset of radicular pain with *no* back pain.
3. The patient will describe nonmechanical leg pain; the patient is extremely uncomfortable at rest.
4. The pain is usually more severe than the pain associated with lateral recess stenosis or spinal stenosis and of equal severity to the leg pain associated with a herniated nucleus pulposus.
5. The paresthetic discomfort often has a burning or uncomfortable characteristic to it.
6. Although the sensory symptoms predominate, it is my experience that mononeuropathy affecting the femoral or the lumbosacral nerve roots has a more significant motor and reflex component on examination. The diagnosis is supported with abnormal blood sugar readings and electrical studies showing slower nerve conduction velocities and the presence of fibrillation potentials, positive waves at rest, and a decrease in the number of motor unit potentials on electromyography (EMG).

Conclusions

Although there are many other causes of extremity symptoms not listed in this table, it is important to recognize that the table includes most causes of lower-extremity pain. Extremity symptoms such as numbness and weakness, in the absence of pain, should suggest very strongly that a primary neurological disorder is possible rather than a mechanical low back condition.

QUESTION 3

Is this a mechanical low back pain condition, and if so, what is the syndrome?

The two important words are *mechanical* and *syndrome*. Mechanical pain is pain aggravated by activity such as bending and lifting and relieved by rest. There may be specific complaints relative to household chores or specific work efforts. These mechanical pains, again, are usually relieved by rest. Although these statements seem straightforward, clinical assessment is not always easy. A poor historian may not be able to relate a history of mechanical aggravation or relief. In addition, if significant leg pain is present, implying a significant inflammatory response around the nerve root, then much rest will be needed before the patient describes a relief of leg pain. Significant mechanical back pain may sometimes be aggravated by simply rolling over in bed. To the unsophisticated historian,

this may have the appearance of nonmechanical back pain. If one takes a careful history, however, and if a patient is a good historian, it is possible to determine that mechanical back pain is pain aggravated by activity and relieved by rest.

The second important word is *syndrome*. It is much safer to make a syndrome diagnosis for mechanical low back pain and then, after investigation, try matching a structural lesion with the clinical syndrome. There are two reasons for taking this approach: (a) Today's investigative techniques are so sophisticated that it is possible to find MRI abnormalities whether a patient has symptoms or not, and (b) a patient may have an obvious structural lesion such as spondylolisthesis yet may have an acute radicular syndrome due to a disc herniation at a level other than that of the spondylolisthesis. In fact, a patient with spondylolisthesis may have any one of the potential diagnoses discussed in this chapter. To focus on the structural lesion of spondylolisthesis shown on radiograph and ignore the history and physical examination will lead to errors in diagnosis and treatment.

There are basically two syndromes in mechanical low back pain (Table 27-7): (a) lumbago (mechanical instability) and (b) sciatica (radicular syndrome). Before enlarging on these syndromes, it is well to take a moment to reflect on the concept of "referred leg pain." Many state that leg pain that does not go below the knee and is associated with good SLR ability is likely referred leg pain. This idea is further entrenched if there is an absence of neurological symptoms or signs. The gate control theory of pain is one of the theories used to explain referred pain. The phenomenon is thought to occur when painful stimuli are reflexively shifted around at the cord level. This shunting results in pain being felt in a myotomal or dermatomal distribution away from the back origin of the pain, such as in the leg. The concept is altogether too simplistic and needs to be reworked in light of new investigative techniques such as CT scanning and MRI. I predict that referred leg pain will be a lot less common than originally thought. It is more likely that patients labeled as having referred pain for their leg radiations have various degrees of radicular pain due to nerve root encroachment by either bone or chronic disc herniations.

The diagnosis of referred leg pain should be reserved for the patient who has the following clinical presentation:

1. There is significant mechanical back pain present as the source of referral.
2. The leg pain affects both legs, is vague in its distribution, and has no radicular component.

TABLE 27-7. *Syndromes in mechanical low back pain*

1. Lumbago—mechanical instability
2. Sciatica—radicular pain
   a. Unilateral acute radicular syndrome
   b. Bilateral acute radicular syndrome
   c. Unilateral chronic radicular syndrome
   d. Bilateral chronic radicular syndrome

3. The degree of referred leg discomfort varies directly with the back pain. When the back pain increases in severity, the referred leg pain occurs or increases in severity. Conversely, a decrease in back pain results in a decrease in the referral of pain. Referred pain is less likely to radiate below the knee.
4. There are no neurological symptoms or signs in concert with the complaint of referred leg pain.

It is safer to assume that any patient with radiating leg pain, especially unilateral leg pain, has a radicular syndrome until proven otherwise.

Lumbago-Mechanical Instability

The lumbago-mechanical instability syndrome is easy to recognize. These patients present exclusively with lumbosacral backache aggravated by activities such as bending, lifting, and sitting. The pain may radiate toward either iliac crest but does not radiate down into the buttock or legs. The pain is almost always relieved by various forms of rest, for example, reduced activity, weight reduction, corset support, or bedrest. Most patients have no trouble describing these relieving efforts.

Most importantly, there are no associated leg symptoms or signs.

Unilateral Acute Radicular Syndrome

Before describing the unilateral acute radicular syndrome, it is important to note that the leg includes the buttock and sacroiliac joint areas proximally (Fig. 27-3). In fact, the younger patient may lateralize discomfort off the midline as high as the top of the sacroiliac joint or iliac crest region. Even this is considered leg pain in the young patient. Obviously, any pain below the buttock crease is to be considered

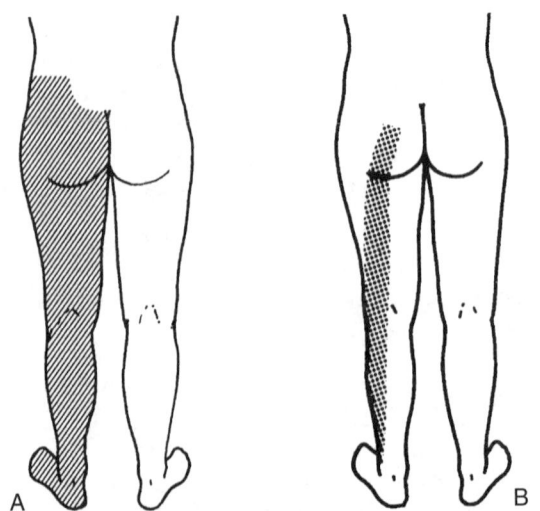

FIG. 27-3. A. When a spine surgeon talks of leg pain, he also includes any pain located in the buttock. **B.** The usual radicular distribution for L-5 or S-1 root lesion.

leg pain. A radicular distribution to leg pain is just what it implies—not a diffuse, but a specific distribution to the pain that follows a radical distribution.

History

Approximately half the patients will attribute the onset of their acute radicular syndrome to some traumatic experience. This may be retrograde rationalization on the part of the patient. Experimental studies and careful statistical analysis of case histories do not support the concept that direct trauma or sudden weight-loading of the spine is routinely the causal agent of disc rupture, although they may aggravate a preexisting lesion. This aspect in the history becomes important when litigation or compensation is involved.

The younger the patient, the more likely sciatica is the only symptom. When asked specifically, many patients may state that they noted numbness in the calf or foot before the pain developed. This is a stage of root compression before the inflammatory radiculitis begins. The majority of patients, however, develop back pain that subsequently radiates to the buttock and then down the leg. Most patients report that as the sciatic pain increases, the back pain decreases in severity. The history of pain is spondylogenic in character—that is to say, the pain is aggravated by general and specific activities and is relieved by rest. Bending, stooping, lifting, coughing, sneezing, and straining at stool will intensify the pain. Infrequently, referral patterns of pain occur, such as perineal or testicular discomfort (pain or paresthesia) and lower abdominal discomfort. The former symptoms are likely due to irritation of lower sacral roots laterally or at the midline, and the latter may be due to muscular splinting of the pelvis.

Patients with acute radicular syndrome may complain of a dermatomal distribution to the paresthetic discomfort. It is interesting to note that although pain occurs in the buttock, thigh, and calf, the symptom in the foot is almost exclusively paresthesia.

Physical Examination

The Back   The posture is characteristic. The lumbar spine is flattened and slightly flexed. The patient often leans away from the side of his pain, and this sciatic scoliosis becomes more obvious on bending forward. The patient is more comfortable standing with the affected hip and knee slightly flexed, a manner accentuated by asking the patient to flex forward (Fig. 27-4). He walks in obvious discomfort, sometimes holding his loin with his hands. The gait is slow and deliberate and is designed to avoid any unnecessary movement of the spine. With gross tension on the nerve root, the patient may not be able to put his heel on the ground and walks slowly and painfully on tiptoe. Forward flexion may be permitted, so the hands reach the knees by virtue of flexion of the hip and knee joint. If the examiner keeps his fin-

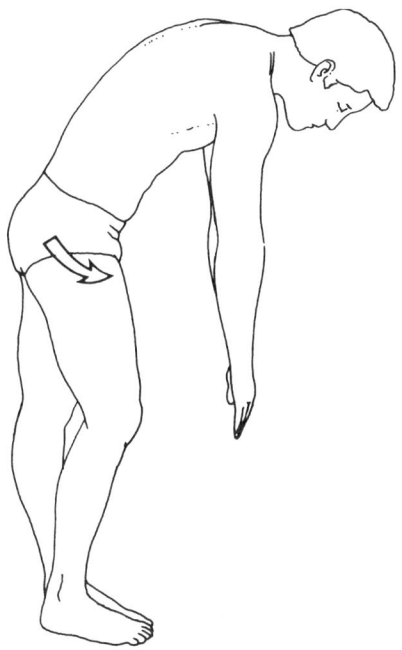

FIG. 27-4. Typical posture assumed by patient with herniated nucleus pulposus when forward flexion is attempted—flexion of knee on affected side and forward rotation of pelvis to affected side.

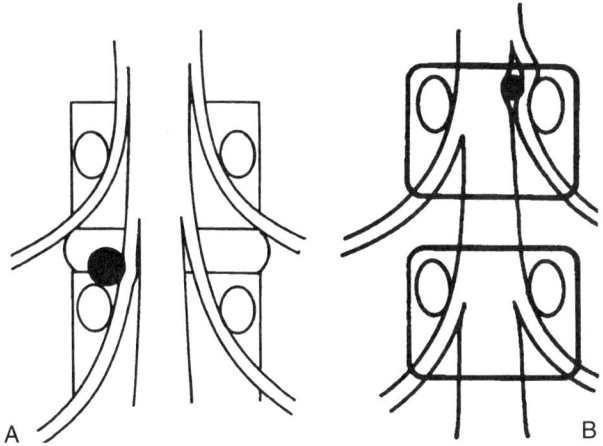

FIG. 27-5. A. Relationship oɪ ╷ ̄niated nucleus pulposus (HNP) lateral to nerve root such that flex. ɔn to affected side increases pain. B. Not unusual location of HNP in axilla of nerve root such that flexion to opposite side increases pain.

gertips on the spinous processes, it is observed that the lumbar spine is splinted and nonmobile. Limitation of flexion in such instances is therefore the result of root tension. The degree of flexion should be recorded by measuring the distance between the fingertips and the floor.

Extension is not significantly limited. A complaint of radiating leg pain on backward extension is usually indicative of a sequestered or extruded disc rupture.

Lateral flexion may be full and free, but in the presence of sciatic scoliosis, lateral flexion toward the convexity of the curve (side of sciatica) is limited.

The phenomenon of sciatic scoliosis and the relief of aggravation of pain on lateral flexion have been attributed to the position of the protrusion in relation to the nerve root (Fig. 27-5). This may be a simplistic explanation in view of the fact that the sciatic scoliosis disappears on recumbency, however. This observation, the loss of lateral curvature of the lumbar spine on recumbency, differentiates the sciatic list from structural scoliosis. On further assessment of the degree of root involvement present, it is imperative to test the extremities specifically for root tension, root irritation, and impairment of root conduction. These are the cardinal signs of lumbar root compromise.

Back Tenderness and Muscle Spasm   In the standing position, especially in the presence of scoliosis, muscle spasm can be observed. At rest, however, the spasm often subsides, and there is little tenderness to be found in the back musculature. Selectively palpating and applying a lateral thrust to the spinous process may cause some back pain and on

rare occasions may produce leg pain. By and large, when the patient with acute radicular syndrome is at rest on the examining table, there is little to find in the back. The patient's major complaint is leg pain, and the majority of physical findings are in the extremity.

Extremities

Root Tension and Irritation   The term *root tension* denotes distortion of the emerging nerve root by an extradural lesion. The three most useful tests for the presence of root tension are limitation of SLR, crossover pain, and the bowstring sign, the latter also arising in part from root irritation.

When testing SLR, it is important not to hurt the patient. Never suddenly jerk the leg up in the air. The standard for SLR testing is a fully extended knee with the hip in slight internal rotation and adduction.

Figure 27-1A demonstrates a good way of doing the SLR test. An SLR test is considered "positive" when the test reproduces pain in the buttock or leg, which limits SLR ability to something less than the normal of 90 degrees. SLR in the acute radicular syndrome is significantly reduced (less than 50% of normal).

Two additional maneuvers are useful to support the finding of limitation of SLR:

1. Aggravation of pain by forced dorsiflexion of the ankle at the limit of SLR
2. Relief of pain by flexion of the knee and hip

Physiogenic sciatic pain due to nerve root compromise is always relieved by flexion of the knee and hip. Continuing to flex the patient's hip with the knee bent does not reproduce and aggravate sciatic pain. This phenomenon is seen only in the emotionally destroyed patient.

If SLR is permissible to 70° before leg pain is produced, the finding is equivocal for the acute radicular syndrome.

Below this level the reproduction of leg pain on SLR, aggravated by dorsiflexion of the ankle and relieved by flexion of the knee, is strongly suggestive of tension on the L-5 or S-1 nerve roots. Reproduction of the sciatic pain in the affected extremity by raising the unaffected leg is irrefutable evidence of root tension in the acute radicular syndrome. This is known as *contralateral* or *crossed SLR pain*.

False-Positive SLR Test   Hamstring tightness may cloud the assessment of the SLR test. These patients generally have a tight body build (e.g., inability to fully extend the elbow). Their hamstring tightness-limiting SLR is bilateral, and the discomfort they feel is distal in the thigh in the region of the hamstring tendons. Hamstring tightness does not produce pain radiating below the knee. Finally, other physical findings of root tension, irritation, and compression are absent when hamstring tightness is the sole cause of decreased SLR ability.

False-Negative SLR Test   On occasion you will encounter a loose-jointed individual with sciatica due to an herniated nucleus pulposus. On SLR testing you may not be impressed with the minor degree of impaired SLR ability until you examine the unaffected leg and see the patient's ability to straight leg-raise well beyond 90 degrees.

Bowstring Sign   The bowstring sign is an important indication of root tension and irritation. To perform the test the examiner carries out SLR to the point at which the patient experiences some discomfort in the distribution of the sciatic nerve. At this level, the knee is allowed to flex and the patient's foot is allowed to rest on the examiner's shoulder (Fig. 27-6). The test demands sudden, firm pressure applied to the tibial nerve in the popliteal fossa. Do the test in the following stages: Apply firm pressure to the hamstrings—this will not hurt. Then, move your thumbs over to the tibial nerve. Apply sudden, firm pressure with your thumb over the nerve. A positive bowstring test is reproduction of radiating leg discomfort. Most commonly the radiating discomfort is pain felt proximally in the thigh and even into the back. Less commonly, radiating discomfort will travel distally, and this discomfort is more often paresthetic in nature than painful. It is important to emphasize that if the test produces local pain only in the popliteal fossa, it is of no significance. This demonstration of root irritation is probably the single most important sign in the diagnosis of tension and irritation of a nerve root by a ruptured intervertebral disc; unfortunately, it is not always present in patients with herniated nucleus pulposus.

Tests to Verify SLR Reduction   When the patient sits with the legs dangling over the side of the bed, the hip and knee are both flexed to 90 degrees. If the knee is now extended fully, the position assumed by the leg is equivalent to 90 degrees of SLR. If the patient is suffering from root compromise, this will cause sudden, severe pain, and the patient will lean backward to avoid tension on the nerve (Fig. 27-7). This is commonly referred to as the "positive flip test." With the psychogenic regional pain syndrome, the patient will permit the examiner to extend the knee of the painful leg without showing any response.

Sometimes crossover pain can be demonstrated only in the sitting position. If one crosses over pain from the asymptomatic leg to the symptomatic leg in the sitting position, this is also considered a positive crossover sign and almost certainly indicative of an acute radicular syndrome.

Patients with acute radicular syndrome may also have tenderness over the sacroiliac joint and down the course of the sciatic nerve. This tenderness has led to the erroneous

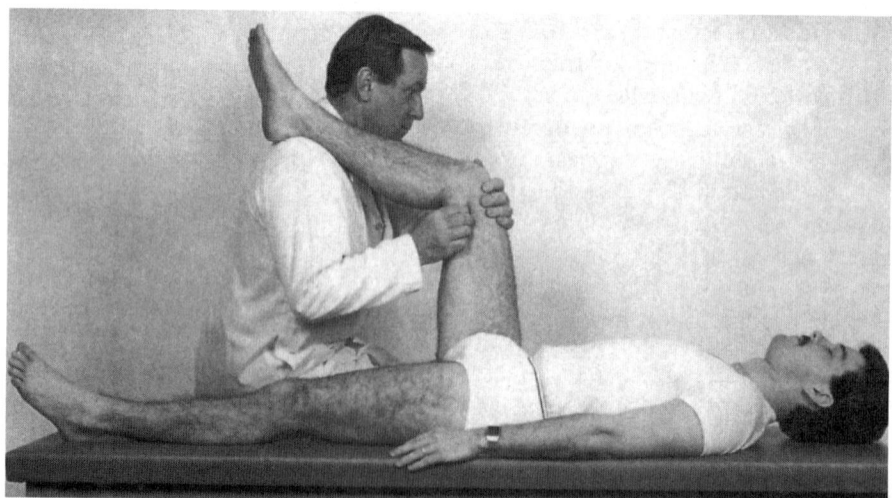

FIG. 27-6. Bowstring test. First do the medial hamstrings (a), then the tibial nerve (b), then the lateral hamstrings (c), then the lateral popliteal nerve (d). A positive response at (b) and (d) equates with organic root irritation. A negative response at all four test sites is a negative test. A positive test at (a) and (c) is indicative of nonorganic reaction.

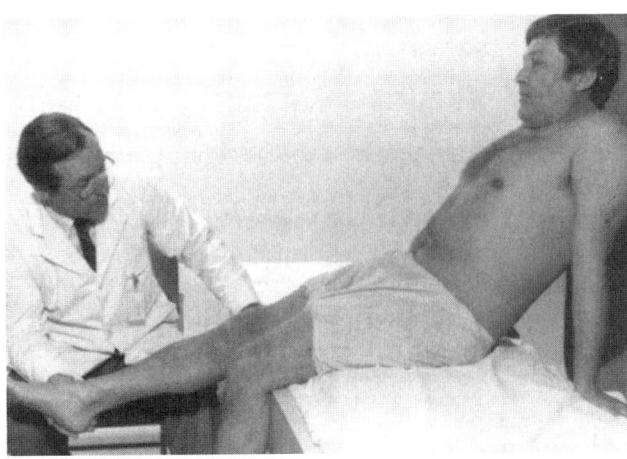

FIG. 27-7. A positive flip test. Because of root tension, an attempt to straight-leg raise in the sitting position causes buttock or leg pain, and the patient flips back on the examining table to relieve the increased tension.

diagnosis of sacroiliac joint strain. It is very unusual in these patients to see any clinical or radiologic evidence of damage to the sacroiliac joint.

Femoral Nerve Stretch   With higher lumbar disc herniations and acute radicular syndromes, the SLR test may be negative, but the femoral stretch test will be positive. Figure 27-8 shows the femoral nerve stretch test. It is not nearly as satisfactory as an SLR test, but if this test reproduces radiating thigh pain, aggravated by knee flexion, then the test is considered positive.

Summary

Table 27-8 summarizes the historic and physical foundation on which to build the diagnosis of an acute radicular syndrome. Table 27-9 shows the differences in the acute radicular syndrome in the various age groups.

TABLE 27-8. *Criteria for the diagnosis of acute radicular syndrome*[a]

1. Leg pain (including buttock) is the dominant complaint when compared to back pain
2. Neurological symptoms that are specific (e.g., paresthesia in a typical dermatomal distribution)
3. Significant SLR changes (any one or a combination of these)
   a. SLR less than 50% of normal
   b. Bowstring discomfort
   c. Crossover pain
4. Neurological sign (see section on anatomical level)

[a]Three or four of these criteria must be present, the only exception being the young patients who are very resistant to the effects of nerve root compression and thus may not have neurological symptoms (criterion 2) or signs (criterion 4).

Bilateral Acute Radicular Syndrome (Cauda Equina Syndrome)

Fortunately, the bilateral acute radicular syndrome is rare. It is usually due to a massive midline sequestered disc. The syndrome is manifested by the sudden onset of bilateral leg pain usually accompanied by bladder and bowel impairment. Perineal numbness is a predominant symptom. It is obviously an emergency and is a diagnosis that is rarely missed.

Unilateral Chronic Radicular Syndrome

The difference between acuteness and chronicity in a radicular syndrome is often difficult to measure. The severity and the duration of the syndrome usually combine to distinguish acute from chronic radicular pain. Chronic unilateral radicular pain is usually a complaint for many months or more. It follows a typical radicular distribution, including pain below the knee, and is usually associated with much in the way of mechanical back pain. Both pains are usually aggravated by walking. Neurological symptoms are less prevalent than in acute radicular syndrome and are sometimes extremely diffuse and nonlocalizing. Straight leg-raising ability is usually

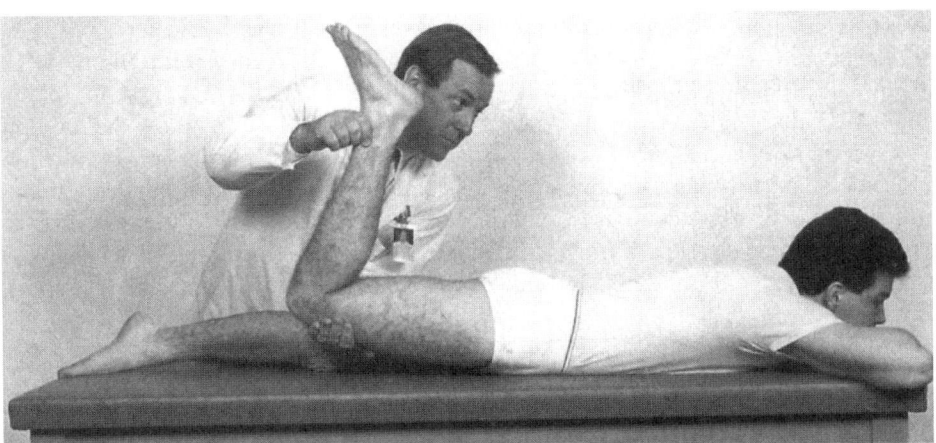

FIG. 27-8. Method of doing femoral stretch.

TABLE 27-9. *Difference in presentation of the acute radicular syndrome in various age groups*

Presentation	Young (< 30 years old)	Adult (35–55)	Older (60+)
Symptoms			
Leg pain	Usually the only symptom	Some back pain (BP), but leg pain (LP) dominates	Usually BP, but LP still dominates
Paresthesia	Often absent	Usually present	Almost always present
Signs			
SLR	Very positive (often 10–20%)	Less than 50% of normal	Occasionally good ability
Neurological signs	Absent in at least 50% of patients	Sometimes absent	Rarely absent

much better than 50% of normal, and bowstring discomfort and crossover pain are not seen in this syndrome. Neurological findings are very few and usually not helpful in localizing the degree of nerve root involvement.

Bilateral Chronic Radicular Syndrome

To many, the bilateral chronic radicular syndrome is known as *neurogenic claudication,* which was summarized in Table 27-6. The structural lesion that causes neurogenic claudication is almost always spinal canal stenosis. This syndrome differs from the unilateral radicular syndrome in two ways:

1. Both legs are affected rather than one leg.
2. The pain of the bilateral radicular syndrome may not be a typical radicular-type pain. Some patients describe typical claudicant leg pain in a radicular distribution. Other patients describe a diffuse type of claudicant leg discomfort that cannot be localized to a radicular distribution.

Many other symptoms are present in this syndrome, including weakness, "heaviness," and "rubberiness" in the legs. Numbness is also prevalent in this syndrome and is often of no value in localizing which nerve roots are compromised. There is a typical march phenomenon with the chronic bilateral radicular syndrome. Symptoms get much worse with prolonged walking, radiate further down the leg, and ultimately interfere with the ability of the patient to ambulate. Some patients may report noticing that if they attach themselves to a shopping cart and walk in the flexed position, they can get more distance before their leg symptoms appear. Characteristically, physical examination in chronic bilateral radicular syndrome reveals little. Straight leg-raising is usually very good, and if the syndrome is due entirely to canal narrowing rather than lateral recess narrowing, there are limited neurological findings except where the syndrome has significantly progressed. These patients will have significant weakness and are often wheelchair bound.

QUESTION 4

Are there clues to an anatomical level on history and physical examination?

Is there an anatomical level clinically? This is an important intermediate question to consider between a syndrome diagnosis (question 3) and a structural diagnosis (question 5). If it is possible to determine an anatomical level clinically, then any structural lesion has to be at the appropriate level or else it cannot be considered a significant defect. A patient who has an anatomical level of S-1 root involvement rarely should have a structural diagnosis localized to the L-3–L-4 interspace!

There are three ways to determine an anatomical level: distribution of leg pain, neurological symptoms, and neurological signs.

Distribution of Leg Pain

Pain in the posterior thigh and posterior calf distribution incriminates the fifth lumbar root or the first sacral root. Whether this pain is posterior or posterolateral in the thigh and calf is of little use in separating fifth lumbar root lesions from first sacral root lesions. Pain down the anterior thigh, however, almost certainly incriminates the fourth lumbar nerve root or higher lumbar nerve roots and excludes involvement of the fifth lumbar or first sacral roots.

Neurological Symptoms

A paresthetic discomfort with a dermatomal distribution is the most helpful historic feature in localizing an anatomical level. Paresthetic discomfort along the lateral edge of the foot incriminates the first sacral nerve root, paresthetic discomfort over the dorsum of the foot and the lateral calf incriminates the fifth lumbar nerve root, and paresthetic discomfort down the medial shin incriminates the fourth lumbar nerve root. In trying to use neurological symptoms to determine an anatomical level, remember the following rule: The more distal the symptom, the more valuable it is as a determinant of an anatomical level.

Neurological Signs

The diagnosis of acute radicular syndrome is in no way totally dependent on the demonstration of root impairment as reflected by signs of motor weakness or changes in sensory appreciation or reflex activity. The presence of such changes reinforces the diagnosis, however. The common neurological changes are summarized in Table 27-10.

Changes in Reflex Activity

The ankle jerk may be diminished or absent with an S-1 lesion. This is tested with the patient kneeling on a chair or sitting comfortably. (If a patient's sciatica is so severe that she cannot sit comfortably, then testing of the reflexes in the sitting position is invalid because the guarding and posturing will depress the reflexes.) This explains the occasional depressed knee reflex seen in the presence of sciatica due to an L-5–S-1 disc protrusion. If the patient has suffered a previous attack of sciatic pain, with compression of the first sacral nerve sufficient enough to obliterate the ankle jerk, this may not return to normal. The absence of the ankle reflex therefore may be merely a remnant of a previous episode of disc rupture, and the present attack may be due to a disc rupture at another level.

With an L-5 root compression, the tibialis posterior reflex (obtained by striking the tendon of the tibialis posterior near its point of insertion) may be absent. Diminution of the lateral hamstring jerk is also seen on occasion with an L-5 root compromise, but multiple innervation of this muscle group makes this an unreliable reflex. With L-4 and L-3 lesions, the knee jerk may be diminished.

Wasting

Muscle wasting is rarely seen unless the symptoms have been present for more than 3 weeks. Very marked wasting is more suggestive of an extradural tumor or other neurological diagnosis than of a disc rupture.

Always measure the girth of the thigh and the girth of the calf. This is a useful baseline from which to assess the progress of the lesion. Remember that if there is gross weakness of the gastrocnemii, the main venous pump of the affected extremity is no longer working, and these patients may even show some measure of ankle edema. The combination of calf tenderness due to S-1 root irritation and the observation of a swollen ankle may give rise to the erroneous diagnosis of thrombophlebitis. For reasons unexplained this phenomenon is more common in far

lateral disc herniations that must affect sympathetic postganglionic fibers.

Motor Loss

The weakness of the gastrocnemii is best demonstrated by getting the patient to rise on tiptoe five or six times. The patient is then asked if it requires more effort to do this on the affected extremity. If the quadriceps is weak, the physician must be aware of this before ascribing the difficulty of tiptoe rising to weakness of the calf muscles; also, if sciatic pain is severe, the test cannot be performed by the patient.

The power of ankle dorsiflexion is best tested by applying full body weight to the dorsiflexed ankle. Testing the dorsiflexors by asking the patient to walk on his heels will demonstrate only marked weakness in this muscle group. Weakness of the flexor hallucis longus (S-1) or weakness of the extensor hallucis longus (L-5) is often the first evidence of motor involvement. The evertors of the foot may be weak with an L-5 lesion. The gluteus maximus may become weak with lesions involving the first sacral nerve root and may be demonstrated by the sagging of one buttock crease when the patient stands. Weakness of the gluteus medius is seen with an L-5 lesion and occasionally is marked enough to produce a Trendelenburg lurch, particularly noticeable when the patient is tired. When the gluteus medius is involved, there is frequently marked tenderness on pressure over the muscle near its point of insertion, and this may be confused with trochanteric bursitis or with gluteal tendonitis.

Quadriceps weakness is seen with an L-4 lesion and can be assessed by the examiner placing his arm under the patient's knee and asking the patient to extend the knee against the resistance of the examiner's hand.

Sensory Impairment

The regions of sensory loss are reasonably constant. Within the sensory dermatomes, there appear to be areas more vulnerable to sensory loss than others. Loss of appreciation of pinprick is first noted in an S-1 lesion below and behind the lateral malleolus and in an L-5 lesion in the cleft between the first and second toes. Sensory appreciation is a subjective response and, as such, may sometimes be difficult to assess. Certain precautions must be followed. Sensory perception varies in different parts of the limb. Identical areas

TABLE 27-10. *Common neurological changes in acute radicular syndrome*

	Root		
Change	L-4	L-5	S-1
Motor weakness	Knee extension	Ankle dorsiflexion	Ankle plantar flexion
Sensory loss	Medial shin to knee	Dorsum of foot and lateral calf	Lateral border of foot and posterior calf
Reflex depression	Knee	Tibialis posterior	Ankle
Wasting	Thigh (no calf)	Calf (minimal thigh)	Calf (minimal thigh)

in each limb must be tested consecutively. The examination must be carried out as expeditiously as is compatible with accuracy because the patient will soon tire of this form of examination, and his answers may not be accurate. When the skin is pricked with a pin, the physiological principle of recruitment is present. Thus, the overall sensory appreciation depends not only on the action of the pinprick, but also on the number of pinpricks experienced.

A sensory examination is interpreted as positive only when the sensory loss approximates one dermatomal distribution and when the loss is not present in the adjacent dermatomes or the same contralateral dermatome.

QUESTION 5

After reviewing the results of investigation, what is the structural lesion, and does it fit with the clinical syndrome?

The potential structural lesion diagnoses are listed in Table 27-11. This table covers only degenerative conditions of the spine; it omits postoperative scarring of arachnoid or nerve roots and fractures and dislocations. It is important to stress here that it is possible to have multiple syndromes related to a single structural lesion. For example, a degenerative spondylolisthesis can cause both mechanical instability (back pain) and bilateral claudicant leg pain as a result of encroachment on the spinal canal. Table 27-12 links syndromes with structural lesions.

Conclusions

It is important to make a clear-cut syndrome diagnosis on the basis of a history and physical examination and to match it to a clear-cut bona fide structural lesion on investigation. Failure to do this leads to wrong diagnoses and futile treatment interventions.

METHODS USED TO DOCUMENT THE STRUCTURAL LESION

Steps to document the presence of a structural lesion in mechanical low back pain should be taken only after a satisfactory answer has been obtained for questions 1, 2, and 3 earlier. Seeking a structural lesion in a patient with an

TABLE 27-11. *Structural lesions in mechanical low back pain*

1. Instability
    a. Intrinsic to disc—degenerative disc disease (DDD)
    b. Extrinsic to disc
        Facet joint disease (FJD)
        Spondylolisthesis
2. Soft tissue lesions—muscle spasm, ligamentous strain
3. Herniated nucleus pulposus (HNP)
4. Narrowing of spinal canal
    a. Spinal canal stenosis (SCS)
    b. Lateral recess stenosis (LRS)

TABLE 27-12. *Relationship of syndromes and structural lesions*

1. Lumbago
    Degenerative disc disease (DDD)
    Facet joint disease (FJD)
    Spondylolysis/spondylolisthesis
    Soft tissue
2. Unilateral acute radicular
    Herniated nucleus pulposus (HNP)
    HNP + lateral recess stenosis (LRS)
3. Unilateral chronic radicular
    LRS
    HNP
4. Bilateral acute radicular
    Central HNP
5. Bilateral chronic radicular
    Spinal canal stenosis (SCS)

unrecognized nonorganic problem is usually a waste of time and money and is a danger to the patient.

False-positive investigative findings are easy to come by with today's sophisticated techniques. Before discussing each of these possible investigative procedures, it is assumed that a thorough history, physical examination, and other necessary investigations have satisfactorily answered questions 1 and 2.

Plain Radiographs

It may not be necessary on the first assessment to do lumbar spine films, but if a patient does not quickly respond to treatment, anteroposterior, lateral, and oblique films should be obtained. Plain radiographs may demonstrate a narrowed disc space, facet joint disease, or spondylolisthesis, but one must not assume that one of these is the causative structural lesion.

In reading plain radiographs, look at the nonskeletal areas first. Review the retroperitoneal area in specific regard to the kidneys and ureters and the abdominal aorta. Be sure that the psoas shadows are intact.

After reviewing the nonskeletal part of a lumbar spine radiograph, consider the skeleton. Look at the sacroiliac joints, survey the pedicles and vertebral bodies for erosions, and finally consider the structural defects that are potential causes of the patient's syndrome. Such things as narrowing of the disc space and translation of vertebral bodies are important to note. Various measurements of plain radiographs are not helpful in assessment of canal or recess narrowing.

Myelography

This test is considered the gold standard by many. To me it is of historic importance only, having been replaced by MRI. Myelography should be considered only when adequate conservative treatment has failed, surgery is contemplated, and the clinician is unskilled in the interpretation of MRI.

Myelography has three purposes:

1. To rule out higher spine pathology
2. To localize the exact level of root involvement
3. To determine if any migration of disc material has occurred

It is not the purpose of this text to discuss in detail the radiological changes that may be seen on myelography, but some general principles regarding interpretation of myelograms will now be described.

Myelography was introduced in 1921 by Sicard using iodized poppyseed oil injected into the epidural space (4). This is a logical place to put radiopaque material because the lesion is, indeed, an epidural lesion and should be demonstrated more easily by a radiopaque substance introduced into the epidural space. Difficulty in aspirating the radiopaque material at the conclusion of the epidural myelography, however, and the suggestion that this might give rise to root irritation at a later date persuaded surgeons to use the intrathecal injection of oil-soluble radiopaque compounds. Because these compounds are emulsified with the cerebrospinal fluid, it is not possible in the majority of instances to aspirate all of the dye injected.

Although many surgeons ordered oil myelograms, few themselves would undergo the procedure because of its difficulty and the postmyelographic complications. With the advent of water-soluble opaque materials and their refinement, however, myelography has become a much safer procedure.

The most popular water-soluble contrast material was metrizamide, but more recently this has been replaced by iohexol and iopamidol. These water-soluble compounds have several advantages over oil-soluble myelography in that the water-soluble contrast material is easier to inject and flows more readily through the nerve root sheaths. Obviously, it has a higher degree of sensitivity in documenting extradural lesions. Figure 27-9 is an example of oil- and water-soluble myelography.

Some neuroradiologists have popularized dynamic myelography. This entails flexion and extension of the patient on the fluoroscopic table with pictures being taken in these positions. Flexion supposedly opens up the spinal canal and reduces the degree of spinal stenosis encroachment on the contrast column. Conversely, extension decreases the dimensions of the spinal canal, and, if a spinal stenotic lesion is present, more constriction of the contrast column will be evident on extension radiographs.

Myelography is still accompanied by some complications such as headache, nausea, and vomiting. More severe complications such as convulsions and infections have also been reported after myelography.

Computed Tomography

A few years ago, CT started to replace myelography. The tenure of CT was short lived because of the advent of MRI, such that CT scanning is also mentioned as a historic footnote to the emergence of MRI as the test of first choice for

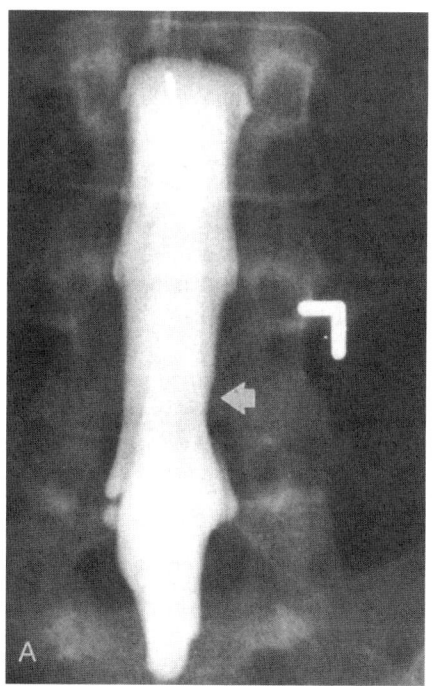
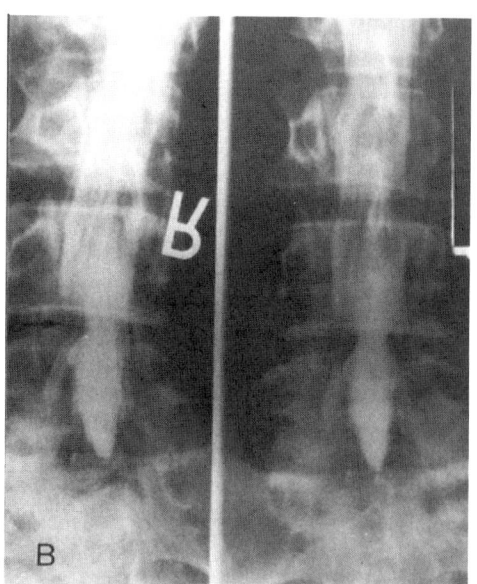

FIG. 27-9. A. Oil-soluble contrast myelography showing defect in contrast column at L-4–L-5 left (arrow). Notice the lack of filling of nerve roots that made interpretation of apparent defect of L-5–S-1 left difficult (ultimately found to be not significant). **B.** Water-soluble contrast myelography showing large HNP central and left L-4–L-5. Notice how well nerve roots fill.

investigation of degenerative conditions in the lumbar spine. Some might view this as a strong statement; it will soon be fact. Bell and others have published excellent articles on the overuse and pitfalls of routine CT scanning (1). Axial images are the most valuable and should be cut from L-3 to the midportion of the sacrum. Therefore any lesion above or below these levels will not be documented by the CT scan. Many neuroradiologists believe that reconstructions are of value, but I am not convinced. Crude measurements from the CT scan can also give some impression as to the integrity of the spinal canal and the lateral recesses. Figure 27-10 demonstrates a narrowed spinal canal.

CT scanning is so simple, so readily available, and so nice to look at that many pitfalls await the unwary. Before embarking on treatment, especially surgery, be sure that the patient's clinical syndrome fits the structural lesion on CT scan. Remember that you see nothing above L-3 on routine scanning and that you do not have sagittal sections of the spine. If there is any doubt, a myelogram must be combined with the CT scan to further document the structural lesion.

Magnetic Resonance Imaging

Magnetic resonance imaging is now the test of first choice for investigation of the patient with degenerative conditions of the spine. The procedure requires no x-ray radiation, and with the development of surface coils, the technique of MRI has improved to the point where it has become extremely sensitive in demonstrating soft tissue abnormalities in the lumbar spine. The major drawbacks to MRI are its cost, its time consumption, its propensity for false-positive results, and the claustrophobic effect it has on patients lying in the chamber for imaging purposes. These drawbacks have been overcome, however, and MRI is so useful in the investigation of a patient with mechanical low

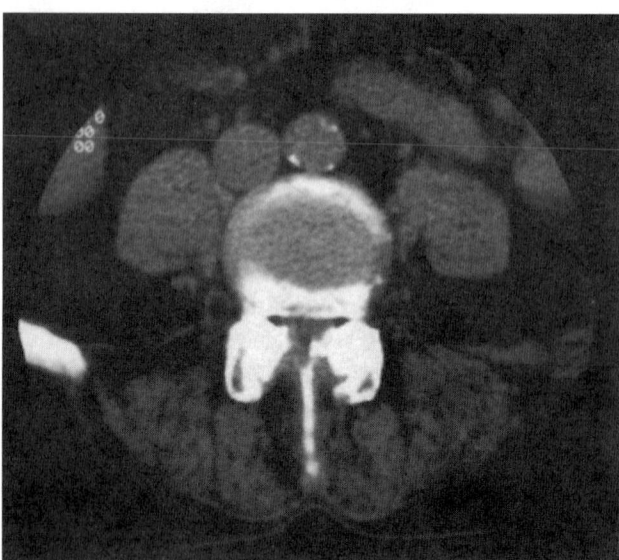

FIG. 27-10. CT showing subluxation of facet joints (left more than right) and canal stenosis.

back conditions that it has replaced CT scanning and myelography. Figure 27-11 is an MRI scan demonstrating a lumbar disc herniation. MRI is limited in its outline of bony detail, a handicap not encountered with the CT scan. In the future a patient who has a mechanical low back pain syndrome, failing to respond to conservative treatment, will be investigated with an MRI scan, and if a clear-cut diagnosis is not evident the choice will be CT with myelography. Myelography by itself will be rarely ordered.

Nerve Root Infiltration

Nerve root infiltration is a procedure that involves blocking the anterior primary ramus of a single nerve root. It is usually the fifth lumbar or first sacral nerve root that is blocked, but any root can be blocked. As a diagnostic procedure it is useful when one is sure that a radicular syndrome is present but unsure of which nerve root is affected. It is of no value in trying to separate referred pain from radicular pain, or a herniated nucleus pulposus from lateral recess stenosis. Most often the procedure is used in chronic unilateral radicular syndrome (due to lateral recess stenosis) when structural recess stenosis lesions are noted at the level of the fifth lumbar and first sacral nerve roots and there are no clinical clues as to the anatomical level. The second indication for a nerve root infiltration is in the presence of scarring or arachnoiditis when trying to decide which root is most symptomatic.

The technique is accomplished in the prone position under image-intensifier control. A paraspinal approach is used to the fifth lumbar nerve root, catching it just as it exits under the pedicle of L-5. The S-1 nerve root is blocked through the posterior first sacral foramen. Under image-intensifier control, a long needle is slowly advanced toward the nerve root. When the nerve root is encountered, radiating discomfort down the leg will result. Usually this radiating discomfort is typical enough that the block can then be accomplished with 1.5–2 mL of 0.5% or 0.75% Marcaine, a long-acting anesthetic agent. On occasion, the radiating discomfort will not be striking, and water-soluble contrast material must be injected to be sure of needle placement.

Although radiography is used to assist in accomplishing a nerve root infiltration, the procedure is not a radiographic evaluation procedure. The first principle of nerve root infiltration is to obtain a good root block. That is to say, if a fifth lumbar nerve root is blocked, the patient should have a drop foot and numbness over the dorsum of the foot when the procedure is finished. Similarly, if the first sacral root is blocked, the patient should have numbness to pinprick sensation along the lateral border of the foot and weakness of plantar flexion. After a good nerve root block is obtained, the patient is asked to participate in the activity that was most aggravating to her. Usually, the patient needs a cane for support because of the profound nature of the root block. Long-acting anesthetic agents last 4–6 hours, and at the end of that time the patient should record her impres-

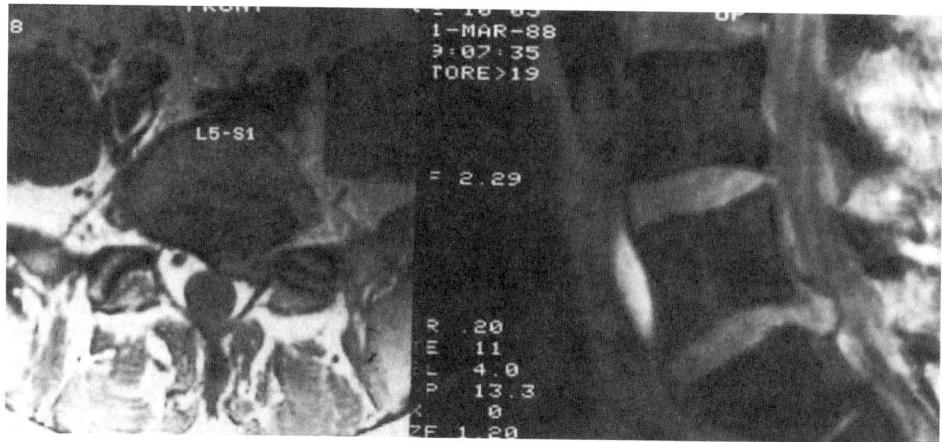

FIG. 27-11. MRI demonstrating a lumbar disc herniation. L-5–S-1 left axial view is T-1–weighted, and sagittal view is gradient echo.

sions of relief or lack of relief of her symptoms with the root block. If you suspected the fifth lumbar nerve root as the culprit, and a good fifth lumbar nerve root block relieves the patient's pain, then the procedure has satisfactorily pinpointed the fifth lumbar nerve root as the source of symptoms. The appropriate surgical procedure can then be carried out with confidence.

Facet Joint Block

A facet joint block is a local anesthetic procedure to temporarily denervate the facet joint. This is accomplished by blocking the facet joint itself and the posterior primary ramus supply to the facet joint. Facet joint innervation from the posterior primary ramus is from multiple segments, and thus multiple blocks are required. It is routine to block the facet joint and posterior primary ramus at L-3–L-4, L-4–L-5, and L-5–S-1 and also to block the ascending posterior primary ramus branch coming out of the S-1 foramen. Also, the procedure is done bilaterally.

Again, an image intensifier is used to guide needle placement. There is little in the way of radiating discomfort to help localize the block, and thus anatomical placement of the needle is important. Figure 27-12 shows such needle placement

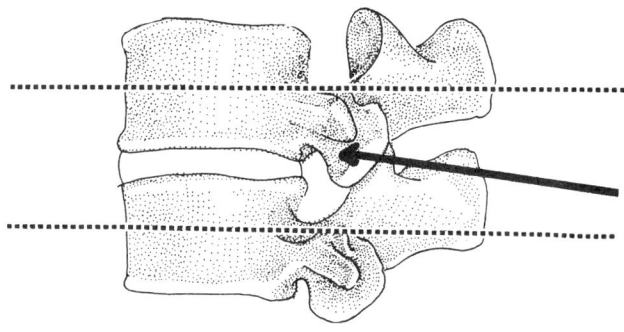

FIG. 27-12. Schematic rendering showing needle tip in correct location for block of facet joint nerve supply (see text).

at the junction of the lateral edge of the superior facet and the superior edge of the transverse process. Here, the posterior primary ramus comes through a ligamentous tunnel to supply the facet joint at that level and send branches to adjacent levels. Next, a needle should be placed within the facet joint itself so that the joint can be blocked. Long-acting anesthetic agents are also used for this procedure. After a satisfactory block is obtained, the patient is asked to participate in the activities that aggravated his pain and, at the end of 4 to 6 hours, to sit down and record his impressions of the effect of the procedure. If a patient has mechanical low back pain prior to the procedure that is abolished by the procedure, this suggests that the facet joints are the source of symptoms, and appropriate procedures can be prescribed.

Both nerve root infiltration and facet joint blocks are procedures that depend on patient response for evaluation. Obviously, if the patient is an abnormal responder (e.g., a patient with nonorganic pain), these two procedures are useless. Both will misguide you if you have missed the diagnosis of a nonorganic syndrome.

Electrodiagnosis

There are three electrodiagnostic procedures that are used in the investigation of a patient with lumbar disc disease: electromyography (EMG), nerve conduction tests (NCTs), and sensory-evoked potentials.

Electromyography

EMG is a motor unit examination. Any disruption in the anterior horn, the nerve fiber, or the muscle fiber has the potential of producing an abnormal EMG. Thus, an abnormal EMG is indicative of lower motor dysfunction. Electromyographic examination for a lumbar spine abnormality includes needle electrode placements in the paraspinal muscles and specific extremity muscles. Electrical activity is recorded on insertion, at rest, and with voluntary contraction or stimulation. Normally, there is unsustained electrical discharge on insertion of the needle and no signal discharge (a silent EMG) at rest. With voluntary contraction, biphasic or triphasic forms of action potentials are seen. Theoretically, with lower motor nerve root dysfunction, insertional activity is abnormal in that more positive sharp waves appear; at rest, there are fibrillation potentials and positive sharp waves; and with stimulation, the quantity of motor units recorded decreases, and multiple polyphasic waves are seen. Extending the theory further, in a herniated nucleus pulposus with single root involvement, the EMG findings will be localized to a single root. With spinal stenosis (multiple root involvement), there will be multiple root findings on EMG. In fact, EMG has a very low sensitiv-ity and specificity in evaluating patients with lumbar disc disease. More blinded studies are required to determine the value of EMG in diagnosing lumbar disc disease. At present, there is overreliance on EMGs when, instead, a good clinical history and physical examination can be more helpful.

Nerve Conduction Tests

Nerve conduction tests measure the speed at which nerve fibers conduct. They are useful in separating peripheral neuropathy from a radiculopathy (trying to answer question 2). In radiculopathy one should see normal NCT velocities, whereas in peripheral neuropathy NCT velocities are often slowed.

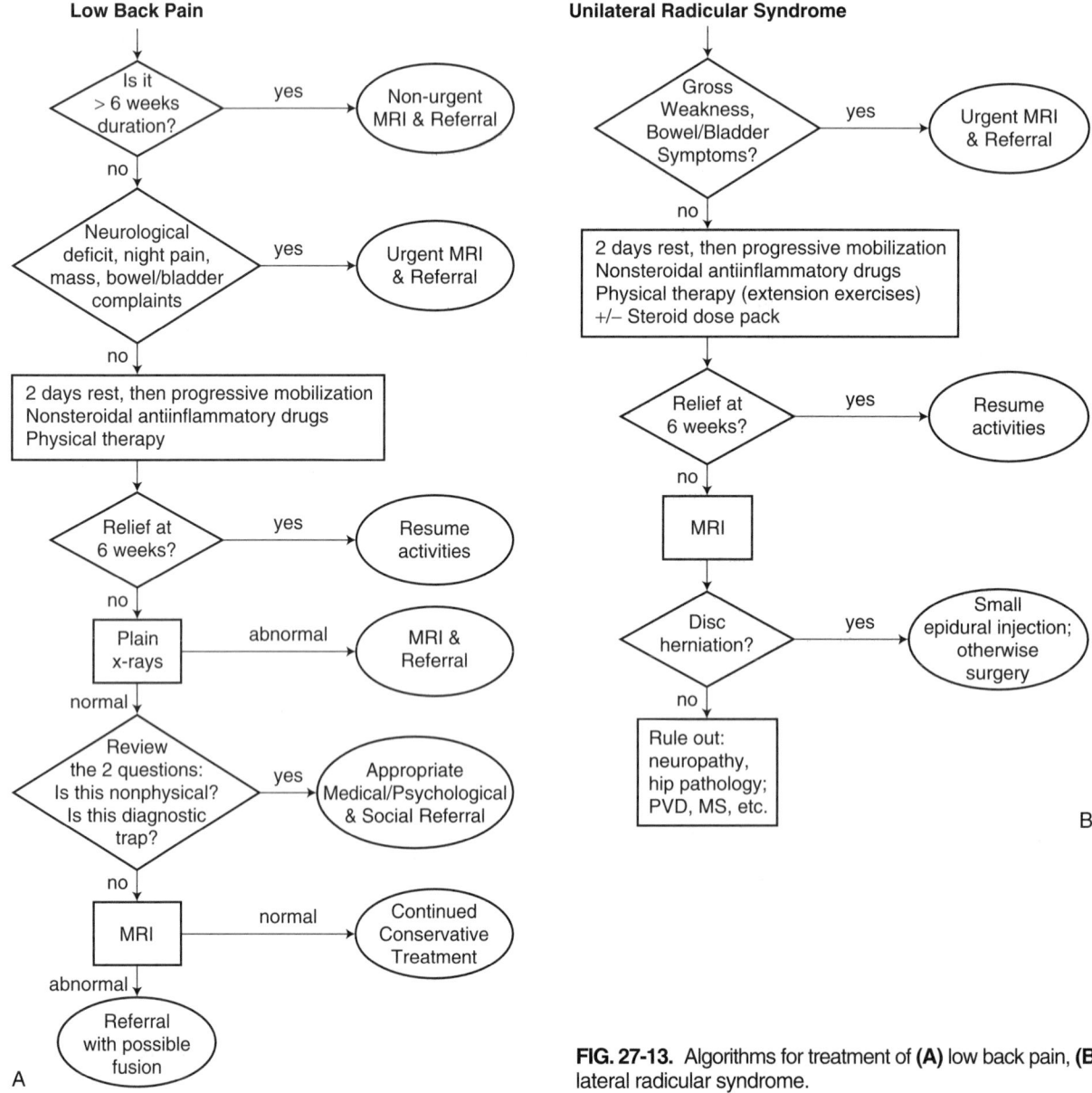

FIG. 27-13. Algorithms for treatment of **(A)** low back pain, **(B)** unilateral radicular syndrome.

Sensory-Evoked Potentials

With the failure of EMG to play a significant role in the evaluation of lumbar disc disease, a search began for new electrodiagnostic fields. Probably the most interesting to date is somatosensory-evoked potentials, which focus on the sensory side of the nerve fiber. These highly sophisticated evaluations have been used for some time in scoliosis and major spine reconstructive surgery. The spinal-evoked potential is transmitted through the dorsal column and is detectible with receptors in the spine or on the skull. Theoretically, lesions of peripheral nerves will prolong the latency response of the sensory input, and root and cord lesions cause change in the wave form. Conflicting evaluations of this technique have appeared in the literature (5). Some authors see great promise in this approach to the evaluation of patients with lumbar disc disease.

Other Tests of Limited or No Value

There are three tests that I place in this classification: epidural venography, thermography, and ultrasonography.

Epidural Venography   In the early 1970s, epidural venography enjoyed a brief popularity. It represented an attempt at a more accurate diagnosis of disc lesions at the L-5–S-1 level, where an oil-based myelogram had at least a 25% false-negative rate. A secondary reason was the false-positive rate of oil-based myelography at the L-4–L-5 level. Epidural venography turned out to be a difficult technical exercise, however, and also stressful for the patient. Limitations resulting from previous surgery also detracted from its value. Eventually, epidural venography was displaced by the advent of water-soluble myelographic compound and CT scanning. It is largely unheard of as a test today.

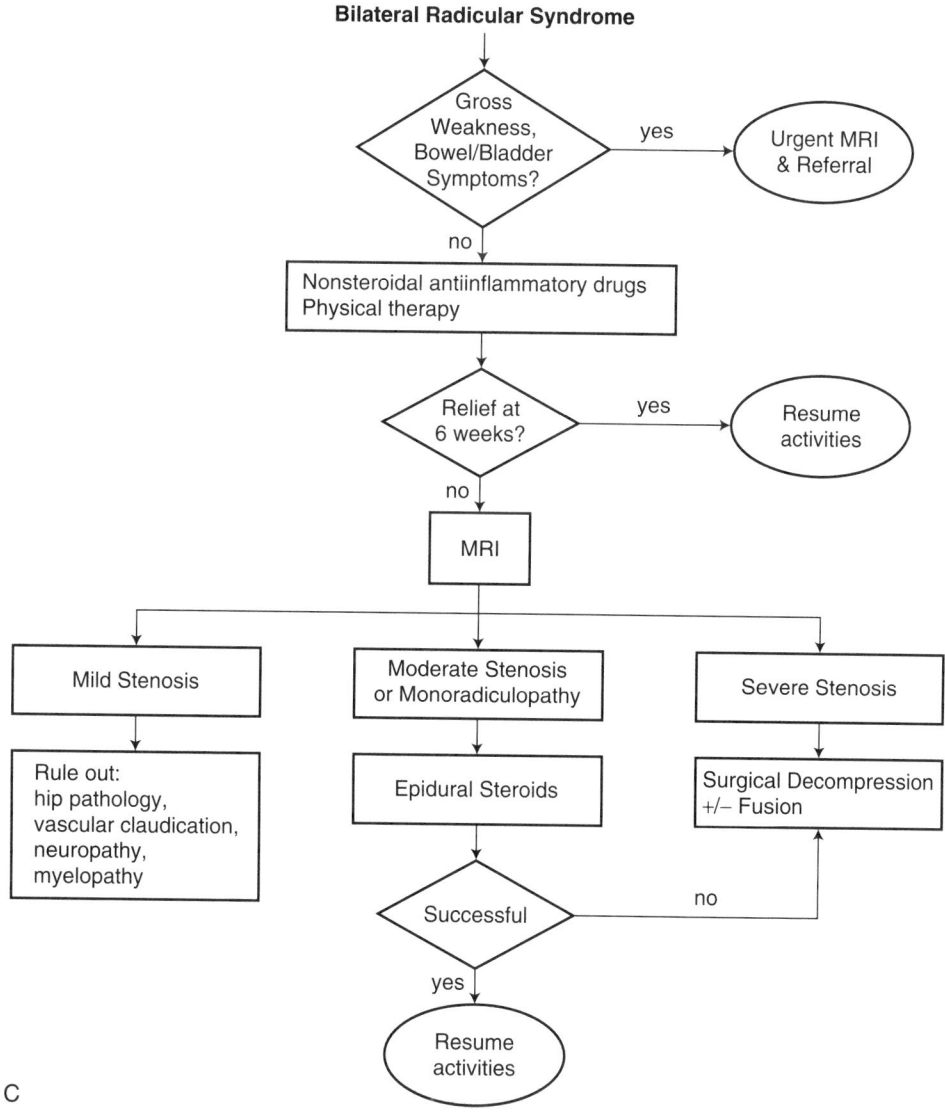

C

FIG. 27-13. Continued   (C) Bilateral radicular syndrome.

Thermography Many doctors have promoted and popularized thermography as a test of nerve root physiology. In theory, it states that pathology causing nerve root irritation will result in changes in skin temperature that can be detected with liquid cholesterol crystals or infrared photography. Although the principle is simple and attractive, there are limited blinded studies to support the claims of thermographers. In fact, a number of very good blinded studies seriously question the clinical value of thermography (6,7). Until thermography is submitted to more blinded studies on specificity and sensitivity, its use should be limited to experimental medicine only. Unfortunately, thermography has found its way into the courts and is being used extensively by judges and juries to determine financial awards. This is an unfortunate occurrence and one that should be halted until further blinded studies are completed.

Ultrasonography In spite of excellent scientific efforts by Porter et al. in England (8), the use of ultrasonography for the evaluation of patients with mechanical low back pain has severe limitations. The technique is exacting and difficult because the bony cover of the spinal canal interferes with visualization of its soft tissue contents. It has become a useful tool during spine surgery for spine trauma in detecting residual fragments anterior to the dura. At this point, however, it is not a useful investigative tool for the ambulatory patient with mechanical low back pain.

Conclusions

The assessment of a patient with a low back disability does not need to be difficult. By keeping a simple system in mind, it is possible to arrive at a good clinical impression by asking yourself the five questions discussed at length in this chapter and committing yourself, eventually, to sequential answers.

Do not commit yourself to any major investigative step until questions 1 and 2 have been adequately answered. Then, if you are satisfied that you have a mechanical low back pain problem, dissect it into a syndrome first, an anatomical level second, and a structural lesion third. The structural lesion diagnosis should fully support the clinical syndrome and the anatomical level. If not, take one step back and repeat the history and physical examination. Listening to the patient's story, doing a thorough physical examination, and supporting your diagnosis with investigation are the best way to avoid erroneous diagnoses and ill-fated surgery.

Treatment

After a diagnosis has been established, treatment can be undertaken as outlined in the algorithms in Fig. 27-13.

REFERENCES

1. Bell GR, Rothman RH, Booth RE et al. A study of computer-assisted tomography. *Spine* 1984;9:552–556.
2. Hitselberger W, Witten R. Abnormal myelograms in asymptomatic patients. *J Neurosurg* 1968;28:204–206.
3. Waddell G, McCulloch JA, Kummel EC et al. Nonorganic physical signs in low back pain. *Spine* 1980;5:117–125.
4. Sicard JL. Roentgenologic exploration of the central nervous system with iodized oil (Lipiodol). *Arch Neurol Psychiatry* 1926;16:420–426.
5. Aminoff MJ, et al. Dermatomal somatosensory evoked potentials in unilateral lumbosacral radiculopathy. *Ann Neurol* 1985;17:171–176.
6. Mahoney L, McCulloch JA, Czima A. Thermography as a diagnostic aid in sciatica. *J Am Acad Thermol* 1985;1:51–54.
7. Mills GH, Davies GK, Getty CJM, Conay J. The evaluation of liquid crystal thermography in the investigation of nerve root compression due to lumbosacral lateral spinal stenosis. *Spine* 1986;11:420–432.
8. Porter RW, Hubbert CS, Wicks M. The spinal canal in symptomatic lumbar disc lesions. *J Bone Joint Surg* 1978;60:485–487.

CHAPTER 28

Spinal Disc Disease

Judson Jeffrey Somerville

In this chapter, we will focus on a brief history of disc disease, reviewing the anatomy, pathophysiology, and diagnosis of disc disease as well as considering both current and future treatments. The majority of treatments for "back pain" are initiated due to unrelenting pain, not muscle wasting, sensory loss, or onset of a cauda equina syndrome. Unfortunately, the symptom of pain is elusive, and the common symptoms of low back pathology, which are based on pain (e.g., sciatica, pain on sitting, standing, or extending the back) do not localize the pain generator. Treatment and diagnostic decisions most often are based on pain symptoms. Consequently, it is no wonder that treating all types of spinal ailments is so difficult. Add to this the natural changes of the spine, and in particular the disc, that come with age, and there develops an even greater complexity in the understanding of painful spinal disease.

There are many causes of spinal pain. However, we shall argue that most back pain, with its associated symptoms, is related to a pain generating disc (PGD) and pain generating facet joints (PGFJs). It is essential to have a full understanding of what causes back pain because this directs diagnostic tests and treatments. Throughout this chapter, an attempt will be made to clearly explain these concepts to improve our understanding of painful versus nonpainful disc disease. Furthermore, we will review treatment options for patients who suffer from PGD. An effort will also be made to clarify the correlation of anatomical changes of the disc (as found on imaging studies) with findings on history, physical examination, and nerve function tests to more accurately diagnose a PGD. Exploring this correlation will simplify indications for treatment, which should improve the quality of outcome the patient receives by removing confusion as to what treatment the patient should undergo and by whom (i.e., pain specialist or orthopedic and/or neurosurgeon). With a better understanding of the history, anatomy, pathophysiology, and diagnosis, as well as treatment indications for a PGD, clinical outcome should improve.

HISTORY OF DIAGNOSIS AND TREATMENT OF SPINAL DISC DISEASE

Back pain has been a plague to society since the beginning of time. As humankind has evolved, so, too, has our awareness of this difficult problem and the complexity of treatment. An Italian anatomist, Domenico Cotunio, first distinguished sciatica from generalized low back pain in 1764 (1). Then, in 1934, the Mixter and Barr classic article, which described a herniated lumbar disc as the cause of radiculopathy, reinvigorated interest in the lumbar disc as a cause of sciatica (2). In 1944, Lindblom was the first to report his observations on the injection of a disc with dye and record the leakage of the dye from the nucleus into the annulus (3). Later, in 1948, Hirsch confirmed the disc as the cause of sciatica by injecting procaine into a patient's disc, which calmed the sciatica (4).

From these early pioneers, the field of diagnosing the pain generating disc (PGD) has progressed, but not without roadblocks. First, Holt, in 1964, reported a 100% incidence of false-positive cervical discograms in 50 prison inmates (5). Then, in 1968, Holt reported that 37% of lumbar discograms were falsely positive (6). Holt's methods were later shown to have major flaws, particularly in regard to subject selection and the lack of fluoroscopic guidance (7). His work slowed the field and cast doubt on the value of discograms for decades. Fortunately, recent studies have reinvigorated the field by verifying the high sensitivity and specificity of discograms (8–18). A more extensive history of disc disease and discography can be found elsewhere (8).

The history of treatment for a PGD began with an effort to stabilize the painful spinal level in the late 1800s. Spinal fusion for disc disease was first attempted in 1891 by Hadra

(19). The use of facet screws for lumbar stabilization was attempted by King in 1948 (20). Soon after, Boucher, using a slightly different technique from King, achieved a 100% fusion rate, but both techniques resulted in morbidity secondary to screw encroachment into the neural foramen 209. In 1984, Magerl modified the techniques of King and Boucher with less risk of neuroforaminal encroachment (21). Others have tried to maintain interbody height with a prosthetic disc (22). Fernstrom was the first to clinically trial an artificial disc in the early 1960s (23). This was unsuccessful due to subsidence of the artificial disc into the intervertebral body (24). Today, the most commonly used artificial disc is the Link intervertebral prosthesis; however, this technique has limited applicability (24). Still others have tried anterior interbody fusions (25). All of these methods have met with mixed results. The prevailing thought is that spinal fusion is a palliative rather than curative procedure and carries significant comorbidity (24). In an effort to maintain the anatomy without performing a fusion the Saul brothers developed the Intradiskal Electrothermal Annuloplasty (IDET) catheter, which preserves disc height and biomechanics when treating painful lumbar disc disease (26,27,28,29).

As it became apparent that the disc was a major source of spine pain, and treatment results were mixed, efforts were made to correlate the diagnosis of disc pathology with a PGD in an effort to improve outcome. By correlating abnormal characteristics of the disc, as found on imaging studies and nerve test results, with physical examination and historical findings, the disc can be pinpointed as a pain generator.

Several imaging techniques, such as CAT scan, MRI, and discograms, have helped to examine the architecture of the disc, but only discograms allow correlation of the patient's symptoms with the architecture of the disc. Newer techniques, such as the current perception test (CPT) (30) and skeletal muscular ultrasound, which capitalize on the symptom of radiculopathy caused by a PGD, allow diagnosis and measurement of this symptom quantitatively and qualitatively. Skeletal-muscular ultrasound can image inflamed nerves roots, and the CPT measures nerve function. These techniques help to more accurately diagnose and locate a PGD and may improve treatment outcomes.

We have come to a time when these newer techniques allow spinal pain due to a PGD to be accurately diagnosed, which should, and has, stimulated more specific treatments and better clinical outcomes. For the most part the current method of treatment for PGD depends on a physician's residency training. Traditional surgeons (e.g., orthopedic and neurosurgeons) typically have a much different approach from the traditional pain specialists (e.g., anesthesiologists, physiatrists, and neurologists). The current treatment approach used by the majority of traditional surgeons for a PGD is laminectomy with discectomy and/or fusion, depending on the patient's symptoms and the anatomical location (i.e., cervical, thoracic, lumbar) of the PGD. Until recently there were no good options for the traditional pain specialist to treat a PGD. With the extraordinarily high cost of open surgery to treat a PGD and the mediocre outcome, at best, for the most prevalent source (lumbar PGD), it was only a matter of time before a less expensive, more effective, and less invasive method was developed that would be usable by a wider range of physicians. Two of these newer percutaneous techniques are the IDET to treat lumbar discogenic and radicular pain and the laser-assisted disc decompression (LADD) technique to treat lumbar radiculopathy (31–33). These techniques are less expensive and less invasive with a high success rate when used for appropriate indications.

As these less invasive techniques have shown success in the lumbar spine, research is now underway to apply these techniques to treat the next most common area of spinal pain, the cervical spine, and, in particular, a cervical PGD (34,35). Although interbody fusion is the current treatment of choice for a cervical PGD, and is much more effective than in the lumbar spine, it is still a very expensive and invasive technique (36–38). With the recent advent of these less expensive and invasive techniques, which are used by both surgeons and pain specialists and which may quickly supplant the older open techniques, there may be less distinction in the future between these groups of physicians.

ANATOMY

The human spine consists of the cervical, thoracic, lumbar, sacral, and coccygeal segments. Of these segments, the cervical, lumbar, thoracic, and superior aspects of the sacrum have discs in the normal anatomy of an adult human. There are 6 cervical, 12 thoracic, and 5 lumbar discs, which progressively increase in volume, height, weight bearing, and, to a lesser extent, width as one progresses caudally from the C-2–3 disc to the L-5–S-1 disc. The anterior longitudinal ligament and the posterior longitudinal ligament run the length of the spine and give structural support to the disc anteriorly and posteriorly, respectively. The posterior longitudinal ligament becomes progressively thinner as it goes from cervical to lumbar, with the L-5–S-1 disc level being the thinnest. The cervical and lumbar regions allow lateral rotation as well as flexion and extension in all planes. For the thoracic segment of the spine, the rib cage and sternum prevent flexion, extension, or rotation. The musculature of the spine is essential for movement of the cervical and lumbar spine and helps keep all of the discs and vertebrae of the spine in line. The areas of the spine that allow movement in a physically fit person are narrower than the adjacent regions. For instance, the head, trunk, and hips have a larger circumference than the neck and waist.

The disc consists of an annulus, nucleus pulposus, and vertebral endplates. The annulus itself consists of fibrous material with layers of lamellae that run at a 45° angle to each other to give further support. The center of the disc, the nucleus pulposus, consists of semifluid glycoproteins.

At the superior border and inferior border of the disc are the vertebral endplates. A disc combines with the two facet joints to form a three-joint structure that is called a spinal level. These three joints give weight-bearing support and coastal movement in the lumbar and cervical regions. The disc functions like a ball-bearing type of joint, whereas the two facet joints function like hinges.

Discs of a newborn contain a high water content (approximately 88%), which progressively dehydrates with age (39). The nutrient supply of the disc is by direct vascularization up until the second decade, when the disc becomes avascular, thereafter depending solely on diffusion for its nutrients and thus has a high metabolic turnover (40).

A spinal disc can be divided into three regions of innervation. The first region is the posterior annulus of the disc, which is innervated by the sinuvertebral nerve. The sinuvertebral nerve is a union of the autonomic root of the gray rami communicans and a somatic branch from the ventral ramus (41,42,43). Each sinuvertebral nerve innervates one spinal segment above and two below (49). The second region of innervation is the lateral and anterior annulus, consisting of a series of nerves derived from the ventral rami and sympathetic nerves (45). The third region is the posterolateral aspect of the annulus, innervated by either or both ventral rami at each level and the terminal portion of the gray rami communicans (46). In a healthy disc, innervation is found only in the outer third of the annulus (45–47). One study indicates, for the lumbar disc, that pain is transmitted via the L-2 nerve root, presumably via the sympathetic afferents from the sinuvertebral nerves (48). This suggestion that the sympathetic nervous system is responsible for back pain is supported by other studies (49,50,51).

PATHOPHYSIOLOGY

Two important questions are: How do discs progress from healthy to degenerative, and what does this mean? However, the key question is: What makes a disc become a pain generating disc (PGD)? Is it structural, innervation, chemical, autoimmune, aging, anatomy, or environment (52)? In varying degrees, it is possibly a combination of all of these effects that causes a PGD with each individual, and what we may find is that there are several disease processes involved in causing a PGD. The fact that approximately 40% of the population have no history of activity-limiting low back pain but have spinal disc abnormalities of degenerative disc disease and/or herniation further complicates the picture (53–57). What follows is an attempt to shed some light on these questions.

As discs age, they lose vascularity and are subject to compressional, tensional, as well as rotational stresses. Apparently these factors lead to disc degeneration (58,59). Disc degeneration is the process by which the disc becomes progressively dehydrated with necrosis of the nucleus pulposus and deterioration of the annulus (60). The disc itself, if

healthy when it suffers a traumatic injury, typically will form a Schmorl's node where the disc material is herniated through the vertebral endplate into the vertebra and not through the annulus (61,62). Several studies have suggested that excessive rotational stress accelerates the process of disc degeneration and the potential of disc herniation (63–65). Farfan found that congenital misalignment of the L-5–S-1 facets causes accelerated degenerative disc disease secondary to abnormal rotation of the L-5–S-1 disc (64). As one progresses up the lumbar spine from the sacrum, the facets assume a more saggital orientation, which reduces torsional stress, possibly protecting the disc (66). Pars intraarticularis defects may increase the incidence of lumbar symptoms because there are several studies that show an approximately 25% increased incidence of lumbar symptoms in those with this defect (66–69), although one study showed no increase in symptoms (70). During the process of degeneration, disc height is often, although not always, lost (71,72). Thus, with degeneration, there is not always an external structural change, and, in fact, Twonney and Taylor found that, at postmortem examination, 72% of lumbar discs in patients under 60 years of age were of normal size (72a). The transition of a disc from healthy to fully degenerated makes the disc susceptible to pain (73), but once fully degenerated the disc does not appear to have as much risk of becoming a pain generator (25,74). Several studies show no correlation with disc height and symptoms (75,76).

With repetitive motion, degeneration of the disc is accelerated, which likely leads to a deterioration of the annulus, causing further disc degeneration (66,77,78,79). The fact that the areas of the spine with the greatest movement (e.g., cervical and lumbar spine) develop degeneration the earliest supports this finding (80). The annulus, which has become weak and fissured by this process, will have a propensity for extrusion of the nuclear contents, forming what we know as a herniated disc and leading to structural changes of the disc. This may or may not precipitate the disc to become a PGD (80a). The process of fissuring of the disc may start in the central portion of the annulus outward (81) or from the annulus inward (82), or a combined external and internal migration (79). Others think increased intradiscal pressure causes this disruption (83). This was demonstrated experimentally by Nachemson (84,85). However, the process of loss of integrity of the annulus and intervertebral endplates will expose the surrounding tissues to the contents of the disc (79,86). These contents may have undergone chemical change in the years since direct vascularization was lost, potentially leading to alteration of the immunological profile of the contents setting up, upon exposure to the body, both a chemical (87,88) and immunological response (87–89,90–92,93). This autoimmunity to disc contents has been show in animals (86,94,95). Another possible precipitator of a PGD, secondary to degeneration of the disc, is fissuring of the disc, which is the best predictor of pain reproduction on discograms (96). During the process of degeneration, the fissuring of the annulus allows in-growth of nerve and vascular tissue often to the center of the disc (77,86,90). This in-growth may also occur from vertebral endplate microfractures (61) and Schmorl's nodes (89). Apparently this in-growth of new tissue makes the disc more susceptible to pain provocation (97). It is not clear whether this in-growth of nervous and vascular tissue is a normal process in an attempt by the body to heal the disc gone bad, or if the disc was never intended to have this in-growth like other types of wounds. Regardless, this in-growth of nervous and vascular tissue is present in PGDs. Perhaps individually or in combination these changes lead to symptoms of a PGD, and the immunological reaction may lead to alteration of the structure of the disc by accelerating the degeneration process of the disc.

When a degenerated disc herniates, whether from acute injury or progressive deterioration, it is more likely to do so through the annulus due to deterioration. Herniations are of several patterns. First, herniated discs occur more frequently in the posterior and posterolateral aspect of the disc. However, they can occur laterally or anteriorly, although this is relatively rare. Lumbar discs are most likely to herniate, in particular the L-5–S-1 disc, due to the anatomical thinning of the posterior longitudinal ligament, the increased weight supported, and rotational stresses around this disc. The process of disc disease, no matter what the cause, may lead to instability of the vertebral levels (98). If the herniation is sufficient it may compress and bathe the nerve root in substances that activate the nerve, which can lead to symptoms of a PGD: muscle spasm, radiculopathy, and low back pain (97). Possibly the herniation of the nuclear contents, with compression of the nerve roots and sensitization of them to pain with irritation from caustic disc substances that leak through the annulus fissures, is the source of radiculopathy. Several studies have shown that compression of the nerve root itself will not cause pain but may sensitize the nerve root to pain (100,101). The contents of the nucleus pulposus are full of substances that activate the nerves and have been shown to precipitate inflammation and cause pain in the nerve roots in both animal models and humans (87,88). The disc has a somatotropic referral pattern, and radiculopathy has a dermatomal referred pattern (18,102–104). The herniation of nuclear contents also reduces the volume of the disc, increasing the pressure on the facets and altering the load on the spine. Some think of the disc and facet joints as a single structure when referring to pathology (105). Whatever the cause, once the disc has become a PGD it can cause paraspinal muscle spasm, particularly if the facet joints are involved, either independently or as a result of the disc space narrowing (105,106–108). Regardless, if it is only the discs or the disc and facet joints, with persistent paraspinal muscle spasm, the patient develops paraspinal trigger points due to muscle ischemia. This process sets up a self-perpetuating pain cycle as the disc cannot heal, the paraspinal muscles become ischemic in an attempt to immobilize the painful segment (disc and facets), and the patient develops behavioral changes to cope with these new physical conditions.

The degeneration of the disc can also lead to spondylolisthesis. Spondylolisthesis results from disruption of the contents of the disc, laxity of the facet joints (to a minor degree), and laxity of the surrounding muscles and ligaments (to a greater degree). Spondylolisthesis is graded in four grades, according to Meyerding (109). With this instability there can be associated osteophyte formation along with subchondral sclerosis. This occurs as the body tries to stabilize the disc to prevent the abnormal motion with associated pain (69,110). Other sources of disc disease that can occur in the disc—such as infection, among others—are beyond the scope of this chapter. Overall, the degeneration of a disc with annulus fissuring, whether or not it produces visible changes and regardless of its cause, appears to be the key in the process that causes a disc to become a PGD.

DIAGNOSIS

Distinguishing discs that are PGD from those that are not can be complicated and challenging. As with all forms of human disease, an accurate diagnosis is predicated on performing a thorough physical examination and taking a detailed history. When taking the history of a patient who may have a PGD it is important to know the family history of disc disease and the patient's response to any prior treatment, including medications, injections, or physical therapy. On physical exam the strength of muscles, integrity of nerves, and areas of tenderness are evaluated. Copies of any studies done to evaluate the patient's pain should be obtained. In particular it is important to know the findings on MRI (soft tissue imaging), CT (bone imaging), ultrasound (inflammation of nerves and paraspinal muscles), and nerve studies, such as EMG, nerve conduction velocity, or current perception test (nerve function). The natural history of the ailment is also important; in particular, what precipitated the patient's pain should be obtained. Is the condition improving, worsening, or the same? Does any particular maneuver exacerbate the pain? What are the referral patterns of the pain, keeping in mind the dermatomal, myotomal, and sclerotomal (111,112) patterns as well as atlantoaxial, cervical (113), thoracic (114), and lumbar facet joint pain referral patterns (115,116). All three types of pain referral patterns (sclerotomal, dermatomal, and myotomal) may occur at the same time and can easily be confused (117). It is important to remember that disc pain is somatotropic, not dermatomal (45,102–104). Along with information obtained with the history and physical, imaging studies, nerve function tests, and discometric injections, if not previously done, may need to be performed to come to an accurate diagnosis. When evaluating patients who complain of neck, thoracic, or low back pain, other potential causes of pain having little or nothing to do with the disc must be considered. Examples include cardiac ischemia with referred pain to the neck and arm, empyema with thoracic pain, or low back referred pain caused by urinary tract infection, peptic ulcer disease, or abdominal aortic aneurysm, just to name a few. It is important to guard against becoming narrow in our thinking and considering every patient with back pain as having a spinal source. In the following sections, the diagnosis of cervical, thoracic, and lumbar PGD will be covered.

Let us digress for a moment on an important point concerning nomenclature. Once a diagnosis is made, it must be more than a description of symptoms, such as back pain or neck pain. In the CPT, for billing purposes, terms like *cervicalgia* and *lumbago* are used, but these terms do not truly define the problem. A correct diagnosis would be, for instance, L-5–S-1 herniated lumbar disc with impingement of the left S-1 nerve root and left S-1 radiculopathy, not lumbago with sciatica. Nomenclature is important to reduce confusion and advance the field by allowing all professionals to speak the same language.

CERVICAL PAIN GENERATING DISCS

In approaching a patient who potentially suffers from a cervical PGD it is important to pay close attention to the symptoms. A patient with cervical PGD may have symptoms of cephalgia, neck pain, and/or radiculopathy in the upper extremities. If the patient suffers from headaches, what is the location of the cephalgia: "migraine pattern," occipital, or tension-type headaches? Does the patient have symptoms of a Horner's syndrome, pain only to the neck, or also to the trapezius muscle region? How frequent is the pain? How long does the pain last? Are symptoms consistent or variable? It is important to determine pain severity because this will influence treatment. Always consider that the patient could suffer from more than one diagnosis related to head pain, such as a cervical PGD and tension headaches. Symptoms of difficulty swallowing also leave one to think of cervical spine pathology, possibly disc related. Sometimes a disc irritating a cervical nerve root will cause unique and unexpected symptoms such as complex regional pain syndrome type symptoms or unilateral facial pain. This unilateral facial pain is often misdiagnosed as migraine. The difficulty is that a clinician will often make the diagnosis of migraine based on known symptoms of this type of headache, not considering cervical spine disease as a possible cause. Thus, if the head hurts worse than the neck, it is a headache even though the headache is due to neck disease. A high level of suspicion for a cervical PGD must be maintained by clinicians when they come across a patient with headache and neck pain. Rarely, the only symptoms for a higher central disc may be those of anterior chest pain.

As discussed earlier, each spinal level consists of three joints (two facet joints and the disc). To make an accurate diagnosis in the patient with neck pain, all three potential pain generators must be considered. The facets, when stimulated in a painful manner, produce a consistent referral pattern (113). An understanding of the referral pattern will improve the clinician's diagnostic skills. A cervical nerve root radiculopathy, which is a symptom of cervical PGD, may have symptoms of weakness, sensory loss, or pain in the upper extremities. In the neck and upper extremities, understanding the dermatomal sensory pattern, innervation required for reflexes, and motor strength, as well as sclerotomal and myotomal referred pain patterns, is critically important in order to make an accurate diagnosis. By practicing the art of clinically differentiating dermatomal, myotomal, and sclerotomal referral patterns over time, the individual varieties of these different patterns can be mastered and allow a more accurate diagnosis of the level of the PGD and PGFJ.

On physical exam, one examines nervous function of the muscles and reflexes, and two tests, which may be positive if a cervical nerve root is irritated, will give useful information. The tests are palpation of Erb's fossa, which places tension on the brachial plexus, and hyperextension of the arm at the shoulder while in 90° of abduction. Both tests will increase the patient's typical pain in a dermatomal pattern if the patient suffers from nerve root irritation. Palpation of the posterior and lateral cervical spine should be done because one may find muscle spasms and tenderness indicating a possible underlying disc injury. The trapezius muscles should also be examined for spasm or reproduction of the patient's pain. Reduced range of motion of the cervical spine secondary to reactive muscle spasm may also be found with discogenic problems or facet problems. Having the patient perform a Valsalva maneuver, if a disc is involved, may also reproduce the patient's pain. The distraction and compression test of the cervical spine may also be useful.

The greater, lesser, and least occipital nerves, which innervate the occipital region of the skull, are also palpated posteriorly at the base of the skull for tenderness and reproduction of the patient's symptoms of occipital headache. These nerves may be irritated by a PGD.

All of this must be kept in mind when examining the cervical spine. Obviously, other medical conditions can occur at the same time a patient suffers from a PGD, such as sinusitis, which may present with overlapping symptoms but is a different disease calling for different treatments.

THORACIC PAIN GENERATING DISC

Disc disease of the thoracic spine, which is symptomatic from a pain perspective, is uncommon. This may be due to the lack of motion in these segments, which protects these discs. Certainly older patients with severe thoracic degenerative disc and severe kyphosis can have cardiac and pulmonary problems, but these discs rarely cause pain. Patients with thoracic spine pain due to a PGD can be of three types: two with radiating pain and one with localized pain. The first type of patient with a thoracic PGD will have symptoms of dermatomal referred pain to the anterior chest or upper abdomen. Often these patients present with abdominal pain, having signs and symptoms consistent with complex regional pain syndrome (CRPS). Their pain is burning in nature, with some or all of the following signs and symptoms: allodynia, inflammation, temperature changes to the skin, sensitivity, and hot and cold in a dermatomal pattern. It is not uncommon to have a patient who presents with severe right, left, or bilateral upper quadrant pain who has had a "million dollar" workup for abdominal pain. These workups are usually completely negative or have only minor findings but nothing of a degree to cause the amount of pain the patient suffers. On careful examination, the patient's symptoms are consistent with thoracic nerve root irritation with referred pain to the upper abdomen. MRI of the thoracic spine may show a disc herniation or disc disease, but frequently the MRI is negative. If there is an injury to the disc it frequently does not show up on MRI. Plain x-rays of the thoracic spine may show loss of disc height, but, again, this is usually not the rule. A current perception test to test the nerve function may help to localize the vertebral level.

On physical exam, palpating along the "track" of the pain around to the involved vertebral level can help to localize the disc. The second type of pain is a PGD with paraspinal muscle spasm and tenderness without radiculopathy. Again this is most probably related to a PGD at that level with a negative MRI. The third type may involve a herniation with nerve root impingement and the expected spectrum of symptoms. Other findings in the thoracic spine may or may not cause symptoms. On MRI, Schmorl's nodes or degenerative disc disease, as well as a herniated nucleus pulposus (either posteriorly, posterolaterally, or anteriorly) in the thoracic spine may be found, which may or may not be symptomatic. If symptomatic, the pain is paraspinal without radiation and/or, with radiation, in a dermatomal pattern, often with paraspinal muscle spasms and "trigger points."

LUMBAR PAIN GENERATING DISCS

In the history we need to assess these questions: When did the pain start? Was it gradual or abrupt? Was there an initiating event (e.g., trauma)? Is there a nerve root injury with radiation of the pain and/or sensory loss down the leg in a dermatomal pattern and/or muscle weakness? Is the pain resolving, unchanged, or getting worse? Has anything helped reduce pain intensity?

The L-3–4, L-4–5, and L-5–S1 discs are the most frequent locations of lumbar PGD. When taking a thorough history it is important to know the most common signs and symptoms of these PGDs. Symptoms of an L-4 nerve root irritation will be pain or decreased sensation starting in the low back running down the leg to the big toe. Symptoms of an L-5 nerve root irritation are referred pain or decreased sensation from the lumbar spine to the middle two or three toes. An S-1 nerve root irritation will present with referred pain or decreased sensation from the lumbar spine to the

lateral foot, including the small toe. These symptoms could be present unilaterally or bilaterally. Occasionally an L-5–S-1 PGD will cause symptoms in the inguinal area consisting of pain in the labia majora in women or in the testicles in men. This referred pain can have CRPS-like symptoms. Rarely will this be the only symptom of an L-5–S-1 PGD. Pain in the lumbar spine due to a PGD will be exacerbated by prolonged sitting or standing but should resolve by lying in the supine position. This increased pain when sitting or standing is physiologically due to increased pressure on the disc when the lumbar spine is in flexion and decreased by extension (118). A PGD can also cause symptoms of referred pain in a sclerotomal and myotomal pattern (111,112). For instance, an L-5–S-1 disc can cause sclerotomal referred pain with hypersensitivity to the sacroiliac joints (117,119). Radiculopathy is one symptom of a PGD but does not need to be present for a patient to have a PGD. When patients complain of leg pain, one should consider the sclerotomal, dermatomal, and myotomal pain referral patterns that will help categorize the type. Burning and shooting pain are consistent with nerve root irritation. Dull pain is more consistent with a sclerotomal or myotomal referral pattern. Thus, by understanding the nature of the pain and the structures involved, we can locate the PGD.

When examining the lumbar spine we also look for scoliosis and scars consistent with previous surgery. When a patient has symptoms of low back pain and pain in one or both extremities we look for a sensory deficit, reflex deficit, and/or motor weakness to help localize the PGD. Loss of the reflex at the patella tendon is consistent with an L-4 nerve root deficit, and loss of reflex at the Achilles tendon is consistent with an S-1 nerve root deficit. There is no reflex test for L-5. The muscle test for the L-4 nerve root is the anterior tibial muscle. For L-5, it is the extensor hallucis longus, and for S-1 it is the peroneus longus and brevis muscles. Patients with lumbar discogenic pain will have a positive Somerville sign (i.e., if they sit for long periods of time on a hard surface they have to elevate one hip or the other or stand to alleviate the pain in their back). Other physical exam findings are also beneficial. The straight leg-raising test can help to support the diagnosis of nerve root irritation and, thus, a PGD. Positive cross straight leg-raising and straight leg-raising tests may also help to diagnose intrathecal pathology. The Kernig, Millgram, Naffinger, and Valsalva tests may also help rule in or rule out intrathecal pathology (120). Occasionally the only symptom of a PGD is deep pain in the lumbar region or occasional lumbar pain with radiation down to the knee. Patients will, however, have a positive Somerville sign and negative straight leg-raising test. The MRI may or may not show abnormalities of the disc. A CT myelogram may show compression of a nerve root, or it may not, but if the MRI is negative it is very unlikely that a CT myelogram will detect it. However, the MRI is not effective in picking up posterolateral disc herniations. On the heavily weighted T-2

MRI images a high-intensity zone may show up indicative of a disc disruption, which may be a sign of a PGD (121–124).

One important point is the need for immediate referral to a spine surgeon if the patient develops rapid progressive weakness, loss of sensation in a leg or the legs, or bowel or bladder incontinence.

Patients who have had previous spinal surgery certainly confuse the picture. Patients who have undergone a lumbar spinal fusion have a 10% to 70% chance of no improvement. One possible reason may be that the "pathological" disc, as imaged by MRI or CT myelogram, was assumed to be the PGD and surgically treated without any spinal diagnostics to further substantiate if the pathological disc was in fact the PGD. This increases the chance that a nonpainful disc was operated on.

Lumbar PGDs frequently occur with pain generating facet joints (PGFJ). The lumbar PGFJ must be differentiated from lumbar PGD because both may occur concordantly or independently at the same or different vertebral levels. PGD and PGFJ demand totally different treatments. Lumbar PGFJs are usually the cause of paraspinal muscle spasm and tenderness, referred pain down to the ankles, and increased pain on extension and lateral flexion of the lumbar spine, whereas a PGD may have symptoms of radiculopathy and a positive Somerville sign. If hyperextending the lumbar spine reduces the pain, this maneuver also points to a lumbar PGD. A skeletal muscular ultrasound can help in diagnosing paraspinal inflammation (consistent with PGFJs) and/or inflammation of the nerve root (consistent with PGD) (125). A current perception test can help localize nerve root deficiencies, if any, by measuring the function of the A-beta, A-delta, or C fibers (126). Deficiencies of these nerves will help make the case of a PGD, but obviously there are other causes of nerve dysfunction. With practice, molding all of this information together will improve the clinician's ability to diagnosis a PGD.

DIAGNOSING DISC PAIN

Discograms

A major advance in the field of spinal diagnostics has been the use of discograms, not only to ascertain pain provocation, but also to delineate the internal disc architecture. Once the appropriate patient has been selected and the workup is consistent with one or more PGDs, then discograms, to confirm the diagnosis and interrogate the discs, are done. Because there are risks with this procedure, including inadvertent dural puncture, nerve root injury, bleeding, and infection, the risks should always be discussed with a patient prior to the procedure. A bleeding time and a CBC should be checked prior to doing discograms to evaluate for preexisting infection or bleeding diathesis. The patient should also be warned that this procedure, which is diagnostic in nature, may exacerbate pain. To obtain the most information from discograms they should be done on the suspected PGD and at least one but preferably two others. This is done to identify a nonpainful disc as a control and to increase the chance of not missing a PGD because more than one disc may be a pain generator. Occasionally, more than three discs will need to be interrogated. Typically, first approach the disc above or below the suspected PGD. This is done to stimulate the most painful disc last, reduce the patient's suffering, and subsequently allow easier cannulation of the PGD. In other words, if the patient is uncomfortable due to stimulating the most painful disc first, it will be technically more challenging to cannulate the other discs. Discograms should be used to diagnose and localize the PGD for fusion or other surgical treatment. Discograms, as with other diagnostic tests, should be used as a tool to direct further treatment. To diagnose a PGD without any further intention to use this information clinically is inappropriate.

Discograms should be done under fluoroscopy, otherwise the risk of complications and a poor quality study is greatly increased. A water-soluble, nonionic contrast is used, such as Omnipaque 240 or Isoview M200 or M300. The patient has an IV started with appropriate IV fluids, depending upon the health of the patient. The amount of sedation and analgesia the patient receives should not be so great as to produce an unresponsive patient. The patient should be stress free, but not somnolent. Reassurance of, and communication with, the patient will decrease the need for sedation. The disc should be approached from the side opposite the patient's pain, if possible, so that if there is any leakage of the contrast around the needle it will not obscure the CT image. Then, under fluoroscopic guidance, the vertebra are counted and the disc(s) in question is (are) located. As with all spinal injections, the injection should be done with both hands. The nondominant hand is used to stabilize the needle by placing it in contact with the patient's body so that, if there is any sudden movement by the patient, the hand and the needle go in the same direction, i.e., away from the patient. The dominant hand is used to advance the needle with resistance from the nondominant hand, which controls advancement of the needle. As with all injections, Dr. Racz's advice of checking the needle's "depth, direction, depth" under fluoroscopy should be observed to reduce the risk of complications (127). The fluoroscopy unit should be aligned to allow maximum visualization of the disc. This is done by lining up the anterior and posterior borders of the inferior vertebral endplate and obliquing the unit to have a view of the disc lucency (from the anterior to posterior portion of the disc) as large as possible and such that the line of the x-ray beam through the SEP, DEP, and DIP does not transverse any vital structures (Fig. 28-1). Then, using a radiopaque marker, the skin entry point (SEP) is located. This is the point in the skin lined up under the x-ray beam such that it overlies the center of the disc to be cannulated. The needle is then directed toward the disc in line with the x-ray "beam." The needle will then

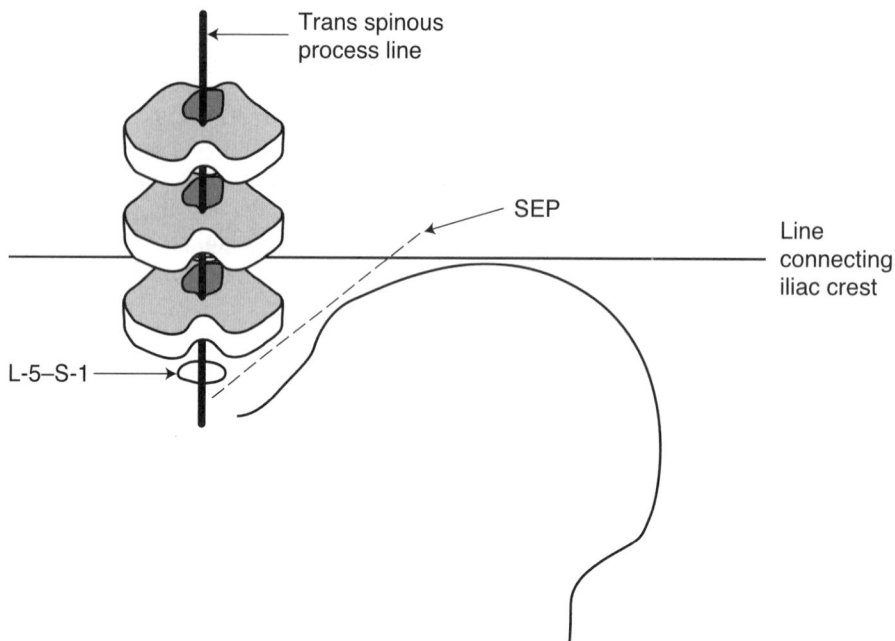

FIG. 28-1. Right-sided approach for L-5–S-1 discogram using Dr. Mironer's approach.

come in line with the "center" of the lucency, which is the disc. This is the disc entry point (DEP). The needle is then advanced under fluoroscopy into the center of the disc. The disc injection point (DIP) is the location where the tip of the needle is centered as much as possible in the center of the disc from AP and lateral views as well as in proportion to the vertebral endplates. The contrast is then injected.

When a discogram is performed, a record is kept of the amount of contrast injected for each disc, the nuclear pattern of the disc, pain provocation pattern, and quality of

the terminal resistance. Additionally, the most painful disc, quality of pain, and any extravasation of contrast are recorded. If an injection of local anesthesia into the disc is done to calm the patient's pain, this is recorded. The amount of sedation and analgesic used, as well as pain tolerance, should be recorded (Table 28-1). A CT scan with 3-mm horizontal cuts of the spinal region where the discograms were performed should follow within 2 hours of the procedure to delineate the disc's internal structures, any derangement to the annulus, and as a permanent

Table 28-1. *Discographic diagnostic categories*

Disc classification (sensitivity)	Intradiscal pressure at pain provocation (above opening pressure)	Pain severity (VAS)	Pain type	Determination
Chemical	Immediate onset of familiar pain occurring as <1 mL of contrast is visualized reaching the outer annulus*, or pain provocation at up to 15 PSI (103.5 KPA)	.>6/10	Concordant	Positive
Mechanical	15 to 50 PSI (103.5–344.7 KPA)	>6/10	Concordant	Positive (but other pain generators may be present; further investigation may be warranted)
Indeterminate	51 to 90 PSI (346.2–620.5 KPA)	>6/10	Concordant	Further investigation warranted
Normal	>90 PSI (620.5 KPA)	No pain		Negative

*Typically, contrast will be visualized reaching the outer annulus at <10 PSI above opening pressure. Consequently, a disc generating familiar/concordant pain as contrast is visualized reaching the outer annulus may be deemed chemically sensitive as defined within the context of this study. Adapted from Derby R et al. Predictive pressure controlled discography. *Spine* 1999;24: 4:365.

record. The continuous fluoroscopy method or intermittent picture technique can be used. A hard copy of the fluoroscopic images (AP and lateral) should also be saved because they will show any extravasation of the contrast from the disc. Because the cervical discs are very narrow, and a CT scan will produce 3-mm slices, the quality of cervical CT disc images may be poor. For this reason, it is more important to keep hard copies of the AP and lateral views of the fluoroscopic images of cervical discograms. Depending upon the patient's future treatment plan, these images will be helpful to the pain specialist and/or spine surgeon.

Using a discometric device to measure the pressure in the disc is a newer technique and may be of greater value in the future as we better understand the usefulness of this information. Derby has written extensively on this subject (128–131). This technique uses a special measuring device that records the pressure reading during injection of the disc and will print a graph of this pressure over time. Contrast is loaded into the specialized syringe and is then connected to the needle cannulating the disc. The pressure is increased by slowly twisting the handle. Each turn causes the injection of 0.5 cc of contrast. The current injection device, due to its large size, is much easier to use for a lumbar disc than a cervical disc. The average volume used during discography for a cervical disc is 0.3 to 1 cc, for a thoracic disc 0.5–1 cc, and for a lumbar disc 1–2 cc. If the disc is incompetent, it will not maintain a constant pressure on pressurization, and contrast extruded out of the disc can be visualized under fluoroscopy. As an additional check on pain provocation with pressurization, the disc can be anesthetized by injecting into the painful disc or discs a small volume of preservative-free (PF) local anesthetic, such as 0.25% Bupivacaine PF. The connecting tubing, if used to connect the syringe to the needle, should be removed because the injection of further volume, depending on the length of the connecting tubing, into the disc can be painful, and overpressurizing the disc should be avoided. If the disc is incompetent, local anesthetic should not be injected because it will leak on the adjacent neural tissue and can obscure the clinical picture. If the disc is not incompetent and the injection of local anesthetic into the painful disc calms the patient's pain, this further confirms that a PGD has been found. There is a chance during discograms that the injected disc is so incompetent that, although it is the PGD, not enough pressure is obtained with the injected dye on the disc to stimulate the patient's pain. This must always be considered when dealing with a very incompetent disc.

Infection is always a concern with discograms. Administration of antibiotics prior to the discogram, such as one gram of a third-generation cephalosporin (or any other antibiotic with activity against skin organisms) may help to reduce the chance of infection. Also, mixing 20 mg of Kefzol per cc of contrast to be used for injection may also reduce the incidence of infection. There is no literature to support giving intradiscal antibiotics, although it is a common practice.

Interpretation of Discograms

To improve the science of pain management and improve the understanding of disc disease it is important to have a nomenclature to describe the discogram radiographic findings. One possible method is the Dallas discogram description (132) with the modification as suggested by Dullerud and Johansen (133). With the Dallas description, two pain and one radiographic parameters were measured. The pain parameters were intensity, which was grouped in four categories: no pain, slight pain, moderate pain, severe pain, and how the pain correlated with the usual pain sensation: sensation of pressure/no pain, dissimilar pain, similar pain, exact reproduction of pain. Then, within 15 minutes of the discogram, a CT of the discogram disc is done with contiguous 3-mm slices (132). From these images degeneration of the circumference of the annulus is assessed and divided into four groups: no change, local degeneration affecting a sector of less than 10%, partial degeneration involving 10% to 50%, and total degeneration affecting more than 50%. The modification of the Dallas description by Dullerud and Johansen consists of grading the annulus disruption by the depth of the tear. They grouped it into no tear, tear confined to annulus, tear through the annulus with contrast opacification of the hernia, subligamentous leak of contrast, and leak through the posterior longitudinal ligament (133). Derby et al.'s manometric interpretation of discograms is another avenue to categorize a PGD. The pressure needed to cause the appearance of contrast in the disc under fluoroscopy is called the opening pressure, and this is recorded. For discometry, the protocol for chemical, mechanical, and indeterminate sensitivity as described by Derby et al. is seen in Table 28-2 (131). Continuing to inject contrast, the pressure at which the patient experiences pain is recorded. If no pain occurs upon reaching 90 PSI in the disc, the discometry is terminated for that disc, and the disc is recorded as nonpainful. As more experience is gained with the taxometry systems a combination will emerge that will be useful in treatment outcome.

Cervical Discograms

Cervical discograms are more challenging, technically, than lumbar, with more potential for complications secondary to the high number of vital organs in close proximity to the cervical spine and the small structure of the neck. The injectionist should have extensive experience with spinal injections, in particular lumbar discograms, before attempting cervical discograms. The risk in performing cervical discograms comes from the fact that the hypopharynx lies in close proximity to the upper cervical discs with the esophagus in close proximity to the anterior cervical spine along its entire length, increasing the possibility of inadvertently traversing these structures while approaching the cervical disc. If these structures were to be inadvertently entered, bacteria could be introduced into the disc, causing an infection.

Table 28-2. *Discogram results form*

Patient		Date			Referring physician			Operating physician		
Level	Contrast pattern normal or abnormal	Extravasation or bulging or degeneration	Total volume accepted by the disc	Terminal resistance	Pain provocation	Intensity of pain	Concordant or atypical pain	Pressures (mmHg) 1. Opening 2. Pain provocation	Location of pain
	___ Normal ___ Abnormal		___ cc	___ Little ___ Moderate ___ Firm	___ Positive ___ Negative	___ Mild ___ Moderate ___ Severe ___ N/A	___ Concordant ___ Atypical	1 _____ 2 _____	
	___ Normal ___ Abnormal		___ cc	___ Little ___ Moderate ___ Firm	___ Positive ___ Negative	___ Mild ___ Moderate ___ Severe ___ N/A	___ Concordant ___ Atypical	1 _____ 2 _____	
	___ Normal ___ Abnormal		___ cc	___ Little ___ Moderate ___ Firm	___ Positive ___ Negative	___ Mild ___ Moderate ___ Severe ___ N/A	___ Concordant ___ Atypical	1 _____ 2 _____	
	___ Normal ___ Abnormal		___ cc	___ Little ___ Moderate ___ Firm	___ Positive ___ Negative	___ Mild ___ Moderate ___ Severe ___ N/A	___ Concordant ___ Atypical	1 _____ 2 _____	
	___ Normal ___ Abnormal		___ cc	___ Little ___ Moderate ___ Firm	___ Positive ___ Negative	___ Mild ___ Moderate ___ Severe ___ N/A	___ Concordant ___ Atypical	1 _____ 2 _____	

Most painful Disc: _____   Note: Intradiscal 0.75% Marcaine at : _____

Total Medication   Versed: _____mg

   Demerol: _____mg

For a cervical discogram, the patient is moved to the procedure room and placed in the supine position on a surgical table compatible with fluoroscopy. Cervical discs should be approached anteriorly given that this position gives better exposure to the cervical discs. A small wedge is then placed under the patient's neck. This will hyperextend the neck, allowing improved access to the cervical disc. Proper positioning is critical because it will greatly enhance the ability to perform this procedure quickly and safely. Following positioning, a sterile prep and drape of the neck are done to the exposed anterior and lateral neck on both the right and left sides. Prep up to the point of the chin, over to the ear and the mastoid process, down to the edge of the table laterally, out to the deltoid on the right and left side, and down to the table on the trapezius muscle and to approximately the second intercostal space on the chest. This broad prep is done to give a comfortable working space.

After the patient is properly positioned, sterile prep and drape are performed, and the instrument field arranged, the discograms are performed. The appropriate disc is located by counting the cervical vertebral bodies down from the atlas. To cannulate the center of the cervical disc for a discogram, it is approached from an oblique angle using fluoroscopy. With the patient in the supine position, a radiopaque marker (such as the tip of a Kelly clamp) is placed on the skin of the anterior neck over the intended disc to be cannulated to establish the correct horizontal plane. The fluoroscopy unit is placed in an oblique angle so that a straight line drawn between the two ends of the C-arm imaging unit would connect the center of the disc and tip of the clamp. On this view of the cervical disc, the location of the clamp tip, which will eventually be used as the marker for the skin entry point (SEP), is positioned so as not to overlap the "air bubble" of the esophagus nor overlap the neural foramen. The esophagus itself extends laterally from the "air bubble," and this must be taken into consideration when approaching the disc. The disc entry point (DEP) is the point on the disc surface in line with the two ends of the C-arm "beam" that travels through the SEP and disc injection point. The DIP is the center of the disc as determined under fluoroscopy by AP and lateral views with the needle tip located at the center of the disc in relation to anterior, posterior, superior posterior, and coronal planes. For safety, the DEP should be midway between the esophagus and the neural foramen and midway between the vertebral endplates. The fluoroscopy unit is then rotated in the cephalocaudad plane while still in the oblique angle until the disc space lucency is as large as possible. With each cervical disc this will be a different angle. This should correlate with the lining up of the borders of the anterior and posterior endplate of the caudad vertebra. This position will give the easiest and safest access to the disc. Then, with the nondominant hand, retract the sternocleidomastoid muscle and carotid neurovascular structures laterally. Then anesthetize the skin at the location of SEP and direct the needle to the DEP to reach the DIP. A 25-gauge, 3-inch Quinke needle can be used, but if one does not have extensive experience with this more flimsy needle, a 22-gauge 3-inch Quinke needle should be used. Although a small-caliber needle will be more comfortable for the patient, it is more likely to misdirect, resulting in a misadventure. For those who do not have extensive experience with a smaller needle (i.e., 25 gauge), then using this needle in a more forgiving area, such as with the facets in the lumbar spine to develop experience with this needle, is recommended prior to approaching the cervical disc. Occasionally, even in the most experienced hands, a 22-gauge needle will be needed to enter the disc due to osteophytes. The C-2–3 and C-3–4 discs will need to be entered from a more lateral-oblique approach. This is needed to reduce the chance of entering the oropharynx and trachea. After identifying the appropriate disc with a radiopaque marker under fluoroscopy one moves lateral in the horizontal plane. While moving the marker laterally fluoroscopic pictures are taken to find the optimal position where the SEP, DEP, and DIP line up. Again the cephalocaudad oblique angle of the fluoroscopy unit is adjusted to "open up" the disc space. Then, after the most medial location laterally is found to assure that the structures just mentioned will not be entered, this is the SEP. The tip of the needle should then, under fluoroscopic guidance, pass through the DEP to the DIP. As the disc is entered from the anterior aspect, care should be taken on advancing the needle using "depth, direction, depth" to assure that the spinal cord is not entered.

Thoracic Discograms

As in the cervical spine, discograms at three levels should be done: the painful disc in question and the discs above and below to reduce the risk of a missed PGD and the need for a second operation if a PGD is missed. The thoracic discs are difficult to access for discograms due to their close proximity to the pleura, which mandates a more medial and steeper approach. With thoracic discs the patient is placed in the prone position, and a posterior approach is used. A sterile prep and drape over the thoracic spine and lateral rib cage are done. One starts at the intervertebral disc in question, which is located by counting under fluoroscopy down from the C-7–T-1 disc and up from T-12–L-1. After the suspected disc is located the caudad and cephalad discs are cannulated first. The disc space should be as transparent (i.e., as wide) as possible. This is done by placing the fluoroscopy unit in the oblique angle within the cephalocaudad plane. A 22-gauge 6- or 8-inch Chiba needle is the most

appropriate to give the best balance between accuracy and comfort because one needs a stiff needle for control of the needle tip and a small-diameter needle for patient comfort. A small 15-degree, 1-cm bend in line with the bevel is then made in the needle. The stylet should easily withdraw from the cannula prior to placing the needle in the disc. The fluoroscopy unit is placed in the oblique angle but only approximately 15 degrees off midline; then, on cephalocaudad oblique views, the disc space is "opened up" by lining up the anterior and posterior borders of the caudad vertebral endplate. Using the tip of a Kelly clamp as a marker to determine the SEP, make sure the pleura is avoided while the needle approaches at the DEP, then the DIP. Again, following anesthetizing the SEP, slowly approach the desired disc using the bend in the needle to steer the needle. A discogram information sheet is used to record data on all of the discs cannulated. A postdiscogram CT is done following the procedure. A hard copy of the fluoroscopic images should be kept. Discometry can be used on these discs as well to record the opening pressure and the pain provocation pressure. Giving IV antibiotics and mixing antibiotics with the contrast may help reduce the chance of infection.

Lumbar Discograms

Lumbar discs are larger and thus easier to cannulate than cervical or thoracic discs. Lumbar discs are approached with the patient in the prone position. A lateral approach to the disc is used with farther lateral placement of the SEP as one progresses from cephalad to caudad in the lumbar spine. For all lumbar discs, except the L-5–S-1 disc, this lateral placement of the SEP holds. A sterile prep and drape of the lumbar, lower thoracic, and sacral/gluteal region laterally to the midaxillary line on both sides are performed. The disc in question should be located by counting down from the T-12–L-1 disc and up from the L-5–S-1 disc. Discograms of three discs should be done to most accurately assess the PGD and/or PGDs. With the fluoroscopy unit in the oblique angle on the side of choice, the angle is increased off midline until the anterior aspect of the facet articulating process bisects the midline of the disc. Then, adjust the cephalocaudad angle of the fluoroscopy unit to "open up" the disc space, which is optimally obtained when the anterior and posterior borders of the inferior endplate of the disc line up. Using a radiopaque marker, the SEP is determined, and a needle for the discogram is selected. The skin is then anesthetized at the SEP. The needle used is a 22-gauge 6- or 8-inch Chiba needle, depending on the size of the patient. A 25-gauge needle can be used but with greater difficulty due to its flexibility. Using "depth, direction, depth" under fluoroscopic guidance, the needle is directed to the DEP by passing the needle tip just inferior to the ventral border of the junction of inferior and superior facet articulating processes. Of note, if the disc is severely narrowed it will be difficult to cannulate. After the needle has transversed the DEP to the DIP, contrast is injected into the disc. Lumbar discs will usually take 1–2 cc of contrast. As for cervical and thoracic discs, a discogram information sheet should be filled out. Again, a postdiscogram CT of the lumbar spine within 2 hours is needed for optimal visualization. Hard copies of the AP and lateral fluoroscopic images of the discograms should be made. As with cervical discograms, giving IV antibiotics and mixing antibiotics with the contrast may help reduce the chance of infection.

A special case is the L-5–S-1 disc. This disc can be very difficult to cannulate due to its unique anatomical location. Its inferior location, frequently overriding the iliac crest, as well as large transverse processes at the L-5 vertebra, creates the difficulty. There are three techniques that have good success, and all three can also be used on the more cephalad lumbar discs to help refine the skills of the injection. The first is the coaxial technique. This technique involves using a 3½-inch 18- or 20-gauge Quinke spinal needle as an introducer. The patient is situated in the prone position, sedated, and the lumbosacral area prepped and draped. Then, from the AP position under fluoroscopy, the cephalocaudad line formed by the spinous processes is lined up an equal distance between the pedicles to give a true AP position and to have a consistent and most effective starting point. Then, by positioning the fluoroscopic unit in a cephalocaudad angle, the anterior and posterior borders of the inferior vertebral endplate are lined up. The SEP of the spinal introducer needle, as determined with a radiopaque marker under AP fluoroscopy, is just lateral to the junction of the superior and inferior articulating processes, in line on lateral view with the caudad third of the neural foramen and the center of the disc. Then, on the lateral fluoroscopic view the introducer is advanced anteriorly past the neural foramen to the posterior border of the disc. On AP view, the introducer needle should pass the lateral aspect of the neural foramen. The stylet of the spinal introducer needle is removed. The Chiba needle, which is to be used to cannulate the disc, is modified. This modification is performed, with a cotton 4 × 4 wrapped around the needle, by taking the index finger and middle finger on one side of the Chiba needle and the thumb on the opposite side at the midportion of the needle. At the same time, the hub is pulled away from the midportion of the needle, separating the fingers and thumb. The needle is pulled between the 4 × 4 and fingers and thumb as the needle is bent. This will give a gentle bend to the needle. This should be done so the curve of the needle is in line with the bevel. Because the catch on the hub of the stylet is in line with the bevel, knowing this allows advancement of the needle while tracking the direction of the curvature of the needle and the bevel. Then, using the modified 22-gauge Chiba needle through the 18-gauge spinal introducer needle or a 25-gauge Chiba through the 20-gauge spinal introducer needle, the Chiba needle is inserted. The stylet of the Chiba needle is then removed, and contrast can be injected at the DIP. A discogram information sheet should be filled out. Hard copies of the fluoroscopic images should be kept. This is a simple technique, and the only technique needed to do L-5–S-1 discograms by our surgical colleagues.

For those who will do the IDET (Intradiscal Electrothermal Annuloplasty) procedure, the following two L-5–S-1 discogram cannulation techniques will also be useful as a learning exercise for the placement of the introducer needle for the IDET catheter in the L-5–S-1 disc. Although these two techniques have a steep learning curve, once mastered, the L-5–S-1 disc can be cannulated as fast or faster than, and as safe as, the previously mentioned technique. The first technique, as described by Mironer, uses a straight 6- or 8-inch 22-gauge Chiba needle (134). With the patient in the prone position under fluoroscopy, a horizontal line is drawn on the skin to connect the points at the superior aspect of the iliac crests. This horizontal line should transect at a right angle the cephalocaudad spinous process line, as determined under fluoroscopy on a true AP. Then, on the side of the spine the disc is to be cannulated, a line is drawn on the skin from a point at the center of the L-5–S-1 disc, as determined under fluoroscopy from a true AP view, to transect the horizontal line connecting the superior points of the iliac crests. This transection should occur midway between the spinous process cephalocaudad line and the most superior point of the ipsilateral iliac crest. The point where the two lines cross is the SEP point. Then, under fluoroscopy using a radiopaque object such as the tip of a clamp to mark it, the SEP is lined up so it overlaps a point posterior and caudad to the lateral edge of the L-5–S-1 disc. On this view, the needle is steered toward the posterolateral caudad edge of the disc or where this point on the disc should be if not visualized under fluoroscopy. By steering the needle toward the caudad portion of the posterolateral aspect of the disc, the nerve root will be avoided. The needle should be advanced slowly with the patient able to respond because this will reduce the chance of nerve injury. The needle tip is then "worked" cephalad along the superior-lateral disc to enter at the DEP, then to the DIP.

The third technique uses a bent needle. This is done by taking a 22-gauge 6- or 8-inch Chiba needle and placing a 1-cm 15-degree bend in the needle in line with the bevel. The stylet should be easily withdrawn before trying to position this needle. Then, line up the fluoroscopy unit on the side of the lumbar spine to be approached, in the lateral, cephalocaudad oblique angle to "open up" the L-5–S-1 disc interspace as much as possible. In patients with a high-riding iliac crest, large transverse process, and/or severe degenerative disc disease with disc height loss it may not be possible to "see the disc." With practice and frequent reference to a skeleton it will quickly become apparent where the disc "should be," improving the ability to cannulate a "difficult" disc. Then, after anesthetizing the skin at the SEP, the needle is placed through the SEP. With the bend in the needle it can be steered to the DEP using fluoroscopy with frequent reference to its position on AP and lateral views. The needle should "ride" down the beam of the x-rays to the DEP and then the DIP. Sometimes, despite the best technique and positioning, it will not be possible to place the needle at the DIP. In this case the contrast should be injected into the annulus. Although not giving as much information as placing the needle at the DIP and not obtaining a nucleogram, it can help determine if there is provocation of the patient's pain, which will be helpful in determining the need for surgery or IDET.

Complications

When performing a procedure it is critically important to be able to diagnose a complication and institute appropriate treatment. For example, if a patient, following discograms, were to develop discitis, a low threshold for making this diagnosis is needed, and appropriate treatment and followup must be instituted. If not, it could be catastrophic. Worsening of the patient's radicular symptoms, worsening back pain, or cauda equina syndrome several days following the procedure could occur with discitis. To work up a patient with suspected discitis an MRI and/or CT scan of the involved disc or discs should be done and may be helpful in localizing the inflammation and infection. An elevated white count and sedimentation rate may or may not be present. After the diagnosis is made, the patient should be admitted to the hospital, blood cultures should be taken, consultation with an infectious disease specialist and spine surgeon will be helpful, and appropriate antibiotics and supportive measures should be started.

Other potential complications can be avoided if it is clear what information is needed. A discogram on a patient with a small spinal canal or with moderate to severe neuroforaminal stenosis may be a relative contraindication to a discogram as a worsening radiculopathy or frank sensory or motor loss may be precipitated. Spondylolisthesis may also precipitate nerve injury on discogram. These conditions, with a narrow spinal canal, can precipitate complications, as pressurizing the disc may cause compression of the spinal cord or nerve roots. This can cut off blood flow with resultant ischemia. Other complications include "spearing" a nerve root, which can cause a transient paresthesia, which may quickly pass; however, if severe damage to a nerve root occurs, then aggressive treatment is needed. An intravenous loading dose of Solumedrol 4 mg/kg and then 125 mg q 8 hours IV for 24 hours should be administered and the patient then placed on a Medrol dose pack. This may prevent long-term sequelae.

TREATMENT OF SPINAL DISC DISEASE

In general, like all physicians, we want to do what is best for our patients. This involves listening to our patients and understanding their expectations of treatment and their level of understanding of their condition to assure the best outcome. Future treatment of disc disease, as always, depends on many things: history, physical findings, results

of imaging and nerve studies, response to previous medical and invasive treatments, as well as physical therapy. Sometimes the best treatment is to do very little, particularly if the patient has a poor understanding of the disease and unrealistic expectations. Aggressively treating this type of patient is fraught with frustration and disappointment on the part of both patient and physician. For our part, to be a complete physician, we need to understand the patient's diagnosis, prognosis, and treatment options. As a specialist it is important to know which diagnoses are treatable and will give significant long-term improvement and which we are unable to treat appropriately. Not referring patients we cannot help will only worsen their condition.

The next important question, after the patient's diagnosis is considered treatable, is when to initiate therapy. The guidelines put forth by the North American Spine Society for the treatment of back pain state that one must have at least 6 weeks of therapy and analgesics prior to more invasive treatment. But what happens to the patient who has too much pain to start physical therapy and for whom analgesics do not work? Certainly, under these circumstances, this patient will not receive any benefit from physical therapy. One must judge every patient individually. Do what is right, not necessarily what guidelines deem appropriate.

If the patient's pain is in the 5–10/10 VAS range and oral medications, injections, and physical therapy have not worked, then more appropriate aggressive treatment is warranted. The pain specialist, compared with the surgeon, had few available treatment options in patients with a PGD until recently. As might be expected, treatment options for a PGD started for the pain specialist in the area with the highest incidence of complaints and the greatest allowance for error: the lumbar spine. Treatments for the cervical spine, however, are in development (34–35,135). Due to the rapid rate of advancement of treatment options and an understanding of what constitutes a PGD, an opportunity to develop an algorithm for treatment of pain in the lumbar spine has developed. What follows is an overview of the treatment options for cervical and thoracic PGD, then one possible treatment algorithm for the lumbar spine.

Treatment of a PGD will be divided into percutaneous invasive treatment and open surgical treatments. The percutaneous treatments will be discussed in detail, whereas only a cursory overview of the effectiveness of the open procedures will be discussed. It is important that the pain specialist have some understanding of the open surgical options for a PGD. If the patient's pain is not calmed with percutaneous techniques, he/she may need to be referred to a spine surgeon for further treatment. Just as an invasive cardiologist works with and has some understanding of what treatment options a cardiothoracic surgeon can provide to treat patients, a pain specialist, in order to make appropriate referrals, should have the same type of relationship with spine surgeons. For simplicity it will be assumed that appropriate conservative measures such as physical therapy, chiropractic treatment, oral medication, and injections were exhausted without improvement in the patient's condition. However, it must be remembered that patients with significant and/or rapid neurological loss or cauda equina syndrome should be referred immediately to a spine surgeon.

TREATMENT OF CERVICAL DISC PAIN

After one has established that a patient is suffering from cervical PGD, whether it be from internal disruption, spondylolisthesis, or frank herniation, the method of treatment must be determined. For the pain specialist, options are few. Currently, research is underway to use a technique similar to the IDET, but instead of using resistive heat it uses radiofrequency energy to heat the cervical disc to a sufficient temperature to denature the collagen with resultant volume reduction and denervation of the disc (34,135). The advantage of this technique is that, although the potential for complications exists, the risks and the invasiveness are less than with an open surgical procedure. Another advantage is the patient is able to have surgical treatment of the disc if this procedure fails. Several clinicians are currently using the LASE technique (see the lumbar treatment section) to treat cervical radiculopathy (43). Both percutaneous techniques are in their early stages but are important developments to watch. From a traditional surgical perspective, the treatment of a cervical PGD is an anterior cervical discectomy and interbody fusion. On review of the literature, an anterior cervical fusion has a high success rate (136,137). The pain specialist should consider two perioperative factors that may affect the outcome of the surgery and will improve understanding: Smokers do have a poorer outcome than nonsmokers, although it is close but not statistically significant, and the use of a cervical collar postoperatively has not correlated with significant improvement in outcome (136,137).

THORACIC DISC

The only treatment for a thoracic PGD is surgical excision of the disc. Fusion is not commonly done for a thoracic PGD. The open surgical approaches with morbidity and mortality rates (138) are listed in Table 28-3.

From this table it can be gathered that laminectomy, to a mid-upper-thoracic PGD in particular, is fraught with a very high rate of morbidity and mortality.

The treatment of a painful thoracic herniated disc depends on the location of the herniation. Lateral herniation in the mid- to upper-thoracic spine should use the transpedicular, costotransversectomy or lateral extracavitary approaches. The choice should depend on the surgeon's experience and the health of the patient (138). For a centrally herniated disc in the thoracic spine, the lateral extracavitary and transthoracic approaches offer the best exposure and are the procedures of choice for more difficult lesions (138). Fortunately, thoracic disc lesions are rare because the only therapy for PGD, beyond conservative

TABLE 28-3. Open surgical approaches with morbidity and mortality rates

	Total patients	Mortality %	Morbidity %
Laminectomy	63	13	59
Transpedicular	11	0	9
Costotransversectomy	17	0	12
Lateral extracavitary	76		12
Transverse arthropediculectomy	88	0	11
Anterolateral thoracotomy	35		3
Thoracoscopy	7	0	0

Adapted from reference 152.

therapy and injections, is open surgery (28,29,138,139). Thoracic discs may be treated like lumbar discs. Thoracoscopy may be the best open percutaneous technique to treat thoracic PGD, but more experience is needed. Percutaneous techniques using radiofrequency and laser are in development.

TREATMENT OF LUMBAR PAIN GENERATING DISC

The potential treatment options for a lumbar PGD are broad. Due to the high incidence of lumbar PGD, larger anatomy, and huge economic cost of this disease, there has been greater opportunity for the development of percutaneous and open surgical treatments for this disease. What follows is a discussion of both open and percutaneous treatments of lumbar PGD with a focus on the percutaneous techniques with adequate references for those who want to learn more about open techniques.

Results of open techniques, including posterolateral interbody and anterior fusions for internal disc disruption (IDD), have been mediocre at best (140–142,146–152). Because IDD makes up 40% of chronic low back pain, the IDET was developed. A consensus statement was published that stated that the strong indications for surgery for lumbar disc herniation include cauda equina syndrome with bowel and/or bladder dysfunction. At a minimum these patients should have symptoms and signs that include a neurogenic bladder and sacral hypesthesia. A second strong indication for surgery is severe and/or progressive motor deficit. Relative indications include severe leg pain for 6 weeks and back pain that is disabling for greater than 3 months and has not responded to aggressive conservative therapy. Because what constitutes a PGD is not fully understood, it is not surprising that the outcome for open surgery is poor.

Percutaneous techniques can be broken into two groups: widely used and selectively used. The widely used techniques include the Intradiscal Electrothermal Annuloplasty therapy (IDET) and the LASE technique. A selectively used technique is epiduroscopy with laser to ablate the disc, which will not be discussed. Contraindications to the widely used techniques include spinal stenosis, severe neuroforaminal stenosis, bleeding diathesis, and infections. Relative contraindications for the IDET include an extruded fragment and severely degenerated disc and patients with concordant facet disease. IDET has a 50% to 85% success rate (153). The patients who receive the best results are those who have a chemically sensitive disc and who on CT discogram have internal herniation with disc disruption or third-degree annular fissures. Chemically sensitive discs are those that may appear totally normal on discogram but produce severe concordant pain on low pressurization. Patients with PGFJ do poorly because there appears to be instability to the vertebral level. In such situations, even though the PGD is alleviated by the IDET, the PGFJs continue to destabilize the spinal level even when the median branches of the posterior rami, which innervates the facets, are ablated with radiofrequency. The IDET works well with discogenic pain and radicular pain. It is critically important for patients who receive this treatment to refrain from lifting more then 10 pounds for the first 6 weeks and, depending on their general health and physical limitations, to start an aerobic exercise program consisting of continuous walking for 20–30 minutes a day 3–5 days per week. They could alternatively start a gradual exercise program consisting of light weights and low-impact exercise such as a stationery bicycle or swimming. Usually after 6 weeks they can slowly progress to normal exercise.

IDET

IDET involves placing an introducer needle into the desired disc, then introducing a special catheter. As far as placing the introducer into the disc for the IDET procedure, it has many similarities to doing a lumbar discogram. The IDET introducer needle is stiffer than a Chiba needle and easier to steer. Of note, the MRI should be reviewed if there are doubts concerning the anatomy of the disc prior to attempting this procedure. This will improve the positioning of the needle because the presence of a bulging disc will be appreciated. First, the DEP, as described earlier in the lumbar discogram section, is the same as for the IDET introducer needle entry point. However, for the IDET introducer needle, the catheter entry point (CEP) into the disc is under the shadow of the superior and inferior articulating processes, as viewed on AP fluoroscopic view, and greater than the needle bevel length below the posterior border of the disc on lateral view (Fig. 28-2). Typically, for physicians well versed in doing discograms, the L-1–2, L-2–3, L-3–4, and L-4–5 discs can be easily cannulated. Cannulating the L-5–S-1 disc with the IDET introducer, as in discograms, is more difficult. (Please review the lumbar discogram section for proper needle placement techniques.) If the bent needle technique is used, it is important to make sure the stylet can

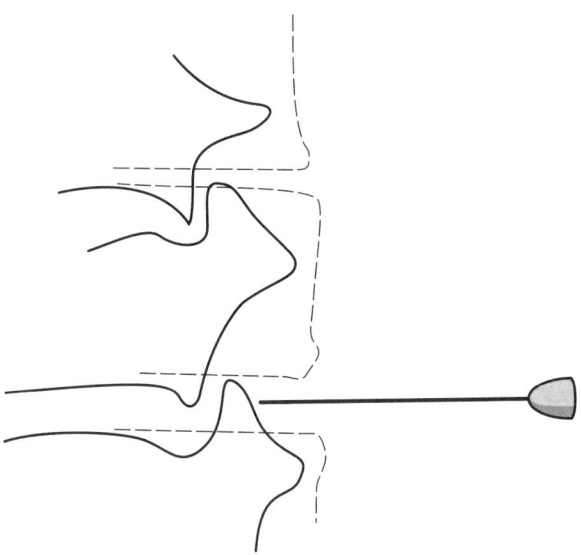

FIG. 28-2. Closeup of AP view, with the needle approaching lumbar disc during discogram.

easily be withdrawn prior to starting the procedure. If the stylet can be easily withdrawn from the needle, then the IDET catheter can also be easily withdrawn. There are two sizes of IDET catheter: 30 cm and 34 cm. The size of the patient and of the disc will determine which size catheter is used. The IDET catheter has a small 2-mm bend, which is in line with the white marker line on the catheter connector, allowing tracking of the position of the catheter tip (Fig. 28-3).

After the introducer needle is at the CEP, the stylet is removed and the IDET catheter is introduced. The bevel of the introducer needle, which is in line with the catch of the introducer stylet hub, is turned so that the bevel faces toward the anterior aspect of the disc. This will help direct

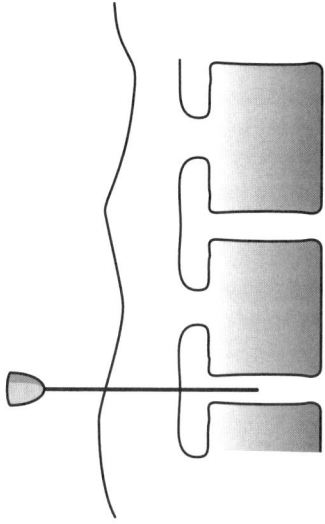

FIG. 28-3. Lateral view of lumbar spine showing correct position of needle in disc.

the catheter into the anterior disc. The white marker line on the IDET catheter should also face anteriorly. The catheter is placed through the introducer, and, when it comes in contact with the disc, a putty-like resistance will be felt. The catheter is advanced under continuous fluoroscopy or with frequent fluoroscopic imaging. The frequent fluoroscopic imaging technique is as effective as continuous fluoroscopy in placing the catheter with less radiation exposure to the patient and staff. The catheter should be placed as superficial as possible in the annulus to attain maximum effect. During the process of placing the catheter it should circle anteriorly and ipsilaterally in the disc on AP and lateral fluoroscopic views, then travel posteriorly in the anterior disc along the contralateral annulus and cross the midline of the posterior disc and pass posterior to the ipsilateral side of the introducer. The catheter heating element, which is seen under fluoroscopy as two darker points (one at the tip of the catheter and the other 6 cm proximally on the catheter) should cover as much of the posterior annulus of the disc as possible. Because the catheter follows the shape of the disc, if the disc is severely bulging, then the catheter may appear, on the lateral view, to be bulging into the epidural space. This will give the impression that the catheter is not in correct position when in fact it is.

In manipulating the catheter care must be taken when the catheter is withdrawn, particularly if it is kinked, because it can get caught on the edges of the introducer bevel, shearing off or damaging the catheter. If, during withdrawal, the catheter does get caught, slightly advance the catheter into the needle, then rotate the introducer needle, taking care not to advance or retract it. This may free the catheter. Another method to free the catheter is to advance the catheter through the introducer needle while twisting the catheter, then attempting to withdraw it. Depending on how far the catheter has advanced through the introducer needle into the disc, it may be difficult or impossible to rotate the catheter. The farther the catheter has advanced into the disc, the more difficult to rotate due to a combination of the viscosity of the disc material and the surface area of the catheter. Finally, slightly withdrawing the introducer needle with the catheter firmly held in place, then attempting to withdraw it may be successful. If all else fails to free the catheter, both the introducer and catheter will have to be removed together to prevent damage to the catheter.

When advancing the catheter, a gentle complete twist or two in the catheter may allow it to advance in more difficult cases. Often the catheter tip will track to one vertebral endplate or the other, blocking its advancement. Placing a twist in the catheter will allow it to negotiate the disc. There will be cases where there are multiple fissures in the disc, and, as the IDET catheter is advanced in the disc, these fissures will be appreciated as "pockets" of resistance. By applying gentle slow pressure it is frequently possible to advance the catheter through these areas. Other times the catheter will kink. Where it is not possible to push the catheter in the

disc, as visualized on an AP fluoroscopic view, past the posterior midline of the disc, and the patient has bilateral lumbar pain, the disc should be cannulated from both sides. That is, after the treatment has been completed on the contralateral side (location of the heating element of catheter), the ipsilateral side must then be treated in a like manner by cannulating the disc from the contralateral side. The IDET catheter will then be directed, as described earlier, around the lateral, anterior, and posterior annulus as far as possible across the midline from the contralateral side.

After the IDET catheter has been placed, its position should be checked on AP and lateral fluoroscopic views to assure that the catheter is properly positioned and that it has not migrated outside the disc and potentially into the spinal canal. After proper position has been assured, the impedance readout on the generator should be checked. A normal reading is 85–230 ohms. If it reads over or below this level, the placement of the catheter must be checked. If the catheter is properly placed, then the cable and generator must be checked to assure proper connection and no sign of damage. If this is checked, and there are no abnormalities, then (while disconnected from the patient) the machine is turned off and then back on. If the situation (low or high impedance) does not correct with turning the machine off and on, then the procedure should be abandoned for fear of harming the patient. If the IDET generator does not read an impedance, the cable as well as the connection must be checked. Rarely will the problem be with the IDET catheter. If the connections and cable look okay, then a new catheter should be tried. If that still does not correct the problem, the procedure should be rescheduled and the equipment sent to the company for evaluation.

After the machine and position of the catheter are correct, the treatment is almost ready to proceed. First, the operator must ensure that the patient is adequately responsive to communicate any changes in pain level or neurological changes. The mode button of the IDET generator is pushed once to read P90. Then the treatment is begun by pushing the RF button. The P90 mode will rapidly raise the temperature of the IDET active catheter tip to 65° Centigrade, then, in 30 seconds, increase the temperature by 1° and continue to raise the temperature of the active catheter tip 1° every 30 seconds until it reaches 90° Centigrade, at which time it will maintain this temperature for 4 minutes. The generator also allows using the P80 and P85 modes, which automatically heat the active catheter tip to 80° and 85° Centigrade, respectively. As the temperature rises, the patient is checked for any new pain different from the usual pain or neurological changes. Quite frequently, as the temperature of the catheter rises, the patient will complain of increasing intensity of the usual pain. This is a good sign because it confirms that one is treating the PGD. Additional analgesics will be needed to treat this increased pain; however, the patient's level of consciousness must be sufficient to communicate with the physician. Occasionally, despite adequate analgesics, the patient's pain will be too great to tolerate any increase in temperature. If this occurs above 80°, the mode button on the IDET generator should be pushed to change the program to the manual, P80, or P85 mode. If the manual mode is used, the IDET temperature guide should be followed to determine the recommended length of time, at this temperature, that the disc should be treated. If at any time the patient complains of neurological changes such as weakness to the legs, increased pain that is different from the usual pain, or a new sensory deficit, the procedure must be halted immediately, the position of the catheter and the impedance rechecked, and the patient observed to see if the neurological changes are resolving. After the appropriate adjustments are made and the patient's symptoms resolved, then heating the IDET catheter can be reattempted. If the symptoms return and no problems were found within the catheter or the generator, then the heating is stopped immediately, and the catheter must be repositioned. If the problem persists after repositioning of the catheter or if the neurological symptoms do not resolve, then the procedure should be abandoned. The IDET generator and cable should then be evaluated by bioengineering for defects if it appears that the generator was the source of the problem. If everything (i.e., impedance, temperature, and visual inspection of the cable and catheter) is normal, then one can conclude that the patient's anatomy or placement of catheter caused the problem.

After the heating is completed, the catheter is allowed to cool to 45° and then carefully removed, leaving the introducer needle in place. Finally, 1 cc of 20 mg of Kefzol or equivalent antibiotic is injected into the disc, and the introducer needle is removed. This injection of antibiotics will cause the patient some pain. The remaining antibiotic is then given IV. After the patient has recovered from anesthesia, precautions are given to the patient and family.

LASER ASSISTED DISC DECOMPRESSION (LADD)

LADD is used for contained herniated discs in the lumbar spine in patients with radicular pain. The laser ablates the disc, reducing its pressure and symptoms (33). The contained herniation should be consistent with symptoms found on history and physical examination and verified by MRI and provocative discograms. CPT nerve testing will help diagnose true radiculopathy, which occurs in only 1% to 2% of patients with back pain. Success rates in the literature run as low as 59% and as high as 88% (31–33). As experience is gained with this technique, the indications may be expanded. It is, however, a useful tool to have in your armamentarium.

The Procedure

The patient is placed in the prone position, and sterile prep and drape are applied. The procedure is done under monitored anesthesia care with IV sedation. This procedure

should be done under fluoroscopy to identify proper location of the LADD introducer and the laser during the procedure. The desired disc is located, then visualized in the lumbar oblique, disc-open position on the side of radiculopathy. The skin is anesthetized over the SEP, and, with a no. 11 blade, a 4-mm incision is made. The LADD needle is then directed to the DEP. The trephine is then placed over the LADD needle down to the annulus, and the annulus is incised. After removal of the trephine, the dilator and introducer are passed over the LADD needle into the disc. The dilator is then removed. The skin stop is placed to prevent movement of the introducer. The endoscope is advanced through the introducer into the mid disc. A Holmium:YAG laser is used. Irrigation for the laser is started through the endoscope port and should run at all times to prevent overheating of the disc and bone. The disc tissue is ablated with laser pulses of 1.4–2.0 joules. Initially 10 pulses per second should be used, but up to 12 pulses per second can be used. The total energy used is about 1–2 kilojoules. Kilojoules are calculated by multiplying joules times the pulses per second. Laser safety is of concern, and proper understanding of laser safety is necessary prior to attempting this procedure. Throughout the procedure the patient should be monitored for changes in neurological or vital signs. Following the procedure, the disc space should close up when the patient coughs, which is an indication of sufficient ablation.

FUTURE OF TREATMENT OF PGD

The spinal disc, like the rest of the human body, is subject to the insults of an abusive environment as well as the process of natural aging. Additionally, the disc, like the body, requires maintenance in the form of good nutrition, exercise, and the avoidance of injuries, both physical (such as trauma) and chemical (such as alcohol and smoking) to maintain optimal performance. Although currently disc disease, by most standards, is considered a single entity, as more effort is put forth to understand it, it will become clear that in fact a PGD is a broad spectrum. Perhaps the natural aging process puts one at risk for a PGD. There are definitive studies to support a conclusion either way. Another source of a PGD is in-growth of neurovascular structures into the fissured disc, but does this occur in all fissured discs or only those that are PGDs? If it does occur in all fissured discs, then why are not all fissured discs painful? Are there sequestered, altered proteins in the disc that may set up autoimmune responses, or is it leakage of disc contents onto traumatized nerve roots following herniation that causes radiculopathy and back pain? The answers will evolve from a continuation of the current treatments and the changing to a new paradigm as well as better diagnostic techniques. In the distant future, with the Human Genome Project having mapped the genome, it will be to medicine as the Apollo program was to technology: a watershed with the appearance of genetic treatments to maintain the "youth" of the disc and reduce the chance of injury. Several companies are now developing percutaneous invasive treatments to treat cervical disc disease. These treatments of cervical discs should be forthcoming, and it will be only a matter of time before these techniques will be applied to the thoracic spine (33). Further improvement will be made in diagnosis by greater experience with discograms and discometry and correlating the results with imaging studies and surgical (IDET and open procedures) outcomes. Many of the tools we have to treat a PGD are primitive, as are the current studies available, which have not been done under physiological conditions, such as MRI of the disc in a supine nonweight-bearing position. We are in a very dynamic age, progressing from current thinking to greater science to treat disc disease, which will continue to plague us for generations to come.

CONCLUSION

It is important to understand the history, diagnosis, pathophysiology, anatomy, invasive and noninvasive studies, and treatment of a PGD. By understanding these aspects of a spinal disc, improvement in the care of the patient is likely. There are still many questions concerning the cause, natural history, and treatment of a PGD. It must be remembered that spinal disc disease is a continuum, a chronic disease. Current treatments are only a patch, not a cure. We don't truly understand the cause, and more study is needed in order to develop more effective treatments.

REFERENCES

1. Cotunio O FA. *De Ischiade Nervosa Canmentarius.* Naples: Simoncos. Brothers, 1764.
2. Mixter WJ, Barr JS. Ruptures of the intervertebral disc with involvement of the spinal canal. *N Eng J Med* 1934;211:210.
3. Lindblom K. Protrusions of the discs and nerve compression in the lumbar region. *Acta Radiol Scand* 1944;25:195–212.
4. Hirsch C. An attempt to diagnose level of disc lesion clinically by disc puncture. *Acta Orthop Scand* 1948;18:131–140.
5. Holt EP Jr. Fallacy of cervical discography report of 50 cases in normal subjects. *JAMA* 1964;188:799–801.
6. Holt EP Jr. The question of lumbar discography. *J Bone Joint Surg (AM)* 1968;50:720–726.
7. Simmons JW, Aprill CN, Dwyer AP, Bradsky A. A reassessment of Holt's data on "The question of lumbar discography." *Clin Orthop Related Research* 988;237:120–124.
8. Fortin JD. Precision diagnostic disc injections. *Pain Physician* 2000;3(3):271–288.
9. Guarino AH. Discography a review. *Current Review of Pain* 1999;3:473–480.
10. Wetzel FT, La Rocca SH, Lowery GL, Aprill CN. The treatment of lumbar spinal pain syndromes diagnosed by discography. *Spine* 1994;19:792–800.
11. Birney TJ, White JJ Jr, Bevens D, Kuhn G. Comparison of MRI and discography in the diagnosis of lumbar degenerative disc disease. *J Spinal Disord* 1992;5:417–23.
12. Simmons JW, Emery SF, McMillin JW, et al. Awake discography a comparison study with magnetic resonance imaging. *Spine* 1991;16(Supp):5216–5221.
13. Walsh TR, Weinstein JN, Spratt KF, et al. Lumbar discography in normal subjects. *J Bone Joint Surg (AM)* 1990;72:1081–1088.
14. Kornberg M, Discography and magnetic resonance imaging in the diagnosis of lumbar disc disruption. *Spine* 1989;14:1368–1372.
15. Zucherman J, Derby R, Hsu K, et al. Normal magnetic resonance imaging with abnormal discography. *Spine* 1988;13:1355–1359.
16. Calhoun E, McCall IW, Williams L, et al. Provocation discography as a guide to planning operation on the spine. *J Bone Joint Surg (BR)* 1988;70:267–271.
17. Mooney V, Haldeman S, Nasca RJ, et al. Position statement on discography. The Executive Committee Of The North American Spine Society, *Spine* 1988;13:1343.
18. Hudgins WR. Diagnostic accuracy of lumbar discography. *Spine* 1977;2:305–309.
19. Hadra BE. Wiring of the spinous processes in Pott's disease. *Trans American Orthop Association* 1891;4:206–211.
20. King D. Internal fixation of lumbosacral fusion. *J Bone Joint Surg (AM)*,1994;30:560–565
20a. Boucher HH. A method of spinal fusion. *J Bone Joint Surg (BR)* 1959;41:248–59.
21. Magerl F. Stabilization of the lower thoracic and lumbar spine with external skeletal fixation. *Clin Orthop* 1984;189:125–141.
23. Fernstrom U. Arthroplasty with intercorporal endoprosthesis in herniated disc and in painful disc. *Act Chi Scand* 1966;355(Suppl):154–159.
24. Griffith SL, Shelokev AP, Buttner-Jan K et al. A multicenter retrospective study of the clinical results of the link ® SB Charite interverbral prosthesis. *Spine* 1994;19(16):1842–1849.
25. Chow SP, Leang JCY, Ma A, et al. Anterior spinal fusion for deranged lumbar intervertebral disc. *Spine* 1980;5:452–458.
26. Saul J, Saul J. *A novel approach to painful internal disc derangement collagen modulation with thermal percutaneous navigable intradiscal catheter- a prospective trial.* Presented at the meeting of The International Society For Study of Lumbar Spine, Kona, Hawaii, June 21-25, 1999.
27. Saul JA. *Intradiscal electrothermal annuloplasty (IDET) treatment for chronic multilevel discogenic pain prospective one-year follow up outcome study.* Presented at combined IITS/ISMTSS Meeting, Cambridge, UK, August 1–5, 1999.
28. Benson MKD, Byres DP. The clinical syndromes and surgical treatment of thoracic intervertebral disc prolapse *J Bone UJT Surg (BR)* 1975;57B:471–477.
29. Mainran DJ, Larson JJSJ, Luck E, et al. A lateral extracavitary approach to the spine for thoracic disc herniation report of 23 cases. *Neurosurgery* 1984;14:178–182.
30. Mironer YE, Somerville JJ. The current perception threshold evaluation in radioculopathy; efficacy in diagnosis and assessment of treatment results. *Pain Digest* 1998;8:37–38.
31. Casper GD, Hartman VL, Mullins LL. Results of clinical trial of the molmium:YAG laser in disc decompsession utilizing a side firing fibers, a two year follow up. *Lasers in Surgery and Medicine* 1996;19:90–96.
32. Bosacco SJ, Bosacco DN, Bermon AT, et al. Functional results of percutaneous laser discectomy. *Journal of Orthopedics (AM)* 1996;12: 825–828.
33. Choy DSJ. Percutaneous laser disc decompression (PLDD): twelve years experience with 752 procedures in 518 patients. *J Clinical Laser Medicine and Surgery* Dec 1998.
34. Personal Communications with Cinchy S. Oratech.
35. Personal Communications with Finn MA. Clarus Medical.
36. Carthen JC, Kinard RE, Vogler JB, et al. Outcome analysis of noninstrumented anterior cervical discectomy and interbody fusion in 348 patients. *Spine* 1998;23(2):188–191.
37. Whitecloud III TS. Modern alterations and techniques for one level discectomy and fusion. *Clinical Orthopedic and Related Research* 1999;359:67–76.
38. Martin GJ, Haid RW, et al. Anterior cervical discectomy with freeze-dried fibula allograft. *Spine* 1999;24(9):852–859.
39. Vlok GJ, Hendrix MRG. The lumbar disc: evaluating the causes of pain. *Orthopedics* 1991;14(4):421
40. Parson D. The structure and function of the intervertebral disc. In: *orthopedics*, Oxford; 1970:7.
41. Bogduk N, Wilson AJ, Tynon W. The human lumbar dorsal rami. *J Anat* 1982;1345:383–397.
42. Edgar MA, Ghadially JA. Innervation of the lumbar spine. *Clin Orthop* 1976;115:35–41.
43. Pederson HE, Blunck CFJ, Gardner E. The anatomy of lumbosacral posterior rami and meningeal branches of spinal nerves (sino-vertebral nerves). *J Bone Joint Surg* 1956;38A:377–391.

44. Edgar MA Nundy S. Innervation of the spinal dura mater. *J Neurol Neuro Surg Psychiat* 1966;29:530–534.
45. Bogduk N, Tynan W, Wilson AJ. The innervation of the human lumbar intervertebral discs. *J Anat* 1981;132:39–56.
46. YoshIzawa, H, O'Brien JP, Smith WT, Trumper M. The neuropathology of intervertebral discs removal for low back pain. *J Pathology* 1980;132:95–104.
47. Malinsky J. The ontogenetic development of nerve terminations in the intervertebral discs of men. *Acta Anat* 1959;38:96–113.
48. Nakamura SI, Takaltashi K, Takahashi Y, et al. The afferent pathways of discogenic low back pain. *Journal of Bone and Joint Surgery* 1996:78.B:4:606–612.
49. White JC, Sweet WH. Pain its mechanics and neurosurgical control. Springfield CC Thomas, 1955:67–98.
50. El Mahdi MA, Abdel Latif FY, Jankom. The spine nerve root intervention, and a new concept of the Clinicopathological inter-relations in back pain and sciatica. *Neuro Chivuvgia stutty* 1981;24;137–141.
51. Takahashi Y, Nakajima K, Sakomoto T, et al. Capsaicin applied to rat lumbar intervertebral disc causes extravasation in the groin skin a possible mechanism of referred pain of the intervertebral disc neuroscilett. 1993;161:1–3.
52. Kurunlahti M Terwonen V, Vanharanto H, et al. Association of Atherosclerosis with low back pain and the degree of disc degeneration. *Spine* 1999;24:2080–2084.
53. Powell MC, Wilson M. Szypryt P, et al. Prevalance of lumbar disc degeneration observed by magnetic resonance in symptomless women. *Lancet* Dec 1986:1366–1367.
54. Weinreb JC, Welbarsht LB, Chen J, et al. Prevalance of lumbosacral intervertebral disk abnormality on MR images in pregnant and symptomless women. *Radiology* 1989;170:125–128.
55. Boden S, Davis D, Dina T, et al. Abnormal magnetic resonance scans of the lumbar spine in symptomatic subjects. *J Bone Joint Surg (Am)* 1990;72:400–403.
56. Jensen M, Brant-Zawadzki M, Obuerowski N, et al. Magentic resonance imaging of the lumbar spine in people without back pain. *N Engl J Med* 1994;331:69–73.
57. Buivski G, Silberstein M. The symptomatic lumbar disc in patients with low back pain: Magentic resonance imaging appearances in both symptomatic and central population. *Spine* 1993;18:1808–1811.
58. Crock HV. A reapprasial of intervertebral disc lesions. *Med J Australia* 1970:183.
59. Powel MC, Wilson M, et al. Prevelance of lumbar disc degeneration observed by magnetic resonance in symptomless women. *Lancet* Dec 1986:1366.
60. Crock HU. Internal disc disruption: a challenge to discs prolapse fifty years on the presidents address: International Society for the study of lumbar spine. *Spine* 1988;11:650–653.
61. Brown T, Haasen RT, and Yorra AJ. Some mechanical tests on the lumbosacral spine with particular reference to the intervertebral discs. *J Bone Joint Surg* 1957;39A:1135.
62. Rolander SD, Blair WE. Deformation and fracture of lumbar vertebral endplate. *Orthop North American* 1975;6:75–81.
63. Farfan HF. Mechanical disorders of the low back. Philadelphia: Lea S Febiger, 1973:199–211.
64. Farfan HF, Sullivan JD. The relation of facet orientation to the intervertebral disc failure. *Can J Surg* 1967;10:179.
65. Farfan HF, Cossette JW, Robertson GH, et al. The effects of torsion on the lumbar intervertebral joints. *J Bone Joint Surg* 1970;52A:468–497.
66. Hult L. The munk fors investigation. *Acta Orthop Scand* 1954;(Supp)16.
67. Wiltse L. The effect of the common anomalies of the lumbar spine upon disc degeneration and low back pain. *Orthop Clinics of North America* 1971;2:571.
68. Wilse LL, Hutchinson RH. Surgical treatment of spondylolisthesis. *Clin Orthop* 1964;35:116.
69. Kettelkamp DB, Wright DG. *Spondylolisthesis in Alaskan eskimo.* Paper presented at the meeting of The Western Orthopaedic Association, Portland, Oregon, October 6, 1970.
70. Splittoff, CA. Roentgenographic comparison of patients with and without backache. *JAMA* 1953;152:1610.
71. Nachemson A, Schultz AB, Berkson MH. Mechanical properties of human lumbar spine segments. *Spine* 1979;4:1–8.
72. Nachemson A. The lumbar spine. The orthopedic challenge. *Spine* 1976;1:1.
72a. Pope M. Measurement of IUD space heights. *Spine* 1977;2: 282–328.
73. Williams PC. *The Lumbosacral Spine.* New York: McGraw-Hill Book Co, 1965.
74. Smith I, Brown JE. Treatment of lumbar intervertebral discs by direct injection with chymopapain. *J Bone Joint Surg* 1967;29B:502–519.
75. Pope M. Measurement of IUD space height, narrowing and low back pain. *Spine* 1977;2:282–286.
76. Dabbs VM, Dabbs LG. Correlation between disc height, narrowing and low back pain. *Spine* 1990;15(12):1366–1369.
77. Brown MD. The pathophysiology of disc disease. *Orthop Clinic North America* 1971;2:359.
78. Allbrook D. Movements of the lumbar spinal column. *J Bone Joint Surg* 1957;39B:339–345.
79. Osti OL, Vernon-Roberts B, Moorer Fraser RD. Annular tears and disc degeneration in the lumbar spine. *J Bone Joint Surg (BR)* 1992;74-B:678–82.
80. Eie N. Load Capacity of the low back. *J Oslo City Hosp* 1966;16: 73–78.
80a. Coppes, MH, Marani E, Thomeer RTWW, et al. Innervation of the "painful" lumbar disc. *Spine* 1997;20:2342–2350.
81. Friberg S, Hirsch C. Anatomical and clinical studies on lumbar disc degeneration. *Acta Orthop Scand* 1950;19:222–42.
82. Balante JO. Tensile properties of the human lumbar annulus fibrosus. *Acta Orthop Scand* 1967;(Suppl):100.
83. Kirkaldy Willis WH. The pathology and pathogenesis of low back pain In: Kirkaldy-Willis WH, ed. *Managing low back pain.* Edinburgh: Churchill Livingstone, 1983:23–43.
84. Nachemson AL. The influence of spinal movement on the lumbar intradiscal pressure and on the tensile stresses in the annulus fibrosus. *Acta Orthop Scand* 1963;33:183–207.
85. Nachemson A. In vivo discometry in lumbar disc with irregular nucleograms. *Acta Orthop Scand* 1965;36:418–34.
86. Butler WF. Histological age changes in the ruptured intervertebral disc of the cat. *Res Vet Sci* 1968;9:130.
87. Marshall LL, Trethewie FR, Luvtein LU. Chemical radiculitis a clinical physiological and immunological implications. *Clin Orthop* 1977;129:61.
88. Gertzbein SD. Degenerative disc disease of the lumbar spine immunological implications. *Clin Orthop* 1977;129:66.
89. Bisla RS, Marchisello PJ, et al. Auto-immunological basis of disk degeneration. *Clinical Orthop and related research* 1976;121:210.
90. Gertzbein SD, Tile M, Gross A, Falk, R. Auto immunity in degenerative disc disease of the lumbar spine. *Orthop Clin North America* 1975;6(1):67.
91. Weissman G. *Rheumatoid arthritis.* W. Muller, ed. London, New York: Acad Press, 1971:141.
92. Naylor A. The biophysical and biochemical aspect of intervertebral disc herniation and degeneration. *Ann Royal Coll Surg Engl* 1962;31:91.
93. Elves MW, Bucknill T, Sullivan MF. In vitro inhibition of leucocyte migration in patients with intervertebral disc lesions. *Orthop Clin North Amer* 1975;6(1):59.
94. Kawakami, M, Tamaki T, Weinstein J, et al. Pathomechanism of pain related behavior produced by allografts of intervertebral disc in rats. *Spine* 1996;21:2101–2107.
95. Kawakami M. Tamaki T, Weinstein J et al. Disc materials produce related behavior in the rat: The role of ph, immune response and chemicals. *Trans Orthop Res Soc* 1995;20:666.
96. Moneta GB, Videmen T Kaivantek, et al. Reported pain during lumbar discography as a function of annular ruptures and disc degeneration. *Spine* 1994;19(17):1968–1974.
97. Yoshizawa H, O'Brian JP, Smith WT, Trumper M. The neuropathology of intervertebral disc removed for low back pain. *J Pathol* 1980;132:95–104.
98. Kirdaldy-Willis WH. A more precise diagnosis for lowback pain. *Spine* 1979;4:102.
99. Coppes MH, Marani E, Thomeer RTWW, et al. Pathomechanism of pain related behavior in the rat: The role of ph, immune response and chemicals. *Trans Orthop Res Soc* 1995;20:666.
100. Gordon SL, Weinstein JN. A review of basic science issues in low back pain, physical medicine and rehabilitation. *Clinics of North*

America 1998;9(2):325.

101. Pedowitz RF, Ryderic BL, Hargens, AR et al. *Motor and sensory nerve conduction deficit induced by acute graded compression of the pig cauda equina.* presented at the 34th Annual meeting of the Orthopedic Research Society, 1988.

102. Hirsch C, Inglemark BF, Miller M. The anatomical basis for low back pain. *Acta Orthop Scand* 1963;33:1–17.

103. Jinkins JR, Whitemore AR, Bradley WG. The anatomic basis of vertebrogenic pain and the autonomic syndrome associated with lumbar disc extrusion. *AJR* 1989;152:1277–1289.

104. Weinstein, J, Claverie W. Gibson S. The pain of discography. *Spine* 1988;13:1344–1348.

105. Kirkaldy-Willis WH, Wedge JH, Yong-Hing K, Reilly J. Pathology and pathogenesis of lumbar spondylosis and stenosis. *Spine* 1978;3:319–328.

106. Brinckmann P, Horst M. The influence of vertebral body fracture, intradiscal injection and partial discectomy on the radial bulge and height of human lumbar discs. *Spine* 1985;10:138–145.

107. Dunlop RB. Pain space narrowing and the lumbar facet joint. *J Bone Joint Surg* 1984;66B:706–710.

108. Lindbolm K. IVD degeneration considered a pressure atrophy. *J Bone Joint Surg* 1957.

109. Meyerding HW. Spondylolisthesis. *Surg Gynecol Obstet* 1932;54:374.

110. Pope MH, Frymoyer JW, Krag MH. Diagnosing instability. *Clin Orthop* 1992;279:60–67.

111. Inman VT, Saunders JB. Referral pain from skeletal structures. *J Nerv Ment Dis* 1944;99:660–667.

112. Walsh NE, Ramamurthy S. *Practical management of pain.* Mosby, 2nd ed. 1992:273–276.

113. Dwyer A, Aprill C, Bogduk N. Cervical zygapophysial joint pain patterns, a study in normal volunteers. *Spine* 1990;15:45.

114. Dreyfuss P, Tibilette. Pain patterns: a study in normal volunteers. *Spine* 1994;19:807.

115. Marks R. Distribution of pain provoked from lumbar facet joints and related structures during diagnostic spinal infiltration. *Pain* 1989;39:37.

116. Ray CD. Percutaneous radiofrequency facet nerve blocks: Treatment of the mechanical low back syndrome radionics. 1982;1:1.

117. Rothman RH. The clinical syndrome of lumbar disc disease. *Ortho Clinic of North America* 1971;2(2):463–475.

118. Nachemson AL. The lumbar spine: an orthopedic challenge. *Spine* 1976;1:59–71.

119. Dejerine J. Semiologie du, systeme nerveux. *Paris Masson* 1914:23.

120. Hoppenfeld S. Physical examination of the spine and extremities. Appleton and Lange, 1976;258–260.

121. Bogduk N. Point of view. *Spine* 1998;23(11):1259–1260.

122. Aprill C, Bogduk N. High intensity zone diagnostic sign of painful lumbar disc on magnetic resonance imaging. *J Radiol (BR)* 1992;65: 361–369.

123. Hauser BO. Letter to the editor. *Spine* 1997;22:1538.

124. Schellhas KP, Pollei SR, Gundry CR, Heithoff KB. Lumbar disc high-intensity zones correlation of magnetic resonance imaging and discography. *Spine* 1996:2179–2186.

125. Yrjama M. Tervonen O, Vanhananta H. Ultrasonic imaging of the lumbar discs combined with vibration pain provocation compared with discography in the 1996 diagnosis of internal annular fissures of the lumbar spine. *Spine* 21(5):571–575

126. Katims JJ, NG LKY. Transcutaneous electrical nerve stimulation (TNS) evokes frequency and wave form dependent subjective sensations in humans. *Society of Neuroscience* 1981;11(7):1818

127. Racz G. Personal communication.

128. Derby R. Lumbar discometry newsletter of the International Spinal Injections Society 1993;1:8–17.

129. Derby R. The relationship between intradiscal pressure and pain provocation during discography. *J Bone Joint Surg (BR)* 1995;19: 59–60.

130. Derby R, Schwarzer A, Bogduk N. *Discography can predict surgical outcome.* Proceedings of the 4th Annual International Spinal Injections Society, Vancouver, Canada, August 1996.

131. Derby R, Howard MW, Grant JM, et al. The ability of pressure controlled discography to predict surgical and non-surgical outcomes *Spine* 1999;24(4):364–371.

132. Sachs BL, VanHaranta H, Sipvey MA, et al. Dallas Discogram description, A new classification of CT/discography in low back disorders. *Spine* 1987;12:287.

133. Dullerud R, Johansen JG, Johnsen ULH, Maganes B. Differentiation between contained and noncontained lumbar disk hernias by CT and MRI imaging. *Acta Radiol* 1995;36:491.

134. Mironer E. Newsletter of the National Forum of Independent Clinicians. Fall 1999:2.

135. Elizabeth personal communication Radionics

136. Cauthen JC, Kinard RE, Vogler JB, et al. Outcome analysis of non-instrumented anterior cervical discectomy and interbody fusion in 134 patients. *Spine* 1998;23(2):188–192.

137. Martin GJ, Heid RW, Macmillian M, et al. Anterior cervical discectomy with freeze dried fibulas allograft. 1999;24(9):852–859.

138. Fessler RG, Sturgill M. Review, complications of surgery for thoracic disc disease. *Surg Neurol* 1998;49:609–618.

139. Carson J, Grumpert J. Jefferson A. Diagnosis and treatment of thoracic intervertebral disc protrusions. *J Neurol Neurosurg Psychiat* 1971;34:68–71.

140. Flynn JC, Hoque MA. Anterior fusion of the lumbar spine. *J Bone Joint Surg* 1979;61A:1143–1150.

141. Hoover NW. Methods of lumbar fusion. *J Bone Joint Surg* 1968; 50A:194-210

142. Morscher E. Indikation und Technik der vordere interkorporelle spondylose bei neurologische symptomen einer spondylolisthesis. *Z Orthop* 1979;117:172–178.

143. Stauffer RN, Coventry, MB. Anterior interbody spine fusion. *J Bone Joint Surg* 1972;54A:756–768.

144. Sorensen, KH. Anterior interbody lumbar spine fusion for incapacitating disc degeneration and spondylolisthesis. *Acta Orthop Scand* 1978;49:269–277.

145. Tunturi T, Kataja M, Keski-Nisula et al. Posterior fusion of the lumbosacral spine. *Acta Orthop Scand* 415–425.

146. Werlinich M. Anterior interbody fusion and stabilization with metal fixation. *Int Surg* 1974;59:269–273.

147. Zimmerman H. Beitrag zur ventralen interkorporelle spondylodese des lumbosacralbereiches. *Z Orthop* 1968;105:303–315.

148. Blumenthal SL, Baker J, Dossett A, Selby DK. The role of anterior lumbar fusion for internal disc disruption. *Spine* 1988;13: 566–569.

149. Frazer RD. Interbody, posterior and combined lumbar fusions. *Spine* 1993;20(Suppl):1675.

150. Knox BD, Chapman TM. Anterior lumbar interbody fusion for discogram can conduct pain. *J Spinal Disord* 1993:242–244.

151. Penta M, Fraser RD. Anterior lumbar interbody fusion a minimum 10 year follow up. *Spine* 1997;22:2429–2434.

152. Schwarzer AC, Aprill CN, Derby R, et al. The prevalence and clinical features of internal disc disruption in patients with chronic lumbar pain. *Spine* 1995;20:1878–1883.

153. Karasek M, Bogduk N. Twelve month follow up of a controlled trial of intradiscal electrothermal annuloplasty for back pain due to intervertebral disc disruption. *Spine* 2000;25(20):2601–2607.

CHAPTER **29**

Neuropathic Pain in Peripheral Neuropathies

Marco Pappagallo

Nociception represents a physiological response to noxious stimuli that arise from the activation and sensitization of tissue nociceptors, also known as A-delta and C nerve fibers. Pain is the human awareness of nociception and has been defined as "an unpleasant sensory and emotional experience associated with tissue damage or described in terms of such damage" (1). A much more complex phenomenon than simple nociception, pain may arise in two ways: (a) as a response to a pathophysiological process occurring within the tissues, e.g., inflammation, or (b) as a response to a pathological process occurring along and within the nervous system pain pathways. In the first instance the pain signal generates from "healthy" tissue nociceptors sensitized by an ongoing release of algogenic molecules (e.g., protons, prostaglandins, bradykinin, serotonin, adenosine, cytokines, etc.). This type of pain has been called *nociceptive*. In the second instance the pain signal is generated ectopicly and spontaneously by abnormal nociceptors and has been appropriately called *neuropathic* (2). However, the separation between nociceptive and neuropathic pain states is at times blurred. For example, inflammatory pain may also be neuropathic. Once released, some proinflammatory cytokinines (e.g., tumor necrosis factor alpha) can structurally damage nerve axons and induce a neuropathic pain state (3,4).

Neuropathic pain may result from peripheral or central nervous system (PNS or CNS) pathological events (e.g., trauma, ischemia, infections) or ongoing metabolic diseases, infections, or structural disorders (e.g., diabetes mellitus, amyloidosis, human immunodeficiency viral infection, nerve entrapment, etc.).

The complex interplay of PNS and CNS pain mechanisms is exemplified in Fig. 29-1. It highlights how physiological and pathological processes easily interact to link central and peripheral events (e.g., sensitization and activation of nociceptors) to dorsal horn/CNS plastic phenomena (e.g., central sensitization) as well as to long-term

pathological changes within the peripheral and central pain pathways (e.g., ectopic discharge, dorsal horn/CNS reorganization).

The topics of this chapter are painful neuropathies and the contemporary treatment of neuropathic pain.

CLINICAL ASSESSMENT OF NEUROPATHIC PAIN

A comprehensive assessment of the patient affected by a neuropathic painful state is imperative and includes:

1. Medical history
2. General, neurological, and regional examinations
3. Diagnostic workup

Medical History

The clinical interview should be focused on questions about onset, duration, progression, and nature of complaints suggestive of *neurological deficits* (e.g., persistent numbness in a body area or limb weakness, such as tripping episodes, the progressive inability to open jars, etc.) as well as complaints suggestive of *sensory dysfunction* (e.g., touch-evoked pain, intermittent abnormal sensations, spontaneous burning and shooting pains) (5).

A variety of painful neuropathies are related to systemic diseases. The presence of complaints such as urinary frequency, nocturia, weight loss, fatigue, edema, somnolence, skin discoloration (e.g., icterus), fever, persistent cough, dry eyes, joints swelling, skin rash, tremors, gait unsteadiness, nail changes, and hair loss should suggest underlying systemic medical conditions. These conditions can include diabetes mellitus, hypothyroidism, chronic renal failure, intestinal malabsorption, malignancy, connective tissue diseases, chronic infections (e.g., human immunodeficiency virus, hepatitis B and C virus, Lyme disease, leprosy), intra-

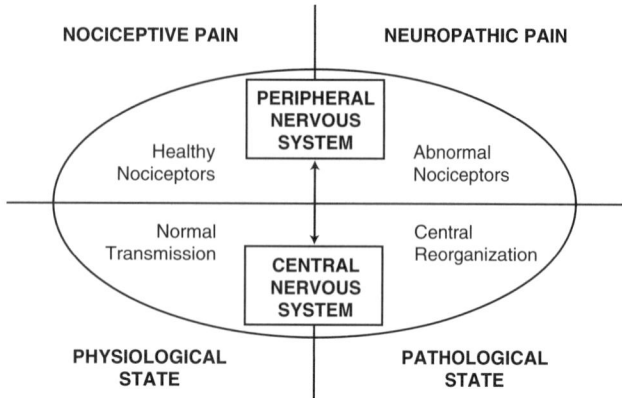

NOCICEPTIVE PAIN | NEUROPATHIC PAIN

PERIPHERAL NERVOUS SYSTEM

Healthy Nociceptors | Abnormal Nociceptors

Normal Transmission | Central Reorganization

CENTRAL NERVOUS SYSTEM

PHYSIOLOGICAL STATE | PATHOLOGICAL STATE

FIG. 29-1. Activation of "healthy" nociceptors with a normal CNS transmission represents the physiological process of pain. Tissue inflammation gives rise to nociceptive pain, which is characterized by peripheral and central sensitization of pain pathways. The entire process may remain within the physiological boundaries of pain transmission. However, given the appropriate conditions, a nociceptive state may evolve into a pathological neuropathic state. Afferent fibers may acquire ectopic activity. Abnormal structural changes may occur within the dorsal horn. Peripheral and central events easily interact during pain transmission and interplay between physiological and pathological states.

venous use of illicit drugs, alcoholism, abnormal dietary habits, or exposure to heavy metals (Table 29-1).

Physical Examination

Some diagnostic clues may derive from the general examination of the patient (5). Examination of the hair can show alopecia, which is seen in thallium poisoning. Wide transverse nail bands called Mees' lines are observed in arsenic and thallium intoxications. Telangiectasias over the abdomen, inguinal, and gluteal regions are found in Fabry's disease. Purpuric skin eruptions of the legs are observed in cryoglobulinemia and in some vasculitidies. Inspection of the extremities can show *pes cavus* and "hammertoes," which are suggestive of Charcot-Marie-Tooth (CMT) disease.

Inspection of the symptomatic region is essential. For example, complex regional pain syndromes (CRPSs) usually involve a single distal extremity, and, at the time of the evaluation, the affected limb may show the classic CRPS abnormalities, such as skin color and temperature changes, edema, and sweating. Light tapping and palpation along the course of the peripheral nerves are also an important part of the examination. A positive *Tinel's sign* (i.e., shooting dysesthesias elicited by finger tapping along the course of a nerve) is evidence for mechanoreceptor sensitivity and suggests the presence of a neuroma or nerve entrapment. Hypertrophy of a nerve trunk suggests either a nerve tumor (e.g., neurofibroma) or a localized hypertrophic neuropathy. Multifocal nerve hypertrophies are found in some peripheral nerve disorders, including leprosy, neurofibromatosis, CMT disease, and acromegaly.

TABLE 29-1. *Etiologies of painful neuropathies*

Metabolic and endocrinologic disorders
  Diabetic neuropathies
  Liver disease
  Renal dysfunction and hemodialysis
  Hypothyroidism
  Acromegaly

Infections
  Human immunodeficiency virus (HIV)
  Varicella Zoster virus (VZV)
  Hepatitis B and C virus (HBV, HCV)
  Human T-cell lymphotrophic virus (HTLV-1)
  Leprosy
  Lyme disease

Demyelinating inflammatory disorders
  Guillain-Barré syndrome (GBS)
  Chronic inflammatory demyelinating polyneuropathy (CIDP)

Malignancies

Entrapment neuropathies

Autoimmune and granulomatous disorders
  Sjögren's syndrome (SS)
  Systemic lupus erythematosus (SLE)
  Rheumatoid arthritis (RA)
  Sarcoidosis
  Polyarteritis nodosa (PAN)
  Churg-Strauss vasculitis (CGV)
  Wegener's granulomatosis (WG)
  Giant cell arteritis or temporal arteritis

Immunoglobulinemias
  Monoclonal (M) proteins
  Primary and secondary amyloidosis
  Cryoglobulinemia

Dietary or absorption abnormalities
  Alcoholic neuropathy
  B_{12}, thiamine, and other vitamin deficiencies
  Strachan's syndrome

Toxic neuropathies
  Heavy metals
  Chemotherapeutic agents
  Nonchemotherapeutic drugs

Hereditary neuropathies
  Charcot-Marie-Tooth disease (CMT)
  Fabry's disease
  Familial amyloid polyneuropathy (FAP)
  Porphyric neuropathy

Cryptogenic painful neuropathies
  Idiopathic polyneuropathy
  Complex regional pain syndromes (CRPSs)
  Essential trigeminal and glossopharyngeal neuralgias

Abnormal Sensory Findings Associated with Neuropathic Pain

Patients with neuropathic pain states usually present with a spontaneous ongoing or intermittent pain characterized by a typical burning and/or shooting, electric-shock quality. They also present with some or all of the following abnormal sensory symptoms and signs (6):

1. *Paresthesias,* which are spontaneous intermittent pain-less abnormal sensations
2. *Dysesthesias,* which are spontaneous or evoked unpleasant sensations, such as annoying sensations elicited by cold stimuli or pinprick testing. Of note, patients with acquired neuropathies complain of dysesthesias more often than patients with inherited PNS diseases.
3. *Allodynia,* which is pain elicited by nonnoxious stimuli (i.e., clothing, air movement, tactile stimuli) when applied to the symptomatic cutaneous area. Allodynia may be *mechanical,* static (e.g., induced by a light pressure), dynamic (induced by moving a soft brush), and *thermal* (e.g., induced by a nonpainful cold or warm stimulus).
4. *Hyperalgesia,* which is an exaggerated pain response to a mildly noxious (mechanical or thermal) stimulus applied to the symptomatic area.
5. *Hyperpathia,* which is a delayed and explosive pain response to a noxious stimulus applied to the symptomatic area.

Allodynia, hyperalgesia, and hyperpathia represent positive abnormal findings, as opposed to the negative findings of the neurological sensory examination, i.e., hypesthesia and anesthesia. The positive and negative sensory findings follow neuroanatomical patterns of distribution. For example, with a distal symmetrical polyneuropathy the sensory symptoms occur first according to a stocking distribution, with numbness and pain in the feet and ankles. Therefore, a careful assessment of both positive and negative sensory findings can provide important information on the anatomical diagnosis and nature of the condition.

Dynamic mechanical allodynia is elicited by stroking the painful region with a cotton swab or a soft brush. Cold allodynia and cold hyperalgesia are assessed by placing a cold stimulus, such as a cold tuning fork, on the painful region for a few seconds. Dynamic mechanical allodynia and cold allodynia/hyperalgesia are findings commonly present in the zone surrounding the cutaneous epicenter of the pain generator (e.g., inflammation). They are also indicative of CNS sensitization (i.e., secondary hyperalgesia), a phenomenon that often complicates neuropathic pain states. Of note, patients affected by sympathetically maintained pain (SMP; see later) are typically affected by cold allodynia and hyperalgesia in the affected limb (7). Static mechanical allodynia (i.e., tenderness), mechanical pinprick hyperalgesia, warm allodynia, and heat hyperalgesia are findings commonly present in the primary zone, at the epicenter of a pain generator. They are indicative of PNS sensitization (i.e., primary hyperalgesia) and most often related to a local inflammatory state.

Diagnostic Workup

A thorough workup of patients with neuropathic pain is essential in delineating the etiology and potential mechanisms of neuropathic pain. Laboratory studies, analysis of

tissue samples from skin and nerve, anatomical studies, and functional neurophysiological studies all have a role to play in the evaluation of patients with chronic neuropathic pain.

Laboratory Assessments

A thorough diagnostic laboratory work up (Table 29-2) includes complete blood cell count (CBC), sedimentation rate, general chemistry profile, thyroid function tests, vitamin B12 and folate serum levels, fasting blood sugar and glycosylated hemoglobin, sero-protein electrophoresis with immunofixation, Lyme disease antibody titers, hepatitis virus B and C screening titers, antinuclear antibodies (ANA), rheumatoid factor (RF), Sjögren titers (SS-A, SS-B), cryoglobulins, anti-sulfatide IgM antibody titer, anti-HU titers, heavy metal serum and urine screening, HIV testing, and cerebral spinal fluid study for ruling out demyelinating neuropathies (i.e., Guillain-Barre syndrome), and polyradiculopathies related to meningeal carcinomatosis (5,8).

It is important to screen for monoclonal proteins in all patients with a chronic neuropathy of undetermined etiology, particularly those individuals over 60 years of age, because a portion of these patients may have a monoclonal gammopathy. Several autoantibodies with reactivity to various components of the peripheral nerve have been associated with peripheral neuropathies. However, despite all diagnostic efforts, chronic neuropathies remain with an idiopathic cause in up to 30% of the affected patients (9).

Analysis of Tissue Biopsy Specimens

The sural nerve is the usual selected nerve for biopsy because the sensory deficit following the procedure is limited to a small area along the dorsolateral aspect of the ankle and foot. The biopsy is useful for the diagnosis of

TABLE 29-2. *Diagnostic laboratory workup*

Cell blood count (CBC)
Sedimentation rate
General chemistry profile
Thyroid function tests
Vitamin B12 and folate serum levels
Fasting blood sugar and glycosylated hemoglobin
Serum protein electrophoresis with immunofixation
Lyme disease antibody titer
Hepatitis virus B and C screening titers
Antinuclear antibodies (ANA)
Rheumatoid factor (RF)
Sjögren titers (SS-A, SS-B)
Cryoglobulins
Anti-sulfatide IgM antibody titer
Anti-HU titers
Heavy metal serum and urine screening
HIV testing
Cerebrospinal fluid study (for demyelinating neuropathies and meningeal carcinomatosis)

vasculitis, amyloidosis, sarcoidosis, leprosy, tumor infiltration, IgM monoclonal gammopathies, Charcot-Marie-Tooth disease, chronic inflammatory demyelinating polyradiculopathies, and small fiber neuropathies. Skin biopsy (10) is a promising technique to evaluate the density of unmyelinated fibers within the dermis and epidermis. Immunostaining with a panaxonal marker has been used to demonstrate the intraepidermal network of C fibers. Patients with diabetic sensory neuropathies, idiopathic neuropathies, and HIV-associated neuropathies have been found to have a significantly diminished intraepidermal density of small fibers.

Anatomical Studies

Magnetic resonance imaging (MRI) studies have become an essential tool in the diagnosis of structural pathologies causing neuropathic pain states. MRI can help with the anatomical evaluation of central and peripheral nervous system structures, including spinal cord, nerve roots, plexuses, and major peripheral nerves.

Electrodiagnostic Studies

Electromyography (EMG) and nerve conduction velocity (NCV) studies help with the localization of the lesion and can indicate an axonal versus a focal segmental demyelinating process. For example, the EMG-NCV study may identify a radiculopathy or mononeuropathy, i.e., a focal process affecting a specific root or nerve. A traumatic injury, compression or nerve entrapment, ischemia, and neoplastic infiltration are common causes of mononeuropathy. The study may also reveal a *mononeuropathy multiplex*, a pathology of multiple but noncontiguous nerves. Mononeuropathy multiplex is often the result of vasculitis and microangiopathy causing axonal disease in multiple noncontiguous nerves. EMG-NCV studies may also help to detect diffuse abnormalities, indicating a polyneuropathy. Of note, diabetes mellitus, hypothyroidism, and hereditary neuropathy with liability to pressure palsy may cause neuropathies that predispose affected patients to the development of superimposed entrapment neuropathies.

ETIOPATHOLOGIES OF NEUROPATHIC PAIN DISORDERS

In this section the etiopathology of peripheral neuropathies that are most commonly associated with neuropathic pain will be discussed (5,8). As shown in Table 29-1, neuropathic pain may have numerous etiologies, including metabolic or endocrinologic disorders, infections, inflammation, malignancy, autoimmune disorders, immunoglobulinemias, dietary or absorption abnormalities, entrapment due to anatomical abnormalities, or exposure to toxins or drugs. In addition, neuropathic pain may arise as a result of hereditary abnormalities.

Metabolic and Endocrinologic Disorders Associated with Neuropathic Pain

Abnormalities in energy metabolism, liver and kidney function, or endocrine regulation may be associated with neuropathic pain states. The most common of these conditions is neuropathy associated with diabetes mellitus.

Diabetic Neuropathies

Several types of neuropathies are associated with diabetes mellitus, including a distal symmetrical polyneuropathy; asymmetrical neuropathies; mononeuropathies due to infarction or entrapment; thoracic radiculopathy; and femoral amyotrophy. The diagnosis of diabetic neuropathy is based on the evidence of hyperglycemia, clinical symptoms, and objective neurological signs. Fasting plasma glucose levels greater than 125 mg/dL on more than one occasion and any plasma glucose level higher than 200 mg/dL (or sustained plasma glucose of more than 200 mg/dL at 2 hours after a 75-gram oral glucose load) confirm the diagnosis of diabetes mellitus. Glycosylated hemoglobin (hemoglobin A1c) is a useful indicator of long-term control of blood sugar levels. EMG-NCV studies can confirm the examination findings (11).

Many mechanisms have been proposed for the pathogenesis of neuropathy in the setting of diabetes mellitus. In general, metabolic factors, microvascular abnormalities, deficiencies of specific neurotrophic factors, and inflammatory changes (e.g., autoimmune process) have all been proposed. Several factors may interplay in causing diabetic neuropathy. The majority of individuals with diabetic polyneuropathy have a pathological involvement of both large- and small-diameter sensory fibers as well as autonomic fibers. However, a distal neuropathy primarily affecting small-diameter axons, i.e., A-delta and C fibers, may occur, and patients affected by this condition present with "burning feet."

Asymmetrical neuropathies include single or multiple cranial mononeuropathies, single or multiple somatic mononeuropathies, or asymmetrical lumbosacral plexopathies. The most common cranial neuropathy syndrome is the painful pupil-sparing diabetic third nerve palsy. Involvement of single nerves in diabetes mellitus may occur either from infarction or entrapment. Entrapment neuropathies of the median and ulnar nerves occur with greater frequency in diabetics. Thoracic radiculopathy usually affects roots or intercostal nerves from T-4 to T-12 causing pain and dysesthesias in the chest and abdomen. The term *diabetic femoral amyotrophy* implies an acute painful asymmetrical proximal lower limb syndrome. Severe unilateral pain develops in the anterior thigh. Weakness develops over days to weeks, affecting the proximal lower extremity muscles. Reduction or absence of the patellar reflex occurs. Weight loss arises in more than one half of the patients. Pain usually subsides spontaneously over weeks or months before motor strength begins to improve. However, a comprehensive evaluation to rule out any concurrent and perhaps treatable pathology affecting the lumbar plexus or femoral nerve must be carried out.

Liver Disease

Several neuropathic syndromes have been associated with acute and chronic liver diseases (5,8). Hepatitis B has been linked with both demyelinating neuropathies and with polyarteritis nodosa (see following). Most patients with neuropathy-associated cryoglobulinemia have hepatitis C infection. Patients with primary biliary cirrhosis may develop a sensory polyneuropathy or dorsal root ganglionopathy.

Renal Failure and Hemodialysis

Peripheral neuropathy develops in a large majority of patients with *renal failure* who require chronic dialysis (5). The pathogenesis of uremic neuropathy is likely secondary to the accumulation of systemic toxins, although no specific factors have been identified. The clinical features are those of a slowly progressive sensory polyneuropathy, characterized by a constellation of symptoms, including burning feet, muscular cramps, dysesthesias, and a restless leg syndrome picture. Accumulation of beta 2-microglobulin amyloid in the carpal ligament and complications of vascular shunts may cause painful median nerve neuropathies.

Hypothyroid and Acromegalic Neuropathy

Patients suffering from hypothyroidism may develop neuropathy characterized by a polyneuropathy with paresthesias and muscle cramps. It can be observed in approximately 30% to 40% of patients with hypothyroidism. Thyroid hormone replacement may improve the neuropathy-associated symptoms. Patients with *hypothyroidism* are also predisposed to develop carpal tunnel syndrome and other entrapment neuropathies (8). Carpal tunnel syndrome may be a complication of *acromegaly*. A generalized neuropathy may also develop independently from the concomitant acromegaly-associated diabetes mellitus.

Infections Often Associated with Neuropathic Pain

Painful peripheral neuropathies occur in a number of infectious diseases, including viral, bacterial, and parasitic infections (5,8).

Human Immunodeficiency Virus (HIV)

HIV infection is associated with a wide variety of peripheral neuropathy syndromes, including distal symmetric or axonal polyneuropathy, inflammatory demyelinating neuropathy, mononeuropathies, and polyradiculopathies. HIV-related neuropathies might also be caused by nutritional deficiencies (see later) or the use of antiviral or antibacterial drugs (e.g., didioxynucleosides, dapsone, isoniazid, etc.) (12). The most common neuropathy related to HIV infection is distal symmetrical polyneuropathy. The onset occurs often with burning feet, distal sensory loss combined with a mild distal weakness, and autonomic dysfunction. It is advisable to test for HIV antibodies in those patients who present with a demyelinating neuropathy and are known to have HIV risk factors or some laboratory results, such as positive hepatitis B serology, polyclonal hypergammaglobulinemia, and CSF pleocytosis. Painful mononeuropathy and multiple mononeuropathies may be secondary to superimposed infections, including herpes zoster, hepatitis C, cytomegalovirus (CMV), and syphilis. Multiple mononeuropathies with severe deficits are more likely to occur in immune-compromised AIDS patients with a CD4+ T-lymphocyte count below 200 cells/mcL. A subset of HIV positive patients with distal symmetrical polyneuropathy has been found to have necrotizing vasculitis. Acute lumbosacral polyradiculopathy is often associated with CMV infection and is one of the most devastating neurological complications in AIDS. In CMV-related lumbosacral polyradiculopathy CSF examination shows a pleocytosis with more than 40% of cells of the polymorphonuclear type, a high level of proteins, and a low concentration of glucose. An MRI with gadolinium may demonstrate enhancement of the cauda equina nerve roots.

Varicella Zoster Virus (VZV)

Varicella Zoster virus can cause a variety of neuropathic conditions. Postherpetic neuralgia is the pain that persists beyond the time of normal healing of the acute skin rash (shingles). PHN occurs in approximately 50% of patients age 60 and older following shingles. The VZV infection can cause extensive inflammatory, hemorrhagic, and necrotic changes in the dorsal root ganglia as well as in the corresponding dorsal horns of the spinal cord.

Hepatitis B Virus (HBV) and Hepatitis C Virus (HCV)

Infections with *HBV* and *HCV* have been reported in association with demyelinating Guillain-Barré syndrome, multiple painful neuropathies secondary to vasculitis, and cryoglobulinemia. The combination of hepatitis C virus infection and cryoglobulinemia has been recognized recently as a cause of painful neuropathy (13).

Human T-cell Lymphotrophic Virus Type 1 (HTLV-1)

Infection with *HTLV-1* can cause a painful neuropathy. Although the majority of the patients affected by human T-cell lymphotrophic virus Type 1 present with spastic paraparesis, many patients may develop a painful neuropathy (14). Because the syndrome is much more common in tropical regions, the term *tropical spastic paraparesis* has also been used to define patients affected by this virus.

Leprosy

The *mycobacterium leprae* can cause a painful neuropathy (15). Leprous neuritis is a very prevalent neuropathy worldwide, especially in tropical and subtropical regions. *Mycobacterium leprae* is likely transmitted through the upper respiratory tract. Once the nasal mucosa is colonized, the organism spreads slowly throughout the body. The skin and superficial nerve trunks are particularly vulnerable. In all forms of leprous neuritis (i.e., tuberculoid, dimorphous, and lepromatous) the fundamental neurological manifestation is anesthesia. However, neuropathic pain occurs and may be quite excruciating. The complication is thought to be due to a vasculitis affecting nerve trunks. Clinically, there is a nodular inflammation of the skin and painful, swollen nerve trunks.

Lyme Disease

The spirochete of Lyme borreliosis (16) can cause a variety of neurological conditions. Infection of the tick-borne spirochete *borrelia burgdorferi* can induce a painful polyradiculopathy and neuropathy. This may present with distal sensory symptoms (i.e., burning feet) or proximal radicular pains. EMG-NCV studies may reveal a multifocal widespread axonal process. A sural nerve biopsy should show axonal loss as well as perivascular and perineural mononuclear inflammation. Serological confirmation of Lyme disease documents previous exposure, but it is not sufficient to establish a causal relationship between infection and neuropathy because at least 10% of asymptomatic individuals are seropositive. High CSF titers of anti-borrelia burgdorferi antibodies are helpful to link the peripheral neurological manifestations to Lyme disease.

Demyelinating Inflammatory Painful Disorders

Guillain-Barré syndrome (GBS) is an acute inflammatory multifocal demyelinating disease affecting spinal roots and peripheral nerves, supposedly caused by an autoimmune disorder initiated by T-lymphocytes and maintained by antibodies against peripheral nerve antigens (15). Approximately 50% of the patients during the acute stage of GBS experience pains in their muscles and spine (17). During the clinical course of GBS, however, pain usually subsides. In contrast, burning, aching pains very rarely occur in patients with chronic inflammatory demyelinating polyneuropathy (CIDP). CSF examination and electrophysiological studies are essential to confirm the diagnosis of both GBS and CIDP. In GBS and CIDP, the CSF study typically shows albuminocytological dissociation (i.e., high levels of proteins and normal cell counts). Electrophysiological workup reveals a pattern of nerve conduction abnormalities supporting the diagnosis of acquired multifocal demyelination.

Malignancies as a Cause of Neuropathic Pain

Neuropathy may result from one or more cancer-related mechanisms (18). Compression, mechanical traction, inflammation, infiltration of nerve trunks or plexuses caused by the primary growing cancer or by metastatic disease affecting bone, soft tissues, or meninges with involvement of adjacent spinal roots, plexuses, and peripheral nerves. Nasopharyngeal carcinomas and skull-based tumors can cause painful cranial neuropathies by direct nerve compression. Salivary gland cancers may induce painful facial neuropathies. Breast or lung cancers can infiltrate the brachial plexus and cause a painful plexitis. Pelvic or retroperitoneal cancers may invade the lumbosacral plexus. Metastatic disease or lymphoma can cause meningeal carcinomatosis and affect multiple spinal roots. Iatrogenic painful neuropathic disorders can be caused by antineoplastic chemotherapy, radiation, or surgical procedures. Antineoplastic therapeutic agents such as cisplatinum, taxoids, and vincristine may cause painful neuropathies. Postradiation plexopathies may arise when more than 60 GY (6000 RAD) of irradiation are given to the patient. Surgical resection of cancers may result in traumatic injuries to peripheral nerves with development of painful neuromas. For example, postthoracotomy pain can be caused by injury to the intercostal nerves and postmastectomy pain by injury to the intercostal brachial nerve.

Compression or entrapment neuropathies occur in the presence of cachexia. For example, patients who have lost substantial fat and muscle body weight because of cancer are prone to develop peroneal neuropathy.

Paraneoplastic autoimmune syndromes due to antineuronal antibodies may present as painful neuropathies. Patients who complain of burning dysesthesias in their feet, hands, and face (in the setting of diagnosed or undiagnosed carcinoma) may have antineuronal nuclear antibodies type 1 (ANNA-1), also known as anti-HU. The vast majority of patients who present with sensory neuronopathy and small cell carcinoma of the lung have significantly elevated titers of ANNA-1. All patients with burning dysesthesias of the face, hands, and legs and positive titers for ANNA-1 should have a chest CT or MRI because the tumor may remain undetected by plain chest x-ray. In any case, ANNA-1 positivity should prompt a careful search for malignancy, especially for a small cell carcinoma of the lung. Painful dysesthesias develop first in one limb and then progress to involve all four limbs and occasionally the face, scalp, and trunk either acutely or over many months. In these patients deep tendon reflexes are reduced or absent, and muscle strength is preserved. Patients may be disabled in their ambulation because of the sensory ataxia that is often associated with the painful symptoms. Peripheral neuropathies are also observed in the presence of lymphomas. Acute inflammatory demyelinating polyneuropathy of the GBS type may occur with lymphomas, particularly Hodgkin's disease.

Painful Neuropathies Associated with Autoimmune and Granulomatous Disorders

Peripheral nerves, including cranial nerves, can be affected by connective tissue disorders (19). The pathogenesis of peripheral neuropathy in connective tissue disorders is complex and may vary according to the specific disorder. Circulating immunocomplexes and ischemic lesions represent the most likely pathogenetic mechanisms of these disorders.

Sjögren Syndrome (SS)

SS is an autoimmune disorder primarily affecting exocrine glands. It is characterized by reduced lacrimal and salivary gland secretion, resulting in dry eyes and dry mouth (*sicca complex*). The *sicca complex* is due to lymphocyte infiltration, inflammation, and consequent dysfunction of lacrimal and salivary glands. SS has 90% prevalence for women. Laboratory tests for autoantibodies to extractable nuclear antigens (ENA, also called SS-A, SS-B), elevated sedimentation rate, rheumatoid factor, and hypergammaglobulinemia may be positive. A sensory neuropathy occurs in almost a third of patients with Sjögren syndrome (20). Painful symptoms may be the major and only complaint in SS-affected patients. If the laboratory tests are negative, a biopsy of the salivary glands of the lower lip is necessary for diagnostic confirmation. This should show lymphocytic infiltrates. A nerve biopsy can also demonstrate perivascular lymphocytic infiltrates.

Systemic Lupus Erythematosus (SLE)

SLE is an autoimmune connective tissue disease where CNS more than PNS manifestations occur. PNS involvement develops in less than a third of SLE-affected patients. Painful cranial nerve neuropathies, painful brachial plexopathy, GBS, or CIDP have been observed in association with SLE. Autoantibodies against peripheral nerve antigens or an immune-mediated vasculitis have been proposed as pathogenetic mechanisms underlying the SLE-related PNS involvement.

Rheumatoid Arthritis (RA)

RA is a chronic syndrome characterized by joint inflammation. The cause is unknown. However, there is a genetic predisposition to RA, and an abnormal immunological response characterized by activated T-lymphocytes and macrophages infiltrating the synovium and releasing proinflammatory cytokines (e.g., tumor necrosis factor alpha, interleukin-1, etc.) occurs. Rheumatoid vasculitis can complicate the overall clinical picture. Painful polyneuropathy or painful mononeuropathies or mononeuropathy multiplex may occur in rheumatoid arthritis. Also, entrapment neuropathies secondary to nerve compression due to joint inflammation may develop. The sedimentation rate is elevated. The rheumatoid factor (RF) titer, i.e., corresponding to a serum titer of antibodies to abnormal gammaglobulins, is often present and elevated. The C4 complement level is frequently low. The synovial fluid is cloudy, rich in neutrophils, but sterile. Cutaneous nerve or muscle biopsies demonstrate a necrotizing vasculitis.

Sarcoidosis

Sarcoidosis is a granulomatous disease affecting multiple organs, including peripheral nerves. Sarcoidosis can cause cranial neuropathies, truncal sensory mononeuropathies, a GBS-like polyradiculopathy, cauda equina syndrome, or mononeuropathy multiplex. Although rare, painful symptoms may accompany the more common motor and sensory deficits. The nerve damage is probably related to granulomas affecting the vasa nervorum. An elevated serum level of angiotensin-converting enzyme (ACE), as well as positive biopsies of lymph nodes, muscles, and sural nerves confirms the diagnosis.

Vasculitidies

A number of immune-based vascular conditions may affect the peripheral nervous system (21). Polyarteritis nodosa (PAN) is the most common vasculitis characterized by necrotizing inflammation of medium-size and small-size arteries. Hepatitis B antigens are found in one third of the PAN cases. Painful mononeuritis multiplex is characteristically associated with PAN. Churg-Strauss vasculitis (CGV) typically presents with asthma, pulmonary infiltrates, and eosinophilia and may be associated with a painful neuropathy. A high titer of antineutrophilic cytoplasm antibodies (ANCA) is important for the diagnosis of CGV. Wegener's granulomatosis (WG) is a necrotizing granulomatous vasculitis that affects the upper and lower respiratory tracts and may be accompanied by glomerulonephritis. The peripheral nervous system is involved in up to one third of WG cases. Patients may present with severe facial pain secondary to cranial nerve neuropathy. Of note, ANCAs are almost constantly present in WG. Giant cell arteritis or temporal arteritis affects large- and medium-size arteries. The vasculitis may affect arteries of peripheral nerves causing ischemic neuropathies or mononeuritis multiplex. The sedimentation rate is usually markedly elevated.

Vasculitic neuropathies may occur in the course of malignancies, such as myeloproliferative or lymphoproliferative disorders, and infections, such as hepatitis C and HIV.

Neuropathic Pain Associated with Immunoglobulinemias

Painful neuropathies may be associated with the presence of excessive amounts of circulating monoclonal proteins, with amyloidosis, or with cryoglobulinemia.

Monoclonal (M) Proteins

Patients undergoing evaluation for chronic peripheral neuropathies of unknown cause should be screened for the presence of monoclonal immunoglobulins (IgG, IgM, IgA, IgD, IgE), also called M proteins (22). A subset of the patients with idiopathic painful peripheral neuropathy has an associated monoclonal gammopathy. Routine serum or urine protein electrophoresis frequently lacks the sensitivity required to detect small amounts of M protein. Serum immunoelectrophoresis (or immunofixation) is then required to detect little amounts of M proteins and to confirm the monoclonal nature. Free monoclonal immunoglobulin light chains (i.e., Bence-Jones protein) can be excreted in the urine and detected by testing a quantitative 24-hour urine collection. Bence-Jones protein is associated to multiple myeloma and amyloidosis.

The pathophysiological relationship between M proteins and neuropathy is unclear, but some specific M proteins may have antibody properties directed against the components of the myelin or axolemma. Some IgM M proteins have been implicated in the pathogenesis of painful neuropathies (23,24). For example, IgM anti-sulfatide and anti-chondroitin sulfate M proteins have been associated with a painful sensory neuropathy and IgM M proteins that react with a myelin-associated glycoprotein (MAG) with a sensory demyelinating neuropathy. Finding an M protein among patients with a neuropathy may lead to the discovery of underlying disorders such as primary systemic amyloidosis, multiple or osteosclerotic myeloma, macroglobulinemia, cryoglobulinemia, lymphoma, or a malignant proliferative disease. Waldenström's macroglobulinemia (WM) is characterized by a malignant plasma cell dyscrasia producing monoclonal IgM proteins; it typically affects elderly men and may cause a sensory neuropathy. A sensory polyneuropathy occurs in approximately 30% of patients with WM.

However, in more than 50% of patients with an M protein, no detectable underlying disease is found. These patients are described as having a monoclonal gammopathy of undetermined significance (MGUS). The underlying mechanism of nerve fiber damage in MGUS neuropathy remains unknown, although an immune-mediated etiology is suspected. Of these patients, a subset may be found to have malignant plasma cell dyscrasia at long-term followups.

Amyloidosis

Primary amyloidosis is a systemic disorder characterized by tissue deposition of abnormal fibrillar proteins (25). In primary systemic amyloidosis, clonal plasma cells synthesize light chain peptides that accumulate in the extracellular spaces of tissues as amyloid. In both primary amyloidosis and amyloidosis complicating multiple myeloma or WM, the extracellular amyloid is made of fragments of immunoglobulin light chains. Primary amyloidosis has a median patient age of onset of 65 years. The neuropathy usually begins with painful dysesthesias in the feet and follows a slowly progressive spreading course. Most patients develop autonomic dysfunction, such as postural hypotension, gastrointestinal disturbances, impaired sweating, and loss of bladder control. Some patients develop a superimposed carpal tunnel syndrome caused by amyloid infiltration of the flexor retinaculum of the wrist. The combination of painful dysesthesias, autonomic dysfunction, and a history of carpal tunnel syndrome should direct the pain physician to the possible diagnosis of amyloidosis. An M protein (light chains) can be diagnosed in 90% of patients by means of serum or urine immunoelectrophoresis. In patients with suspected amyloid neuropathy, a nerve/muscle biopsy represents the most sensitive diagnostic technique.

Cryoglobulinemia

Cryoglobulins are immunoglobulins that precipitate on cooling. Cryoglobulinemia may occur as a primary condition without any apparent underlying disease (*essential cryoglobulinemia*). Alternatively, cryoglobulinemia may be secondary to autoimmune diseases, infections (e.g., hepatitis C), or lymphoproliferative disorders. Cryoglobulins are classified into three types: (a) M proteins associated with myeloma, macroglobulinemia, and other lymphoproliferative disorders, (b) M proteins with antirheumatoid factor activity, and (c) polyclonal IgM and IgG. Hepatitis C viral infection appears to be the most common cause of type II cryoglobulinemia. Cryoglobulinemia is often associated with painful vasculitis and mononeuritis multiplex (26,27). In most cases the nerve biopsy shows myelinated fiber loss, axonal degeneration, and necrotizing vasculitis.

Painful Neuropathies Associated with Dietary or Absorption Abnormalities

Alcoholic Neuropathy and Vitamin Deficiencies

Neuropathy usually begins insidiously in patients affected by alcoholism and likely associated nutritional deficiencies. Patients complain of painful burning feet and numbness. Leg cramps and gait difficulty are common. Nerve biopsy may reveal axonal loss of both small and large fibers (8,15). Deficiencies of thiamine and other B vitamins, which are due to inadequate dietary intake, impaired absorption, or perhaps a higher metabolic demand in alcoholic patients, are other causes of polyneuropathy. The clinical constellation of painful neuropathy, orogenital dermatitis, and amblyopia has been named *Strachan's syndrome*. This syndrome was originally referred to as Jamaican neuritis and appears to occur in malnourished individuals and occasionally in alcoholic patients (28). The prevention and treatment of this syndrome are reportedly based on a high intake of thiamine, vitamin B12, riboflavin, niacin, and antioxidant agents. *Pyridoxine (vitamin B6) deficiency* can cause a painful neuropathy. Deficiency of pyridoxine, however, may occur during treatment with isoniazid (INH), hydralazine, or rarely penicillamine. These drugs structurally resemble vitamin B6 and interfere with pyridoxine coenzyme activity. When using INH, supplementary pyridoxine (100 mg daily) is recommended. Paradoxically, mega doses (e.g., more than 200–300 mg/day) of pyridoxine have also been found to cause a painful sensory polyneuropathy. *Vitamin B12 and folate deficiency* can cause a sensory polyneuropathy, as well as spasticity secondary to myelopathy. Acquired malabsorption of vitamin B12 and folate may occur following gastric and/or ileum surgical resections for the treatment of a wide range of gastrointestinal diseases. Strict vegetarians and individuals affected by intestinal parasites (e.g., tapeworms) may also develop B12 and folate deficiency. Low serum levels of vitamin B12 and/or folate confirm the diagnosis of vitamin deficiency. Individuals who abuse or are often exposed to nitrous oxide (which inactivates some vitamin B12 dependent enzymes, perhaps in the setting of low serum levels of B12) may develop signs of neuropathy and myelopathy. Pernicious anemia is an autoimmune process directed against the parietal cells of the gastric mucosa that causes malabsorption of vitamin B12. The full-blown clinical picture of vitamin B12 deficiency consists of megaloblastic anemia, glossitis, and neurological signs such as painful neuropathy and myelopathy (29).

Painful Entrapment Neuropathies

Entrapment neuropathies are caused by a focal chronic compression of a peripheral nerve. Traditionally the term *entrapment* has not been used for nerve compressions due to pathological masses or tumors. The compression of entrapment neuropathies, therefore, is caused by anatomical structures (e.g., carpal tunnel, cubital groove, etc.) surrounding the course of a nerve. Patients with entrapment neuropathies complain of sharp shooting pains often radiating along the distribution of the affected nerve. Motor and sensory findings arise over time. A positive Tinel's sign or tenderness at the site of nerve compression can be elicited during the neurological examination. Electrophysiological testing and diagnostic peripheral nerve blocks are useful in confirming the clinical diagnosis of entrapment neuropathy (30).

Painful Toxic Neuropathies

Peripheral neuropathy is one of the most common reactions of the nervous system to toxic chemicals. Some drugs, heavy metals, and industrial, environmental, and biological agents are known to cause toxic neuropathies (5,31).

Heavy Metal Toxicity

Thallium and arsenic consistently induce a painful neuropathy, as well abnormal lines in nails (Mees' lines) and systemic effects. Alopecia occurs with thallium intoxication.

Serum, urine (24-hour collection), and hair testing confirm the diagnosis of heavy metal neuropathy.

Neuropathy Secondary to Drug Exposure

Some drug-induced painful neuropathies are caused by: (a) *amiodarone,* a class III antiarrhythmic agent used in the management of refractory ventricular arrhythmias. A painful polyneuropathy may develop in patients receiving long-term amiodarone therapy; (b) *cisplatinum,* an agent used in the treatment of ovarian, bladder, and testicular malignancies. Peripheral neuropathy is the cisplatinum dose-limiting side effect. The neuropathy may develop several months after discontinuation of the drug. (c) *Colchicine* is an agent used in the treatment of gout. A distal axonal neuropathy can occur in patients receiving chronic colchicine therapy, especially if the patients are affected by renal insufficiency; (d) *metronidazole,* an antibiotic used in the treatment of protozoa and anaerobic bacterial infections. It may cause a painful polyneuropathy; (e) *pyridoxine,* or vitamin B6. It can cause a severe, painful sensory neuropathy when taken at mega doses (higher than 200–300 mg/day, see earlier section on dietary abnormalities associated with neuropathy); (f) *taxoids,* alkaloids used in the treatment of ovarian cancer. These agents disrupt microtubule assembly and axonal transport. A painful sensory neuropathy develops with doses above 200 mg/m^2; (g) *vincristine,* a vinca alkaloid used in chemotherapeutic regimens. It can cause a painful polyneuropathy. Vincristine, when used at the conventional doses, invariably causes a mild polyneuropathy. Of note, paresthesias and dysesthesias often start in the fingers and hands.

Hereditary Painful Neuropathies

Eliciting a history of long-standing complaints of numbness and limb weakness, obtaining a detailed family history, looking for musculoskeletal abnormalities such as hammertoes, high arches in the feet, or spinal scoliosis, and performing a neurological evaluation in relatives are some clinical ways of identifying hereditary neuropathies (5,32).

Charcot-Marie Tooth Disease (CMT)

CMT is the most common inherited neuropathy, with an estimate of 1 patient to every 2500 people in the United States (33). Painful symptoms of CMT disease (34) have been reported to occur in the hypertrophic or demyelinating form (CMT-1). In this form there is a marked reduction in nerve conduction velocities (NCVs) as well as "onion bulb" formation on nerve biopsy findings (corresponding to a progressive process of large fiber demyelination and subsequent remyelination). In the axonal form (CMT-2), NCVs are minimally impaired, and nerve biopsy findings show axonal loss without "onion bulb" formation. Both CMT type 1 and 2 have an autosomal dominant inheritance. Of note, CMT disease is also known to have a third clinical form, a severe demyelinating neuropathy with onset in early childhood. This form has been called CMT type 3 (or Dejerine-Sottas disease). Patients with CMT-1 develop their initial complaints, such as difficulties in walking or running, during the first or second decade. Adult patients have absent ankle jerks. Enlarged hypertrophic peripheral nerves can be found on regional exam. In CMT-2, clinical symptoms begin later than in CMT-1. They might begin in middle age or later. Peripheral nerves are not enlarged. Neuropathic pain appears to be a relevant and underrecognized problem in patients with CMT disease. Patients may complain of shooting, sharp, burning pains in their toes, feet, ankles, and knees.

Fabry's Disease (FD)

FD is an x-linked recessive disorder in which a deficiency of the lysosomal enzyme alpha-galactosidase causes accumulation of the glycolipid ceramide-trihexoside in the endothelial cells of blood vessels (5). The typical cutaneous angiokeratomas are telangiectasias mainly located over the lower part of the trunk, glutei, and scrotum. A painful small fiber neuropathy develops in childhood or adolescence. Fever and hot environments may intensify distal dysesthesias and lancinating pains. Autonomic dysfunction occurs and includes anhidrosis, impaired lacrimation and salivation, and decreased intestinal motility. Deposition of the glycolipid in vascular structures leads to vascular disease affecting heart, kidneys, and brain. Leukocytes or skin fibroblasts are used to test the activity of the lysosomal enzyme alpha-galactosidase and determine the diagnosis of Fabry's disease.

Familial Amyloid Polyneuropathy (FAP)

FAP is a group of autosomal dominant disorders characterized by the extracellular deposition of amyloid along and within peripheral nerves and visceral organs (8). The majority of patients with FAP have mutations of the plasma protein transthyretin. This is a transport protein for thyroxin and is synthesized in the liver. The neuropathy begins insidiously in the third and fourth decades, often presenting with lancinating pains and paresthesias. Patients also develop signs of autonomic dysfunction, such as postural hypotension, bladder dysfunction, and anhidrosis. A restricted form of FAP, also called FAP type 2, presents with carpal tunnel syndrome in the fourth or fifth decade. Autonomic manifestations are absent. Surgical decompression of the carpal tunnel may provide not only pain relief, but also the diagnosis. In fact, the biopsy of the flexor retinaculum taken at the time of the surgery demonstrates amyloid infiltration. Another variant of the disease, called apolipoprotein A1 amyloidosis (FAP type 3), presents with neuropathy, early renal involvement, and duodenal ulcers. A fourth variant of FAP, called gelsolin amyloidosis (FAP type 4), begins in

the third decade with corneal clouding and neuropathy. This is followed in the fifth decade by progressive cranial neuropathies and facial skin changes producing a "saggy" face. The diagnosis of amyloidosis is established by confirming the presence of amyloid in nerve and muscle biopsies. In order to differentiate FAP from the more common nonfamilial forms of amyloidosis, a search for an M protein (light chains) should be conducted by testing serum and urine with immunoelectrophoresis. If no evidence of plasma cell dyscrasia is found, serum electrophoresis should be focused on transthyretin. The finding of a variant transthyretin should prompt genetic testing.

Porphyric Neuropathy

High serum levels of porphyrins have toxic effects on the autonomic, peripheral, and central nervous systems (5). Porphyrias are dominant inherited disorders and include acute intermittent porphyria (AIP), variegate porphyria (VP), and hereditary coproporphyria (HCP). Porphyrins accumulate because of hereditary enzyme defects affecting the synthesis of heme. These partial enzyme defects remain latent until precipitating factors trigger acute attacks, often characterized by neuropsychiatry manifestations. Precipitating factors include certain drugs, alcohol, or unbalanced dieting during prolonged fasting. Porphyric attacks usually occur during the second and third decades of life and are more common and severe in women. All clinical symptoms can be explained by dysfunction of the autonomic, peripheral, and central nervous systems. Patients may present with abdominal pain, nausea, vomiting, tachycardia, and difficulty with urination. A subacute neuropathy characterized by paresthesias, dysesthesias, sharp pains, and cramps may affect the extremities or the trunk. Patients with VP and HCP may also develop cutaneous photosensitivity during adult life. High concentrations of ALA (aminolevulinic acid) and PBG (porphobilinogen) in blood and urine confirm the diagnosis of porphyria.

Cryptogenic Painful Neuropathies

Idiopathic Polyneuropathy

Idiopathic neuropathy commonly afflicts patients in the sixth decade of life. Patients with idiopathic painful axonal neuropathy are commonly affected by burning feet. Most patients have elevated sensory thresholds on examination and impaired distal sweating, which can be measured by the quantitative sudomotor axon reflex test. A skin biopsy may show a reduced density of nerve fibers in the epidermis. This finding provides evidence of distal small fiber neuropathy.

Complex Regional Pain Syndromes

In 1994 the International Association for the Study of Pain (IASP) renamed the disorder formerly called reflex sympathetic dystrophy (RSD) as *complex regional pain syndrome (CRPS) type 1* and the disorder previously called causalgia as *CRPS type 2* (1).

The term *CRPS* implies the presence of regional pain and sensory findings after a noxious event. Associated abnormalities, such as regional edema and changes in skin color, temperature, and sudomotor activity, appear to be out of proportion to the physical damage from the noxious event.

CRPSs may be secondary to an abnormal neuroimmunologic inflammatory process. Inflammatory cytokines such as tumor necrosis factor alpha (TNF-alpha), interleukin (IL) 1-beta, IL-6, and IL-8 are known to induce significant changes in nociceptors, including sensitization, activation, or even axonal damage. An outgrowth of the concept that immunological changes may result in the occurrence of CRPSs is the number of observations addressing the role of macrophages and macrophage-released cytokines and NGF in the genesis of hyperalgesia (4,35). The release of neurotrophic factors from damaged tissue and activated macrophages may also play a role in CRPSs (36). Neurotrophic factors, including nerve growth factor, induce the development of miniature axon sprouts from the endings of small nerve afferent fibers as well as from the sympathetic efferent nerves.

It also appears that there may be a genetic predisposition to the development of CRPS type 1, with a higher incidence in certain HLA types, e.g., HLA DQ 1 (37). Pathological studies in patients affected by intractable CRPS type 1 demonstrated a microangiopathic process and the presence of C fiber axonal sprouts, suggesting the occurrence of a small fiber neuropathy (38).

Although the multiple pathogeneses of CRPS have not been defined, it appears that a traumatic injury to the distal extremity of genetically predisposed individuals may initiate a process that results in a neuropathic "stalemate" state in the affected limb. Of interest is that in several instances CRPSs appear to be maintained by plastic mechanisms that can be switched off by early and aggressive therapeutic interventions.

Sympathetically Maintained Pain

Abnormal changes in the axons of A-delta and C fibers give rise to ectopic discharges, mechanosensitivity, and, at times, *alpha-adrenoreceptor excitability* (3). These abnormalities have been noted not only in the axons of A-delta and C fibers but also in the dorsal root ganglion (DRG) cells of the affected afferent fibers and paradoxically in the cell bodies of uninjured axons within the same DRG (4,39,40). Alpha-adrenoreceptor excitability likely represents the pathophysiological basis of what has been called *sympathetically maintained pain* (SMP). SMP is a pathogenetic mechanism (and not a clinical entity), and it may complicate the pathogenesis of CRPSs. In the past, it was often "misunderstood" that all patients with RSD had an abnormal sympathetic

nervous system involvement. On the contrary, the majority of patients with CRPSs do not have SMP. SMP may occur only temporarily and complicate CRPSs as well as other painful disorders, including shingles, neuralgias, and metabolic or autoimmune neuropathies (41).

Essential Trigeminal and Glossopharyngeal Neuralgias

Idiopathic trigeminal neuralgia or *tic douloureux* is a neuropathic painful state characterized by severe, lancinating, brief (less than 60 seconds), unilateral facial pains. The paroxysmal symptoms follow the distribution of one or two branches of the trigeminal nerve. Facial trigger points are commonly present, and chewing or talking can induce the attacks. The onset is after age 50 in the vast majority of patients. The etiology of the condition may be related to a vascular structure, e.g., a tortuous artery, compressing the preganglionic segment of the trigeminal nerve within the posterior cranial fossa. Secondary trigeminal neuralgia should be suspected in young patients. Etiologies include multiple sclerosis, meningioma, or other posterior fossa tumors. Diagnostic evaluation includes an MRI of the posterior fossa with gadolinium.

Idiopathic glossopharyngeal neuralgia appears to have a vascular mechanical pathogenesis similar to tic douloureux. However, the clinical features of the attacks are more variable, including more prolonged pains that may radiate to the tongue, throat, ear, or along the lateral and anterior aspects of the neck. The pain may be accompanied by autonomic symptoms such as salivation or syncope. Trigger points may be located in the tonsil or posterior one third of the tongue, and swallowing may induce the painful attacks. Secondary glossopharyngeal neuralgia can be caused by oropharyngeal carcinoma, retropharyngeal or paratonsillar abscess, or elongated styloid process. Diagnostic evaluation includes imaging studies of the posterior fossa, skull base, and neck.

THERAPEUTIC INTERVENTIONS FOR NEUROPATHIC PAIN

The Pharmacology of Pain

The pain signal is transmitted from the peripheral nociceptors, through the dorsal horn of the spinal cord, through the thalamus, and up to the cortex. In the periphery, nociceptors can be activated by the chemical products of tissue damage and inflammation, which include prostanoids, serotonin, bradykinin, cytokines, adenosine, adenosine-5'-triphosphate (ATP), histamine, protons, free radicals, and neurotrophins. These agents can directly activate afferent fibers and induce pain or sensitize them to a range of mechanical, thermal, and chemical stimuli. Of note, a proportion of the afferent fibers that are normally unresponsive to noxious stimuli ("silent" or "sleeping" nociceptors) can be "awakened" by inflammatory chemicals and contribute to pain and hyperalgesia (2). The products of tissue damage and inflammation interact with receptors located on the A-delta and C fibers to initiate membrane excitability and intracellular transcriptional changes.

Membrane components recently identified and supposed to be relevant to the development of pathological pain and potential targets for analgesic drugs include (3,42,43): (a) the sensory neuron specific (SNS and SNS-2) tetrodotoxin-resistant (TTX-r) voltage gated sodium channels; (b) the vanilloid receptor-1 (VR-1) involved in the transduction of heat; VR-1 is activated by noxious heat and low pH; (c) the acid-sensing ion channels (ASICs). These are *amiloride*-sensitive channels activated by low pH. ASICs are possibly involved in the transduction of mechanical stimuli; (d) the tyrosine kinase (TrkA) receptor for nerve growth factor (NGF). The TrkA-NGF complex is internalized and retrogradely transported to the DRG cell body, where it initiates gene transcription that gives rise to up-regulation of channels involved in pain transmission. However, a very recent study (44) indicates that another growth factor, the glial cell line-derived neurotrophic factor (GDNF), may have potent analgesic effects in neuropathic pain models. It seems that following a nerve injury, GDNF can prevent and abolish ectopic discharges from afferent fibers by blocking the expression of certain subtypes of sodium channels involved in pain transmission; (e) the interleukin (IL)-1 receptor for IL-1 beta, which also promotes gene transcription for fiber excitability; (f) the sensory neuron-specific ATP receptor (P2X3); (g) T-type currents calcium channels; (h) bradykinin receptors; and (i) alpha-adrenergic receptors.

The pharmacology of peripheral analgesics still relies on the use of antiinflammatory agents such as the cyclooxygenase (COX)-1 and -2 inhibitors and steroids. Emerging peripheral analgesics for neuropathic inflammatory states include the new generation bisphosphonates, which appear to block the recruitment of macrophages at the site of a nerve injury as well as induce macrophagic depletion of proinflammatory cytokines (e.g., IL-1 beta, TNF alpha, IL-6, leukemia inhibitory factor) (45,46). The sodium channel blockers *lidocaine, mexiletine, carbamazepine,* and *lamotrigine* (which suppress abnormal ectopic discharges) and the neurotoxin *capsaicin* (which induces nociceptor desensitization by acting on the VR-1 receptors) are some peripheral analgesics utilized for neuropathic pain. Topical *clonidine,* an alpha-2 adrenergic agonist, is analgesic in SMP. Clonidine causes local inhibition of noradrenaline release by acting on the adrenergic alpha-2 autoreceptors of the sympathetic endings (47). Neurotransmitters of nociception within the dorsal horn of the spinal cord include the excitatory amino acids (EAAs) glutamate and aspartate, as well as a number of neuropeptides (e.g., substance P, calcitonin gene-related peptide, cholecystokinin, neurokinin A). EAAs can induce central sensitization. They act on several receptors, including N-methyl D-aspartate (NMDA), alpha-amino-3-hydroxy-5-methyl-4-isoxazole-propionic acid (AMPA), kainate, and the metabotropic receptors. The NMDA receptors seem to play a relevant role in pain modulation. Neuropeptides such as substance P act on the NK receptors. Substance P has been shown to be the preferred transmitter for the NK-1 receptor. Of note, the incoming C fibers entering the dorsal horn contain EAAs and neuropeptides. Noxious stimuli induce the release of both EAAs and neuropeptides. These neurotransmitters cooperate to sensitize the spinal sensory neurons involved in the transmission of the pain signal (2).

A variety of central analgesic substances have been identified. Some have antagonistic or inhibitory effects and others powerful agonistic effects. The central action of the pure opioid agonists (e.g., morphine, methadone, fentanyl, oxycodone, hydromorphone, etc.) has been well known and utilized clinically. Among all the analgesic medications currently available, the most powerful and effective drugs are still the agents acting on the mu-, kappa-, and delta-opioid receptors. Opioid receptors are located not only in the CNS (primarily in the dorsal horn) but also peripherally in the nociceptors (2). It seems that opioids may have more relevant central as well as peripheral analgesic effects during painful inflammatory states (48,49). Of note, recent studies have indicated that the addition of an extremely low dose of an opioid receptor antagonist (e.g., naltrexone) to morphine in a ratio of 1:1000 (or less) can strikingly enhance the analgesic efficacy of morphine (50).

Drugs acting on the alpha-2-adrenergic spinal receptors (e.g., *clonidine, tizanidine*) have been clinically recognized as being powerful analgesic adjuvants (2,51). NMDA receptor antagonists (e.g., *dextromethorphan, ketamine*) suppress central sensitization and stabilize membrane excitability of the dorsal horn pain-signaling neurons (52).

Blockade of the N-type calcium channels within the dorsal horn gives rise to analgesia and represents a novel alternative for intrathecal analgesia with opioids or local anesthetics. Ziconotide is a peptide analgesic derived from the venom of the predatory marine snail *Conus magellaris.* Ziconotide is a neuron-specific (N-type) calcium channel blocker that may soon be available for clinical use (53,54).

Recent studies indicate a central analgesic action of a number of emerging substances. The activation of the CNS adenosine A1 receptors is relevant to pain control, and intrathecal *adenosine* appears to induce analgesia (55,56). Similarly, agents acting on the N-acetylcholine receptor (e.g., *epibatidine,* ABT-594) (57,58) and on the cannabinoid receptors (CB1 and CB2) (59) have shown promising analgesic properties. Of note, endogenous cannabinoids have been identified. Recent studies suggest a potential role of cannabinoids not only as antiallodynic/antihyperalgesic agents but also in the potentiation of opioid analgesia (60,61). Unfortunately, most of the emerging analgesics appear to have a narrow therapeutic window. This will likely limit their utilization as first- or even second-line therapeutic agents for pain control.

Pharmacologic Agents with Some Established Efficacy for Neuropathic Pain

Antiepileptic Drugs (AEDs)

Antiepileptic drugs (AEDs) are becoming the most promising agents for the management of neuropathic pain. The efficacy of gabapentin for postherpetic neuralgia (i.e., a neuropathic state characterized by allodynia and spontaneous burning pain) and painful diabetic neuropathy (i.e., a state characterized predominantly by spontaneous burning pain) has been shown in two recent controlled trials (62,63).

Gabapentin acts on neither GABA receptors nor sodium channels, and its analgesic mechanism of action is unclear. Trigeminal neuralgia (i.e., a neuropathic condition characterized by brief, excruciating, lancinating facial pains) responds well to carbamazepine, whereas another AED, lamotrigine, has shown some efficacy for carbamazepine-resistant trigeminal neuralgia (64). Topiramate has been anecdotally used in the treatment of CRPS type 1 (65). Several new AEDs (levetiracetam, zonisamide, oxcarbazepine, tiagabine) have become available for medical use in the United States. Some of these agents may have potential analgesic properties. For example, preliminary data suggest that the AED zonisamide, a blocker of sodium and T-type calcium channels, may have an antineuropathic analgesic effect (66).

Opioids

Opioids are currently the most potent and effective analgesics utilized to treat acute and chronic painful states, and as such they have been prescribed to patients suffering from intractable pain states. Morphine, a mu agonist, represents the mainstay for the treatment of moderate to severe nociceptive cancer pain (2,67). Evidence from animal studies and recent controlled trials has also shown the efficacy of opioid analgesics in the treatment of neuropathic pain (68–71). The pure opioid agonists, morphine, fentanyl, methadone, levorphanol, oxycodone, hydromorphone, and hydrocodone, are the mainstay for opioid therapy. The treatment of chronic pain should rely on the use of long-acting agents (i.e., methadone, levorphanol) or controlled-release preparations of morphine, fentanyl, oxycodone, and hydromorphone. Among the pure opioid agonists, methadone has peculiar properties. It has an intrinsic N-methyl D-aspartate (NMDA) receptor antagonistic effect, which may add adjuvant analgesia in neuropathic pain (see following).

Unlike antiinflammatory drugs, opioid agonists have no analgesic "ceiling dose" and do not cause direct organ damage. Except for constipation, tolerance occurs for most of the opioid-related side effects (e.g., nausea, vomiting, respiratory depression, and drowsiness). *Opioid titration* and *opioid rotation* are essential concepts in the management of neuropathic pain. In order to determine adequate opioid responsiveness, a careful and persistent titration of the opi-

oid is needed (2). However, opioid-related side effects and the degrees of analgesia and tolerance are extremely variable among patients receiving these medications. Neuropathic pain may respond well to morphine, but in some patients it responds only to methadone, and in some others to fentanyl (67). Trials of different opioids (i.e., opioid rotation) have strongly been encouraged, especially when, during the initial drug trial, severe pain persists or side effects become intolerable. *Tramadol* is an analgesic agent with a weak mu opioid agonistic effect. Its potency is comparable to that of a codeine-acetaminophen preparation. Of note, in controlled trials tramadol has shown efficacy for neuropathic pain (72,73).

Studies indicate that patients on a stable opioid analgesic regimen do not report significant impairment in their driving ability, attention, mood, and general cognitive functioning (74). Addiction (i.e., a pattern of abnormal drug-seeking and -taking behaviors for nontherapeutic purposes) and clinically relevant analgesic tolerance (67,75,76) are rarely seen in patients who receive these medications for pain control. Clinical experience and recent animal studies indicate that genetics (and not acute or chronic administration of opioid analgesics for pain control) represents the foremost predisposing factor to the development of addictive behaviors (75,77). Therefore, addiction in pain medicine is not iatrogenic in origin, and a trial of opioid analgesics should never be precluded in patients with incapacitating neuropathic pain.

Tricyclic Antidepressants

Antidepressants also have an important role as adjuvants in the treatment of chronic pain. These agents are useful in the management of several comorbidities, such as anxiety, depression, and insomnia (2), that frequently affect patients with chronic neuropathic pain. Tricyclic antidepressants (TCAs), such as amitriptyline, nortriptyline, and desipramine (78), have established efficacy for neuropathic pain. They have been used successfully for painful diabetic neuropathy and postherpetic neuralgia. TCAs may provide pain relief in nondepressed patients affected by neuropathic pain. TCAs have frequent adverse effects to which tolerance poorly develops. The side effects include cardiotoxicity, confusion, urinary retention, orthostatic hypotension, nightmares, weight gain, drowsiness, dry mouth, and constipation.

Venlafaxine is a newer antidepressant that lacks the anticholinergic and antihistamine effects of the TCAs. Venlafaxine appears to possess an analgesic mechanism of action, with similar TCA-like beneficial properties, but fewer side effects (79,80). Selective serotonin reuptake inhibitors (SSRIs) such as paroxetine and fluoxetine are effective antidepressants. While also used for neuropathic pain, paroxetine and other SSRIs have not been as efficacious as the TCAs (78).

Local Anesthetics and Topical Analgesics

Local anesthetics, such as intravenous lidocaine and oral mexiletine, have been utilized in patients with neuropathic pain (54). The antiarrhythmic local anesthetic mexiletine is a sodium channel blocker with analgesic properties for neuropathic pain similar to those of some AEDs (e.g., lamotrigine, carbamazepine). Mexiletine is contraindicated in the presence of second- and third-degree atrioventricular conduction blocks. Also, the incidence of gastrointestinal side effects (e.g., diarrhea, nausea) is quite high in patients taking mexiletine. Intravenous lidocaine has been shown to decrease pain in patients with postherpetic neuralgia.

Topical analgesics for neuropathic pain include: (a) lidocaine, which can be administered as a patch and has established efficacy for postherpetic pain (81) and anecdotal benefit for other neuropathic pain states (82); (b) transdermal clonidine, that has an antiallodynic effect at the site of its application in patients with SMP (46); and (c) capsaicin, which needs to be compounded at high concentrations (> 1%) and administered topically under local or regional anesthesia (83). Capsaicin is the natural substance present in hot chili peppers. Recently, a capsaicin-activated neuronal membrane receptor has been cloned (84) and named the vanilloid receptor. It is located exclusively on small nerve fibers. After an initial depolarization, the single administration of a large dose of capsaicin appears to produce a prolonged deactivation of the capsaicin-sensitive nociceptors. The analgesic effect is dose-dependent and may last for several weeks. Over-the-counter creams need to be applied several times a day for many weeks. Of note, controlled studies of capsaicin at low concentrations (i.e., 0.075% or less, corresponding to the doses found in over-the-counter preparations) have given mixed results, and this likely is because of the initial burning pain induced by each application. In fact, patient compliance has been poor, and during clinical trials dropout rates have been high.

Pharmacologic Adjuvants for Neuropathic Pain

In addition to the agents discussed earlier, many drugs from a variety of pharmacologic classes can be used in patients with chronic neuropathic pain as adjuvant therapy, to "boost" or increase the effectiveness of an analgesic regimen. In many cases, the mechanisms supporting this enhancement of analgesic response are unclear.

Alpha-2 Adrenergic Agonists

Alpha-2 adrenergic agonists are known to have a spinal antinociceptive effect. Controlled trials have shown the effectiveness of intraspinal clonidine for pain control (85,86). Clonidine has been found to potentiate intrathecal opioid analgesia (2). Moreover, transdermal clonidine was found to have a local antiallodynic effect in patients affected by sympathetically maintained neuropathic pain (47).

Tizanidine is a relatively short-acting oral alpha-2 adrenergic agonist with a much lower hypotensive effect than clonidine. Tizanidine has been used for the management of spasticity. However, animal studies and clinical experience indicate the usefulness of tizanidine for a variety of painful states, including neuropathic pain disorders (87,88,89). The most common side effects of the alpha-2 adrenergic agonists are somnolence and dizziness (to which tolerance usually develops) and, with clonidine, hypotension.

NMDA Antagonists and Cannabinoids

Animal experiments and clinical observations indicate that NMDA receptors play an important role in the central mechanisms of hyperalgesia and chronic pain (52). Ketamine and the oral agent dextromethorphan are NMDA antagonists that may be used in conjunction with opioids in the management of severe neuropathic states characterized by allodynia and hyperalgesia. However, these agents, in particular ketamine, have a very narrow therapeutic window. Ketamine can easily cause intolerable side effects, such as hallucinations and memory impairment. Of interest is also the possibility that NMDA antagonists may prevent or counteract opioid analgesic tolerance (90). These agents may be used at subclinical, and therefore safe, dosages in order to block the progression of opioid tolerance. This approach should be considered any time analgesic tolerance has developed and its management is necessary for optimal pain control (28).

Animal studies and clinical observations indicate that cannabinoids, including the currently available antiemetic dronabinol, have analgesic properties (59). Interestingly, the addition of inactive doses of cannabinoids to low doses of opioid mu agonists appears to potentiate opioid antinociception. Moreover, cannabinoids appear to have a predominant antiallodynic/antihyperalgesic effect (60,61). This may be quite advantageous in the treatment of some incapacitating neuropathic pain states.

Antiinflammatory Drugs and Bisphosphonates

Nonsteroidal antiinflammatory drugs, e.g., cyclooxygenase (COX) type 1 and 2 inhibitors and acetaminophen, have been of little benefit in the treatment of neuropathic pain. *Steroid* therapy may be considered for severe inflammatory pain to due cancer infiltrating structures like the brachial or lumbosacral plexi, roots, or nerve trunks.

High doses of intravenous bisphosphonates were reported to be efficacious in the treatment not only of bone pain secondary to metastatic disease, but also of CRPSs (46,91). Their analgesic effect may be related to the depletion of activated macrophages and decreased release of proinflammatory cytokines in the area of nerve inflammation. In the animal model of neuropathic pain (sciatic nerve ligature), bisphosphonates reduced the number of activated macrophages infiltrating the injured nerve, reduced Wallerian nerve fibers degeneration, and decreased experimental hyperalgesia (39).

GABA Agonists

Baclofen is an analog of the inhibitory neurotransmitter gamma-aminobutyric acid (GABA) and has a specific action on the GABA-B receptors. It has been used for many years as an effective spasmolytic agent. Baclofen has also shown effectiveness in the treatment of trigeminal neuralgia (2). Clinical experience supports the use of low-dose baclofen to potentiate the antineuralgic effect of carbamazepine for trigeminal neuralgia. Of note, baclofen has also been used intrathecally to relieve intractable spasticity, and it may have a role of adjuvant when added to spinal opioids for the treatment of intractable neuropathic pain and spasticity. The most common side effects of baclofen are drowsiness, weakness, hypotension, and confusion. Of note, discontinuation of baclofen always requires a slow tapering in order to avoid the occurrence of seizures and other severe neurological manifestations.

Benzodiazepines (e.g., alprazolam, lorazepam, diazepam, etc.) are GABA-A agonists. Their clinical use in patients with chronic pain is controversial (2,92). In a controlled trial, patients with postherpetic neuralgia did worse on lorazepam than placebo or amitriptyline (93). Benzodiazepine-related side effects include the onset of depression and disruption of physiological sleep. In combination with opioids, benzodiazepines cause significant cognitive impairment, whereas opioid analgesics alone do not (74). Moreover, benzodiazepines when added to an opioid regimen may even favor the development of true tolerance to opioid analgesia (94), and clinical experience seems to support this notion.

Invasive Treatment Interventions

Implantable devices, such as intrathecal pumps or spinal cord, motor cortex (95), and deep brain stimulators, have recently become available for the treatment of neuropathic pain poorly responding to standard pharmacological and conservative therapeutic modalities. Among the most commonly utilized implantable devices are intrathecal pumps (IPs) and spinal cord stimulators (SCSs). SCSs have been successfully used in patients with intractable limb pain that is not treatable by conventional methods. A recent randomized trial (96) showed the efficacy of spinal cord stimulation for CRPSs. Patients who received spinal cord stimulation and physical therapy demonstrated a significant decrease in pain intensity when compared to those receiving physical therapy alone. However, although significant pain relief was obtained in the SCS-treated patients, no significant improvement in the functional status was observed. IPs are used to deliver into the cerebrospinal fluid analgesics such as opioids, clonidine, local anesthetics, and baclofen and will likely be utilized in the near future for other emerging analgesic agents (e.g., ziconotide, adenosine) (97). Clin-

ical experience and several reports indicate that clonidine and/or local anesthetics intrathecally can potentiate opioid analgesia for neuropathic pain (98). Intrathecal morphine is currently the most commonly used analgesic administered by pump. However, prior to implant of an intrathecal morphine pump, opioid trials need to be performed to show that the patient's pain is somewhat opioid responsive. Pumps can be implanted in a permanent fashion after trials are successful. For some specific intractable neuropathic pain disorders, neuroablative procedures might be considered. For example, the dorsal root entry zone (DREZ) lesion has been recommended for the treatment of intractable pain from brachial plexus avulsions (99,100). The decision to perform neuroablative surgery should come only after a thorough assessment has been carried out by a multidisciplinary team of pain medicine specialists and after conservative management has failed to produce improvement in the patient's quality of life.

ANALGESIC STEPLADDER FOR NEUROPATHIC PAIN

The number and variety of options for analgesic treatment in neuropathic pain can be confusing and daunting, even for physicians specializing in the treatment of pain. Polypharmacy and combination treatment employing agents from a variety of pharmacologic classes are the rule, and specific agents can be employed in an escalating regimen that matches the intensity and nature of the neuropathic pain state. Table 29-3 provides a systematic algorithm for selection and implementation of different analgesics and adjuvant regimens, based on the clinical experience and concepts such as the primary quality (i.e., burning, lancinating, allodynic) of neuropathic pain, its level of intensity, and type of syndrome.

CONCLUSIONS

Neuropathic pain states are difficult disorders to treat. Although not yet fully understood, advances are being made in the comprehension of the various mechanisms and etiologies underlying the neuropathic pain syndromes. Patients suffering from these disorders need to have treatment plans tailored to their individual problems. As indicated, a trial of a single medication is considered initially if the patient presents with mild neuropathic pain and with an overall high level of function. However, as the patient becomes less functional or presents with incapacitating pain, a more aggressive intervention based on a combination of pharmacological therapies is necessary. Medications such as AEDs, opioids, antidepressants, and topical agents, along with a rehabilitation medicine program, can help a major portion of patients suffering from these disorders. Implantable devices can aid the patient with intractable disease. Although progress is being made in treating patients with neuropathic pain, it is important to remember that the

TABLE 29-3. *Analgesic stepladder for neuropathic pain*

Primary quality	Proposed steps of analgesic intervention (see text for treatment rationale)
	Step 1
Burning pain	Gabapentin or an antidepressant (e.g., TCA, venlafaxine, paroxetine); *start treatment from step 2 if intensity of pain is moderate to severe* (> 5 on the scale 0–10, where 0 = no pain and 10 = worst pain imaginable)
Lancinating pain	Carbamazepine or lamotrigine; *start treatment from step 2 if intensity of pain is moderate to severe* (> 5 on the scale 0–10, where 0 = no pain and 10 = worst pain imaginable)
Allodynia/ hyperalgesia[a]	Lidocaine 5% patch + gabapentin; *start treatment from step 2 if intensity of pain is moderate to severe* (> 5 on the scale 0–10, where 0 = no pain and 10 = worst pain imaginable)
	Step 2
Burning pain	Opioid + gabapentin or antidepressant
Lancinating pain[b]	Opioid + carbamazepine or lamotrigine
Allodynia/ hyperalgesia[a]	Opioid + gabapentin
	Step 3
Burning pain	First opioid rotation or methadone + gabapentin or antidepressant +/– alpha-2 adrenergic agonist (e.g., tizanidine)
Lancinating pain[b]	First opioid rotation or methadone + carbamazepine or lamotrigine +/– baclofen
Allodynia/ hyperalgesia[a]	First opioid rotation or methadone + gabapentin + oral NMDA antagonist (e.g., dextromethorphan)
	Step 4
Burning pain[c]	Second opioid rotation + antidepressant + gabapentin or new AED +/– alpha-2 adrenergic agonist (e.g., tizanidine)
Lancinating pain[c]	Second opioid rotation + mexiletine or new AED + baclofen
Allodynia/ hyperalgesia[a]	Second opioid rotation + gabapentin + NMDA antagonist and/or dronabinol
	Step 5
Burning pain[c]	Intervention: intrathecal opioid +/– local anesthetic +/– clonidine or emergent analgesic (ziconotide) or neurostimulatory procedure
Lancinating pain[c]	Intervention: intrathecal opioid +/– local anesthetic +/– clonidine or emergent analgesic (ziconotide) or neurostimulatory procedure
Allodynia/ hyperalgesia[c]	Intervention: intrathecal opioid +/– local anesthetic +/– clonidine or emergent analgesic (ziconotide) or neurostimulatory procedure

[a]If SMP, add topical clonidine and sympatholytic interventions.

[b]Consider a combination of carbamazepine and lamotrigine or baclofen without opioids for essential trigeminal/glossopharyngeal neuralgias.

[c]If neuropathic pain is severe, consider the following trials on a compassionate basis: (a) using intravenous bisphosphonates or steroids if neuropathic pain is related to severe inflammation, CRPSs, or cancer; (b) adding an extremely low dose of oral naltrexone (in 1:1000 ratio with morphine) to potentiate morphine analgesia; (c) if appropriate, using a large dose of topical capsaicin under regional blockade; and (d) if intrathecal or neurostimulatory interventions fail or are contraindicated, consider, when appropriate, a neuroablative procedure (e.g., DREZ for brachial plexus avulsion).

goals of care are always to: (a) perform a comprehensive diagnostic evaluation of the patients, (b) determine the cause of the pain syndrome, if necessary by obtaining appropriate consultations, (c) assess and reassess the clinical and psychosocial status of the patients longitudinally throughout the various treatment trials, (d) be supportive without patronizing or telling the patients to "learn how to live with their pain," and (e) strive for the maximal amount of pain relief that will hopefully allow the patients to have as functional a lifestyle as possible.

REFERENCES

1. Merskey H, Bogduk N. International Association for the Study of Pain (IASP). *Classification of chronic pain* (2nd ed). Seattle: IASP Press, 1994.
2. Pappagallo M. Aggressive pharmacologic treatment of pain. In: Pisetsky DS, Bradley L, eds. Pain management in the rheumatic dis-

eases. *Rheumatic Disease Clinics of North America* Feb 25 1999;1: 193–213.

3. Baron R. Peripheral neuropathic pain: from mechanisms to symptoms. *Clin J Pain.* June 2000;16(2 Suppl):S12–20.

4. Bennett GJ. Scientific basis for the evaluation and treatment of RSD/CRPS syndromes: laboratory studies in animals and man. In: Max M, ed. *Pain* 1999—An updated review. Seattle: IASP Press, 1999: 331–337.

5. Asbury AK. Diseases of the peripheral nervous system. In: Isselbacher KJ, et al., eds. *Harrison's Principles of Internal Medicine,* 14th ed. New York: McGraw-Hill, 2000:2457–2469.

6. Backonja MM, Galer BS. Pain assessment and evaluation of patients who have neuropathic pain. *Neurol Clin* Nov 1998;16(4):775–790.

7. Campbell JN. Complex regional pain syndrome and the sympathetic nervous system. In: Campbell, JN, ed., *Pain* 1996—An updated review. Seattle: IASP Press, 1996:89–96.

8. Bosch EP, Smith BE. Disorders of peripheral nerves. In: Bradley WG, Daroff RB, Fenichel GM, Marsden CD, eds., *Neurology in Clinical Practice,* 3rd ed, Boston: Butterworth-Heinemann, 2000:2045–2130.

9. Wolfe GI, Barohn RJ. Cryptogenic sensory and sensorimotor polyneuropathies. *Semin Neurol* 1998;18:105–111.

10. Holland NR, Stocks A, Hauer P, et al. Intraepidermal nerve fiber density in patients with painful sensory neuropathy. *Neurology* 1997;48: 708–711.

11. Waldman SD. Diabetic neuropathy: diagnosis and treatment for the pain management specialist. *Curr Rev Pain* 2000;4(5):383–387.

12. Sadler M, Nelson M. Peripheral neuropathy in HIV. *Int J STD AIDS* Jan 1997;8(1):16–21.

13. Tembl JI, Ferrer JM, Sevilla MT, et al. Neurologic complications associated with hepatitis C virus infection. *Neurology* Sept 11 1999;53(4):861–864.

14. Douen AG, Pringle CE, Guberman A. Human T-cell lymphotropic virus type 1 myositis, peripheral neuropathy, and cerebral white matter lesions in the absence of spastic paraparesis. *Arch Neurol* July 1997;54(7):896–900.

15. Asbury AK. Pain in generalized neuropathies In: Fields HL, ed., *Pain Syndromes in Neurology, Butterworths Neurology Medical Reviews Vol 10.* London: Butterworths, 1990.

16. Logigian EL. Peripheral nervous system Lyme borreliosis. *Semin Neurol* 1997;17:25–30.

17. Moulin DE, Hagen N, Feasby TE, et al. Pain in Guillain-Barre syndrome. *Neurology* 1997;48:328–331.

18. Amato AA, Collins MP. Neuropathies associated with malignancy. *Semin Neurol* 1998;18:125–144.

19. Olney RK. Neuropathies associated with connective tissue disease. *Semin Neurol* 1998;18:63–72.

20. Grant IA, Hunder GG, Homburger HA, et al. Peripheral neuropathy associated with sicca complex. *Neurology* 1997;48:855–862.

21. Moore PM. Vasculitic neuropathies. *J Neurol Neurosurg Psychiatry.* Mar 2000;68(3):271–274.

22. Kissel JT, Mendell JR. Neuropathies associated with monoclonal gammopathies. *Neuromuscul Disord* Jan 1996;6(1):3–18.

23. Latov N. Pathogenesis and therapy of neuropathies associated with monoclonal gammopathies. *Ann Neurol* May 1995;37(Suppl 1): S32–42.

24. Dabby R, Weimer LH, Hays AP, et al. Antisulfatide antibodies in neuropathy: clinical and electrophysiologic correlates. *Neurology* April 11 2000;54(7):1448–1452.

25. Falk RH, Comenzo RL, Skinner M. The systemic amyloidosis. *N Engl Med J* 1997;337:898–909.

26. Caniatti LM, Tugnoli V, Eleopra R, et al. Cryoglobulinemic neuropathy related to hepatitis C virus infection. Clinical, laboratory and neurophysiological study. *J Peripher Nerv Syst* 1996;1(2):131–138.

27. Authier FJ, Pawlotsky JM, Viard JP, et al. High incidence of hepatitis C virus infection in patients with cryoglobulinemic neuropathy. *Ann Neurol* Nov 1993;34(5):749–750.

28. Roman GC. An epidemic in Cuba of optic neuropathy, sensorineural deafness, peripheral sensory neuropathy and dorsolateral myeloneuropathy. *J Neurol Sci* Dec 1 1994;127(1):11–28.

29. Toh BH, van Driel IR, Gleeson PA. Pernicious anemia. *N Engl J Med* Nov 3 1997;337(20):1441–1448.

30. Williams VB, Pappagallo M. Entrapment neuropathies. In: Benton HT, et al., eds., *Essentials of Pain Medicine and Regional Anesthesia.* New York: Churchill-Livingston, 1999:295–298.

31. Schaumburg HH, Kaplan JG. Toxic peripheral neuropathies. In: AK Asbury, PK Thomas, eds., *Peripheral nerve disorders 2.* Oxford: Butterworth-Heinemann, 1995:238–261.

32. Dyck PJ, Chance PF, Lebo RV, et al. Hereditary motor and sensory neuropathies. In: Dyck PJ, Thomas PK, Griffin JW, et al., eds., *Peripheral neuropathy,* 3rd ed. Philadelphia: Saunders, 1993:1094–1136.

33. Martyn CN, Hughes RA. Epidemiology of peripheral neuropathy. *J Neurol Neurosurgery Psychiatry* 1997;62:310–318.

34. Carter GT, Jensen MP, Galer BS, et al. Neuropathic pain in Charcot-Marie-Tooth disease. *Arch Phys Med Rehabil* Dec 1998;79(12): 1560–1564.

35. Bennett GJ. Does a neuroimmune interaction contribute to the genesis of painful peripheral neuropathies? *Proc Natl Acad Sci USA.* July 6 1999(b);96(14):7737–7738.

36. Woolf CJ, Safieh-Garabedian B, MA Q-P, et al. Nerve growth factor contributes to the generation of inflammatory sensory hypersensitivity. *Neuroscience* 1994;62:327–331.

37. Kemler MA, van de Vusse AC, van den Berg-Loonen EM, et al. HLA-DQ1 associated for reflex sympathetic dystrophy. *Neurology* Oct 12 1999; 53(6):1350–1351).

38. Van der Laan L, ter Laak HJ, Gabreels-Festen A, et al. Complex regional pain syndrome type I (RSD): pathology of skeletal muscle and peripheral nerve. *Neurology* 1998;51:20–25.

39. Liu CN, Michaelis M, Amir R, Devor M. Spinal nerve injury enhances subthreshold membrane potential oscillations in DRG neurons: relation to neuropathic pain. *J Neurophysiol* July 2000;84(1):205–215.

40. Shinder V, Govrin-Lippmann R, Cohen S, et al., Structural basis of sympathetic-sensory coupling in rat and human dorsal root ganglia following peripheral nerve injury. *J Neurocytol* Sep 1999;28(9): 743–761.

41. Pappagallo M. Complex regional pain syndromes. In: Galer B, ed., *A supplement to Neurology Reviews, Clinical Trends & News in Neurology.* March 2000:25–29.

42. Costigan M, Woolf CJ. Pain: molecular mechanisms. *The Journal of Pain,* 2000;1(3)(Suppl 1): 35–44.

43. Hill RG. Peripheral analgesic pharmacology—an update. In: Max M, ed., *Pain* 1999—An updated review. Seattle: IASP Press, 1999:391–395.

44. Boucher TJ, Okusek K, Bennett DL, et al. Potentanalgesic effects of GDNF in neuropathic pain states. *Science* Oct 6 2000;290(5489): 124–127.

45. Liu T, van Rooijen N, Tracey DJ. Depletion of macrophages reduces axonal degeneration and hyperalgesia following nerve injury. *Pain* May 2000;86(1–2):25–32.

46. Varenna M, Zucchi F, Ghiringhelli D, et al. Intravenous clodronate in the treatment of reflex sympathetic dystrophy syndrome. A randomized, double blind, placebo controlled study. *J Rheumatol* June 2000;27(6):1477–1483.

47. Davis KD, Treede RD, Raja SN et al. Topical application of clonidine relieves hyperalgesia in patients with sympathetically maintained pain. *Pain* 1991;47:309–317.

48. Maekawa K, Minami M, Masuda T, Satoh M. Expression of mu- and kappa-, but not delta-, opioid receptor mRNAs are enhanced in the spinal dorsal horn of the arthritic rats. *Pain* Feb 1996;64(2):365–371.

49. Zhang Q, Schaffer M, Elde R, Stein C. Effects of neurotoxins and hindpaw inflammation on opioid receptor immunoreactivities in dorsal root ganglia. *Neuroscience* July 1998;85(1):281–291.

50. Crain SM, Shen KF. Antagonists of excitatory opioid receptor functions enhance morphine's analgesic potency and attenuate opioid tolerance/dependence liability. *Pain* Feb 2000; 84(2–3):121–131.

51. Khan ZP, Ferguson CN, Jones RM. Alpha-2 and imidazoline receptor agonists. Their pharmacology and therapeutic role. *Anaesthesia* Feb 1999;54(2):146–165.

52. Bennett GJ. Update on the neurophysiology of pain transmission and modulation: focus on the NMDA-receptor. *J Pain Symptom Manage* Jan 2000;19(Suppl 1):S2–6.

53. Wang YX, Pettus M, Gao D, et al. Effects of intrathecal administration of ziconotide, a selective neuronal N-type calcium channel blocker, on mechanical allodynia and heat hyperalgesia in a rat model of postoperative pain. *Pain* Feb 2000;84(2–3):151–158.

54. Wallace MS. Calcium and sodium channel antagonists for the treatment of pain. *Clin J Pain* June 2000;16(2 Suppl):S80–85.

55. Khandwala H, Zhang Z, Loomis CW. Inhibition of strychnine-allodynia is mediated by spinal adenosine A1- but not A2-receptors in the rat. *Brain Res* Oct 12 1998;808(1):106–109.

56. Gomes JA, Li X, Pan HL, Eisenach JC. Intrathecal adenosine interacts with a spinal noradrenergic system to produce antinociception in nerve-injured rats. *Anesthesiology* Oct 1999;91(4):1072–1079.

57. Kesingland AC, Gentry CT, Panesar MS, et al. Analgesic profile of the nicotinic acetylcholine receptor agonists, (+)-epibatidine and ABT-594 in models of persistent inflammatory and neuropathic pain. *Pain* May 2000;86(1–2):113–118.

58. Meyer MD, Decker MW, Rueter LE, et al. The identification of novel structural compound classes exhibiting high affinity for neuronal nicotinic acetylcholine receptors and analgesic efficacy in preclinical models of pain. *Eur J Pharmacol* Mar 30 2000;393(1–3):171–177.

59. Richardson JD. Cannabinoids modulate pain by multiple mechanisms of action. *The Journal of Pain* 2000;1(1):2–14.

60. Richardson JD, Aanonsen L, Hargreaves KM. Antihyperalgesic effects of spinal cannabinoids. *Eur J Pharmacol* Mar 19 1998;345(2):145–153.

61. Pugh G Jr, Smith PB, Dombrowski DS, Welch SP. The role of endogenous opioids in enhancing the antinociception produced by the combination of delta 9-tetrahydrocannabinol and morphine in the spinal cord. *J Pharmacol Exp Ther* Nov 1996;279(2):608–616.

62. Baconja M, Beydoun A, Edwards K, et al. Gabapentin for the symptomatic treatment of painful neuropathy in patients with diabetes mellitus: a randomized controlled trial. *JAMA* 1998;280:1831–1836.

63. Rowbotham M, Harden N. Stacey B, et al. Gabapentin for the treatment of post herpetic neuralgia: a randomized controlled trial. *JAMA* 1998;280:1837–1842.

64. Zakrzewska JM, Chaudhry Z, and Nurmikko TJ, et al. Lamotrigine in refractory trigeminal neuralgia: results from a double-blind placebo controlled crossover trial. *Pain* Nov 1997; 73(2):223–230.

65. Pappagallo M. *Preliminary experience with topiramate in the treatment of chronic pain syndromes.* Poster presented at the 17th Annual Meeting, American Pain Society, San Diego, CA 1998.

66. Tomlinson DR, Malcangio M. et al., *Effects of zonisamide on mechanically induced nociception in rats with streptozotocin-diabetes.* Abstract. American Pain Society. Ft. Lauderdale, FL Oct 1999.

67. Portenoy RK. Opioid therapy for chronic nonmalignant pain: a review of the critical issues. *J Pain Symptom Manage* Apr 1996;11(4):203–217.

68. Suzuki R, Chapman V, Dickenson AH. The effectiveness of spinal and systemic morphine on rat dorsal horn neuronal responses in the spinal nerve ligation model of neuropathic pain. *Pain* Mar 1999;80(1–2):215–228.

69. Watson CPN, Babul N. Efficacy of oxycodone in neuropathic pain: a randomized trial in post-herpetic neuralgia. *Neurology* 1998;50:1837–1841.

70. Dellimijn P, Vanneste J. Randomized double-blind active-placebo-controlled crossover trial of intravenous fentanyl in neuropathic pain. *Lancet* 1997;349:753–758.

71. Raja SN, Haythornthwaite J, Pappagallo M, et al. *Controlled trial on the efficacy of opioids and tricyclics antidepressants in postherpetic neuralgia (PHN).* Abstract #286, presented at the 9th World Congress on Pain, August 22-27, Vienna, Austria, 1999

72. Haythornthwaite JA, Menefee LA, Quatrano-Piacentini AL, et al. Outcome of chronic opioid therapy for non-cancer pain. *J Pain Symptom Manage* 1998;15:185–194.

73. Pappagallo M, Heinberg LJ. Ethical issues in the management of chronic nonmalignant pain. *Semin Neurol* 1997;17:203–211.

74. Pappagallo M. The concept of pseudotolerance. *J Pharm Care Pain Sympt Control* 1998;6:95–98.

75. Portenoy RK. Current pharmacotherapy of chronic pain. *J Pain Symptom Manage* Jan 2000;19(1 Suppl):S16–20.

76. Harati Y, Gooch C, Swenson M, et al. Double-blind randomized trial of tramadol for the treatment of the pain of diabetic neuropathy. *Neurology* June 1998;50(6):1842–1846.

77. Sindrup SH, Madsen C, Brosen K, and Jensen TS. The effect of tramadol in painful polyneuropathy in relation to serum drug and metabolite levels. *Clin Pharmacol Ther* Dec 1999;66(6):636–641.

78. Max MB, Lynch SA, Muir J, et al. Effects of desipramine, amitriptyline and fluoxetine on pain in diabetic neuropathy. *N Engl J Med* 1992;326:1250–1256.

79. Lang E, Hord AH, Denson D. Venlafaxine hydrochloride (Effexor) relieves thermal hyperalgesia in rats with an experimental mononeuropathy. *Pain* Nov 1996;68(1):151–155.

80. Schreiber S, Backer MM, Pick CG. The antinociceptive effect of venlafaxine in mice is mediated through opioid and adrenergic mechanisms. *Neurosci Lett* Oct 1 1999;273(2):85–88.

81. Galer BS, Rowbotham MC, Perander J, Friedman E. Topical lidocaine patch relieves postherpetic neuralgia more effectively than a vehicle topical patch: results of an enriched enrollment study. *Pain* Apr 1999;80(3):533–538.

82. Devers A, Galer BS. Topical lidocaine patch relieves a variety of neuropathic pain conditions: an open-label study. *Clin J Pain* Sep 2000; 16(3):205–208.

83. Robbins WR, Staats PS, Levine J, et al. Treatment of intractable pain with topical large doses of capsaicin: Preliminary report. *Anesth Analg* 1998;86:579–583.

84. Caterina MJ, Schumacher MA, Tominaga M, et al: The capsaicin receptor: a heat-activated ion channel in the pain pathway. *Nature* 1997;389:816–824.

85. Eisenach JC, DuPen S, Dubois M, et al. Epidural clonidine analgesia for intractable cancer pain. The Epidural Clonidine Study Group. *Pain* June 1995;61(3):391–399.

86. Khan ZP, Ferguson CN, Jones RM. Alpha-2 and imidazoline receptor agonists. Their pharmacology and therapeutic role. *Anaesthesia* Feb 1999;54(2):146–165.

87. Fromm GH, Aumentado D, Terrence CF. A clinical and experimental investigation of the effects of tizanidine in trigeminal neuralgia. *Pain* June 199;53(3):265–271.

88. McCarthy RJ, Kroin JS, Lubenow TR, et al. Effect of intrathecal tizanidine on antinociception and blood pressure in the rat. *Pain* Mar 1990;40(3):333–338.

89. Fogelholm R, Murros K. Tizanidine in chronic tension-type headache: a placebo controlled double blind crossover study. *Headache* Nov 1992;32(10):509–513.

90. Price DD, Mayer DJ, Mao J, Caruso FS. NMDA-receptor antagonists and opioid receptor interactions as related to analgesia and tolerance. *J Pain Symptom Manage* Jan 2000;19(Suppl 1): S7–11.

91. Cortet B, Flipo RM, Coquerelle P, et al. Treatment of severe, recalcitrant reflex sympathetic dystrophy: assessment of efficacy and safety of the second generation bisphosphonate pamidronate. *Clin Rheumatol* Jan 1997;16(1):51–56.

92. Dellemijn PL, Fields HL. Do benzodiazepines have a role in chronic pain management? *Pain* May 1994;57(2):137–152.

93. Max MB, Schafer SC, Culnane M, et al. Amitriptyline, but not lorazepam, relieves postherpetic neuralgia. *Neurology* Sep 1988;38(9): 1427–1432.

94. Gear RW, Miaskowski C, Heller PH, et al. Benzodiazepine mediated antagonism of opioid analgesia. *Pain* May 1997; 71(1):25–29.

95. Garcia-Larrea L, Peyron R, Mertens P, et al. Electrical stimulation of motor cortex for pain control: a combined PET-scan and electrophysiological study. *Pain* Nov 1999;83(2):259–273.

96. Kemler MA, Barendse GA, van Kleef M,. Spinal cord stimulation in patients with chronic reflex sympathetic dystrophy. *N Engl J Med* Aug 31 2000;343(9):618–624.

97. Bennett G, Deer T, Du Pen S, et al. Future directions in the management of pain by intraspinal drug delivery. *J Pain Symptom Manage* Aug 2000;20(2):S44–50.

98. Katz N. Neuropathic pain in cancer and AIDS. *Clin J Pain* June 2000;16(Suppl 2):S41–48.

99. Campbell JN, Solomon CT, James CS. The Hopkins experience with lesions of the dorsal horn (Nashold's operation) for pain from avulsion of the brachial plexus. *Appl Neurophysiol* 1988;51(2–5): 170–174.

100. Thomas DG, Kitchen ND Long-term follow up of dorsal root entry zone lesions in brachial plexus avulsion. *J Neurol Neurosurg Psychiatry* June 1994;57(6):737–738.

CHAPTER **30**

Neuropraxic Injuries

Sarah E. DeRossett

The concept of *neuropraxia,* originally defined by Seddon in 1943 (1), refers to nerve dysfunction lasting from several hours to 6 months after a nonpenetrating injury. Demyelination with associated conduction slowing or even conduction block is seen in neuropraxic injuries, but the nerve axons and surrounding structures remain intact; by contrast, in *axonotmesis,* there is physical disruption of axons within an intact epineurium, and in *neurotmesis,* there is complete transection of the entire nerve and all the connective tissue structures, including the epineurium (1–3). In the latter two types of injuries, Wallerian degeneration occurs in response to axonal injury, and recovery occurs by means of collateral sprouting and the slow process of axonal regeneration. Recovery from neuropraxic damage is by remyelination and is relatively rapid by comparison.

CLINICAL SPECTRUM

Injuries to peripheral nerves are not rare in modern society and constitute a major medical and public health problem. Injuries resulting in axonotmesis or neurotmesis are encountered most commonly following trauma resulting in laceration, crush, angulation, or stretch injuries to the nerve. Neuropraxic injuries, on the other hand, are more likely to occur following blunt trauma or in the setting of nerve compression or entrapment. The prognosis for recovery from neuropraxia is excellent with return to normal or near normal function within weeks to months with tincture of time and appropriate treatment of any perpetuating factors such as compression. By contrast, nearly all cases of neurotmesis will require surgical repair to ensure optimal recovery of function.

ELECTROPHYSIOLOGICAL CONFIRMATION AND CLASSIFICATION

Electrodiagnostic studies provide the most objective and quantitative means of classifying nerve injuries as to loca-

tion and severity and also provide critical information relevant to prognosis (4,5). With regard to the latter, the principal determinant of outcome is the extent and severity of axonal degeneration (4). Because complete loss of clinically detectable nerve function can occur with both demyelinating and axonal insults, the strategy utilized in distinguishing between the different types of nerve injuries is to demonstrate the presence of functioning axons electrophysiologically by one of several possible methods (5). Perhaps the most straightforward technique is to stimulate the nerve above the level of the lesion while recording at a site below the lesion. If a response is obtained, the nerve has not been severed. If no response is obtained the nature of the injury remains unclear, and loss of function could be due to axonotmesis, neurotmesis, or severe neuropraxia. An alternative technique for detecting the presence of intact axons within an injured nerve is to have the patient attempt voluntary contraction while the electromyographer records from the muscle innervated by the damaged nerve with an EMG electrode. The demonstration of motor unit potentials signals the preservation of intact axons even in the absence of clinically detectable muscle contraction. Thus, electrophysiological studies may be useful in demonstrating preservation of nerve axons following injury despite complete lack of clinically detectable function. Inability to demonstrate the functional integrity of axons immediately following an acute nerve injury does not prove that the nerve has been severed, on the other hand. Axonal degeneration and demyelination cannot be discriminated reliably in the acute setting, and surgical exploration may be necessary to distinguish between complete transection and lesser injuries when electrophysiological studies fail to demonstrate the presence of functioning axons (4).

In addition to being useful in characterizing the nature of the lesion, electrodiagnostic testing can be invaluable in localizing the site of the nerve injury when clinical data are inconclusive in distinguishing between a nerve root or plexus injury and in the setting of injury to multiple nerves or nerve injury remote to the site of trauma (4).

Finally, electrodiagnostic studies may provide key information useful in assessing recovery during the course of treatment, be it conservative or surgical. For example, electrophysiological evidence of reinnervation may be seen in muscles long before clinical improvement is apparent, providing relevant information regarding the appropriateness of the prescribed treatment plan. Alternatively, failure to demonstrate reinnervation may be an indication for surgical exploration and intervention.

Although the utility of electrodiagnostic studies in characterizing acute nerve injuries should be apparent from the foregoing, it cannot be overemphasized that the timing and interpretation of these studies require considerable expertise; hence, the diagnosis and management of acute nerve trauma should be undertaken only at a center with high-quality electrodiagnostic capabilities.

RECOVERY FROM INJURY

Recovery from nerve injury takes place primarily in the form of remyelination in the case of neuropraxia and reinnervation in the case of axonotmesis and neurotmesis. Remyelination after paranodal demyelination occurs as a result of elongation of the original myelin lamellae with restoration of normal conduction velocities. In the setting of more extensive demyelination, Schwann cells proliferate and lay down new myelin. The newly formed intercalated internodes are usually shorter than the original internode, and conduction velocities may not be restored fully to normal (5–7).

Reinnervation after axonal injury occurs by the processes of collateral sprouting from surviving axons and axonal regeneration. Collateral sprouting occurs immediately following a partial nerve injury and may result in effective restoration of normal or near normal function within 3 to 6 months, provided that fewer than 80% of the axons to a particular muscle are injured (4). If the nerve injury is complete or exceeds the ability of the muscle to reinnervate by collateral sprouting, axonal regeneration occurs. In axonotmesis injuries, the basal laminal tubes of the original nerve fibers remain intact for the most part and form conduits along which the injured axon can regenerate (5,8). Regeneration in this setting is relatively efficient and results in normal or near normal function. By contrast, regeneration following complete transection is highly variable and inefficient, and much depends on the degree of separation between the severed nerve ends. Oftentimes the nerve must be surgically repaired if reasonable function is to be assured. Aberrant regeneration and the formation of painful neuromas are frequent outcomes of ineffective regeneration after neurotmesis. Though more widely recognized as a potential complication of Bell's palsy, aberrant regeneration of injured median or ulnar nerves may result in decreased dexterity in the hand and serious functional consequences (5,9).

Rate of clinical recovery following acute nerve injury varies according to the severity and nature of the injury. In neuropraxic injuries, such as acute compressive neuropathies, recovery takes place typically over 2 to 12 weeks and in some instances may take as long as 6 months (5,10–12). The rate at which recovery takes place in nerve injuries that rely on axonal regeneration for recovery depends on many factors and cannot be predicted with exact certainty. In a crush injury (axonotmesis), axonal regeneration takes place at a rate of approximately 8 mm/day in the upper arm, 1 to 2 mm/day at the wrist, and 1 to 1.5 mm/day in the hand (5). More severe injuries, such as a laceration injury requiring suturing, may result in growth rates as slow as 1 to 2 mm/day (5,13).

COMPRESSIVE AND ENTRAPMENT NEUROPATHIES

Compressive neuropathy is defined as a focal mononeuropathy due to damage to a peripheral nerve as a result of pressure. The compression may be internal or external and may occur anywhere along the course of the nerve, although it is more common at specific sites where individual nerves are especially vulnerable. An entrapment neuropathy is a focal mononeuropathy caused by mechanical impingement at a vulnerable anatomical site, for example, as the nerve courses through a fibrous tunnel or passes over a muscular band (14,15).

Distal Median Neuropathy and Carpal Tunnel Syndrome

Median neuropathy affecting the distal portion of the nerve is the most common entrapment neuropathy affecting the upper extremity (16). Typically, the nerve is compressed at the wrist as it passes through the carpal tunnel, comprised of carpal bones on three sides and the transverse carpal ligament above. Nine flexor tendons to the digits and thumb also course through the carpal tunnel with the median nerve. Patients with distal median neuropathy may manifest carpal tunnel syndrome, a constellation of clinical signs and symptoms caused by nerve compression. It is important to remember that electrodiagnostic abnormalities indicative of median neuropathy are not sufficient to establish the clinical diagnosis of carpal tunnel syndrome (16). For example, not infrequently patients with polyneuropathy who undergo electrodiagnostic studies are noted to have distal median neuropathy. In the absence of clinical signs or symptoms of carpal tunnel syndrome, this constitutes an incidental finding that does not warrant directed treatment.

The constellation of signs and symptoms indicative of carpal tunnel syndrome includes a wide variety of clinical findings, any one of which is nonspecific when considered alone. Patients usually present with wrist and arm pain associated with intermittent paresthesias in the hand, often precipitated by repetitive movements and especially prominent at night. Pain and paresthesias are almost always the symptoms that bring the patient to medical attention. Motor signs, such as thenar weakness or atrophy, usually develop long after sensory symptoms have become manifest. Although the clinical presentation may be variable, findings highly suggestive of carpal tunnel syndrome include nocturnal paresthesias that awaken the patient from sleep, pain or paresthesias when driving or holding an object such as a telephone or book, sensory disturbance of digits 1, 2, 3, and 4, weakness or wasting of the thenar eminence, and symptoms reproduced by Phalen's maneuver (16,17). Pain and paresthesias may be provoked by tapping over the median nerve at the wrist in many instances (Tinel's sign), but Phalen's maneuver is considered to be both more sensitive and specific (16,18). Phalen's maneuver is performed by holding the wrist in a passively flexed position for 30 seconds to 2 minutes, and a positive provocative test is indicated by the production of paresthesias in the middle or index fingers (16).

Electrodiagnostic Studies

Electrodiagnostic confirmation of clinically apparent carpal tunnel syndrome is accomplished by demonstrating distal median neuropathy while excluding other conditions included in the differential diagnosis, chiefly C-6–C-7 radiculopathy and brachial plexopathy in the proper clinical setting. In most cases of distal median neuropathy, demyelination is present at the site of compression with secondary axonal loss when severe. Despite that fact, initial routine studies may be normal in as many as 25% of patients, necessitating that internal comparison studies of adjacent nerves in the same hand be performed to confirm the diagnosis (16). Thus, it is important to recognize that electrodiagnostic studies may be negative at first glance in a significant minority of patients, necessitating a detailed comprehensive assessment to confirm the diagnosis.

Etiology

Distal median neuropathy is most often an isolated mononeuropathy due to repetitive use of the extremity. Less commonly, it is symptomatic of a variety of medical conditions in which there is compromise in the size of the carpal tunnel with resultant compression of the median nerve (13). Examples of medical conditions in which distal median neuropathy and carpal tunnel syndrome may be seen include pregnancy, rheumatoid arthritis, hypothyroidism, diabetes, acromegaly, gout, tenosynovitis, and amyloidosis (17,19–23). The routine use of screening tests such as thyroid function tests or rheumatoid factor are of low yield, however, and indicated only in the presence of risk factors or other associated symptoms (16). Rarely, the median nerve may be affected by schwannomas, neurofibromas, and ganglion cysts, and MRI or CT may be useful in these select instances. Structural lesions such as these typically result in palpable fullness in the wrist or slowly progressive deficits without symptom-free intervals (17–18).

Differential Diagnosis

Distal median neuropathy may be confused with entrapments of the proximal median nerve (anterior interosseous syndrome, pronator syndrome, entrapment at the ligament of Struthers), but, fortunately, such entrapments are uncommon. Clues on the physical examination that suggest a more proximal lesion include sensory symptoms over the thenar eminence and weakness of median muscles proximal to the wrist, most notably flexor pollicis longus (distal thumb flexion), pronator teres and pronator quadratus (arm pronation), and flexor carpi radialis (wrist flexion) (16). More often relevant is differentiating distal median neuropathy from cervical radiculopathy at the C-6 and C-7 levels. Nerve root lesions at these levels may produce pain and paresthesias in a distribution similar or identical to the symptoms of distal median neuropathy, and the two diagnoses may be difficult to differentiate in mild or early cases. Symptoms suggestive of cervical radiculopathy include neck pain, radiation of symptoms from the neck to the shoulder and/or arm, and precipitation or exacerbation of symptoms by movement of the neck. Similarly, physical signs that further support the diagnosis of radiculopathy include weakness or atrophy of muscles innervated by the C-6 and C-7 nerve roots and asymmetry of the muscle stretch reflexes that they subserve.

Treatment

The treatment of carpal tunnel syndrome is intuitive and straightforward. In patients with isolated sensory symptoms or reversible conditions such as pregnancy, conservative measures are instituted. These include removal of provoking factors and use of a neutral wrist splint. If conservative treatment is unsuccessful, surgical decompression of the median nerve by sectioning the transverse carpal ligament may be warranted. Surgical decompression is also indicated in the presence of thenar weakness or atrophy (24). The success rate of surgery depends on the duration and severity of symptoms, but, overall, surgical decompression is highly successful (85% to 97% response rates) (25–27). Failure rates after surgery increase significantly in patients with longstanding symptoms. Open surgical decompression via a longitudinal incision extending from the wrist to the palm allows direct visualization of the transverse carpal ligament and decreases the risk of damaging adjacent structures. This technique also decreases the risk of surgical failure due to incomplete sectioning of the ligament (23). Another treatment technique sometimes employed in the treatment of carpal tunnel syndrome is the injection of corticosteroids locally. Such injections may provide relief lasting for several weeks but rarely result in definitive resolution of the problem and carry the attendant risk of tendon or nerve damage.

Ulnar Neuropathy at the Elbow

Ulnar neuropathy at the elbow is the second most common entrapment neuropathy affecting the upper extremity (28). The motor portion of the ulnar nerve derives from the C-8 and T-1 ventral roots, whereas the sensory component originates from the eighth cervical dorsal root ganglion. Given off by the medial cord of the brachial plexus, the ulnar nerve enters the condylar groove formed by the medial epicondyle of the humerus and the olecranon process of the ulna. The nerve passes beneath a retinaculum connecting the humeral and ulnar heads of the flexor carpi ulnaris, known as the cubital tunnel or humeroulnar aponeurotic arcade (29). Distal to the elbow, the nerve exits the cubital tunnel, which, together with the condylar groove, constitutes the two most common sites of ulnar nerve compression, after which it courses through the flexor carpi ulnaris muscle. Both anatomical variations of the cubital tunnel as well as aspects of elbow joint mechanics predispose the ulnar nerve to potential compression at this juncture in its course (30).

The clinical diagnosis of ulnar nerve entrapment at the elbow is oftentimes straightforward. Typical symptoms include numbness and paresthesias in the fourth and fifth digits of the affected extremity. In addition, pain localized to the elbow or radiating from the elbow into the ulnar side of the hand is frequently encountered, as are symptoms at night provoked by flexion of the elbow for extended periods of time. Motor signs in more severe cases include weakness or atrophy of the intrinsic muscles of the hand and the formation of a claw hand due to weakness of the third and fourth lumbricals, although the latter is seen more commonly with distal lesions. Weakness of abductor digiti minimi is seen in more than 75% of cases, although weakness of the first dorsal interosseus is present even more frequently (31).

Provocative maneuvers aimed at increasing the sensitivity of the neurologic examination have been described and include the reproduction of pain and paresthesias by tapping or exerting sustained manual pressure proximal to the cubital tunnel, maintaining the elbow in sustained flexion, or combining sustained flexion with manual pressure (30,32). The latter maneuver reportedly has the highest sensitivity (32). In addition, a motor sign in which an involuntary twitch in the ulnar-innervated finger flexors and intrinsic hand muscles is produced by tapping over the ulnar nerve proximal to the groove, termed a motor Tinel sign, has been described (33).

Electrodiagnostic Evaluation

Ulnar neuropathies at the elbow may be either demyelinating or axonal in nature. However, many patients with symptoms suggestive of ulnar neuropathy have normal electrophysiologic studies, and electrodiagnostic confirmation of the clinical diagnosis may present a number of chal-

lenges (30). First, the fact that the ulnar nerve gives off no branches in the upper arm impedes electrophysiologic localization of some lesions. Second, anatomical variations in the composition and course of the nerve are common. Third, the degree of slack in the nerve at the elbow creates the potential for nerve length-surface distance discrepancies, which may differ depending on the position of the arm and which may contribute meaningfully to the outcome of the test results. Thus, when routine studies are negative or equivocal, more detailed comprehensive electrodiagnostic studies are warranted (30).

Etiology

As with distal median neuropathy, ulnar neuropathy at the elbow may be idiopathic or due to a wide variety of identifiable causes. Structural and mechanical factors include bony deformities as a result of old fractures or diseases such as rheumatoid arthritis, external compression, soft tissue tumors and masses, prolapse of the ulnar nerve, abnormal muscles, and leprosy, which results in hypertrophy of the ulnar nerve and is the leading cause of neuropathy worldwide (5). Rheumatoid arthritis, uremic polyneuropathy, and diabetic polyneuropathy are common associated conditions (30). External compression, particularly in the anesthetized patient, may result in iatrogenic ulnar neuropathies that can be severe (34). Similarly, comatose or bed-bound patients are also at risk of developing ulnar neuropathies as a result of prolonged immobility (33).

Differential Diagnosis

The differential diagnosis of ulnar neuropathy at the elbow includes C-8 radiculopathy and brachial plexopathy involving the lower trunk or medial cord. Although the sensory disturbance of a C-8 radiculopathy may closely resemble that of an ulnar neuropathy, C-8 radiculopathy produces muscle weakness outside the distribution of ulnar-innervated muscles. In addition, the presence of neck pain, especially radiating pain or sensory symptoms, supports the diagnosis of radiculopathy. Similarly, brachial plexopathy is distinguished from ulnar neuropathy by involvement of radial- and median-innervated muscles and sensory impairment extending outside the distribution of the ulnar nerve. Horner's syndrome may also be a sign of lower trunk plexopathy, and care should be taken to examine the size and reactivity of the pupils, particularly if neoplastic infiltration of the brachial plexus is a diagnostic possibility.

Treatment

As with median nerve entrapment, the management of ulnar nerve entrapment may be medical or surgical, although the appropriate surgical treatment of ulnar neuropathy is more controversial. In general, patients with only intermittent sensory symptoms and normal clinical examinations can be managed conservatively (30,35). Conservative management strategies include avoiding activities that result in prolonged elbow flexion or pressure on the elbow and splinting during sleep. Patients with fixed sensory loss, weakness, or significant denervation on electrodiagnostic studies should be considered for surgical decompression (30). A variety of procedures have been championed by different authors, and some authors espouse tailoring the choice of surgical procedure to the specific site of nerve entrapment, e.g., simple decompression in the setting of cubital tunnel entrapment and nerve transposition in condylar groove entrapment (36). Intraoperative electroneurography may be required for optimal management in some cases (36). As with distal median neuropathy, the most consistent predictor of outcome is duration of symptoms prior to surgery; in this regard, half of patients with symptoms present for less than one year recover with surgery (37).

Radial Neuropathy

Although the radial nerve is the nerve most frequently injured in trauma to the upper extremity (38), it is a target of compression far less often than the median and ulnar nerves (39–41). The radial nerve is derived primarily from the C-5–C-8 cervical roots, with T-1 contributing to the radial nerve in 11% of the population (42). The radial nerve, a continuation of the posterior trunk of the brachial plexus, gives off motor and sensory branches throughout the arm and is vulnerable to compression at four different sites: (a) proximal to the spiral groove, (b) at or distal to the spiral groove, (c) during its course as the posterior interosseous nerve as it passes through the supinator muscle, and (d) during its course as the superficial radial nerve in the forearm, wrist, and hand (43). The clinical presentation of radial neuropathies at these different sites has been well reviewed elsewhere (43) and includes patterns of weakness and sensory loss in addition to salient changes in reflex patterns that differ according to the level of the lesion. For example, a high-radial neuropathy proximal to the spiral groove results in decreased or absent brachioradialis and triceps reflexes, whereas a high-radial neuropathy at or distal to the spiral groove results in a decreased or absent brachioradialis reflex with preservation of a normal triceps reflex. By contrast, in both posterior interosseous and superficial radial neuropathies, the triceps and brachioradialis reflexes are normal.

Electrodiagnostics

Electrodiagnostic studies are useful in confirming and localizing a radial neuropathy and distinguishing it from radiculopathy or plexopathy (5). Specifically, electromyographic abnormalities confined to radial-innervated muscles confirm the diagnosis, whereas abnormalities in the paraspinal and C-7–innervated muscles support the diagnosis of radiculopathy. In lesions involving the posterior cord of the brachial plexus, studies of the deltoid, teres major, and latissimus dorsi may be abnormal.

Etiology

Trauma constitutes the most common cause of high-radial neuropathies proximal to the spiral groove (39). Nontraumatic compressive injuries have been associated with the use of crutches (17) and with the windmill pitching motion used in competitive softball (44). Compression of the radial nerve at or distal to the spiral groove usually occurs during sedation sufficient to prevent the patient from being awakened by painful paresthesias, hence the name "Saturday night palsy" (5,45). Other causes of radial nerve compression in the upper arm include tourniquet-induced neuropathy, improper positioning of immobile parkinsonian or nursing home patients, and "Honeymooner's palsy" (5,42,46–48).

As with radial neuropathies in the upper arm, trauma is a common cause of posterior interosseous neuropathy, usually as a result of fractures or dislocations of the radius or ulna. In addition, the posterior interosseous nerve can be compressed by a wide variety of soft tissue masses, including enlarged bursae, rheumatoid synovium, lipomas, and neuromas, to name a few (5). The nerve may also be entrapped in the radial tunnel that extends from the lateral intermuscular septum of the arm to the proximal surface of the supinator muscle (42,49).

Superficial radial neuropathy may be caused by injury or nerve entrapment in the forearm, wrist, or hand, but extrinsic compression at the wrist is the most common etiology by far (5,50). Causes of superficial radial neuropathy include compression by watchbands, bracelets, handcuffs, roping together of the hands, tight plaster casts, and even meeting badges (5,50–54). In addition, the superficial radial nerve can be compressed by lymphatic vessels and a variety of benign tumors (55–57).

Differential Diagnosis

Proximal radial neuropathies must be distinguished from C-7 radiculopathy, as well as from lesions involving the posterior cord of the brachial plexus from which it originates. The sensory abnormalities of a C-7 radiculopathy may involve the dorsum of the hand and lateral fingers but also may involve the palmar aspect of the middle finger, unlike radial neuropathies. In C-7 root lesions resulting in motor weakness, median-innervated muscles, such as pronator teres, flexor carpi radialis, flexor digitorum superficialis, and flexor pollicis longus, will be affected in addition to some of the radial-innervated muscles, such as the triceps and extensors of the wrist and fingers. In addition, although the triceps reflex may be diminished in both C-7 radiculopathies and radial neuropathies, the brachioradialis reflex should be normal in the setting of radiculopathy.

Motor signs that may be present in posterior cord brachial plexopathy and absent in radial neuropathy include weakness in abduction, adduction, and internal rotation of the shoulder. In addition, brachial plexopathy involving the posterior cord results in impaired sensation over the posterior arm and forearm and over the lateral shoulder in addition to the hand.

Besides electrodiagnostic studies, imaging studies of the cervical spine and brachial plexus may be useful in excluding other conditions such as foraminal stenosis or compressive lesions of the brachial plexus.

Treatment

Radial nerve compression during sleep or anesthesia is almost always neuropraxic in nature and recovers spontaneously within a few weeks (12,58). In comatose or immobile patients with prolonged external compression, recovery may take several months if axonal degeneration has occurred. Severe traumatic radial neuropathies associated with fracture of the humerus may require surgery, either to release the nerve, which may have become entrapped at the fracture site, or to repair by surgical graft a nerve that has been transected (5). Surgery may also be indicated in the management of posterior interosseous neuropathies in the setting of compressive mass lesions, fractures, or dislocations. Regardless of the etiology of a radial or posterior interosseous neuropathy, the function of the hand can be improved by the use of a splint that holds the wrist and fingers in dorsiflexion (5). In superficial radial neuropathies presumed to be due to repetitive movement, conservative measures consisting of restricting wrist activities and splinting at night are instituted; subsequent exploration and decompression should be considered when patients have traumatic injury and when conservative measures fail (59).

Peroneal Neuropathy

Peroneal mononeuropathy is the most common compressive neuropathy of the lower extremity (60–62). The common peroneal nerve and the separate and distinct tibial nerve together make up the sciatic nerve, which originates from the L-4 through S-2 nerve roots (62). The common peroneal and tibial nerves separate in the upper popliteal fossa and follow different paths. Near the fibular head, the most common site of peroneal compression, the common peroneal nerve divides into the deep peroneal nerve, which is mainly motor, and the superficial peroneal nerve, which is mainly sensory.

Although most peroneal neuropathies are unilateral, bilateral lesions are encountered 10% of the time (61). The most common clinical presentation is partial or complete foot drop, which may develop acutely or over several days or weeks (62). There may be associated numbness involving the dorsal surface of the foot and the lower lateral leg, but pain is rare. Formal strength testing reveals isolated weakness of ankle and toe dorsiflexion and ankle eversion. Apparent weakness of ankle inversion, due to the fact that

inversion is best tested with the foot dorsiflexed, is a common source of confusion and misdiagnosis (61). Thus, it is important to remember to passively dorsiflex the ankle when testing inversion in patients with foot drop to avoid this pitfall (62). Both knee and ankle reflexes are normal in peroneal neuropathy.

Electrodiagnostic Evaluation

As with other peripheral nerve lesions, electrodiagnostic studies in patients with foot drop are useful in confirming the presence of suspected peroneal neuropathy, excluding other possible diagnoses, and specifying the site and nature of the lesion, which, in turn, provide useful information regarding the expected course of recovery (62). Electrodiagnostic studies are particularly useful in eliminating other lower motor neuron lesions that may result in foot drop, such as L-5 radiculopathy, lumbosacral plexopathy, and sciatic mononeuropathy, and in establishing the alternative diagnosis of motor neuron disease in the appropriate setting.

Etiology

External compression is the most frequent cause of peroneal neuropathy and occurs for a variety of reasons, including anesthesia, coma, prolonged bedrest, habitual leg crossing, prolonged squatting, and with the application of plaster casts and the use of leg braces (5,61). Predisposing medical conditions associated with the development of compressive peroneal neuropathy include diabetes and polyneuropathy (61). After compression, the next most common cause of peroneal neuropathy is trauma, including fracture of the fibula, knee dislocation or surgery, laceration injuries, and stretch injuries associated with severe ankle sprains (62). Rare causes of peroneal nerve lesions include mass lesions such as ganglia, Baker's cysts, osteomas, nerve sheath tumors, and lipomas (5,62). Unlike carpal tunnel and cubital tunnel entrapment neuropathies in the upper extremity, peroneal nerve entrapment at the fibular tunnel is extremely rare (62).

Differential Diagnosis

Foot drop is a common presenting symptom in many disorders, including both upper and lower motor neuron lesions. In addition to the disorders already described, unilateral foot drop may be seen as a manifestation of vasculitis, and bilateral foot drop occurs in a wide variety of disorders, including distal myopathy, peripheral neuropathy, cauda equina syndrome, thoracolumbar myelopathy, and parasagittal mass lesions, such as meningiomas. Establishing the correct diagnosis depends on careful integration of clinical and electrophysiologic data, along with appropriate imaging studies when indicated. In addition, patients with an established diagnosis of peroneal neuropathy that is progressive in nature should be investigated for the presence of systemic illness or a local mass lesion, especially in the absence of an identifiable source of external compression (5).

Treatment

Protective knee pads placed over the fibular head to prevent compression in vulnerable patients is often helpful. An ankle-foot orthosis is useful in preventing contractures when the foot drop is complete or when a protracted recovery is expected. In patients with trauma as the etiology of the peroneal neuropathy, incomplete lesions are usually treated conservatively and resolve spontaneously, whereas complete transections mandate nerve repair (5).

Tarsal Tunnel Syndrome

Entrapment neuropathies of the tibial nerve are rare. Tarsal tunnel syndrome, with entrapment of the tibial nerve behind and below the medial malleolus, is the most common tibial nerve entrapment encountered in clinical practice (63). The tibial nerve is susceptible to compression in the narrow tarsal tunnel, which is covered by a thick ligament, analogous to the way in which the median nerve is compressed in the carpal tunnel. Likewise, tarsal tunnel syndrome is associated with many of the same conditions that predispose to distal median neuropathy, including sports-related repetitive stress, diabetes, arthritis, tenosynovitis, hypothyroidism, and acromegaly, although systemic disease is encountered more frequently in association with carpal tunnel syndrome (63–65).

The clinical features of tarsal tunnel syndrome include foot and ankle pain with tingling and numbness in the distribution of the tibial nerve (5,63). Motor symptoms are consistently absent. The two most commonly reported objective findings are sensory loss in the distribution of the terminal branches of the plantar nerve and Tinel's sign at the tarsal tunnel (63,66).

Electrophysiologic Studies

The nerve conduction study confirms the diagnosis of tarsal tunnel syndrome in the vast majority of cases (63). Specifically, sensory nerve conduction studies utilizing surface electrodes and signal averaging have been found to be superior to terminal motor latency studies, confirming the diagnosis in 90% to 100% of cases (63,66–67).

Differential Diagnosis

The two major entities that can mimic the sensory complaints of tarsal tunnel syndrome are distal sensory neuropathy and L-5 or S-1 radiculopathy. Unlike tarsal tunnel syndrome, which is usually unilateral, distal sensory neuropathy is bilateral and characterized by objective sensory

loss in a stocking distribution, including the dorsal and lateral aspects of the foot, territories that lie outside the distribution of the tibial nerve. Signs and symptoms that help to differentiate lumbosacral radiculopathy from tarsal tunnel syndrome include sensory abnormalities in a dermatomal distribution, pain radiating from the low back, and weakness in any of the calf muscles, all of which favor radiculopathy. In addition, certain medical conditions, such as tenosynovitis and plantar fasciitis, can cause pain in the region of the medial ankle, resulting in diagnostic confusion in some instances. The absence of objective sensory loss in these conditions helps to differentiate them from tarsal tunnel syndrome, however (63).

Treatment

As with carpal tunnel syndrome, surgery is extremely effective in relieving symptoms in patients for whom an external source of compression such as tight shoes or boots cannot be found. The usual surgical technique includes exploration of the tarsal tunnel with surgical release of the flexor retinaculum along with removal of any masses or tortuous blood vessels that may serve to compress the tibial nerve (63,68).

Plantar Interdigital Neuropathy

Interdigital neuropathies result from damage to an interdigital nerve as it lies between the heads of adjacent metatarsal bones just before it divides into two digital nerves. Interdigital neuropathy was first described by Morton in 1876 and represents the first clinically described entrapment neuropathy (69). Although widely referred to as Morton's neuroma, the fibrous nodule that forms in the interdigital nerve is composed of fibrous connective tissue and supporting stroma (70–71).

Interdigital fibromas may affect any of the interdigital nerves but form most frequently between the third and fourth metatarsal bones. Women are affected far more frequently than men, most likely as a result of wearing high-heeled shoes with narrow toe boxes. Most commonly, patients complain of pain on the plantar surface of the foot that is precisely localized between the two metatarsal heads and that often radiates into the toes.

Diagnostic Evaluation

Sensory nerve conduction studies of the interdigital nerves of the foot can be helpful in confirming the diagnosis of interdigital neuropathy in unclear circumstances (72–73). In most cases, however, the diagnosis can be established clinically with subsequent demonstration of the fibroma by ultrasound, CT, or MRI imaging. The most useful clinical test is the web-space compression test in which the dorsal and plantar surfaces of the involved web space are compressed by the examiner's thumb and index finger while the metatarsal heads are squeezed together simultaneously with the other hand (63,74). Reproduction of the patient's pain using this maneuver is considered a positive test. In addition, a palpable click, termed a Mulder's sign, said to be almost diagnostic, may be produced using this maneuver (63,75). Further confirmation of a suspected fibroma may be accomplished by ultrasound, which is the most convenient and least expensive means of determining the precise location, size, and shape of the lesion (74).

Treatment

Patients with mild symptoms are usually treated conservatively at first. Advocating that patients change from high-heeled shoes to flat shoes with a wide toe box may be useful in preventing the further evolution of symptoms but is rarely sufficient to treat symptoms that have already developed. Injection of local anesthetics and steroids at the site of entrapment may provide some symptomatic relief, but the majority of patients will require surgery for definitive treatment. Several treatment approaches have been advocated, including open excision of the fibrous nodule along with incision of the transverse metatarsal ligament, endoscopic excision of the ligament, decompression of the fibroma without excision of the nodule either with or without internal neurolysis, and percutaneous electrocoagulation (63,77–79).

PHARMACOLOGIC MANAGEMENT OF NEUROPATHIC PAIN

Medications from a variety of pharmacologic classes have been reported to be safe and effective in producing significant pain relief in patients with peripheral neuropathic pain and may be helpful in managing symptoms associated with the above described condition. Much of the objective data that have been derived in this regard come from patients with a diagnosis of painful polyneuropathy associated with diabetes. The management of peripheral neuropathic pain in other conditions remains largely anecdotal or unsupported. Nonetheless, it is clear that many commercially available preparations are being prescribed for the control of neuropathic pain, albeit in some instances more frequently than for Food and Drug Administration-approved indications. The current method of arriving at an optimal pharmacologic regimen involves sequential drug trials, and, not infrequently, patients are labeled as treatment failures as a result of inadequate therapeutic trials. The two most common reasons for unsatisfactory treatment results are (a) failure to titrate the dosage of the medication and (b) initiation of more than one drug at a time (80). Similar to the guidelines for pharmacotherapy that have been recommended for the treatment of painful polyneuropathy (80), a set of recommended guidelines for treatment of neuropathic pain in other conditions is presented in Table 30-1.

TABLE 30-1. *Pharmacotherapy guidelines*

1. Select the initial drug based on consideration of coexistent/comorbid conditions/symptoms that need treatment (e.g., mood disturbance, sleep disruption).
2. Initiate one drug at a time, observing the following:
   a. begin with the lowest possible dose
   b. titrate slowly according to tolerance and effectiveness
   c. continue to titrate until moderate or better pain relief is achieved or intolerable side effects are encountered
3. Continue any drug that results in moderate or better pain relief with an acceptable side-effect profile.
4. Add a second drug, if necessary, after the patient has been optimized on the first, taking into consideration the side-effect profiles of the new drug in the context of the patient's other medications.

Currently, the most useful drugs in treating neuropathic pain are the so-called adjuvant analgesics, drugs whose primary indication is not for the treatment of pain. These medications clearly possess antinociceptive properties, however, both in animal models and in clinical practice. Table 30-2 lists the major categories of clinically useful adjuvant analgesics with representative examples of each. It is worth noting that traditional analgesics may provide additional pain relief in patients already optimized on an appropriate regimen of first-line agents.

Adjuvant Analgesics

The tricyclic antidepressants are the best studied and most widely prescribed drugs for the treatment of neuropathic pain, at least at the present time. Controlled trials have demonstrated moderate relief of pain by this class of drugs (81). By contrast, controlled trials with serotonin selective

TABLE 30-2. *Drugs used to treat neuropathic pain*

First Line
Adjuvant analgesics
  Tricyclic antidepressants
    amitriptyline
    nortriptyline
    desipramine
    imipramine
  Anticonvulsants
    gabapentin
    carbamazepine
    phenytoin
    clonazepam
    topiramate
    lamotrigine
  Local anesthetics
    mexiletine

Second line
Traditional analgesics
  tramadol
  combination analgesics
  potent opioids

reuptake inhibitors have yielded mixed results, and currently there is no strong evidence to commend their use in the treatment of neuropathic pain (80,82–83).

A number of anticonvulsants have been used in the treatment of neuropathic pain with varying degrees of evidence-based support. Several controlled trials have demonstrated efficacy for carbamazepine and phenytoin, although side effects are frequent (84). Gabapentin, on the other hand, is frequently considered as a first-line agent in the treatment of neuropathic pain because of perceived efficacy in conjunction with a favorable side-effect profile and the lack of drug-drug interactions (85). Clonazepam is an anticonvulsant with sedating side effects that may prohibit its use as monotherapy, although it may be used as a second agent at night for improved control of nocturnal pain. Other newer anticonvulsants, such as lamotrigine and topiramate, are also being used for the treatment of neuropathic pain, but data to commend their use are lacking at the present time.

Attempts to use local anesthetic agents to treat neuropathic pain date back several decades. Intravenous lidocaine and oral mexiletine have been shown in controlled clinical trials to be efficacious in painful polyneuropathy (86–87), though only mexiletine is a practical treatment option in this regard. Despite demonstrated efficacy in controlled trials, the clinical utility of mexiletine is limited by frequent intolerable side effects and potentially serious effects on cardiac conduction.

CONCLUSIONS

Peripheral nerve problems, including traumatic nerve injury and the entrapment neuropathies, are encountered in all specialties of medicine. Optimal diagnosis and treatment of the underlying problem, as well as management of associated symptoms, such as neuropathic pain, often require a comprehensive multidisciplinary approach. Fortunately, the clinical features and underlying pathophysiology are well understood in many instances, and the directed use of appropriate diagnostic tests such as electrophysiologic studies successfully establishes a definitive diagnosis most of the time. Conservative treatment measures may suffice in some instances, and highly successful surgical techniques can be used in cases that fail to respond to lesser measures and in special cases that mandate surgical intervention. In addition, medications that are moderately effective in treating the pain associated with these conditions may be useful in managing patients acutely and in treating residual symptoms that remain after appropriate treatment.

REFERENCES

1. Seddon HJ. Three types of nerve injury. *Brain* 1943;66:236–288.
2. Sunderland S. A classification of peripheral nerve injuries producing loss of function. *Brain* 1951;74:491–516.
3. Lundborg G. *Nerve injury and repair.* Edinburgh: Churchill Livingstone, 1988.
4. Parry GJ. Electrodiagnostic studies in the evaluation of peripheral nerve and brachial plexus injuries. In: Evans, RW, ed. *Neurologic clinics,* Vol. 10, No. 4, Philadelphia: W.B. Saunders Company, 1992: 921–934.
5. Stewart JD. *Focal Peripheral Neuropathies,* 2nd ed. New York: Raven Press, 1993.
6. Allt G. Repair of segmental demyelination in peripheral nerves: an electron microscope study. *Brain* 1969;92:639–646.
7. Spencer PS, Weinberg HJ, Rinae CS. The perineurial window—a new model of focal demyelination and remyelination. *Brain Res* 1975;96: 323–329.
8. Haftek J, Thomas PK. Electron-microscope observations on the effects of localized crush injuries on the connective tissues of peripheral nerves. *J Anat* 1968;103:233–243.
9. Ford FR, Woodhall B. Phenomena due to misdirection of regenerating fibers of cranial, spinal and autonomic nerves. *Arch Surg* 1938; 36:480–496.
10. Fowler TJ, Danta G, Gilliatt RW. Recovery of nerve conduction after a pneumatic tourniquet: observations on the hind-limb of the baboon. *J Neurol Neurosurg Psychiatry* 1972;35:638–647.
11. Denny-Brown D, Brenner C. The effect of percussion of nerve. *J Neurol Neurosurg Psychiatry* 1944;7:76–95.
12. Trojaborg W. Rate of recovery in motor and sensory fibres of the radial nerve: clinical and electrophysiological aspects. *J Neurol Neurosurg Psychiatry* 1970;33:625–638.
13. Sunderland S. *Nerves and nerve injuries,* 2nd ed. Edinburgh: Churchill Livingstone, 1978.
14. Kopell HP, Thompson WAL. *Peripheral entrapment neuropathies.* Baltimore: Williams & Wilkins, 1963.
15. Dawson DM. Entrapment neuropathies of the upper extremities. *N Engl J Med* 1993;329:2013–2018.
16. Preston DC. Distal median neuropathies. In: Logigian, EL, ed. *Neurologic clinics,* Vol.17, No.3. Philadelphia: W.B. Saunders Company, 1999:407–424.
17. Preston DC, Shapiro BE. *Electromyography and neuromuscular disorders.* Boston: Butterworth-Heinemann, 1998.
18. Kuschner SH, Ebramzadeh E, Johnson D, et al. Tinel's sign and Phalen's test in carpal tunnel syndrome. *Orthopedics* 1992;15:1297–1302.
19. Massey EW. Carpal tunnel syndrome in pregnancy. *Obstet Gynecol Surv* 1978;33:145–148.
20. Murphy F, Beetham WP Jr, Torgerson WR Jr. Carpal tunnel syndrome caused by tophaceous gout: report of two cases with review of the literature. *Lahey Clin Found Bull* 1974;23:18–23.
21. Mahloudji M. Familial carpal-tunnel syndrome due to amyloidosis (letter). *Lancet* 1968;1:1374.
22. O'Duffy JD, Randall RV, MacCarty CS. Median neuropathy (carpal-tunnel syndrome) in acromegaly: a sign of endocrine overactivity. *Ann Intern Med* 1973;78:379–383.
23. Conway SR, Jones HR Jr. Entrapment and compression neuropathies. In: Tollison CD, ed. *Handbook of pain management,* 2nd ed. Baltimore: Williams & Wilkins, 1994:470–483.
24. Kaplan SJ, Glickel SZ, Eaton RG. Predictive factors in the non-surgical treatment of carpal tunnel syndrome. *J Hand Surg (Br)* 1990;15: 106–108.
25. Semple JC, Cargill AO. Carpal-tunnel syndrome: results of surgical decompression. *Lancet* 1969;1:918–919.
26. Campbell WW. Entrapment neuropathies. In: Gilchrist J, ed. *Prognosis in neurology.* Boston: Butterworth-Heinemann, 1998:307–312.
27. Clarke AM, Stanley D. Prediction of the outcome 24 hours after carpal tunnel decompression. *J Hand Surg (Br)* 1993;18:180–181.
28. Miller RG. Ulnar nerve lesions. In: Brown, WF, Bolton CF, eds. *Clinical electromyography.* Stoneham, MA: Butterworths, 1987:99–116.
29. Campbell WW, Pridgeon RM, Riaz G, et al. Variations in anatomy of the ulnar nerve at the cubital tunnel: pitfalls in the diagnosis of ulnar neuropathy at the elbow. *Muscle Nerve* 1991;14:733–738.
30. Bradshaw DY, Shefner JM. Ulnar neuropathy at the elbow. In: Logigian EL, ed. *Neurologic clinics,* Vol.17, No.3. Philadelphia, W.B. Saunders, 1999:447–461.
31. Stewart JD. The variable clinical manifestations of ulnar neuropathies at the elbow. *J Neurol Neurosurg Psychiatry* 1987;50:252–258.
32. Novak CB, Lee GW, MacKinnon SE, et al. Provocative testing for cubital tunnel syndrome. *J Hand Surg* 1994;19A:817–820.
33. Montagna P. Motor Tinel sign. A new localizing sign in entrapment neuropathy. *Muscle Nerve* 1994;17:1493–1494.

34. Miller RG, Camp PE. Postoperative ulnar neuropathy. *JAMA* 1979; 242:1636–1639.

35. Dellon AL, Hament W, Gittelshon A. Non-operative management of cubital tunnel syndrome: an eight year prospective study. *Neurology* 1993;43:1673–1677.

36. Campbell WW, Pridgeon RM, Sahni KS. Short segment incremental studies in the evaluation of ulnar neuropathy at the elbow. *Muscle Nerve* 1992;15:1050–1054.

37. LeRoux PD, Ensign TD, Burchiel KJ. Surgical decompression without transposition for ulnar neuropathy: factors determining outcome. *Neurosurgery* 1990; 27:709–714.

38. Barton NJ. Radial nerve lesions. *Hand* 1973;5:200.

39. Dawson DM, Hallett M, Millender LH. Radial nerve entrapment. In: *Entrapment neuropathies,* 2nd ed. Boston: Little, Brown, and Co., 1990;199–231.

40. Eaton CJ, Lister GD. Radial nerve compression. *Hand Clin* 1992; 8:345.

41. Kleinert JM, Mehta S. Radial nerve entrapment. *Orthop Clin North Am* 1996;27:305.

42. Dumitru D. *Electrodiagnostic medicine.* Philadelphia: Hanley and Belfus, 1995; 891–898.

43. Carlson N, Logigian EL. Radial neuropathy. In: Logigian EL, ed. *Neurologic clinics,* Vol.17, No.3. Philadelphia: W.B. Saunders Company, 1999:499–523.

44. Sinson G, Zager EL, Kline DG. Windmill pitcher's radial neuropathy. *Neurosurgery* 1994;34:1087.

45. Sunderland S. Traumatic injuries of peripheral nerves: simple compression injuries of the radial nerve. *Brain* 1945;68:56–72.

46. Bolton FB, McFarlane RM. Human pneumatic tourniquet paralysis. *Neurology* 1978;28:787–793.

47. Preston DN, Grimes JD. Radial compression neuropathy in advanced Parkinson's disease. *Arch Neurol* 1985;42:695.

48. Sloane PD, McLeod MM. Radial nerve palsy in nursing home patients: association with immobility and haloperidol. *J Am Geriatr Soc* 1987;35:465.

49. Barnum M, Mastey RD, Weiss AC, et al. Radial tunnel syndrome. *Hand Clin* 1996;12:679.

50. Dawson DH, Hallett M, Millender LH. *Entrapment neuropathies,* 2nd ed. Boston: Little, Brown, 1990.

51. Rask MR. Watchband superficial radial neuropraxia. *JAMA* 1979; 241:2702.

52. Lanzetta M, Foucher G. Entrapment of the superficial branch of the radial nerve (Wartenberg's syndrome): a report of 52 cases. *Int Orthop* 1993;17:342.

53. Appel H. Handcuff neuropathy. *Neurology* 1991;41:955.

54. Preston DC, Shapiro BE. Meeting badge neuropathy. *Neurology* 1997;48:289.

55. Fossati E, Irigaray A, Asurey N, et al. Lymphatic compression of the superficial branch of the radial nerve—a case report. *J Hand Surg* 1984;9A:898.

56. Jacob RA, Buchino JJ. Lipofibroma of the superficial branch of the radial nerve. *J Hand Surg (Am)* 1989;14A:704–706.

57. Gillies RM, Burrows C. Nerve sheath ganglion of the superficial radial nerve. *J Hand Surg (Br)* 1991;16B:94-95.

58. Watson BV, Brown WF. Quantitation of axon loss and conduction block in acute radial nerve palsies. *Muscle Nerve* 1992;15:768–773.

59. Dellon AL. Musculotendinous variation about the medial humeral epicondyle. *J Hand Surg (Br)* 1986;11B:175–181.

60. Berry H, Richeardson PM. Common peroneal nerve palsy, a clinical and electrophysiological review. *J Neurol Neurosurg Psychiatry* 1976;39:1162–1171.

61. Katirji MB, Wilbourn AJ. Common peroneal mononeuropathy: a clinical and electrophysiologic study of 116 lesions. *Neurology* 1988;38:1723–1728.

62. Katirji B. Peroneal Neuropathy. In: Logigian, EL, ed. *Neurologic clinics: entrapment and other focal neuropathies,* Vol.17, No.3. Philadelphia: W.B. Saunders, 1999:567–591.

63. Oh SJ, Meyer RD. Entrapment neuropathies of the tibial (posterior tibial) nerve. In: Logigian, EL, ed. *Neurologic clinics: entrapment and other focal neuropathies,* Vol.17, No.3. Philadelphia: W.B. Saunders, 1999:593–615.

64. Cimino WR. Tarsal tunnel syndrome: review of the literature. *Foot Ankle Int* 1990;11:47–52.

65. Radin EL. Tarsal tunnel syndrome. *Clin Orthop* 1983;181:167–170.

66. Oh SJ, Sarala PK, Kuba T, et al. Tarsal tunnel syndrome: electrophysiological diagnosis. *Ann Neurol* 1979;5:327–330.

67. Galardi G, Amadio S, Maderna L, et al. Electrophysiologic studies in tarsal tunnel syndrome. Diagnostic reliability of motor distal latency, mixed nerve and sensory nerve conduction studies. *Am J Phys Med Rehabil* 1994;73:193–198.

68. Lam SJS. Tarsal tunnel syndrome. *J Bone Joint Surg* 1990;49B:87–92.

69. Morton TG. A peculiar and painful affection of the fourth metatarsophalangeal articulation. *Am J Med Sci* 1876;71:37–45.

70. Lassman G. Morton's toe. Clinical, light and electron microscopic investigations in 133 cases. *Clin Orthop* 1979;142:73–84.

71. GuiloffRJ, Scadding JW, Klenerman L. Morton's metatarsalgia: Clinical, electrophysiological and histological observations. *J Bone Joint Surg BR* 1984;66B:586–591.

72. Oh SJ, Kim HS, Ahmad BK. Electrophysiological diagnosis of interdigital neuropathy of the foot. *Muscle Nerve* 1984;7:218–225.

73. Falck B, Hurme M, Hakkarainen S, et al. Sensory conduction velocity of plantar digital nerves in Morton's metatarsalgia. *Neurology* 1984;34:698–701.

74. Wu KK. Morton's interdigital neuroma: a clinical view of its etiology, treatment, and results. *J Foot Ankle Surg* 1996;35:112–119.

75. Mulder JD. The causative mechanism in Morton's metatarsalgia. *J Bone Joint Surg* 1951;33B:94–95.

76. Shapiro PP, Shapiro SL. Sonographic evaluation of interdigital neuroma. *Foot Ankle Int* 1995;16:604–605.

77. Barrett S, Pignetti T. Endoscopic decompression for intermetatarsal nerve entrapment—the EDIN technique: early clinical results. *J Foot Ankle Surg* 1994;33:503–508.

78. Finney W, Wiener SN, Catanzariti F. Treatment of Morton's neuroma using percutaneous electrocoagulation. *J Am Podiatr Med Assoc* 1989;63:470–474.

79. Gauthier G. Thomas Morton's disease: A nerve entrapment syndrome: a new surgical technique. *Clin Orthop* 1979;142:90–92.

80. Galer BS. Painful Polyneuropathy. In: Backonja M, ed. *Neurologic clinics,* Vol.16, No.4. Philadelphia: W.B. Saunders, 1999; 791–811.

81. McQuay HJ, Tramer M, Nye BA, et al. A systemic review of antidepressants in neuropathic pain. *Pain* 1996;68:217–227.

82. Max MB, Lynch SA, Muir J, et al. Effects of desipramine, amitriptyline, and fluoxetine on pain in diabetic neuropathy. *N Engl J Med* 1992;326:1250–1256.

83. Sindrup SH, Gram LF, Brosen K, et al. The selective reuptake inhibitor paroxetine is effective in the treatment of diabetic neuropathy symptoms. *Pain* 1990.

84. McQuay H, Carroll D, Jadad AR, et al. Anticonvulsant drugs for management of pain: a systemic review. *BMJ* 1995;311:1047–1052.

85. Rosner H, Rubin L, Kestenbaum A. Gabapentin adjunctive therapy in neuropathic pain. *Clin J Pain* 1996;12:56–58.

86. Dejgard A, Petersen P, Kastrup J. Mexiletine for treatment of chronic diabetic neuropathy. *Lancet* 1988;2:9–11.

87. Galer BS, Miller KV, Rowbotham MC. Response to intravenous lidocaine differs based on clinical diagnosis and site of nervous system injury. *Neurology* 1993;43:1233–1235.

CHAPTER 31

Gynecologic Pain

Fred M. Howard

Through love all pain is turned to healing.

Rumi

Chronic pelvic pain (CPP) is a common and significant affliction of women during the peak of their productive years. The mean age of occurrence is about 30 years of age. In the United Kingdom it is estimated to have an annual prevalence of 3.8% in women aged 15 to 73, which is higher than migraine (2.1%) and similar to asthma (3.7%) and back pain (4.1%) (1). In a U.S. study of women in primary care offices in a university setting, 12% of women reported current CPP and 33% reported a past history of CPP (2). In another study of women of reproductive age in primary care private practices, 39% had pelvic pain at least some of the time, and 12% had pain on more than 5 days per month or lasting a full day or more each month (3). A Gallup poll in the United States found that 16% of women reported pelvic pain problems and that 11% limited home activity because of it, 16% took medications for it, and 4% missed at least one day of work per month because of it (4). CPP is estimated to account for 10% of all referrals to a gynecologist (5) and is the indication for 12% of all hysterectomies and over 40% of gynecologic diagnostic laparoscopies (6). It is estimated that direct and indirect costs of CPP in the United States are over two billion dollars per year. CPP often leads to years of disability and suffering, with loss of employment, marital discord and divorce, as well as numerous untoward and unsuccessful medical misadventures. Clearly, pelvic pain is an important part of the practice of any clinician who provides health care for women.

Pelvic pain may be acute, recurrent, or chronic. A criterion of greater than 6 months' duration is usually used to diagnose pelvic pain as chronic (7,8). This is somewhat arbi-

trary because acute pelvic pain rarely lasts more than one month without crisis, resolution, or cure (6). Part of the rationale for a 6-month criterion is that after months of pelvic pain, pain itself can become an illness rather than a symptomatic manifestation of some other disease (9). The cyclic pain of dysmenorrhea and the episodic pain of dyspareunia are sometimes considered criteria for CPP, but it is probably better to consider dysmenorrhea and dyspareunia separately because the diagnoses and treatments of these symptoms frequently differ from those of CPP. However, women with CPP often have dysmenorrhea or dyspareunia as part of their symptom complex (10).

Women suffering from CPP are a heterogeneous group, and the possible diagnoses are numerous and varied (Table 31-1). Occasionally, one of these disorders is the only diagnosis, and curative treatment is possible. More often, the pain is long-standing with numerous prior diagnoses and treatments, and a number of contributing factors may need evaluation and treatment. Because of this a multidisciplinary approach is often ideal. For example, endometriosis, irritable bowel syndrome, poor posture, and emotional stresses may all be contributing factors in a single patient, with the need for simultaneous gynecologic, gastroenterologic, and physical therapy and psychological treatment. Such care is probably best accomplished via a multidisciplinary clinic, but that is not always possible or necessary. Often a multidisciplinary approach to diagnosis and treatment provided by the woman's internist, urologist, family physician, gynecologist, or gastroenterologist, using consultants as indicated, provides optimal continuity, confidence, and personal attention. However, this requires sufficient time, interest, and knowledge by the primary physician.

This chapter will be limited to a discussion of gynecologic disorders that cause or contribute to CPP. Nongynecologic

459

TABLE 31-1. *Diseases that may cause or contribute to chronic pelvic pain in women*

Gynecological—Extrauterine
  Adhesions
  Adnexal cysts
  Chronic ectopic pregnancy
  Chlamydial endometritis or salpingitis
  Endometriosis
  Endosalpingiosis
  Ovarian retention syndrome (residual ovary syndrome)
  Ovarian remnant syndrome
  Ovarian dystrophy or ovulatory pain
  Pelvic congestion syndrome
  Postoperative peritoneal cysts
  Residual accessory ovary
  Subacute salpingo-oophoritis (chronic PID)
  Tuberculous salpingitis
 	
Gynecological—Uterine
  Adenomyosis
  Atypical dysmenorrhea or ovulatory pain
  Cervical stenosis
  Chronic endometritis
  Endometrial or cervical polyps
  Intrauterine contraceptive device
  Leiomyomata
  Symptomatic pelvic relaxation (genital prolapse)
 	
Urologic
  Bladder neoplasm
  Chronic urinary tract infection
  Interstitial cystitis
  Radiation cystitis
  Recurrent, acute cystitis
  Recurrent, acute urethritis
  Stone/Urolithiasis
  Uninhibited bladder contractions (detrusor dyssynergia)
  Urethral diverticulum
  Urethral syndrome
  Urethral caruncle
	Gastrointestinal
	  Carcinoma of the colon
	  Chronic intermittent bowel obstruction
	  Colitis
	  Constipation
	  Diverticular disease
	  Hernias
	  Inflammatory bowel disease
	  Irritable bowel syndrome
	
	Musculoskeletal
	  Abdominal wall myofascial pain (trigger points)
	  Chronic coccygeal pain
	  Compression of lumbar vertebrae
	  Degenerative joint disease
	  Disc
	  Faulty or poor posture
	  Fibromyositis
	  Hernias: ventral, inguinal, femoral
	  Spigelian
	  Low back pain
	  Muscular strains and sprains
	  Neoplasia of spinal cord or sacral nerve
	  Neuralgia of iliohypogastric, ilioinguinal, and/or
	    genitofemoral nerves
	  Pelvic floor myalgia (levator ani spasm)
	  Piriformis syndrome
	  Rectus tendon strain
	  Spondylosis
	
	Other
	  Abdominal cutaneous nerve
	  Entrapment in surgical scar
	  Abdominal epilepsy
	  Abdominal migraine
	  Bipolar personality disorders
	  Depression
	  Familial Mediterranean fever
	  Neurologic dysfunction
	  Porphyria
	  Shingles
	  Sleep disturbances
	  Somatic referral

disorders important in women with CPP are discussed elsewhere.

TAKING A HISTORY

A thorough history is crucial to diagnostic evaluation, but it also represents a powerful therapeutic tool. Compassionately taken, with the patient talking and the clinician listening, it establishes rapport and allows the patient to leave the physician's office feeling better. Although pain questionnaires are useful in evaluating women with CPP, they must be used to supplement, not replace, allowing the patient to tell her story. Not only does this allow the chance to obtain a more detailed history, but also it allows observation of the patient's reaction to critical aspects of the history and enhances establishment of rapport and trust. It is important that the initial interview occur while the patient is fully clothed because personal and intimate questions

about psychosocial issues such as abuse or dyspareunia need to be asked.

Often the diagnostic approach to the woman with CPP is directed more by the specialty of the clinician than the woman's clinical characteristics. Clearly, the diversity of potential diagnoses (Table 31-1) demands a more general approach. Although the history is directed to the patient's pain, a thorough review of systems, with particular attention to the gastrointestinal, urologic, and musculoskeletal systems and the reproductive tract, must not be neglected. This chapter reviews some of the basic questions about pain related to the reproductive tract (Table 31-2).

How old are you?

Age may be a helpful part of the history in regard to reproductive tract involvement. Women with CPP associated with reproductive system disease tend to be of reproductive

TABLE 31-2. *Some of the most important questions to ask in the history of women with suspected gynecologic pelvic pain*

How old are you?
How many pregnancies have you had?
Where does it hurt?
How much does it hurt?
What is the quality or character of your pain?
When and how did your pain start, and how has it changed? Did pain start initially as menstrual cramps (dysmenorrhea)?
Do you have pain with your periods? Does your pain worsen with menses or just before menses? Is there any cyclic pattern to your pain? Is it the same 24 hours a day, 7 days a week? Is your pain constant or intermittent?
What makes your pain better? What makes your pain worse?
Do you have pain with deep penetration during intercourse? If so, does it continue afterward?
Have you ever been diagnosed with or treated for a sexually transmitted disease or pelvic inflammatory disease?
Do you have rectal pain, especially with bowel movements?
What form of birth control do you use or have you used in the past?
What prior evaluations or treatments have you had for your pain? Have any of the previous treatments helped?
How has the pain affected your quality of life?
Are you depressed or anxious?
Are you taking any drugs?
In the past have you been or are you now being abused physically or sexually? Are you safe?
What other symptoms or health problems do you have?
What do you believe or do you fear is the cause of your pain?

age, that is, 15 to 50 years of age (11–13). Women with CPP who are older than reproductive age are much less likely to have abnormalities of the reproductive tract, other than malignancies.

How many pregnancies have you had?

Pregnancy and childbirth are traumatic events to the musculoskeletal system, especially the pelvis and back, and may lead to CPP. Additionally, the hormonal changes of pregnancy cause laxity of ligaments, and this may lead to pain. Historical risk factors associated with pregnancy and pain include lumbar lordosis, delivery of a large infant, muscle weakness and poor physical conditioning, a difficult delivery, vacuum or forceps delivery, and use of gynecologic stirrups for delivery (14).

Pelvic floor relaxation with prolapse of the bladder (cystocele), uterus (uterine descensus), cul-de-sac (enterocele), and rectum (rectocele) may occasionally be a cause of CPP. A history of prior pregnancy, especially multiparity, is a risk factor for pelvic floor relaxation. Parity may also be a contributor or cause of pelvic congestion syndrome.

Women with a history of no pregnancies may have disorders that cause infertility and CPP, such as endometriosis, chronic PID, or pelvic adhesive disease.

Where does it hurt?

It is useful to have the patient mark the location of her pain on a pain map (Fig. 31-1). Pain maps often show that the patient has more than just pelvic pain. For example, up to 60% of women with chronic pelvic pain also have headaches, and up to 90% have backaches (15). Sometimes the pain map may show a distribution of pain suggesting a nonvisceral source, such as a dermatomal distribution or a myotomal pattern.

Most gynecologic pain is of visceral origin, and true visceral pain is not well localized. The cervix, uterus, and adnexae have the same metameric innervation as the bladder, distal ureter, lower ileum, colon, and rectosigmoid, so patients have difficulty differentiating if visceral abdominopelvic pain is of gynecologic, urologic, or intestinal origin (16). About 60% of women with CPP have unilateral pain, and about 40% have bilateral or diffuse pain (17). Lateral pelvic pain is commonly of adnexal or sigmoid colonic origin (18). Midline or central infraumbilical pain may be secondary to the uterus, uterosacral ligaments, posterior cul-de-sac, or cervix but may also be due to mild distention of either the left or right hemicolon. Pain from the bladder or vagina may localize over the mons pubis, pubic bone, or groin. Back pain in the lower sacral and midline areas may be from the uterosacral ligaments, posterior cul-de-sac, or cervix. Complaints of pain both ventrally and dorsally often suggest intrapelvic pathology, whereas only dorsal low back pain suggests an orthopedic or musculoskeletal origin.

Asking about radiation of pain can be helpful, also. It is not uncommon for the lateral pain of adnexal origin to radiate down the anterior or anteromedial thigh. Pain of uterine or cervical origin, including dysmenorrhea, may

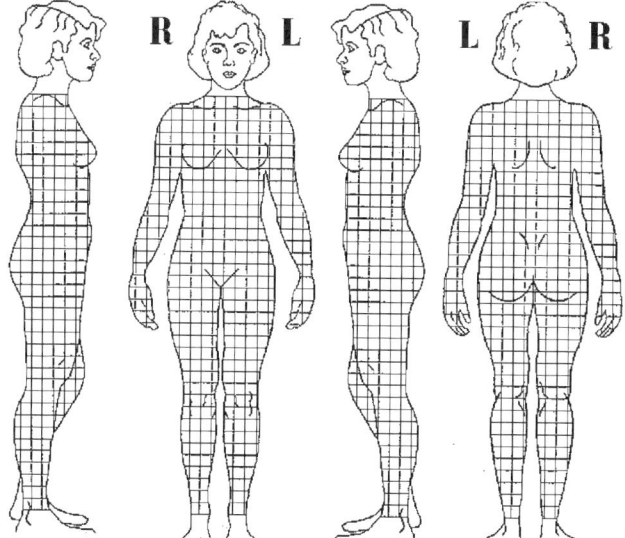

FIG. 31-1. Example of a human figure on which the patient may "map" her areas of pain.

also radiate down the anteromedial thigh. Radiation down the posterior thigh is often associated with musculoskeletal problems.

How much does it hurt?

Severity should be assessed with some type of rating system to obtain some degree of objectivity and reproducibility. In clinical practice, a simple rating system of "no pain, mild pain, moderate pain, severe pain" is often used, but this is not very sensitive to smaller changes in pain severity and may not be very useful in following patients' responses during treatment. The Society of Reproductive Medicine (Birmingham, Alabama) has suggested that endometriosis-associated pain be rated using the descriptors from the McGill Pain Questionnaire, that is, "mild, discomforting, distressing, horrible, and excruciating." The visual analog scale (VAS), which uses a 10-cm line with descriptive labels of pain severity at the ends, is also a widely used rating system. A commonly used adaptation of the VAS, which simplifies the measurement and the scale, is shown in Figure 31-2. This adaptation allows the patient to directly give a numerical rating to her pain and facilitates conversion to a verbal numerical rating system.

What is the quality or character of your pain?

The quality of pain should be sought because such descriptors sometimes help in diagnosis. Patients frequently have difficulty describing their pain, and the physician may need to supply possible descriptive terms for the nature of the pain.

Visceral pain is usually described as being a "deep" or internal aching pain with intermittent sharp and radiating

Pain severity at its *WORST*

0   1   2   3   4   5   6   7   8   9   10

No Pain   Worst Possible Pain You Can Imagine

Pain severity at its *Least*

0   1   2   3   4   5   6   7   8   9   10

No Pain   Worst Possible Pain You Can Imagine

Pain severity at its *AVERAGE* level

0   1   2   3   4   5   6   7   8   9   10

No Pain   Worst Possible Pain You Can Imagine

FIG. 31-2. Example of a modification of the traditional visual analog scale that may be used to evaluate the severity of chronic pain. The patient is asked to circle the number that most appropriately rates her pain severity.

pains. The description of the sensation of pelvic pressure or "that everything is falling out" is classically associated with pelvic floor relaxation defects. However, women with spasm of the pelvic floor muscles (levator ani) also often give the same description.

Do you have pain with your periods? Does your pain worsen with menses or just before menses? Is there any cyclic pattern to your pain? Is it the same 24 hours a day, 7 days a week? Is your pain constant or intermittent?

Any temporal pattern of pain should be sought. Asking the patient to keep a diary is sometimes helpful, with timing and severity of pain, medication use, and other potentially related factors noted (19). Cyclicity related to menses particularly suggests gynecologic pain. Three of the more common gynecologic diagnoses associated with CPP—endometriosis, adenomyosis, and pelvic congestion—correlate with the menstrual cycle and have similar premenstrual patterns of pain or pain severity (Fig. 31-3). Although pain of gynecologic origin often has premenstrual and menstrual exacerbation, this is not pathognomonic of gynecologic disease, and the same pattern may often occur with pain of intestinal, urologic, or musculoskeletal origin, also. For example, symptoms of irritable bowel syndrome frequently increase premenstrually (16).

When and how did your pain start, and how has it changed? Did pain start initially as menstrual cramps (dysmenorrhea)?

On average, women have CPP for 2 to 5 years before they seek medical help (20). Although the duration of pain probably has little diagnostic value, it may have prognostic value. In many patients pain worsens in intensity, changes in nature, and expands to involve larger areas of the body over time. The prognosis is worse in women whose pain has significantly expanded to involve areas not originally involved.

If a specific precipitating factor(s) can be found, it may aid in diagnosis. For example, an immediately antecedent trauma, such as a fall, surgery, or motor vehicle accident, suggests that a musculoskeletal cause is likely rather than a gynecologic disorder. Pain that started with a pregnancy or immediately postpartum may suggest peripartum pelvic pain syndrome. Pain that started at or soon after menarche as dysmenorrhea, progressed to premenstrual pain, and then became constant suggests endometriosis. If pain started soon after a physical or sexual assault, it may have significant musculoskeletal or psychological components.

What makes your pain better? What makes your pain worse? Do you have pain with deep penetration during intercourse? If so, does it continue afterward?

Open-ended questions about provocative and palliative factors should be asked. Examples of pertinent factors that may alter pelvic pain intensity include work, exercise, sitting, standing, lifting, lying down, heat or heating pad, ice

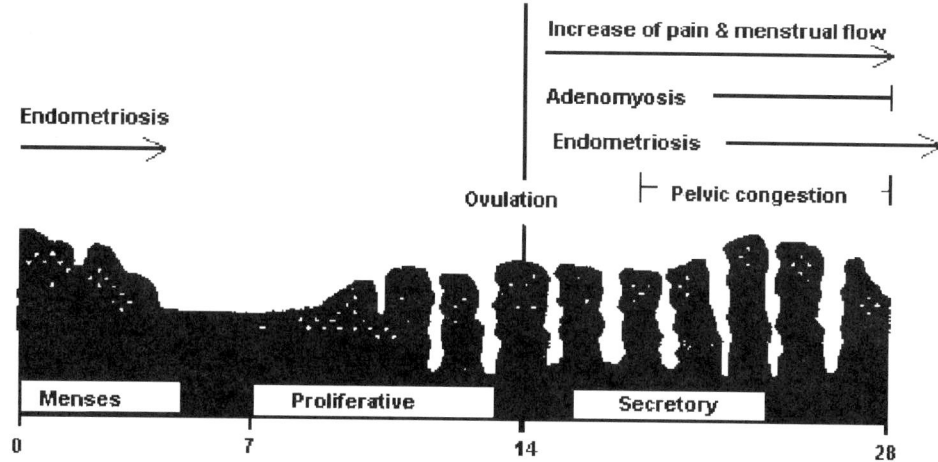

FIG. 31-3. Characteristic patterns of pain with endometriosis, pelvic congestion, and adenomyosis.

packs, eating, menses, intercourse, urination, or defecation. After the patient answers open-ended questions about anything that affects her pain, it is important to ask her specific questions about bowel function, bladder function, and especially intercourse. Many women are shy about revealing these aspects of their histories. The amount, type, and effectiveness of pain medications may be included in this part of the history, too.

Activities that increase or decrease pain sometimes give clues as to possible gynecologic diseases. For example, pain associated with pelvic floor relaxation or prolapse worsens during the course of the day as the woman is on her feet. Similarly, pain of pelvic congestion syndrome, which is also related to posture, is least on arising from sleep or rest and worsens during the day or the longer the woman is on her feet. In contrast, pain associated with adenomyosis or endometriosis is not influenced as much by rest or time of day. Pain related to specific positions may suggest adhesive disease.

A history of pain or increased pain with coitus is frequently interpreted as pathognomonic of psychological disease, marital problems, endometriosis, vulvodynia, and so on. In fact, dyspareunia is present in about 50% of women with CPP. It occurs with all of the preceding as well as with irritable bowel syndrome, inflammatory bowel disease, interstitial cystitis, adhesions, and pelvic floor defects and is not specific for any particular disease. If intercourse is painful, it is important to find out if pain is with entry at the outermost part of the vagina or if it is with deeper penetration high in the vagina or pelvis, or both. Per se, diseases associated with CPP do not cause entry dyspareunia, except as vaginismus secondary to deep dyspareunia. Dyspareunia occurring with deep penetration, lasting for several hours or more after coitus, or precipitating pelvic or abdominal pain may suggest endometriosis, abdominopelvic adhesions, or pelvic congestion syndrome. At laparoscopy, women with these complaints are significantly more likely to have endometriosis or pelvic adhesions than women without such complaints (21).

Have you ever been diagnosed with or treated for a sexually transmitted disease or pelvic inflammatory disease?

It is pertinent to ask about prior sexually transmitted diseases or pelvic inflammatory disease (PID) because it is estimated that 18% to 27% of all women with acute PID develop CPP (22). Epidemiologic studies suggest that PID occurs most frequently among teenagers and women less than 25 years of age, which is about a decade younger than the mean age of women with CPP (5).

Clinically, the pain of chronic PID is usually related to coitus and physical activity and is acyclic, although there may be premenstrual or menstrual exacerbation. The actual mechanisms by which CPP results from PID and why most women with reproductive organ damage secondary to acute PID do not develop CPP are not known (23).

What form of birth control do you use or have you used in the past?

Hormonal contraceptive therapy may mask gynecologic pain associated with diseases such as endometriosis or adenomyosis. Asking about prior use may reveal that onset or exacerbation of pain correlates with discontinuation of hormonal contraception. Also, if hormonal contraception is currently being used, then it is less likely that these medications will offer a therapeutic option.

A history of other contraceptive methods may also be relevant. For example, there is one report of an IUD fragment as a cause of CPP (7). After removal and doxycycline therapy the patient had pain relief.

Have you ever had any kind of surgery?

Obviously a history of surgery for pain may lead to the consideration of recurrence or inadequate surgery of the specific disease that was treated. Surgical history, however, may be pertinent other than for the specific diagnosis for which the surgery was performed. For example, spillage of gallstones at the time of laparoscopic and open cholecystectomy has been reported as a cause of CPP in at least two cases (24,25).

The Marshall-Marchetti-Krantz procedure for urinary incontinence has also been reported as a cause of CPP with localization to the pubic symphysis due to osteitis pubis or osteomyelitis in several cases. These cases present long after surgery without fever but with altered gait and significant pelvic pain. In such cases aggressive diagnostic evaluation with biopsy and needle aspiration guided by computer-assisted tomography is advised (26).

Prior cervical surgery for dysplasia may cause cervical stenosis with resultant hematometra and CPP. A high association of cervical stenosis and endometriosis has also been reported (27).

What prior evaluations or treatments have you had for your pain? Have any of the previous treatments helped?

A thorough history about prior treatments or evaluations can be time consuming in women with chronic pelvic pain because they often have been through extensive prior evaluations and treatments. An accurate compilation of this record may be extremely useful in suggesting associated or etiologic diseases. If nothing else, it avoids repeating invasive and expensive diagnostic and therapeutic procedures. For example, a randomized trial published by Peters et al. showed quite clearly that performing a laparoscopy in women who had prior negative laparoscopies or laparotomies did nothing to improve the outcomes compared to multidisciplinary pain therapy without laparoscopy (28).

Patients should be asked to evaluate their response to prior treatments, including the duration of any positive responses. For example, a good response to gonadotropin-releasing hormone agonist (GnRH-a), followed by a pregnancy and 2 to 3 years of pain relief, suggests that GnRH-a therapy is a good option for the treatment of recurrent CPP. Similarly, a good response to surgical treatment of endometriosis may suggest that repeat surgery is an option for recurrent pain.

How has the pain affected your quality of life?

Although an evaluation of pain's effect on the woman's quality of life is not always helpful in differential diagnosis, it certainly aids in evaluation of the severity of pain, as well as helps set goals for treatment. Many women with CPP have had their lives totally disrupted by their pain, resulting in job loss, marital discord and divorce, isolation from friends and family, and so on. Although distressing, it is important to elicit such information.

PSYCHOSOCIAL HISTORY

A complete psychosocial evaluation involves extensive interviews of the patient and her family or partner, questionnaires, behavioral observation, and psychological testing with instruments like the Minnesota Multiphasic Personality Inventory and Beck Depression Inventory. This usually requires a psychologist, or similarly educated professional, and cannot always be done—nor is it always necessary. However, some psychosocial history is always an important part of the history. The following questions represent a minimum evaluation.

Are you depressed or anxious?

The relationship of depression and chronic pain is complex. For example, there is reasonable evidence to suggest that depression leads to chronic pelvic pain, and there is reasonable evidence to suggest that chronic pelvic pain leads to depression (29). Depression is noted in patients in whom organic pathology can be found and in those in whom no such pathology is noted (30). Depression tends to maintain or increase the level of pain, regardless of the degree of physical disease. It is one of several predictors of pain severity in women with CPP, and also it is a significant indicator of responsiveness to treatment. Furthermore, major depressive illness sometimes develops in chronic pain patients, with a cycle of pain, depression, and withdrawal. Thus it is important to seek evidence of depression in women with CPP.

In addition to simply asking the patient if she is depressed, she should be asked about associated symptoms consistent with depression such as (a) diminished interest in or pleasure from daily activities, (b) poor appetite, (c) weight loss, (d) overeating, (e) weight gain, (f) insomnia, (g) trouble falling asleep, (h) awakening during the night with inability to fall back to sleep, (i) sleeping too much or much more than usual, (j) feeling tired or having little energy, (k) feeling bad about oneself, (l) feelings of letting oneself or one's family down, (m) feelings of worthlessness, (n) feelings of excessive guilt, (o) inability to concentrate normally, (p) inability to make decisions, and (q) thoughts about death or committing suicide.

Are you taking any drugs?

It is important to find out about medication use, as well as self-medication with street or illegal drugs. Alcohol use should also be included in this questioning. The patient needs to understand that this information is important in trying to seek medical ways to control or alleviate pain while avoiding untoward drug and medication interactions. A history of substance abuse may be particularly useful in planning treatment. Such women have a significant risk of noncompliant overuse of prescription opioid pain medication if this is part of their treatment.

In the past have you been or are you now being abused physically or sexually? Are you safe?

It has been suggested that sexual abuse might in some way be specifically related to the development of chronic pelvic pain. Although it is mechanistically tempting to etiologically link sexual abuse with pelvic pain, current data do not support an association with major sexual abuse any more specifically than they do an association with major physical (nonsexual) abuse. In other words, there appears to be an association between physical and/or sexual abuse and chronic pelvic pain. It may be that a history of both physical and sexual abuse serves as a marker for a greater magnitude of abuse and that the greater the magnitude of abuse, the stronger the correlation with chronic pelvic pain (31,32).

With the correlation of abuse and chronic pain, and with the high prevalence of domestic violence, it is important to ask women with CPP if they are in a safe environment. This question should be asked in a private setting without the spouse or significant other present. Satisfaction or dissatisfaction with marital or family relationships and support may be explored at this time, also (33).

What other symptoms or health problems do you have?

Although this question is a part of every patient's history and review of systems, in this context it is included as a clue to somatization disorders. Table 31-3 gives a series of symptoms that can be sought and then used as a way to evaluate somatization. In a small study of this "somatization scale," women with CPP and a nonsomatic diagnosis had on average two more symptoms than those with a somatic diagnosis for their pain (10). If the patient had eight or more symptoms and also had a history of sexual abuse, there was a 78% chance of a nonsomatic diagnosis after thorough evaluation of her pain. Seeking evidence of somatization is important because its presence complicates treatment and suggests that psychological evaluation and treatment are needed.

What do you believe or do you fear is the cause of your pain?

The patient's cognitive perspectives on her pain can be explored by asking for her ideas of the cause of her pain.

TABLE 31-3. *Example of a somatization scale that has been used to evaluate women with chronic pelvic pain. High score is eight or more symptoms*

A	Headache
B	Low back pain
C	Pain with urination
D	Sleeplessness
E	Weight loss or gain
F	Dizziness
G	Passing out
H	Depression
I	Premenstrual syndrome
J	Shortness of breath
K	Joint pain
L	Nausea
M	Bloating
N	Vomiting
O	Diarrhea
P	Constipation
Q	Fatigue

A goal of this exploration is especially to evaluate and discern fears the patient may have about the etiology of her pain, such as cancer, pelvic infection due to remote past sexual acts, arguments with her spouse, divine retribution, and so on. This question may also include an exploration of the patient's concerns about what will happen to her during the evaluation and treatment of her pain.

PHYSICAL EXAMINATION

The physical examination is comparable to the patient history as a powerful diagnostic and therapeutic tool. Guided by a thorough history, the examination can lead to an accurate diagnosis that directs therapy or further testing. As a therapeutic tool, a gently and meticulously performed physical examination, especially if it follows a compassionately taken history, establishes trust that the physician is caring and competent. Because the examination is often uncomfortable and painful for the woman with CPP, it is important that the physician go slowly enough to allow her to recover and relax between various portions of the examination. In some cases this can be time consuming. Additionally, during the physical examination it is not uncommon for the patient to remember aspects of her history that she previously omitted, and time must be allowed for her to relate these additions to the history. Patience and kindness go a long way in establishing rapport with the patient, especially during the initial evaluation. The importance of establishing rapport with the patient at the initial visit cannot be overstated—it may well be the most important objective of the initial encounter.

During the examination a patient with CPP sometimes exhibits behavior that seems exaggerated or even hysterical, or she may relate sensations or pain distributions that seem nonanatomic or nonphysiologic. In spite of this, it is crucial that the patient be taken seriously and that her behavior and descriptions not be dismissed as ridiculous, impossible, or unimportant. Such reactions by the physician are counterproductive and create only mistrust and anger. Tolerance and an open mind are important in evaluating the woman with CPP and go a long way in establishing rapport. It is important to remember that even a "routine" pelvic examination is very emotionally stressful for many patients with CPP (34).

A major goal of the examination is to detect, inasmuch as possible, the exact anatomic locations of tenderness and correlate these with areas of pain. At each tender or painful area palpated, the patient should be asked whether this pain reproduces the complaint for which she is being evaluated. This requires a systematic and methodical attempt to duplicate the pain by palpation or positioning. The physician may find it useful to record these findings on a human anatomy diagram.

Although this chapter is limited to gynecologic aspects of CPP, it must be stressed that a thorough examination addressing all potential systems that can cause pelvic pain must be performed. For simplicity, I divide the examination into (a) standing, (b) sitting, (c) supine, and (d) lithotomy components. Some of the important parts of each of these components of the examination are summarized in Tables 31-4 to 31-7. Only the lithotomy part of the examination is reviewed in this chapter.

After the patient is in lithotomy position, initially inspect the external genitalia for redness, discharge, abscess formation, excoriation, perineal fistula, ulcerations, pigment changes, condylomata, atrophic changes (thinning, paleness, loss of vaginal rugae, protruding urethral mucosa), or signs of trauma. Look for fistulas and fissures because they may occasionally be the first objective evidence of inflammatory bowel disease.

Perform basic sensory testing to sharpness, dullness, and light touch, and test the bulbocavernosus and anal wink reflexes. Use a cotton-tipped swab to evaluate the

TABLE 31-4. *Components of the standing physical examination of the woman with chronic pelvic pain and some of the general problems or diagnoses that may be suggested based on these components of the examination. Examination components in parentheses are not always a necessary part of the examination.*

Standing examination	Possible problems diagnosed
Gait	Short leg syndrome Herniated disc General musculoskeletal problems
Posture with and without forward bending	Typical pelvic pain posture Scoliosis One-leg standing
Standing on one leg with and without hip flexion	Laxity of the pubic symphysis Laxity of pelvic girdle Weakness of the hip and pelvis
Iliac crest symmetry	Short leg syndrome One-leg standing
Groin evaluation with and without Valsalva	Inguinal hernia Femoral hernia
(Incisional evaluation with and without Valsalva)	Incisional hernia
Pubic symphysis evaluation, including trigger points	Peripartum pelvic pain syndrome Trigger points Osteitis pubis Osteomyelitis pubis
Hip and sacroiliac evaluation, including trigger points	Arthritis of hip Trigger points
Buttocks (gluteus and piriformis) evaluation, including trigger points	Piriformis syndrome Pelvic floor pain syndrome Gluteal trigger points
(Fibromyalgia tender point evaluation)	Fibromyalgia
(Pelvic floor relaxation evaluation)	Enterocele Rectocele Cystocele Uterine descensus

TABLE 31-5. *Components of the sitting physical examination of the woman with chronic pelvic pain and general problems or diagnoses that may be suggested based on these components of the examination*

Sitting examination	Possible problems diagnosed
Posture	Levator ani spasm Pelvic floor pain syndrome
Palpation of the upper and lower back	Trigger points Myalgia Arthritis
Palpation of sacrum	Trigger points Sacroiliitis
Palpation of gluteal and piriformis muscles	Trigger points Myalgia
Palpation of the posterior superior iliac crests	Peripartum pelvic pain syndrome
Basic sensory testing to sharpness, dullness, and light touch	Herniated disc
Muscle strength testing and deep tendon	Herniated disc

TABLE 31-6. *Components of the supine physical examination of the woman with chronic pelvic pain and general problems or diagnoses that may be suggested based on these components of the examination. Examination components in parentheses are not always a necessary part of the examination.*

Supine examination	Possible problems diagnosed
Posture for lordosis or pelvic tilt	Lordosis Pelvic tilt Abdominal weakness Stiffness of the lumbar spine
Active leg flexion, knee to chest	Low back dysfunction Low back pain Abdominal muscle weakness Deconditioning
Obturator and psoas sign testing	Shortening, dysfunction, or spasm of the obturator or iliopsoas muscles or fascia
Head raise and leg raise	Herniated disc Abdominal muscle weakness Deconditioning
Light abdominal palpation	Referred visceral pain Nerve entrapment Neuropathy
Gentle pinching	Referred visceral pain Nerve entrapment Neuropathy
Head's maneuver	Referred visceral pain Nerve entrapment Neuropathy

(Continued)

TABLE 31-6. *Continued*

Supine examination	Possible problems diagnosed
Dermographism evaluation	Referred visceral pain Nerve entrapment Neuropathy
Single digit palpation	Trigger points Myofascial pain Hernias Nerve entrapments
Abdominal wall tenderness test	Abdominal wall pain Visceral pain
Groin and abdominal evaluation with and without Valsalva	Inguinal hernia Spigelian hernia Epigastric hernia Diastasis recti
(Incisional evaluation with and without Valsalva)	Incisional hernia
Pubic symphysis evaluation	Trigger points Osteitis pubis Osteomyelitis pubis
Traditional abdominal examination for distention, masses, ascites, bowel sounds, shifting dullness, vascular bruits, deep tenderness, guarding, or rigidity	Acute disease

TABLE 31-7. *Components of the lithotomy physical examination of the woman with chronic pelvic pain and general problems or diagnoses that may be suggested based on these components of the examination. Examination components in parentheses are not always a necessary part of the examination.*

Lithotomy examination	Possible problems diagnosed
Visual inspection of the external genitalia	Inflammatory and infectious diseases Vulvar abscess Trauma Fistula Ulcerative disease Pigmented lesions (neoplasias) Condylomata Atrophic changes Fissure
Basic sensory testing to sharpness, dullness, and light touch	Nerve entrapment Neuropathy Spinal cord lesion
Cotton-tipped swab evaluation of the vestibule	Vulvar vestibulitis
Single digit palpation of vulva and pubic arch	Trigger points

TABLE 31-7. *Continued*

Supine examination	Possible problems diagnosed
(Colposcopic evaluation of the vulva and vestibule)	Neoplasia
Sims retractor or single blade speculum examination of vagina and pelvic muscles	Enterocele Cystocele Rectocele Uterine descensus
Cotton-tipped swab evaluation of cervical os, paracervical, and cervical tissues	Trigger points
(Cotton-tipped swab evaluation vaginal cuff)	Trigger points Neuroma
Single digit pelvic examination of introitus	Vulvar vestibulitis Vaginismus Trigger points
Single digit pelvic examination of levator ani	Pelvic floor pain syndrome Trigger points
Single digit pelvic examination of coccygeus	Pelvic floor pain syndrome Trigger points
Single digit pelvic examination of piriformis with and without abduction	Piriformis syndrome
Single digit pelvic examination of anterior vaginal urethral and trigonal evaluation	Chronic urethral syndrome Urethritis Cystitis Interstitial cystitis Trigonitis Urethral diverticulum Vaginal wall cyst
Single digit pelvic examination of cervix, paracervical areas, and vaginal fornices	Trigger points Endometriosis Cervicitis Repeated cervical trauma Pelvic infection Pelvic infection Ureteral pain
Single digit pelvic examination of uterus	Adenomyosis Pelvic congestion syndrome Pelvic infection Premenstrual syndrome Adhesions
Single digit pelvic examination of coccyx	Coccydynia
Single digit pelvic examination of adnexa	Pelvic congestion syndrome Endometriosis
Bimanual pelvic examination	See text
Rectovaginal examination	See text

(Continued)

vestibule for the localized tenderness of vulvar vestibulitis. To do this hold the labia apart and gently palpate the vestibule, vulva, hymen, and the area of the minor vestibular glands with a cotton-tipped swab. Patients with vulvar vestibulitis demonstrate exquisite tenderness in localized areas at the minor vestibular glands just external to the hymen, with normal sensation in adjacent vestibular and vulvar areas (Fig. 31-4). Use a cotton-tipped applicator or single digit palpation to evaluate the vulva and pubic arch for trigger points and for skin or mucosal lesions that reproduce the patient's symptoms. Pay particular attention to areas of previous vulvar or vaginal trauma and scars from surgeries or deliveries.

Show any areas of abnormality of the external genitalia to the patient using a hand mirror to allow her to see her genitalia while demonstrating the lesions or areas of tenderness. This not only educates the patient as to the findings, but also allows her a sense of increased control during the examination. This technique also allows the patient to guide the physician in localizing areas of tenderness during the examination when there is entrance dyspareunia or vulvar pain (35).

Assess the pelvic floor muscles for pain or tension by insertion of a Sims retractor or a single blade of the speculum into the posterior vagina while asking the patient to relax. The resistance to downward or posterior pressure can be evaluated to reveal increased muscle tone, tension, or spasm (36). This maneuver may also reproduce part of the patient's symptom complex. Single speculum blade or Sims retractor examination may also reveal evidence of pelvic relaxation, with uterine descensus, cystocele, enterocele, or rectocele.

Of course, the traditional speculum examination is done to allow full visual inspection and to obtain requisite cytologic and bacteriologic specimens. Note the position of the cervix because lateral displacement suggests possible ipsilateral uterosacral endometriosis (37). Use a cotton-tipped swab to evaluate the cervical os and the paracervical and

cervical tissues for tenderness, especially at one, three, six, and nine o'clock. In posthysterectomy patients palpate the full vaginal cuff for tenderness with a cotton-tipped applicator. If localized tender points are elicited, it may be worthwhile to block them with 0.25% bupivacaine and reevaluate for tenderness after 5 minutes (38).

Always initiate the manual portion of the pelvic examination with a single index finger, first noting any introital tenderness or spasm. Vaginismus can be identified by involuntary introital spasm at this point in the examination in 75% of women with this diagnosis (35). Next, directly palpate the levator ani muscles for tone and tenderness. The levator ani muscles are easily palpated during vaginal or rectal examination. They lie adjacent to the lateral vaginal walls just above the hymeneal ring. The medial margins of the muscles are slightly thicker than a standard pencil, running in an anteroposterior direction. Identification may be confirmed by having the patient contract her pelvic muscles. The anus simultaneously elevates when the levators are contracted. Normally this palpation causes only a pressure sensation, but in patients with pelvic floor pain syndrome (PFPS) it may cause pain consistent with at least part of the patient's clinical pain symptoms. In some patients with PFPS, there will also be tenderness of the coccyx, lateral sacrum, or sacrococcygeal ligaments. Digital pressure on the involved muscle characteristically reproduces or intensifies the patient's pain symptoms. It is not unusual for the tenderness to be unilateral. Also palpate the insertion of the levators if possible, both laterally at the arcus tendinei and anteriorly at the pubic rami.

Gently palpate the piriformis, coccygeus, and obturator internus muscles bilaterally seeking tenderness that reproduces the patient's pain. The piriformis muscles are somewhat more difficult to palpate than the levators. Rectal examination may allow an easier evaluation than vaginal examination. Transvaginally or transrectally the examining finger is pressed posterolaterally just superiorly to the ischial spine. In the lithotomy position, if the patient is asked to abduct the thigh against resistance (hold the patient's knee laterally on the same side being examined) as the piriformis is palpated, the muscle may be more easily palpated, and there is exquisite tenderness of the muscle if there is spasm or tension myalgia involving the piriformis (piriformis syndrome).

Gently palpate the anterior vaginal urethral and trigonal areas to elicit any areas of tenderness, induration, or thickening. Also, massage the urethra to elicit any secretions. Urethral tenderness with or without discharge is consistent with chronic urethritis or chronic urethral syndrome. Next, evaluate the "gutter" on either side of the urethra for any fullness, fluctuance, or discomfort that might suggest a urethral diverticulum or vaginal wall cyst (36). Also evaluate the bladder base for tenderness. Tenderness is consistent with trigonitis or interstitial cystitis.

Next, still using a single digit, palpate the cervix, paracervical areas, and vaginal fornices for tenderness or trigger

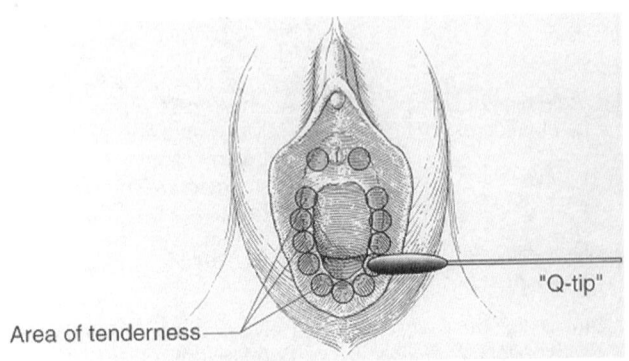

Area of tenderness ———

FIG. 31-4. Patients with vulvar vestibulitis demonstrate exquisite tenderness to palpation with a cotton-tipped applicator in localized areas at the minor vestibular glands just external to the hymen, shown by the shaded circles. Sensation is normal in adjacent vestibular and vulvar areas.

points. Cervical tenderness may suggest problems such as cervicitis, repeated cervical trauma (usually from intercourse), or pelvic infection. Vaginal forniceal tenderness may suggest problems such as pelvic infection, endometriosis, ureteral tenderness, or trigger points.

Compress the uterus against the sacrum to evaluate uterine tenderness (Fig. 31-5). Uterine tenderness may be consistent with diseases such as adenomyosis, pelvic congestion syndrome, pelvic infection, or premenstrual syndrome. A uterus that is immobile and fixed in position, especially a retroflexed position, may suggest endometriosis or adhesions. Next, palpate the coccyx with the single digit and attempt to move it 30 degrees or less. This part of the examination may also be done during the bimanual or rectovaginal examination. Normally the coccyx moves 30 degrees without eliciting pain, but in patients with coccydynia this movement elicits pain.

Palpate the adnexal areas next, still using a single digit without the use of the abdominal hand. This is often a more accurate manner of assessing intrinsic tenderness of the ovaries or tube than the traditional bimanual examination, especially in patients with abdominal wall tenderness or trigger points. All ovaries are tender, so it is the degree of tenderness and the similarity to the chief pain complaint that are clinically useful.

All of the preceding are "monomanual-monodigital" evaluations, that is, only one finger of one hand is used. No abdominal palpation with the other hand is involved. The traditional bimanual examination is the last portion of the pelvic examination in the pelvic pain patient. It is the least sensitive portion of the evaluation because it involves stimulation of all layers of the abdominal wall, the parietal peritoneum, and the palpated organ or organs. Evaluate the uterus for size, shape, tenderness, and mobility. A fixed, retroverted uterus may suggest endometriosis or cul-de-sac adhesions. Endometriosis is also suggested by tenderness

of the posterior uterus, nodularity of the uterosacral ligaments and cul-de-sac, and narrowing of the posterior vaginal fornix. Pelvic nodularity is, however, not diagnostic of endometriosis and may occur with other conditions, particularly ovarian carcinoma.

Examine the adnexae for thickening, mobility, or enlargement. Asymmetric, enlarged ovaries, particularly if fixed to the broad ligament or pelvic sidewall, may imply the presence of endometriosis. Bilateral or unilateral ovarian tenderness almost always occurs with pelvic congestion syndrome.

Palpate the ureters for abnormal tenderness and possible reproduction of pain complaints, particularly at the uterovesical junctions. They are not infrequently a source of pain and tenderness. Figure 31-6 illustrates the technique used to examine the ureters.

Palpate the cecum on the right and the rectosigmoid on the left for masses, hard feces, and tenderness. Either or both may be abnormally tender with irritable bowel syndrome.

Perform a rectal or rectovaginal examination last. Marked discomfort with digital rectal examination often accompanies irritable bowel syndrome or chronic constipation, as may hard feces in the rectum. Evaluate function of the internal and external anal sphincter by reflex wink and voluntary constriction. Carefully examine the rectovaginal septum for nodularity and tenderness, suggestive of endometriosis. It is useful to reevaluate the pelvic floor muscles during the rectovaginal examination. Start in the posterior midline and sweep laterally and anteriorly so the rectal finger passes over the piriformis, the coccygeus, and then the levator ani muscles. Rectal examination should also include evaluation for rectal masses because many colorectal carcinomas are palpable this way. Tenderness of the anal canal may suggest abscess or fissures in the canal. Test for occult fecal blood.

In many women with endometriosis-associated pelvic pain there is detectable tenderness only during menses. For

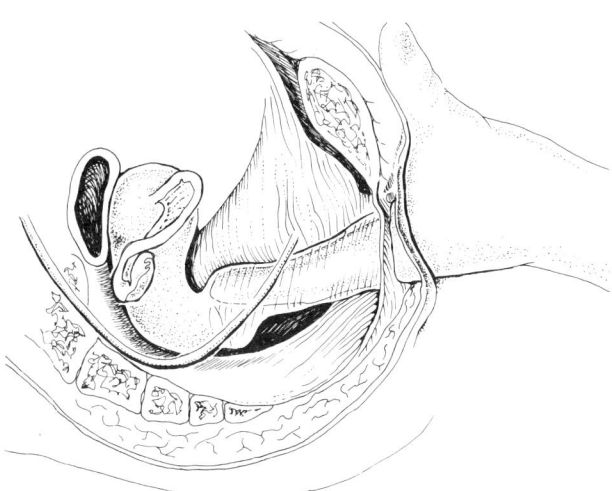

FIG. 31-5. Evaluating the uterus for tenderness during single-digit examination by compressing it against the sacrum.

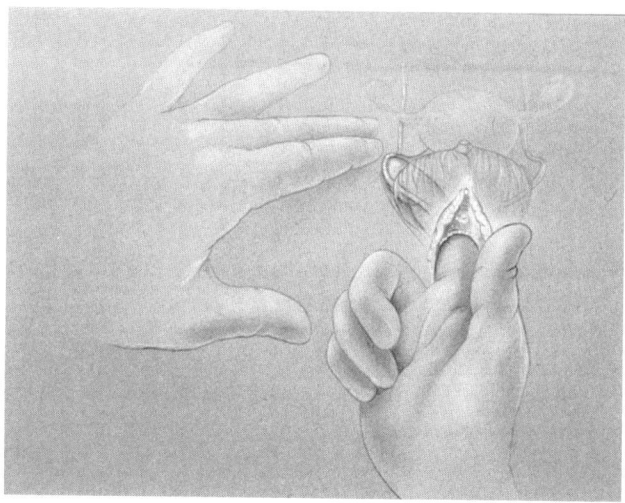

FIG. 31-6. Illustration showing the technique used to examine the ureters.

this reason it is sometimes helpful to do the examination during the first day or two of menstrual flow in women with suspected endometriosis. This may also increase the likelihood of finding tender endometriotic nodules in the pelvis or rectovaginal septum.

Although findings can be briefly explained during the physical examination, after completion the physician should fully explain any positive or negative findings. Any tentative diagnoses should be explained as well. Any further testing or evaluations recommended should be discussed, described, and justified. Finally, any questions should be answered.

LABORATORY AND IMAGING STUDIES

Although this chapter is limited to a discussion of diagnostic tests somewhat specific to the genitourinary tract, some general comments about the use of "routine" tests in women with CPP are warranted. All too often all women with CPP are routinely put through a barium enema and upper gastrointestinal series to "rule out" gastrointestinal disease, an intravenous pyelogram to "rule out" urinary tract disease, a pelvic ultrasound to "rule out" gynecologic disease, a complete blood count and sedimentation rate to "rule out" infection, and so on. Such routine or algorithmic approaches are not worthwhile, especially because such general tests rarely accomplish their intended purpose of "ruling out" the involvement of organ systems or inflammatory or infectious processes. Diagnostic tests should be obtained when indicated by the history and physical examination and when the results will change the diagnosis, change the further evaluation, or change the treatment. Table 31-8 lists diagnostic tests relevant to many of the possible diagnoses in women with CPP. A full discussion of these tests is beyond the scope of this chapter, and only some of those specific to the genitourinary tract will be reviewed.

It is reasonable for the physician to test for sexually transmitted diseases. Cervical cultures or smears for gonorrhea and chlamydia, syphilis serology, hepatitis B surface antigen screening, and HIV testing are all appropriate as part of primary health care for the patient. In patients with dyspareunia, testing for sexually transmitted diseases, especially with urethral and cervical gonorrhea cultures and chlamydial PCR testing (which can also be done on urine), is advisable regardless of risk factors or history. Other specific infectious causes of painful intercourse should also be ruled out. This requires vaginal cultures, urine cultures, vaginal wet preps, and vaginal pH. These tests for infectious etiologies are advisable in almost all cases of dyspareunia.

Although urinalysis and urine culture are relatively inexpensive and are noninvasive, they are not always necessary. However, in the woman who has any urinary tract symptoms or who is to undergo invasive procedures that include bladder catheterization, it is advisable to perform them. Persistent irritative bladder symptoms of frequency and urgency associated with chronic pelvic pain may suggest interstitial cystitis, but neoplasia must also be ruled out, especially if the woman is a smoker. Urine cytology should be done in such cases, in addition to urinalysis and culture. Urinary oxalate levels are often measured in women with vulvar vestibulitis because oxalate crystals are the most commonly mentioned irritant in association with vulvar vestibulitis (39). Although the usefulness of urinary oxalate testing has been seriously questioned by many investigators, it may still be worthwhile in certain cases. Sometimes a urine drug screen is indicated in the woman with CPP, especially if there is a history of substance abuse or significant psychological symptoms.

Hormonal levels generally are not useful, but estradiol and FSH levels may be helpful in suspected cases of ovarian remnant syndrome as evidence of continuing ovarian activity helps to establish the diagnosis. In women with depression, thyroid stimulating hormone, thyroxin, triiodothyronine levels (TSH, T4, T3), and sometimes antithyroid antibody assays should be measured to rule out thyroid conditions that may manifest as depression. Other tests that may be indicated in the depressed woman include blood counts to rule out anemia and infection, renal and hepatic function tests, electrolytes, rapid plasma reagen (RPR) to rule out neurosyphilis, and human immunodeficiency virus (HIV) testing to rule out autoimmune deficiency syndrome.

Ca-125 levels may be elevated with diseases associated with pelvic pain, such as endometriosis. Ca-125 has been evaluated as an aid to diagnosis and followup of patients with endometriosis, but as a diagnostic test it has a low sensitivity and specificity (40). A major concern with the use of Ca-125 levels for diagnosis is that levels are also elevated with cancers of the ovary, endometrium, gastrointestinal tract, fallopian tube, and breast. They are also increased with pelvic inflammatory disease, pregnancy, menses, and leiomyomata (41).

Ultrasonography can be a helpful diagnostic test. In patients with a pelvic mass it may help identify the origin as uterine, adnexal, gastrointestinal, or bladder. If an adnexal mass is found, sonography may show the location, size, and solid or cystic components and aid in nonoperative or preoperative diagnosis. If endometriosis is suspected, ultrasonography is useful to identify possible endometriomas prior to laparoscopic evaluation and treatment. It can also be used to follow patients after treatment and identify any recurrence of endometriomas.

In cases of suspected uterine pathology, ultrasonography can be valuable in women with leiomyomata, both to confirm the diagnosis and to document the number of fibroids, their location, degree of calcification, and rate of growth. Transvaginal sonography, in particular, may identify and distinguish leiomyomas from adenomyomas (42). Ultrasound is not as reliable for the diagnosis of adenomyosis without adenomyoma formation (43). In some cases ultrasonography may detect endometrial polyps or an unsuspected intrauterine device (44). Hysterosonography is

TABLE 31-8. *Some of the laboratory tests and imaging studies that may be useful with different disorders associated with chronic pelvic pain*

Symptom, finding, or suspected diagnosis	Potentially useful tests
Abdominal epilepsy	Electroencephalography
Adenomyosis	Ultrasonography Hysterosalpingography Magnetic resonance imaging
Chronic intermittent bowel obstruction	Flat and upright abdominal x-rays Computerized tomography
Chronic pelvic pain—general	Complete blood cell count Sedimentation rate
Chronic urethral syndrome	Urodynamic testing
Colorectal cancer	Barium enema radiography Computerized tomography
Compression or entrapment neuropathy	Nerve conducting velocities Needle electromyographic studies
Constipation	Anorectal balloon manometry Colonic transit time
Depression	Thyroid stimulating hormone Thyroxin Triiodothyronine levels Antithyroid antibody Complete blood count Renal function tests Hepatic function tests Electrolytes Rapid plasma reagen Human immunodeficiency virus testing
Diarrhea	Stool specimens for ova and parasites Stool polymorphonuclear leukocytes and red blood cells Stool cultures Stool for C. difficile toxin Stool guiaic testing Barium enema radiography
Diverticular disease	Barium enema radiography
Dyspareunia	Urethral and cervical gonorrhea cultures Chlamydial PCR testing Vaginal cultures Urine cultures Vaginal wet preps Vaginal pH
Endometrial polyps	Ultrasonography Sonohysterography Hysterosalpingography
Endometriosis	Ca-125 Ultrasonography Barium enema radiography Hysterosalpingography Computerized tomography Magnetic resonance imaging
Hematuria	Urine culture Urine cytology Cystourethroscopy Computerized tomography
Hernia of the linea alba	Abdominal wall ultrasonography Computerized tomography

(Continued)

TABLE 31-8. *Continued*

Symptom, finding, or suspected diagnosis	Potentially useful tests
Inflammatory bowel disease	Barium enema radiography Upper gastrointestinal series with follow through Computerized tomography
Inguinal hernia	Herniography
Internal supravesical hernia	Ultrasonography Computerized tomography
Interstitial cystitis	Urine cytologies Urodynamic testing
Leiomyoma uteri	Ultrasonography Hysterosalpingography
Musculoskeletal disorders (some)	Plain film radiography Computerized tomography
Obstructive cervical stenosis	Ultrasonography
Obturator hernia	Herniography Computerized tomography
Osteomyelitis	Bone scan
Ovarian cancer	Ca-125 Ultrasonography Computerized tomography
Ovarian remnant syndrome	Follicle-stimulating hormone Estradiol Gonadotropin releasing hormone agonist stimulation test Ultrasonography ± clomiphene stimulation Barium enema radiography Computerized tomography
Ovarian retention syndrome	Ultrasonography Computerized tomography
Pelvic congestion syndrome	Pelvic venography Ultrasonography ± Doppler
Pelvic floor relaxation	Vaginal sonography Perineal ultrasound Introital sonography Rectosonography Colporectocystourethrography Magnetic resonance imaging Anal electromyography Pudendal nerve terminal latency
Pelvic mass	Ultrasonography Computerized tomography
Pelvic tuberculosis	Chest x-ray
Perineal hernia	Herniography
Porphyria	Urine porphobilinogen
Richter hernia	Computerized tomography
Sciatic hernia	Computerized tomography
Spigelian hernia	Abdominal wall ultrasonography Computerized tomography Herniography
Spinal disc pathology	Magnetic resonance imaging
Stress fracture	Bone scan
Substance abuse	Drug screen

TABLE 31-8. *Continued*

Symptom, finding, or suspected diagnosis	Potentially useful tests
Umbilical hernia	Abdominal wall ultrasonography Computerized tomography Herniography
Uncertain intrauterine device	Ultrasonography
Urethral diverticulum	Vaginal sonography Voiding cystourethrography Double balloon cystourethrography Magnetic resonance imaging
Urinary tract infection	Urinalysis Urine culture
Uterine anomalies	Hysterosalpingography
Vesical-sphincter dyssynergia	Urodynamic testing
Vulvar vestibulitis	Urinary oxalate

particularly effective in distinguishing endometrial thickening from endometrial polyps (45).

Transvaginal ultrasonography can be used to diagnose cervical stenosis if it is obstructive; sonography may show fluid or debris, or a fluid-debris level in the endometrial cavity (46). A lobulated or distorted cervix may suggest an occult carcinoma or fibroids as the cause.

Ultrasonography can also be useful in the diagnosis of ovarian retention syndrome and ovarian remnant syndrome. Vaginal ultrasound shows a pelvic mass in 50% to 85% of cases of ovarian remnant syndrome. The mass is usually cystic or multiseptated with a well-defined solid tissue ring surrounding it. The diagnostic accuracy of ultrasound may be improved by pretreatment with clomiphene citrate (47). Not all ovarian remnants have functional follicles that respond and enlarge with clomiphene, so this technique is not invariably helpful.

Ultrasound can be used to identify pelvic varicosities and to suggest a diagnosis of pelvic congestion syndrome (48,49), although the technology has not yet reached the stage where it can be used to definitively diagnose pelvic congestion syndrome (50–52).

In patients in whom intestinal endometriosis is suspected, evaluation of the intestinal tract is usually normal because most patients have involvement of the serosa or muscularis, not the mucosa. Sigmoidoscopy may show a bluish submucosal mass in some of these cases. Mucosal lesions may be diagnosed by sigmoidoscopy, colonoscopy, or barium enema studies, but these evaluations are certainly not necessary on a routine basis (53).

Pelvic venography is performed in women with possible pelvic congestion syndrome and currently is the only reliable way to diagnose this syndrome. Transuterine venography has been the most commonly employed method due to its relative ease, low risk of complications, and relatively low cost (54–58). Water-soluble contrast medium is introduced into the uterine venous system via injection into the myometrium of the uterine fundus with a special single-lumen needle (Rocket Needle, Rocket Co., London, England). Several images are taken during the first minute after injection (59). The images are scored based on the maximum diameter of the ovarian veins, time of disappearance of contrast, and the degree of congestion of the ovarian plexus (see Table 31-9). The score can range from 3 to 9, with 3 or 4 being normal and 5 to 9 suggesting increasingly severe pelvic congestion. This method has a sensitivity of 91% and specificity of 89% and a likelihood ratio of 8.3 for a positive test and a likelihood ratio of 0.1 for a negative test.

Selective ovarian venography has also been used to diagnose pelvic congestion syndrome and can be performed either via a jugular venous approach or via the much more commonly used transfemoral approach (60,61). Special Teflon catheters are passed under fluoroscopic guidance into the ovarian veins and nonionic water-soluble contrast

TABLE 31-9. *Scoring system for assessing pelvic venography*

	Score		
	1	2	3
Maximal diameter of ovarian veins (mm)	1–4	5–8	> 8
Time to disappearance of contrast medium after end of injection (seconds)	0	20	40
Ovarian plexus congestion	Normal	Moderate	Extensive

medium injected. Because the right ovarian vein drains directly into the inferior vena cava, it is more difficult to cannulate and usually involves using a different type or size catheter than the left side. Some consider this invasive technique to be the method of choice for diagnosis of pelvic varicosities (62). Criteria that suggest venous congestion are maximum ovarian vein diameter of 10 mm, congestion of the ovarian venous plexus, filling of veins across the midline, or filling of vulvar and thigh varicosities (63,64).

In patients with suspected urinary tract involvement by endometriosis, ovarian remnant syndrome, ovarian retention syndrome, pelvic masses, and so on, intravenous pyelography has traditionally been used, but computerized tomography (CT) with intravenous contrast is a more accurate and informational technique and is preferable in most cases. In addition to evaluating for possible obstruction of the ureters, CT should be done to identify any effects that previous operations or the current condition have had on ureteral location. This is important because dense pelvic adhesions are usually encountered in these cases and may distort the anatomy and make the ureters difficult to identify during surgery (65). Serum urea nitrogen and creatinine levels should be obtained if there is evidence of ureteral dilation, hydronephrosis, or ureteral deviation.

Magnetic resonance imaging (MRI) has not been extensively used in women with CPP, but it holds great promise because of the superb anatomic images it provides. For the preoperative diagnosis of adenomyosis, MRI provides excellent soft tissue contrast, is minimally invasive, and avoids ionizing radiation (66). Magnetic resonance imaging is also helpful in the evaluation for obstructive uterine anomalies in adolescents with endometriosis. MRI has been investigated as a noninvasive diagnostic modality for pelvic congestion syndrome, but it is not yet clear if it will be of diagnostic value (67,68). Theoretically, magnetic resonance imaging should be very accurate in detecting an ovarian remnant, but, as with pelvic congestion, there have not been published reports to allow an evaluation of its utility.

Urodynamic testing is indicated if chronic urethral syndrome is suspected. This can identify patients with abnormal voiding patterns due to dyssynergic voiding. Voiding and electromyographic studies reveal prolonged or intermittent voiding patterns and hyperactivity of the pelvic floor or external urethral sphincter. Mean urinary flow rates are notably decreased, and mean flow times are increased with intermittent and prolonged flow rate patterns (69). Maximal urethral closure pressure is increased by twofold over normal in women with chronic urethral syndrome. In spite of the common symptom of incomplete emptying, women with chronic urethral syndrome do not have an increase in residual volume. Maximal intravesical pressure is normal, as is functional bladder capacity. Not all patients with clinical evidence of chronic urethral syndrome have urodynamic abnormalities.

Urodynamics may reveal uninhibited bladder contractions. Uroflowmetry when the patient experiences stranguria demonstrates the erratic prolonged flow characteristic of vesical-sphincter dyssynergia (70). Pelvic floor electromyography and pressure studies can also objectively document muscle spasm and inability to relax during voiding.

LAPAROSCOPY

Laparoscopy is liberally used by gynecologists in the evaluation of pelvic pain—over 40% of gynecologic diagnostic laparoscopies are done for CPP (6,71). Although laparoscopy sometimes is considered a routine part of the evaluation of gynecologic pain, ideally the decision about laparoscopy should be based on the patient's history and physical examination findings. This approach avoids unnecessary risks, expense, and false expectations by the patient.

In a review of 1524 laparoscopies for CPP, endometriosis was the most commonly diagnosed disorder (33%), followed by adhesive disease (24%), chronic PID (5%), ovarian cysts (3%), pelvic varicosities (less than 1%), leiomyomata (less than 1%), and a variety of other diagnoses (4%) (72). No visible pathology was detected in 35% of patients.

Unfortunately, many physicians consider laparoscopy the ultimate or definitive diagnostic evaluation of CPP and, when the findings are negative, may make one or more of the following statements to their patients.

1. There is nothing wrong.
2. The pain is in your head, and you should see a psychiatrist or psychologist.
3. You should have a neurolytic procedure, such as uterine nerve transection or presacral neurectomy.
4. The only thing that is left to do is a hysterectomy.
5. Nothing can be done, and you must learn to live with the pain.

Although statements 2, 3, and 4 may at times be appropriate, generally speaking all five statements are inappropriate without significant knowledge about the patient and evaluations other than a laparoscopy. A negative laparoscopy is not synonymous with no diagnosis or no disease. Laparoscopy must not be viewed as a final, definitive test. Realistically, the major role of laparoscopy for CPP is to diagnose endometriosis or adhesive disease. A meticulously performed negative laparoscopy means that a woman does not have endometriosis-associated or adhesion-associated pain; it does not mean that a woman has no physical basis for her pain.

There is evidence that telling the patient she does not have a life-threatening disease (e.g., ovarian cancer) or a serious gynecologic disease (e.g., endometriosis or apparent sterility) may be helpful, resulting in a decrease of subsequent pain in some women (73). However, this aspect of a negative laparoscopy is probably of limited benefit in most CPP patients. Indeed, in a randomized clinical trial, Peters et al. showed that omitting laparoscopy from the evaluation of women with long-standing CPP neither improves nor worsens their outcomes (28).

Conscious laparoscopic pain mapping (CLPM) is a diagnostic laparoscopy under local anesthesia, with or without conscious sedation, directed at the identification of sources of pain. CLPM has been reported to lead to the treatment of subtle or atypical areas of disease that might have been overlooked if the procedure had been done under general anesthesia (74). However, scant data have been presented to confirm this claim (75–78).

The technique used to map the pelvis is a gentle probing or tractioning of tissues and organs with a blunt probe or forceps passed through the secondary trocar site. There should be a systematic evaluation in this manner of the entire pelvis, seeking the presence or absence of tenderness and pain. Diagnosis of an etiologic lesion or organ should be based on the severity of pain elicited and on replication of the pain that is the patient's presenting symptom. Applying or injecting local anesthetic to sites of focal tenderness may block the pain response and possibly improve the predictability that surgical excision will be therapeutic. CLPM is not always successful. A successful CLPM occurs when all areas of the pelvis can be systematically inspected, including the base of the cul-de-sac, both fallopian tubes, and bilateral ovarian fossae, allowing for limitations due to adhesions. Unsuccessful CLPM has been reported in 0% to 30% of cases.

The results of published series of CLPM procedures have given inconsistent results. For example, endometriosis has been diagnosed in 10% to 85% of successfully mapped patients. This wide range may reflect differences in populations or may reflect differences in procedural techniques. It is clear that much more work needs to be done to define the role of CLPM in CPP. For example, one concern regarding CLPM is that the tenderness elicited by probing or traction is in response to a nonstandardized mechanical stimulus and hence may not be physiological or reproducible. This raises the question of whether the findings at CLPM using this methodology have any relevance to the patient's CPP. Furthermore, it remains to be seen whether the source of pain as identified at CLPM is indeed responsible for the symptom.

GYNECOLOGIC DISEASES: DIAGNOSES AND TREATMENTS

Accessory and Supernumerary Ovaries

Women can have extra ovarian tissue that is ectopic in its location, which may be a supernumerary or an accessory ovary. Accessory ovary is extra ovarian tissue that is invariably situated near a normally placed ovary, may be connected to it, and seems to have developed from it as tissue that was split from the embryonic ovary during early development. Supernumerary ovary is an extra ovary that is entirely separate from the normally placed ovaries and apparently arises from a separate primordium or anlage. Ectopic ovaries, either accessory or supernumerary, are

exceedingly rare. They normally produce no symptoms (79) but can occasionally be associated with CPP if they undergo cystic or neoplastic transformation.

Pelvic and lower abdominal pain are reported in 40% of cases of supernumerary ovary. The complaints range from dyspareunia to deep-seated chronic pelvic pain. Acute pain is sometimes a symptom and has been reported in cases of hemorrhage within a cyst. With accessory ovary symptoms are somewhat vague, including dysmenorrhea, metrorrhagia, and pelvic tenderness. Acute abdominopelvic pain occurred in one patient as a result of accessory ovarian torsion.

Ultrasonography is a noninvasive diagnostic tool that may be helpful in cases with a mass, but no cases of ectopic ovary have actually been diagnosed sonographically. Laparoscopic findings have directed the surgeons to the diagnosis in some cases. In suspected cases, a thorough examination of the pelvis and peritoneal cavity may locate the ectopic ovary. In particular, accessory ovaries are usually very small in size and are easily missed.

Adenomyosis

Adenomyosis is an ingrowth of endometrial glands and stroma into the myometrium at least one or two low power fields from the endometrium, at least 2 to 3 mm below the endometrial surface (80,81). If adenomyosis forms a nodule of hypertrophic myometrium and ectopic endometrium it is called an adenomyoma. Adenomyomas may be confused with intramural leiomyomas. The reported incidence of adenomyosis ranges from 5% to 70% (82–88), varying with the scrutiny of histologic evaluation and the patient's symptoms, age, and parity. About 80% of cases of adenomyosis are reported in women in their fourth and fifth decades of life.

Although the usual profile of a patient with adenomyosis is a parous woman with menorrhagia and dysmenorrhea, the presence of associated pelvic pathology in 60% to 80% of cases makes accurate diagnosis based only on symptoms and history very difficult. Not all women with adenomyosis are symptomatic. Of women complaining of menstrual disorders or pelvic pain, 22% and 24%, respectively, are found to have adenomyosis, frequencies not different from that of incidental adenomyosis.

The physical examination of the woman with adenomyosis who is symptomatic with pelvic pain, dysmenorrhea, and menorrhagia shows a symmetrically enlarged, tender uterus in 60% to 80% of cases, but it rarely exceeds a size of 12 weeks' gestation. The uterus is diffusely boggy to palpation, or it may have a nodular consistency, reminiscent of multiple small intramural fibroids.

Magnetic resonance imaging (MRI) may be useful for the preoperative diagnosis of adenomyosis. On T_2 weighted images, diffuse adenomyosis distorts normal zonal anatomy of the uterus, causing enlargement of the functional zone, seen as a wide band with low signal intensity adjacent to the endometrium.

Diagnostic hysteroscopy may show small diverticula when there is a connection between the ectopic sites of adenomyosis in the endometrial cavity (89). In symptomatic patients with a normal-appearing endometrial cavity, a hysteroscopic myometrial biopsy may be helpful.

Gonadotropin suppression with GnRH agonists may give temporary relief of symptoms, but medical therapy with GnRH agonists does not provide a definitive cure (90–92). There may be a role for endometrial ablation or resection in some patients with adenomyosis. Adenomyosis penetrating to a depth of 3 mm may be adequately treated with such uterine-preserving therapies, but more deeply penetrating disease may be left under a scar and may cause recurrent bleeding and pain. The principal method of diagnosis and therapy of adenomyosis is still hysterectomy.

Adhesions

An adhesion is fibrous tissue by which anatomic structures abnormally adhere to one another. Adhesions are well accepted as causes of intestinal obstruction (93,94) and infertility (95). However their role as a cause of CPP is controversial (6).

Adhesions are believed to cause pelvic pain that generally is exacerbated by sudden movements, intercourse, or certain physical activities. Often the pain is consistent in its location, although over time the area of involvement may expand. A history of one of the classic causes of adhesions—pelvic inflammatory disease, endometriosis, perforated appendix, prior abdominopelvic surgery, or inflammatory bowel disease—makes this a more likely diagnosis. At least one of these historical factors is present in 50% of women with adhesions (96).

Laparoscopy is the gold standard for diagnosing pelvic adhesive disease. Due to the uncertainty about the role of adhesions as a cause of CPP, it seems reasonable that women suspected of having pain associated with adhesive disease should undergo conscious laparoscopic pain mapping whenever possible. This could determine not only the presence of adhesions but also whether they are likely to be responsible for the pain.

Laparoscopy is not only the gold standard for the diagnosis of adhesion, but also in the hands of a skilled laparoscopic surgeon is the preferred method of treatment. Because patients with adhesions have significant risk of anterior abdominal adhesions many experts recommend open laparoscopy (97). This may not necessarily prevent injury to any bowel adherent at the umbilicus, however (98,99). Because of this we recommend a left upper quadrant trocar insertion. This allows insertion of the umbilical trocar under direct vision. Occasionally, adhesions will have to be cleared from the anterior abdominal wall or alternate insertion sites selected before other trocars can be inserted (100). Preoperative bowel preparation is recommended for all patients undergoing laparoscopic adhesiolysis.

Uncontrolled, observational studies show that laparoscopic lysis of adhesions is beneficial in reducing the pain level in 60% to 90% of patients with chronic pelvic pain (101–104). However, the only randomized trial of adhesiolysis (performed by laparotomy, not laparoscopy) failed to show any significant improvement in pain symptoms after lysis of adhesions, compared to a control group who did not undergo adhesiolysis (105). Only when a subgroup analysis of the 15 women with severe, stage IV adhesions was done was there any detectable improvement in pain that could be attributed to adhesiolysis. At the current time the best that can be stated is that adhesions are thought to produce chronic pain by some investigators but to be coincidental by others. Possibly a more accurate opinion might be that some adhesions produce pain sometimes, but not all adhesions produce pain all the time. This is an area where conscious laparoscopic pain mapping may prove to be especially valuable in future research.

Adnexal Cysts

Except for endometriomas, ovarian cysts usually do not produce CPP. This is not surprising because most other ovarian cysts capable of causing pelvic pain, such as hemorrhagic corpora lutea or follicle cysts, are usually asymptomatic, and when they cause pain, it is almost always acute. These cysts generally resolve spontaneously within one or two cycles and thus are rarely causes of CPP.

However, this does not mean that ovarian cysts never cause CPP. There are published cases of young women with recurrent functional cysts and CPP in whom prolonged ovarian suppression with oral contraceptives and repeated surgical interventions with laparotomies were necessary (106,107). The issue of when or if ovarian cysts are a cause of CPP is clinically important because the ovaries tend to form significant adhesions when surgically manipulated (108), and such adhesions may cause CPP (or infertility). Clearly, surgery on the ovary is best avoided unless benefits are likely, a judgment that is not always easy.

Bimanual pelvic examination usually establishes the location and size of adnexal cysts. Pelvic ultrasonography can show the location, size, and solid or cystic components. Computerized tomography may also be diagnostically helpful in some cases but is more expensive and not always necessary.

Hormonal suppression of nonfunctional, chronic ovarian cysts is generally unsuccessful. In the uncommon circumstance of cyclical, recurrent pelvic pain associated with functional cysts, hormonal suppression may be successful. Aspiration of adnexal cysts guided by ultrasound is possible, but the recurrence rate is almost 100% if they are of ovarian origin. Therefore, surgical extirpation or cystectomy remains the treatment of choice if hormonal suppression is unsuccessful. Unless contraindicated by sonographic evidence of malignancy, surgery may be performed laparoscopically. Patients who are candidates for laparoscopic treatment of adnexal cysts experience a more rapid recovery, less postoperative pain, and decreased adhesion formation (109,110).

Dysmenorrhea

Dysmenorrhea is the term applied to severe, cramping pain in the lower abdomen, lower back, and upper thighs that occurs during menses (111). It may be a symptom of reproductive tract disease, but it can also be a diagnosis in itself. It is termed *primary dysmenorrhea* when it is not a symptom of another disorder. *Secondary dysmenorrhea* is the term used when dysmenorrhea is a symptom of pelvic pathology. Dysmenorrhea is frequently a component of CPP. It is a common complaint of both adolescent and adult women and in the United States is estimated to cost 600 million work-hours and two billion dollars per year due to absenteeism (112).

Primary dysmenorrhea appears to be due principally to prostaglandins, in particular $F_{2\alpha}$ and E_2, released from the endometrium at menses (113–119). There are two major pathways of synthesis of prostaglandins. In the cyclooxygenase pathway, arachidonic acid is converted into cyclic endoperoxides, then into PGE_2, $PGF_{2\alpha}$, prostacyclin, or thromboxane A_2. It has been shown that both estradiol and progesterone levels influence the synthesis and levels of endometrial $PGF_{2\alpha}$ (120–122). The other metabolic pathway for arachidonic acid metabolism, the lipoxygenase pathway, leads to the formation of leukotrienes. Leukotrienes cause uterine muscle contractions and are potent vasoconstrictors and bronchoconstrictors. Many nonsteroidal antiinflammatory drugs (NSAIDs) block the cyclooxygenase pathway, but they do not block the lipoxygenase pathway (123,124). This observation may explain why these drugs do not relieve primary dysmenorrhea in all patients.

In addition to prostaglandins, several other factors may play a role in the etiology of dysmenorrhea. One is vasopressin, a powerful stimulant of the uterus, particularly at the onset of menstruation. There is a fourfold increase in circulating vasopressin levels during menstruation in women with dysmenorrhea over the levels in asymptomatic women. The effect of vasopressin is not thought to be mediated by prostaglandins because vasopressin levels are not decreased when dysmenorrhea is relieved by prostaglandin synthetase inhibitors (125).

Primary dysmenorrhea usually begins 6 to 12 months after menarche and coincides with the onset of ovulatory cycles. However, a large percentage of patients also complain of pain from the first cycle (126). Patients complain of spasmodic or cramping lower abdominal pain that may radiate suprapubically, to the low back, and to the anteromedial aspect of the thighs. The pain may also be of continuous dull aching character. Other symptoms, such as headache, nausea, vomiting, diarrhea, and fatigue, often accompany the menstrual pain. Symptoms typically last 72

hours or less. They may also start 1 or 2 days prior to the onset of menses. Occasionally, the accompanying vasoconstriction in the acute phase may be so marked that the patient appears to be shocky.

A careful pelvic examination should be performed to look for findings that suggest secondary dysmenorrhea, such as uterine enlargement or irregularity, pelvic masses, or pelvic tenderness. A rectal examination should be done to assess nodularity and tenderness along the uterosacral ligaments and cul-de-sac, findings suggestive of endometriosis. The presence of an intrauterine device may be confirmed by finding its string at the cervix. Primary dysmenorrhea is a diagnosis of exclusion. Sometimes a laparoscopy may have to be performed to rule out pelvic pathology, particularly endometriosis.

No laboratory tests are diagnostic or specific to primary dysmenorrhea. Although prostaglandin levels have been measured experimentally in menstrual fluid, this is not a clinically useful test.

Successful management of dysmenorrhea can be challenging. A healthy lifestyle, including nutritional supplements, and aerobic exercise such as walking, swimming, and bicycling may produce an overall benefit and decrease the impact of dysmenorrhea on the patient's daily activities. For appropriate selection of treatment, it is usually helpful to determine if dysmenorrhea is primary or secondary.

Oral contraceptives provide significant relief of primary dysmenorrhea. They suppress ovulation, resulting in lower levels of prostaglandins, and also markedly reduce spontaneous uterine activity. Oral contraceptives are a good first-line therapy for many young women, especially if contraception is also needed.

The NSAIDs that inhibit prostaglandin synthetase have had a pivotal role in treating primary dysmenorrhea (127–131). In a review of 51 published trials of primary dysmenorrhea treated with NSAIDs (132), 72% of patients had significant relief with NSAIDs compared to 15% with placebo. Unlike oral contraceptives, NSAIDs need to be taken only 2 to 5 days per month and do not suppress the hypothalamic-pituitary-ovarian axis. The choice of a particular NSAID depends on the clinical efficacy, side effects, patient acceptance, and individual clinical experience. NSAIDs should be started at or just before the onset of pain and continued regularly during the symptomatic period. They should be taken on an "as-needed" basis initially. If pain control with an as-needed regimen is insufficient, it is sometimes worth a trial of scheduled, regular dosing. Also, when pain is inadequately controlled, the initial or loading dose may be increased by up to 50% during the next cycle, but the maintenance dose should be kept the same. A trial of up to 3 to 6 months may be needed to demonstrate effective relief of symptoms. If a particular NSAID is ineffective, it is worth trying a different one because there is significant variability of individual responsiveness to NSAIDs. The side effects of NSAIDs include gastric irritation, heartburn, abdominal pain, nausea, vomiting, headache, occasional visual disturbances, allergic reactions, and blood disorders. However, these are unusual when these drugs are used on an intermittent basis for dysmenorrhea. The NSAIDs are contraindicated in patients with asthma or hypersensitivity to aspirin.

Calcium antagonists such as verapamil and nifedipine reduce uterine activity and contractility. They have produced relief in some resistant cases of dysmenorrhea. They may provide a different approach by decreasing the severity of myometrial contractions, decreasing intrauterine pressure and the resultant pain (133). They have no effect on other symptoms such as vomiting or diarrhea (134).

Transcutaneous electrical nerve stimulation can be used to treat dysmenorrhea. It relieves primary dysmenorrhea without any significant reduction of uterine activity and represents a nonpharmacologic treatment option (135). One study using TENS in two consecutive cycles in 61 sufferers reported 30% marked relief, 60% moderate relief, and 10% no relief of pain (136). Acupuncture also effectively treats primary dysmenorrhea (137).

Surgical interruption of neural pathways from the uterus may be done to decrease the pain of primary or secondary dysmenorrhea. Presacral neurectomy consists of transection of the sympathetic nerves of the superior hypogastric plexus at the sacral promontory. It has an efficacy of about 75% in relieving midline dysmenorrhea. Uterine nerve ablation by transecting the uterosacral ligaments may be more easily performed than a presacral neurectomy, but there are less reliable data regarding its efficacy. Cervical dilatation has been historically used to relieve dysmenorrhea thought to be secondary to cervical stenosis. Its value is debatable.

Endometriosis

Endometriosis is the presence of ectopic tissue that possesses the histological structure and function of the uterine mucosa (138–151). By definition it requires histological documentation of ectopic endometrial glands and stroma, that is, endometrium located outside of the endometrial cavity. It represents one of the most common causes of gynecologic pain (152–154). The prevalence of endometriosis in the general population is believed to be 1% to 7% (155–158). Because it is accurately diagnosed only by surgical biopsy with histologic confirmation, the true prevalence and incidence of endometriosis have been difficult to determine. In women who undergo a laparoscopy to evaluate chronic pelvic pain, the prevalence of endometriosis is about 33% (6). It remains an enigmatic disorder in that the etiology, the natural history, and the precise mechanisms by which it causes pain are not completely understood (159). In some patients it behaves almost like a malignancy, yet in others it is a seemingly irrelevant and insignificant finding; in some it is associated with incapacitating symptoms, but in others it is just an incidental histologic diagnosis; and in some cases it recurs "like dandelions in the grass," whereas in others excision results in its total and permanent elimination. It is truly a disease of contrasting characteristics.

Most women diagnosed with endometriosis-associated pain are 20 to 45 years of age, but it has been reported in girls as young as 10 years, and it may be a more common cause of pain in teenagers than is generally recognized. It may also occur in postmenopausal women, particularly if they are on estrogen replacement (160–162). About 70% of women with endometriosis and CPP are nulligravida, with a history of infertility or prior miscarriages.

Classically the woman with endometriosis presents with one or more of the following triad: an adnexal mass (endometrioma), infertility, or pelvic pain (163). Estimates are that 5% to 40% of women with endometriosis have chronic pelvic pain. Endometriosis-associated pelvic pain most often starts as dysmenorrhea, and about 75% of women with endometriosis-associated pelvic pain have dysmenorrhea as a component of their pain symptoms. Classically the dysmenorrhea pain of endometriosis is worst during the first several days of menses but also may be significant for several days prior to menses. Dyspareunia with deep penetration is also a frequent component of endometriosis-associated pain, occurring in 8% to 33% of cases. It may also continue postcoitally for several hours. Sometimes there is point tenderness with intercourse. When this occurs women may describe pain when a specific area is hit during coitus. When dyspareunia is referred to the rectum or lower sacrococcygeal area it may suggest rectovaginal septum or uterosacral ligament involvement. Although CPP, dyspareunia, and dysmenorrhea are characteristic symptoms of endometriosis, they are not as specific nor diagnostic as is commonly thought and by themselves do not justify a diagnosis of endometriosis.

Endometriosis involves the intestinal tract in 12% to 37% of women. Symptoms that may occur with intestinal involvement are tenesmus, dyschezia, constipation, diarrhea, and, rarely, hematochezia or symptoms of bowel obstruction. Severity of symptoms may not correlate with the extent of involvement or fluctuate with menses.

Urinary tract involvement occurs in 10% to 20% of women, most often at the bladder peritoneum and anterior cul-de-sac. Involvement of the distal one third of the ureter is possible and may lead in rare cases to obstruction. Often there are no symptoms secondary to bladder involvement, but frequency, pressure, dysuria, or hematuria occasionally are present.

Endometriosis may rarely cause significant pulmonary symptoms with lung involvement, such as dyspnea on exertion, pleural effusion, and lung collapse. Catamenial hemothorax has been reported. A cyclically bleeding or a cyclically tender mass in an incisional scar may also occur with endometriosis.

Treatment of endometriosis-associated pelvic pain is complex, and none of the options for therapy are ideal for all patients (Table 31-10) (164,165). Many factors must be considered in planning treatment, and the patient should

TABLE 31-10. *General treatment options for women with endometriosis-associated pelvic pain*

Observation with palliative treatment
Conservative surgery
Hormonal suppression
Combined medical and surgical treatments
Definitive extirpative surgery

be actively involved in the decisions. Her understanding of the disease will influence decisions about treatment. It is important to consider the location and extent of endometriosis, as well as severity of symptoms and any other pelvic pathology in planning treatment. The patient's age, reproductive plans, duration of infertility, and attitude toward surgery or toward hormonal medications may be vital components of the patient's needs or concerns. The patient's motivation and her emotional state may influence options and choices. Plans may need to be modified based on the tolerance of drug therapies or persistence or worsening of symptoms.

Ideally, the efficacy of any therapy is substantiated by data from randomized clinical trials, and fortunately such studies are available for medical and surgical treatment of endometriosis-associated pelvic pain.

Danazol, a 17-ethinyl-testosterone derivative, is one of the most commonly used medical treatments and has been used as the "gold standard" or control treatment for the evaluation of most other medical treatments (166). Danazol is contraindicated in patients with abnormal uterine bleeding, pregnancy, breastfeeding, or impaired renal, cardiac, or hepatic function. It is mildly androgenic and anabolic, activities that account for many of its side effects. It does not significantly affect LH and FSH levels in premenopausal women but lowers estrogen levels by directly inhibiting steroidogenesis at the ovarian and adrenal levels. It induces atrophic changes in the endometrium and endometriosis by its effect on estrogen levels. Its half-life is about 4 to 5 hours, so it must be dosed at least twice a day. Side effects are acne, edema, weight gain, hirsutism, voice changes, hot flashes, abnormal uterine bleeding, decreased breast size, decreased libido, vaginal dryness, nausea, weakness, and muscle cramps. From a placebo-controlled study, the absolute risk of side effects were acne 57%, edema 41%, muscle cramps 32%, and irregular spotting 63% (167). Weight gain averaged 2.6 kg in the danazol-treated patients. Exercise may decrease the number of side effects reported by patients receiving danazol by as much as one half. However, it has no effect on relief of pain or time to recurrence over that obtained with danazol only without an exercise program (168).

There is only one placebo-controlled, double-blind randomized clinical trial of danazol for the treatment of endometriosis-associated pelvic pain (167). Thirty-five patients with stage I or II endometriosis completed the trial. Danazol, given at a dose of 600 mg/d for 6 months, showed a decrease of mean pain scores of 80% at the end of 6 months' treatment, and 6 months after discontinuation of medication the average decrease of pain scores was 65%. At the end of the 6 months of danazol therapy, 3 (17%) of 18 patients treated with danazol had severe painful symptoms (including pelvic pain, low back pain, diarrhea, dysuria, and dyspareunia), compared to 12 (75%) of 16 in the placebo group (169). This means that there is about a 58% decrease in the number of patients with severe pain symptoms due to danazol treatment (absolute risk reduction) or that about two patients need to be treated with danazol to eliminate severe pain in one patient (number needed to treat [NNT] of 2).

Medroxyprogesterone acetate (MPA) has been a recommended treatment for many years. Suggested doses of MPA have been 10 mg three times a day orally or 100 mg intramuscularly every 2 weeks for 3 months, then 200 mg per month for 4 months. However, the only placebo-controlled, randomized clinical trial showing efficacy used a dose of 100 mg/d orally for 6 months. The efficacy of MPA at this high dosage was not statistically different from that of danazol. After 6 months of treatment there was a 71% decrease of pelvic pain scores and a 47% decrease 6 months after discontinuation of treatment. The number needed to treat for MPA for severe pain symptoms was 2, the same as that for danazol. Side effects of MPA include breakthrough bleeding, mood changes, depression, irritability, weight gain, and prolonged amenorrhea and anovulation after discontinuation of depot-MPA (167). Bone mineral density is decreased in women who use depot medroxyprogesterone acetate, even in the lower doses used for contraception (150 mg every 3 months) (170).

Gestrinone, a 19-nortestosterone derivative with mostly progestogenic and low androgenic activity, has been studied in at least two large randomized clinical trials, one comparing it to danazol (171) and one to leuprolide acetate (172). The dose of oral gestrinone was 2.5 mg twice weekly. Pain was relieved in 70% to 75% of patients treated with gestrinone and was not different from the control treatments. Side effects were similar to danazol, although more patients experienced hirsutism with gestrinone (about 40% vs. 10%) and leg cramps with danazol (about 25% vs. 15%). The randomized study of gestrinone versus leuprolide compared gestrinone to intramuscular leuprolide acetate 3.75 mg every 4 weeks for 6 months. Nonmenstrual pelvic pain was not different between the gestrinone and leuprolide groups pretreatment (VAS scores of 4.1 and 4.7, respectively) or at the end of 6 months of treatment (VAS scores of 1.2 and 1.6, respectively). However, 6 months after completion of treatment there was a lower pain level in the gestrinone group (VAS scores of 1.1 vs. 3.4, respectively). Bone density evaluations in this study showed that there was a decrease of 3.0% ± 4.8% at the end of treatment with leuprolide compared to a slight increase of 0.9% ± 2.1% with gestrinone. Gestrinone lowered HDL-lipoprotein levels by about 35%, whereas leuprolide caused no significant change.

Gonadotropin releasing hormone (GnRH) agonists are analogs of naturally occurring gonadotropin-releasing hormone. The GnRH agonists currently available for use in the United States are nafarelin, leuprolide, and goserelin. They all work at the hypothalamic-pituitary level to shut down LH and FSH production and release, although their initial effect is stimulation of activity. This "down-regulation" leads to a dramatic decline in estradiol levels. GnRH agonists may also have efficacy related to their effect on the immune system. For example, GnRH agonists have been shown to increase natural killer cell numbers and T-cell mitogenic activity (173).

Nafarelin is administered intranasally at a dose of 200–400 µg twice a day. Leuprolide is most often given intramuscularly in a depot form at a dose or 3.75 µg or 7.5 µg every 28 days. There is also a 3-month depot form. Goserelin is administered as a depot subcutaneous insertion or implant, 3.6 mg every 28 days. GnRH analog treatment is usually continued for 6 months. Side effects of the GnRH agonists are loss of bone density, hot flashes, vaginal dryness, decreased libido, headaches, emotional lability, acne, and reduced breast size. Nafarelin may cause nasal irritation. In a placebo-controlled trial of leuprolide, the absolute risk of side effects was hot flashes in 59% and headaches in 24%. Bone density loss was 11.8% after 6 months (174).

Only depot leuprolide acetate and triptorelin have been evaluated in randomized, placebo-controlled clinical trials (174,175,176). In a small randomized trial of leuprolide acetate treatment of women with stages I, II, III, or IV endometriosis, at 3 months there was a mean decrease of pelvic pain scores of 1.2 (on a 0-to-3 scale) compared to a 0.3 decrease in the placebo group. In a larger randomized clinical trial of 3 months of depot leuprolide, the objective was to demonstrate that empiric treatment based on a preoperative diagnosis of endometriosis was beneficial. However, the design of the study affords a placebo-controlled evaluation of the efficacy of 3 months of depot leuprolide acetate for treatment of women with CPP, dyspareunia, and dysmenorrhea, both with and without endometriosis. Leuprolide relieved dysmenorrhea in 100% of women in the study, compared to 41% with placebo (number needed to treat of 1.7). Leuprolide relieved dyspareunia in 86% of the women, compared to 39% with placebo (number needed to treat of 2.1). Pelvic pain was relieved in 80% of those treated with leuprolide, compared to 37% treated with placebo (number needed to treat of 2.3). When the analysis is separated by whether or not endometriosis was confirmed at the time of subsequent laparoscopy, in women with endometriosis pain was relieved in 81% treated with leuprolide, compared to 39% treated with placebo (number needed to treat of 2.3). In women without endometriosis, the corresponding responses were 73% and 17%, respectively (number needed to treat of 1.8).

In the triptorelin trial women with disease of mild to moderate stage were studied, and there was a mean decrease in visual analog scale pain scores of 4.9 (84%) in the treated group and 2.1 (34%) in the placebo group at the end of treatment at 6 months. Dysmenorrhea was totally relieved, as all women receiving triptorelin were amenorrheic during treatment. Dyspareunia was relieved in 77% of triptorelin-treated women and 45% of placebo-treated women. This gives an absolute risk reduction of 32% and a number needed to treat of 3 for dyspareunia.

There are a number of randomized clinical trials comparing the GnRH agonists leuprolide (177), goserelin (178,179), and nafarelin (180–182) to danazol. They show that there is no significant difference in efficacy of treatment of pelvic pain, dysmenorrhea, and dyspareunia between the GnRH agonists and danazol, with relief of symptoms in 50% to 70% of patients with either treatment (183). With either GnRH analog or danazol pain symptoms begin to return within the first year after discontinuation of treatment (184). For example, one trial of leuprolide versus danazol showed return of pelvic pain within one year in 30% to 60% and of dysmenorrhea in 65% to 75% of patients. As an aside, this study also looked at analgesic usage and did not show any change in the use of analgesics with either leuprolide or danazol.

When patients have a recurrence of pain within one year of treatment, retreatment with GnRH analogs appears to be fairly effective, with about two thirds of patients showing a significant reduction of pain levels during retreatment (185). However, retreatment with GnRH analogs within one year of completing a course of treatment results in further loss of bone density that is additive. For example, mean bone density loss with 3 to 6 months of nafarelin treatment at 400 µg/day was 1.4 ± 0.4%, loss with retreatment within one year was 0.6 ± 0.4%, and total loss of bone density with treatment and retreatment was 1.9 ± 0.8%.

Because of concerns about loss of bone density, studies have been done looking at less than 6 months of treatment and at add-back treatment with estrogen or progestogen. For example, Hornstein et al. (186) compared 3 months of nafarelin (plus 3 months of placebo) to 6 months of nafarelin in a double-blind, randomized clinical trial and found that about 74% of women had at least some improvement in pain in both groups. Less than one half of the patients completed the full 18 months of the study, but in those completing the study there were no significant differences in pain levels (although pain levels steadily increased during the 12 months of followup after discontinuation of treatment). An interesting aside from this study was that the degree of suppression of estradiol levels correlated with relief of dysmenorrhea but did not correlate with or predict relief of dyspareunia or pelvic pain.

In a randomized clinical trial of estrogen add-back therapy, patients with endometriosis-associated pelvic pain were assigned to one of four treatment groups for one year: (a) leuprolide, 3.75 mg every 28 days and oral placebo daily; (b) leuprolide, 3.75 mg every 28 days, and oral norethindrone acetate, 5 mg daily; (c) leuprolide, 3.75 mg every 28 days, and norethindrone acetate, 5 mg daily, plus conjugated equine estrogen, 0.625 mg daily; or (d) leuprolide, 3.75 mg every 28 days, and norethindrone acetate, 5 mg daily, plus conjugated equine estrogen, 1.25 mg daily (187). There were significant differences in loss of bone density between the groups. Those who received only leuprolide lost 6.3% of their mean bone density over the 52 weeks of the trial, in contrast to mean bone density losses in the lower and higher estrogen add-back groups of only 0.2% and 0.7%, respectively. Mean bone density loss in the group who received only norethindrone acetate add-back was 1.0%. Hot flashes were significantly decreased by about 50% in all three add-back groups. Suppression of menses also differed between the groups, with 100% suppression in both the leuprolide-only group and the norethindrone acetate-only add-back group, compared to 70% and 40% suppression in the lower and higher estrogen add-back groups, respectively. Differences in efficacy of treatment of dysmenorrhea, pelvic pain, and pelvic tenderness did not reach statistical significance. However, the higher estrogen add-back group approached significance for less effectiveness for dysmenorrhea and pelvic pain. Also, this group had more patients who dropped out of the trial prior to the completion of one year due to lack of improvement of symptoms than did the other groups. This study supports add-back therapy with 5 mg per day of norethindrone acetate, with or without 0.625 conjugated equine estrogen, for GnRH analog treatment of endometriosis-associated pelvic pain without any significant effect on efficacy but with notable improvement of safety for up to one year of treatment.

Oral contraceptive treatment was popularized by Kistner (188). He used high-dose pills such as Enovid and induced "pseudopregnancy" with the high levels of estrogen and progesterone. It is more common now to use low-dose pills in a cyclical manner to decrease dysmenorrhea or in a continuous method to induce amenorrhea. If breakthrough bleeding occurs with the continuous method, then the dose is doubled for 5 days to stop the bleeding and then decreased back to one per day for 6 to 9 months. No more than three or four pills per day should be used in trying to maintain amenorrhea. Side effects are weight gain, breast tenderness, nausea, chloasma, abnormal uterine bleeding, enlargement of myomas, thrombophlebitis and thromboembolism, increased appetite, irritability, depression, edema, hypertension, and increased vaginal discharge. Oral contraceptives are contraindicated in women with a history of or high risk of thrombosis or a history of breast cancer and relatively contraindicated with diabetes, collagen vascular disease, or hypertension.

There appears to be only one randomized clinical trial of oral contraceptives used for endometriosis-associated pain (189). This was a small study of 6 months' treatment with either low-dose contraceptive pills (0.02 mg ethinyl estradiol with 0.15 mg desogestrel daily taken cyclically) or monthly subcutaneous injections of goserelin 3.6 mg. The dose of ethinyl estradiol was increased to 0.03 mg if break-

through bleeding occurred in the contraceptive group. Although goserelin was more effective at relieving dysmenorrhea and possibly dyspareunia during treatment, there was no difference in relief of nonmenstrual pelvic pain. Six months after discontinuation of treatment, symptoms had recurred in all patients.

Not surprisingly, *conservative surgical treatment* is very common because symptomatic endometriosis often can be surgically treated at the same time as the laparoscopic diagnosis is done (190). The technical objectives of conservative surgery are to restore normal pelvic anatomy and to resect, coagulate, or vaporize all endometriosis implants. The clinical objective is to relieve pelvic pain. Surgery for endometriosis can be challenging, tedious, and frustrating, rivaling that for invasive carcinoma. The surgeon must be well versed in pelvic surgery, especially retroperitoneal dissection. Tissue planes are often obliterated, and lesions may involve vital viscera. Injuries to bowel, bladder, or ureter may be necessary components of the surgery in some patients. Inadvertent injuries to these organs, especially without recognition, are complications that obviously must be guarded against vigorously.

There is only one placebo-controlled, double-blind, randomized clinical trial of surgical treatment, and it was limited to women with stage I, II, or III endometriosis (191). Blinding was accomplished in this study by using a three-puncture technique in all procedures and not telling patients until 6 months postoperatively whether they had laser ablation or simply diagnostic laparoscopy. Followup data were collected by a study nurse also blinded to treatment group. At 3 months there was no statistical difference between the placebo and control groups. At 6 months 40% of women had alleviation of pain that could be attributed to treatment with laser laparoscopy. From this it is possible to calculate a number needed to treat (NNT) of 2.5. This means that to obtain pain relief at 6 months in one woman it was necessary to surgically treat two to three women. It is important to note that this study, the only published, placebo-controlled, double-blind, randomized clinical trial of surgical treatment, excluded women with stage IV endometriosis. Although there seems to be no reason *a priori* to assume that similar results would not occur in women with stage IV disease, it must be stated that there is no similar evidence regarding the efficacy of conservative, laparoscopic surgical treatment of endometriosis-associated pelvic pain in women with stage IV disease.

Both presacral neurectomy (192–195) and uterosacral neurectomy (uterine nerve resection or transection of the uterosacral ligament) (196–198) have been recommended for relief of CPP associated with endometriosis. For both procedures the evidence for efficacy is mostly from observational studies, although *presacral neurectomy* (PSN) has been evaluated in at least two randomized clinical trials. In the first study only eight patients with dysmenorrhea—four with PSN and four without PSN—were randomized (199). However, due to results in 18 nonrandomized patients combined with the results in the eight randomized patients, the monitoring committee stopped the study because of the marked difference in relief of dysmenorrhea between the groups. In the larger randomized trial it was shown that only midline dysmenorrhea was affected by adding PSN to conservative surgery for moderate or severe endometriosis (200). Presacral neurectomy had no statistically significant effect on the frequency and severity of dysmenorrhea, pelvic pain, or dyspareunia. Taken together these trials suggest that presacral neurectomy has a role in conservative surgery for endometriosis but is most effective for the treatment specifically of midline dysmenorrhea. There appears to be a small effect, if any, on nonmenstrual pelvic pain or dyspareunia. In women with failure or recurrent pain after PSN it is unwise to repeat the PSN due to retroperitoneal fibrosis and distorted anatomy.

The only published randomized trial of *uterosacral neurectomy* (USN), also called laparoscopic uterosacral nerve ablation or LUNA, was of central dysmenorrhea in women without endometriosis (201). It showed no improvement in any patient in the control group and relief in 45% of the USN group at one year of followup.

It seems very important to note that the data from all of the placebo-controlled trials suggest that, whether treatment of endometriosis-associated pelvic pain is with surgery or with medication, about one woman out of every two treated will obtain a clinically significant decrease in her pain that can be attributed to the treatment. The data do not suggest that there is any difference in the efficacy of medical or surgical treatment.

Based on this observation it seems appropriate to ask if combining surgical and medical treatments might improve the 50% absolute benefit obtained with either alone. Unfortunately, the results of two well-designed randomized, placebo-controlled clinical trials of postoperative medical treatment suggest little additional benefit of combination therapy (202,203). One study of women with stage III or IV endometriosis debulked via laparotomy and then treated with 3 months of nafarelin (400 ug per day) or placebo nasal spray showed that at 12 months postoperatively there was no difference in pain levels between the groups. The other study included women with stages I–IV endometriosis who underwent "reductive" laparoscopic surgery followed by 180 days of treatment with nafarelin, 200 µg b.i.d., or placebo nasal spray b.i.d. Although at 6 months, while still on medical treatment, the nafarelin group had lower pain levels, at 12 months (6 months after discontinuation of nafarelin) there was no statistically or clinically significant difference in pain scores between the nafarelin- and placebo-treated groups.

In summary, the evidence appears to suggest that 6 months of treatment postoperatively with GnRH analogs lowers mean pain levels while the patients are on the medication but does not affect pain levels at 12 months postoperatively. A reasonable way to interpret and apply these data is to initiate medical treatment after conservative sur-

gical debulking therapy if patients have persistent or recurrent pain, rather than treat all patients postoperatively.

In summary, gynecologists must recognize that the finding of endometriosis in women with CPP does not ensure that medical and/or surgical treatment of endometriosis will result in effective relief of pain. To the contrary, although treatment of endometriosis in women with pelvic pain is clearly indicated based on randomized, placebo-controlled, double-blind clinical trials, pain relief of 6 or more months' duration due to treatment can be expected in only about 50% of women with endometriosis-associated CPP.

If fertility is not desired, then hysterectomy, with or without bilateral salpingo-oophorectomy, is often recommended for endometriosis-associated pelvic pain. There is no consensus as to the advisability of removal of both ovaries if one or both are not directly involved by endometriosis. In one study evaluating this dilemma, recurrence of pain when one or both ovaries are preserved has been reported to occur in 62% of cases, compared to 10% when both ovaries are removed, giving a relative risk for pain recurrence of 6.1 (204). Reoperation for pain was also more likely with ovarian preservation, with 31% requiring reoperation, compared to 4% if both ovaries were removed at the time of hysterectomy for endometriosis. Although uncommon, endometriosis has been reported to recur after hysterectomy and bilateral salpingo-oophorectomy, with and without estrogen replacement therapy (205–207).

Endosalpingiosis

Endosalpingiosis is the presence of ectopic oviduct epithelium. Typical locations of endosalpingiosis are similar to those of endometriosis: pelvic peritoneum, uterus, fallopian tubes, ovaries, cul-de-sac, omentum, bladder serosa, bowel serosa, periaortic area, and skin (208). Endosalpingiosis is probably underreported because much of the surgery for endometriosis consists of ablation of all recognized peritoneal abnormalities without histological evaluation. Endosalpingiosis is thought to be commonly associated with previous tubal surgery such as tubal ligation or salpingectomy, as well as with "chronic salpingitis." Grossly, endosalpingiosis usually appears as punctate, 1–2 mm, white to yellow, opaque or translucent, fluid-filled, cystic lesions that give a granular appearance to the involved peritoneum. Histologically, endosalpingiosis is diagnosed by the presence of benign ciliated and nonciliated columnar cells along with peg cells in abnormal locations.

Endosalpingiosis-associated pelvic pain has been treated like endometriosis, with danazol, GnRH analogs, and surgery (208).

Endocervical and Endometrial Polyps

Cervical polyps are hyperplastic tumor-like formations of the cervix formed of epithelium and stroma. They are not true neoplasms. They are pedunculated, roughly pear-shaped, soft, smooth, and red or purple and vary from a few millimeters to 3 cm long. The pedicle almost always rises from the cervical canal but occasionally may arise from the external surface of the cervix (209). Endometrial polyps are pedunculated tumorous formations of the endometrium that are a hyperplastic phenomenon of the epithelium and stroma rather than a true neoplasm. They are found in up to 27% of all patients who have a cervical polyp and in 57% of postmenopausal women with cervical polyps. All cervical polyps present during tamoxifen treatment have been found to be associated with endometrial polyps.

About 40% of women with cervical polyps are symptomatic, with menometrorrhagia in 40% of those with symptoms, postmenopausal bleeding in 30%, postcoital bleeding in 12%, and abnormal vaginal discharge in 18%. Occasionally, women with endocervical polyps present with dysmenorrhea or with intermittent cramping pelvic pain.

All menopausal patients with a cervical polyp should have a diagnostic hysteroscopy or sonohysterography to demonstrate the presence or absence of an associated endometrial polyp.

Removal of cervical polyps is recommended for the asymptomatic patient. Polypectomy and endometrial sampling are recommended for the symptomatic patient. Endometrial polyps found by sonography, hysterosonography, or hysteroscopy should be removed hysteroscopically.

Leiomyomata

A leiomyoma is a benign tumor of smooth muscle; other names are *fibroid, fibromyoma,* or *myoma.* Uterine leiomyomas are the most common tumors of the female pelvis and occur in one in every four to five women, with the highest incidence in the fifth decade (210).

One of three women with myomas experiences pain, but it is usually dysmenorrhea. CPP in women with leiomyomata is more likely to be produced by associated pathology (e.g., endometriosis or adhesions) than by the uterine fibroid. Occasionally, pressure-type pain from myomas may present as CPP (211). In addition to pressure-type pain, leiomyomata may impinge on surrounding structures and cause pain. The onset of pain in such cases is usually gradual. Collision dyspareunia, rectal pressure, and pelvic discomfort are likely with a fixed retroverted fibroid that fills the cul-de-sac. Ureteral compression from very large myomas can produce hydronephrosis and back pain. Intermittent torsion of a pedunculated leiomyoma can cause sharp pelvic pain.

Leiomyomata can be diagnosed by finding an enlarged, firm, irregularly shaped uterus at the time of pelvic examination. With degeneration, the consistency of the myomas may become softer, or even cystic, to palpation. Rarely, the uterus may be tender. Sometimes it is difficult to differentiate uterine myomata from an adnexal tumor.

Ultrasonography can usually distinguish uterine from ovarian tumors. It also is valuable to document the number of fibroids, their location, degree of calcification, and rate of growth. Other imaging techniques such as computerized tomography and magnetic resonance imaging are too expensive to be routinely used but may sometimes be helpful in distinguishing ovarian from uterine masses. Laparoscopy is helpful to discover associated pathology in chronic pelvic pain patients.

Treatment of chronic pelvic pain associated with uterine fibroids includes expectant management, medical therapy, radiologic embolization, surgical removal or destruction of the myomas, and hysterectomy. Expectant management is an option if symptoms are not severe, the patient is approaching menopause, and repeat examinations can be performed every 6 months to assure there is no rapid growth. Nonsteroidal antiinflammatory drugs can be used to treat dysmenorrhea, and iron therapy may be necessary to treat anemia. Oral contraceptives and progesterone may be of limited benefit in treatment of dysmenorrhea or menorrhagia associated with myomas. Gonadotropin releasing hormone agonists (GnRH-a) have been effective in reducing the size and symptoms of leiomyomata. By creating a hypoestrogenic environment, the smooth muscle cellular component is reduced up to 50% in volume (212). Maximum reduction in size occurs after 3 months of therapy, but long-term control can be produced by prolonging the hormonal suppression. Unfortunately, regrowth to pretreatment size will occur within 12 weeks after cessation of GnRH-a. Therapy has been useful to reduce blood loss, treat iron deficiency anemia, and convert an abdominal to a vaginal hysterectomy.

Hysterectomy is usually the optimal way to ensure successful treatment with complete removal of all myomas and no recurrences. The vaginal route is preferred, either after GnRH-a, or by morcellation in skilled surgical hands. Laparoscopic hysterectomy or laparoscopically assisted vaginal hysterectomy may be performed with some of the advantages of a transvaginal hysterectomy. Laparoscopic supracervical hysterectomy is also an option in those patients with good pelvic support who wish to avoid a laparotomy.

Myomectomy is an option for those patients wishing to retain their reproductive potential. Myomectomy is sometimes discouraged due to a belief of an inordinate risk of blood loss and adhesion formation. There is no evidence that complications are increased with myomectomy versus hysterectomy. Use of dilute vasopressin, limited uterine incisions, and careful hemostasis assure reasonable blood loss and reduce postoperative adhesions. Laparoscopic myomectomy can now be performed with little blood loss and decreased recovery (213). However, uterine incision closure can be difficult and requires a surgeon skilled in laparoscopic suturing.

Hysteroscopic transcervical resection of submucous myomas is becoming more common in the surgical approach to infertility and abnormal uterine bleeding, but little is known regarding its benefit in those patients with pain. Other nonmedical therapies, including myolysis by electrodesiccation or cryotherapy, are under investigation. Arterial embolization has been demonstrated to decrease the size of fibroids, but long-term results are lacking (214).

Mittelschmerz

As described by Fehling in 1881, mittelschmerz is the lower abdominal pain that occurs at mid-cycle associated with ovulation. It is believed to be due to the release of fluid and blood from the ovarian follicle with ovulation. It is self-limiting and rarely lasts longer than 12–24 hours (215). However, it may recur on a monthly basis and present as CPP. Mittelschmerz is rarely a cause of severe recurrent pelvic pain, but in the rare cases where it is, treatment with oral contraceptives to suppress ovulation is usually effective.

Ovarian Retention Syndrome (Residual Ovary Syndrome)

Ovarian retention (or residual ovary syndrome) is the presence of pelvic pain, dyspareunia, or a pelvic mass after intended conservation of one or both ovaries at the time of hysterectomy (216,217). The reported incidence of ovarian retention syndrome ranges from 0.9% to 4.9% (218–222). It is proposed that adhesions interfere with ovarian function and ovulation, leading to a pelvic mass composed of multiple cystic, atretic, or hemorrhagic follicles and producing pelvic pain due to the ovary's inability to cyclically expand because of its encapsulation in dense adhesions (223,224).

Chronic lower abdominal or pelvic pain is the presenting symptom in at least two thirds of patients with ovarian retention syndrome. The intensity and cyclicity of pain may vary, with some patients suffering cyclically, whereas others suffer continuously. The quality of pain also differs and can range from a bothersome ache to recurrent colicky pain and incapacitating cramps. Pelvic pain is often referred to the site of the retained ovary. The pain can also radiate to the lower back and into the legs. Deep dyspareunia occurs in at least one fifth of patients.

On physical examination most patients have a tender pelvic mass at the vaginal vault. Diagnosis may be aided by the use of abdominal or vaginal ultrasound or computerized tomography (225). Intravenous pyelography may be important prior to surgical treatment because of the frequency of dense pelvic adhesions encountered with resultant distortion of ureteral anatomy (226). A diagnostic approach using GnRH agonists has been suggested based on the theory that because functional ovaries are an integral part of ovarian retention syndrome, suppressing their function should produce an amelioration of symptoms (227). Laparoscopy may also be used as a diagnostic test and has the advantage of being diagnostically and therapeutically beneficial. Conscious laparoscopic pain mapping may be useful in cases where the diagnosis is not clear.

Medical treatment with hormonal replacement therapy, continuous medroxyprogesterone, oral contraceptives, or GnRH agonists, rather than difficult surgery, has been suggested, but published results of such treatment are scarce. Salpingo-oophorectomy is the most common treatment and can sometimes be performed laparoscopically (228). Surgery usually involves extensive adhesiolysis, and because of that most reported series have been with abdominal laparotomy as the surgical approach.

Ovarian Remnant Syndrome

Ovarian remnant syndrome is the persistence of functional ovarian tissue inadvertently not removed at the time of intended extirpation of one or both ovaries, with or without hysterectomy. It is one of the least considered and least recognized conditions in the patient with pelvic pain who has had an oophorectomy (229–233). It has been shown experimentally that incompletely excised, devascularized ovarian tissue can reimplant and function (234). The diagnosis of ovarian remnant syndrome should be considered in any woman with lower abdominal pain or an ipsilateral pelvic mass several months or more after an oophorectomy. This is especially true in those with prior hysterectomy and bilateral salpingo-oophorectomy because too often it is assumed to be impossible for these women to have a gynecologic disease. This is unfortunate because up to 30% of such women may have ovarian remnant syndrome (11).

The major predisposing factor to ovarian remnant syndrome is a difficult oophorectomy due to prior pelvic inflammatory disease, adhesive disease from prior surgery, endometriosis, difficulty in hemostasis due to increased pelvic vascularity, and alteration of the anatomy by a neoplasm (235). Ovarian remnant syndrome is a disorder that usually occurs in the reproductive years (236). It usually presents as chronic pain of varying quality and severity in the abdominopelvic area, with or without a palpable pelvic mass. Because most of these patients have undergone multiple surgeries, including a hysterectomy and bilateral salpingo-oophorectomy, the possibility of a gynecologic cause is usually not recognized. The absence of hot flashes in a woman not receiving hormonal replacement following bilateral oophorectomy should be a signal to investigate carefully for ovarian remnant. Of reported cases, 70% to 100% have had no history of postmenopausal vasomotor symptoms in spite of not receiving hormonal replacement therapy.

Ovarian remnants are usually too small to be palpated abdominally. Tenderness to deep palpation may be present and if present is usually on the same side as the remnant. Pelvic palpation may reveal tenderness in one or both fornices. Bimanual pelvic exam may reveal a palpable mass, although its absence does not preclude the diagnosis. It is usually tender, small (less than 5 cm), and located on the pelvic sidewall (close to the ureters) or at the lateral vaginal apex, lateral to the vaginal fornices.

Vaginal ultrasound shows a pelvic mass in 50% to 85% of cases. The diagnostic accuracy of ultrasound may be improved by pretreatment with clomiphene citrate (237). A 5- to 10-day course of clomiphene citrate, 100 mg daily, appears to stimulate follicular formation in up to 90% of cases, and this may permit easier sonographic visualization. Not all ovarian remnants have functional follicles, so this technique is not consistently helpful.

Measurement of follicle-stimulating hormone (FSH) levels can be useful in cases of suspected ovarian remnant syndrome (230,232,236). If the woman is not on hormonal replacement, or it is withheld for 3 weeks or more, premenopausal FSH levels lower than 40 mIU/mL are present in about 50% to 75% of women with an ovarian remnant. A postmenopausal level of FSH does not absolutely exclude an ovarian remnant because it may have low metabolic activity and simply fail to produce estrogen levels sufficient to suppress FSH.

GnRH agonists initially stimulate gonadotropin production and therefore ovarian estrogen production, and this property offers another method for diagnosing ovarian remnant syndrome. A baseline level of estradiol is measured, and GnRH agonist (depot-leuprolide, 3.75 mg intramuscularly once, or leuprolide, 1 mg a day for 3 days subcutaneously) is administered, followed by a repeat measurement of estradiol 4 to 7 days later. If hormonally responsive ovarian tissue is present, then a significant rise in estradiol occurs. This test may not be reliable if exogenous hormones are being taken. The advantages of this test include the ease with which the marker can be detected, its widespread availability, and its ability to produce a response even when the remnant is extremely small.

Ovarian remnant syndrome is usually difficult to treat. Properly performed surgical excision appears to be the optimum treatment for the woman with chronic pelvic pain who has an ovarian remnant (231,232,238,239). Having said this, there is a postoperative recurrence rate of 8% to 15%, and multiple surgeries for remnants are not uncommon. Alternatives include medical treatment and radioablative therapy. Sonographically directed aspiration of cysts has also been suggested (240).

Medical therapy usually consists of hormonal suppression with depot-medroxyprogesterone acetate (150 mg intramuscularly each month), danazol (600 mg per day orally), depot-leuprolide acetate (3.75 mg intramuscularly each month), or combined estrogen-progestogen therapy. Radioablation of the ovarian remnant with 1000–2000 rads has been successfully used in a limited number of cases (241).

Pelvic Congestion Syndrome

Pelvic congestion syndrome is characterized by pelvic pain and dyspareunia associated with pelvic varicosities (pelvic veins that are consistently dilated to 5 mm or more) and congestion (slow drainage of dilated pelvic veins with resultant stasis). Congestive dysmenorrhea, or premenstrual cramping pain, is one of the most common symptoms and occurs in at least 90% of cases. Women with pelvic congestion tend to have episodes of severe, acute pelvic pain in addition to their underlying dull, aching chronic pain—94% of patients with pelvic congestion have this symptom. They tend to complain of moving pelvic pain locations, whereas patients with other pelvic pathology tend to complain of consistent pain locations. They also have exacerbation of pain by walking, standing, lifting, bending, and experiencing stress. Deep dyspareunia occurs in greater than 70% of cases. Postcoital ache, lasting in some cases up to 24 hours, is reported in 65% of cases.

Deep abdominal palpation at the *ovarian point,* which lies at the junction of the upper and middle thirds of a line drawn from the anterior superior iliac spine to the pubic symphysis, reproduces the pelvic pain complained of by the patient. On pelvic examination pelvic congestion patients usually have bilateral ovarian tenderness. The finding of both ovarian tenderness and postcoital aching is present in 94% of pelvic congestion patients. Superficial vulvar and paravulvar varices are sometimes observed in women with pelvic congestion (242). These may involve only the immediate medial aspect of the thigh or, in more severe cases, extend into the posteromedial thigh and buttock and spread down over the posterior aspect of the legs.

Although none of these clinical clues is specific enough to be diagnostic, they may still be useful to the clinician in planning the diagnostic evaluation. For example, if a woman with CPP gives a history of moving pelvic pain that is increased by most normal activities, has episodes of severe and acute pelvic pain, has aching pain after intercourse, has "congestive" dysmenorrhea, and has tenderness over both ovaries, then the likelihood of finding a pathologic abnormality at laparoscopy is less than 1%. In such a case evaluations other than laparoscopy, especially pelvic venography, may be more appropriate (243–249).

Pelvic venography has proved to be an invaluable tool in the diagnosis of pelvic varicosities. The two most common techniques used are selective retrograde ovarian venography and transuterine venography. These were discussed in the previous section on diagnostic tests.

Appropriate therapy for pelvic congestion is uncertain. One of the first treatments for PCS was surgical ovarian vein ligation. Ligations may now be performed laparoscopically using titanium clips or suture ligation to occlude the veins (242). Radiologic transcatheter embolization of the ovarian veins has been suggested as an alternative to surgical ligation (250–252). With followup ranging from 6 months to 4 years, pain relief has been reported in 58% to 100% of patients. All reports of ligation and embolization have been observational.

Medroxyprogesterone acetate (MPA) has been evaluated in a randomized controlled trial, with and without psychotherapy. The results showed that MPA was effective after 2 months and that its efficacy was increased by psychotherapy. However, pain returned when treatment was stopped. The combination of GnRH agonist with add-back (estradiol valerate and MPA) also showed some efficacy (253). Hormonal treatment generally has not been a feasible long-term approach, particularly in the younger woman.

Surgical treatment with hysterectomy and bilateral salpingo-oophorectomy has shown efficacy in women with venographically documented PCS who had failed to obtain relief with long-term medical therapy (254). Because the majority of such women are in their reproductive years, the benefits of extirpative surgery must be carefully weighed against the drawbacks of loss of fertility and the necessity of long-term hormone replacement therapies. Also, the use of objective diagnostic criteria is crucial.

Pelvic Floor Pain Syndrome

Pelvic floor pain syndrome (PFPS) is caused by or associated with pain and tenderness of the levator ani, coccygeus, or piriformis muscles or their associated fascia or insertions. As a major component of the musculoskeletal system of the pelvis, the pelvic floor is not infrequently a contributor to chronic pelvic pain (CPP) and in some cases may be the primary cause (255). It may be a form of tension myalgia that mechanistically produces pain much as tension headaches produce pain (256). CPP due to pelvic floor dysfunction was first brought to "modern" attention by Thiele in the 1930s (257). He termed the syndrome *coccygodynia*, but numerous other names (e.g., pelvic floor myalgia, piriformis syndrome, levator ani spasm syndrome, and diaphragma pelvis spastica) have been used for pain thought secondary to the levator ani, coccygeus, and piriformis muscles (258,259).

PFPS occurs predominantly in women in their 40s and 50s. Most have been treated for numerous other problems, such as endometriosis, pelvic inflammatory disease, low back pain, lumbar disc disease, or degenerative joint disease, prior to the diagnosis of PFPS.

Abnormalities of posture are probably more important than generally appreciated in the etiology of this syndrome. Many of the women are "slumpers" or "slouchers" who sit with pressure on the upper buttocks, coccyx, and base of the spine rather than on the ischial tuberosities. Prolonged sitting in this posture may result in fatigue and spasm of the supporting pelvic muscles. Also, a particular abnormal posture, termed "typical pelvic pain posture," has been noted in a majority of women with CPP. This is a kyphosis-lordosis or occasionally just a marked lordosis. PFPS may also result from trigger points of one or more of the muscles of the pelvis.

Symptoms are usually vague and poorly localized. Pain may be diffuse within the pelvis, more localized about the rectum or the anterior pelvis, or unilateral. Low back pain and radiation to the sacrum at the area of insertion of the

levator ani are not uncommon (greater than 80% of patients). Radiation to the hip and down the back of the thigh, like sciatica, may also be noted and is particularly characteristic of piriformis spasm. Pain is most often described as aching, throbbing, or heaviness. Similarly to patients with pelvic relaxation disorders, patients may describe the sensation as one of "everything falling out or dropping." Pain may be quite severe and in some patients has a characteristic of acute attacks that awake the patients from sleep with rectal pain ("proctalgia fugax") or vaginal pain ("colpalgia fugax"). Characteristically, pain from spasm of the levator ani starts in the afternoon and becomes progressively worse. Pain is increased by long sitting or prolonged standing in one position. Characteristically, it is not worsened by bowel movements. However, dyspareunia is a common symptom.

The most common finding with PFPS is tenderness and spasm of one or more of the levator muscles (puborectalis, pubococcygeus, and iliococcygeus). Digital pressure on the involved muscle characteristically reproduces or intensifies the patient's pain. It is not unusual for the tenderness to be unilateral. In some patients with PFPS, there is also tenderness of the coccyx, lateral sacrum, or sacrococcygeal ligaments.

The diagnosis of PFPS is by clinical history and physical findings. No imaging or laboratory evaluations are useful in establishing the diagnosis. However, because PFPS may frequently occur secondary to other pelvic pathology, evaluations may be needed to rule out diagnoses such as endometriosis or adhesions. This is especially true if PFPS does not respond to appropriate physical therapy and medical treatment.

The classic treatment for PFPS is Thiele's massage. This is done with the rectal finger massaging the involved, tender muscles with a firm sweeping motion. Fifteen to twenty strokes, taking about 5 minutes, are done at each treatment. Treatments are repeated daily for 4 to 5 days, then every other day until improvement. Most often, about six sessions are needed. The initial sessions are usually quite uncomfortable, and most patients note an exacerbation of pain after the first one or two treatments. Many women find it less unpleasant if the technique is modified to transvaginal massage rather transrectal.

Hot sitz baths may also be helpful, either as an adjunct to Thiele's massage or as an initial therapy prior to starting massage. Vaginal and rectal diathermy, ultrasound, bedrest, relaxation exercises, biofeedback training, analgesics, Kegel exercises, TENS unit, acupuncture, vaginal electrical stimulation, and infiltration with steroid and/or local anesthetic (especially if trigger points are present) are all treatments for PFPS. Treatment with muscle relaxants, particularly diazepam, may be helpful for acute control of spasm and pain. There are no well-performed studies that allow a recommendation of any specific treatment modality or combination at this time. Coccygectomy is sometimes done for this syndrome but probably has little if any role in the modern management of the problem.

Peritoneal Cysts

Peritoneal mesothelial cysts are rare, but when present they may be a cause of CPP. The proper nomenclature for these cysts is not clear, nor is it clear if the diverse cases reported with varied names represent the same process (260). There are probably at least two distinct types that are associated with CPP. One is related to surgical adhesive disease and is probably best termed *postoperative peritoneal cysts* or *peritoneal inclusion cysts* (261–264). The other is a reactive mesothelial proliferation and may or may not be related to surgery and adhesive disease. It is probably best termed *benign cystic mesothelioma* or *multicystic peritoneal mesothelioma*. Neither is a neoplasm nor premalignant.

Postoperative peritoneal cysts (POPC) may occur months to years after surgery and occur after a variety of operative procedures (265). POPCs are loculated areas between adherent viscera in which fluid accumulates. Although they have been reported after removal of both ovaries, they appear to be more common if one or both ovaries remain. They have been reported only in women. Almost all women with these cysts present with abdominopelvic pain and a palpable pelvic mass (266). The mean age at presentation is 38 years, with a range of 24 to 46 years (267).

Benign cystic mesotheliomas (BCMs) have been reported more frequently than postoperative peritoneal cysts (268). BCMs represent a nonneoplastic reactive mesothelial proliferation. Many, but not all, patients have a history of endometriosis, pelvic inflammatory disease, or prior abdominal surgery. Benign mesothelial cysts have been reported in men but are much more common in women. Although BCMs may occur anywhere in the peritoneum, they are most commonly found in the pelvis.

More than 80% of patients with either POPC or BCM present with chronic or recurrent abdominopelvic pain. Pain often starts as a gradual development of lower abdominal fullness, bloating, or distention. There may be associated dysuria and constipation (269). Most of the cases without pain have presented with asymptomatic abdominopelvic masses.

At the time of physical examination, tenderness in the area of a POPC or PCM is usually present, although a mass is not always palpable. When present, a mass is generally located in the pelvis and is soft, cystic, and tender, with sizes ranging from 4 to 24 cm.

Ultrasonography almost always reveals POPCs and PCMs as complex, cystic masses with thin walls and septations. In patients with ovaries, ovarian fluid may produce cysts around the ovaries, causing the sonographic appearance of a complex adnexal mass. By transvaginal ultrasound it may be distinguished from a malignancy by the appearance of an intact ovary amid septations and fluid.

Several medical treatments have shown varying degrees of success in case reports. Tamoxifen, 20 mg per day, has been used to treat one case of benign cystic mesothelioma in a 19-year-old woman (270). Depot leuprolide, 3.75 mg per month, also has been used to treat a patient symptomatic with recurrent benign cystic mesothelioma, but response was insufficient, and surgery was still necessary (271).

Surgical treatment is often necessary and is usually difficult and complicated. POPCs are invariably adherent to adjacent structures, and tissue planes are poorly defined. It is usually not feasible to perform the surgery laparoscopically. Laparoscopic excision has been reported for benign cystic mesotheliomas (272). With POPCs and BCMs the risk of recurrence is 30% to 50% after surgical resection (273).

Transvaginal or percutaneous aspiration with ultrasound guidance is also a treatment option (265,267). Aspiration is not always successful, especially with large masses, and about 50% of cases recur (268). In cases that recur, repeat drainage followed by ethanol instillation may be an option. Cystic mesothelioma has also been successfully treated by using tetracycline, 25 mL of 1.3% solution, as a sclerosing agent (274).

Symptomatic Pelvic Relaxation (Genital Prolapse)

The pelvic floor is the supportive layer that prevents the abdominal and pelvic organs from falling through the opening of the bony pelvis (275,276). With damage or loss of strength of the fascia and muscles of the pelvic floor, relaxation or support defects may occur. Pelvic support disorders are common and account for almost 400 000 surgical procedures annually in the United States (277). Most of these procedures are for correction of function, not for the relief of pelvic pain. However, relaxation disorders of the pelvic floor can cause pelvic and back pain and should be considered as possible causes or contributors during the evaluation of the woman with chronic pelvic pain (CPP). Because the diagnosis is usually apparent from the physical examination, and pain is most often mild in intensity, it is common to neglect the potential role of pelvic floor support defects in CPP.

Most often, women with pelvic floor relaxation have a painful, dragging sensation where the tissues connect to the pelvic wall (usually identified by the patient as occurring in the groin and pelvis) and sacral backache caused by traction on the uterosacral ligaments. The symptoms may subside when the patient is lying down and seem minimal in the morning but increase progressively the longer she is erect and active (278). Most patients also have an underlying sense of heaviness, fullness, or insecurity that it is difficult for them to describe and is often expressed as a feeling that "something is just not right." Although this is difficult for patients to put into words, it causes significant distress and should not be ignored. There may be pain during sexual intercourse, or penetration may be obstructed because of tissue protruding outside the introitus. The frequency of intercourse may be diminished because of anxiety on the part of the partner.

Therapy of pelvic floor relaxation with physiotherapy may recover some muscle function. Biofeedback-assisted pelvic floor rehabilitation exercises have reduced reports of pain by an average of 83% and allowed three fourths of patients to resume intercourse (279,280). Neuromuscular electrical stimulation has been used to excite motor and sensory fibers of the pudendal nerves, produce a pelvic floor muscle contraction, and thus increase the strength of the muscles and treat pelvic floor relaxation syndromes (281). None of these treatments is able to restore the pelvic floor to its original structure and function.

Surgical therapy for pelvic floor relaxation addresses specific defects in the fascial layers that have been disrupted. The appropriate surgical reapproximation of this fascial layer depends upon the accurate diagnosis of the fascial layer involved. Details of surgical repair are not discussed in this chapter because such reconstructive surgery constitutes a major component of gynecological surgical education and training and is discussed in depth in many surgical texts.

Tuberculous Pelvic Inflammatory Disease

Although not a common diagnosis in the United States, tuberculous PID must be remembered as a potential diagnosis in women with CPP, especially because the incidence of tuberculosis (TB) has increased in association with human immunodeficiency virus-autoimmune deficiency disease (HIV-AIDS). As many as 25% of women with pulmonary TB have pelvic TB (282), and about 25% of women with pelvic tuberculosis have CPP (283).

Acute Diseases

It must be remembered that women with chronic pelvic pain are no less likely than the rest of the population to develop acute and serious illnesses, such as appendicitis or cystitis. Thus, with acute exacerbations of pain it is important to remember to review the symptoms and reevaluate the patient as appropriate to rule out the possibility of acute medical or surgical conditions.

REFERENCES

1. Zondervan KT, Yudkin PL, Vessey MP et al. Prevalence and incidence in primary care of chronic pelvic pain in women: evidence from a national general practice database. *Br J Obstet Gynaecol* 1999;106:1149–1155.
2. Walker EA, Katon WJ, Jemelka RP, et al. The prevalence of chronic pelvic pain and irritable bowel syndrome in two university clinics. *J Psychosom Obstet Gynecol* 1991;12(Suppl):65–75.
3. Jamieson DJ, Steege JF. The prevalence of dysmenorrhea, dyspareunia, pelvic pain, and irritable bowel syndrome in primary care practices. *Obstetr Gynecol* 1996;87:55–58.
4. Mathias SD, Kuppermann M, Liberman RF, et al. Chronic pelvic pain: prevalence, health-related quality of life, and economic correlates. *Obstet Gynecol* 1996;87:321–7.
5. Reiter RC. A profile of women with chronic pelvic pain. *Clin Obstet Gynecol* 1990;33:130–138.
6. Howard FM. The role of laparoscopy in chronic pelvic pain: promise and pitfalls. *Obstet Gynecol Survey* 1993;48:357–387.
7. Reiter RC, Gambone JC. Nongynecologic somatic pathology in women with chronic pelvic pain and negative laparoscopy. *J Reprod Med* 1991;36:253–259.
8. Steege JF, Stout AL. Resolution of chronic pelvic pain after laparoscopic lysis of adhesions. *Am J Obstet Gynecol* 1991;165:278–281.
9. Steege JF. Assessment and treatment of chronic pelvic pain. *Telinde's operative gynecology updates* 1992;1:1–10.
10. Reiter RC, Shakerin LR, Gambone JC, Milburn AK. Correlation between sexual abuse and somatization in women with somatic and nonsomatic chronic pelvic pain. *Am J Obstet Gynecol* 1991;165:104–109.
11. Howard FM. Laparoscopic evaluation and treatment of women with chronic pelvic pain. *J Amer Assoc Gynecol Laparoscopists* 1994;1:325–331.
12. Walker E, Katon W, Harrop-Griffiths J, et al. Relationship of chronic pelvic pain to psychiatric diagnoses and childhood sexual abuse. *Am J Psychiatry* 1988;145:75–80.
13. Longstreth GF, Preskill DB, Youkeles L. Irritable bowel syndrome in women having diagnostic laparoscopy or hysterectomy. Relation to gynecologic features and outcome. *Digest Dis Sci* 1990;35:1285–1290.
14. Mens JMA, Vleeming A, Stoeckart R, et al. Understanding peripartum pelvic pain: implications of a patient survey. *Spine* 1996;21:1363–1370.
15. Reiter RC. Chronic pelvic pain. *Clin Obstet Gynecol* 1990;33:117.
16. Rapkin AJ, Mayer EA. Gastroenterologic causes of chronic pelvic pain. *Obstet Gynecol Clin NA* 1993;20:663–683.
17. Rapkin AJ. Adhesions and pelvic pain: a retrospective study. *Obstet Gynecol* 1986;68:13–15.
18. Malinak LR. Pelvic pain—when is surgery indicated? *Contemp Ob/Gyn* 1985;26:43–50.
19. Rapkin AJ, Karnes LD. New hope for patients with chronic pelvic pain. *The Female Patient* 1988;31:100–117.
20. Low WY, Edelmann RJ, Sutton C. Short term psychological outcome of surgical intervention for endometriosis. *Br J Obstet Gynaecol* 1993;100:191–192.
21. Mahmood TA, Templeton AA, Thomson L, Fraser C. Menstrual symptoms in women with pelvic endometriosis. *Br J Obstet Gynaecol* 1991;98:558–563.
22. Westrom L. Effect of acute pelvic inflammatory disease on fertility. *Am J Obstet Gynecol* 1975;121:707–712.
23. Ranaer M., ed. *Chronic pelvic pain in women.* New York: Springer-Verlag, 1981: 93.
24. Dulemba JF. Spilled gallstones causing pelvic pain. *J Amer Assoc Gynecol Laparoscopists* 1996;3;309–311.
25. Pfeifer ME, Hansen KA, Tho SPT, et al. Ovarian cholelithiasis after laparoscopic cholecystectomy associated with chronic pelvic pain. *Fertil Steril* 1996;66:1031–1032.
26. Sexton DJ, Heskestad L, Lambeth WR, et al. Postoperative pubic osteomyelitis misdiagnosed as osteitis pubis—report of 4 cases and review. *Clin Infect Dis* 1993;17;695–700.
27. Barbieri RL. Stenosis of the external cervical os: an association with endometriosis in women with chronic pelvic pain. *Fertility & Sterility* Sep 1998;70(3):571–573.
28. Peters AAW, van Dorst E, Jellis B, et al. A randomized clinical trial to compare two different approaches in women with chronic pelvic pain. *Obstet Gynecol* 1991;77:740–744.
29. Walker EA, Sullivan MD, Stenchever MA. Use of antidepressants in the management of women with chronic pelvic pain. *Obstet Gynecol Clin NA* 1993;20:743–751.
30. Rapkin AJ, Kames LD. The pain management approach to chronic pelvic pain. *J Reprod Med* 1987;32:323–327.
31. Rapkin AJ, Kames LD, Darke LL, et al. History of physical and sexual abuse in women with chronic pelvic pain. *Obstet Gynecol* 1990;76:92–96.
32. Walling MK, Reiter RC, O'Hara MW, et al. Abuse history and chronic pain in women: I. Prevalences of sexual abuse and physical abuse. *Obstet Gynecol* 1994;84:193–199.

33. Stout AL, Steege JF, Dodson WC, Hughes CL. Relationship of laparoscopic findings to self-report of pelvic pain. *Am J Obstet Gynecol* 1991;164:73–79.

34. Thompson TL. Managing the "difficult" Ob/Gyn patient. *The Female Patient* 1990;15:81.

35. Steege JF, Ling FW. Dyspareunia. a special type of chronic pelvic pain. *Obstet Gynecol Clinics NA* 1993;20:779–793.

36. Bavendam TG. Irritable bladder—a commonsense approach. *Contemporary Ob/Gyn* April 1993:70–77.

37. Propst AM, Storti K, Barbieri RL. Lateral cervical displacement is associated with endometriosis. *Fertility & Sterility* Sept 1998;70(3):568–570.

38. Slocumb JC. Neurologic factors in chronic pelvic pain: trigger points and the abdominal pelvic pain syndrome. *Am J Obstet Gynecol* 1984;149:536–543.

39. Solomons CC, Melmed MH, Heitler SM. Calcium citrate for vulvar vestibulitis: a case report. *J Reprod Med* 1991;36:879–882.

40. Lanzone A, Marane R, Muscatello R, et al. Serum Ca-125 levels in the diagnosis and management of endometriosis. *J Reprod Med* 1991;36:603.

41. Adamson GD. Diagnosis and clinical presentation of endometriosis. *Am J Obstet Gynecol* 1990;162:568.

42. Fedelle L, Bianchi S, Dorta M. Transvaginal ultrasonography in the differential diagnosis of adenomyoma versus leiomyoma. *Am J Obstet Gynecol* 1992;167:603–606.

43. Bohlman ME, Ensor RE, Saunders RC. Sonographic findings in adenomyosis of the uterus. *Am J Roentgenal* 1987;148:765–766.

44. Bonilla-Musoles F, Raga F, Osborne NG, et al. Three-dimensional hysterosonography for the study of endometrial tumors: comparison with conventional transvaginal sonography, hysterosalpingo-sonography, and hysteroscopy. *Gynecol Oncol* 1997;65:245–252.

45. Cohen JR, Luxman D, Sagi J, et al. Sonohysterography for distinguishing endometrial thickening from endometrial polyps in postmenopausal bleeding. *Ultrasound Obstet Gynecol* 1994;4:227–230.

46. Hall DA, Yoder IC. Ultrasound evaluation of the uterus. In: Callen PW, ed., *Ultrasonography in obstetrics and gynecology.* Philadelphia: WB Saunders, 1994:586–614.

47. Kaminski PF, Sorosky JI, Mandell MJ, et al. Clomiphene citrate as an adjunct in locating ovarian tissue in ovarian remnant syndrome. *Obstet Gynecol* 1990;76(5 Part 2):924–926.

48. Montanari GD, Alfieri G, Grella P, et al. Ultrasonic tomography in the diagnosis of pelvic congestion. *Minerva Ginecologica* 1975;27(3):219–223.

49. Frede TE. Ultrasonic visualization of varicosities in the female genital tract. J *Ultrasound Med* 1984;3(8):365–369.

50. Taylor KJW, Burms PN, Woodcock JP. Blood flow in deep abdominal and pelvic vessels: ultrasonic and pulsed Doppler analysis. *Radiology* 1985;154:487–493.

51. Fleischer AC, Kepple DM. *Transvaginal color duplex sonography: clinical potentials and limitations.* Seminars in Ultrasound, CT and MR 1992;13(1):69–80.

52. Smith MR. Pulsatile pelvic masses: options for evaluation and management of pelvic arteriovenous malformations. *Am J Obstet Gynecol* 1995;172(6):1857–1863.

53. Rapkin AJ, Mayer EA. Gastroenterologic causes of chronic pelvic pain. *Obstet Gynecol Clin NA* 1993;20:663–683.

54. Hammen R. The technique of pelvic phlebography. *Acta Obstet Gynecol Scand* 1965;44:370–374.

55. Bellina JH, Dougherty C, Michal A. Transmyometrial pelvic venography. *Obstet Gynecol* 1969;34(2):194–199.

56. Beard RW, Highman JH, Pearce S, Reginald PW. Diagnosis of pelvic varicosities in women with chronic pelvic pain. *Lancet.* 1984;ii:946–949.

57. Hammen R. The technique of pelvic phlebography. *Acta Obstet Gynecol Scand* 1965;44:370–374.

58. Bellina JH, Dougherty C, Michal A. Transmyometrial pelvic venography. *Obstet Gynecol* 1969;34(2):194–199.

59. Murray E, Comparato MR. Uterine phlebography. *Am J Obstet Gynecol* 1968;102(8):1088–1093.

60. Tarazov PG, Prozorovskij KV, Ryzhkov VK. Pelvic pain syndrome caused by ovarian varices. Treatment by transcatheter embolization. *Acta Radiologica* 1997;38:1023–1025.

61. Sichlau MJ, Yao JST, Vogelzang RL. Transcatheter embolotherapy for the treatment of pelvic congestion syndrome. *Obstet Gynecol* 1994;83(5)part 2:892–896.

62. Capasso P, Simons C, Trotteur G, et al. Treatment of symptomatic pelvic varices by ovarian vein embolization. *Cardiovasc Intervent Radiol* 1997;20:107–111.

63. Kennedy A, Hemmingway A. Radiology of ovarian varices. *Br J Hosp Med* 1990;44:38–43.

64. Kennedy A, Hemmingway A. Radiology of ovarian varices. *Br J Hosp Med* 1990;44:38–43.

65. Berek JS, Darney PD, Lopkin C, Goldstein DP. Avoiding ureteral damage in pelvic surgery for ovarian remnant syndrome. *Am J Obstet Gynecol* 1979;133:221–222.

66. Mark AS, Hricak H, Heinrich LW. Adenomyosis and leiomyoma: differential diagnosis with MR imaging. *Radiology* 1987;168:527–529.

67. Joja I, Asakawa M, Motoyama K, et al. Uterine cirsoid aneurysm: MRI and MRA. *Journal of Assisted Tomography* 199620(2):290–294.

68. Gupta A, McCarthy S. Pelvic varices as a cause for pelvic pain, MRI appearance. *Magnetic Resonance Imaging* 1994;12(4):679–681.

69. Summit Jr RL. Urogynecologic causes of chronic pelvic pain. *Obstet Gynecol Clin NA* 1993;20:685–698.

70. Kaplan WE, Firlit CF, Schoenberg HW. The female urethral syndrome: external sphincter spasm as etiology. *J Urol* 1980;124:48–49.

71. Roseff SJ, Murphy AA. Laparoscopy in the diagnosis and therapy of chronic pelvic pain. *Clin Obstet Gynecol* 199033:137.

72. Howard FM. The role of laparoscopy in the evaluation of chronic pelvic pain: pitfalls with a negative laparoscopy. *J Am Assoc Gynecol Laparosc* 1996;4:85–94.

73. Baker PB, Symonds EM. The resolution of chronic pelvic pain after normal laparoscopic findings. *Am J Obstet Gynecol* 1992;166:835–856.

74. Almeida Jr OD, Val-Gallas JM. Conscious pain mapping. *J Am Assoc Gynecol Laparosc* 1997;4:587–590.

75. Demco LA. Effect on negative laparoscopy rate in chronic pelvic pain patients using patient assisted laparoscopy. *J Soc Laparoendosc Surg* 1997;1:319–321.

76. Palter SF, Olive DL. Office microlaparoscopy under local anesthesia for chronic pelvic pain. *J Am Assoc Gynecol Laparosc* 1996;3:359–364.

77. Demco L. Mapping the source and character of pain due to endometriosis by patient-assisted laparoscopy. *J Am Asssoc Gynecol Laparosc* 1998;5:241–245.

78. Howard FM, El-Minawi A, Sanchez R. Conscious laparoscopic pain mapping in women with chronic pelvic pain. *Obstet Gynecol* 2000;96:934–939.

79. Wharton LR. Two cases of supernumerary ovary and one of accessory ovary, with an analysis of previously reported cases. *Am J Obstet Gynecol* 1959;78(5):1101–1118.

80. Cullen TS. *Adenomyoma of the uterus.* Philadelphia: WB Saunders, 1908.

81. Azziz R. *Adenomyosis: current perspectives.* Obstetrics and Gynecology Clinics of North America 1989;16:221–235.

82. Benson RC, Sneeden VD. Adenomyosis: a reappraisal of symptomatology. *Am J Obstet Gynecol* 1958;76:1044.

83. Bird CC, McElin TW, Manalo-Estrella P. The elusive adenomyosis of the uterus revisited. *Am J Obstet Gynecol* 1972;112:582–593.

84. Israel SL, Woutersz T. Adenomyosis a neglected diagnosis. *Obstet Gynecol* 1959;13:168.

85. Mathur BBL, Shah RS, Bhende YM. Adenomyosis uteri: a pathologic study of 290 cases. *Am J Obstet Gynecol* 1962;84:1820.

86. Molitor JJ. Adenomyosis: a clinical and pathologic appraisal. *Am J Obstet Gynecol* 1971;110:275.

87. Nikkanen V, Punnonen R. Clinical significance of adenomyosis. *Ann Chir Gynaecol* 1980;69:278.

88. Owolabi TO, Strickler RC. Adenomyosis: a neglected diagnosis. *Obstet Gynecol* 1977;50:424.

89. McCausland AM. Hysteroscopic myometrial biopsy: its use in diagnosing adenomyosis and its clinical applications. *Am J Obstet gynecol* 1992;166:1619–1628.

90. Grow DR, Filer RB. Treatment of adenomyosis with long-term GnRH analogues: a case report. *Obstet Gynecol* 1991;78:538–39.

91. Nelson JR, Corson SL. Long-term management of adenomyosis with gonadotropin releasing hormone agonist: a case report. *Fertil Steril* 1993;39:441–443.

92. Hirata JD, Moghissi KS, Ginsburg KA. Pregnancy after medical therapy of adenomyosis with gonadotropin releasing hormone agonist. *Fertil Sterile* 1993;59:444–445.

93. Miller EM, Winfield JM. Acute intestinal obstruction secondary to postoperative adhesions. *Arch Surg* 1959;78:148–153.

94. Stricker B, Blanco J, Fox HE. The gynecologic contribution to instestinal obstruction in females. *J Am Coll Surg* 1994;178:617–620.

95. Drake TS, Grunert GM. The unsuspected pelvic factor in the infertility investigation. *Fertil Steril* 1980;34:27–31.

96. Stovall TG, Elder RF, Ling FW. Predictors of pelvic adhesions. *J Reprod Med* 1989;34:345–348.

97. Brill AI, Nezhat FR, Nezhat CH et al. The incidence of adhesions after prior laparotomy: a laparoscopic appraisal. *Obstet Gynecol* 1995;85:269–272.

98. Hasson HM. Open laparoscopy versus closed laparoscopy: a comparison of complication rates. *Adv Plan Parent* 1978;13:41.

99. Penfield AJ. How to prevent complications of open laparoscopy. *J Reprod Med* 1985;30:660.

100. Howard FM, El-Minawi AM, DeLoach VE. Direct laparoscopic cannula insertion at the left upper quadrant. *J Am Assoc Gynecol Laparosc* 1997;4:595–600.

101. Steege JF, Stout A. Resolution of chronic pelvic pain after laparoscopic lysis of adhesions. *Am J Obstet Gynecol* 1991;165:278–283.

102. Sutton C, MacDonald R. Laser laparoscopic adhesiolysis. *J Gynecol Surg* 1990;6:155–159.

103. Fayez JA, Clark RR. Operative laparoscopy for the treatment of localized chronic pelvic-abdominal pain caused by postoperative adhesions. *J Gynecol Surg* 1994;10:79–83.

104. Duffy DM, diZerega GS. Adhesion controversies pelvic pain as a cause of adhesions, crystalloids in preventing them. *J Reprod Med* 1996;41:19–26.

105. Peters AAW, Trimbos-Kemper GCM, Admiraal. C, Trimbos JB. A randomized clinical trial on the benefit of adhesiolysis in patients with intraperitoneal adhesions and chronic pelvic pain. *Br J Obstet Gynaecol* 1992;99:59–62.

106. Stone SC, Swartz WJ. A syndrome characterized by recurrent symptomatic functional cysts in young women. *Am J Obstet Gynecol* 134:310,1979.

107. Hasson HH. Laparoscopic management of ovarian cysts. *J Reprod Med* 1990;35:863.

108. Wiskind AK, Toledo AA, Dudley G, Zusmanis K. Adhesion formation after ovarian wound repair in New Zealand white rabbits: a comparison of ovarian microsurgical closure with ovarian nonclosure. *Am J Obstet Gynecol* 1990;163:1674.

109. Perry CP, Upchurch JC. Pelviscopic adnexectomy. *Am J Obstet Gynecol* 1990;162;70–81.

110. Righi RV, McComb PF, Fluker MR. Laparoscopic oophoropexy for recurrent adnexal torsion. *Hum Reprod* 1995;10:3136–3138.

111. Smith RP. Cyclic pain and dysmenorrhea. *Obstet Gynecol NA.* 1993;20:753–64.

112. Sundell G, Milson I, Andersch B. Factors influencing the prevalence and severity of dysmenorrhea in young women. *Br J Obstet Gynaecol* 1990;97:588.

113. Pickles VR. A plain-muscle stimulant in the menstruum. *Nature* 1957;180:1198–1199.

114. Pickles VR, Hall WJ, Best FA, Smith GN. Prostaglandin in endometrium and menstrual fluid from normal and dysmenorrheic subjects. *Br J Obstet Gynecol* 1965;72:185–187.

115. Smith OW, Mass B. Menstrual toxin. *Am J Obstet Gynecol* 1947;54:201.

116. Kurzok R, Lieb CC. Biochemical studies of human semen. II. The action of semen on the human uterus. *Proc Soc Exp Biol Med* 1930; 28:268–272.

117. Goldblatt MW. Properties of human seminal fluid. *J Physiol* 84: 208–218, 1935

118. von Euler US. On the specific vasodilating and plain muscle stimulating substance from accessory genital glands in man and certain animals (prostaglandin and vesiglandin) *J Physiol* 1936;88:213–234.

119. von Euler US. Some aspects of the actions of prostaglandins. The first Heymans Memorial lecture. *Arch Int Pharmacodyn Ther* 1973; 202(Suppl):295–307.

120. Jordan VC, Pokoly TB. Steroid and prostaglandin relations during the menstrual cycle. *Obstet Gynecol* 1971;49:449–451.

121. Wilson L, Cendella RJ, Butcher RL, Inskeep EK. Levels of prostaglandins in the uterine endometrium during the ovine estrous cycle. *J Anim Sci* 1972;34:93–96.

122. Pickles VR. Prostaglandin in the human endometrium. *Int J Fertil* 1967;12:335–337.

123. Chan WY, Dawood MY, Fuchs F. Relief of dysmenorrhea with the prostaglandin synthetase inhibitor Ibuprofen: effect on prostaglandin levels in menstrual fluid. *Am J Obstet Gynecol* 1979;135:102–104.

124. Pickles VR, Hall WJ, Bes FA, Smith CN. Prostaglandins in endometriosis and menstrual fluid from normal and dysmenorrheic subjects. *Br J Obstet Gynaecol* 1965;72:185.

125. Akerlund M, Stromberg P, Forselin MD. Primary dysmenorrhea and vasopressin. *Br J Obstet Gynaecol* 1979;86:484.

126. Widholm OM, Kantero RA. A statistical analysis of the menstrual patterns of Finnish girls and their mothers. *Acta Obstet Gynecol Scand* 1971;14(Suppl):1–2.

127. Dawood MY. Ibuprofen and dysmenorrhea. *Am J Med* 1984;77(1A): 87–94.

128. Kajanoja P, Tuulikki V. Naproxen and indomethacin in the treatment of primary dysmenorrhea. *Acta Obstet Gynecol Scand* 1979;87 (Suppl):87–90.

129. Corson SL, Bolognese RJ. Ibuprofen therapy for dysmenorrhea. *J Reprod Med* 1978;20:246–248.

130. Kapadia L, Elder MD. Flufenamic acid in treatment of primary spasmodic dysmenorrhea; a double-blind crossover study. *Lancet* 19781:348–349.

131. Smith RP. The dynamics of nonsteroidal antiinflammatory therapy for primary dysmenorrhea. *Obstet Gynecol* 1987;70:785–787.

132. Owen PR. Prostaglandin synthetase inhibitors in the treatment of primary dysmenorrhea: outcome trials reviewed. *Am J Obstet Gynecol* 1984;148:96–99.

133. Anderson KE, Ulmsten U. Effects on nifedipine on myometrial activity and lower abdominal pain in women with primary dysmenorrhea. *Brit J Obstet Gynaecol* 1978;85:142–144.

134. Forman A, Anderson KE, Ulmsten U. Combined effects of diflunisal and nifedipine on uterine contractility in dysmenorrheic patients. *Prostaglandins* 1982;23(2):237–239.

135. Milsom I, Hedner N, Mannheimer C. A comparative study of the effect of high-intensity transcutaneous nerve stimulation and oral naproxen on intrauterine pressure and menstrual pain in patients with primary dysmenorrhea. *Am J Obstet Gynecol* 1994;170: 123–126.

136. Kaplan B, Peled Y, Pardo J, et al . Transcutaneous electrical nerve stimulation (TENS) as a relief for dysmenorrhea. *Clin Exp Obstet Gynecol* 1994;21:87.

137. Helms JM. Acupuncture in the management of primary dysmenorrhea. *Obstet Gynecol* 1987;69:51–56.

138. Sampson JA. Peritoneal endometriosis due to dissemination of endometrial tissue into the peritoneal cavity. *Am J Obstet Gynecol* 1927;14:422.

139. Sampson JA. Benign and malignant endometrial implants in the peritoneal cavity and their relationship to certain ovarian tumors. *Surg Gynecol Obstet* 1924;38:287.

140. Sampson JA. Perforating hemorrhagic (chocolate) cysts of the ovary. *Arch Surg* 1921;3:245.

141. Nunley WC. Medical management of endometriosis: a review. *Hosp Formul* 1985;20:704.

142. Droegemueller W, Herbst AL, Mishell DR, Stenchever MA. Comprehensive Gynecology. St. Louis, MO: CV Mosby, 1987:493.

143. Barbieri RL. Etiology and epidemiology of endometriosis. *Am J Obstet Gynecol* 1990;162:565.

144. Martin DC, Berry JD. Histology of chocolate cysts. *J Gynecol Surg* 1990;6:43.

145. Jansen RP, Russell P. Nonpigmented endometriosis: clinical, laparoscopic, and pathologic definition. *Am J Obstet Gynecol* 1986;155:1154.

146. Sampson JA. Peritoneal endometriosis due to dissemination of endometrial tissue into the peritoneal cavity. *Am J Obstet Gynecol* 1927;14:422.

147. Sampson JA. Benign and malignant endometrial implants in the peritoneal cavity and their relationship to certain ovarian tumors. *Surg Gynecol Obstet* 1924;38:287.

148. Sampson JA. Perforating hemorrhagic (chocolate) cysts of the ovary. *Arch Surg* 1921;3:245.

149. Nunley WC. Medical management of endometriosis: a review. *Hosp Formul* 1985;20:704.
150. Droegemueller W, Herbst AL, Mishell DR, Stenchever MA. *Comprehensive gynecology*. St. Louis, MO: CV Mosby, 1987:493.
151. Barbieri RL. Etiology and epidemiology of endometriosis. *Am J Obstet Gynecol* 1990;162:565.
152. Sampson JA. Peritoneal endometriosis due to dissemination of endometrial tissue into the peritoneal cavity. *Am J Obstet Gynecol* 1927;14:422.
153. Sampson JA. Benign and malignant endometrial implants in the peritoneal cavity and their relationship to certain ovarian tumors. *Surg Gynecol Obstet* 1924;38:287.
154. Sampson JA. Perforating hemorrhagic (chocolate) cysts of the ovary. *Arch Surg* 1921;3:245.
155. Barbieri RL. Etiology and epidemiology of endometriosis. *Am J Obstet Gynecol* 1990;162:565.
156. Mahmood TA, Templeton AA, Thomson L, Fraser C. Menstrual symptoms in women with pelvic endometriosis. *Br J Obstet Gynaecol* 1991;98:558–563.
157. Barbieri RL. Etiology and epidemiology of endometriosis. *Am J Obstet Gynecol* 1990;162:565.
158. Mahmood TA, Templeton AA, Thomson L, Fraser C. Menstrual symptoms in women with pelvic endometriosis. *Br J Obstet Gynaecol* 1991;98:558–563.
159. Koninckx PR, Lesaffre E, Meuleman C, et al. Suggestive evidence that pelvic endometriosis is a progressive disease, whereas deeply infiltrating endometriosis is associated with pelvic pain. *Fertil Steril* 1991;55:759.
160. Hajjar LR, Kim WS, Nolan GH, et al. Intestinal and pelvic endometriosis presenting as a tumor and associated with tamoxifen therapy: report of a case. *Obstet Gynecol* 1993;82:642–644.
161. Redwine DB. Endometriosis persisting after castration: clinical characteristics and results of surgical management. *Obstet Gynecol* 1994;83:405–413.
162. Kempers RD, Dockerty MB, Hunt AB, Symmonds RE. Significant postmenopausal endometriosis. *Surg Gynecol Obstet* 1960;3:348–356.
163. Adamson GD. Diagnosis and clinical presentation of endometriosis. *Am J Obstet Gynecol* 1990;162:568.
164. Adamson GD, Nelson HP. Surgical treatment of endometriosis. *Obstet Gynecol Clinics NA* 1997;24:375–409.
165. Kettel LM, Hummel WP. Modern medical management of endometriosis. *Obstet Gynecol Clinics NA*. 1997;24:361–373.
166. Greenblatt RB, Dmowski WP, Mahesh VB, Scholer HFL. Clinical studies with an antigonadotropin—danazol. *Fertil Steril* 1971;22:102.
167. Telimaa S, Puolakka J, Ronnberg L, Kauppila A. Placebo-controlled comparison of danazol and high-dose medroxyprogesterone acetate in the treatment of endometriosis. *Gynecol Endocrinol* 1987;1:13.
168. Carpenter SE, Tjaden B, Rock JA, Kimball A. The effect of regular exercise on women receiving danazol for treatment of endometriosis. *Int J Gynecol Obstet* 1995;49:299–304.
169. Farquhar C, Sutton C. The evidence for the management of endometriosis. Current opinion. *Obstet Gynecol* 1998;10:321.
170. Cundy T, Cornish J, Roberts H, et al. Spinal bone density in women using depot medroxyprogesterone acetat contraception. *Obstet Gynecol* 1998;92:569–573.
171. Bromham DR, Booker MW, Rose GL, et al. Updating the clinical experience in endometriosis—the European perspective. *Br J Obstet Gynaecol* 1995;102(Suppl 12):12–16.
172. The Gestrinone Italian Study Group. Gestrinone versus a gonadotropin-releasing hormone agonist for the treatment of pelvic pain associated with endometriosis: a multicenter, randomized, double-blind study. *Fertil Steril* 1996;66:911–919.
173. Hsu CC, Lin YS, Wang ST, Huang KE. Immunomodulation in women with endometriosis receiving GnTH agonist. *Obstet Gynecol* 1997;89:993–998.
174. Dlugi AM, Miller JD, Knittle J. Lupron depot (leuprolide acetate for depot suspension) in the treatment of endometriosis: a randomized, placebo-controlled, double-blind study. *Fertil Steril* 1990;54:419–427.
175. Ling FW. Randomized control trial of depot leuprolide in patients with chronic pelvic pain and clinically suspected endometriosis. Pelvic pain study group. *Obstet Gynecol* 1999;93:51–58.
176. Bergqvist A, Bergh T, Hogstrom L, et al. Effects of triptorelin versus placebo on the symptoms of endometriosis. *Fertil Steril* 1998;69:702.
177. Wheeler JM, Knittle JD, Miller JD. Depot leuprolide versus danazol in treatment of women with symptomatic endometriosis. I. Efficacy results. *Am J Obstet Gynecol* 1992;167:1367–1371.
178. Rock JA, Truglia JA, Caplan RJ. The Zoladex Endometriosis Study Group. Zoladex (goserelin acetate implant) in the treatment of endometriosis: a randomized comparison with danazol. *Obstet Gynecol* 1993;82:198–205.
179. ANZ Zoladex Group. Goserelin depot versus danazol in the treatment of endometriosis. The Australian/New Zealand experience. *Fertil Steril* 1995;63:504–507.
180. Henzyl MR, Corson SL, Moghissi K, et al. Administration for nasal nafarelin as compared with oral danazol for endometriosis. A multicenter double-blind clinical trial. *N Engl J Med* 1988;318:485–489.
181. Kennedy SH, Williams IA, Brodribb J, et al. A comparison of nafarelin acetate and danazol in the treatment of endometriosis. *Fertil Steril* 1990;53:998–1003.
182. Nafarelin European Endometriosis Trial Group. Nafarelin for endometriosis: a large-scale, danazol-controlled trial of efficacy and safety, with 1-year follow-up. *Fertil Steril* 1992;57:514–522.
183. Adamson GD, Kwei L, Edgren RA. Pain of endometriosis: effects of nafarelin and danazol therapy. *Int J Fertil* 1994;39:215–217.
184. Waller KG, Shaw RW. Gonadotropin-releasing hormone analogues for the treatment of endometriosis: long-term follow-up. *Fertil Steril* 1993;59:511–515.
185. Hornstein MD, Yuzpe AA, Burry K, et al. Retreatment with nafarelin for recurrent endometriosis symptoms: efficacy, safety, and bone mineral density. *Fertil Steril* 1997:1013–1018.
186. Hornstein MD, Yuzpe AA, Burry KA, et al. Prospective randomized double-blind trial of 3 versus 6 months of nafarelin therapy for endometriosis associated pelvic pain. *Fertil Steril* 1995;63:955–962.
187. Hornstein MD, Surrey ES, Weisberg GW, Casino LA, for the Lupron Add-Back Study Group. Leuprolide acetate depot and hormonal add-back in endometriosis: a 12-month study. *Obstet Gynecol* 1998;91:16–24.
188. Kistner R W. Treatment of endometriosis by inducing pseudo-pregnancy with ovarian hormones. *Fertil Steril* 1959;10:539–554.
189. Vercellini P, Trespidi L, Colombo A, et al. A gonadotrophin-releasing hormone agonist versus a low-dose oral contraceptive for pelvic pain associated with endometriosis. *Fertil Steril* 1993;60(1):75–79.
190. Howard FM. Laparoscopic evaluation and treatment of women with chronic pelvic pain. *J Amer Assoc Gynecol Laparosc* 1994;1:325–331.
191. Sutton CJG, Ewen SP, Whitelaw N, Haines P. Prospective, randomized, double-blind trial of laser laparoscopy in the treatment of pelvic pain associated with minimal, mild, and moderate endometriosis. *Fertil Steril* 1994;62:696–700.
192. Polan ML, DeCherney A. Presacral neurectomy for pelvic pain in infertility. *Fertil Steril* 1980;34:557.
193. Lee RB, Stone K, Magelssen D, et al. Presacral neurectomy for chronic pelvic pain. *Obstet Gynecol* 1986;68:517.
194. Tjaden B, Schlaff WD, Kimball A, Rock JA. The efficacy of presacral neurectomy for the relief of midline dysmenorrhea. *Obstet Gynecol* 76:89,1990.
195. Black WT. Use of presacral sympathectomy in the treatment of dysmenorrhea. A second look after twenty-five years. *Am J Obstet Gynecol* 1964;89:16.
196. Doyle JB, Des Rosiers JJ. Paracervical uterine denervation for relief of pelvic pain. *Clin Obstet Gynecol* 1963;6:742.
197. Lichten E. Three years experience with LUNA. *Am J Gynecol Health* 1989;5:9.
198. Lichten EM, Bombard J. Surgical treatment of primary dysmenorrhea with laparoscopic uterine nerve ablation. *J Reprod Med* 1987;32:37.
199. Tjaden B, Schlaff WD, Kimball A, Rock JA. The efficacy of presacral neurectomy for the relief of midline dysmenorrhea. *Obstet Gynecol* 1990;76:89–91.
200. Candiani GB, Fedele L, Vercellini P, et al. Presacral neurectomy for the treatment of pelvic pain associated with endometriosis: a controlled study. *Am J Obstet Gynecol* 1992;167:100–103.
201. Lichten EM, Bombard J. Surgical treatment of primary dysmenorrhea with laparoscopic uterine nerve ablation. *J Reprod Med* 1987;32:37–41.

202. Parazzini F, Fedele L, Busacca M, et al. Postsurgical medical treatment of advanced endometriosis: results of a randomized clinical trial. *Am J Obstet Gynecol* 1994;171:1205–1207.

203. Hornstein MD, et al. Use of nafarelin versus placebo after reductive laparoscopic surgery for endometriosis. *Fertil Steril* 1997;68:860–864.

204. Namnoum AB, Hickman TN, Goodman SB, et al. Incidence of symptom recurrence after hysterectomy for endometriosis. *Fertil Steril* 1995;64:898–902.

205. Metzger DA, Lessey BA, Soper JT, et al. Hormone-resistant endometriosis following total abdominal hysterectomy and bilateral salpingo-oophorectomy: correlation with histology and steroid receptor content. *Obstet Gynecol* 1991;78:946.

206. Redwine DB. Endometriosis persisting after castration: clinical characteristics and results of surgical management. *Obstet Gynecol* 1994;83:405–413.

207. Dmowski WP, Radwanska E, Rana N. Recurrent endometriosis following hysterectomy and oophorectomy: the role of residual ovarian fragments. *Int J Gynecol Obstet* 1988;26:93.

208. Davies SA, Maclin VM. Endosalpingiosis as a cause of chronic pelvic pain. *Am J Obstet Gynecol* 1991;164:495–496.

209. DiSaia PJ. Disorders of the uterine cervix. In: Scott JR, DiSaia PJ, Hammond CB, Spellesy WN, eds. Danforth, Philadelphia: JP Lippincott, *Obstet and Gynecol*, 1994:892–924.

210. Buttram VC, Reiter RC. Uterine leiomyomata: etiology, symptomatology, and management. *Fertil Steril* 1981;36:433–445.

211. Hutchins FL. Uterine fibroids. *Obstet Gynecol Clinics N Amer* 1995;22:659–665.

212. Kawamura N, Shibata S, Ito F, et al. Correlation between shrinkage of uterine leiomyoma treated with buserelin acetate and histopathologic findings of biopsy specimen before treatment. *Fertil Steril* 1997;68:632–636.

213. Reich H. Laparoscopic myomectomy. *Obstet Gynecol Clin NA* 1995;22:757–759.

214. Ravina JH, Herbreteau D, Ciraru-Vigneron N, et al. Arterial embolisation to treat uterine myomata. *Lancet* 1995;346:671–672.

215. Hann LE, Hall, DA, Black EB, Ferrucci, JT. Mittelschmerz: Sonographic demonstration. *JAMA* 1979;241:2731–2732.

216. Grogan RH. Residual ovaries. *Obstet Gynecol* 1958;12(3):329–332.

217. Christ JE, Lotze EC. The residual ovary syndrome. *Obstet Gynecol* 1975;46(5):551–556.

218. Ranney B, Abu-Ghazaleh S. The future function and fortune of ovarian tissue which is retained in vivo during hysterectomy. *Am J Obstet Gynecol* 1977;128(6):626–634.

219. Grogan RH, Duncan CJ. Ovarian salvage in routine abdominal hysterectomy. *Am J Obstet Gynecol* 1955;70:1277–1283.

220. De Neef JC, Hollenbeck ZJR. The fate of ovaries preserved at the time of hysterectomy. *Am J Obstet Gynecol* 1966;96(8):1088–1097.

221. Gevaerts POH. Abdominale totale uterus extirpatie of supravaginale uterus amputatie. Thesis, Leiden, Holland, 1963. Quoted in De Neef JC and Hollenbeck ZJR: the fate of ovaries preserved at the time of hysterectomy. *Am J Obstet Gynecol* 1966;96(8):1088–1097.

222. Mckenzie LL. On discussion of the frequency of oophorectomy at the time of hysterectomy. *Am J Obstet Gynecol* 1968;100:724–725.

223. Sidall-Allum J, Rae T, Rogers V, et al. Chronic pelvic pain caused by residual ovaries and ovarian remnants. *Br J Obstet Gynaecol* 1994;101:979–985.

224. Grogan RH. Reappraisal of residual ovaries. *Am J Obstet Gynecol* 1967;97(1):-124–129.

225. Price FV, Edwards R, Buchsbaum HJ. Ovarian remnant syndrome: difficulties in diagnosis and management. *Obstet Gynecol Suurv* 1990;45(3):151–156.

226. Berek JS, Darney PD, Lopkin C, Goldstein DP. Avoiding ureteral damage in pelvic surgery for ovarian remnant syndrome. *Am J Obstet Gynecol* 1979;133:221–222.

227. Carey MP, Slack MC. GnRH analogue in assessing chronic pelvic pain in women with residual ovaries. *Br J Obstet Gynecol* 1996;103:150–153.

228. Perry CP, Upchurch JC. Pelviscopic adnexectomy. *Am J Obstet Gynecol* 1990;162:79.

229. Webb MJ. Ovarian remnant syndrome. *Aust NZ J Obstet Gynecol* 1989;29(4):433–435.

230. Nelson DC, Avant GR. Ovarian remnant syndrome. *Southern Med J* 1982;75(6):757–758.

231. Symmonds RE, Petit PDM. Ovarian remnant syndrome. *Obstet Gynecol* 1979;54(2):174–177.

232. Pettit PD, Lee RA. Ovarian remnant syndrome: diagnostic dilemma and surgical challenge. *Obstet Gynecol* 1988;71(4): 580–583.

233. Shemwell RW, Weed JC. Ovarian remnant syndrome. *Obstet Gynecol* 1970;36:299–303.

234. Minke T, DePond W, Winkelmann T, Blythe J. Ovarian remnant syndrome: study in laboratory rats. *Am J Obstet Gynecol* 1994;171(6): 1440–1445.

235. Mattingly RF, Frederick EG. Difficult hysterectomy. *Clin Obstet Gynecol* 1972;15:877–801.

236. Sidall-Allum J, Rae T, Rogers V, et al. Chronic pelvic pain caused by residual ovaries and ovarian remnants. *Br J Obstet Gynaecol* 1994; 101:979–985.

237. Kaminski PF, Sorosky JI, Mandell MJ, et al. Clomiphene citrate as an adjunct in locating ovarian tissue in ovarian remnant syndrome. *Obstet Gynecol* 1990;76(5:2):924–926.

238. Howard FM. Laparoscopic treatment of ovarian remnant and ovarian retention syndrome. *JAAGL* 1995;2(Suppl):S20.

239. Kamprath S, Possover M, Schneider A. Description of a laparoscopic technique for treating patients with ovarian remnant syndrome. *Fertil Steril* 1997;68(4):663–667.

240. Fleischer AC, Tait D, Mayo J, et al. Sonographic features of ovarian remnants. *J Ultrasound Med* 1998;17(9):551–555.

241. Thomas WW, Hughes LL, Rock J. Palliation of recurrent endometriosis with radiotherapeutic ablation of ovarian remnants. *Ferhl Steril* 1997;68(5):938–940.

242. Mathis BV, Miller JS, Lukens ML, Paluzzi MW. Pelvic congestion syndrome: a new approach to an unusual problem. *The American Surgeon* 1995;61:1016–1018.

243. Beard RW, Belsey EM, Lieberman BA, Wilkinson JCM. Pelvic pain in women. *Am J Obstet Gynecol* 1977;128:566–570.

244. Renaer M, Nijs P, van Assche A, Vertommen H. Chronic pelvic pain without obvious pathology. Personal observations and a review of the problem. *Eur J Obstet Gynaecol Reprod Biol* 1980;10:415–463.

245. Renaer M. Chronic pelvic pain without obvious pathology. In: *Chronic pelvic pain in women*. New York: Springer-Verlag, 1981: 162–175.

246. El-Minawi MF, Mashhor N, Reda MS. Pelvic venous changes after tubal sterilization. *J Reprod Med* 1983;28(10):641–648.

247. Beard RW, Reginald PW, Wadsworth J. Clinical features of women with chronic lower abdominal pain and pelvic congestion. *Br J Obstet Gynaecol* 1988;95:153–161.

248. Beard RW, Reginald PW, Pearce S. Psychological and somatic factors in women with pain due to pelvic congestion. *Adv Exp Biol Med* 1988;245:413–421.

249. Beard RW, Kennedy RG, Gangar KF, et al. Bilateral oophorectomy and hysterectomy in the treatment of intractable pelvic pain associated with pelvic congestion. *Br J Obstet Gynaecol* 1991;98:988–992.

250. Edwards RD, Robertson IR, MacLean AB, Hemmingway AP. Case report: pelvic pain syndrome—successful treatment of a case by ovarian vein embolization. *Clin Radiol* 1993;47:429–431.

251. Florio F, Balzano S, Nardella M, Villani G. Varicocele ovarico trattato con scleroembolizzazione percutanea. Descrizione di un caso. *Radiol Med* 1993;85:295–297.

252. Abbas FM, Currie JL, Mitchell S. Selective vascular embolization in benign gynecologic conditions. *J Reprod Med* 1994;39:492–496.

253. Gangar KF, Stones RW , Saunders C, et al. An alternative to hysterectomy? GnRH analogue combined with hormone replacement therapy. *Br J Obstet Gynaecol* 1993;100:360–364.

254. Beard RW, Kennedy RG, Gangar KF, et al. Bilateral oophorectomyand hysterectomy in the treatment of intractable pelvic pain associated with pelvic congestion. *Br J Obstet Gynaecol* 1991;98:988.

255. Baker PK. Musculoskeletal origins of chronic pelvic pain. *Obstet Gynecol Clin NA* 1993;20:719–742.

256. Smith WT. Levator spasm syndrome. *Minnesota Medicine* Aug 1959; 1076–1079.

257. Thiele GH. Coccygodynia and pain in the superior gluteal region. *JAMA* 1937;109:1271–1275.

258. McGivney JQ, Cleveland BR. The levator syndrome and its treatment. *Southern Med J* 1965;58:505–510.

259. Sinaki M, Merritt JL, Stillwell GK. Tension myalgia of the pelvic floor. *Mayo Clin Proc* 1977;52:717–722.

260. Ross JM, Welch WR, Scully RE. Multilocular peritoneal inclusion cysts (so-called cystic mesotheliomas). *Cancer* 1989;64:1336–1346.

261. Gussman D, Thickman D, Wheeler JE. Postoperative peritoneal cysts. *Obstet Gynecol* 1986;68:535.

262. Monafo W, Goldfarb W. Postoperative peritoneal cysts. *Surgery* 1963;53:470.

263. Falk HC, Bunkin IA. Intraperitoneal cysts simulating ovarian cysts. *Obstet Gynecol* 1953;1:18.

264. Lees RF, Feldman PS. Brenbridge ANAG, et al. Inflammatory cysts of the pelvic peritoneum. *Am J Roentgenol* 1978;131:633.

265. Gussman D, Thickman D, Wheeler JE. Postoperative peritoneal cysts. *Obstet Gynecol* 1986;68:53S–55S.

266. Lipitz S, Seidman DS, Schiff E, et al. Treatment of pelvic peritoneal cysts by drainage and ethanol instillation. *Obstet Gynecol* 1995;86:297–299.

267. Sohaey R, Gardner TL, Woodward PJ, Peterson M. Sonographic diagnosis of peritoneal inclusion cysts. *J Ultrasound Med* 1995; 14:913–917.

268. Birch DW, Park A, Chen V. Laparoscopic resection of an intra-abdominal cystic mass: a cystic mesothelioma. *Canadian J Surg* 1998;41:161–164.

269. Birch DW, Park A, Chen V. Laparoscopic resection of an intra-abdominal cystic mass: a cystic mesothelioma. *Canadian J Surg* 1998; 41:161–164.

270. Letterie GS, Yon JL. The antiestrogen tamoxifen in the treatment of recurrent benign cystic mesothelioma. *Gynecol Oncol* 1998;70:131–133.

271. Letterie GS, Yon JL. Use of a long-acting GnRH agonist for benign cystic mesothelioma. *Obstet Gynecol* 1995;85:901–903.

272. Navarra G, Occhionorelli S, Santini M, et al. Peritoneal cystic mesothelioma treated with minimally invasive approach. *Surg Endosc* 1996; 10:60–61.

273. Carpenter HA, Lancaster RJ, Lee RA. Multilocular cysts of the peritoneum. *Mayo Clin Proc* 1982;57:634–638.

274. Benson RC, Williams TH. Peritoneal cystic mesothelioma: successful treatment of a difficult disease. *J Urol* 1990;143:347–348.

275. DeLancey JOL Anatomy and biomechanics of genital prolapse. *Clinical Obstetrics and Gynecology* 1993;36:897–909.

276. DeLancey JOL Pelvic organ prolapse. In: Scott JR, DiSaia PJ, Hammond CP, Spellacy WN, eds. *Danforth's obstetrics and gynecology* 7th ed. Philadelphia: JB Lippincott Co., 1994:803–825.

277. Norton PA. Pelvic floor disorders. The role of fascia and ligaments. *Clinical Obstet & Gynecol* 1996;36:926–938.

278. Shull BL. Clinical evaluation of women with pelvic support defects. *Clinical Obstet and Gynecol* 1993;36:939–951.

279. Glazer HI, Rodke G, Swencionis C, et al. Treatment of vulvar vestibulitis syndrome with electromyographic biofeedback of pelvic floor musculature. *J Reprod Med* 1995;40:283–290.

280. Travel J, Simons D. *The trigger point manual*. Baltimore: Williams and Wilkins, 1983(1).

281. Pigne A, Oudin G. Treatment of sexual dysfunction. In: Schussler B, Laycock J, Norton P, Stanton S, eds. *Pelvic floor reeducation principles and practices*. London: Springer-Verlag, 1994:126–129.

282. Anthuber C, Pigne A. Neuromuscular electrical stimulation. In: Schussler B, Laycock J, Norton P, Stanton S, eds. *Pelvic floor reeducation principles and practices*. London: Springer-Verlag. 1994: 163–167.

283. Charles D. Pelvic tuberculosis: Not gone, but sometimes forgotten. *Contemp Ob/Gyn* July 1991:97.

284. Ranaer M, ed. *Chronic pelvic pain in women*. New York: Springer-Verlag, 1981:91.

CHAPTER 32

Concepts in Male Genitourinary Pain

Richard A. Schmidt and Dirk Zerman

Male genitourinary pain is a significant medical problem that is often descriptively elusive, difficult to diagnose, and even more difficult to treat. It includes a number of labels that are interesting in their lack of findings other than sensitivity. Presently, male genitourinary pain is generally viewed as isolated to a peripheral locus or tissue site. This is implied in the descriptive, rather than pathodiagnostic, labels that are applied—e.g., the terms *prostatodynia, orchalgia, testalgia, painful granuloma, epididymo-orchalgia, glans hypersensitivity,* and *nonspecific urethritis.* When there is identifiable pathology, such as a prostatic abscess, stone caught in the urethra, a granuloma, or an epididymal cyst, treatment may lead to relief, but a complete cure from pain is unusual. Surgical approaches to pain rarely result in true resolution of the pain. For example, a painful scrotum often persists after removal of a testis for orchalgia, an epididymectomy for epididymitis, or the excision of a granuloma after vasectomy. There thus would appear to be a need to reexamine the approaches taken toward management of male pelvic pain. Therefore, a more global view of the painful male pelvis is taken in the following discussion. Neurological explanations are offered to underscore the role of the nervous system in the etiology and maintenance of pain and to provide an appreciation of conditions and circumstances that predispose to permanent pain syndromes.

INNERVATION OF PELVIC STRUCTURES

All visceral organs of the pelvis share the same innervated source (1,2). This gives rise to the notion that the pelvis is just one neurological organ system with some variance in the CNS representation of the various organ systems (3,4). The viscera are parasympathetically innervated via S-3–4 and sympathetically innervated via T-12–L-2. Even the testes are now considered to receive source innervation via the sacral nerves. This is based on tracer mapping studies

and the referred sensations described by patients having S-3 stimulation therapy. Sympathetic nerves have an important role in the male genital system. Its responsibilities are primarily concerned with transport of the gene pool. Stimulation of the hypogastric nerves is known to produce contraction of the epididymis, vas, seminal vesicles, prostate, and bladder neck. However, because of the importance of sympathetic nerves in sensitization and neurogenic inflammation, there may indeed be an important role played by these nerves in the generation and sustenance of male genitourinary pain. Sites rich in sympathetic influence (the bladder neck, prostate, vas, and epididymis) are all tissues prone to hypersensitivity in the male.

These findings are important in the interpretation of male genital pain syndromes. For example, referred pain must be differentiated from site or organ specific pain. The key to this differentiation lies in the physical exam.

The anatomy of the pelvic floor encompasses two functional layers: (a) the deeper levator layer, innervated via S-3–4 and (b) a superficial layer innervated via S-2 and the pudendal nerve. This separation is readily apparent in the muscle contractions of the pelvic floor observed with stimulation of the various sacral nerves. Contraction of the levator produces a very visible deepening and flattening of the gluteal crease as the pelvic organs are pulled inward and upward toward the pubis. Visually, the perineum moves with a bellows-like action that should be very apparent. This dynamic should be readily identifiable in everyone with voluntary tightening and relaxation efforts.

The second functional layer to the pelvis is composed of all of the muscles below the levator: the transversus peronei, ileo-, and bulbocavernosus muscles, the urethral sphincter, and the superficial anal sphincter. These muscles are innervated by the pudendal nerve, which is primarily derived from S-2. Stimulation of the pudendal nerve produces an anterior-posterior squeezing, a vise-like or clamp-like movement.

These two motions, the bellows and the clamp, are distinctly different from a functional perspective. Normally the two motions will blend together, with the bellows response much more evident and easy to appreciate. In many of the pelvic pain syndromes encountered these motions become fractionated or dyssynergic relative to each other and to the bladder.

CNS Consequences of Persistent Nociception

Tendonitis and myalgia are classic consequences of inappropriate muscle behavior. This is a rule played out within all striated muscles of the body. Thus, it can be expected that repetitive dysfunctional behavior of the pelvic floor muscles would have the potential to predispose to, or trigger, at some point in time, a neuroinflammatory cascade within the involved CNS circuits (Fig. 32-1) (5). This cascade of events involves architectural and communicative changes within the CNS, increased numbers of dendritic buttons on motor neurons, and enhanced afferent responses to a variety of peripheral sensations (6). These related phenomena are maintained by an up-regulation in the production of facilitating peptides in the dorsal root ganglia and dorsal horns (e.g., glutaminergic facilitation) (7). Permissive crosstalk from inappropriate convergence-projection, dichotomized sensory C fibers, and windup can occur within the dorsal horn laminations, brainstem, and at other relevant levels of the CNS. Motor neurons end up receiving enhanced afferent input from a variety of competing sources. The progressive chaos in sensory processing, the associated release of excitotoxic transmitters, and the aberrant sympathetic reflex activity (8,9) eventually result in the emergence of sensitized peripheral tissues, irritative voiding symptoms, dyssynergic voiding efforts, and neurogenically mediated inflammation changes within sensitized issue.

Sensitization, windup, and expansion of receptive fields are classic response properties of the CNS to nociceptive input (10,11). The symptoms of urethral allodynia, referred pain, frequency, and urgency are consistent with these CNS events, as are the signs of sphincter hyperalgesia (local pain), pelvic floor tenderness, rigidity of movement, and dyssynergic voiding. Any breakdown in the pathway (i.e., loss of gated regulation) that normally assures a coordinated CNS regulation of pelvic floor behavior only reinforces pathophysiological behavior.

THE IMPORTANCE OF THE PELVIC FLOOR IN MALE GENITOURINARY PAIN

A vicious circle of pain and dysfunction is often the result of many factors at play over years but perhaps realized with only one triggering event. It is very important to appreciate that inappropriate or nociceptive somatic afferent bombardment of delicate central regulatory micturition circuits

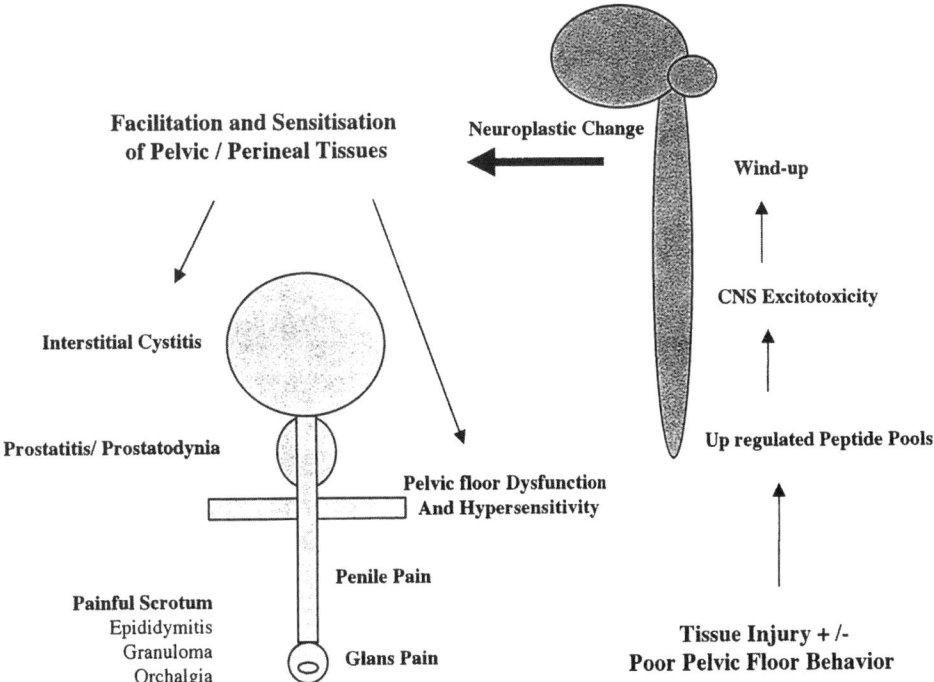

Genesis of Male Genito Urinary Pain

Facilitation and Sensitisation of Pelvic / Perineal Tissues

Neuroplastic Change

Wind-up

Interstitial Cystitis

Prostatitis/ Prostatodynia

CNS Excitotoxicity

Pelvic floor Dysfunction And Hypersensitivity

Up regulated Peptide Pools

Penile Pain

Painful Scrotum
Epididymitis
Granuloma
Orchalgia

Glans Pain

Tissue Injury + /- Poor Pelvic Floor Behavior

FIG. 32-1. CNS events triggered by peripheral nociception.

can be extremely harmful, over time, to the integrity of central pelvic organ regulation. A constant or repetitive noxious behavior can lead to gradual breakdown of normal gating within these CNS centers. There are numerous examples of retentive voiding habits learned in childhood and continued into adulthood, toileting shyness, intolerance of parents toward bedwetting, excessive exercise routines, and chronic postural imbalance. Instrumentation and surgical and psychological distress (12,13) can then compound the neural stress associated with these behaviors. Eventually, a cascade of neural events, normally intended to repair traumatized tissue, is triggered (14–17). A variety of dysfunctional and autonomic symptoms logically follow. It is not surprising, therefore, that chronic pelvic floor dysfunction is often combined with hypersensitivity of lower urinary tract structures. Both are maintained by an up-regulated production of mediators of inflammation and sensitization.

Based on this understanding, it is not surprising that many patients with pelvic pain syndromes do not demonstrate an ability to properly contract and relax the perineum on command. The urethral sphincter and levator muscles often have a distinct hypersensitivity to physical exam, and resting tone is exaggerated. Whether this behavior is predisposing to pain or is a consequence of pain remains to be determined. However, restoration of proper pelvic floor dynamics is one of the important parameters in the management of pain. The reason for this is rooted in CNS responses to persistent nociception.

Referred Pain

Levator myalgias, pain associated with levator hypersensitivity on rectal palpation, can present as a referred pain to the scrotum because of the S-3 link with the viscera. Urethral sphincter pain can present as pain at the tip of the penis, symphysial region, the inner thigh, or groin (inguinal region) (18–20).

In addition to the somatic relationships between referred pain in the pelvis there are extremity relationships. S-2 mediated pain refers to the soles of the feet. Occasionally, tingling of the fingers or achiness in the wrists will be described. S-3 mediated pain will refer to the large toe. S-4 pain generally refers into the rectum. Patients should be queried as to sensitivity or discomforts that may be present in the feet. Hypersensitivity in any of these pathways should be relegated to that specific dermatome.

The Physical Exam

It is logical that all patients presenting with a pain disorder of the genitourinary system should be queried as to their toileting habits. Any recollection of problems in early childhood, adolescence, or adulthood should be noted. A voiding diary is recommended to check for unrecognized voiding irregularities. A patient may not be aware of the fact that his voiding effort is inefficient or less than optimal. This historical exploration should then be followed by a careful clinical examination of the perineum.

Particular interest should be taken in sorting out the dynamics of the pelvic floor. The first step should always be an observation of voluntary attempts to tighten and relax the perineum. This is done with the patient in lithotomy or standing but stooped over and leaning against an examination table. With a "hold" effort, contraction and relaxation of the pelvic floor muscles should be clearly evident. There should be an instantaneous, unhesitating identity with the perineal muscles. The movement should be effortless and free of extraneous muscular activity (i.e., abdominal tightening, Valsalva, pelvic tilt, etc.). The "bellows"-like movement of the levator should be repeatable with consistency, and the contraction should be sustainable for 2–3 seconds before relaxation is permitted. Often the effort is flawed dynamically. Contraction or relaxation or both may be absent or weak. For a more careful exam, the gluteal crease should be slightly separated and the anal region observed for "clamp-like" wrinkling on the hold effort. Occasionally, one may see fibrillations in the superficial anal muscle fibers or the clamp-like movement of the sphincter to the exclusion of the levator bellows-like movement. An alternative recruitment of the pudendal innervated perineal muscles is to observe contraction at the base of the penis during the hold and relaxation effort.

An assessment of pelvic sensation, rectal tone, strength of the lower limbs and feet, and the lability of reflexes involving the bulbocavernosus, anal, knee, and ankle muscles should then be carried out. Brisk lower extremity, urethral, anal, and bulbocavernosal reflexes are useful markers of a hyperexcitable state within specific sacral dermatomes. This examination provides useful insight into the functional integrity of the sacral nerve roots controlling bladder and sphincter behavior. The tonus of the deep (i.e., levator shelf) and superficial anal sphincter should be quantified as normal, weak, or high. Tenderness should be assessed over the levator body, the prostate apex and base, the bladder neck, and the external urethral sphincter. Lastly, the patient is asked to contract on the examining finger, and again the movement is assessed for fluidity, consistency, and repeatability.

The logic for this approach lies in the fact that pain symptoms can result from an abnormality expressed throughout a dermatome. Even if pain appears to be site specific, normalization of voiding effort should be assured in order to help down-regulate aberrant CNS activity contributing to the pain symptoms.

Lastly, sites of specific tenderness should be examined and a quantification scheme applied to the reflex excitability and sensitivity of all relevant tissues—soles of the feet, levator body, urethral sphincter, prostate, bladder neck, and perineal sensation. This approach is recommended in all pelvic pain conditions.

Urodynamics

Urodynamic studies are used to provide an objective documentation of dynamic behavior of the whole lower urinary tract. Traditionally, urodynamic testing includes a cystometrogram, a urethral pressure profile, a urinary flow rate check, and a documentation of residual urine by ultrasound. Additional tests include leak point pressure and various neurologic tests—EMG monitoring of the pelvic floor, pudendal motor term latencies, and evoked potential studies. Radiologic tests include video monitoring of the bladder during filling and emptying (i.e., a voiding cystourethrogram or VCUG). Of the entire test, the most useful information will be obtained from the urethral pressure profile (UPP).

Recording of Urethral Sphincter Activity

The urethral pressure profile (UPP) is recorded with the bladder filled to roughly 25% and 75% of suspected capacity. Sensitivity to the presence of the catheter is especially noted (hypersensitive urethras are most often associated with labile activity and with irritative voiding symptoms). Each time the profile is repeated, changes in urethral tone, reflex excitability of the pelvic floor striated muscles, and triggering of an unstable bladder contraction are noted. The real value of the UPP is achieved only when the data are collected and viewed with a dynamic perspective. Static pressure readings have limited value. They are, however, useful in cases of pure anatomical weakness.

There are a number of syndromes whose underlying symptoms are consistent with the urodynamic findings of a hyperpathic urethra. There are two principal features common to all of these syndromes.

Voiding Dysfunction

Symptoms of voiding dysfunction include urgency, frequency, dribbling, occasional incontinence, and chronic urinary retention, primarily due to a failed micturition reflex secondary to inefficient sphincter relaxation.

Genitourinary Hypersensitivity (Tables 32-1 and 32-2)

Symptoms include localized tenderness and referred discomforts primarily to the lower abdomen, pubic region, and inner thigh and secondarily to the feet, flanks, jaws, shoulders, and hands.

Many diagnoses assigned to patients have little to do with the origin of the symptoms. Without proper assessment, the true cause of symptoms will not be appreciated.

Treatment

The approaches to management of pain follow three lines of care: (a) management of pelvic floor behavioral and/or psychological stress that adds to pain; (b) medications to reduce pain, anxiety, and memoried muscle tone; (c) surgery for identifiable abnormalities. All three are important. Surgery has its place but should not be viewed as the primary therapy. In fact, surgery for male genitourinary pain is rarely definitive and should be undertaken only when there is a reasonable expectation of benefit. Orchiectomies, epididymectomies, prostatectomies, and nerve ligations, purely to relieve pain, are of particular concern in this regard.

There is a host of medications from which to chose (21) (Table 32-3). But the primary medication protocol should be a tricyclic (e.g., elavil 25–50 mg qid), an analgesic (e.g., oxycodone Tabs I-II q6h prn), an anxiolytic (e.g., xanax 0.5 mg qid), and an alpha blocker (minipress I-II tabs HS) in some combination. This is a very inexpensive protocol that often is successful in relieving pain, especially when used simultaneously with pelvic floor biofeedback. One can graduate the strength of the medication if there is no pain relief. Marcaine, ropivicaine, or lidocaine, mixed with a steroid and given as site-specific injections once a week for

TABLE 32-1. *Descriptive diagnosis for chronic pelvin pain (CPP)*

Chronic abacterial prostatitis	Epididymitis
Prostatodynia	Vasectomy "granuloma" pain
Orchalgia/testalgia	Coccyxodynia
Penile pain	Tension floor myalgia
Interstitial cystitis	Urethritis/urethralgia

TABLE 32-2. *Chronic pain syndromes*

What's in		What's out
Dedicated pelvic care centers	Vs.	Solo MD pain management
The pelvis is a neurobiological unit	Vs.	Isolated pelvic organ inflammatory disease
Neuromediated inflammatory theories	Vs.	"Psychological" pain
Nondestructive care—medication, biofeedback, neuromodulation	Vs.	Destructive care—urethrotomy, neurolysis, adhesiolysis, diversion
Combination drug regimes: tricyclics, alpha blockers, anxiolytics, antiseizure, nonnarcotic/narcotic medications	Vs.	Solo dependence on opioids/astringent intravesical instillation, e.g., silver nitrate, chlorpactin
Preemptive anesthesia (epidural, spinal, wound)	Vs.	Solo general anesthesia
Long-term care programs using symptom scores/ void diaries/ flow rates	Vs.	Short-term limited followup postdiagnostic or surgical procedures

TABLE 32-3. *Medications*

Presently used	Efficacy to be determined
Tricyclic antidepressants/SSRI Elavil, Nortriptyline/Paxil	Neurotoxins Capsaicin, Resiniferotoxin, Botox, cone snail toxin
Adrenergic blockers Minipress, Flomax, Hytrin, Cardura	Channel drugs Na, K, NMDA blockers
Anticonvulsants Dilantin, Tegretol, Neurontin, Clonazepam	Autoimmune BCG
Anticholinergics Detrol, Ditropan-XL	Antiinflammatory Hyaluronic acid, COX-2/leukotriene inhibitors
Short-acting analgesics Vicodin, Percocet	Commercial combinations e.g., Vicoprofen, morphine + dextromethorphan
Long-acting analgesics Oxycontin, Durgesic, MS-Contin	New immune suppressants
Nonnarcotic analgesia	H2 blockers—rantidine, cimetidine
Implantable drug delivery morphine/clonidine	

2 or 3 weeks, can also be tried. Subsequently, local Botox injections can follow (22), but appropriate trials for this approach have yet to be done, and no conclusions as to the efficacy are available.

For more generalized pain, refractory to medication and biofeedback, a trial of sacral nerve stimulation can be tried (23). Good responses are associated with a reduction in tenderness of the levator muscles. After these approaches have failed, point surgery can be considered. Surgery, however, should always be preceded by the more conservative options because there are inherent risks in windup and metabolic disturbances of peripheral nerve integrity. Symptom scores, void diaries, and urodynamic studies are recommended as a means to follow effectiveness of therapy and should be done periodically, even after a period when pain seems to have been controlled, stabilized, or cured. These are relatively easy to obtain and will help quantify the motor/sensory disturbances in neural regulation of pelvic organs. They will also provide a baseline guide for response to therapy.

Neurotoxins—Botulinum Toxin A

Botulinum toxin type A (BTX) is a potent neurotoxin with a high affinity toward acetylcholine (ACh) receptors. It is produced by the gram-negative, rod-shaped anaerobic bacterium *Clostridium botulinum*. Although the neurotoxin is most potent at somatic neuromuscular junctions, it does have the ability to inhibit autonomic cholinergic transmission (21). BTX is therefore capable of inhibiting transmitter release from pre- and postganglionic cholinergic nerve endings of the autonomic nervous system as well as interfering with smooth muscle visceral function. Injected BTX will be quickly attached to ACh receptors when injected into the target tissue. There is very little risk that the BTX will adversely affect neighboring striated or visceral smooth muscle or even ganglionic transmission. BTX does not penetrate the blood-brain barrier in doses used therapeutically, nor does it affect cardiac muscle. For these reasons, BTX, in doses used clinically, is considered a highly selective and safe neurotoxin.

Effects of Botulinum Toxin

Whether pelvic muscular dysfunction is a root cause of pain or an integral part of the CNS failure that underlies pain, addressing the muscular dysfunction directly makes sense. It is a logical step toward reducing the neurogenic cascade of events that can feed inflammation and hypersensitivity in tissue. It has been shown that BTX can not only weaken injected muscle, but also affect neighboring muscle within the same dermatome (24). This may occur by local diffusion of the BTX or by its impact on the spinal reflex regulation of muscle within the dermatome. The latter, indirect effect of BTX on spinal cord circuit could occur via BTX action at the intrafusal (25) and/or extrafusal neuromuscular junction (26,27). An observed change in muscle activity pattern after BTX injection suggested that a central reorganization is induced by the therapy. This position is supported by results from a positron emission tomography (PET) study, which showed an increased activation within the parietal cortex and the caudal supplementary motor area after BTX therapy of writer's cramp. The changes that did occur reflected changes in muscle movement strategy and in the associated CNS activation patterns that controlled these muscle activities. These changes could also be explained by a cortical reorganization secondary to loss of motor neurons and decreased sensory afferent input (28).

BTX selective urethral sphincter injection can reduce the hypertonic and hyperreflexic sphincter activity, with the potential to provide pain relief and improvement of lower urinary tract symptoms. Thus, by selectively influencing the contractile tension in the striated urethral sphincter, one can assess, with little risk, the impact on pain and bladder emptying.

CONCLUSION: A BEHAVIORAL PHILOSOPHY TOWARD PELVIC PAIN CONDITIONS

The CNS is composed of a delicately balanced (i.e., gated) circuitry, with a built-in predisposition toward instability. Tissue and/or nerve injury and/or chronic behavioral dysfunction can trigger a release of excitotoxic transmitters.

These in turn can create prolonged changes in central neural circuitry, with resultant permanent change in the way in which nociceptive sensory information is processed.

The concept of abnormal muscular dynamics, mirroring, or driving aberrations in CNS regulation of the lower urinary tract should be considered when there is an obvious disconnect of conscious control of pelvic floor behavior, and there is no explainable cause of chronic pain, regardless of the location of complaint. Therapeutically, the goal is to "wind down" CNS excitability first and foremost before moving to surgical treatments. Preemptive anesthesia (29,30) is recommended for all surgeries performed where there is evidence of pelvic neural dysregulation. This approach should minimize the risk of aggravating symptoms and result in a marked improvement of patient care and satisfaction.

This is a neurological perspective of the problem and requires a more behavioral-based neurodiagnostic evaluation. The approach is consistent with the present shift in emphasis of care toward modulation-based treatments.

REFERENCES

1. Schmidt RA. Pelvic pain. *Problems in Urology* 1989;3:270.
2. Curhan GC, et al. Epidemiology of interstitial cystitis: a population-based study. *J Urol* Feb 1999:549–552.
3. Vizzard MA, Erickson VL, Card JP, et al. Transneuronal labeling of neurons in the adult rat brainstem and spinal cord after injection of pseudorabies virus into the urethra. *J Comp Neurol* 1995;355:629–640.
4. Zermann D, Doggweiler R, Ishigooka M, Schmidt RA. Central autonomic innervation of the lower urinary tract—a neuroanatomic study. *World J Urol* 1998;16:417–423.
5. Woolf CJ, Thompson SW. The induction and maintenance of central sensitization is dependent on NMDA receptor activation; implications for the treatment of post-injury pain hypersensitivity states. *Pain* 1991;Mar 44(3):293–299.
6. Dubner R, Ruda MA. Activity-dependent neuronal plasticity following tissue injury and inflammation. *Trends Neurosci* 1992;15:96–103.
7. Price DD, Mao I, Mayer DJ. Central consequences of persistent pain states. In: Jensen TS, Turner JA, Wiesenfeld-Hallin Z, eds. *Proceedings of the 8th World Congress on pain, progress in pain research and management*, Seattle: IASP Press, 1997;8:155–184.
8. Wesselmann U, Lai J. Mechanism of referred visceral pain: uterine inflammation in the adult virgin rat results in neurogenic plasma extravasation in the skin. *Pain* 1997;73:309–317.
9. McMahorn SB, Wall PD. Receptive field of lamina I projections cells move to incorporate a nearby region of injury. *Pain* 1984;19:235–247.
10. Coderre TJ, Katz J, Vaccarino AL, Melzack R. Contribution of central neuroplasticity to pathological pain: review of clinical and experimental evidence. *Pain* 1993;52:259–285.
11. Hylden JLK, Nahin RL, Traub RJ, Dubner R. Expansion of receptive fields in spinal lamina I projections in rats with unilateral adju-vant-induced inflammation: the contribution of dorsal horn mechanism. *Pain* 1989;37:229–243.
12. Zermann DH, Ishigooka M, Doggweiler R, Schmidt RA. Chronic pelvic pain and bladder dysfunction—wind-up and central sensitization—so we need a more neurourological approach in pelvic surgery? *J Urol* 1998;160:102–105.
13. Rygh IJ, Svendsen F, Hole K, Tjolsen A. Natural noxious stimulation can induce long term increase in spinal nociceptive responses. *Pain* 1999;82:305–309.
14. Dubner R, Basbaum AI. Spinal dorsal horn plasticity following tissue or nerve injury. In: Wall PD, Melzack R, eds. *Textbook of pain*. New York: Churchill Livingstone, 1994:225–241.
15. Lembeck F, Holzer P. Substance P as neurogenic mediator of antidromic vasodilation and neurogenic plasma extravasation. *Naunyn-Schmiedeberg's Arch Pharmacol* 1979;310:175–183.
16. Bennet GJ, Me YK. A peripheral mononeuropathy in rat that produces disorders of pain sensation like those seen in man. *Pain* 1988;33:87–107.
17. Levine JD, Dardick SJ, Basbaum AI, Scipio E. Reflex neurogenic inflammation I: contribution of the peripheral nervous system to spatially remote inflammatory responses that follow injury. *J Neuro* 1985;5:1380–1386.
18. Ishigooka M, Zerman D, Doggweiler R, Schmidt RA. Similarity of distribution of spinal c-fos and plasma extravasation after acute chemical irritation of the bladder and the prostate. *J Urol* Nov 2000;164:1751–56.
19. Zermann DH, Ishigooka M, Doggweiler, R, Schmidt RA. Neuro-urological insights to the etiology of genitourinary pain in men. *J Urol* (1999a; 161:903–908.
20. Zermann DH, Schmidt RA. *Neurophysiology of the pelvic floor and its role in prostate disorders and pelvicpain*. Book chapter. ISIS Medical Media, 1999.
21. Jankovic J, Brin MF. Therapeutic uses of botulinum toxin. *New Engl J Med* 1991; 324 :1186–1194.
22. Nuutinen L, Prithvi R. Overview of current and investigational non-narcotic drugs for treatment of acute and chronic pain. *Current Review of Pain* 1998;2:187.
23. Schmidt RA. Neurostimulation and neuromodulation: a guide to selecting the right urologic patient *Eur. Urol* 1998;34(Suppl 1).
24. Eleopra R, Tugnoh V, Caniatti L, DeGrandis D. Botulinum toxin treatment in the facial muscles of humans: evidence of an action in untreated near muscles by peripheral local diffusion. *Neurology* 1996; 46:1158–1160.
25. Priori A, Berardelli A, Mercuri B, Manfredi M. Physiological effects produced by botulinum toxin treatment of upper limb dystonia. Changes in reciprocal inhibition between forearm muscles. *Brain* 1995; 118:801–807.
26. Bertolasi L, Priori A, Tomelleri G, et al. Botulinum toxin treatment of muscle cramps: a clinical and neurophysiological study. *Ann Neurol* 1997;41:181–186.
27. Gelb DJ, Yoshimura DM, Olney RK, et al. Change in pattern of muscle activity following botulinum toxin injections for torticollis. *Ann Neurol* 1991;29:370–376.
28. Ceballos-Baumann AO, Sheean G, Passingham RE, et al. Botulinum toxin does not reverse the cortical dysfunction associated with writer's cramp. A PET study. *Brain* 1997;120:571–582.
29. Lascelles BDX, Waterman AE, Cripps PJ, et al. Central sensitization as a result of surgical pain: investigation of the pre-emptive value of pethidine for ovariohysterectomy in the rat. *Pain* 1995;62:140–142.
30. Pockett S. Spinal cord synaptic plasticity and chronic pain. *Anesth Analg* 1995;80:173–179.

CHAPTER 33

Complex Regional Pain Syndrome

Allen H. Hord and Linda H. Wang

A regional pain disorder associated with autonomic disturbances, as well as motor and sensory abnormalities, was described many years ago and named causalgia by Weir Mitchell (1). Later, the term *reflex sympathetic dystrophy* (RSD) became commonly used (2). Because of the different clinical presentations and the difficulty in diagnosing and treating the unique pain states, many other terms are used to describe different clinical manifestations of this disorder (Table 33-1). The major reason for the many (and often confusing) terms is that the root causes of the disease and its true pathophysiology are not yet completely understood.

In 1986, the International Association for the Study of Pain (IASP) tried to simplify the terms into RSD and causalgia (3). Dissatisfaction remained over the term *RSD*, since the presence of sympathetic dysfunction and dystrophic changes were not uniform and there was no evidence of a reflex arc. In 1994, the IASP adopted the term *complex regional pain syndrome* (CRPS) to replace RSD and causalgia, where CRPS Type I is equivalent to RSD and CRPS Type II to causalgia (4).

TABLE 33-1. *Other terms used to describe CRPS*

Acute atrophy of bone
Acute peripheral trophoneurosis
Algodystrophy mineures
Algodystrophy reflexes
Algodystrophy
Algoneurodystrophy
Causalgia
Clenched fist syndrome
Chronic traumatic edema
Mimo-causalgia
Minor-causalgia
Neurodystrophy
Pain-dysfunction syndrome
Posttraumatic dystrophy
Posttraumatic osteoporosis
Reflex neurovascular dystrophy
Reflex sympathetic dystrophy
Shoulder hand syndrome
Spreading neuralgia
Sudeck's atrophy
Sympathalgia
Sympathetically maintained pain
Sympathetic overdrive syndrome
Thermalgia
Traumatic angiospasm
Traumatic vasospasm

TYPES OF CRPS

CRPS Type I (RSD)

CRPS Type I or RSD is a syndrome that usually develops after an initiating noxious event, is not limited to the distribution of a single peripheral nerve, and is usually disproportionate to the inciting event. It is associated with evidence of edema, changes in skin blood flow, abnormal sudomotor activity, and allodynia and/or hyperalgesia (4). Cold hyperalgesia is a common patient complaint, whereas heat hyperalgesia is often evident on testing. Mechanical allodynia is also a frequent complaint. In our clinical experience, vibratory allodynia is also commonly present.

CRPS Type II (Causalgia)

CRPS Type II or causalgia is burning pain, allodynia, and hyperpathia usually in the hand or foot after partial injury of a major peripheral nerve (4). Vasomotor and sudomotor changes are common as in CRPS Type I. The most common injuries associated with CRPS Type II are of the median and sciatic nerves.

INITIAL CAUSES OF CRPS

CRPS is typically initiated by a traumatic injury to the limb such as sprain, dislocation, fracture, crush injury and laceration, or surgery (5), or a peripheral nerve injury. It has also been reported following minor procedures such as routine venipuncture (6), central line placement (7), or epidural steroid injection (8). No correlation exists between the severity of the injury and the resultant intensity of the patient's symptoms. In addition, the syndrome has been associated with medical conditions such as diabetic neuropathy, multiple sclerosis (9), cerebral vascular accidents (10), myocardial infarction, and cancerous infiltration a nerve plexus (11). Sometimes, no cause can be identified (Table 33-2).

TABLE 33-2. *Initial causes of CRPS*

Trauma

Accidental injury
Sprain, dislocations, fracture (usually of the hands, feet, or wrists)
Minor cuts or pricks, lacerations, contusions
Crush injury of fingers, hands, or wrists; traumatic amputation of fingers or toes
Burn

Surgery
Procedures in the extremities
Excision of small tumors ganglia of wrist
Forceful manipulation, tight casts
Surgical scars
Damage to small peripheral nerves with a needle
Injections or irritants

Medical conditions

Visceral diseases
Diabetic neuropathy, myocardial infarction

Neurologic diseases
Cerebral vascular accidents, tumors
Poliomyelitis, combined degeneration, tumors
Spinal nerves or their roots: herpes zoster, radiculitis
Brachial plexus, spinal cord injury
Infiltrating carcinoma from the breast, apex of the lung (upper extremity), or pelvis (lower extremity)

Other diseases
Multiple sclerosis

Infections
Extremity skin and other soft tissues
Periarticular

Vascular disease
Polyarteritis nodosa, diffuse arteritis
Arteriosclerosis
Peripheral thrombophlebitis, tissues

Musculoskeletal disorders
Postural defects
Myofascial syndromes
Idiopathic

Because CRPS has different clinical presentations and is often misdiagnosed, its actual incidence is unknown. Little data has been published assessing the epidemiology of CRPS. In the United States, most clinical studies have indicated that higher incidence of this disease appears at middle age, but it occurs in almost every age group, including children (12–16). The higher incidence in working age groups may reflect an association with work-related trauma. This disorder affects all races, although it appears that CRPS has a higher incidence in females (17), Caucasians, and northern Europeans (18).

Mailis and Wade were the first to suggest a possible genetic predisposition to CRPS (18). Recently, the results from a clinical study in Netherlands suggest that HLA-DQ1or HLA-DQ13 (the human leukocyte antigen) may be associated with CRPS Type I and Type II (19–21).

ETIOLOGY/PATHOGENESIS OF CRPS

While theories abound, the definitive etiology/pathogenesis of CRPS remains unclear (22,23). The following paragraphs summarize several theories of the pathophysiology of this disorder.

Hyperdynamic Sympathetic Activity

CRPS may be caused by a prolonging of the normal sympathetic response to injury. A sympathetic reflex arc is the normal response to any traumatic injury. Painful afferent impulses from the periphery travel along A-delta and C fibers from the peripheral nerves to enter the spinal cord through the dorsal roots and synapse in the dorsal horn with interneurons carrying the impulses to the ascending spinothalamic tract to the somatosensory cortex; the anterior horn, where a motor reflex may be initiated by efferent motor fibers causing muscle contraction; and the intermediolateral cell column, where the painful message is relayed to the sympathetic nerve cell bodies.

After injury, a sympathetic reflex is activated in response to pain whereby efferent sympathetic impulses are sent out of the spinal cord through the white rami communicantes and then into the sympathetic chain to synapse in the sympathetic ganglion. The impulses are carried by postganglionic sympathetic fibers (the gray rami communicantes) as they leave the ganglia and travel with the peripheral nerve and/or blood vessels to the extremity, producing vasoconstriction. This is a normal fight-or-flight reflex, which gives way to vasodilatation as part of the orderly progression toward healing (24). If this sympathetic reflex arc does not shut down but continues to function and/or accelerate, a sympathetic hyperdynamic state ensues. This results in increased vasoconstriction and tissue ischemia, causing persistent nociception. Persistent nociception continues to increase afferent pain impulses traveling to the spinal cord and reactivate the sympathetic reflex (24). Why a hyperdynamic sympathetic state continues after the initial tissue injury has healed is unknown. Most recent reviews of hypotheses for this syndrome have been focusing on the site of origin of the pain impulses.

This hypothesis was popular for many years. However, not only is it simplistic, but there is little evidence for increased sympathetic nerve stimulation. In animals, there is evidence that sympathetic denervation occurs after injury (25) even though peripheral receptors may remain sensitive to circulating catecholamines.

Sensitization of Peripheral Mechanoreceptors and Nociceptors

Clinical and animal studies suggest that there may be sympathetic-afferent coupling at sensory nerve endings, by expression of alpha-adrenergic sensitive receptors on injured nerves (26). Norepinephrine may be released from sympathetic terminals or denervation hypersensitivity to circulatory catecholamines may occur. Sympathetic stimulation may directly activate the peripheral sensory nerves of the afferent spinothalamic tract, which transmit intense pain and temperature signals to the somatosensory cortex.

Alteration of Input to the Central Nervous System

Constant and normal sensory input is thought to suppress sympathetic activity. When an extremity becomes painful, it is used less. In the case of CRPS, allodynia and hyperalgesia cause the patient to minimize contact, which eventually results in decreased afferent activity. This decreased afferent activity limits the normal inhibition of the sympathetic system, allowing increased sympathetic discharge. Such a mechanism can explain the positive clinical results seen with massage, desensitization, and stress loading of a body part affected by CRPS.

Neurogenic Inflammatory Process

In its early phase, CRPS Type I has an inflammatory component. Substance P and other neuropeptides are considered to be the cardinal mediators of neurogenic inflammation (27). Analysis of joint fluid and synovial biopsies in CRPS patients (28) has shown increases in protein concentration, synovial hypervascularity, and neutrophil infiltration. Such a mechanism can explain the positive clinical results seen with corticosteroids in early CRPS (stage 1).

Altered Central Processing

CRPS is characterized by spontaneous burning pain and pain from gentle mechanical stimulation (allodynia). During light touch, afferents signal gentle mechanical stimulation, but never signal pain in normal patients. Therefore, the abnormal touch-evoked pain sensations strongly implicate altered central processing of the signal from peripheral mechanoreceptors.

Some earlier studies (29,30) proposed that the essential dysfunction in CRPS might be an abnormal sensitivity in spinal nociceptive neurons, or in higher centers (31). Tahmoush (32) specifically suggested that there might be abnormal discharge of wide-dynamic-range (WDR) neurons in the dorsal horn of the spinal cord. Furthermore, Roberts (33), based on reviewing studies, hypothesized that sensitization of WDR neurons plays an important role in altered central processing in CRPS.

Initiation of Sensitization of WDR Neurons

WDR neurons (also called multireceptive neurons or class 2 cells), second-order neurons associated with sensory processing, exist in high concentration in Lamina V of the dorsal horn. Roberts (33) proposed that trauma in some peripheral tissue first activates unmyelinated (C) nociceptors. This activity excites WDR neurons in the spinal cord and also causes these neurons to become more responsive to all subsequent afferent input (sensitized). This sensitization of WDR neurons results in an abnormally high rate of firing in response to afferent input (34). The supporting evidence can be found in several studies (35–40). However, there is no study that indicates the onset time for the initiation of this sensitization of WDR neurons. In addition, it is still unclear why this sensitization of WDR neurons does not take place in all noxious events.

Maintenance of the Sensitization of WDR Neurons

The initiation of sensitization of WDR neurons may be induced by all injuries in peripheral tissue. However, this sensitization of WDR neurons may be persistent or may be transient. WDR neurons with persistent sensitization may be involved in the development of CRPS.

Gracely et al. (41) propose that altered central processing in CRPS is maintained dynamically by ongoing activity from nociceptive afferents. Rygh et al. (42), based on studies using a single-unit extracellular recording technique, reported that long-term changes could be induced in WDR neurons in the spinal dorsal horn of rats after either tetanic stimulation to the sciatic nerve or a severe natural stimulus. Continuous sensitization of WDR neurons may be also due to activation of A fiber alpha-2 adrenoceptors. It has been demonstrated that after a peripheral nerve lesion, noradrenaline released by activity of sympathetic postganglionic axons excites primary afferent neurons. Thus, by activating alpha-adrenoceptors, signals are generated that enter the "pain pathways" of the central nervous system (43). In addition, inflammation due to peripheral tissue injuries can result in the sensitization of primary nociceptive afferent fibers by prostanoids that are released from sympathetic fibers (44). The site of coupling, however, is unclear.

Sympathetic Actions on Primary Afferents that Project on the Sensitized WDR Neurons

Roberts also proposed that the spontaneous burning pain associated with CRPS results from sympathetic activity on mechanoreceptors that project onto sensitized WDR neurons. Following chronic constriction injury of the sciatic nerve in the rat, rapid sprouting of adrenergic fibers in the dorsal root ganglia grows in the distribution of the injury (26). WDR neurons may respond to sympathetic efferent actions on the sensory nerves in the absence of cutaneous stimulation. One of the cutaneous receptors, called slowly adapting type I (SAI) receptors, has been reported to be responsive to light touch and to maintained pressure (45). SAI receptors have been shown to make excitatory monosynaptic connections with WDR neurons (45). Using spinal recording techniques in cats, Roberts and Foglesong (46) found that nearly half of WDR neurons tested were activated by sympathetic stimulation, but none of the nociceptor-specific neurons and only 17% of the low-threshold neurons were activated.

In summary, the essential dysfunction in CRPS is a persistent sensitization of spinal WDR neurons, resulting in an abnormally high rate of firing in response to nonnociceptive afferent input. Although the initiation of sensitization may be due to action potentials in C-nociceptors, the spontaneous pain and ongoing sensitization associated with the syndrome may be caused by sympathetic activation of mechanoreceptors that project onto sensitized WDR neurons.

CLINICAL PRESENTATION OF CRPS

The major clinical symptoms, forming a triad of sensory, autonomic, and motor dysfunction, show a great variability as to expression and time course.

Sensory Dysfunction

Pain

Pain associated with CRPS is the most prominent and disabling symptom. The pain is usually constant and spontaneous but with recurrent paroxysmal aggravations by physical or psychological stress. It may vary in severity from mild discomfort to excruciating and intolerable pain. The pain is most severe at night (47). Pain may be described as burning, aching, tearing, crushing, stabbing, or lancinating in nature. Most patients have multiple qualities to their pain. Initially, the pain may be localized to the site of injury, but later presents in a nonanatomical distribution that does not follow the distribution of a single peripheral nerve. The pain often is described in a stocking or glove distribution (48). With time, it may spread to involve the entire extremity. Pain spreading beyond the affected extremity to the contralateral limb, and sometimes even to the ipsilateral extremity or the entire side of the body, have been described.

Altered Sensation

Hyperesthesia (increased sensation upon stimulation) is almost invariably a part of CRPS (49). The patient characteristically protects the involved extremity. Not infrequently, a patient will appear for treatment with the involved extremity wrapped in a protective cloth. If the examining physician attempts to touch the affected extremity, the patient characteristically withdraws and refuses to allow anything to make contact with it. In addition, hyperalgesia (increased pain response to a slightly painful stimulus) in CRPS is often an important clinical finding. Allodynia (pain that is produced by a nonpainful stimulus) may be present, such as pain with the light touch of a bedsheet. Patients with CRPS usually also complain about an unpleasant or uncomfortable, but not painful, feeling after application of cold (ice pack, fluoromethane), vibration (tuning fork), or light touch on the affected extremity. The IASP defines this abnormal sensation as dysesthesia. There also may be hyperpathia, which is a delayed overreaction and after-sensation to a stimulus.

Autonomic Symptoms

Disturbance of autonomic function is a common finding for CRPS. It may manifest either as vasoconstriction, which produces pallor or cyanosis and coldness of the skin, or as vasodilatation, which results in a warm and erythematous extremity. Not infrequently, edema and sudomotor disturbances (hyperhidrosis or hypohidrosis) are also evident (50,51). As the disease progresses, trophic changes develop insidiously and include thin, glossy skin; atrophy of muscle; decalcification of bones; thickened and brittle nails; coarsened hair; and a decrease in the rate of hair and nail growth.

Motor Dysfunction

Stiffness is the most distressing physical finding for CRPS patients, and it is much worse than that found in usual cases of trauma, surgery, or other diseases (52–54). The CRPS patients are often unable to initiate movement. Without treatment, the stiffness becomes progressively worse throughout the course of the disease. Other dyskinetic symptoms or signs (53) include muscle spasm, intention or postural tremor, weakness, and hyperreflexive movement (55).

Other

Another group of clinical findings includes reactive psychological disturbances. These include anxiety, depression, and the state of hopelessness experienced by the patient (56).

Although the majority cases of CRPS are reported in extremities, facial pain syndromes are also reported (57) after maxillofacial surgery for cancer, penetrating trauma such as bullet wounds, head injury, and difficult dental procedures. The clinical presentations of facial CRPS may be similar to those in CRPS of an extremity.

COURSE OF CRPS

CRPS progresses in phases. DeTakats (24) initially defined the three stages of CRPS, and Bonica (24) later modified them. Stage I is the acute, hyperemic, or traumatic stage. It occurs immediately after injury and may last several weeks or months. Stage II is the dystrophic or ischemic stage and usually takes place within 2 to 6 months from the onset of symptoms. Its duration is extremely variable. Finally, stage III is the atrophic stage. This usually occurs greater than 6 months after onset and may be permanent (24). However, patients do not necessarily fit into a particular stage. One may have a mixed clinical picture. It is not critical to stage the patient with CRPS, but it may be useful in determining treatment options (Table 33-3).

Stage I (Acute/Hyperemic Stage)

The acute or hyperemic stage begins at the time of injury or may be delayed by several days or weeks. It is characterized by moderate constant burning pain, which is usually localized to the area of injury. The pain is aggravated by movement and is associated with hyperesthesia, allodynia, and hyperpathia. Hypoesthesia (diminished sensitivity to

noxious stimulation) may also be present. Local edema is a major component of CRPS during stage I. At this stage the skin is usually warm, red, and dry because of presumed vasodilatation. However, an animal study has shown that nutritional blood flow to the skin may be decreased despite abnormally high flow through thermoregulatory AV shunts, which causes the increase in temperature immediately following nerve injury (58).

In cases involving an injured arm, the patients hold the hands and fingers in a slightly flexed position. The grip is weak. An affected leg is also weak, and the patient may use a cane or crutch to walk. Limitation of range of motion or strength is primarily due to pain in this stage. Radiographs taken in this stage usually show slight, if any, osteoporosis, but bone scans show increased total flow to the limb and increased bone metabolism. This stage can last from a few weeks to as long as 6 months. Most clinical studies suggest that recognition of stage I is important, since the syndrome can be more easily reversed by exercise, corticosteroids, or sympathetic blockade.

Stage II (Dystrophic/Ischemic Stage)

The stage is characterized by the spreading of edema, increasing stiffness of the joints, and muscular wasting. Pain remains the major symptom and is usually spontaneous and burning in nature. Pain in the affected limb can be increased by any stimulus. The pain may radiate proximally or distally from the site of injury and may involve the whole extremity. Hyperpathia and allodynia are usually more pronounced than in stage I. Redness begins to diminish, and eventually skin color is more likely to be pale or cyanotic. The skin is moist at the early phase of stage II. Hyperhidrosis may give way to dryness later in the second stage. The hair is coarse, and the nails show ridges and are brittle. Signs of atrophy become more prominent, and radiographs usually reveal patchy osteoporosis. During this stage, sympathetic blocks may still be effective in reversing the process.

Stage III (Atrophic Stage)

The third stage implies irreversible trophic changes and intractable pain involving the limb. The skin becomes smooth, glossy, cold, and tight; and it appears pale or cyanotic in color. The hair may be long and course at the beginning of this stage and may later be thin or absent. The subcutaneous tissues are atrophic, as are the muscles, particularly the interossei. The affected limb may have flexor tendon contractions and marked atrophy of the muscles leading to severe limitations in joint and limb mobility. Marked osteoporosis is present and radiographs show subperiosteal resorption of bone. Since the effects of CRPS at this stage are mostly irreversible, the patient is left with not only a permanent disability, but also constant pain and emotional distress. The spreading of pain within the limb

TABLE 33-3. *Clinical presentations of CRPS*

Clinic presentations	Stage I	Stage II	Stage II
Burning pain	Moderate	Severe	Severe
Allodynia	Moderate	Severe	Severe
Edema	Severe	Moderate to severe	Mild
Skin temperature	Warm	Cold	Cold
Skin discoloration	Redness	Mild cyanotic/pale	Severe cyanotic/pale
Sudomotor disturbance	Mild	Moderate	Severe
Stiffness	Mild (due to pain)	Moderate	Severe
Trophic changes	None	Mild to moderate	Severe
Location of symptoms	Around injured site	Radiate proximally/distally from the injured site	Entire extremity
Sympathetic blocks	Effective	May be effective	Usually ineffective

is common and spread to other limbs has been described (59). The mechanism of spread to other limbs is unknown.

DIAGNOSTIC STUDIES

There is no confirmatory test or procedure available for CRPS (60). The following studies may help the physician make a proper diagnosis or determine the best course of treatment.

Temperature Measurement

Temperature changes in the affected extremity are a simple but important observation to record during examination of the patient with suspected CRPS. Skin temperature depends on thermoregulatory blood flow, which is under the control of the sympathetic nervous system. Early in the course of CRPS (hyperemic stage), the affected extremity may be warmer than other tissues, whereas later in the course, skin blood flow and temperature may be reduced.

Thermography

Thermography is a noninvasive procedure that images the temperature distribution of the body surface. This test measures thermoregulatory blood flow and is useful for measuring temperature differences between the affected and unaffected limbs. The temperature of a limb with CRPS in the early stages of this disease will be about 2°C higher than an unaffected limb (61), while in the later stages, the affected limb will have a lower temperature than the unaffected limb. This has also been shown in animals with an experimental neuropathy (25,62). Potentially confounding variables have to be considered, including room temperature, emotions, tobacco, and alcoholic or caffeinated beverages. Thermography is valuable in recording a precise skin temperature at a precise time, but does not measure dynamic changes. Therefore, it cannot diagnose CRPS with a great degree of accuracy or specificity. However, it is a rapid, noninvasive, sensitive technique for early detection of CRPS (63).

Plain Radiographs

The radiological aspects of CRPS have often been reviewed with much attention directed to the patchy demineralization (patchy osteoporosis) found in later stages of CRPS (64). Genant et al. (65), using fine detailed radiography, described five types of bone resorption in CRPS patients: metaphyseal regional resorption, subperiosteal resorption, intracortical resorption, endosteal bone resorption, and surface erosions of subchondral and juxta-articular bone. However, patchy osteoporosis is not a diagnostic finding, since other medical conditions and diseases may show the same radiographic change, and these changes may not be observed in all patients with CRPS.

Radionuclide Imaging (Three-Phase Radionuclide Bone Scanning)

The technique uses intravenous 99mTc-methylene diphosphonate in three phases of exposure: angiographic, immediate postinjection blood-pool image, and delayed images at 3 or 4 hours (66). In the first phase, serial images demonstrate arterial blood flow. The second phase reveals the vascular and soft tissue distribution of radionuclide. The third (late or delayed) phase shows uptake of technetium into bone in response to an increase in blood flow, inflammatory reaction, osteogenic activity, and/or increase in bone metabolism. The scan pattern most commonly associated with CRPS includes increased flow to the involved extremity in the angiographic and/or blood-pool phases and diffuse periarticular uptake in delayed images (67–69). Blood flow on bone scan returns to normal as the disease progresses. Sensitivity and specificity of the three -phase bone scan appears to be high, although lack of common diagnostic criteria for CRPS prevents comparison to other techniques (67,70). In addition, similar scans may be seen in several other medical conditions, such as disuse osteoporosis, cellulitis, degenerative joint disease, recent trauma, and osteomyelitis (67).

Hoffman and colleagues (71) evaluated the effect of stellate ganglion block on the three-phase radionuclide bone scanning. They reported that all of their 15 patients with upper extremity CRPS had significant relief with the stellate ganglion block with 0.5% bupivacaine. There was a significant linear relationship between change in counts from baseline to postsympathetic block on the blood-pool image and bone-uptake image. As blood-pool and bone-uptake counts increased following sympathetic blockade, the likelihood of CRPS findings on bone scan also increased. The study suggests that sympathetic blocks may increase the sensitivity of the three-phase bone for diagnosis of CRPS.

Sudomotor Testing

The sympathetic postganglionic neuron may be involved in CRPS. A useful index of sympathetic innervation is the integrity of exocrine sweat gland function, because these glands are innervated by sympathetic cholinergic fibers whose function is abolished by sympathectomy. The resting sweat output (RSO) test and the quantitative sudomotor axon reflex test (Q-SART) are used to assess the sudomotor system (51). The findings that correlate best with the diagnosis of CRPS are an increase in RSO and a depressed Q-SART.

Chelimsky and his colleagues (51) suggest the use of multiple autonomic functions tests, including the quantitative sudomotor axon reflex test (Q-SART), the resting sweat output test (RSO), and the resting skin temperature test (RST), for the evaluation of the diagnosis of CRPS. They found that increased RSO predicted the diagnosis of CRPS with 94% specificity, and the specificity was 98% when RSO was considered in conjunction with reduction in Q-SART.

Sympathetic Blocks

In the past, sympathetic blockade was considered both diagnostic and therapeutic for CRPS. This procedure involves injection of a local anesthetic at the sympathetic ganglia to temporarily block sympathetic innervation in the extremity supplied by those ganglia. However, the response to sympathetic blockade is not 100%, even in otherwise classic CRPS (72–74), which suggests that the pain with CRPS may or may not be mediated by the sympathetic nervous system.

Temporary sympathetic blockade usually is used clinically to determine whether pain is, in whole or in part, due to activity in the sympathetic nervous system. When substantial pain relief occurs following sympathetic blockade, the pain syndrome is referred to as sympathetically maintained pain (SMP) (75), in contrast to sympathetic independent pain (SIP) if little or no pain relief occurs (76). Thus, a response to sympathetic blockade should not be used to confirm or rule out a diagnosis of CRPS, but to determine which patients have SMP.

There are a variety of ways in which the sympathetic nervous system can be temporarily blocked. The efficacy and selectivity of the sympathetic block is crucial for accuracy in the diagnosis of the sympathetic nervous system involvement, although the adequacy of sympathetic blockade in SMP does not consistently correlate with the degree of pain relief obtained (77). The most popular method for diagnostic sympathetic block is injection of local anesthetics at the level of the paraspinal sympathetic chain of ganglia, which blocks both preganglionic and postganglionic fibers. Intravenous systemic phentolamine is another method used diagnostically to block both alpha-1 and alpha-2 adrenergic receptors (78). Meanwhile, intravenous regional (IVR) blocks, such as with guanethidine or bretylium, can produce a sympathetic block by preventing release of noradrenaline from sympathetic postganglion neurons (79). Intrathecal and epidural administration of local anesthetics, which block sympathetic preganglionic fibers, are also used for sympathetic blockade (80). However, somatic blockade cannot be excluded with neuraxial regional blocks, and they should not be used to diagnose SMP (although they can be used for treatment).

Pain Relief in the Absence of Sympathetic Block (False Positives)

Patients may report significant pain relief following sympathetic blocks. However, there may be no clinical findings indicating that sympathetic blockade occurred. One explanation is a placebo response (74), because saline injections may give pain relief in some patients. However, pain relief from local anesthetic lasted significantly longer than saline control in the same study of patients with SMP (81). When interpreting the results of sympathetic block, both degree of pain relief and duration of relief must be considered.

Pain relief may also occur due to spread of the anesthetic to nearby somatic afferent nerves and dorsal root ganglia. This can occur with stellate ganglion injections and is unavoidable with epidural and intrathecal local anesthetic injections (82). Another possibility for false positive results is that systemic distribution of locally injected anesthetics occurs and produces analgesia through actions distant from the injection site (83). Recently Linchitz and Raheb (84) reported subcutaneous infusion of lidocaine provided effective pain relief for CRPS patients. Their results suggest that a local anesthetic's systemic action may inhibit the hyperalgesic component of CRPS. Dellemijn et al. suggest correlating phentolamine results with stellate ganglion block results to rule out pain relief from local anesthetic uptake (85).

Lack of Pain Relief Because of Inadequate Sympathetic Blockade (False Negatives)

Obviously, if the pain is truly independent of activity in the sympathetic nervous system, no pain relief is expected. Procedural accuracy is also one of the key factors determining the value of diagnostic sympathetic blocks. A traditional stellate ganglion block at the level of C-6 may give a high incidence of false negative pain relief in SMP of the upper extremity (86), because only cervical sympathetic blockade and partial upper extremity sympathetic blockade may occur. Hogan et al. (86) recommend the injection be done at the T-1 level if using an anterior paratracheal approach in order to block all sympathetic fibers arising from upper thoracic ganglia. Malmquist et al. (87) suggest monitoring upper extremity sympathetic blockade by four criteria: a Horner's syndrome, skin temperature rise to 34°C or higher, greater than 50% increase in skin blood flow, and complete abolition of skin resistance response.

Similarly, lumbar sympathetic block needs to encompass anterolateral prevertebral spread over low segmental levels in order to include the wide diversity in anatomic distribution of sympathetic fiber to the lower extremity. Using imaging methods, such as fluoroscopy or CT, should improve the success of complete lumbar sympathetic block.

Like the problems with sympathetic ganglion blocks, intravenous systemic phentolamine also may have false negative responses. Raja et al. (88) found neither 0.5mg/kg nor 1.0mg/kg of phentolamine caused complete sympathetic block as measured by capillary blood flow changes, abolition of sympathetically induced vasoconstriction, and temperature responses. Therefore, the sensitivity and specificity of response to sympathetic blocks and their value as diagnostic aids will not be fully established without further clinical study.

CLASSIFICATION AND CRITERIA FOR CRPS

RSD and causalgia were the most broadly used terms to describe this regional pain problem before 1994. RSD had become a nondiscriminating diagnosis for patients with many other pain conditions, such as neuropathic pain, myofascial pain, neuralgias, and joint disorders. In 1994, the IASP developed the new nomenclature, CRPS, to replace RSD and causalgia (3). The IASP criteria for CRPS Types I and II are shown in Tables 33-4 and 33-5. Wong and Wilson (89) emphasized that the new classification by IASP was based on a descriptive method that would allow modifications in the future, if indicated by new scientific findings. They summarized:

(1) Complex denotes the varied and dynamic nature of the clinical presentation within a single person over time, and among persons with seemingly similar disorders. It also includes the features of inflammation, autonomic, cutaneous, motor, and dystrophic changes, which distinguish this from other forms of neuropathic pain.
(2) Regional, as in the wider distribution of symptoms and findings beyond the area of the original lesion, is a key characteristic of the disorder.
(3) Pain is the hallmark characteristic of the syndrome. It is out of proportion to the inciting event and includes spontaneous pain, which is often described as burning in quality, and thermal or mechanical allodynia.

The terms *SMP* and *SIP* were not considered as separate disorders but as descriptors of types of pain that can be found in a variety of pain disorders, including CRPS Types I and II. The presence or absence of SMP is not one of the criteria for CRPS.

Few or only mild symptoms may occur in the early stages of CRPS, making the diagnosis difficult. Since many other medical conditions have a similar presentation, it is important to obtain a detailed history, perform a careful physical examination, and order selected laboratory tests. During the examination, the affected extremity should always be compared with the contralateral extremity.

Many other medical conditions have symptoms in common with CRPS Type I and Type II. The examiner must exclude other diagnoses such as unrecognized local pathology (e.g., fracture, strain, sprain), traumatic vasospasm,

TABLE 33-4. *Diagnostic criteria for CRPS Type I*

1. The presence of an initiating noxious event, or a cause of immobilization.
2. Continuing pain, allodynia, or hyperalgesia with the pain disproportionate to any inciting event.
3. Evidence at some time of edema, changes in skin blood flow, or abnormal sudomotor activity in the region of the pain.
4. This diagnosis is excluded by the existence of conditions that would otherwise account for the degree of pain and dysfunction.

Note: Criteria 2–4 must be satisfied. (From Classification of chronic pain: descriptions of chronic pain syndromes and definitions of pain. Merskey H, Bogduc N, eds, 2nd ed: IASP Press, p.42 1994.)

TABLE 33-5. *Diagnostic criteria for CRPS Type II*

1. The presence of continuing pain, allodynia, or hyperalgesia after a nerve injury not necessarily limited to the distribution of the injured nerve.
2. Evidence at some time of edema, changes in skin blood flow, or abnormal sudomotor activity in the region of the pain.
3. This diagnosis is excluded by the existence of conditions that would otherwise account for the degree of pain and dysfunction.

Note: All three criteria must be satisfied. (From Classification of chronic pain: descriptions of chronic pain syndromes and definitions of pain. Merskey H, Bogduc N, eds, 2nd ed: IASP Press, p.42 1994.)

Raynaud's disease, thromboangiitis obliterans, and venous thrombosis (3). In addition, vasoconstriction, edema, and hyperhidrosis may occur as a normal response to localized injury or pain.

TREATMENT

Methods of treatment of CRPS vary widely (Table 33-6), leading to confusion and lack of coordination in treatment. In choosing treatments for CRPS, the inciting pathology, symptoms and physical findings, stage of the disease, and risk-benefit ratio of the treatment for the individual patient must be considered.

Physical Therapy

One of the more common methods of managing CRPS has been multiple-modality physical therapy (PT) (90–92). It is possible that most cases of early CRPS resolve with PT in the postinjury period, so the diagnosis of CRPS is never made. PT aims to improve or maintain mobility and function of the affected limb so the severe osteoporosis, contractures, and muscular atrophy seen in the second and third stages will be avoided. Unfortunately, some patients are intolerant of joint manipulation because of the pain associated with even the mildest levels of PT. In these patients, pain should be controlled with medication or sympathetic or somatic blocks to facilitate PT.

Active and passive exercises are the most important physical treatment. The rationale of this treatment is that active and passive exercises produce a flood of large fiber input to T cells in the substantia gelatinosa, thereby "closing the gate" to the small unmyelinated C fibers transmission of pain. However, Oerlemans et al. (90) recently reported a prospective study of 135 CRPS patients in whom those undergoing PT did not differ significantly from those treated with control treatment (social work) regarding permanent impairment 12 months after treatment.

Watson and Carlson (93) suggested a regimen for CRPS of the hand that they proposed would avoid the pain of joint movement. The regimen consisted of traction and compression, without the joint movement, produced by

TABLE 33-6. *Published treatments for CRPS*

Physical therapy
    Compress application, hot and cold
    Deep friction massage
    Electroacupuncture
    Immobilization with splints
    Range-of-motion exercises
    Transcutaneous nerve stimulation
    Ultrasound

Pharmacologic therapy
    Corticosteroids
    Reserpine (oral)
    Local anesthetics (ganglion block)
    Alpha-adrenergic stimulation (central)
        Methyldopa
        Clonidine
    Alpha-adrenergic antagonism (peripheral)
        Phenoxybenzamine
        Prazosin
        Phentolamine
        Terazosin
    Calcium channel block
        Nifedipine
        Diltiazem
        Verapamil
        Isradipine
    Intravenous regional
        Reserpine
        Guanethidine
        Bretylium
        Ketanserin
        Ketorolac
        Labetalol
    Smooth muscle relaxation
        Griseofulvin
    Alteration of rheology or platelet
        Dazoxiben
        Dextran
        Plasma exchange
        Stanozolol
    Increased serotonin
        Hydroxytryptophan (oral)
        Tricyclic antidepressants

Surgical therapy
    Preganglionic sympathectomy
    Postganglionic sympathectomy
    Periarterial sympathectomy
    Dorsal root entry zone destruction
    Thalamotomy
    Spinal cord stimulation
    Peripheral nerve stimulation

Other
    Hypnosis
    Psychotherapy
    Biofeedback
    Relaxation therapy
    Behavioral modification
    Radiation therapy

scrubbing and carrying exercises. This program of "stress loading" was shown to decrease pain, edema, and vasomotor symptoms while increasing the range of motion and grip strength in series of 41 patients. Most patients were able to perform normal activities, and only 6% failed to return to work after treatment.

Hand and wrist splints commonly have been used in the therapy of upper extremity CRPS. In the latter two stages of the disease, splints may limit contracture formation in some patients but exacerbate pain and disease progression in others.

Transcutaneous electrical nerve stimulation (TENS) is another form of therapy that has been used to control pain in patients with CRPS. Stimulation of A fibers may cause decreased activity of wide-dynamic-range (WDR) neurons in the spinal cord and thus a decrease in pain. Although several investigations involving the use of TENS in children with CRPS have reported excellent results, most studies of adult patients have reported long-lasting relief in only 25% of patients (94). However, Robaina and colleagues (95) reported good to excellent results with TENS in 20 of 29 patients with longstanding CRPS. On the other hand, reports of exacerbation of CRPS pain during TENS therapy are not unusual (96,97).

Daily ultrasonic stimulation has been reported to be effective in a small series of patients (98). Heat therapy (whirlpool, paraffin, or radiant heat) has also been used, although it may cause increased swelling in some patients.

Occupational Therapy

Occupational therapy, alone or in addition to PT, has also been recommended. However, few published studies demonstrate how PT and occupational therapy contribute in different ways to the treatment of CRPS. However, PT has an advantage over occupational therapy regarding cost-effectiveness (90).

Psychological Therapy

Although there is no evidence that CRPS is a psychiatric illness, personality traits and behavioral patterns in patients with CRPS have been noted to be strikingly similar (99). More specifically, patients with CRPS report high levels of anxiety (100,101) and increasing disability caused by CRPS pain in stressful situations. These observations should be regarded as important factors in patient care. A cycle of pain leading to self-perceived stress and disability, which leads to "learned helplessness" followed by behavioral reinforcement, may develop (102). Interruption of this cycle through behavior modification may prove to be a valuable part of therapy. In addition to common psychosocial problems that accompany chronic pain, patients with CRPS also experience exacerbation of their pain with periods of anxiety and stress. It is believed that the release of endogenous catecholamines in response to anxiety and stress result in direct stimulation of sensitized alpha-adrenergic receptors in the affected extremity. Reducing anxiety by minimizing family conflicts and stressful work and social situations is therapeutic. A regimen of thermal biofeedback coupled with guided imagery has been used in the treatment of pain and cold intolerance in patients with CRPS (103). Gainer (104) reported complete resolution of severe symptoms, including pain, dystonia, cold intolerance, and discoloration, with the use of hypnotherapy.

Full discussion of the psychological aspects of CRPS can be found elsewhere (105), but the importance of routine psychological evaluation of patients with CRPS should be emphasized so that individualized therapy can be instituted early in the course of the disease.

Pharmacological Therapy

Corticosteroids

Steroid therapy usually involves the use of oral prednisone given initially at a high dose, followed by rapid tapering. Numerous corticosteroid agents also have been used in patients with CRPS (106–108). Steinbrocker and colleagues (109) used loading doses of corticotropin and cortisone (100 mg and 200 mg/day, respectively) for 3 to 10 days before reducing the dose by small increments for the treatment of "shoulder-hand syndrome." Therapy was continued for approximately 6 months, and pain relief was reported in 9 of 13 patients, whereas 2 of 13 had therapy-related complications. One group from Denmark reported excellent results with oral prednisone at 30 mg/day for no more than 12 weeks in a double-blind, randomized, placebo-controlled study (110). The majority of studies showing efficacy of corticosteroids have selected patients with warm hands, suggesting that the patients were treated early after injury where inflammation may play a greater role than later. Kingery (111) critically reviewed 22 controlled clinical trials for treatment of CRPS. He emphasized that the trial data showed long-term effectiveness only for corticosteroids.

Epidural steroids have been used for the treatment of CRPS in some centers, despite the lack of controlled trials. Dirksen and colleagues (112) reported a patient with a brachial plexus injury who, after failing to get relief from stellate ganglion blockade or intravenous (IV) regional guanethidine, had relief of symptoms of CRPS after treatment with epidural methylprednisolone 60 mg weekly for 4 weeks.

The mechanism of action of corticosteroids in the treatment of CRPS is unknown. Although inflammatory changes occur in CRPS, NSAIDs have not demonstrated therapeutic effects comparable to those of steroids. It has been speculated that immunologic factors may work in CRPS, but no specific findings to support this theory have been published.

Nonsteroidal Antiinflammatory Drugs (NSAIDs)

As noted, systemic NSAIDs are not usually effective in CRPS and other neuropathic pain states. However, there has been one report of the use of ketorolac in an IV regional technique for the treatment of CRPS (113). Vanos (113) and colleagues reported seven patients in whom 60 mg ketorolac was given in saline or 0.5% lidocaine (113). All patients had significant pain relief lasting from 1 to 60 days. There was increased duration of effect with repeated blocks. A recent report by Faria (22) suggests that intramuscular ketorolac may also improve the pain associated with CRPS.

Smooth Muscle Relaxant

Because the vasoconstriction seen in CRPS may lead to tissue or nerve ischemia, medications that produce vasodilatation have been used. A target of pharmacological manipulation has been the smooth muscle of blood vessel walls. Direct relaxation, achieved with griseofulvin in doses of less than 2 mg/day, has been beneficial to some patients, but side effects, such as headache, diarrhea, nausea, and vomiting, are common.

Calcium Channel Blockers

The calcium channel blockers (nifedipine, verapamil, and diltiazem) (114) have proved to be effective in producing vasodilation with minimal side effects in patients with Raynaud's phenomenon. Although nifedipine was shown to be effective in relieving symptoms of CRPS in a preliminary report (115), the investigators were unable to show efficacy in a double-blind study. A study by Muizelaar and colleagues (114) emphasizes that treatment with a calcium channel blocker, such as nifedipine, is more successful in the early stage of CRPS than in the chronic (late) stage. In our experience, some patients have decreased pain or cold intolerance when taking nifedipine. However, the response is unpredictable and appears to be less pronounced with extended-release preparations.

Alpha-adrenergic Agonists and Antagonists

Central alpha-2-receptor agonists, such as clonidine, which cause decreased sympathetic outflow and vasodilatation, have been used for the treatment for CRPS (116). Rauck et al. (117) published a randomized, blinded, placebo-controlled trial of epidural clonidine for treatment of CRPS. Cervical or lumbar epidural catheters were inserted in 26 patients with upper or lower extremity CRPS, respectively. Patients who responded to a single dose of epidural clonidine, but not placebo, received an open-label trial of continuous epidural clonidine for 43 days. They reported that extensive analgesia was obtained in patients receiving epidural clonidine. However, sedation and hypotension may limit epidural clonidine administration for CRPS.

Clonidine also can be applied to the affected skin areas (118,119). Application of clonidine to the skin of patients with CRPS or SMP causes a decrease in stimulus-evoked hyperalgesia (118). The effect appears to be attributable to local presynaptic inhibition of norepinephrine release because injection of intradermal norepinephrine or phenylephrine causes return of the hyperalgesia (118,119). Transdermal clonidine may be useful in patients with CRPS limited to a small area.

Alpha-1 receptor blockade, with agents such as prazosin, terazosin (120), and phenoxyben zamine (72), has been shown to help some patients, but in many, alpha-adrenergic blockade results in hypotension, reflex tachycardia, fatigue, and dizziness. The IV administration of phentolamine has been recommended as diagnostic test for SMP. Phentolamine is a mixed alpha-1/alpha-2 adrenergic antagonist that does not cross the blood–brain barrier. It is not known whether its beneficial effects in patients with SMP are from its alpha-1 or alpha-2 blockade. In our experience, administration of a pure alpha-1 antagonist, such as prazosin, does not always relieve pain, even if the patient does respond to phentolamine. If a trial of prazosin or terazosin is initiated, the dose needs to be titrated upward until pain is relieved or symptoms, such as orthostasis, become limiting. Patients with CRPS seem to tolerate prazosin well, although care should be exercised in normotensive elderly patients and in young women.

Chronic oral use of phenoxybenzamine has been reported to be successful in the management of CRPS, but there is a high incidence (43%) of orthostatic hypotension (121). The rationale for the use of phenoxybenzamine is that it causes noncompetitive, irreversible blockade of alpha-adrenergic receptors, resulting in long-lasting sympathetic blockade. Phenoxybenzamine also has been used for treatment of CRPS by the IVR technique. Malik and colleagues (122) reported that IVR blockade with phenoxybenzamine produced long-term symptom relief (7 days to 18 months) in five patients with CRPS. However, it was not a controlled, randomized, double-blind study.

The results from a recent study of nifedipine and phenoxybenzamine (114) indicate there is no significant difference in efficacy between the two drugs and they are beneficial only for early CRPS. Choices between calcium channel blockers or alpha-adrenergic blockers have been based more on practical considerations.

Calcitonin

Calcitonin is a 32-amino acid hormone of the thyroid "C" cells that lowers plasma inorganic calcium concentration and greatly reduces osteoclastic and osteoblastic activity in the bone. This results in a decrease of the rate of bone remodeling and an increase in the amount of calcium salts deposited in the bone. Possibly the most beneficial effect seems to be the improvement of osteoporosis as seen on radiographs.

Calcitonin has been used experimentally in patients with CRPS, and the results have been encouraging (123,124). Rico and colleagues (125) administered 100 units of salmon calcitonin in a treatment group, while control patients were treated with naproxen 500 mg every 12 hours. Patients treated with calcitonin showed decreased isotope uptake on three-phase bone scan during the treatment period. A synthetic amino analogue of eel calcitonin, carbocalcitonin (carboCT), has been shown to improve pain, edema, mobility, and uptake on three-phase bone scan (126). CarboCT was given intramuscularly (40 units) on a daily basis for 2 to 10 months with no adverse effects. Calcitonin directly constricts bone blood vessels and may prevent osteolytic and osteoclastic activities (127,128). In addition, calcitonin has an analgesic effect. Hamamci and colleagues (123) also reported that 4 weeks of intramuscular salmon calcitonin treatment might be beneficial in decreasing pain and joint tenderness and improving passive range of motion of hemiplegic patients with stages I and II CRPS.

Intranasal calcitonin has had encouraging results in patients with Paget's disease and osteoporosis. Thus, Bickerstaff and Kanis (129) performed a randomized, double-blind trial of calcitonin in 40 patients with CRPS. Calcitonin (200 IU) or placebo was given intranasally twice daily. Measurements of tenderness, hand volume, grip strength, presence of pain, sudomotor changes, swelling, and stiffness were recorded. Although intranasal calcitonin caused a significant decrease in serum calcium, both groups improved, and there was no difference between groups. In another study, Gobelet and colleagues (130) compared treatment with intranasal calcitonin (100 IU three times a day) to a placebo spray. All patients underwent passive PT during the 3-week study period. The authors reported a significant decrease in pain scores and an increase in mobility in all patients, with a larger increase in those receiving calcitonin than in those receiving placebo. Unfortunately, the statistical analyses are incorrectly done, and no conclusions can be drawn from the data.

Antidepressants

Antidepressants are believed to exert their analgesic effects through the enhancement of transmitter activity in central pain-modulating systems, including the descending serotonergic and noradrenergic systems. Most of the evidence supporting the use of antidepressants in the treatment of CRPS/neuropathic pain has focused on the tricyclic antidepressants, including the tertiary amine compounds amitriptyline, imipramine, doxepin, and clomipramine, and the secondary amine compounds desipramine and nortriptyline. The selection of a tricyclic antidepressant for the treatment of CRPS is influenced by the side-effect profile of these drugs. For example, a concern about the potential for orthostatic hypotension suggests the use of a less hypotensive compound, such as nortriptyline. However, amitriptyline is considered the drug of first choice, if tolerated, since it is the most extensively studied agent.

Some investigators recommend obtaining plasma concentrations of tricyclic antidepressants (131). In nonresponders, low levels suggest either poor compliance or rapid metabolism. At relatively high doses, monitoring of plasma concentration can reassure the clinician that further dose increments are safe.

Evidence in support of the analgesic efficacy of the "newer" antidepressants, such as trazodone, fluoxetine, sertraline, maprotiline, and paroxetine, is relatively scant. However, given the favorable side-effect profiles of some of these newer antidepressants, one or more of these agents may be considered for therapeutic trials if the tricyclics are contraindicated or poorly tolerated.

Opioids

Regional opioids are frequently used in the treatment of CRPS. Azad and colleagues (132) reported that continuous axillary brachial plexus analgesia with low-dose morphine (0.16 mg /hour, 3.84 mg /day) might be beneficial in patients with upper extremity CRPS. Epidural opioids combined with local anesthetics or intrathecal opioids also have been successfully used in treatment of CRPS (56,111,133–136). Systemic opioids can be only considered as the last resort of treatment for CRPS, because it appears the pain associated with CRPS often is poorly responsive to them. Meanwhile, the use of opioids tends to lead to drug dependence, depression, and tolerance. Opioids are often used as an adjunct to other treatments, such as controlling pain to allow PT.

Anticonvulsants

Anticonvulsants are usually considered to be first-line drugs for the treatment of neuropathic pain. The presumed mechanism of analgesic action of anticonvulsants is their suppression of afferent electrical activity, although the mechanisms of each drug may vary (137). Carbamazepine is one of the most frequent anticonvulsants used for trigeminal neuralgia. Phenytoin 300 mg per day was reported to give 75% to 80% pain relief in a patient with CRPS of the knee (137,138). The patient was weaned from phenytoin after 1 year with no increase in pain. However, there are no controlled clinical trials of phenytoin in the treatment for CRPS.

Gabapentin (Neurontin) is more popularly used in the treatment of neuropathic pain than other anticonvulsant drugs (e.g., phenytoin, carbamazepine, and valproic acid) because of its better side-effect profile. Mellick and Mellick (139) successfully used gabapentin alone to treat six CRPS patients. The investigators emphasized that gabapentin specifically reduced hyperpathia, allodynia, hyperalgesia, and skin and soft tissue changes. There are no published controlled clinical trials of the use of gabapentin for treatment of CRPS pain, although two double-blind, randomized controlled studies have indicated that gabapentin is effective at high dose (3600

mg/day) for diabetic neuropathic pain and postherpetic neuralgia (140).

Topical Drugs

Available topical therapies fall into four types: capsaicin preparations (141), clonidine (118,119), nitroglycerine ointment (142,143), and dimethyl sulfoxide cream (144). However, controlled studies of these drugs are very limited and clinical experience is minimal. The potential advantages of the topical route for some patients are substantial and empirical use of many drugs, including anticonvulsants, is commonplace. We have frequently used phenytoin or carbamazepine ointments (compounded locally) for patients with small areas of allodynia or hyperalgesia who do not tolerate the side effects of systemic gabapentin or other anticonvulsants.

Capsaicin Topical capsaicin has been suggested as treatment for certain neuropathic pain states since it may deplete substance P in small primary afferent nociceptive neurons. However, there are two major limitations to its use. First, efficacy is low at the doses that are commercially available (0.075% or less) (145). Second, compliance is poor because of intense initial burning effects. Robbins and colleagues (145) reported a trial of topical, high-dose capsaicin (5% to 10%) in 10 CRPS patients with intractable foot pain. The individuals received a one-time topical application of 15 ml of capsaicin cream under regional anesthesia (either lumbar epidural or lower extremity peripheral nerve block). The large-dose capsaicin administered with regional anesthesia significantly reduced pain from 1 week to 50 weeks after the procedure (145).

Clonidine Topical application of a clonidine transdermal patch may also substantially reduce hyperalgesia to mechanical and cold stimuli in CRPS patients, indicating that the pain with CRPS may be mediated via alpha-1 adrenergic receptors located in the affected tissue (118,119). This study suggests that transdermal clonidine may be useful in patients with CRPS limited to a small area.

Nitroglycerine Ointment In 1993, Manahan and colleagues (142) found that topical nitroglycerine might be used as an adjuvant in the management of stage III CRPS. They observed increased level of function, as well as subjective improvement in pain and reduction of edema in their patients.

Dimethyl Sulfoxide Cream A prospective, randomized, and double-blind study of 32 patients showed that dimethyl sulfoxide 50% in a fatty cream (DMSO 50%) could significantly reduce the symptomatic pain at stage I CRPS (144).

Antispastic Agents

The manifestations of motor involvement in CRPS patients are stiffness, fixed dystonic posturing, weakness, tremor, or myoclonic jerks. The dystonia in CRPS patients is often unresponsive to treatment.

In a series of 200 patients, Schwartzman and Kerrigan (46) reported 43 had weakness, spasm, inability or difficulty in initiating movement, or dystonic posturing. Some patients have large amplitude tremors on electromyography. The authors reported that sympathetic blockade or sympathectomy gave relief in most patients, and two patients had relief of symptoms with as much as 120 mg per day of baclofen. We have seen some subjective clinical improvement in tremors after the administration of intravenous phentolamine or with treatment with oral tizanidine.

Baclofen, a specific γ-aminobutyric acid (GABA)-receptor (type B) agonist, inhibits sensory input to the neurons of the spinal cord. Intrathecal baclofen therapy has proved effective in patients with spasticity. The technique also has been used to treat CRPS patients with dystonia since oral baclofen is sedating and has low penetration into the spinal cord. In a small-sample-size study of intrathecal baclofen for treatment of dystonia in CRPS (147), 6 of 7 patients receiving 50 and 75 µg of intrathecal baclofen had complete or partial resolution of focal dystonia in a double-blind, randomized, controlled crossover trial. Four patients also experienced long-term improvement (0.5 to 3 years) in their dystonia with a subcutaneous pump for continuous intrathecal administration of baclofen. Some of the patients also reported reductions in pain, sensory symptoms, and autonomic symptoms during continuous intrathecal baclofen.

Other Medications

There have been reports of successful treatment of CRPS with propranolol (148,149). In both reports, pain and hyperalgesia were relieved by a relatively high dose. Labetalol also has been used by IVR technique as described below.

Agents that decrease blood viscosity increase tissue blood flow; thus, the use of low-molecular weight dextran, stanozolol, and plasma exchange have been evaluated in patients with CRPS (150,151). None of these therapies has demonstrated consistent efficacy, and they are not considered primary therapeutic modalities (152,153).

Recently, several recent studies (154–156) reported that the administration of oral vitamin C in patients with wrist fracture was associated with a lower frequency of RSD.

There is considerable evidence that N-methyl-D-aspartate (NMDA) receptor antagonists, such as ketamine, can abolish nociceptor hypersensitivity in animals. Lin and colleagues (133) reported that long-term low dose of epidural ketamine combined with morphine and bupivacaine could attenuate neuropathic pain in RSD. Their two patients diagnosed with lower extremity RSD failed to respond to conventional treatment with NSAIDs, steroids, anticonvulsants, antidepressants, epidural lidocaine, sympathectomy,

and rehabilitation. However, epidural injection of this combination three times a day for several courses of treatment over 3 to 6 months provided significant pain relief in both patients. They suggest that synergy from this combination may give an alternative treatment for CRPS. Although there are no further clinical trials published for the treatment of CRPS with NMDA antagonists, ketamine and dextromethorphan have been examined in neuropathic pain in general (157).

NERVE BLOCKS

Although the causal mechanisms of CRPS are not limited purely to sympathetic hyperactivity, selective sympathetic ganglion block with local anesthetic is still the mainstay of therapeutic management for those patients with SMP (158).

Anatomy of Sympathetic Ganglia

The paravertebral sympathetic trunk extends from the base of the skull to the coccyx. From the cervical to the lumbar regions, the trunks are located bilaterally on the anterolateral surface of the vertebral body. At the level of the coccyx, the trunks meet anterior as the ganglion impar. The cervical sympathetic trunk is generally divided into the superior, middle, and cervicothoracic (stellate) ganglia. The superior cervical ganglion is the largest of the three. It is located at the level of the second and third cervical vertebrae. The middle cervical ganglion is the smallest and is usually found at the level of the sixth cervical vertebra. The stellate (cervicothoracic) ganglion is a fusion of the lower cervical and first thoracic ganglia and is located anterolateral to the longest colli muscle at the level of the seventh cervical vertebra and first rib. The ganglion is located in close proximity to the lung apex inferior, the carotid artery anterior, the longest colli muscle posteromedially, and the anterior scalene muscle laterally. Preganglionic sympathetic fibers destined for the superior and middle cervical ganglia traverse the stellate ganglion without interruption.

Sympathetic innervation of the head and neck is derived mostly from T-1 to T-3, whereas preganglionic fibers supplying the upper limbs are derived from T-2–6. Postganglionic fibers travel with the brachial plexus to the upper extremity. The blood vessels of the upper extremity receive their sympathetic innervation from the adjacent brachial plexus.

The lumbar portion of sympathetic chain is found in the retroperitoneal connective tissue on the anterolateral surface of the vertebral column at the anteromedial surface of the psoas major. It passes posterior to the iliac arteries to reach the pelvic area where it is located anteriorly to the sacrum and medially to the anterior sacral foramina. Four branches, the lumbar splanchnic nerves, leave the lumbar sympathetic trunk to join the celiac, mesenteric, and superior hypogastric plexuses. Branches from the sacral portion of the sympathetic trunk give off branches to the inferior hypogastric plexus and to the roots of the somatic nerves, which form the sacral plexus. Preganglionic sympathetic fibers to the lower limb originate in the lower three thoracic and upper two to three lumbar segments of the spinal cord. Because the preganglionic fibers travel caudad through the sympathetic trunk, a surgical sympathectomy can be accomplished by removing the lumbar sympathetic trunk and ganglia between L-1 and L-3.

Local Anesthetic Blocks

Local anesthetic blockade of selective sympathetic chain can be used for treatment of CRPS or to predict the response to sympathectomy. More than 80% of patients with CRPS have been reported to respond to a series of the selective sympathetic chain blocks combined with PT (158–160). Lower recovery rates are seen in patients with longstanding pain or partial major peripheral nerve injury (CRPS Type II, causalgia) (74). Another study (74) reports a 50% long-term success rate with the use of sympathetic block for treatment of CRPS Type II. Pain relief usually lasts longer than the duration of local anesthetic blockade, although patients rarely experience permanent pain relief from a single block. A series of blocks usually is performed as long as pain continues to decrease, or the period of pain relief after each block continues to increase. When intermittent sympathetic ganglion blockades fail to give long-term relief, an IV regional block or a continuous sympathetic block should be tried. If pain is not relieved by sympathetic blockade, the diagnosis of CRPS should be reevaluated. Although it is possible that the patient has CRPS in which pain is independent of the sympathetic nervous system (SIP), other possible causes of pain should be considered and excluded.

Stellate Ganglion Block

The stellate ganglion block, or cervicothoracic sympathetic block, is usually carried out by injection of local anesthetic on the anterior tubercle (Chassaignac's tubercle) of C-6 or on the transverse process of C-7. The stellate ganglion is used most for diagnostic and prognostic purposes in upper extremity CRPS because sensory blockade is avoided (details of techniques of this block are not reviewed in the chapter). For a series of therapeutic blocks, stellate ganglion, brachial plexus, or cervical epidural block can be used. Some authors recommend the use of brachial plexus block for producing a more complete sympathetic blockade to the arm. Theoretically, sympathetic innervation from as low as T-4 may be missed with stellate ganglion block, especially with low-volume injections. However, temperature or other measures of sympathetic function can be used to ensure adequate sympathetic blockade, as described below.

Lumbar Sympathetic Ganglion Block

For the reasons stated, lumbar sympathetic ganglion block for lower extremity CRPS is preferred to epidural block for

diagnostic and prognostic purposes. Unlike stellate ganglion blockade, for which a Horner's syndrome usually accompanies a successful blockade, there are no obvious physical signs accompanying sympathetic blockade. Thus, it is important to document successful needle placement with fluoroscopy or objective measurements of sympathetic blockade. If fluoroscopic guidance is used, injection of contrast should confirm placement of the needle tip in the retroperitoneal space, anterior and lateral to the vertebral body. Although some authors have recommended that three separate needles be used at L-2, L-3, L-4, a single injection at L-2 or L-3 is sufficient if enough volume is injected (Fig. 33-1).

Skin temperature measurement is used most often to monitor the adequacy of sympathetic blockade. A 1°C increase in temperature is commonly considered the minimum expected change, but Rauck suggests that a minimum of 2°C should accompany sympathetic blockade unless there is a fixed arterial obstruction (161). The sympathogalvanic response, or sweat test with ninhydrin or cobalt blue, can be used to test for sympathetic interruption. These tests are described elsewhere (161). They are reliable but time consuming to use routinely. Irazuzta and colleagues (162) described the use of laser Doppler to monitor sympathetic blockade. The investigators found that laser Doppler was able to detect a tenfold increase in skin blood flow within 4 minutes, whereas an average of 11 minutes was required for 1° C temperature increase. The equipment is expensive but easy to use and may be a worthwhile investment for the busy clinician.

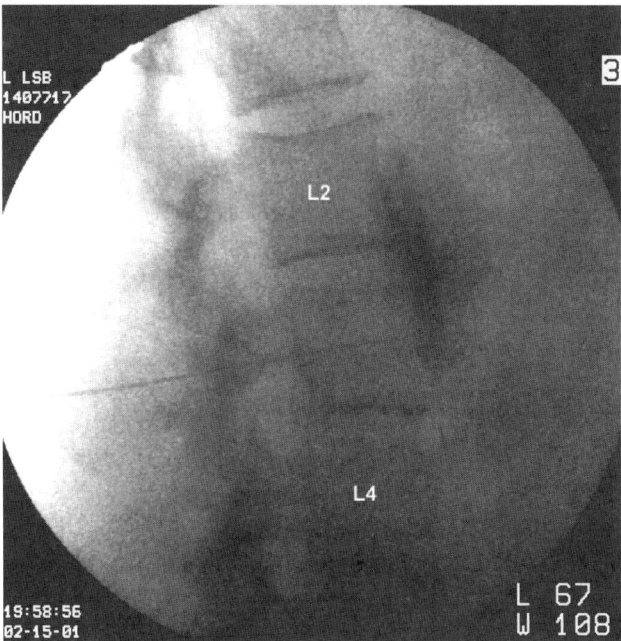

FIG. 33-1. Lumbar sympathetic block performed at L-3 showing the pattern of spread after injection of 15 ml of local anesthetic and contrast. Note the needle tip near the anterolatera border of the L-3 vertebral body and the spread of the injectate from L-2 to L-3 in the prevertebral space.

Continuous Infusions/Continuous Paravertebral Sympathetic Block

Continuous infusions of local anesthetic may provide prolonged relief, and continuous paravertebral sympathetic block has been recommended for the treatment of CRPS since 1953 (163). Catheters can be placed anywhere along the sympathetic chain to block preganglionic (i.e., epidural) or postganglionic (i.e., brachial plexus) fibers and sympathetic ganglia. The infusion is continued for 1 to 3 weeks while active and passive PT is performed. Linson and colleagues (164) used a similar technique to treat upper extremity CRPS in 29 patients. A catheter was placed near the stellate ganglion, and patients were given intermittent doses of bupivacaine 0.5% to maintain sympathetic blockade. Treatment was continued for as long as 14 days and combined with PT. At follow-up in 6 months to 6 years, 19 of the patients maintained the improvement obtained by the procedure. Although more clinical trials are needed, Stanton-Hicks (165) has recommended that continuous sympathetic blockade be performed at the first sign of resistance to treatment with intermittent blockades. If the patient has too much pain to perform PT once the infusion is discontinued, a catheter for long-term home infusion can be implanted. Paravertebral sympathetic catheters may be hard to maintain; Linson et al. (164) had to replace half of the catheters in their study within 2 to 4 days. We find that an epidural catheter is easier to keep in place and the use of a dilute concentration of local anesthetic (less than 0.125% bupivacaine) will avoid loss of sensation and motor function in patients who do not need it. The placement of an epidural catheter also allows the physician to provide sensory analgesia when needed.

Somatic Blocks

Somatic peripheral nerve blocks, such as the brachial plexus, lumbar plexus, and the epidural blockade also have been evaluated for the treatment of CRPS pain. Patients with stage II and stage III CRPS may not obtain adequate analgesia for PT with sympathetic blockade alone because pain from manipulation of fibrotic joints and muscles is carried by A-alpha nerve fibers. Although this pain is difficult to control, continuous somatic nerve blockade combined with PT offers the only hope of rehabilitation (134). Any patient with a range-of-motion deficit when tested during general or regional anesthesia should be considered for continuous somatic blockade (Fig. 33-2). In addition, there may be patients with sympathetically dependent and independent pain who need sensory analgesia to tolerate PT. These patients will need intermittent or continuous somatic blockade.

Intermittent Somatic Blockade

Intermittent somatic blocks with local anesthetic have sometimes been used for treatment of refractory cases of CRPS.

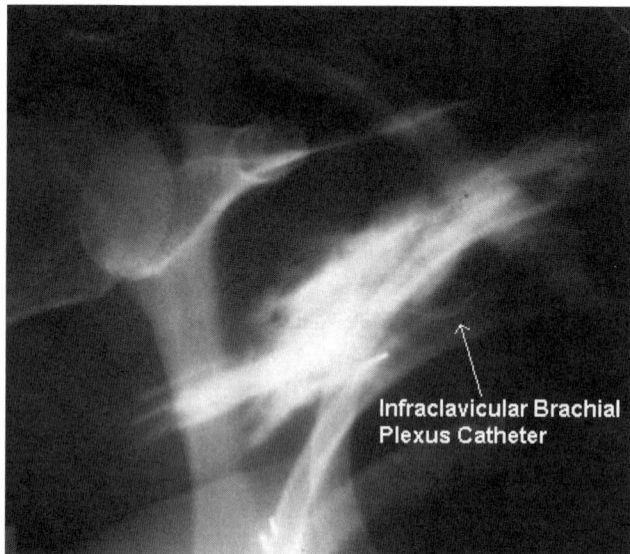

FIG. 33-2. Pattern of contrast spread after injection through an infraclavicular brachial plexus catheter. Note the extension of contrast medially and laterally within the brachial plexus. The filling defects noted in the axillary region represent the axillary artery and nerves of the brachial plexus. Also note the S-shaped pattern of the catheter caused by contraction of the pectoralis muscles.

Gibbons and colleagues (166) reported a series of 25 patients who were treated with interscalene blockades for upper extremity pain. Of the 25 patients, 17 had CRPS. Eleven of the patients with CRPS had significant pain relief on follow-up. Nine of the 11 had increased range of motion. Stellate ganglion block had previously been performed in eight of the patients. Although six patients had some response to stellate block, none had obtained long-term relief of pain. Thus, somatic blockade of the brachial plexus should be considered in patients who are refractory to sympathetic blockade or have restricted range of motion.

Continuous Somatic Blockade

Continuous somatic blockade is an alternative in patients who need prolonged analgesia for PT. Stanton-Hicks (165) has recommended the addition of an opioid to provide epidural analgesia for PT when a dilute concentration of local anesthetic is not sufficient. When a sensory blockade is needed, we try to place the epidural catheter laterally in the epidural space to limit the spread of local anesthetic to the unaffected side. This can be done blindly or with fluoroscopic guidance. A unilateral sensory block usually can be obtained on the affected side so that PT can be performed without the addition of opioid to epidural solution. Alternatively, a catheter may be placed in the brachial or lumbar plexus on the affected side. Initially an infusion of bupivacaine that results in motor and sensory blockade may be required (0.25% to 0.5% at 6 to 10 ml/hour). Additional decreases in concentration are made as long as the patient continues to have full active range of motion. If active motion is maintained without sensory analgesia, the patient usually can be treated with local anesthetic blocks or intermittent bolus IV regional guanethidine or bretylium on an as-needed basis. However, a most recent case report by Maneksha et al. (167) suggests that CRPS patients may develop a resistance to epidural local anesthetic blockade.

Sensory analgesia may also be useful in patients with active CRPS or a history of sympathetic dysfunction who require surgery. Continuous epidural or peripheral nerve blockade can be used perioperatively. Hobelmarn and Dellon (168) have reported 20 patients with CRPS who were treated with continuous brachial plexus blockade after surgery for nerve entrapment, neuroma resection, or capsulotomy. A plastic catheter was placed in the brachial plexus from an axillary approach, and patients were given 10 ml of 0.5% bupivacaine with epinephrine every 12 hours. None of the patients was reported to experience an exacerbation of CRPS postoperatively.

Numerous other drugs, such opioid, ketamine, clonidine, have been added into the regimen of somatic or epidural blockade to increase or prolong the effect of somatic or epidural blockades (132,133,169). However, there are no systematic evaluations of these combinations for the treatment of CRPS.

Intravenous Regional Blockade (IVR)

IVR blockade is the injection of local anesthetic alone (Bier block) or with other agents (IVR sympathetic block) into the venous system below an occluding tourniquet. This appears to produce anesthesia and/or sympathetic block by direct diffusion of the medications from the blood vessels into the nearby nerves.

Guanethidine

Guanethidine was first used in an IVR technique for Type II CRPS (causalgia) by Hannington-Kiff in 1974 (79). Guanethidine selectively inhibits peripheral sympathetic nerve transmission. It is transported by the norepinephrine reuptake pump into the presynaptic vesicles of the postganglionic adrenergic neurons. After causing an initial release of norepinephrine, guanethidine prevents the reuptake of norepinephrine from the synaptic cleft and inhibits additional release of norepinephrine. This biphasic effect is seen clinically as an initial increase in sympathetic tone, followed by a prolonged decrease in sympathetic activity. Although the oral use of guanethidine for CRPS had been described, systemic side effects such as postural hypotension, dizziness, nausea, and diarrhea are common (170). Administration of intravenous guanethidine (10 to 20 mg) into a limb isolated by a tourniquet produces a high concentration in the adrenergic neurons of the affected extremity while minimizing systemic side effects. The effect of guanethidine is specific to patients with SMP because only

adrenergic neurons are blocked. Wahren and colleagues (171) found that patients with SIP had no change in vibration-produced allodynia after IVR guanethidine. Patients with SMP had normalization of their heat, cold, and vibration-pain thresholds after administration of IVR guanethidine. The mean duration of chemical sympathectomy after IVR guanethidine is 3 days after the first treatment and 6 days after the second. An increasing duration of sympathetic blockade may be seen with a series of treatments. Hannington-Kiff has postulated that repeated administration of guanethidine leads to an accumulation of guanethidine in sympathetic nerve endings, causing retraction of axons from their effected sites. Concurrent administration of tricyclic antidepressants may interfere with the uptake of guanethidine into presynaptic vesicles by interfering with the norepinephrine pump.

Glynn and colleague's (172) single-blind, placebo-controlled clinical trial and Driessens and colleague's (127) prospective, unblinded clinical trial with CRPS patients in the 1980s supported Hannington-Kiff's suggestion that guanethidine is effective in treating CRPS. In 1991, Eulry et al. (173) also recommended IVR bock with guanethidine as second-line treatment after failure of other treatment based on results from their open label study of guanethidine in 118 RSD patients. However, statistical values (p values), if calculated, were not given for the parameters in their article.

Bonelli et al. (174) compared IVR guanethidine and stellate ganglion block in RSD patients in the early 1980s. Ten RSD patients received treatment every other day with stellate ganglion block (SGB) with bupivacaine to a total of 8 blocks (16 days). Nine RSD patients were treated with regional intravenous guanethidine every 4 days for 16 days (total of 4 treatments with IVR guanethidine). Patients were followed up in 1 month and 3 months after treatments. They reported significant sustained reduction in pain scores for up to 3 months for both treatments. Guanethidine produced skin temperature elevation and increased plethysmographic amplitude (24 hours and 48 hours after treatments) for longer duration than SGB. They concluded that IVR guanethidine was a good choice compared to conventional stellate ganglion block, because fewer blocks were needed, sympathetic blockade was longer in duration, and there were negligible risks and contraindications.

Meanwhile, the analgesic effectiveness of IVR block with guanethidine is still controversial. Ramamurthy and Hoffman (175) reported a randomized double-blind, placebo-controlled, multicenter study with IVR guanethidine. They found that therapeutic benefits provided by IVR blockade with guanethidine were not different from those provided by the IVR placebo. While pain and other symptoms tended to decrease over time, there was no relationship between the number of IVR guanethidine blocks and relief of symptoms. However, their study patients were not chosen based on the presence of SMP, so no conclusion can be drawn as to the efficacy of IVR guanethidine in SMP.

Five other randomized double-blind studies (176,177) and an open label and multiple dose study by Kaplan et al. (178) showed no significant analgesic effect of IVR block with guanethidine. However, it is known that guanethidine will be ineffective if patients are on tricyclic antidepressants (TCAs). Of the recently conducted studies, only Rama-murthy and Hoffman's (175) excluded patients on tricyclic antidepressant therapy.

Bretylium

Bretylium, because of its quaternary ammonium structure, has minimal gastrointestinal and psychological effects. Aside from its ability to raise the electrical threshold of ventricular fibrillation, bretylium resembles guanethidine and reserpine in its adrenergic-blocking properties. Bretylium accumulates in postganglionic adrenergic neurons and inhibits conduction by preventing norepinephrine release. Although its effect in low concentration is specific for adrenergic neurons, in high concentration, bretylium has local anesthetic and neuromuscular blocking properties (179). Systemically administered bretylium does not interfere with the receptor response to intravenous catecholamines (180).

Bretylium has been used for malignant ventricular dysrhythmias in doses of 5 to 20 mg/kg. Doses as high as 40 mg/kg have been used occasionally with no reports of toxicity. Its major side effects are hypertension and tachycardia from the initial release of norepinephrine, followed by orthostatic hypotension from chemical sympathetic blockade. Orthostatic hypotension can be prevented by the IV administration of 750 to 1000 ml saline or lactated Ringer's solution after an IV regional blockade.

Ford and colleagues (181) described the use of IVR bretylium for treatment of CRPS. They used 1 mg/kg of bretylium and obtained pain relief and subjective warmth in the extremity for 7 to 21 days after the first treatment in four patients. Subsequent treatments resulted in pain relief lasting 25 days to 7 months. This low dose of bretylium appears to be virtually without side effects. In our experience, sympathetic blockade after IVR bretylium (1.5 mg/kg) lasted 2 weeks to 7 months in patients who received only 6 to 24 hours of relief after multiple sympathetic ganglion blockades with local anesthetic (179). The average duration of pain relief (greater than 30%) was 20 days. Permanent relief of symptoms of CRPS was seen in one patient. Because of its minimal toxicity and apparent efficacy, we use bretylium for IVR chemical sympathectomy when it is commercially available.

Reserpine

Reserpine has been well demonstrated in the treatment of Raynaud's phenomenon. The first published data established the interest of reserpine blockade in the management of CRPS (182). However, it is less effective and its side effects are more prominent than are those of guanethidine (183).

Ketanserin

Ketanserin is an antagonist at 2,5-hydroxytryptamine (5-HT) receptors. Although the possible role of 5-HT in the etiology of CRPS is unknown, ketanserin has been used in two published clinical studies for the treatment of CRPS. In one study, ketanserin 10 mg and placebo were given by intravenous bolus to nine patients with CRPS that had been present for 5 months to 10 years (184). The intravenous injections were given in a double-blind fashion and in randomized order. Digital blood flow, measured by plethysmography, was increased moderately in two patients and markedly in two others. There was no change in blood flow in five of the nine patients; thus, there was no difference between the ketanserin and placebo groups. Because the patient groups were small, it is not known whether intravenous ketanserin is effective or whether a specific subgroup of patients with CRPS is responsive to blockade of serotonin 2 receptors.

Ketanserin does appear to be effective when administered by IVR technique. Hanna and Peat (185) studied 16 patients with peripheral pain described as burning. Nine of the patients had CRPS by criteria that included vasospasm, edema, and trophic changes. In a double-blind manner, patients were given either placebo (saline) or ketanserin (10 mg for arm; 20 mg for leg) for two consecutive treatments, followed by two treatments with the alternate medication in randomized order. In patients with CRPS, but not those with other causes of peripheral burning pain, there was an average of 60% to 70% reduction in pain for longer than 2 weeks. There was a higher incidence of drowsiness, fainting, and shakiness after administration of ketanserin compared with that of placebo. Additional study of IVR ketanserin is needed to confirm these positive results.

Other

Buflomedil is a vasodilator drug that relaxes smooth muscle fibers, increases microcirculation flow rate, and inhibits the influx of calcium ions into smooth-muscle cells. In a report of IVR blocks with buflomedil (186), the results were considered good in 70% of the cases. The most spectacular effect was antiedematous, with improvement of mobility and secondary alleviation of pain (186). The effects last for 24 to 36 hours, requiring repetition of the procedure followed by oral treatment. However, this study was not placebo-controlled or randomized. Multiple moderate side effects occurred, including headache (5%), pruritus, excessive sweating, and increased body odor.

IVR administration of labetalol (alpha and beta adrenergic blocker) (187), atropine (muscarinic cholinergic antagonist) (188), droperidol (alpha-adrenergic antagonist) (189) also have been reported. However, there are no controlled studies of these agents for treatment of CRPS.

NEUROABLATION AND NEUROAUGMENTATION

Surgical Sympathectomy

Paravertebral sympathectomy is used in patients in whom all other methods of therapy have failed to provide long-lasting relief and who remain incapacitated by their disease. Excellent results have been reported in such patients (190,191). Obviously, the potential morbidity of such a procedure warrants an exhaustive trial of physical and pharmacological therapy. Prognostic sympathetic blocks with local anesthetics should be temporarily successful in relieving pain before surgical sympathectomy is considered. Confounding variables, such as the coadministration of analgesics and sedatives, technical failure, and blockade of somatic nerves, should be prevented. The possibility of placebo response should be minimized by repeating sympathetic blocks before considering surgical sympathectomy. Psychological issues should be addressed preoperatively.

The first successful surgical treatment of a patient with causalgia was reported by Spurling in 1930 (192). He performed a sympathetic ganglionectomy and ramisection of the stellate ganglion on a 24-year-old man who had been shot in the right axilla. The surgery improved circulation and stopped the burning pain in his right arm. This single report set the stage for a surgical therapy for CRPS that changed little during the ensuing 50 years. In 1987, Mockus and colleagues (193) reported some degree of relief in 97% of patients after surgical sympathectomy, including 61% with total relief. Pain relief was maintained in 94% of patients who were interviewed an average of 2.9 years after surgery.

Olcott and colleagues (190) performed surgical sympathectomy on a group of 35 patients who had not responded to conservative management but had temporary pain relief after sympathetic blockade. Of the 35 patients, 74% had relief of pain, were fully rehabilitated, and did not require narcotic medications. Another 17% had greater than 50% relief of pain and satisfactory, but not complete return of function. One patient who did not initially obtain pain relief was found to respond to contralateral sympathetic block and underwent a successful contralateral lumbar sympathectomy. Munn and Baker (194) reported that cross-communication of sympathetic fibers from the contralateral side may account for persistence or recurrence of symptoms. This can be easily diagnosed with a contralateral sympathetic blockade. Because the incidence of clinically significant sympathetic fiber crossover is believed to be low, a routine bilateral sympathectomy is not recommended.

Mockus and colleagues (193) reported wound complications (10%) and permanent Horner's syndrome (8%) as the major perioperative problems. Although postsym-

pathectomy neuralgia was present in approximately 40% of patients, it resolved within 10 weeks (average, 5 weeks) (195). Olcott and colleagues (190) also reported spontaneous resolution of postsympathectomy neuralgia. The incidence of neuralgia in their patients was 23% for upper extremity and 67% for lower extremity sympathectomies. In addition, all patients had Horner's syndrome after cervicothoracic sympathectomy; the authors thought this was because an extensive sympathectomy, including the stellate ganglion to T-6 or T-7 *via* a transthoracic approach, was needed for relief of pain. Similarly, they recommend removal of the sympathetic ganglion from L-4 to L-2, or L-1 if possible, when performing a lumbar sympathectomy.

Schwartzman et al. (196) reported long-term outcome (24 to 108 months) following sympathectomy for 29 patients with CRPS Type I. All seven patients who had sympathectomy within 12 months of injury achieved permanent symptom relief. Only nine of 13 patients (69%) who had sympathectomy 13 to 24 months after injury, and four of nine patients (44%) who had sympathectomy after 24 months of injury achieved permanent symptom relief. Another previous similar study by AbuRahma et al. (197) also reported that 20 of 21 patients had long-term satisfactory outcomes by surgical sympathectomy within 12 months following injury.

Radiofrequency Sympatholysis

A radiofrequency lesion is a heat lesion in the target tissue generated by a controlled electric field delivered at the electrode tip. The role of radiofrequency lesion generation for the purpose of making therapeutic lesions in the nervous system has been expanding.

Rocco (176) used lumbar radiofrequency sympatholysis for the relief of pain in two types of patients with CRPS and SMP in the lower extremities. The first group of patients had shown temporary relief with lumbar sympathetic block. The second group had recurrence of CRPS after phenol lumbar sympatholysis or surgical lumbar sympathectomy. Five out of 20 patients continued to be pain free 5 months to 3 years after the radiofrequency lumbar sympatholysis. The remaining 15 patients had temporary relief or no relief at all. The results from this study suggest that individualized patient management is necessary when considering radiofrequency sympatholysis in the treatment of patients with CRPS pain.

Recently we have been using pulsed radiofrequency sympatholysis on a frequent basis. Its duration appears to be considerably longer than with local anesthetic blocks, but the effect is still reversible, avoiding the major complications of neurodestructive procedures. Lesioning of the stellate ganglion or lumbar sympathetic ganglia is relatively easy and the lesioning itself (but not needle placement) is usually painless (Fig. 33-3). Vasodilation from sympathetic blockade is almost immediate. The duration of sympathetic blockade is variable, but it appears that duration increases

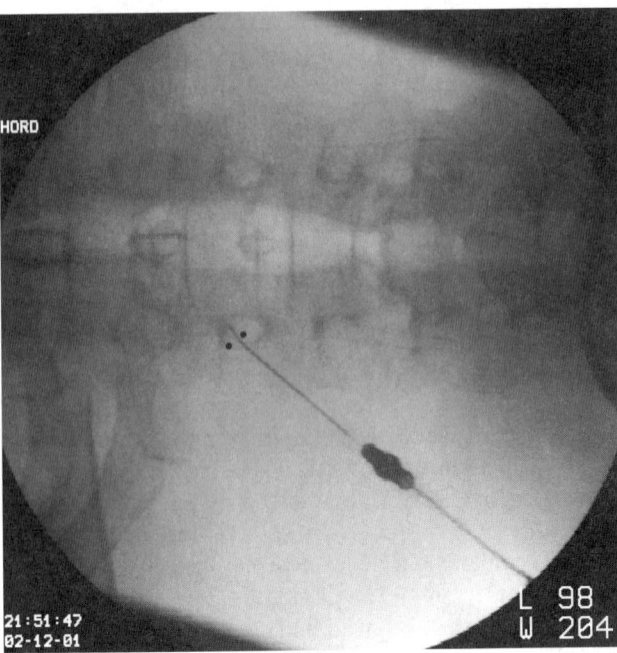

FIG. 33-3. A radiofrequency cannula in proper position for pulsed-RF lesioning of the stellate ganglion. Three lesions are usually made in a triangular pattern. The black dots mark the other two lesion sites.

with repeated lesioning. Therefore, we recommend pulsed radiofrequency lesioning as the second step after local anesthetic sympathetic blocks in patients with SMP. Heat lesions are reserved for those patients who have insufficient duration of sympathetic blockade from pulsed lesioning.

Spinal Cord Stimulation (Dorsal Column Stimulation)

Spinal cord stimulation (SCS) has been used in the treatment of CRPS. SCS seems to be successful in relieving pain in more than 50% of CRPS patients who proved unresponsive to other types of treatment (47,198–202). Little is known about the mechanism behind this beneficial effect. The relief of pain in CRPS due to SCS may be related to vasodilation, since SCS increases local blood flow. However, Kemler and colleagues (203) found that pain relief in CRPS by SCS does not depend on vasodilation. SCS in an animal model of neuropathy indicates that stimulation decreases the excitability of WDR neurons, which spontaneously discharge following partial sciatic nerve injury (204).

Many authors have reported successful treatment of chronic pain syndromes with spinal cord stimulation (SCS), but few have separately studied patients with CRPS. In a study by Barolat and colleagues (205), 18 patients who had failed to obtain pain relief from sympathetic block or surgical sympathectomy underwent a trial of SCS. Fourteen patients had a successful 1 week trial of SCS and one or two permanent leads were implanted in each patient. Initial stimulation settings were variable, but a rectangular pulse of an amplitude sufficient to induce comfortable paresthesia in the affected area was desired. Eleven of the 14 patients had moderate to good pain relief, which was limited to the areas in which paresthesias were produced by SCS. Robaina and colleagues (206) reported six patients with CRPS in whom greater than 50% pain relief was obtained with SCS, whereas five of the six patients had greater than 75% pain relief. Stimulation at the threshold of paresthesia with a 0.05 to 0.2-ms pulse width at 80 to 120 Hz was used by Robaina and colleagues (206). Recently, Kemler and colleagues (203) reported a randomized, controlled trial of spinal cord stimulation for CRPS. The group assigned to receive spinal cord stimulation plus PT (24 patients) had a mean reduction of 2.4 cm in the intensity of pain on a visual-analogue scale at 6 months, as compared with an increase of 0.2 cm in the group assigned to receive PT alone (18 patients). In addition, the proportion of patients with a score of 6 ("much improved") for global perceived effect was higher than in the control group. Spinal cord stimulation led to an 11% improvement in the overall score for the health-related quality of life in those 24 patients.

Outcomes from SCS in patients with CRPS have indicated that with careful selection of patients and successful test stimulation, spinal cord stimulation is safe, reduces pain, and improves the health-related quality of life in those patients.

Peripheral Nerve Stimulation

Racz and colleagues (191) have reviewed peripheral nerve stimulation for the treatment of RSD. A Resume® electrode (Medtronic, Minneapolis, MN) is placed deep to the peripheral nerve, and a layer of fascia is placed between the electrode and the nerve. The most common sites of stimulation are the ulnar, median, saphenous, and tibialis nerves. Bipolar stimulation with 0.8 to 1.2 V at a 400- to 500-ms pulse width and 65 to 80 Hz is used during the 3-day trial period. A pulse generator is implanted if the pain is significantly relieved with stimulation. Racz et al. (191) report a series of 11 patients who had improved sleep patterns, decreased narcotic use, and decreased pain with this method of peripheral nerve stimulation.

RECOMMENDATIONS OF TREATMENT

Boas and colleagues (207) also suggest an algorithm-based proposal for CRPS management. The protocols contain three elements of treatment: psychotherapy, physical and exercise treatment, and analgesic interventions. Within each treatment element there is progression from least-invasive to most-invasive therapies, depending on patient response. Each of the three primary elements is recommended; each helping to facilitate full compliance with the other two objectives.

A PT evaluation should be done before treatment and continued concurrently with other treatments. Psychological examination should be part of the routine initial evaluation of patients with CRPS. If additional intervention is indicated, it can be part of a coordinated treatment program. Late psychological referral or uncoordinated treatment may undermine medical treatment by implying to the patient that his or her pain is believed to be psychosomatic or that his or her psychological problems in coping with the disease are unexpected.

When a series of sympathetic ganglion blocks is begun with local anesthetic, approximately three blocks are done before deciding whether continuation of the series is warranted. If there is no pain relief after any of the blocks, no more are performed. In that case, the diagnosis of CRPS should be reevaluated because SIP secondary to CRPS is a diagnosis that requires exclusion of all other possible causes of pain. If pain relief is obtained, the series is continued as long as the patient has increased periods of pain relief after each block. When a plateau is reached (uniform duration of relief after each block), the clinician must decide whether the duration of relief is sufficient to continue therapy. In general, patients whose pain relief lasts less than 2 weeks should consider IVR bretylium or pulsed-RF lesioning.

Reviews of the treatment of CRPS have indicated that with modern methods of conservative treatment, surgical treatment is infrequently required (165,174). In a review of 17 500 operative procedures, Kleinert and colleagues (208) identified 506 patients with CRPS. This probably is the largest reported series in the literature and indicates an incidence of 2.9% after surgery on the extremities. Of the 506 patients with CRPS, 323 were treated with PT and oral medications, and 183 were treated with sympathetic block. The permanent success rate with sympathetic blocks was 66%. Only 23 patients (4.5%) required surgical sympathectomy, and 19 had permanent pain relief. Thus, surgical therapy for CRPS is required infrequently but may be effective when used appropriately. RF heat lesioning should be considered before surgical sympathectomy.

Somatic sources of pain may be important in perpetuating a cycle that leads to sympathetic overactivity. Thus, coexisting problems, such as tendonitis, carpal tunnel syndrome, and ulnar nerve entrapment, should be treated concurrently. If surgery is indicated, it should be delayed until a series of sympathetic blockades has been initiated. Blocks should be continued through the perioperative period. A long-acting sympathetic blocking technique, such as IVR bretylium, seems ideal if performed preoperatively or intraoperatively.

Patients who are thought to have stage 3 CRPS should have an examination under anesthesia to confirm the presence of decreased passive range of motion caused by contractures and ankylosis. Continuous somatic blockade with local anesthetic is instituted for 2 to 4 weeks. With complete motor neuron blockade, the therapist and patient perform passive exercises until the range of motion is normal. Then, the concentration of the local anesthetic infusion is decreased to allow active range of motion while maintaining sensory blockade to prevent pain. When active range of motion is normal, local anesthetic concentration is further decreased until sensation is normal but sympathetic nerves remain blocked. If active range of motion is maintained, the infusion is discontinued. When pain at rest or evidence of sympathetic overactivity persist, a series of intermittent sympathetic blocks, IVR bretylium blocks, or RF lesioning may be performed on an outpatient basis.

Gabapentin should be considered in all patients, while oral medications, such as corticosteroids, calcium channel blockers, antidepressants, other anticonvulsants, and topical agents can be considered as adjuvant treatments in selected CRPS patients.

CONCLUSION

CRPS is a condition seen by a wide variety of medical personnel. Although research models have been used to investigate the mechanisms behind this disease process, human studies primarily contain reports of clinical presentation and treatment. Spontaneous remission of CRPS is rare, but many cases resolve with proper, early treatment. Since diagnosis and instigation of treatment are the most important factors in the eventual outcome of this disabling condition, every effort should be made to diagnose and treat CRPS as soon as it occurs.

REFERENCES

1. Mitchell SW, Morehous CR, Keen WW. *Gunshot wounds and other injuries of the nerves.* Philadelphia: J.B. Lippincott Publishers, 1864.
2. Evans JA. Reflex sympathetic dystrophy. *Surgical Clinics of North America* 1946;26:780–790.
3. International association for the study of pain subcommittee on taxonomy: classification of chronic pain. Descriptions of chronic pain syndromes and definition of terms (1–5). *Pain* 1986;3(Suppl):S29–S30.
4. Merskey H, Bogduk N. *Classification of chronic pain*, 2nd ed. Seattle: IASP Press, 1994.
5. Wasner G, Backonja MM, Baron R. Traumatic neuralgias: complex regional pain syndromes (reflex sympathetic dystrophy and causalgia): clinical characteristics, pathophysiological mechanisms and therapy. [Review] *Neurologic Clinics* 1998;16(4):851–868.
6. Brock TR. Reflex sympathetic dystrophy linked to venipuncture: a case report. *Journal of Oral & Maxillofacial Surgery* 1989;47(12):1333–1335.
7. Burton AW, Conroy BP, Sims S, et al. Complex regional pain syndrome type II as a complication of subclavian catheter insertion [letter]. *Anesthesiology* 1998;89(3):804.
8. Siegfried RN. Development of complex regional pain syndrome after a cervical epidural steroid injection. *Anesthesiology* 1997;86(6):1394–1396.
9. Das A, Puvanendran K. Syringomyelia and complex regional pain syndrome as complications of multiple sclerosis. *Archives of Neurology* 1999;56(8):1021–1024.
10. Geurts AC, Visschers BA, Van Limbeek J, et al. Systemic review of aetiology and treatment of post-stroke hand oedema and shoulder-hand syndrome. [Review]. *Scandinavian Journal of Rehabilitation Medicine* 2000;32(1):4–10.
11. Ku A, Lachmann E, Tunkel R, et al. Upper limb reflex sympathetic dystrophy associated with occult malignancy. *Archives of Physical Medicine & Rehabilitation* 1996;77(7):726–728.
12. Cimaz R, Matucci-Cerinic M, Zulian F, et al. Reflex sympathetic dystrophy in children. *Journal of Child Neurology* 1999;14(6):363–367.
13. Barbier O, Allington N, Rombouts JJ. Reflex sympathetic dystrophy in children: review of clinical series and description of the particularities in children. *Acta Orthopaedica Belgica* 1999;65(1):91–97.

14. Parrillo SJ. Reflex sympathetic dystrophy in children. [Review]. *Pediatric Emergency Care* 1998;14(3):217–220.
15. Stanton RP, Malcolm JR, Wesdock KA, et al. Reflex sympathetic dystrophy in children: an orthopedic perspective. *Orthopedics* 1993;16(7):773–780.
16. Dietz FR, Mathews KD, Montgomery WJ. Reflex sympathetic dystrophy in children. *Clinical Orthopaedics & Related Research* 1990;258:225–231.
17. Allen G, Galer BS, Schwartz L. Epidemiology of complex regional pain syndrome: a retrospective chart review of 134 patients. *Pain* 1999;80(3):539–544.
18. Mailis A, Wade J. Profile of Caucasian women with possible genetic predisposition to reflex sympathetic dystrophy: a pilot study. *Clin J Pain* 1994;10(3):210–217.
19. Van de Beek WJ, Van Hilten JJ, Roep BO. HLA-DQ1 associated with reflex sympathetic dystrophy [letter]. *Neurology* 2000;55(3):457–458.
20. Van Hilten JJ, Van de Beek WJ, Roep BO. Multifocal or generalized tonic dystonia of complex regional pain syndrome: a distinct clinical entity associated with HLA-DR13. *Annals of Neurology* 2000;48(1):113–116.
21. Kemler MA, Van De Vusse AC, Van den Berg-Loonen EM, et al. HLA-DQ1 associated with reflex sympathetic dystrophy. *Neurology* 1999;53(6):1350–1351.
22. Faria SH, Flannery JC. Reflex sympathetic dystrophy syndrome: an update. [Review]. *Journal of Vascular Nursing* 1998;16(2):25–30.
23. Kurvers HA. Reflex sympathetic dystrophy: facts and hypotheses. [Review]. *Vascular Medicine* 1998;3(3)207–214.
24. Bonica JJ. Causalgia and other reflex sympathetic dystrophies. *Postgrad Med*, 1973;53:143–148.
25. Wakisaka S, Kajander KC, Bennett GJ. Abnormal skin temperature and abnormal sympathetic vasomotor innervation in an experimental painful peripheral neuropathy. *Pain* 1991:46:299–313.
26. Ramer MS, Bisby MA. Rapid sprouting of sympathetic axons in dorsal root ganglia of rats with a chronic constriction injury. *Pain* 1997;70:237–244.
27. Daemen M, Kurvers H, Bullens P, et al. Neurogenic inflammation and reflex sympathetic dystrophy (in vivo and in vitro assessment in an experimental model). *Acta Orthopaedic Belgica* 1998;64(4):441–447.
28. Graif M, Schweitzer M, Marks B, et al. Synovial effusion in reflex sympathetic dystrophy: an additional sign for diagnosis and staging. *Skeletal Radiology* 1998;27(5):262–265.
29. Loh L, Nathan P. Painful peripheral states and sympathetic blocks. *J Neuro. Neurosurgery Psychiat*, 1978;41:664–671.
30. Sunderland, S. Pain mechanisms in causalgia. *J Neurol Neurosurgery Psychiat*, 1976;39(5):471–480.
31. Melzack, R. Phantom limb pain: implications for treatment of pathologic pain. *Anesthesiology* 1971;35:409–419.
32. Tahmoush, AL. Causalgia: redefinition as a clinical pain syndrome. *Pain* 1981;10:187–197.
33. Roberts W. A hypothesis on the physiological basis for causalgia and related pains. *Pain* 1986;24:297–311.
34. Mayer DJ, Price DD, Becker DP. Neurophysiological characterization of the anterolateral spinal cord neurons contributing to pain perception in man. *Pain* 1975;1(1):51–58.
35. Chung JM, Kenshalo Jr DR, Gerhart KD, et al. Excitation of primate spinothalamic neurons by cutaneous C-fiber volleys. *J Neurophysiology* 1979;42(5):1354–1369.
36. Kenshalo DR, Leonard RB, Chung JM, et al. Facilitation of the responses of primate spinothalamic cells to cold and mechanical stimuli by noxious heating of the skin. *Pain* 1982;12(2):141–152.
37. Kenshalo DR, Leonard RB, Chung JM, et al. Responses of primate spinothalamic neurons to graded and to repeated noxious heat stimuli. *J Neurophysiology* 1979;42(5):1370–1389.
38. Price DD, Browe AC. Spinal cord coding of graded nonnoxious and noxious temperature increases. *Experimental Neurology* 1975;48:201–221.
39. Price DD, Hayes RL, Ruda, M, et al. Spatial and temporal transformations of input to spinothalamic tract neurons and their relation to somatic sensations. *J Neurophysiology* 1978;41(4):933–947.
40. Schouenborg J, Sjölund BH. Activity evoked by A- and C-afferent fibers in rat dorsal horn neurons and its relation to a flexion reflex. *J Neurophysiology* 1983;50(5):1108–1121.
41. Gracely RH, Lynch SA, Bennett GJ. Painful neuropathy: altered central processing maintained dynamically by peripheral input. *Pain* 1992;51:175–194.
42. Rygh LJ, Svendsen F, Hole K, et al. Natural noxious stimulation can induce long-term increase of spinal nociceptive responses. *Pain* 1999;82(3):305–310.
43. McLachlan EM, Janig W, Devor M, et al. Peripheral nerve injury triggers noradrenergic sprouting within dorsal root ganglia. *Nature* 1993;363(6429):543–546.
44. Levine JD, Fields HL, Basbaum AI. Peptides and the primary afferent nociceptor. *J Neuroscience* 1993;13(6):2273–2286.
45. Tapper DN, Brown PB, Moraff H. Functional organization of the cat's dorsal horn: connectivity of myelinated fiber systems of hairy skin. *J Neurophysiol* 1973;36:817–826.
46. Roberts WJ, Foglesong ME. I. Spinal recordings suggest that wide-dynamic range neurons mediate sympathetically maintained pain. *Pain* 1988;34:289–304.
47. Oerlemans HM, Oostendorp Ra, De Boo T, et al. Signs and symptoms in complex regional pain syndrome type I/reflex sympathetic dystrophy: judgment of the physician versus objective measurement. *Clinical Journal of Pain* 1999;15(3):224–232.
48. Veldman PH, Reynen HM, Arntz IE, et al. Signs and symptoms of reflex sympathetic dystrophy: prospective study of 829 patients. *Lancet* 1993;342(8878):1012–1016.
49. Sieweke N, Birklein F, Riedl B, et al. Patterns of hyperalgesia in complex regional pain syndrome. *Pain* 1999;80(1-2):171–177.
50. Chan RC, Chuang Ty, Chiu FY. Sudomotor abnormalities in reflex sympathetic dystrophy. *Chinese Medical Journal* 2000;63(3):189–195.
51. Chelimsky TC, Low PA, Naessens JM, et.al. Value of autonomic testing in reflex sympathetic dystrophy. *Mayo Clinic Proceedings* 1995;70(11):1029–1040.
52. Geertzen JH, Dijkstra PU, Stewart RE, et al. Variation in measurements of range of motion: a study in reflex sympathetic dystrophy patients. *Clinical Rehabilitation* 1998;12(3):254–264.
53. Verdugo RJ, Ochoa JL. Abnormal movements in complex regional pain syndrome: assessment of their nature. *Muscle & Nerve* 2000;23(2):198–205.
54. Schwartzman RJ, Kerrigan J. The movement disorder of reflex sympathetic dystrophy. *Neurology* 1990;40(1);57–61.
55. Deuschl G, Blumberg H, Lucking CH. Tremor in reflex sympathetic dystrophy. *Archives of Neurology* 1991;48(12)1247–1252.
56. Arden RL, Bahu SJ, Zuazu MA, et al. Reflex sympathetic dystrophy of the face: current treatment recommendations. *Laryngoscope* 1998;437–442.
57. Jaeger B, Singer E, Kroening R. Reflex sympathetic dystrophy of the face. Report of two cases and a review of the literature. *Archives of Neurology* 1986;43(7):693–695.
58. Hord AH, Denson DD, Huerkampb MJ, et al. Changes in rat paw perfusion after experimental mononeuropathy: assessment laser Doppler fluxmetry. *Anesth Analg* 1999;88(1):103–108.
59. Maleki J, LeBel AA, Bennett GJ, et al. Patterns of spread in complex regional pain syndrome, type I (reflex sympathetic dystrophy). *Pain* 2000;88:259–266.
60. Sandroni P, Low PA, Ferrer T, et al. Complex regional pain syndrome I (CRPS I): prospective study and laboratory evaluation. *Clinical Journal of Pain* 1998;14(4):282–289.
61. Friedman MS. The use of thermography in sympathetically maintained pain. [Review]. *Iowa Orthopaedic Journal* 1994;14:141–147.
62. Bennett GJ, Ochoa JL. Thermographic observations on rats with experimental neuropathic pain. *Pain* 1991;45(1):61–67.
63. Karstetter KW, Sherman RA. Use of thermography for initial detection of early reflex sympathetic dystrophy. [Review] *Journal of the American Podiatric Medical Association* 1991;1(4):198–205.
64. Arriagada M, Arinoviche R. X-ray bone densitometry in the diagnosis and followup of reflex sympathetic dystrophy syndrome. *Journal of Rheumatology* 1994;21(3):498–500.
65. Genant HK, Kozin F, Bekerman G, et al. The reflex sympathetic dystrophy syndrome. A comprehensive analysis using fine-detail radiography, photon absorptimetry, and bone and joint scintigraphy. *Radiology* 1975;117(1):21–32.
66. Goshen E, Zwas ST. Three-phase Tc-99m MDP bone scan in reflex sympathetic dystrophy. Appearance and resolution of findings in bilateral disease. *Clinical Nuclear Medicine* 1996;21(5):426–428.
67. Zyluk A, Birkenfeld B. Quantitative evaluation of three-phase bone scintigraphy before and after treatment of post-traumatic reflex sympathetic dystrophy. *Nuclear Medicine Communications* 1999;20(4):327–333.

68. Zyluk A. The usefulness of quantitative evaluation of three-phase scintigraphy in the diagnosis of post-traumatic reflex sympathetic dystrophy. *Journal of Hand BR* 1999;24(1):16–21.

69. Schiepers C, Bormans I, De Roo M. Three-phase bone scan and dynamic vascular scintigraphy in algoneurodystrophy of the upper extremity. *Acta Orthopaedica Belgica* 1998;64(3):322–327.

70. Davidoff G, Werner R, Cremer S, et al. Predictive value of the three-phase technetium bone scan in diagnosis of reflex sympathetic dystrophy syndrome. *Archives of Physical Medicine & Rehabilitation* 1989; 70(2):135–137.

71. Hoffman J, Phillips W, Blum M, et al. Effect of sympathetic block demonstrated by three-phase bone scan. *Journal of Hand Surgery* 1993; 18(5):860–864.

72. Baron R, Levine JD, Fields HL. Causalgia and reflex sympathetic dystrophy: does the sympathetic nervous system contribute to the generation of pain? [Review] *Muscle & Nerve* 1999;22(6):678–695.

73. Hennart D, Leon M, Sylin P, et al. Sympathetic nerve blocks in refractory sympathetic dystrophy syndrome. *Acta Orthopaedica Belgica* 1999;65(1):83–85.

74. Boas RA. Sympathetic nerve blocks: in search of a role. [Review] *Regional Anesthesia & Pain Medicine* 1998;23(3):292–305.

75. Roberts WJ. A hypothesis on the physiology basis for causalgia and related pains. *Pain* 1986;24:297–311.

76. Campbell JN, Meyer RA, Srinivasa RN. Is nociceptor activation by alpha-1 adrenoceptors the culprit in sympathetically maintained pain? *Am Pain Xoc J* 1992:1:3–11.

77. Treede RA, Davis KD, Campbell JN, et al. The plasticity of cutaneous hyperalgesia during sympathetic ganglion blockade in patients with neuropathic pain. *Brain* 1992;115:607–621.

78. Arner S. Intravenous phentolamine test: diagnostic and prognostic use in reflex sympathetic dystrophy. *Pain* 1991;46(1):17–22.

79. Hannington-Kiff JG. Intravenous regional sympathetic block with guanethidine. *Lancet* 1974;1:1019.

80. Bowler GMR, Wildsmith JA, Scott DB. Epidural administration of local anesthetics. In: Cousins MJ, Phillips GD, eds., *Acute Pain Management*. New York: Churchill Livingstone, 1986;187–235.

81. Price DD, Long S, Wilsey B, et al. Analysis of peak magnitude and duration of analgesia produced by local anesthetics injected into sympathetic ganglia of complex regional pain syndrome patients. *Clinical J Pain* 1998;14:216–226.

82. Löfström JB, Lloyd JW, Cousins MJ. Sympathetic neural blockade of upper and lower extremity. In: Cousins MJ, Bridenbaugh PO, eds., *Neural blockade in clinical anesthesia and management of pain*. Philadelphia: J.B. Lippincott, 1980:355–382.

83. Rowbotham MC, Fields HL. Topical lidocaine reduces pain in postherpetic neuralgia. *Pain*, 1989;38:297–311.

84. Linchitz RM, Raheb JC. Subcutaneous infusion of lidocaine provides effective pain relief from CRPS patients. *Clinical J Pain*, 1999;15(1): 67–72.

85. Dellemijn PL, Fields HL, Allen RR, et al. The interpretation of pain relief and sensory changes following sympathetic blockade. *Brain* 1994;117(pt 6):1475–1487.

86. Hogan QH, Erickson SJ, Haddox JD, et.al. The spread of solutions during stellate ganglion block. *Reg Anesth* 1992;17:78–83.

87. Malmquist EL, Bengtsson M, Sörensen J. Efficacy of stellate ganglion block: a clinical study with bupivacaine. *Reg Anesthesia* 1992;17: 340–347.

88. Raja SN, Treede RD, Davis KD, et al. Is systemic alpha-adrenergic blockade with phentolamine a diagnostic test for sympathetically maintained pain. *Anesthesiology* 1991;74:691–698.

89. Wong, GY, Wilson PR. Classification of complex regional pain syndromes—new concepts. 1997;13:319–325.

90. Oerlemans HM, Oostendorp RA, De Boo T, et al. Adjuvant physical therapy versus occupational therapy in patients with reflex sympathetic dystrophy/complex regional pain syndrome type I. *Archives of Physical Medicine & Rehabilitation* 2000;81(1):49–56.

91. Oerlemans HM, Goris JA, De Boo T, et al. Do physical therapy and occupational therapy reduce the impairment percentage in reflex sympathetic dystrophy? *American Journal of Physical Medicine & Rehabilitation* 1999;78(6):533–539.

92. Severens JL, Oerlemans HM, Weegels AJ, et al. Cost-effectiveness analysis of adjuvant physical or occupational therapy for patients with reflex sympathetic dystrophy. *Archives of Physical Medicine & Rehabilitation* 1999;80(9):1038–1043.

93. Watson HK, Carlson L. Treatment of reflex sympathetic dystrophy of the hand with an active "stress loading" program. *Journal of Hand Surgery* 1987;12(5 Pt 1):779–785.

94. Wall PD, Sweet WH. Temporary abolition of pain in man. *Science* 1967;155:108.

95. Robaina FJ, Rodrigues JL, De Vera JA, et al. Transcutaneous electrical nerve stimulation and spinal cord stimulation for pain relief in reflex sympathetic dystrophy. *Stereotactic & Functional Neurosurgery* 1989,52(1):53–62.

96. Schutzer S, Gossling H. Current concepts review: the treatment of reflex sympathetic dystrophy O syndrome. *J Bone Joint Surg* 1984;66A:625.

97. Withrington RH, Parry CBW. The management of painful peripheral nerve disorders. *J Hand Surg*, 1984;9B:24.

98. Portwood MM, Lieberman JS, Taylor RG. Ultrasound treatment of reflex sympathetic dystrophy. *Archives of Physical Medicine & Rehabilitation* 1987;68(2):116–118.

99. Adler E, Weiss AA, Zohair D. A psychosomatic approach to reflex sympathetic dystrophy. *Psychiatr Neurol* 1959;138:256.

100. Poplawksi ZJ, Wiley AM, Murray JF. Post-traumatic dystrophy of the extremities: a clinical review and trial of treatment. *J Bone Joint Surg* 1983;64A:642.

101. Sherry DD, Weisman R. Psychologic aspects in childhood reflex neurovascular dystrophy. *Pediatrics* 1988;81:572.

102. Shumacker HB, Abramson DI. Posttraumatic vasomotor disorders: with particular reference to late manifestations and treatment. *Surg Gynecol Obstet* 1949;88:417.

103. Barowsky EI, Zweig JB, Moskowitz J. Thermal biofeedback in the treatment of symptoms associated with reflex sympathetic dystrophy. *J Child Neurology* 1987;2:229.

104. Gainer MJ. Hypnotherapy for reflex sympathetic dystrophy. *American Journal of Clinical Hypnosis* 1992;34(4):227–232.

105. Haddox JD. Psychological aspects of reflex sympathetic dystrophy, pain and the sympathetic nervous system. In: Raj PP, Stanton-Hicks M, eds., *Series, Current management of pain*. Boston: Kluwer Academic Publishers, 1990:207.

106. Grundberg AB. Reflex sympathetic dystrophy: treatment with long-acting intramuscular corticosteroids. *Journal of Hand Surgery Am* 1996;21(4):667–670.

107. Sibley J, Blocka KL. The onset of reflex sympathetic dystrophy despite pretreatment with corticosteroid. *Journal of Rheumatology* 1984;11(6):870–871.

108. Christensen K, Jensen EM, Noer I. The reflex sympathetic dystrophy syndrome response to treatment with systemic corticosteroids. *Acta Chirurgica Scandinavica* 1982;148(8):653–656.

109. Steinbrocker O, Neustadt D, Lapin L. Shoulder-hand syndrome: sympathetic block compared with corticotropin and cortisone therapy. *JAMA* 1953;153:788–791.

110. Ecker A. Thermography in the diagnosis of reflex sympathetic dystrophy. *NY State J Med* 1984;84:6.

111. Kingery WS. A critical review of controlled clinical trials for peripheral neuropathic pain and complex regional pain syndromes. *Pain* 1997;73(2):123–139.

112. Dirksen R, Rutgers MJ, Coolen JM. Cervical epidural steroids in reflex sympathetic dystrophy. *Anesthesiology* 1987;66(1): 71–73.

113. Connelly NR, Reuben S, Brull SJ. Intravenous regional anesthesia with ketorolac-lidocaine for the management of sympathetically-mediated pain. *Yale Journal of Biology & Medicine*, 1995;68 (3–4):95–99.

114. Muizelaar JP, Kleyer M, Hertogs IA, et al. Complex regional pain syndrome (reflex sympathetic dystrophy and causalgia): management with the calcium channel blocker nifedipine and/or the alpha-sympathetic blocker phenoxybenzamine in 59 patients. *Clinical Neurology & Neurosurgery* 1997;99(1):26–30.

115. Prough DS, McLeskey CH, Poehling GG, et al. Efficacy of oral nifedipine in the treatment of reflex sympathetic dystrophy. *Anesthesiology* 1985;62(6):796–799.

116. Kabeer AA, Hardy PA. Long-term use of subarachnoid clonidine for analgesia in refractory reflex sympathetic dystrophy. Case report. *Regional Anesthesia* 1996;21(3):249–252.

117. Rauck RL, Eisenach JC, Jackson K, et.al. Epidural clonidine treatment for refractory reflex sympathetic dystrophy. *Anesthesiology* 1993;79(6):1163–1169.

118. Kirkpatrick AF, Derasari M. Transdermal clonidine: treating reflex sympathetic dystrophy [letter]. *Regional Anesthesia* 1993;18(2):140–141.

119. Davis KD, Treede RD, Raja SN, et al. Topical application of clonidine relieves hyperalgesia in patients with sympathetically maintained pain. *Pain* 1991;47(3):309–317.

120. Stevens DS, Robins VF, Price HM. Treatment of sympathetically maintained pain with terazosin. *Reg Anesth* 1993;18(5):318–321.

121. Carter SA . Finger systolic pressures and skin temperatures in severe Raynaud's syndrome: the relationship to healing of skin lesions and the use of oral phenoxybenzamine. *Angiology* 1981;32(5):298–310.

122. Malik VK, Inchiosa MA Jr, Mustafa K, et al. Intravenous regional phenoxybenzamine in the treatment of reflex sympathetic dystrophy. *Anesthesiology* 1998;88(3):823–827.

123. Hamamci N, Dursun E, Ural C, et.al. Calcitonin treatment in reflex sympathetic dystrophy: a preliminary study. *British Journal of Clinical Practice* 1996;50(7):373–375.

124. Gobelet C, Meier JL, Schaffner W, et al. Calcitonin and reflex sympathetic dystrophy syndrome. *Clinical Rheumatology* 1986;5(3):382–388.

125. Rico H, Merono E, Gomez-Castresana F, et al. Scintigraphic evaluation of reflex sympathetic dystrophy: comparative study of the course of disease under two therapeutic regimens. *Clin Rheumatol* 1987;6:233.

126. Nuti R, Vattimo A, Martini G, et al. Carbocalcitonin treatment in Sudek's atrophy. *Clin Orthop* 1987;215:217.

127. Driessens MF, VanHoutte PM, Mortier G. Effect of calcitonin, hydrocortisone, and parathyroid hormone on canine bone blood vessels. In: Arlet J, Ficat RP, Mungerford DS, eds., *Bone circulation.* Baltimore: Williams & Wilkins, 1984:228.

128. Friedman J, Raisz LG. Thyrocalcitonin: inhibitor of bone resorption in tissue culture. *Science* 1965;150:1465.

129. Bickerstaff Dr, Kanis JA. The use of nasal calcitonin in the treatment of posttraumatic algodystrophy. *Br J Rheumatology* 1991;30:291.

130. Gobelet C, Waldburger M, Meier JL. The effect of adding calcitonin to physical treatment of reflex sympathetic dystrophy. *Pain* 1992;48:171.

131. Belgrade MJ. Following the clues to neuropathic pain. Distribution and other leads reveal the cause and the treatment approach. *Postgraduate Medicine* 1999;106(6):127–132.

132. Azad SC, Beyer A, Romer AW, et al. Continuous axillary brachial plexus analgesia with low dose morphine in patients with complex regional pain syndromes. *European Journal of Anaesthesiology* 2000;17(3):185–188.

133. Lin TC, Wong CS, Chen FC, et al. Long-term epidural ketamine, morphine, and bupivacaine attenuate reflex sympathetic dystrophy neuralgia. *Canadian Journal of Anaesthesia* 1998;45(2):175–177.

134. Brown DL. Somatic or sympathetic block for reflex sympathetic dystrophy. Which is indicated? *Hand Clinics* 1997;13(3):485–497.

135. Berry H. Long-term treatment of intractable reflex sympathetic dystrophy with intrathecal morphine. *Canadian Journal of Neurological Sciences* 1996;23(2):156–157.

136. Becker WJ, Ablett DP, Harris CJ, et al. Long term treatment of intractable reflex sympathetic dystrophy in intrathecal morphine. *Canadian Journal of Neurological Sciences* 1995;22(2):153–159.

137. Falasca FG, Toly TM, Reginato AJ, et al. Reflex sympathetic dystrophy associated with antiepileptic drugs. *Epilepsia* 1994;3(2):394–399.

138. Chateurvedi SK. Phenytoin in reflex sympathetic dystrophy. *Pain* 1989;36(3):379–380.

139. Mellick GA, Mellick LG. Reflex sympathetic dystrophy treated with gabapentin. *Archives of Physical Medicine & Rehabilitation* 1997;78(1):98–105.

140. Mao J, Chen LL. Gabapentin in pain management. *Anesthesia & Analgesia* 2000;91(3):680–687.

141. Cheshire WP, Snyder CR. Treatment of reflex sympathetic dystrophy with topical capsaicin. Case report. *Pain* 1990;42(3):307–311.

142. Manahan AP, Burkman KA, Malesker MA, et al. Clinical observation of the use of topical nitroglycerin in the management of severe shoulder-hand syndrome. *Nebraska Medical Journal* 1993;78(40):87–89.

143. Foley K, Schatz L, Martin RL. Topical nitroglycerin facilitates intravenous regional techniques in patients with reflex sympathetic dystrophy. *Anesthesiology* 1998;69(6)1029.

144. Zuurmond WW, Langendijk PN, Bezemer PD, et al. Treatment of acute reflex sympathetic dystrophy with DMSO 50% in a fatty cream. *Acta Anaesthesiologica Scandinavica* 1996;40(3):364–367.

145. Robbins WR, Staats PS, Levine J, et al. Treatment of intractable pain with topical large-dose capsaicin: preliminary report. *Anesthesia & Analgesia* 1998;86(3):579–583.

146. Schwartzman RJ, Kerrigan J. The movement disorder of reflex sympathetic dystrophy. *Neurology* 1990;40(1):57–61.

147. Van Hilten BJ, Van de Beek WJ, Hoff JI, et al. Intrathecal baclofen for the treatment of dystonia in patients with reflex sympathetic dystrophy. *New England Journal of Medicine* 2000;343(3):625–630.

148. Simpson G. Propranolol for causalgia and Sudeck atrophy. *JAMA* 1974;227:327.

149. Tahmoush AJ. Causalgia. Redefinition as a clinical pain syndrome. *Pain* 1981;10:187.

150. Day TW, Mendoza F. Pharmacologic management of Raynaud's phenomenon. *South Med J* 1984;77:1160.

151. Engkvist O, Wahren LK, Wallin G. Effects of regional intravenous guanethidine block in posttraumatic cold intolerance in hand amputees. *J Hand Surg* 1985;10B:145.

152. Dodman B, Rowell NR. Low molecular weight dextran in systemic sclerosis and Raynaud's phenomenon. *Acta Drm Venereol* 1982;62:440.

153. Klinenberg JR, Wallace D. Plasmapheresis in Raynaud's disease. *Lancet* 1978;1:1310.

154. Zollinger PE, Tuinebrijer WE, Kreis RW, et al. Effect of vitamin C on frequency of reflex sympathetic dystrophy in wrist fractures: a randomized trial. *Lance* 1999;354(9195):2025–2028.

155. Amadio PC. Vitamin C reduced the incidence of reflex sympathetic dystrophy after wrist fracture. *Journal of Bone & Joint Surgery Am* 2000;82(6):873.

156. Misicko NE. Vitamin C prevents reflex sympathetic dystrophy. *Journal of Family Practice* 2000;49(3):268–269.

157. Takahaski H, Miyazaki M, Nanbu T, et al. The NMDA-receptor antagonist ketamine abolishes neuropathic pain after epidural administration in a clinical case. *Pain* 1998;75(2-3):391–394.

158. Abram SE. Pain of sympathetic origin. In: Raj PP ed., *Practical management of pain.* Chicago Yearbook, 1986:451.

159. Bonica JJ. Causalgia and other reflex sympathetic dystrophies, In: Bonica JJ, Liebeskind JC, Albe-Fessart D, eds., *Advances in pain research and therapy.* New York: Raven, 1979(3):141.

160. Carron H, Weller RM. Treatment of post-traumatic sympathetic dystrophy. *Adv Neurol* 1974;4:485.

161. Rauck R. Sympathetic nerve bocks. In Raj PP, ed., *Practical management of pain,* 2nd ed. St. Louis: Mosby Yearbook, 1992:778.

162. Irazuzta JE, Berde CB, Sethna NF. Laser doppler measurements of skin blood flow before, during, and after lumbar sympathetic blockade in children and young adults with reflex sympathetic dystrophy syndrome. *J Clin Monit* 1992;8:16.

163. Betcher AM, Bean G, Casten DF. Continuous procaine block of paravertebral sympathetic ganglions. *JAMA* 1953;151:288.

164. Linson MA, Leffert R, Todd DP. The treatment of upper extremity reflex sympathetic dystrophy with prolonged continuous stellate ganglion blockade. *J Hand Surg* 1983;8:153.

165. Stanton-Hicks M. Upper and lower extremity pain. In: Raj PP, *Practical management of pain,* 2nd ed. St. Louis: Mosby Yearbook, 1992:312.

166. Gibbons JJ, Wilson PR, Lamer TJ. Interscalene blocks for chronic upper extremity pain. *Clin J Pain* 1992;8:264.

167. Maneksha FR, Mirza H, Poppers PJ. Complex regional pain syndrome (CRPS) with resistance to local anesthetic block: a case report. *Journal of Clinical Anesthesia* 2000;12(1):67–71.

168. Hobelmarm CF, Dellon L. Use of prolonged sympathetic blockade as an adjunct to surgery in the patient with sympathetic maintained pain. *Microsurgery* 1989;10:151.

169. Ribbers GM, Geurts AC, Rijken RA et al. Axillary brachial plexus blockade for the reflex sympathetic dystrophy syndrome. *International Journal of Rehabilitation Research* 1997:20(4):371–380.

170. Tabira T, Shibasaki H, Kuroiwa Y. Reflex sympathetic dystrophy (causalgia) treatment with guanethidine. *Arch Neurol* 1983;40:430.

171. Wahren LK, Torebjörk E, Nyström B. Quantitative sensory testing before and after regional guanethidine block in patients with neuralgia in the hand. *Pain* 1991;46:23.

172. Glynn J, Basedow RW, Walsh JA. Pain relief following post-ganglionic sympathetic blockade with I.V. guanethidine. *British Journal of Anaesthesia* 1981;53(12):1297–1302.

173. Eulry F, Lechevalier D, Pats B, et al. Regional intravenous guanethidine blocks in algodystrophy. *Clinical Rheumatology* 1991;10(4): 377–383.
174. Bonelli S, Conoscente F, Movilia PG, et al. Regional intravenous guanethidine vs. stellate ganglion block in reflex sympathetic dystrophies: a randomized trial. *Pain* 1983;16:297.
175. Ramamurthy S, Hoffman J. Intravenous regional guanethidine in the treatment of reflex sympathetic dystrophy/causalgia: a randomized, double-blind study. Guanethidine Study Group. *Anesthesia & Analgesia* 1995;81(4):718–723.
176. Rocco AG. Radiofrequency lumbar sympatholysis. The evolution of a technique for managing sympathetically maintained pain. *Regional Anesthesia* 1995;20(1):3–12.
177. Jadad AR, Carroll D, Glynn CJ, et al. Intravenous regional sympathetic blockade for pain relief in reflex sympathetic dystrophy: a systemic review and a randomized, double-blind crossover study. *Journal of Pain and Symptom Management* 1995;10(1):13–20.
178. Kaplan R, Claudio M, Kepes E, et al. Intravenous guanethidine in patients with reflex sympathetic dystrophy. *Acta Anaesthesiologica Scandinavica* 1996;40(10):1216–1222.
179. Hord AH, Rooks MD, Stephens BO, et al. Intravenous regional bretylium and lidocaine for treatment of reflex sympathetic dystrophy: a randomized, double-blind study. *Anesthesia & Analgesia* 1992;74(6):818.
180. Boura ALA, Green AF. The actions of bretylium: adrenergic neurone blocking and other effects. *Br J Pharmacol* 1959;14:536.
181. Ford SR, Forrest WH Jr, Eltheringon L. The treatment of reflex sympathetic dystrophy with intravenous regional bretylium. *Anesthesiology* 1988;68(1):137–140.
182. Benzon HT, Chomka CM, Brunner EA. Treatment of reflex sympathetic dystrophy with regional intravenous reserpine. *Anesthesia & Analgesia* 1980;59(7):500–502.
183. Chuinard RG, Dabezies EJ, Gould JS, et al. Intravenous reserpine for treatment of reflex sympathetic dystrophy. *Southern Medical Journal* 1981;74(12):1481–1484.
184. Bouameaux HM, Hellemans H, Verhaeghe R. Ketanserin in chronic sympathetic dystrophy: an acute controlled trial. *Clin Rheumatology* 1984;3:556.
185. Hanna MH, Peat SJ. Ketanserin in reflex sympathetic dystrophy a double-blind placebo controlled cross-over trial. *Pain* 1989;38:145.
186. Farcot JM, Gautherie M, Foucher G. Regional intravenous sympathetic nerve blocks. *Hand Clinics* 1997;13(3):499–517.
187. Parris WCV, Harris R, Lindsey K. Use of intravenous regional labetalol in treating resistant reflex sympathetic dystrophy (abstract). *Pain Supplement* 1987;4:5206.
188. Glynn CJ, Stannard C, Collins PA, et al. The role of peripheral sudomotor blockade in the Tx of patients with sympathetically maintained pain. *Pain* 1993;53:39–42.
189. Kettler RE, Abram SE. Intravenous regional droperidol in the management of reflex sympathetic dystrophy: a double-blind, placebo-controlled, crossover study. *Anesthesiology* 1988;69(6):933–936.
190. Olcott C, Eltherington LG, Wilcosky BR, et al. Reflex sympathetic dystrophy: the surgeon's role in management. *J Vasc Surg* 1991; 14:488.
191. Racz GB, Lewis R Jr, Heavner JE, et al. Peripheral nerve stimulator implant for treatment of causalgia. In: Raj PP, Stanton-Hicks M, eds., *Pain and the sympathetic nervous system, Series Current management of pain*. Boston: Kluwer Academic Publishers, 1990:225.
192. Spurling RG. Causalgia of the upper extremity: treatment of dorsal sympathetic ganglionectomy. *Arch Neurol* 1930;23:784.
193. Mockus MB, Rutherford RB, Rosales, C. et al. Sympathectomy for causalgia. *Arch Surg* 1987;122:668.
194. Munn JS, Baker WH. Recurrent sympathetic dystrophy: successful treatment by contralateral sympathectomy. *Surgery* 1987;102:102.
195. Bonica JJ. Causalgias and other reflex sympathetic dystrophies. In: Bonica JJ, ed., *The management of pain*, Vol 1, 2nd ed. Malvern, Pennsylvania: Lea& Febiger, 1990:220.
196. Schwartzman RJ, Liu JE, Smullens SN, et al. Long-term outcome following sympathectomy for complex regional pain syndrome type I (RSD). *Journal of Neurological Sciences* 1997;150(2):149–152.
197. AbuRahma AF, Robinson PA, Powell M, et al. Sympathectomy for reflex sympathetic dystrophy: factors affecting outcome. *Annals of Vascular Surgery* 1994;8(4) 372–379.
198. Barolat G, Sharan AD. Future trends in spinal cord stimulation. *Neurological Research* 2000;22(3):279–84.
199. Kemler MA, Barendse GA, Van Kleef M, et al. Electrical spinal cord stimulation in reflex sympathetic dystrophy: retrospective analysis of 23 patients. *Journal of Neurosurgery* 1999;90(Suppl 1):79–83.
200. Segal R, Stacey BR, Rudy TE, et al. Spinal cord stimulation revisited. *Neurological Research* 1998;20(5):391–396.
201. Kumar K, Toth C, Nath RK, et al. Epidural spinal cord stimulation for treatment of chronic pain-some predictors of success. A 15-year experience. *Surgical Neurology* 1998;50(2): 110–120.
202. Kumar K, Nath RK, Toth C. Spinal cord stimulation in the management of reflex sympathetic dystrophy. *Neurosurgery* 1997:40(3): 503–508.
203. Kemler MA, Barendse GA, Van Kleef M, et.al. Pain relief in complex regional pain syndrome due to spinal cord stimulation does not depend on vasodilation. *Anesthesiology* 2000;92(6):1653–1660.
204. Kemler MA, Barendse GAM, Va Kleef M, et al. Spinal cord stimulation in patients with chronic reflex sympathetic dystrophy. *New England J Med* 2000;343:618–624.
205. Barolat G, Schwartzmann R, Woo R. Epidural spinal cord stimulation in the management of reflex sympathetic dystrophy. *Stereotact Funct Neurosurg* 1989;53:29.
206. Robaina FJ, Rodriguez JL, de Vera JA, et.al. Transcutaneous electrical nerve stimulation and spinal cord stimulation for pain relief in reflex sympathetic dystrophy. *Stereotact Funct Neurosurg* 1989;52:53.
207. Boas RA, FANZCA, Sympathetic nerve blocks: in search of role. *Reg Anesthesia & Pain Medicine* 1998;23(3):292–305.
208. Kleinert HE, Cole NM, Lisle W, et al. Post-traumatic sympathetic dystrophy. *Orthopedic Clinics of North America* 1973;4:917.

CHAPTER 34

Phantom Pain: What It Is and What To Do

Peter G. Wilson

There is a delicious mystery about phantom limb pain (PLP), a combination of fascination and frustration: fascination with possible etiologic mechanisms and frustration with treatments. We have worked with PLP patients over many years and have admired their coping with pain, asking for help, and getting more discouraged (as do we), as many of these techniques fail and occasionally succeed.

As the years roll by, we get a slightly better idea of the mechanisms of phantom pain, but because of the uncertainty and reservations, we still have no single way to treat this very painful phenomenon. It must be stressed that this pain is real and not a figment of the patient's imagination. The patients feel "crazy" enough, and we should not play into this false belief of "craziness and imaginary pain," because of our own ignorance and frustration.

PLP has a long and fascinating history. Paré (1), the great medieval surgeon, writes movingly about this phenomenon; and Mitchell (2) published material, albeit under a fictional account. Both touch on the strangeness of this phenomenon—something that isn't supposed to be there, actually being there. Various cultures have used magic and sorcery to get rid of this troublesome pain, the underlying theme being that there is something unclean, brought on the individual by himself or herself. The resulting exorcisms had as poor results as we might expect, although some of the techniques, such as burying the limb, have become a piece of today's treatment.

We will present three of our cases to show important differences and then go on to a discussion of these differences.

CLINICAL VIGNETTES FOR PHANTOM PAIN

The following three vignettes show patients at different time frames after the amputation. Some will deal with the difference in time, and some will include a differentiation between phantom pain and phantom sensation. We will

not deal with stump pain except in the area of differential diagnosis.

Case 1

Roy, a 19-year-old boy, had been working unloading newspapers from a truck in the early morning when a drunken driver slammed him into the back of the delivery truck, leaving him on the ground, bleeding. An hour later, he was in the hospital. For the next 3 weeks, his leg was in traction with terrible pain, only moderately and intermittently controlled with pain medication, and there was a question as to whether an amputation would be necessary. One day he was told that he would have debridement of the area only to find on awakening that he had a below-the-knee amputation to which he responded with both rage and relief. A few days later, when questioned about pain, he said that he did have some pain, but it seemed to be in a strange place. This was not followed up for a few days until a nurse asked why, if he was in pain, he wasn't asking for pain medication, at which point he timidly mentioned that the pain was in the toes of the foot that he no longer had.

Case 2

Anne was a 67-year-old widow who had a 10-year history of diabetes, which had brought on peripheral vascular problems that caused increasing pain in her lower extremity over the past 2 years. She found herself walking less and less and, over the 6 months before coming into the hospital, less able to sleep at night, gradually ending up in a reclining chair where she was able to sleep for 3 or 4 hours on a good night. Life was becoming intolerable for both her and her family. When she was finally admitted to the hospital, a large gangrenous area had formed on the sole of her foot, which was both smelly and painful. She was informed by her surgeon that they would be trying a by-pass operation to which she readily agreed. A week later, it was obvious to the surgeons that the by-pass was not working; it also was obvious to the patient, because the pain continued unabated even as she was given pain medication. She found herself getting rather droopy on the medication and rather resentful that the medical staff continued to talk to her about possible amputation. Four weeks after her admission to the hospital she was told that an amputation would be necessary, probably a below-the-knee amputation. After the operation, she had numerous complications including infections and poor healing, complained of a lot of stump pain, and needed large doses of pain medication every 3 hours. Because the surgeon felt that she was requesting too much medication, he arranged for a psychiatric evaluation, and Anne admitted to the psychiatrist that the pain was not so much in the stump, but in that "place where there isn't any leg." She was quite sure that she was crazy, in that if she mentioned this to the staff, she would be "put away." On a followup 2 weeks later, the phantom pain was less severe in that it no longer was a constant irritation and would only bubble up every 6 to 7 hours. She had also been taught by the staff to take some medication before the pain built up, so that in a 24-hour span she would actually need less of the medication. Three months later on followup, she was complaining of occasional phantom pain with numerous phantom sensations during the day, and on 1-year followup, was commenting that she was having phantom pain about once a week, and phantom sensation every day. Five years after the operation, she was moving well with a prosthesis, was going through her daily activities roughly as she had before the onset of her crippling symptoms, and upon close questioning reported that she now had phantom pain lasting a number of minutes once every 2 to 3 weeks, and phantom sensations once a week.

Case 3

Kenneth was a 53-year-old self-employed man, married, with his sister-in-law also living in the apartment. A man who had traveled and lived in various parts of the world, he had suffered from periodic depressions from young adulthood to the present. Over the past 2 years, intermittent claudication of both legs had increased to the point where he could go no more than a half a block before he had to stop. He was no longer able to move about and did most of his work at his desk and over the phone. His wife, who had always been careful about his diet and the care of both extremities, was horrified when he began developing ulcers on both lower extremities. Sympathectomy on both sides was done, but 4 months later it was obvious that this wasn't doing the job. Thrombotic episodes in both legs were followed by revascularization and creating new channels, but because of recurrent thrombotic episodes, this proved

not fruitful. His surgeons began talking about possible amputation. Kenneth threatened suicide, so they talked less about it. Further bilateral thromboembolic episodes led to a necessity for quick amputations, and with his surgeon, wife, and sister-in-law insisting, he had bilateral above-the-knee amputations. After the operations, he screamed out in pain, and as a result was given massive amounts of Levo-Dromoran and, because of severe depression, large doses of antidepressants. He had bilateral phantom pain and complained loudly about it being helped "only slightly" by the medication. Although he was sad, the depressive symptoms cleared, but the phantom pain remained intense and steady. He was given TENS treatment in the hope that this would decrease the need for medication, but this only helped for short stretches, right after the treatments. Three months later, on followup, the pain was nearly as intense as previously, and his wife reported that although he was getting around fairly well in his wheelchair, attempts to give him bilateral prostheses had failed. Because the high dosage of Levo-Dromorane was making him drowsy, he tried to take less of the medication but unfortunately found that the pain was "very, very bad." Hypnosis was attempted but he was a poor subject, so progressive relaxation and desensitization were tried, which were also not successful. Another course of antidepressants was initiated, not because the symptoms of depression were so disabling, but in the hope that "it might help with the pain." Doses of up to 300 mg of nortriptyline did not help, either, with mood or for pain. At the end of the year, he was still taking large doses of Levo-Dromoran at times when the pain was "too bad," and he was still complaining of daily ongoing pain and poor sleep at night because of the pain. On a 4-year followup, the pain had decreased so that he was only having pain for about a half hour once or twice a day.

ETIOLOGIC FACTORS

This phenomenon must first be put in context. All three people had a definite loss, sometimes suddenly and sometimes over time, but loss in all cases. Some had pain before the amputation, some did not. Parkes (3) focuses on this loss and the grief that must follow this loss, proposing a sequence that may lead to resolution. How people cope with the loss (4), and a possible effect on the intensity of the PLP, will be discussed later in this chapter.

An amputation is a mutilation and disfiguration of the body, a traumatic event that patients describe as "they cut me up," "they hacked a piece away," and "they butchered me." All our patients, no matter how grateful, felt that an aggressive act had been done to them. Many that were awake during the procedure, had nightmares afterward.

After the procedure, there is a stump, pain in the stump, heavy bandages, and a hospital stay. The body is forever changed and the way one thinks about one's body is changed (5) or strongly denied. One is also seen differently by family, friends, and employers, and there are activities one can no longer do, some forever. One is changed for one's lifetime and perhaps past one's lifetime, according to some religions. Add to this, pain coming at various times, at various intensities, and you can see the further obstacles to the daily quality of life, the quantity of life, and one's functioning.

Why is it that people who lose a limb through amputation will have periods of phantom sensation, followed by phantom pain over varying periods of time? We do know that many patients will have decreasing amounts of pain, as the stump is telescoped and incorporated, but a percentage will be stuck with chronic pain. Now that we educate people—preoperatively, when possible—as to this pain and ask the right questions, both pre- and postoperatively, we know that 60% to 80% of people have pain over time and are willing to talk about it. This is much different from the time, not long ago, when we didn't ask and the patients didn't tell us.

Although there is stump pain, phantom sensations, and PLP, we will concentrate on PLP.

Age is certainly a factor, as is culture, but more important are the coping mechanisms that people use. Does this help with various treatments? Does the primary disease have an impact? Does the relationship with the medical helpers make a difference? Yes to all of the above.

Age and physical shape play a large role. Younger people tend to heal more quickly and frequently are more willing to use a prosthesis, especially if they are in decent physical shape. On the other hand, they tend to be angrier about the loss and as adolescents, frequently go for long periods without being willing to do the necessary prosthesis training. People over 65 who are in poor physical shape and have chronic diseases are harder to get back on their feet with prostheses and have a harder and longer road to healing. Older people are also more prone to depression and, when depressed, less willing to make the necessary adjustments, physically and emotionally.

Culture plays a role, in that Western culture tends to overemphasize youth, beauty, and mobility, which can either spur the person to recovery or make him or her feel that life in the fast lane is over. Therefore, what is the use of trying? This is not so for areas of the world where other qualities, such as wisdom and experience, are of importance.

A primary disease, such as diabetes, may have a large impact. Having a chronic disease that, as one of my patients mentioned, "Takes away pieces of you . . . piece by piece, over time, and makes me hopeless," has a debilitating effect. The situation will not get better, probably worse. A sudden car accident that shears off your leg, although devastating initially, at least may not lead to "losing more parts of me, soon."

Our studies indicate that the relationship with helpers, doctors, nurses, physical therapists, other patients has a large influence on outcomes. Patients who are willing to

trust the helpers, willing to listen to other patients, and be motivated by the helpers generally do better than the depressed, suspicious, help-rejecting patient who feels that this injury and pain, by a hostile world, means that no one and no environment can be trusted.

This hospital and rehabilitation support system is greatly helped by a personal support system, family, and friends. When there is little such support, the rehabilitation road is longer and rougher.

The pain may be reported as burning, shooting, cramping, heated, with many other manifestations. It may be "started" by heat, exertion, stress, and urination among many other apparent "triggers." The pain may start hours after the amputation, or some years after the amputation. It may be constant or intermittent and finally be acute or fall into the chronic category. There are many ways to experience the pain, over variable amounts of time and intensity, and all very real and distressing and disturbing.

Although phenomenologically there is agreement about the nature of phantom limb pain, what causes the pain is not at all well understood. There are many theories concerning its etiology, which can be lumped into three groups: (1) central theories, (2) peripheral theories, and (3) psychological theories.

The central theories include Melzack's gait control theory, which centers around the idea of reverberating circuits and deals mostly with the rostral brain stem. According to Melzack and Loeser (6), it is the reticular activating system that exerts an inhibitory influence on the somatosensory projection system. With an amputation, many peripheral fibers are destroyed, the input is reduced, inhibition is decreased, and synchronous self-sustaining activity develops at all neuronal levels. Pain occurs when output from these self-sustaining neurons reaches the cortical level.

Riddoch (7) hypothesizes that a cortical representational body image develops over time as a result of peripheral input from all the senses. After amputation, this perception remains unaltered and cortical cells, independent of peripheral impulses, are then responsible for the phantom phenomena. Others see the pain owing its existence to a thalamic or subthalamic lesion and indeed phantom pain shows some characteristics identical with thalamic pain (8). Unfortunately none of the medullary or cerebral causes describe all or even most of the phantom pains, and it has not been possible, at present, to duplicate studies that provoke pain by stimulating either the cortex or certain parts of the midbrain.

The peripheral theories (9) hypothesize that the pain is caused by persistent sensation of the nerve endings in the stump. The amputee then feels that these sensations are assigned to the part of the body that was originally innervated by the severed nerves. Not infrequently, abscesses or scar tissues have been found to trigger the pain, but unfortunately the pain persists long after the injury has healed or after the scar tissue has been removed. Again, many questions are not answered by this peripheral theory, including the fact that amputees under 6 years old don't seem to have phantom pain (10) but, more important, that the pain does not follow the distribution of the severed nerves.

Most people do not believe that the psychological factors are the *sole* cause of phantom limb pain, but some studies seem to indicate that emotional factors are among the risk factors causing phantom pain. Many studies have been done looking at the personality structures of patients with phantom pain (11), and many risk factors have been found by various people to have an impact on the presence of pain. Unfortunately, none of these studies has been duplicated, although some, like those by Parkes (3), hold promise. In Parkes's study, the following were highly predictive of persistent phantom pain: (1) the appearance of stump or phantom pain within 3 weeks, (2) illness that had lasted longer than 1 year prior to the amputation and persisted after surgery, (3) unemployment not due to pain, and (4) rigid and compulsively self-reliant personality types. The first three are measurable, the fourth, difficult to measure. Others have looked closely at the concept of denial (12) or the denial of the loss of a body part (4). Here again, there is a question of whether high denial or low denial is very good.

TREATMENT STRATEGIES

Looking at treatment, we know that nothing works all the time or even part of the time. In treatment, we have to move to a model that includes "better," without always being a "cure." As in many medical situations, improving the pain, lessening the disability, and making the patient more comfortable are all laudable and important results.

Since we don't know the etiology of phantom pain, treatment becomes a pick-and-choose kind of a situation. Sherman and Sherman reported 68 treatment methods of which they allege 43 are successful (13). There are, however, a number of areas of agreement as to what will make for a better prognosis.

At the top of the list is preoperative preparation, which should certainly include the warning to patients that phantom sensations are probable and phantom pain occasional. This preparation should also include evaluation of the patient's personality type, previous surgical experiences, and a thorough discussion of the meaning of the loss (3,4). Since the amputated member will have to be buried, there should be a discussion of the care and disposal of the part. The details of the surgical procedure should be left to what the patient wants to hear and not how little or how much the physicians wish to mention. Some patients are most interested in knowing all the details, whereas others will stop you after a number of sentences and say they have had enough. In either case the patient's wishes should be followed, unless there seems to be maladaptive denial. At this preoperative meeting, the rehabilitation program should be stressed, and the prosthetist and/or the rehabilitation team should talk to the patient. We have found that a patient who has gone through rehabilitation and successfully uses and wears the prosthesis is most useful in talking to the preamputation patient. Postoperatively, the patient should be allowed to mourn the loss and counterproductive coping mechanisms using counterphobic and denial mechanisms should be looked for and addressed early. The patient who refuses to look at the stump after a week postoperation is a good example.

Some studies seem to indicate that early return to work and maximal use of the prosthesis reduce the risk of developing phantom limb pain (14,15), and other studies seem to indicate that counseling of the family is helpful to the situation and perhaps may have an impact on phantom limb pain risk.

When trying to decipher the literature of treatments for PLP, it is useful to partition into the following areas: (1) acute and chronic PLP, (2) the route that medication is given (i.e., by anesthesia), (3) whether medication is given before or after the amputation, and (4) the originating country of the study and report. Other ways to look at treatment options include (1) drugs and drug combinations, (2) various kinds of stimulations, (3) miscellaneous group of options from many disciplines, including psychology and nursing.

Preoperatively, medications are given intrathecally, epidurally, or injected locally. There is much interest in having the patient pain-free before the operation (preemptive analgesia); researchers feel that a preoperative pain-free period will lead to less PLP (16,17). Medications include epidural morphine and bupivacaine, either individually or in combinations. Some of the studies seem to give excellent results, but many studies have only a few patients or are anecdotal (18). This is not to say that they are useless, only that a larger number of studies may have to be done. Some are promising and should be followed up.

Postamputation, with the appearance of PLP, there is general agreement that medical treatment and electrical stimulation should be tried before the surgical treatments are attempted.

When medication is given postoperatively, after the PLP has appeared, treatment results universally seem to be less efficacious. Jahangiri (17) has found that epidural infusion of diamorphine has prevented PLP, and Elizaga and colleagues (19) use intraneuronal blocks for the same purpose. Ketamine is found useful by some (20,21) and not useful by others (18). Among classes of drugs, β-blockers, central nervous system serotonin agonists, tricyclic antidepressants, and calcitonin have been tried.

Analgesics, especially salicylates, are frequently used but seem to be more useful in keeping the pain under some kind of control than in eliminating it. Propranolol (22) has been used with some success, and a number of studies have shown that carbamazepine (23) and gabapentin may be of great help. Various neuroleptics have been tried without much success, but the use of tricyclic antidepressants, as a help in chronic pain, is well known. Recent studies with SSRIs show some promise, especially since they seem to have fewer side effects than tricyclic antidepressants.

Transcutaneous stimulation was used with good results in about half of the patients studied by Thoden and colleagues in 1979 (24). Spinal cord stimulation and deep brain stimulation have been tried in a number of patients, sometimes with spectacular results (25). Mundinger and Neumuller (26), in 1981, used a combination of deep brain stimulation and transcutaneous stimulation, which worked in about half the patients. The reasons for using these electrostimulations are that they are nontraumatic and can be repeated. In a number of studies, local anesthetics and nerve blocks have been useful, seeming to work for about one-third to one-half of the patients (27). When electrical stimulation is used, it is frequently in the late stages of PLP, and this may skew the results.

This brings us back to a discussion of pain and the philosophy of pain treatments. Perry (28) has shown that doctors tend to undermedicate patients with pain, partly out of ignorance of pharmacokinetics, partly out of fear of addicting the patient, and sometimes as a way of differentiating themselves from the person in pain. No matter how we look at pain, though, it is real, and although it certainly has both objective and subjective components, it is something that deserves treatment. This becomes especially important in phantom pain because the patient tends to see the pain as "crazy": how can you have pain in an area that isn't there—a viewpoint, which not infrequently, is shared by the surgical staff for their own reasons. Well-known studies by Twycross (29) have shown that pain medication taken regularly, and in adequate doses, means that frequently patients will be taking less of the medication over a 24-hour period and the effect will be greater. Fears of addicting patients have proved to be unfounded. This brings us directly to the point of narcotics and Jensen and Rasmussen's (30) excellent statement that "resistant pains are not to be accepted until narcotics have been tried." They have found that the vast majority of patients can manage on a fixed morphine dose for many years without becoming addicted.

In surgical therapy, both local and central procedures have been done. The peripheral surgical procedures include the excision of neuromata (31), which seems to be most effective for stump pain. Even here the percentage of cure is small and the procedure is only useful when there are very positive indications for the presence of neuromata. Unfortunately, this procedure is frequently used when the signs and symptoms of neuromata are not that clear. Occasionally, more extensive amputation has been tried to see if this will help with the phantom pain, but this is usually ineffective.

Rhizotomy (32) used to be fairly popular but is now almost entirely abandoned.

Cordotomy (33) was fairly popular in the 1940s but, due to rather low numbers of patients improving, the treatment is not done frequently now.

Sympathectomy (34) was done frequently in the 1950s but at least three-quarters of the patients had recurrence of the pain within 6 months.

Midbrain lesions, thalamotomy, prefrontal lobotomies, and cortical ablations have been done in the past, probably out of frustration, and did not prove to be of much use.

Psychological treatments have proved to be of limited and circumscribed use. Relaxation techniques, in our own group, proved to help in the general well-being of the patient, but did not seem to help much with the pain. Biofeedback techniques (35) have been reported as occasionally effective in individual patients but have not been useful in large groups. Hypnosis (36) was one of the treatments of choice in the 1950s and seemed to hold promise. Unfortunately, it does not seem to work over long periods of time and has been reported infrequently.

Psychotherapy (37), by itself, was reported to be of limited help in the 1950s, when there were indications that the treatment improved the general well-being of the patient, but had little effect on the pain. Educational counseling, used in conjunction with tricyclics, frequently is of more use in chronic pain than intensive psychotherapy. It is, nevertheless, important for patients to realize that they are understood and that the doctors feel that the pain is real. Work with the family should follow the same lines.

It is known that PLP patients are more prone to depression, and therefore the diagnosis and treatment of depression is important. We know that patients with pain and depression do less well with rehabilitation, by not following through with needed exercises and care, and that pain perception is greater with depression. Therefore, treatment is important. As the reality of the amputation and pain comes to the forefront, coping, body image, and change in ability to move have to be faced. Symptom-focused psychotherapy, plus antidepressants, in proper dosage over proper time, can lead to a better result. We have often found that physicians use low dosage and give up, before the medications have a chance to work.

Physical therapy started early after the amputation seems to be of great use in keeping the phantom pain within limits (27), and there are studies that seem to indicate that early physical therapy may actually decrease the risk of the phantom pain. Ultrasound, heat, and peripheral stimulation have been reported as useful in certain individuals and certainly are safe enough to use. In many reports, the pain seems to decrease over short stretches of time, and this is not to be denigrated.

CONCLUSIONS

We must continue to study these patients and hopefully more prospective studies like those of Parkes and Sherman will be done. Researchers need to continue to look at the patient through all parameters—physiologically, psychologically, preoperatively—and follow them for many, many years. In our own study, patients interviewed after 12 years report occasionally having phantom sensations; some report phantom pain. It is crucial that we do not denigrate the pain, that we treat it with all the forces that we can marshal, going from one treatment to the other until, hopefully, we hit something that works. With proper studies, perhaps we will be able to predict which people are most at risk for phantom pain and after that use studies of various approaches to match the patient and the appropriate treatment.

These are challenging and difficult therapeutic maneuvers, but we continue to hope as the etiologic factors are further elucidated. When I wrote about this condition 10 years ago, much less was known and there were fewer therapies available. Now, there is more hope, but no one answer, which means that we have to mix and match from the menu of treatments available.

REFERENCES

1. Paré A. *The works of that famous chirurgion, Ambrose Paré*. London: R. Cotes, 1649.
2. Mitchell SW. Phantom limbs. *Lippincott's Magazine of Popular Literature and Science* 1871;8:563–569.
3. Parkes CM. Factors determining the persistence of phantom pain in the amputee. *Journal of Psychosomatic Research* 1973;17:97–108.
4. Zuk GH. The phantom limb: a proposed theory of unconscious origins. *Journal of Nervous and Mental Diseases* 1956;124:510–513.
5. Desjarlais, R. On the vagaries of bodies. *Culture, Medicine and Psychiatry* June 1995;19(2)207–15.
6. Melzack R and Loeser JD. Phantom body pain in paraplegics: evidence for a central pattern generating mechanism for pain. *Pain* 1978;4:195–210.
7. Riddoch G. Phantom limbs and body shape. *Brain* 1941;44:197–222.
8. Tasker R. Pain resulting from nervous systeem pathology. In: Bonica JJ, ed., *The management of pain*, Philadelphia: Lea and Febinger, 1990: 264-280.
9. Livingston WK. *Pain mechanism: a physiologic interpretation of causalgia and its related states.* New York:Macmillan, 1944.
10. Simmel ML. The absence of phantoms for congenitally missing limbs. *Am J Psychology* 74:467-470, 1961.
11. Scott LE, et al. Preoperative predictors of postoperative pain. *Pain* 1983;15:283–293.
12. Schilder P. The image and appearance of the human body. *Studies in the constructive energies of the psyche.* London: Kegan Paul, 1935.
13. Sherman R, Sherman C. Prevalence and characteristics of chronic phantom limb pain among American veterans: results of a trial survey. *Am J Phys Med* 1983;62:227–238.
14. Langer E, Jania IL, Wolfer JA. Reduction of psychological stress in surgical patients. *J Exp Soc Psychol* 1975;11:155–165.
15. Wilson PG, Krebs MJS, Cohen DEI. Risk factors in amputation. (Unpublished study)
16. Bach S, et al., Phantom limb pain in amputees during the first 12 months following limb amputation, after preoperative lumbar epidural blockade. *Pain* 1988;33;297–303.
17. Jahangiri M, et al. Prevention of phantom pain after major lower limb amputation by epidural infusion of diamorphine, clonidine and bupivacaine. *Annals of the Royal College of Surgeons of England* 1994;76;324–326.
18. Nicolajsen L, et al. Randomized trial of epidural bupivacaine and morphine in prevention of stump and phantom pain in lower limb amputation. *Lancet* 1997;350:1353–1357.
19. Elizaga AM, et al. Continuous regional analgesia by intravenous block; *J of Rehabilitation Research and development* 31(3):179–187.
20. Knox DJ. Acute phantom pain limb pain controlled by ketamine. *Anesthesia and Intensive Care* October 1995 ;23(5):620–622.
21. Franks JF, et al. Ketamine for management of intractable phantom limb pain. *Ugeskrift fur Laeger* June 12 1995;157(24);3481–3482.
22. Marsland AR, Weekes JWN, Atkinson RL, Leong MG. Phantom limb pain: a case for beta blockers? *Pain* 1982;12:295–297.
23. Elliott F, Little A, Milbrandt W. Carbamazepine for phantom-limb phenomena. *The New England Journal of Medicine* 1976;295:678.
24. Thoden U, Gruber RP, Krainick J-U, Huber-Muck L. Langzeitergebnisse transkutaner nervenstimulation bei chronish neurogenen schmerzzustanden. *Nervenarzt* 1979;50:179–184.
25. Krainick J-U, Thoden U, Riechert T. Pain reduction in amputees by long-term spinal cord stimulation. *Journal of Neurosurgery* 1980;52:346–350.
26. Mundinger F, Neumuller H. Programmed transcutaneous (*TNS*) and central DBS) stimulation for control of phantom limb pain and causalgia: a new method for treatment. In: Siegfried J, Zimmermann M, eds., *Phantom and Stump Pain*, Berlin:Springer Verlag, 1981:167–178.
27. Sherman RA. Published treatments of phantom limb pain. *American Journal of Physical Medicine* 1980;59:232–244.
28. Perry S. Undermedication for pain. *Psychia Ann* 1984;14:960.
29. Twycross RG. Diseases of the central nervous system: relief of terminal pain. *Br Med J* 1975;4:212.
30. Jensen TS, Rasmussen P. Amputation. In: Wall P, Melzack R, eds. *Textbook of pain*, Churchill Livingstone, 1984.
31. Baumgartner R, Riniker C. Surgical stump revision as a treatment of stump and phantom pains. Results of 100 cases In: Siegfried S, Zimmermann M, eds. *Phantom and stump pain*. Berlin: Springer Verlag , 1981.
32. White J, Sweet W. *Pain and the neurosurgeon: a forty-year experience*. Springfield, Illinois: Charles C. Thomas, 1969.
33. Siegfried J, Cetinalp E. Neurosurgical treatment of phantom limb pain: a survey of methods. In: Siegfried J, Zimmermann M, eds. *Phantom and stump pain*. Berlin: Springer Verlag, 1981:148–155.
34. Kallio KE. Permanency of results obtained by sympathetic surgery in the treatment of phantom pain. *Acta Orthopaedica Scandinavica* 1950;19:391–397.
35. Sherman R. Case reports of treatment of phantom limb pain with a combination of electromyographic biofeedback and verbal relaxation techniques. *Biofeedback and Self Regulation* 1976;1(3):353.
36. Siegel EF. Control of phantom limb pain by hypnosis. *American Journal of Clinical Hypnosis* April 1979;21:285–286.
37. Postone N. Phantom limb pain. *Psychiatry in Medicine* August 1994, 1987;17(1):57–70.

CHAPTER 35

Postherpetic Neuralgia

P. Prithvi Raj

Herpes zoster, an acute infectious disease caused by varicella virus belonging to the DNA group of viruses, primarily affects the posterior spinal root ganglion of the spinal nerves. Varicella and herpes zoster have long been recognized as manifestations of the same infectious agent, and it has been concluded that the same virus causes them. Antigens derived from vesicles of patients with varicella or herpes zoster react similarly, and DNA studies have confirmed biophysical similarities (1).

INCIDENCE

Herpes zoster affects approximately 125 per 100,000 persons annually, striking both sexes equally, with no apparent seasonal variation. While the incidence is only 0.5 in 1000 for children (2), it increases to five to 10 in 1000 for patients in their eighties (2). Waning immune surveillance has been suggested for the increased incidence with age (3). Age is also a major factor in the development of postherpetic neuralgia, which develops almost exclusively in patients older than 50 years. Incidence ranges from 15% to 70% (4,5).

Triggering factors for herpes zoster include surgery (6) or trauma; irradiation and other immunosuppressive agents; malignancies; and infections such as tuberculosis, syphilis, malaria, and acquired immunodeficiency syndrome (AIDS). Stressful life events also reactivate the latent varicella-zoster virus (7). Secondary herpes zoster caused by inflammation, neoplasm, or direct injury to the cranial or peripheral nerve may recur more frequently, clear more rapidly, and result in less scarring and pigmentation than idiopathic zoster.

Herpes zoster is more prevalent and severe in immunosuppressed patients (8–11). It is a major problem following radio or chemotherapy and bone marrow transplantation,

correlating with depressed cell-mediated immunity (12). Patients deficient in T-lymphocyte macrophage-mediated immune defenses are more susceptible to viral spread beyond the ganglion-nerve-dermatome unit and visceral and nervous system complications represent a major threat for these patients (13).

ACUTE HERPETIC STAGE

Herpes zoster can progress in three stages (Table 35-1). Both virus and host interact at each stage to affect the development and course.

Lesions are most often thoracic, trigeminal (mostly ophthalmic), or cervical, with less than 1% bilateral (Fig. 35-1). Recurrences are experienced by approximately 1% to 8% of patients, about half of the time at the site of the previous eruption (Table 35-2).

TABLE 35-1. *Stages of herpes zoster*

Stage I	Viral replication Loss of immune surveillance
Stage II	Clinical syndrome (acute herpes zoster) Viral effect on ganglion-nerve-dermatome Antiviral immune response by the body Cytolysis from virus and host inflammatory reaction
Stage III	Sequelae of herpes zoster Central nervous system and visceral spread Antiviral immune response

(Raj, P. Pain due to herpes zoster. In: Raj P, ed. *Practical management of pain,* 2nd ed. Chicago: Mosby-Year Book, 1992;45, with permission.)

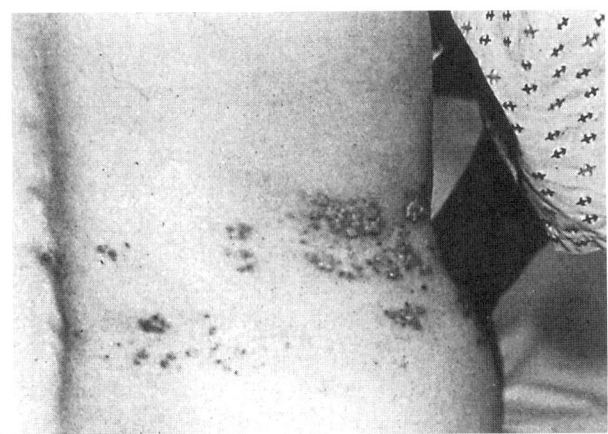 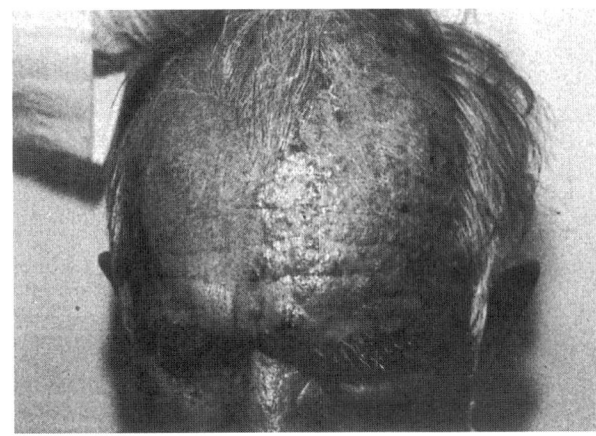

A   B

FIG. 35-1. A. A 38 year-old woman presenting with 14-day-old acute herpes zoster in T-7–10 distribution. She was admitted to the hospital 3 weeks previously for workup with a diagnosis of renal colic prior to the appearance of the rash. **B.** A 76-year-old man with 3-day-old acute herpes zoster in the left ophthalmic nerve distribution.

Pain of Acute Stage

Acute herpes zoster is associated with pain, paresthesia, and dysesthesia in the dermatomal distribution of one or more affected posterior root ganglia, sometimes accompanied by fever, malaise, headache, nausea, stiff neck, and regional or diffuse adenopathy. Pain is usually mild initially but may intensify. A vesicular eruption usually appears within 4 to 5 days, if not sooner.

Presentation of Acute Herpes Zoster

Following localized erythema and swelling, red papules progress through vesicles, blebs, and pustules (Fig. 35-2). Lesions are usually unilateral in part of the dermatome but affect sensation of the entire segment in mild cases. More severe cases involve the entire segment, with larger blebs that tend to coalesce, in addition to continuous burning and sharp pain, burning pain precipitated by movement or change in skin tension.

The erythema gradually resolves; blebs dry up and wrinkle, and the sharp pain recedes. Scales of encrusting

TABLE 35-2. *Site and incidence of acute herpes zoster*

Site of herpes zoster	Incidence (percentage)
Thoracic	50
Face (ophthalmic)	3–20
Cervical	10–20
Bilateral	<1
Recurrent	1–8
Recurrent at the site of previous herpes zoster	50

(From Raj P. Pain due to herpes zoster. In: Raj P, ed. *Practical management of pain,* 2nd ed. Chicago: Mosby-Year Book, 1992, with permission.)

blebs fall off, leaving pink scars that retract and produce pocks without pigment. Hyperesthesia and hyperalgesia gradually resolve, with the patient becoming asymptomatic.

Course of Viral Multiplications and Pathogenesis Caused in the Nervous System

Knowledge of the pathogenesis of varicella and herpes zoster is somewhat limited. Although varicella is exogenous and herpes zoster is endogenous, the varicella zoster virus is present in both lesions and can serve as a source of infection to others.

Characteristically, varicella is associated with no immunity, while herpes zoster possesses partial immunity to the virus. During the course of varicella, the virus may pass from the sensory nerve ending up to the sensory ganglia; there it remains latent until activated and shed from the dorsal root ganglion cell, stimulating the production of antiviral antibody and other immune mechanisms. Antibodies are present only in varicella convalescent serum; however, antibody titers may be high in acute zoster and even higher in convalescent zoster, indicating an amnestic response.

If immunity falls below a critical level, the activated virus can continue to replicate within the sensory ganglion, resulting in neuronal necrosis, inflammation, and neuralgia. It is then spread antidromically to the sensory nerve endings of the skin, causing a vesicular eruption. Varicella-zoster-like particles have been seen in the ganglia of patients who died of varicella-zoster infection.

In acute zoster, hemorrhagic inflammation affects the posterior spinal ganglion, the peripheral nerve of the affected ganglion, and the dorsal spinal nerve root, spreading to the spinal cord and leptomeninges. Demyelinization is associated with Wallerian degeneration,

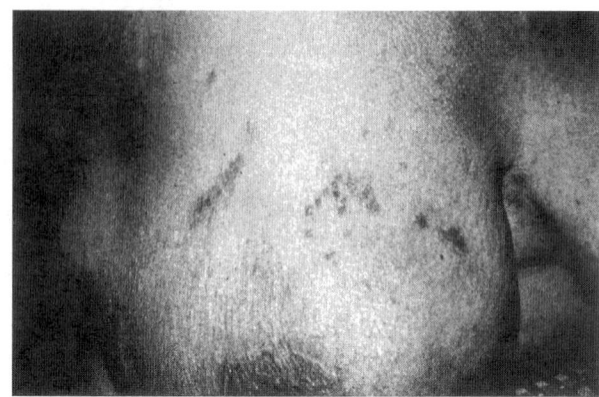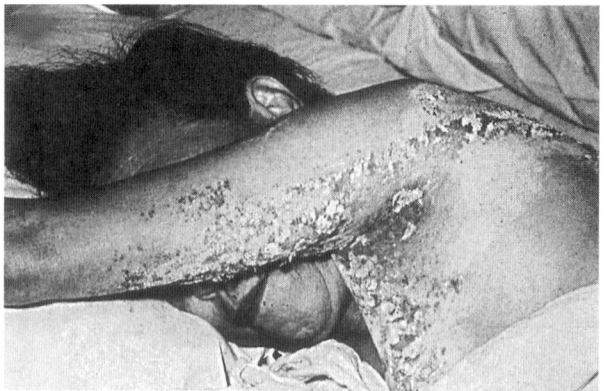

FIG. 35-2. A. A papular formation in the T-3 distribution. This was confirmed as early acute herpes zoster. **B.** A 3-week-old herpes zoster in the T-2–3 distribution in the crusting stage.

fibrosis, and cellular infiltration in the peripheral nerve (Fig. 35-3). Degeneration can reach the ipsilateral posterior spinal cord within 9 days after vesicular eruption and can last 5 to 9 months. Measurement of tissue impedance after herpes zoster indicates lower-than-normal impedance in affected segments (14,15).

If infection spreads along the posterior nerve root to the meninges and spinal cord, local meningitis, cerebrospinal fluid pleocytosis, and myelitis result, and spread to anterior motor roots may cause local palsies. Hematogenous dissemination can cause aberrant vesicles. Although the amnestic response sometimes terminates the infection before vesicles develop, more severe and prolonged local response and more hematogenous dissemination can occur when the immune response is greatly deficient.

Sequence of Immunologic Responses to Varicella

The sequence of immunologic responses to varicella in patients not previously exposed has been summarized (Table 35-3) (16). Mortality and severity of cell-mediated immune deficiency are directly related (9). The status of the immune response is similarly related to the occurrence of herpes zoster and its complications. Although no correlation between antibody and protection against herpes zoster has been indicated, increased antibody levels may correlate with the severity and sequelae of the disease (17).

Symptomatic herpes zoster tends to occur only when cell-mediated immunity to varicella-zoster is depressed; the ability to mount a specific cellular immune response and the incidence of zoster are inversely correlated. The HLA-DR antigen is significantly expressed on T-cell surfaces in herpes zoster, predominantly on suppressor/cytotoxic cells (18). Lymphocyte and monocyte function is impaired, and the normal ratio of helper T cells to suppressor T cells is reversed. The infection is limited by the cell-mediated immune lymphocytic transformation (19), lymphocyte-monocyte inactivation of virus, and local host responses of interferon production and polymorphonuclear inflammatory response within the vesicle. Antibody administration also modifies the disease, perhaps altering membrane antigens and cellular cytotoxicity (20).

The association of specific IgM with acute infection suggests both reinfections with exogenous varicella virus

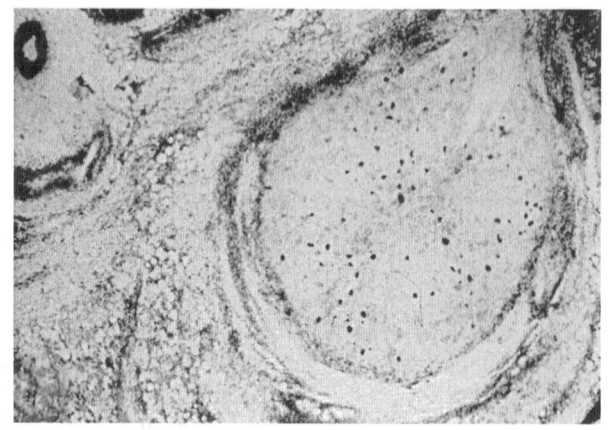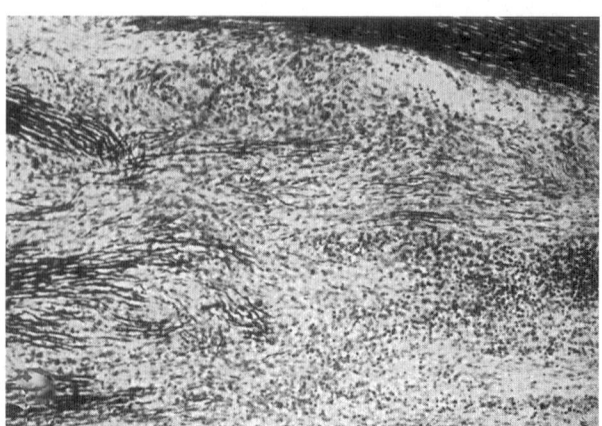

FIG. 35-3. A. Inflammatory reaction in the geniculate ganglion due to acute herpes zoster. Ganglion and satellite cells show intranuclear inclusion. There is also round cell infiltration and neuronal destruction. **B.** The ganglion is swollen and hemorrhagic.

TABLE 35-3. *Sequence of immunologic responses to varicella*

Local and systemic responses to varicella
and herpes zoster virus

Systemic

Varicella zoster infection

| | 2–5 days after rash appears |

IgG, IgA, and IgM induced
(complement-fixing antibody detected)

| | 2–3 wk |

IgG, IgA, and IgM induction reaches maximum
(detected fluorescent antibody
to membrane antigen)

High IgG levels present in childhood after varicella infection

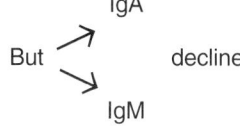

But   IgA ↗   ↘ IgM   decline

(complement-fixing antibody not detected
after 1 to 2 years)

Local
Production of interferon
Influx of neutrophils within the vesicles

(From Raj P. Pain due to herpes zoster. In Raj P, ed. *Practical management of pain,* 2nd ed. Chicago: Mosby-Year Book, 1992, with permission.)

and antigen stimulation caused by exposure to endogenous varicella zoster (21). Repetitive asymptomatic viral activity may be important in enhancing the immunologic system.

Measurement of Immune Responses

Complement-fixing antibody is not very useful in determining the immune status of a general population for herpes zoster. The fluorescent antibody to membrane antigen (FAMA) assay is earlier and more sensitive in diagnosing acute varicella-zoster virus and evaluating humoral immune states in high-risk patients with leukemia. Complement-enhanced neutralizing antibody is equivalent to FAMA for diagnosis and evaluation of humoral immunity in immunosuppressed persons, but immune adherence hemagglutination does not appear to be as sensitive. The enzyme-linked immunosorbent assay is an alternative to FAMA or complement-enhanced neutralizing antibody tests. Radioimmunoassay studies for detecting varicella-

zoster virus-specific IgG antibody show sensitivity but decreased specificity for some children.

Optimal drug treatment depends on early and accurate diagnosis. Appropriate laboratory techniques for diagnosis of acute herpes zoster are shown in Table 35-4. Rapid diagnostic tests allow earlier diagnosis.

Differential Diagnosis

Before the eruption of lesions, herpes zoster can be mistaken for coronary disease, pleurisy, pleurodynia, costochondritis (Tietze's syndrome), pericarditis, cholecystitis, neural disease, acute and subacute abdominal conditions, appendicitis, collapsed intervertebral disk, neuropathies, and myofascial pains.

Distinguishing between herpes simplex and herpes zoster can be difficult, despite their difference (22). Typically, herpes simplex occurs in a young woman as frequent

TABLE 35-4. *Laboratory diagnosis of acute herpes zoster*

Techniques	
Virus recovery from	
Vesicles	
Blood	
Lung	
Liver	
CSF	
Oropharynx	
(only occasionally)	
Scrapings from the vesicles contain cellular material with multinucleated giant cells	Show acidophilic intranuclear inclusions
Tzanck smear	
Hematoxylin and eosin stain	
Giemsa stain	
Papanicolaou stain	
Paragon multiple stain	
Punch biopsy for electron microscopy	More reliable and provides diagnosis before vesicular stage develops
Culture tests (in human epithelioids or fibroblasts) in 3 to 4 days	Focal lesion with swollen refractile cells
Virus specifically identified in culture by intranuclear inclusions after staining and by gel-precipitation techniques	
Staining of cellular material with direct fluorescent antibody of Tzanck smear	Readily identifies infected cells

(From Raj P. Pain due to herpes zoster. In: Raj P, ed. *Practical management of pain,* 2nd ed. Chicago: Mosby-Year Book, 1992, with permission.)

recurrences of either Type 1 (orofacial) or Type 2 (genital) herpes simplex, whereas herpes zoster occurs as a single episode in an older man with a history of chicken pox (22,24). Acute herpes simplex is associated with mild symptoms, few lesion sites, and limited dermatome spread, with postherpetic neuralgia uncommon; acute herpes zoster usually has severe symptoms, many lesion sites, and extensive dermatomal spread, with postherpetic neuralgia a common sequela.

Mechanism of Nociception

Activation of nociceptive primary afferents by direct viral attack and secondary inflammatory changes in skin, peripheral nerve, posterior root ganglion, nerve roots, leptomeninges, and the spinal cord may explain the pain in acute herpes zoster. Postherpetic neuralgia may involve both peripheral and central mechanisms. Impairment of segmental pain-modulating systems may play a role, with diminished large-fiber function allowing increased transmission of nociceptive information through the dorsal horn of the spinal cord. Dysesthetic pain in peripheral nerve lesions may also be due to damaged or regenerating nociceptive afferent fibers whereas aching or stabbing pain may relate to activation of nociceptive nervi nervorum (25). Such central mechanisms may explain why proximal ablative procedures usually fail to provide sustained pain relief.

POSTHERPETIC NEURALGIA

Postherpetic neuralgia is a sequelae of acute herpes zoster. Although spontaneous resolution of herpes zoster may be expected in most patients, a significant number of older patients experience intractable pain. Postherpetic neuralgia has been variably defined as pain persisting beyond the crusting of lesions or beyond 4 weeks, 6 weeks, 2 months, or 6 months. Postherpetic neuralgia occurs in about 10% of patients over 40 years of age and 20% to 50% of patients over 60 years of age. Some young patients may experience postherpetic neuralgia for 1 or 2 weeks after the herpes zoster lesions heal, although hypoesthesia or hyperesthesia may persist.

Postherpetic neuralgia is one of the most difficult problems encountered by physicians. Few other conditions create such agonizing pain and suffering for the patient. Many of these patients consider suicide as a means of relief from the debilitating pain.

Clinical Manifestation

Patients with postherpetic neuralgia complain of unrelenting pain typically associated with depressed affect and vegetative signs, such as sleep disturbances, anorexia, lassitude, constipation, and diminished libido. The pain is often qualitatively similar to that of herpes zoster neuralgia, with some combination of burning, aching, or itching, accompanied by severe paroxysms of stabbing or burning pain. Many patients describe allodynia superimposed on the continuous component of the pain.

Marmikko and Bowsher assessed somatic sensory perception thresholds (warm, cold, hot pain, touch, pinprick, vibration, two-point discrimination), allodynia, and skin temperature in the effected area of 42 patients with unilateral postherpetic neuralgia and 20 patients who have had unilateral shingles not followed by postherpetic neuralgia and compared it to the mirror image on the other side (26). There was no difference between the two groups for age or length of time after the acute herpes zoster infection. The postherpetic neuralgia group showed significant changes in all sensory threshold measurements when the affected area was compared with the mirror-image area on the unaffected side, while the group without postherpetic neuralgia exhibited no threshold changes. The mechanical allodynia was present in 87% of the postherpetic neuralgia group. No differences in skin temperature were recorded. Their findings show a deficit of sensory functions mediated by both large and small primary afferent fibers and also suggest major central involvement in the pathophysiology of the condition.

MANAGEMENT

Pharmacological

Acute Herpes Zoster

The goals of treatment are early resolution of the acute disease and prevention of postherpetic neuralgia. The earlier the institution of treatment, the less likely the development of postherpetic neuralgia (27). Pain should be treated aggressively, especially in elderly patients and immunosuppressed patients, who are prone to postherpetic neuralgia (28,29). After postherpetic neuralgia is established, there is no reliable treatment for this syndrome. Unfortunately, no treatment regimen is fully effective; this has led to many different treatments with varying success rates.

Some physicians do not treat acute herpes zoster because they believe it will resolve spontaneously if left alone. They institute treatment only if postherpetic neuralgia develops. This is a great disservice to the group of patients with intractable pain from postherpetic neuralgia. Treatment during the early stages of acute herpes zoster is the best means of preventing needless pain and suffering (30,31).

There is no available treatment that is effective in all cases. Success is usually limited with any method. Many methods of management have been tried for acute herpes zoster and postherpetic neuralgia.

Postherpetic Neuralgia

A threefold purpose governs the role of drug therapy in the patient with postherpetic neuralgia: (1) to provide analgesia for pain, (2) to reduce depression and anxiety, and (3) to decrease insomnia. Because a considerable degree of depression, anxiety, and insomnia accompany all chronic pain syndromes, hypnotics, tranquilizers, antidepressants, and anticonvulsants frequently have been used as analgesic adjuvants in the management of postherpetic neuralgia. These include the barbiturates, Rauwolfia alkaloids, phenothiazine derivatives, benzodiazepines, amphetamines, tricyclic antidepressants, phenytoin, and carbamazepine.

It is important to warn the patient of the potential side effects of any drug. Patients are less likely to stop taking the prescribed medication if they know that certain unpleasant effects are expected as a normal occurrence and that they usually are not permanent.

However, it is equally important for the physician to adopt a positive approach regarding the medication. On average, 35% of patients benefit significantly from the placebo effect. This can be used to advantage by describing enthusiastically the desirable effects of each drug, which, with time, may be obtained in some patients. They also are less likely to stop taking their medication before it has had time to provide the desired effect.

Specific Drug Therapy

Antiviral Agents

Acute Herpes Zoster   Antiviral agents are now standard therapy for acute herpes zoster. The herpes zoster virus, like all viruses, is a parasite that takes over healthy cells and uses their DNA to reproduce itself. It is believed that, if viral DNA synthesis can be slowed or inhibited, then specific host immune systems might have more time to help control the viral infection. Some substances that grossly inhibit DNA synthesis were developed as possible anticancer drugs and have been found to have a more significant antiviral than anticancer activity. Theoretically, these agents could either kill the virus or alter its replication. To be effective, the agents must be given before significant tissue damage occurs. Such agents include acyclovir, cytarabine, vidarabine, idoxuridine, sorivudine, famciclovir, valacyclovir, and brivudine.

Experimental trials using systemic administration of cytarabine in various dose schedules gave conflicting results, ranging from apparent success in early, uncontrolled studies to no benefit or apparent worsening of infection in controlled trials. Controlled studies of vidarabine in the treatment of herpes zoster in immunosuppressed patients have been promising. Therapy was most successful when administered early to patients younger than age 38 or to those with reticuloendothelial malignancy. Cutaneous healing was accelerated, pain was relieved acutely, and the incidence of postherpetic neuralgia was low.

Acyclovir masquerades as one of the building blocks of the DNA needed by the herpes virus to reproduce itself. This stops the chain, and the virus ceases to replicate. Although acyclovir accelerates cutaneous changes in herpes zoster, the intensity and duration of acute herpetic neu-

ralgia appear to be directly related to time of therapy initiation (not later than 6 days after onset) (30). The author of a metaanalysis of 30 clinical trials in immunocompetent patients found five homogeneous, randomized, placebo-controlled trials that showed oral acyclovir 800 mg/day within 72 hours of rash onset may reduce the incidence of residual pain at 6 months by 46% (31). However, at an estimated cost of from $250 to $300 for 7 days' treatment with oral acyclovir, use of this antiviral may not be economically justified in immunocompetent younger patients, especially in developing countries (32).

Some ophthalmologists have used idoxuridine for treating herpetic lesions of the conjunctiva and cornea. Prompt treatment is necessary, and best results are obtained when used within 4 or 5 days of the onset of infection. This drug's effects are variable, and it will not prevent postherpetic neuralgia. Varying concentrations of idoxuridine in dimethyl sulfoxide have been used in New Zealand to treat patients with herpes zoster, and it has been shown that pain decreased faster and that fewer vesicles developed after topical applications. Early initiation of treatment is necessary. Similar positive results have been reported from Denmark. Idoxuridine in dimethyl sulfoxide 35% to 40% has been used in Great Britain on herpes zoster skin lesions. It is reported that there is faster healing of lesions, there is a shorter duration of postherpetic neuralgia, and late sequelae are uncommon. Success depends on early institution of treatment. The solvent decreases inflammation and edema and has a bacteriostatic action. It is an extremely strong solvent that has not been approved by the Food and Drug Administration for this use. Thymidine analogues have been found to have some inhibitory effect on certain strains of varicella zoster virus.

Newer Viral Agents
Although acyclovir has been shown to be effective in shortening the duration of zoster pain, other newer agents may offer some advantages. Sorivudine has compared favorably with acyclovir in terms of accelerating cutaneous healing (33) and preventing recurrences and new episodes (34). Valacyclovir may be more efficacious than acyclovir in shortening time to complete resolution of herpes zoster-associated pain (35,36) and appears to offer cost benefits (37). Famciclovir has been shown to be efficacious in treating herpes zoster (38–40). It has also been shown to accelerate healing of genital herpes in humans (41–43), in preventing further outbreaks of genital herpes (unpublished data on file, SmithKline Beecham, 1998, Philadelphia) in humans, and in preventing HSV-1 latency in mice (44–46). Famciclovir may be more effective than acyclovir in prevention of latency for genital herpes (47,48). Intravenous foscarnet is the current treatment of choice for acyclovir resistant zoster (49,50).

Other Anti Zoster Agents
Interferon, which is produced by the body's immune system, appears to play a role in the control of disease. It seems to work more effectively in tandem

with other components of the body's immune system. Large doses, however, can cause adverse effects. It has been reported that interferon production in the vesicle fluid of patients with disseminated herpes zoster is delayed in comparison with that of patients with localized disease. When human leukocyte interferon has been administered, it has been shown to increase circulating interferon. It may, therefore, be used in cases where there might be a risk of herpetic dissemination.

Zoster immune globulin is not effective in altering the clinical course of herpes zoster in immunocompromised adults. It is used currently, however, for the passive protection of susceptible leukemia patients who have been exposed to chickenpox. It also is recommended for use in immunocompromised children at risk from chicken pox.

Adenosine monophosphate given intramuscularly also has been used in the treatment of acute herpes zoster. The exact mechanism by which it provides certain therapeutic benefits is not understood. It may correct underlying biochemical imbalances or defects at the cellular level. Beneficial effects also may occur as a result of the vasodilating effect of the drug and its ability to decrease tissue edema and inflammation.

One can speculate that the ultimate answer to the problem of herpes zoster and its sequela, postherpetic neuralgia, lies in the field of antiviral therapy. An antiviral agent is needed to kill the virus safely and reliably before there is neurologic damage. Investigation is still needed to find the most effective antiviral agents against the varicella-zoster virus.

Postherpetic Neuralgia   As a rule, antiviral agents are inappropriate in the treatment of postherpetic neuralgia. An exception may include their use to prevent the possible recurrence of herpes zoster infection in a susceptible patient. For example, the patient with Hodgkin's disease is predisposed to recurrent herpes zoster; antiviral agents may be given before treatment of the primary disease (chemotherapy and radiation therapy) when reactivation of the virus is most likely.

Analgesics

Acute Herpes Zoster   Analgesics are an important adjunctive therapy for acute herpes zoster. They may be categorized as nonaddictive, moderately addictive, or strongly addictive agents. Selecting the optimal agent for a specific patient involves consideration of various factors, the most important of which are quality, intensity, duration, and distribution of pain.

Nonnarcotic, nonaddictive drugs are used for the control of mild pain. Oral aspirin and acetaminophen are effective drugs with a low incidence of side effects. However, they are not effective in controlling severe pain. Evidence suggests that topical application of acetylsalicylic acid markedly reduces the spread of infection and produces an analgesic effect (51,52).

Codeine, propoxyphene, pentazocine, and oxycodone are examples of moderately addicting drugs. The incidence of addiction is relatively low, but dependence may occur with these agents. They are good analgesic agents, but they sometimes produce adverse side effects such as constipation.

When used properly, the strongly addictive narcotics are effective in the treatment of severe pain, providing relief to varying degrees. In acute herpes zoster, strong medication may be needed to control severe pain. Because the acute stage is short, strongly addictive drugs may be used for a limited period. In such cases, the narcotic is tapered off as treatment decreases the degree of pain. When pain is at a level that can be controlled by nonnarcotic drugs, the narcotics should be discontinued. Examples of strongly addictive drugs are morphine, hydromorphone, and meperidine.

Postherpetic Neuralgia   Narcotics may be required to control the severe intractable pain of postherpetic neuralgia. They should be used with extreme caution, however. Postherpetic neuralgia patients usually are not terminally ill. The side effects such as nausea, loss of appetite, and constipation usually make these patients miserable. There may be adverse drug interactions with antidepressants and other drugs. Adequate pain relief may be obtained with other drugs. The temporary initial use of narcotics to relieve extreme pain may be necessary; however, they should be tapered off as soon as possible.

Antiinflammatory Agents   The effects of corticosteroid therapy in acute herpes zoster are still unclear, but reports are encouraging. Results of recent, limited studies suggest that corticosteroids such as prednisone are well tolerated and may significantly reduce the duration of acute neuralgia and improve quality of life; however, they have not been shown to be efficacious in preventing postherpetic neuralgia (53). Inflammation and scarring are reduced with antiinflammatory agents. Despite the uncertain effects of corticosteroid therapy on herpes zoster, these drugs have been used extensively to treat this infection.

The role of antiinflammatory drugs in acute herpes zoster is controversial. If host responses contribute significantly to tissue injury, then attenuation of these responses may be beneficial. Unfortunately, the host defenses that cause tissue injury may be inseparable from those that eliminate or prevent the spread of infection. Currently, dissociation of protective from harmful host responses to the virus has not been demonstrated clearly. However, in the immunocompetent individual, a vigorous antiviral response is altered only very mildly by corticosteroids. Similarly, in the presence of potent antiviral therapy, even in the immunosuppressed patient, a reduction in the inflammatory response eventually may be safe and have a salutary effect. These are important issues for future investigation.

Oral antiinflammatory drugs usually are administered in the first 10 days and continued for as long as 3 weeks. Prednisone is usually the agent of choice. It may be given orally in doses of 60 mg/day the first week, 30 mg/day the second week, and 15 mg/day the third week.

Corticosteroids also have been administered by subcutaneous injection under affected skin, with and without a local anesthetic. Enthusiastic anecdotal reports of large numbers of patients claim 80% to 100% success in treating acute herpes zoster, with a rapid resolution of pain and diminished incidence of postherpetic neuralgia. The experience of others has been less enthusiastic. Corticosteroids administered with nerve blocks will be discussed below. There is no indication for antiinflammatory agents in postherpetic neuralgia.

Antidepressants and Tranquilizers

Acute Herpes Zoster   Major depression has been associated with a marked decline in varicella zoster virus-specific cellular immunity. Antidepressants have two actions: they can relieve pain, and they can relieve depression. Tricyclic drugs are known to block serotonin reuptake. Therefore, they would be expected to enhance the action of this neurotransmitter at synapses, and such enhancement can produce analgesia in laboratory animals. One of the mechanisms active in central pain states is some defect in the transmission system in the neuroaxis, specifically, a deficit in serotonin.

There is a strong consensus among clinical investigators that centrally active antidepressants should be tried in any patient who is not obtaining pain relief, whether he or she appears depressed or not. Tricyclics and anxiolytics frequently are given together because, although depression is not common in acute herpes zoster, many patients experience anxiety along with the severe pain. The most widely used combination is amitriptyline and fluphenazine. Amitriptyline alone has been shown to significantly reduce pain in older patients by more than one-half, making a strong argument for its use with an antiviral in this group of patients (54).

In addition to their antidepressant and analgesic properties, tricyclics are also sedatives. Amitriptyline and doxepin may correct the sleep disturbance, frequent awakening, and early morning awakening that are common in severe chronic pain states. Adverse side effects of tricyclic antidepressants include hypo- or hypertension, tachycardia, arrhythmias, drowsiness, confusion, disorientation, dry mouth, blurred vision, increased intraocular pressure, urinary retention, and constipation.

Postherpetic Neuralgia   Antidepressants and tranquilizers frequently are used in conjunction with analgesics. Some patients become depressed as a reaction to their pain. The signs of depression may be so subtle that they are easily missed. As many as 90% of patients seen may be depressed. Approximately 85% of these patients will respond to antidepressant drugs.

Tricyclic antidepressants are the most commonly used drugs, and they are the most effective single drug class used in the management of postherpetic neuralgia. Antidepressants may act at a higher level than the neurotransmitters, perhaps on pressure molecules in the hypothalamus or pituitary. This could explain why only some depressed patients fit the catecholamine hypothesis (that is, a deficit of serotonin or norepinephrine is the cause of the problem). Both chronic pain and depression may represent neurotransmitter deficiencies, and the antidepressants may restore these to normal levels. These drugs should be given in appropriate doses, and several should be tried before concluding that there is no response.

Topical application of a local anesthetic plus a tricyclic antidepressant can be effective (28,29). Tricyclics and anxiolytics commonly are given together because many patients have anxiety with their depression. This feeling may be caused by anticipation of painful spasms, social obligations that may exacerbate the pain by increasing stress, fear of having a painful episode in public, or fear that the pain may never leave. Many patients who did not obtain relief with tricyclics alone may benefit when a phenothiazine is added. For lasting pain relief, treatment must be continued throughout life. Amitriptyline 50 to 75 mg/day and fluphenazine 1 mg three or four times a day is the usual recommended dose. As a last resort, immediate relief has been obtained in some hospitalized patients who had not responded to any other therapy with a short course of high-dose chlorprothixene 50 mg every 6 hours for 5 days. Because this requires hospitalization and is associated with adverse effects, this treatment is recommended only if all other methods fail and if the pain is severe, because pain often returns in a few weeks or months.

Anticonvulsants, Topical Agents, and Antiarrhythmic Agents

Acute Herpes Zoster   Anticonvulsant agents and antiarrhythmic agents are not usually prescribed for acute herpes zoster.

Postherpetic Neuralgia   Anticonvulsants sometimes are useful when other medications have failed. Phenytoin 100 mg three to four times a day or carbamazepine 500 to 1000 mg daily in three to four divided doses can be used to relieve sharp pain.

Sodium valproate 200 mg twice a day and amitriptyline 10 to 25 mg twice a day have been successful. If the stabbing component of pain continues, the dose of amitriptyline can be increased. The dull-ache component of the pain is most resistant to therapy. If it persists, the scar can be infiltrated with a local anesthetic and corticosteroids, or TENS can be started.

Gabapentin has been shown to effectively reduce pain and sleep interference and improve mood and quality of life in patients with postherpetic neuralgia and in patients with painful neuropathy (55,56). Maximum dosage administered was 3600 mg/day.

The side effects of anticonvulsants tend to limit their use. These include bone marrow depression, ataxia, diplopia, nystagmus, abnormal liver function tests, nausea, lymphadenopathy, confusion, and vertigo. Capsaicin has been used for patients with postherpetic neuralgia with unreliable results. This drug depletes substance P from sensory nerve endings in the skin and has been used topically for various dermatologic diseases.

Intravenous lidocaine has been advocated for the treatment of many types of chronic neurogenic pain, including postherpetic neuralgia. The oral antiarrhythmics (such as mexiletine) have been tried, and reports are encouraging. However, definitive studies on the efficacy of oral antiarrhythmics for the treatment of postherpetic neuralgia are lacking.

Nerve Blocks

Acute Herpes Zoster

Local Infiltration   In a large group of patients, subcutaneous injections of triamcinolone 0.2% in normal saline have been administered under areas of eruption and sites of pain and itching with excellent results and reduction of postherpetic neuralgia. Subcutaneous injections of corticosteroids and local anesthetics offer an effective treatment for acute herpes zoster. The procedure is not associated with any significant complications, the technique is simple and inexpensive, and the response to treatment is fairly predictable (Fig 35-4).

Somatic Nerve Blocks   Because nerve root involvement is suspected in acute herpes zoster, somatic nerve blocks have been used in its treatment. These can include brachial plexus, paravertebral, intercostal, and sciatic blocks. They are of limited value in the acute phase and of no value in the postherpetic stage.

Sympathetic Nerve Blocks   As an understanding of the pathology of herpes zoster developed, attention was directed toward the sympathetic ganglia. Sympathetic blocks have been done to relieve the vasospasm that was thought to cause the pain and nerve damage. Evidence suggests that sympathetic blockade during the acute phase of herpes zoster can help the immediate pain problem, often dramatically. Of greater value, however, is the possibility that it can prevent the development of postherpetic neuralgia. Although the evidence for this is less compelling, it is probably a worthwhile prophylactic measure that should be used as early as possible.

Trigeminal herpes zoster has been treated with a bupivacaine block of the ipsilateral stellate ganglion. Just one block often proves effective. However, success depends on administration within the first 2 or 3 weeks after onset of the outbreak. The incidence of success decreases thereafter. This therapy also apparently prevents lesions from progressing into the postherpetic syndrome, at least in younger patients.

Central Blocks   Epidural blocks using local anesthetic have been successful in acute herpes zoster. The duration of the infection is shorter, the lesions dry faster, and the pain is relieved. Spinal blocks usually are not indicated because they are not as specific as epidural blocks. A patient who has had a laminectomy in the affected area would be an exception to this general rule. The use of lumbar plexus blockade has been reported in relieving pain in an elderly patient for whom other approaches were contraindicated (55).

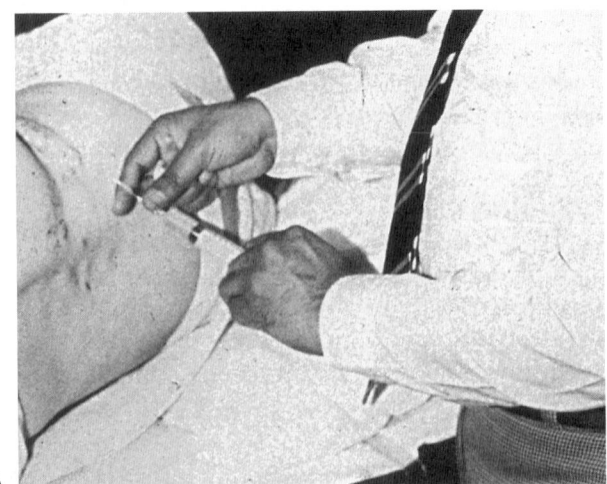 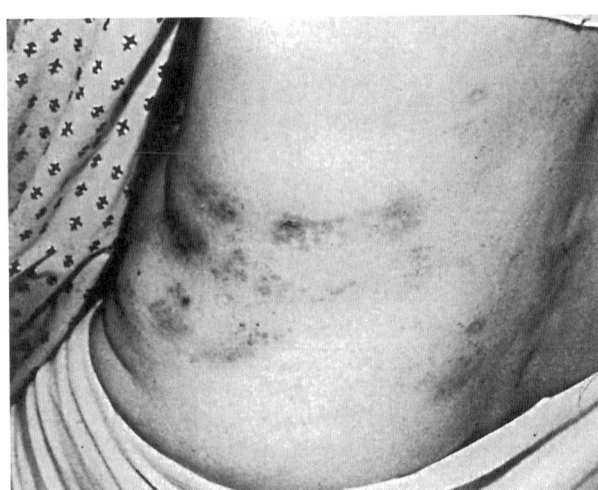

A   B

FIG. 35-4. A. Intracutaneous infiltration of Decadron with 0.125% bupivacaine in the vesicles of the acute herpes zoster, which are 3 weeks old. **B.** Four days after intracutaneous infiltration of Decadron and bupivacaine treatment of the patient shown in (A). Note bruising due to needle penetration, as well as flattening of vesicles and acceleration of healing.

Neurolytic Blocks Neurolytic blocks are not indicated in acute herpes zoster.

Postherpetic Neuralgia

The pathogenesis of postherpetic pain is unknown. Autopsy studies have shown that the entire sensory pathway, including the brain and sympathetic ganglia, may be involved. There appear to be multiple areas along this pathway that can initiate pain. This provides a rationale for the various methods of treatment and an explanation of treatment failures.

Analgesic blocks can be used as prognostic, therapeutic, and prophylactic tools in managing pain. As prognostic tools, blocks help predict the effects of prolonged interruption of nerve pathways achieved through injection of neurolytic agents or surgery. By interrupting pain pathways, therapeutic blocks influence the autonomic response to noxious stimulation. They break the cycle of this disease. Patients with severe intractable pain who are not suited to other treatment regimens may be relieved by blocks with neurolytic agents.

Local Infiltration Subcutaneous infiltration of corticosteroids has been used; pain relief was obtained in approximately 64% of patients. A 0.2% solution of triamcinolone in normal saline was injected daily under all areas of pain, burning, or itching until the desired effect was obtained. Maximum benefit was achieved in the first 12 treatments. In a comparison study, subcutaneous infiltration of bupivacaine 0.25% and triamcinolone 0.2% was used alone or in conjunction with systemic medication and sympathetic blockade. Overall results showed moderate-to-significant improvement in 70% of patients. A difference in response to treatment was noticed in relation to duration of symptoms; patients with symptoms for less than 1 year responded better (85% success) than patients with symptoms for greater than 1 year (55%).

Subcutaneous infiltration of corticosteroids can offer an effective treatment for postherpetic neuralgia. No significant complications have been recorded; the technique is simple and inexpensive; and the response to treatment is fairly predictable. Most importantly, it offers relief for some patients with postherpetic neuralgia of many months' duration.

The total number of such treatments ranges from 1 to 10 (average, 4 to 6 injections). In acute herpes zoster, treatments are usually given two or three times weekly and tapered to one per week, if the patient is responding well.

Somatic Nerve Block Nerve root involvement is an obvious characteristic of postherpetic neuralgia, and sensory nerve blocks were used in early attempts to relieve its pain. The results were limited, depending primarily on the duration of the blocks, although there were some reports of success in managing pain in the early stages of the disease. Coincidental spontaneous resolution may have been responsible. Nerve blocks are primarily used in postherpetic neuralgia for diagnosis and prognosis, especially as a prognostic block before neurolytic block. Corticosteroids injected around the dorsal nerve have had unpredictable and limited success.

Sympathetic Nerve Block Sympathetic blocks are sometimes helpful in alleviating pain, although results are sometimes temporary and may only be obtainable in patients with neuralgia of less than 2 months' duration. Sympathetic blocks of the stellate ganglion and trigeminal branch blocks are often used to treat trigeminal zoster.

Central Blocks Epidural corticosteroid administration has been successful in treating various lumbosacral conditions. For instance, epidural nerve blocks are often used to treat zoster in the fifth cervical dermatome. For patients with postherpetic neuralgia, the pain relief is only temporary. Spinal blocks are not indicated for these patients.

Neurolytic Block Neurolytic blocks may be considered in patients with posterpetic neuralgia when other blocks have not given the patient significant relief. They should only be done after a prognostic block has shown that an effective block of the appropriate area can be achieved. Neurolytic agents are used in cases of prolonged destruction of nerves. These blocks include ethyl alcohol 50% in aqueous solution, absolute alcohol 95% in aqueous solution, and phenol 6%. Ethyl alcohol causes a higher incidence of neuritis than phenol. This is primarily a result of incomplete peripheral nerve block after inaccurate needle placement or spillage of the agent on somatic nerve fibers. The duration of effects may vary from days to years, but usually it ranges from 2 to 6 months (Fig. 35-5).

Ammonium compounds also can be used for peripheral nerve block. Pain relief follows selective destruction of unmyelinated C fibers by the ammonium ion. A solution of ammonium sulfate 10% in lidocaine 1% or ammonium chloride 15% is used. The duration of action ranges from 4 to 24 weeks.

Neuritis does not occur with either ammonium sulfate or chloride. The most annoying side effect is numbness, which can be as bad as the pain for some patients.

Cryoanalgesia also has been used as a means of producing long-term neural blocks with unpredictable results.

Complications that may result from any nerve block procedure include pain, local hemorrhage, infection, needle soreness, sterile abscess (usually in the immunosuppressed patient), vertigo, and Cushing's syndrome.

Psychological Interventions

Acute Herpes Zoster

Because the acute phase of herpes zoster is short, psychological interventions are not mandatory. However, some patients (especially those with severe anxiety and fear) benefit from a support program. Some studies show that

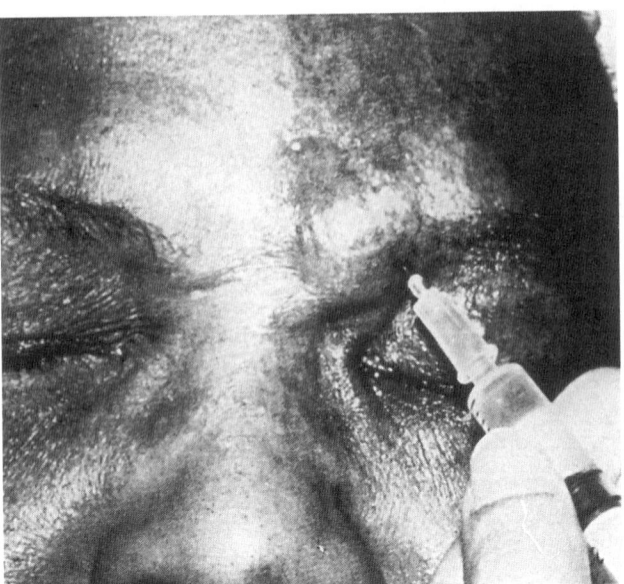

FIG. 35-5. Supraorbital neurolytic block (6% phenol) in a 75-year-old woman suffering from postherpetic neuralgia.

interventions such as psychotherapy can also positively affect certain components of the immune response (56–58). A regimen consisting of psychological support, administration of antiviral agents, and patient education has been described by one author as the best available option for the management of herpes virus infections (59).

Postherpetic Neuralgia

It is especially important in patients with postherpetic neuralgia to treat the whole patient and not just an area of the skin. The emotional stability of the patient almost always is affected, and the stresses involved for the patient and all members of the household require thoughtful management.

Severe depression is seen in more than 50% of these patients, and as previously noted, suicide commonly is considered by those with long-term intractable pain. Counseling by a psychologist or clinical social worker who is experienced in pain management is a valuable adjunct to drug therapy. Training the patient in stress management and relaxation techniques is important. Anxiety and stress can exacerbate and prolong the pain. By practicing these techniques, the patient may be able to control pain to some degree.

In some patients, the pain-tension-anxiety cycle can convert acute pain symptoms into a chronic condition. Often, no matter what is done to treat these patients, the pain is not relieved unless the stress factors are also removed. Basically, two types of persons are susceptible to chronicity: the tense, hard-driving, conscientious perfectionist and the dependent individual unable to cope with life but burdened with repressed anger and hostility. Reinforcement of the patient's response to pain (such as moaning, grimacing, asking for medication, and remaining in bed) or favorable conse-

quences of the pain (such as attention and expressions of sympathy, perhaps also the occasion to manipulate others) may lead to chronic behavior which, eventually, is independent of the original underlying pathologic condition.

The most important guideline in preventing chronicity is complete honesty. Make patients aware of the relationship between the psyche and pain and relieve them of the fear of organic disease. After the patient fully accepts the emotional causes of pain, he or she can learn to relieve the pain by controlling anxiety and tension.

Family and friends should be included in counseling sessions. They, too, must cope with the pain a loved one is experiencing. The counselor not only can ease their anxiety but also can teach them how to provide effective emotional support to help the patient endure an extremely difficult period. Concentrating on the special needs of families may require extra effort on the part of the staff, but it should result in a greater number of patients who recover with the physical and emotional well-being of the family intact.

Many patients are elderly and live alone. They are unable to turn to family and friends to provide the assistance they need for routine daily tasks. The counselor should contact appropriate social service agencies to provide transportation and other necessities (such as prepared meals, grocery shopping, housework, and regular contact with the patient to check on his or her well being).

Other Therapeutic Options

Acute Herpes Zoster

Usually, TENS is not used in the treatment of acute herpes zoster. However, results of a preliminary, randomized, single-blind study suggest that a new form of percutaneous electrical nerve stimulation may be useful in treating acute herpes zoster lesions (60). Ice therapy is a counterirritation technique based on the gate control theory. It is sometimes used alone in the acute stage to cool the area. Acupuncture and hypnosis usually are not used in acute herpes zoster because other conventional methods are more appropriate. Surgery and neurosurgery are not indicated. The acute stage is self-limited and does not require such drastic measures. Autohemotherapy has been shown to be effective in eliminating clinical sequelae of herpes zoster, but this alternative method requires further investigation (61).

Postherpetic Neuralgia

Because many patients continue to have some residual pain of varying degrees that can be aggravating, they may require management with other techniques (62). The following techniques are used when all others fail (Table 35-5).

1. TENS: This has been used in an attempt to relieve the intractable pain of postherpetic neuralgia. Although the success rate is low, relief can be sufficient to permit a return to normal activity without analgesic therapy.

TABLE 35-5. *Therapeutic strategy for acute herpes zoster*

		Treatment		
Type of patient	Age (years)	Antiviral	Antiinflammatory	Pain relief
Young immuno-competent	<50	–	–	Sympathetic block
Old immuno-competent	>50	–	+	Epidural, somatic and/or sympathetic block—infiltration block helpful
Young immuno-suppressed	<50	++ Within 72 hours	-	Systemic narcotics
Old immuno-suppressed	>50	+ Within 72hours	+	Nerve blocks + systemic oral analgesics Adjuvant oral analgesics

–, not required; +, useful; ++, necessary

(From Raj P. Pain due to herpes zoster. In: Raj P, ed. *Practical management of pain,* 2nd ed. Chicago: Mosby-Year Book, 1992, with permission.)

2. Ice and other cold therapies: Ice is applied to the skin for 2 to 3 minutes several times a day, starting with the least sensitive area and approaching the most sensitive area. A vibrator is then used in the same manner in conjunction with psychotropic drugs. Ethyl chloride, or other cold sprays, can be used alone as treatment. Fluid is sprayed over the entire painful area, beginning at the upper area and working down. Evaporation cools the area. The procedure is repeated twice at 1-minute intervals until the skin is thoroughly cooled. When beneficial, these treatments will relieve pain for varying lengths of time. When the pain returns to near its former intensity, the treatment can be repeated. If the patient responds satisfactorily, the pain is relieved by two or three sets of sprays per day. Good-to-excellent pain relief has been maintained in patients with refractory postherpetic pain using cryocautery with a stick of solid carbon dioxide (dry ice) applied directly to the hyperesthetic sites.

3. Acupuncture: Significant pain relief has been obtained in patients with postherpetic neuralgia treated with acupuncture. Further investigation is warranted (Fig. 35-6).

4. Hypnosis: Hypnosis acts at the level of the cerebral cortex. Impulses are sent down from higher centers to close the neurophysiologic gate that controls pain. Pain relief through hypnosis is sometimes complete but, more often, it is not. Hypnotism is reported to be helpful in patients with chronic unbearable pain; this changes to bearable discomfort by breaking up patterns of suffering.

5. Dimethyl sulfoxide: The treatment value of this agent in postherpetic neuralgia is unknown. It may be tried as a benign last resort. Only a few states have approved this solvent for medical use.

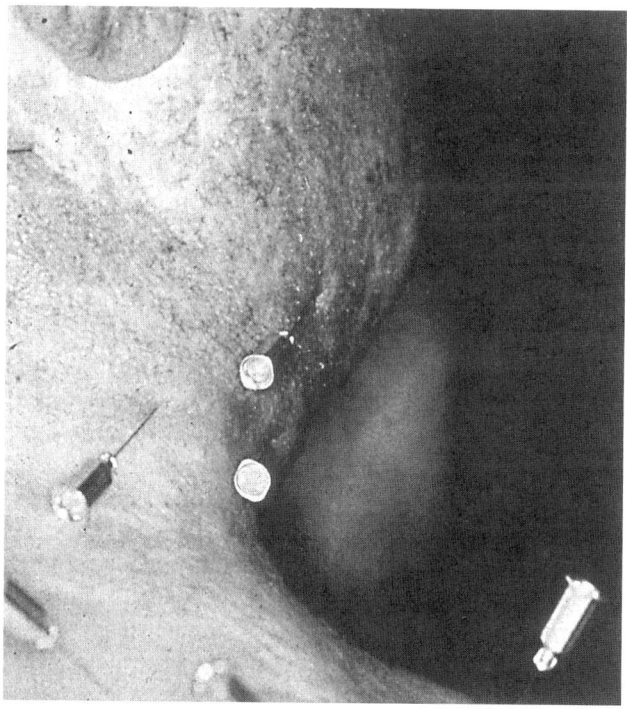

FIG. 35-6. In a patient with postherpetic neuralgia, acupuncture in progress for pain relief.

Surgery and Neurosurgery

Surgery is the last resort for the treatment of severe intractable postherpetic pain. It is not always successful. More effective management techniques learned in recent years have limited this option further.

Surgery usually attacks the pain pathway in stages at progressively higher divisions. Because it was suspected that the origin of the pain lay in the scar and peripheral receptors, wide excision and skin grafting were tried. This was not found to be effective and is rarely used today.

Radiofrequency lesions (rhizotomy) of the somatic afferents and sensory root ganglia has also had poor results. Investigators who have had some success recommended that ablation include several segments above and below the affected area. Sympathectomy has not been successful in treating postherpetic neuralgia.

Cordotomy has been used with good results. In most cases, however, the pain returns. Early recurrence has been blamed on failure to ablate all the nerves in the pathway, which resume function after the swelling has decreased. Stereotactic ablation of the conducting paths in the thalamus and mesencephalon and frontal lobotomy have been used. These should only be tried in patients with short life expectancies who have not had success with any other methods.

Because of the finality of surgery and the unpredictable results, many surgeons in recent years have taken advantage of technologic advances in other areas to replace destructive procedures. These include dorsal column stimulators used to block transmission of nerve impulses. An implantable electrode placed over the dorsal columns of the spinal cord has been tried with some success. Deep brain stimulators, which are patient activated, have been applied to the mesencephalic medial lemniscus to block the pain-conducting systems and stimulate endorphin secretion, the body's natural pain reliever. Good pain relief has been achieved in many patients.

THERAPEUTIC STRATEGY FOR PATIENTS SUFFERING FROM HERPES ZOSTER

It is useful to categorize affected patients according to their immune status and age (Table 35-6). This allows the clinician to direct efforts toward all antiviral, antiinflammatory, or antinociceptive effects, based on the probability of success and risk factors involved. These patients can be categorized into four groups: (1) immunocompetent young, (2) immunocompetent older, (3) immunosuppressed young, and (4) immunosuppressed older patients.

TABLE 35-6. *Complications*

Neuralgia
Facial or oculomotor palsy
Paralysis of motor nerves
Myelitis
Meningoencephalitis
Postherpetic neuralgia
Systemic toxicity or dissemination
Fevers
Chills
Bacteria sepsis
Varicella pneumonia

Immunocompetent Young Patients

Patients in this group have no defined underlying illness, are younger than 50 years of age, and have normal immunologic responsiveness. Although they have acute herpes zoster, their reaction to the infection is brisk, enabling them to confine the rash in the initial unit. Likewise, postherpetic neuralgia does not occur. The acute morbidity is low, and healing is rapid. The rationale for treatment of this group of patients is to relieve their intolerable pain and prevent inflammatory damage of the tissues. Antiviral agents administered during the first 72 hours may be helpful in stopping the replication of the virus and spreading the infection to the peripheral nerves. Antiinflammatory agents (corticosteroids administered locally or systematically) are useful in decreasing tissue damage and keeping the inflammatory reaction of the host to a minimum. The obligatory treatment is to decrease the severe pain of neuralgia. This is best done using sympathetic or epidural blocks in the first 3 to 4 weeks of onset of infection. Antidepressant agents also are helpful as adjuvant agents.

Immunocompetent Older Patients

The major objective of therapy in this group is to prevent postherpetic neuralgia. Although suffering no underlying disease, the response to varicella-zoster virus in this group may be less vigorous than in young patients, leading to a slower viral clearance and perhaps a higher incidence of spread beyond the initial unit of infection. Nonetheless, nervous system and visceral complications are still infrequent and, by themselves, probably do not warrant the use of potentially toxic therapy at this time. However, both antiviral and antiinflammatory therapies may be valuable in preventing postherpetic neuralgia. Of these, the latter has been shown prospectively to be effective in this group of patients. It is reasonable on the basis of the current evidence to treat older patients with acute herpes zoster who are immunologically normal with a limited course of corticosteroids (e.g., 60 mg of prednisone or its equivalent daily for 5 days, tapering the dose over the following 2 weeks).

The value of antivirals in this group of patients has not been tested carefully, although one trial suggested no effect in the incidence of persistent pain in patients treated with acyclovir despite an effect on acute pain. This issue deserves careful study. A four-treatment-arm study of the individual and combined effects of antivirals and corticosteroids is needed. At this point, antiviral therapy in this group probably is indicated only in an investigative setting. Pain relief should be addressed in these patients. Conventional narcotics should be avoided because these patients are usually older and frail. In addition, there is a high incidence of postherpetic neuralgia. Nonnarcotic analgesics in association with nerve blocks (epidural and sympathetic blocks or local intracutaneous infiltration with bupivacaine and corticosteroids) are recommended.

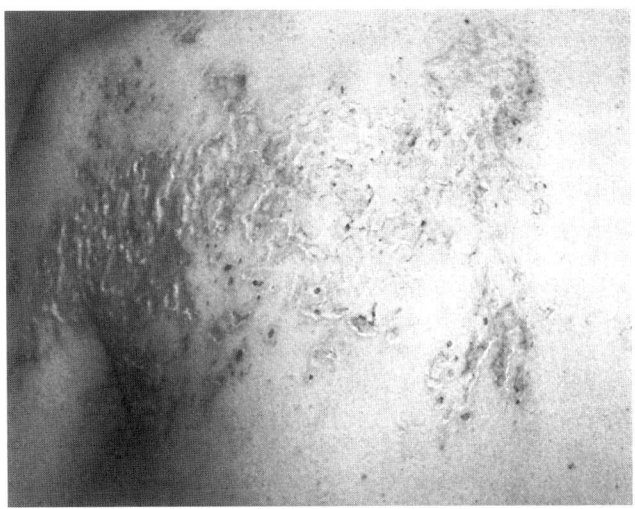

FIG. 35-7. Note the confluence of vesicular response due to herpes zoster in a 30-year-old man suffering from AIDS. These aberrant vesicles can be present at multiple sites and spread with hematogenous dissemination.

Immunosuppressed Young Patients

Our principal concern in immunodeficient younger patients is the spread of the virus in and outside the primary ganglion-nerve-dermatome unit (Fig. 35-7). Postherpetic neuralgia is not a major issue. Therapy, therefore, is directed at confining the viral infection. Currently, acyclovir is available, is of proven efficacy, and can be recommended for patients. It seems reasonable to recommend hospitalization for patients in this group who are at greatest risk of developing complications, particularly those with lymphoproliferative disease or early dissemination. It also must be emphasized that, if therapy is given, every effort should be made to start treatment early. When newer agents become available, they will require similar consideration, with their convenience, cost, and toxicity weighed against the magnitude of their potential benefit. It can be predicted, however, that when other oral drugs are introduced, their efficacy proved, and their toxicity demonstrated to be low, the indications for treatment will expand. The clinical decision to administer these drugs to this group of patients would be an easy one, with virtually all patients in this group routinely receiving such treatment. Pain relief in such patients should be obtained by the techniques that are common for acute pain management.

Immunosuppressed Older Patients

In this group of patients, therapeutic objectives include prevention of both viral spread and postherpetic pain. As discussed previously, antiviral therapy may be helpful in both respects. Acyclovir has been effective in reducing infection, and it may reduce postherpetic pain. The latter requires additional confirmation. More importantly, because of the risk of viral dissemination, patients in this group require

antiviral treatment. However, the use of corticosteroids to prevent postherpetic neuralgia warrants separate comment. In older immunocompetent patients, corticosteroids appear to cause no special risk and to be therapeutically beneficial; but in the immunosuppressed individual, greater caution is required. These patients are more susceptible to viral spread and central nervous system and visceral complications. Corticosteroids may impair their remaining defenses below a critical level, increasing the risk of these complications. Data from a collaborative study suggest that corticosteroids did not protect against postherpetic pain in this group. This issue must be investigated separately, particularly to consider the effects of combined antiviral and steroid therapy. If potent antiviral coverage were available, corticosteroids might be safe. Pain relief is best provided by nerve blocks.

COMPLICATIONS

Acute Herpes Zoster

The most common complications of acute herpes zoster usually appear after eruption of the rash (Table 35-6). They include neuralgia, facial or oculomotor palsy, paralysis of motor nerves, and myelitis. Meningoencephalitis, which has its onset either during or 2 to 4 days after the rash appears, can also be a complication. Postherpetic neuralgia seems to occur more frequently and is more protracted in immunosuppressed patients, especially in Hodgkin's disease or other lymphomas.

There is a marked increase in the incidence of infection in the immunosuppressed or older immunoincompetent patient. The clinical course in these patients is exaggerated. It is acutely disabling in many cases, and it may become life threatening if visceral involvement occurs with dissemination. In the early stages, the infection often spreads segmentally to involve ipsilateral and, less frequently, contralateral dermatomes. It usually is associated with fever and increasing debilitation. While some of the old lesions are healing, new lesions continue to appear. Many patients have dissemination and visceral involvement that ultimately may be fatal.

Generally, patients in whom the disease remains localized for 4 to 6 days do not experience complications. The greatest morbidity and mortality usually occur with visceral involvement through dissemination, especially in patients older than 40 years of age.

Systemic toxicity, fever, chills, and sometimes secondary bacterial sepsis occur. Varicella pneumonia, which is associated with a high mortality, occurs less frequently.

Postherpetic Neuralgia

Although physical complications occur with acute herpes zoster, the complications from the postherpetic stage are primarily emotional. Depression is common and may include suicidal tendencies. Destruction of the patient's life style (inability to work, break-up of the family, and restricted mobility that prohibits former social activities) may be the tragic human consequences that affect the patient with long-term pain. Physical function may be impaired beyond that seen during the acute stage because of the longer period of immobility.

PROGNOSIS

There is a close relationship between the duration of neuralgia and therapeutic efficacy; prompt treatment shortens the progressive course of the disease and also decreases its severity. There also appears to be a correlation between the age of the patient and the response to therapy. Patients younger than 60 years of age generally respond better to therapy and, even untreated, have a lower incidence of postherpetic neuralgia than older patients. In addition, older patients do not respond as well as young patients to therapy and specifically to sympathetic nerve blocks. For unknown reasons, postherpetic neuralgia lesions in the ophthalmic division of the trigeminal nerve are often the most difficult lesions to treat successfully. The psychological make-up of the individual patient is also important. Lastly, one fifth of patients with neoplasms who have had herpes zoster will have this disease at least once again.

REFERENCES

1. Human RW. Structure and function of the varicella-zoster virus genome. In: Nahmias AJ, Dowde WR, Schinazi RF, eds. *The human herpesviruses: an interdisciplinary perspective.* New York: Elsevier Science Publishing; 1981:27–35.
2. Loeser JD. Review article—Herpes zoster and postherpetic neuralgia. *Pain* 1986;25:149–164.
3. Berger R, Florent G, Just M. Decrease of the lymphoproliferative response to varicella-zoster virus antigen in the aged. *Infecf Immun* 1981;32:24–27.
4. Eaglstein WH, Katz R, Brown JA. The effect of early corticosteroid therapy on skin eruption and pain of herpes zoster. *JAMA* 1970;221:1681–1683.
5. Keczkes K, Basheer AM. Do corticosteroids prevent postherpetic neuralgia? *Br J Dermatol* 1980;102:551–555.
6. Dirbas FM, Swain JA. Disseminated cutaneous herpes zoster following cardiac surgery. *J Cardiovasc Surg* 1990;31:531–532.
7. Schmader K, Studenski S, MacMillan J, et al. Are stressful life events risk factors for herpes zoster? *J Am Geriatr Soc* 1990;38:1188–1194.
8. Arvin AM, Pollard RB, Rasmussen LE, et al. Cellular and humoral immunity in the pathogenesis of recurrent herpes viral infections in patients with lymphoma. *J Clin Invest* 1980;;65:869–878.
9. Gershon AA, Steinberg SP. Antibody responses to varicella-zoster virus and the role of antibody in host defenses. *Am J Med Sci* 1981;282:12–17.
10. Miyagawa Y, Miyazaki M, Inutsuka S, et al. Herpes zoster in patients with sarcoidosis. *Respiration* 1992;59:94–96.
11. Rusthoven JJ, Ahlgren P, Elhakim T, et al. Risk factors for varicella-zoster disseminated infection among adult cancer patients with localized zoster. *Cancer* 1988;62:1641–1646.
12. Atkinson K, Meyers JD, Storb R, et al. Varicella-zoster virus infection after marrow transplantation for aplastic anemia or leukemia. *Transplantation* 1980;29:47–50.
13. Price RW. Herpes zoster: an approach to systemic therapy. *Med Clin North Am* 1982;66:1105–1117.
14. Raj PP. *Practical management of pain,* 2nd ed. St. Louis: Mosby Year Book, 1992:517–545.
15. Chen H-J. Measurement of tissue impedance in dorsal root entry zone surgery for pain after brachial plexus avulsion and herpes zoster. *Clin J Pain* 1991;7:323–329.
16. Steele RW. Immunology of varicella-zoster virus. In: Nahmias AJ, O'Reilly RJ, eds. *Immunology of human infection Part II. Viruses and parasites: immunodiagnosis and prevention of infectious diseases.* New York: Plenum Publishing 1982.
17. Higa K, Kenjiro D, Haruhiko M, et al. Factors influencing the duration of treatment of acute herpetic pain with sympathetic nerve block: importance of severity of herpes zoster assessed by the maximum antibody titers to varicella-zoster virus in other wise healthy patients. *Pain* 1988;32:147–157.
18. Yoshiike T, Aikawa Y, Wonghwaisayawan H, et al. HLA-DR antigen expression on peripheral T-cell subsets in pityriasiorosea and herpes zoster. *Dermatologica* 1991;182:160–163.
19. Zanolli MD, Powell BL, McCalmont T, et al: Granuloma annulare and disseminated herpes zoster. *Int J Dermatol* 1992;31:55–57.
20. Gershon AA, Steinberg SP. Inactivation of varicella zoster virus in vitro: effect of leukocytes and specific antibody. *Infect Immun* 1981;33:507–511.
21. Gershon AA, Steinberg SP, Borkowsky W, et al. IgM to varicella-zoster virus demonstration in patients without clinical zoster. *Pediatr Infect Dis* 1982;1:164–167.
22. Straus SE. Clinical and biological differences between herpes simplex virus and varicella-zoster virus infections. *JAMA* 1989;262:3455–3458.
23. Straus SE, Ostrove JM, Inchauspe G, et al. Varicella-zoster virus infections. *Ann Intern Med* 1988;108:221–237.
24. Ragozzino MJ, Melton LJ III, Kurland LT, et al. Population based study of herpes zoster and its sequelae. *Medicine (Baltimore)* 1982;61:310–316.
25. Watson CPN, Morshead C, Van der Kooy D, et al. Postherpetic neuralgia: post-mortem analysis of a case. *Pain* 1988;34:129–138.
26. Marmikko T, Bowsher D. Somatosensory findings in post-herpetic neuralgia. *J Neurol Neurosurg Psychiatry* 1990;53:135–141.
27. Fields HL, Rowbotham MC. *Pathophysiology of postherpetic neuralgia.* Presented at the Herpes Zoster and Postherpetic Neuralgia Satellite Symposium, Whistler Mountain, British Columbia, August 13 and 14, 1996.
28. Bennett GJ. *Animal models and their relation to neuropathic pain: particularly HZ and PHN.* Presented at the Herpes Zoster and Postherpetic Neuralgia Satellite Symposium, Whistler Mountain, British Columbia, August 13 and 14, 1996.
29. Bennett GJ. Hypotheses on the pathogenesis of herpes zoster-associated pain. *Ann Neurol* 1994;35:538–541.
30. Jovanovic J, Cvjetkovic D, Pobor M, et al. Herpes zoster—treatment with a acyclovir. *Med Pregl* 1997;50:305–308.
31. Jackson JL, Gibbons R, Meyer G, et al. The effect of treating herpes zoster with oral acyclovir in preventing postherpetic neuralgia. A meta-analysis. *Arch Intem Med* 1997;157:909–912.
32. Kubeyinje EP. Cost-benefit of oral acyclovir in the treatment of herpes zoster. *Int J Dermatol* 1997;36:457–459.
33. Gnann JW Jr, Crumpacker CS, Lalezari JP, et al. Sorivudine versus acyclovir for treatment of dermatomal herpes zoster in human immunodeficiency virus infected patients: results from a randomized, controlled clinical trial. Collaborative Antiviral Study Group/AIDS Clinical Trials Group, Herpes Zoster Study Group. *Antimicrob Agents Chemother* 1998;42:1139–1145.
34. Bodsworth NJ, Boag F, Burdge D, et al. Evaluation of sorivudine (BV-araU) versus acyclovir in the treatment of acute localized herpes zoster in human immunodeficiency virus-infected adults. The Multinational Sorivudine Study Group. *J Infect Dis* 1997;176:103–111.
35. Wood MJ, Shukla S, Fiddian AP, et al. Treatment of acute herpes zoster: Effect of early (<48 h) versus late (48–72 h) therapy with acyclovir and valacyclovir on prolonged pain. *J Infect Dis* 1998;178 (Suppl 1):S81–84.
36. Stein GE. Pharmacology of new antiherpes agents: Famciclovir and valacyclovir. *J Am Pharm Assoc* 1997;NS37:157–163.
37. Grant DM, Mauskopf JA, Bell L, et al. Comparison of valacyclovir and acyclovir for the treatment of herpes zoster in immunocompetent patients over 50 years age: a cost-consequence model. *Pharmacotherapy* 1997;17:333–341.
38. Stott GA. Famciclovir: a new systemic antiviral agent for herpesvirus. *Am Farr Physician* 1997;55:2501–2504.
39. Tyring S, Barbarash RA, Nahlik JE, et al. Famciclovir for the treatment of acute herpes zoster: effects on acute disease and postherpetic neuralgia. A randomized, double blind, placebo-controlled trial. *Ann Intem Med* 1995;123:89–96.

40. Degreef H. Famciclovir Herpes Zoster Clinical Study Group. Famciclovir, a new oral drug: Results of the first controlled clinical study demonstrating its efficacy and safety in the treatment of uncomplicated herpes zoster in immune competent patients. *Int J Antimicrob Agents* 1994;4:241–246.

41. Sacks SL, Martel A, Aoki F, et al. *Clinic-initiated treatment of recurrent genital herpes using famciclovir: results of a Canadian multicenter study*. Presented at the Sixth International Congress for Infectious Diseases, Prague, Czechoslovakia, 1994.

42. Sacks SL, Aoki FY, Diaz-Mitoma F, et al. Patient-initiated, twice daily oral famciclovir for early recurrent genital herpes: a randomized, double-blind multicenter trial. *JAMA* 1996;276:44–49.

43. Mertz G, Loveless MO, Levin MJ, et al. Oral famciclovir for suppression of recurrent genital herpes simplex virus infection in women. *Arch Intern Med* 1997;157:343–349.

44. Field JH, Thackray AM. The effects of delayed-onset chemotherapy using famciclovir or valacyclovir in a murine immunosuppression model for HSV-1. *Antiviral Chem Chemother* 1995;6:210–216.

45. Field JH, Tewari D, Sutton D, et al. Comparison of efficacious of famciclovir and valacyclovir against herpes simplex virus type 1 in a murine immunosuppression model. *Antimicrob Agents Chemother* 1995;39: 1114–1119.

46. Thackray Am, Field JH. Differential effects of famciclovir and valacyclovir on the pathogenesis of herpes simplex virus in a murine infection model including reactivation from latency. *J Infect Dis* 1996; 173:291–299.

47. Ahmed A, Woolley PD. *Comparison of famciclovir and acyclovir in first episode of genital herpes: possible effect on latency*. Presented at the European Conference on Herpesviruses, Paris, France, 1996.

48. Loveless M, Sacks SL, Harris JRW. Famciclovir in the management of first episode genital herpes. *Infect Dis Clin Pract6* 1997;(Suppl1): S12–16.

49. Breton G, Fillet AM, Katlama C, et al. Acyclovir-resistant herpes zoster in human immunodeficiency virus-infected patients: results of foscarnet therapy. *Clin Infect Dis* 1998;27:1525–1527.

50. Wutzler P. Antiviral therapy of herpes simplex and varicella-zoster virus infections. *Intervirology* 40:343-356, 1997.

51. Bareggi SR, Priola R, De Benedittis G. Skin and plasma levels of acetylsalicylic acid: a comparison between topical aspirin/diethyl ether mixture and oral aspirin in acute herpes zoster and postherpetic neuralgia. *Dur J Clin Pharmacol* 1998;54:231–235.

52. Primache V, Binda S, De Benedittis G, et al. In vitro activity of acetylsalicylic acid on replication of varicella-zoster virus. *New Microbiol* 1998;21:3997–3401.

53. Ernst ME, Santee JA, Klepser TB. Oral corticosteroids for pain associated with herpes zoster. *Ann Pharmacother* 1998;32:1099–1103.

54. Bowsher D. The effects of pre-emptive treatment of postherpetic neuralgia with amitriptyline: a randomized, double-blind, placebo-controlled trial. *J Pain Symptom Manage* 1997;13:327–331.

55. Hadzic A, Vloka JD, Saff GN, et al. The "three-in-one block: for treatment of pain in a patient with acute herpes zoster infection. *Reg Anesth* 1997;22:575–578.

56. Applegate KL, Cacioppo JT, Keicolt-Glaser JK, et al. *The effects of stress on the immune system: Implications for reactivation of latent herpes viruses*. Presented at the Herpes Zoster and Postherpetic Neuralgia Satellite Symposium, Whistler Mountain, British Columbia, August 13 and 14, 1996.

57. Lutgendorf S, Antoni MH, Jumar M, et al. Changes in cognitive copying strategies predict EEBV-antibody titre follows a stresor disclosure induction. *J of Psychosomatic Research* 1994;38:63–78.

58. Esterling BA, Antoni MH, Fletcher MA, et al. Emotional disclosure through writing or speaking modulates latent Epstein-Barr virus antibody titers. *J of Consulting and Clinical Psychology* 1994;62:130–140.

59. Tyring SK. Advances in the treatment of Herpesvirus infection: the role of famciclovir. *Clin Therapeutics* 1998;20:661–670.

60. Ahmed HE, Craig WF, White PF, et al. Percutaneous electrical nerve stimulation: an alternative to antiviral drugs for acute herpes zoster. *Anesth Analg* 1998;87:911–914.

61. Olwin JH, Ratajczak HV, House RV. Successful treatment of herpetic infections by autohemotherapy. *J Altern Complement Med* 1997;3: 155–158.

62. Rowbotham M, Harden N, Stacey B, et al. Gabapentin for the treatment of postherpetic neuralgia. A randomized controlled trial. *JAMA* 1998;280:1837–1842.

*Acknowledgment: A portion of the material in this chapter has been taken from the *Acute Herpes Zoster and Postherpetic Neuralgia* for *Principles and Practice of Pain Management*, ed. 2, edited by Drs. Carol Warfield and Zahid Bajwa to be published by McGraw-Hill.

CHAPTER 36

Chronic Joint and Connective Tissue Pain

Roger B. Traycoff

Successful management of pain in patients with rheumatic diseases requires an awareness that pain is both an experience and a sensation. We observe pain behavior, not pain. The behavior may or may not be appropriate for the intensity of the nociceptive stimulus. It is affected by both past experience and environmental reinforcers. Failure to recognize the importance of these psychological factors may lead to inappropriate therapy. Treatment should be disease, rather than symptom oriented. Empiric therapy is seldom appropriate, often leading to suboptimal results.

The two major determinants of pain behavior are the intensity of the stimulus and the patient's interpretation of the meaning of the pain. When dealing with patients who have rheumatic diseases, the source of nociception is usually obvious. Physicians tend to focus on physical findings, being disease- rather than patient-oriented. The question of somatization is seldom raised, and the emotional component of pain behavior may not be considered.

To optimally manage patients with rheumatic diseases, one must understand the natural history of the disease untreated and the psychological and socioeconomic consequences of having a chronic debilitating illness. Patients are driven by both learned behavior and previous interaction with health care providers. The importance of the patient–physician relationship cannot be overemphasized. Patient satisfaction and compliance with therapy are affected by how they perceive their disease and their expectations regarding treatment and outcome.

Most failures in the management of pain due to rheumatic disease arise from (a) the physician's inability to make a correct diagnosis, (b) the physician's failure to educate the patient, (c) the patient's noncompliance with therapeutic regimens, and (d) the physician's inappropriate use of analgesic drugs. Successful management of pain requires that physicians have an understanding of disease mechanisms, a knowledge of drug pharmacokinetics and pharmacodynamics, and a sense of the patient's beliefs. More importantly, one must recognize the limitations of current treatments and the need for a conservative approach to management. In some instances, a physician may not have enough data to make rational choices regarding treatment. For example, it would be inappropriate to administer potentially toxic drugs to patients early in the course of their disease, when there is a high probability of spontaneous remission. Similarly, it would be incorrect to use symptom-directed therapy in patients with chronic progressive illnesses.

In the most basic construct, pain associated with rheumatic disease can be divided into (a) inflammatory or noninflammatory arthritis and (b) systemic or localized disease, based on pathophysiology. Treatment should be directed at the cause of the pain. Pain arising from inflammation should be treated with antiinflammatory drugs rather than simple analgesics or opiates. Nonsteroidal antiinflammatory drugs (NSAIDs) and the salicylates are prototypic drugs having both antiinflammatory and analgesic properties. They are most effective in treating inflammation arising as a consequence of the release of prostaglandins and leukotrienes, however. In contrast, corticosteroids have no intrinsic analgesic properties. Relief of pain following treatment with corticosteroids is due to their antiinflammatory effects. Disease-modifying agents such as gold compounds, penicillamine, and methotrexate have no intrinsic analgesic properties. Pain relief arises from suppression of inflammation through alteration of the underlying disease process.

NSAIDs are the mainstay of therapy of inflammatory joint disease, having both analgesic and antiinflammatory properties. It appears that the NSAIDs are most effective in the presence of prostaglandin-mediated pain. For this reason, they are more correctly classified as antialgesics than analgesics; NSAIDs act by raising the threshold for the firing of free nerve endings. They do not alter neural transmission or the response to the nociceptive stimulus (1).

One's choice of simple analgesic is usually dictated by individual preference rather than differences among the various classes of drugs. There is little evidence to support the use of simple analgesics such as acetaminophen, codeine, or propoxyphene in the treatment of pain associated with synovitis. There are data, however, that show that acetaminophen is as effective as NSAIDs in the treatment of noninflammatory joint disease (2).

Using opiates to treat the pain of rheumatic origin is inappropriate. Opiates can cause physical dependence and addiction. The short-term benefit of use is far outweighed by problems associated with physical dependence and loss of efficacy over time. Potent opiates such as morphine and meperidine are rarely used for treating rheumatic diseases except in the presence of major trauma. Even then, most musculoskeletal pain will respond to immobilization and therapy with antiinflammatory drugs.

One must establish a doctor–patient relationship that promotes wellness and discourages dependency. In discussions with the patient, physicians should not be overly optimistic or pessimistic. Undue optimism will create unrealistic expectations, whereas excessive pessimism will cause patients to seek alternative care, often becoming prey to the purveyors of unproven remedies.

The major variables when treating pain are the underlying disease process, the patient's expectations regarding both outcome and response to therapy, and the drugs available for use. Having a correct diagnosis is a prerequisite for providing effective care. Pain not associated with inflammation can be treated with acetaminophen, low-dose salicylates, or NSAIDs. Psychotropic drugs such as benzodiazepines and tricyclic antidepressants are used as adjunctive therapy, recognizing that their effects are primarily symptom directed. Tricyclic antidepressants, used to treat depression and "fibrositis-like" symptoms, are particularly useful when treating patients with nonarticular rheumatism (3). Benzodiazepines such as diazepam should only be used for treating patients with "trait anxiety" (3). They are not appropriate for chronic use because of their potential to cause physical dependence. Drug-seeking behavior will increase rather than decrease pain behavior.

When treating patients with rheumatic diseases, the goals are to relieve pain, preserve function, and prevent joint destruction. Pain of inflammatory joint disease is best achieved by controlling inflammation. Educating and encouraging patients to participate in the treatment process will ensure compliance. Emphasis on wellness and promoting the concept of self-help are important adjuncts to pharmacotherapy. Referrals to allied health personnel such as physical therapists and occupational therapists, as well as use of arthritis support groups, should be incorporated into the treatment plan. Reliance on drug therapy alone should be discouraged because outcome may relate to variables other than pain control.

APPROACH TO DIAGNOSIS

The history and physical examination remain the cornerstones of the diagnostic process. Having a correct diagnosis is a prerequisite for optimal therapy. An empiric approach to management is seldom appropriate; it may lead to either over- or undertreatment. Therapy should be disease specific as well as symptom directed.

Being able to localize the anatomic source of pain is invaluable to the diagnostic process. One must determine whether the pain is articular, periarticular, muscular, or neurogenic in origin. The pain of rheumatic disease is most often articular in origin. It is characteristically associated with decreased and painful range of motion. Erythema and swelling are often seen when examining appendicular joints. Axial joints such as hips and shoulders seldom have clinical evidence of synovitis.

The absence of confirmatory physical findings does not preclude a physical basis for pain. The diagnosis of psychogenic pain is suggested by finding inconsistencies in either the history or the physical examination. Although psychogenic pain is rare, somatization with exaggerated pain behavior is not uncommon. Somatoform disorders and somatic pain can coexist. Pain is as much an experience as a sensation, being affected by learned behavior, environmental reinforcers, and secondary gain.

When it is difficult to distinguish articular from periarticular pain syndromes, the patient's response to intraarticular injection of local anesthetic can help define the anatomic source of pain. Failure to relieve pain with intraarticular injection of local anesthetic is evidence against the diagnosis of arthritis, assuming there is no coexistent extraarticular source for pain. When the response to intraarticular injection of local anesthetic is unclear, selective infiltration of extraarticular structures with local anesthetics can be of great diagnostic value, confirming or refuting the presence of tendinitis, bursitis, or enthesopathy.

It is also important to determine whether the patient's response to the nociceptive stimulus is appropriate. The patient's complaints should be taken at face value; pain is whatever the patient says it is. One must always remember that therapy should be disease rather than symptom directed, however. The goals are to decrease suffering and to treat the underlying disease process.

History and Physical Examination

The medical history is the keystone of the diagnostic process. The history will suggest whether the disease is systemic or regional, acute or chronic, inflammatory or noninflammatory, or psychogenic in etiology. The patient's description of his or her pain is important. Articular and bursal pain are usually described as aching, cramping, or throbbing. Neuritic pain is characterized by numbness, tingling, or burning. The presence of hyperesthesia, dysesthesia, and allodynia suggests either deafferentation pain or reflex sympathetic dystrophy.

The relationship of pain to physical activity is also important. Pain that is present only with activity suggests a mechanical or vascular etiology. Pain present both with activity and at rest is often inflammatory. Pain that is worse at night or during periods of rest should suggest the possibility of tumor, infection, or neuropathy. Pain that is unrelated to position or activity and not responsive to therapy should suggest the possibility of deafferentation or psychogenic pain.

A systematic review of systems will provide a basis for distinguishing among the rheumatic diseases. A history of weight loss, photosensitivity, Raynaud's phenomenon, dermatitis, or polyserositis should suggest the diagnosis of systemic lupus erythematosus, or a variant. A history of ocular or genitourinary symptoms should suggest the diagnosis of Reiter's syndrome. A history of diarrhea or abdominal pain should raise the possibility of enteropathic or reactive arthritis. Complaints of back pain or stiffness not relieved by rest should suggest the diagnosis of spondyloarthropathy.

The physical examination can confirm and characterize abnormalities suggested by the history. It should be performed in a systematic and thorough manner. The examiner should look for joint swelling, articular tenderness, decreased range of joint motion, and deformities. Extraarticular manifestations of rheumatic diseases should be sought because of their diagnostic importance. Cutaneous involvement is a feature of psoriatic arthritis, Reiter's syndrome, systemic lupus erythematosus, and systemic vasculitis. Finding subcutaneous nodules should suggest the diagnoses of rheumatoid arthritis, rheumatic fever, or amyloidosis. Conjunctivitis and iritis are features of spondyloarthropathies such as Reiter's syndrome, ankylosing spondylitis, and enteropathic arthritis. Finding tophi is diagnostic of gout. Pitting of the nails is a sign of psoriatic arthritis, and clubbing a clue to hypertrophic osteoarthropathy. The presence of enthesopathy, tenosynovitis, or axial skeleton involvement should suggest the diagnosis of spondyloarthropathy. Decreased range of motion of the lumbar spine and decreased chest expansion are clues to ankylosing spondylitis.

Laboratory Analyses

Laboratory studies should be used to confirm rather than make diagnoses. None of the available serologic tests for rheumatic diseases have perfect sensitivity or specificity. The basic laboratory evaluation should include an erythrocyte sedimentation rate (ESR), hemogram, urinalysis, and chemical profile or its equivalent. In general, an elevated ESR confirms the presence of an inflammatory process. Anemia is both a clue to systemic disease and a marker for chronicity. The finding of autoimmune hemolytic anemia suggests the diagnosis of systemic lupus erythematosus. Leukopenia and thrombocytopenia are features of systemic lupus ery-

thematosus; their presence would be evidence against the diagnosis of rheumatoid arthritis, with the exception of Felty's syndrome. The finding of hypercalcemia in a patient with rheumatic complaints should suggest the diagnosis of hyperparathyroidism, and the possibility of pseudogout. Hyperuricemia, although not diagnostic of gout, is a helpful clue to urate arthropathy. The finding of proteinuria or hematuria on urinalysis should suggest the possibility of glomerulonephritis due to systemic lupus erythematosus or vasculitis. Nephrotic syndrome is also a characteristic feature of amyloidosis, especially when associated with an underlying lymphoproliferative disorder.

Serologic studies such as rheumatoid factors, antinuclear antibodies, tissue typing with human leukocyte antigens (HLAs), and serum complement levels may be helpful in the differential diagnosis of rheumatic diseases. Rheumatoid factors are markers for chronic antigenic stimulation. They are not a specific marker for rheumatoid arthritis, being found in other autoimmune diseases, including systemic lupus erythematosus, scleroderma, Sjögren's syndrome, polyarteritis nodosa, mixed connective tissue disease, and amyloidosis. Rheumatoid factors have also been identified in patients with chronic infections, patients with chronic liver disease, and in the elderly with no identifiable underlying disease process. The major value of the rheumatoid factor is its ability to distinguish rheumatoid arthritis and other connective tissue diseases from the spondyloarthropathies. The presence of a rheumatoid factor in the serum of patients presenting with rheumatic complaints makes the diagnosis of spondyloarthropathy unlikely.

Testing for antinuclear antibodies (ANAs) by indirect immunofluorescence is a useful screen for systemic lupus erythematosus; however, the ANA test lacks specificity. Antinuclear antibodies are found in sera of patients with scleroderma, mixed connective tissue disease, rheumatoid arthritis, and autoimmune liver disease. Antinuclear antibodies are often drug induced, occurring in the absence of disease. A positive test for ANAs is not diagnostic of systemic lupus, but a negative result in a symptomatic patient is good evidence against the diagnosis. Patients whose test for ANAs is positive should have additional studies performed. Testing for antibodies against ribonucleoprotein (RNP), Smith antigen (Sm), and soluble cytoplasmic antigens (SSA and SSB) can be helpful.

Synovial fluid analysis has an important role in the diagnosis of arthropathies. Joint fluid should be routinely sent for white cell and differential counts, and for compensated polarized microscopy to screen for the presence of crystals. Gram's stain of the aspirate as well as culture and measurement of lactic acid levels in the synovial fluid should be ordered when infection is a consideration. Measurements of synovial fluid protein, glucose, and complement levels are of less value, often adding little to the diagnostic process. Tissue typing for the presence of HLA-B27 is of little value as a screening test for the spondyloarthropathies. The high prevalence of HLA-B27 in the normal population limits its specificity. Up to 8% of the white population is HLA-B27–positive. The absence of HLA-B27 also has limited diagnostic value because a significant percentage of patients with spondyloarthropathies are HLA-B27–negative.

Measurements of serum complement levels have limited diagnostic value. In most rheumatic diseases, the serum complement levels are normal or elevated. The presence of hypocomplementemia may be a clue to the presence of immune complex disease. Usually one measures the total hemolytic complement level (CH_{50}), and the C-3 and C-4 component levels. A very low total hemolytic complement level is a marker for hereditary complement deficiencies. A low C-3 level with a normal C-4 level should suggest alternative pathway activation. A low C-4 level with either a normal or low C-3 level should suggest classic pathway activation as seen with immune complex disease.

DRUG THERAPY

Simple Analgesics

Acetaminophen, dextropropoxyphene, and codeine are useful in the treatment of noninflammatory rheumatic pain; however, there is little evidence to support their use in treating inflammatory joint disease. They are often used empirically as single agents or in combination with other drugs. Acetaminophen is frequently used for treating mild to moderate pain. Codeine and propoxyphene are often reserved for treating patients with more severe pain on the mistaken assumption that they are more effective analgesics. When used in recommended doses, they are no better analgesics than either aspirin or acetaminophen.

As a rule, codeine and propoxyphene should not be administered as single agents. Acetaminophen or aspirin combined with codeine or propoxyphene are the favored formulations. A combination of a peripheral-acting drug with a central-acting drug provides better analgesia than either agent used alone (5). Combining aspirin with acetaminophen or aspirin with an NSAID, however, is no more effective than using maximal recommended doses of each agent alone. Pain relief from combining NSAIDs is usually not additive, but the side effects appear to increase in frequency and severity.

Acetaminophen, a central- and peripheral-acting analgesic, has an excellent efficacy–side effect profile (6). It is most often administered to patients who are intolerant of NSAIDs; it has been shown to be as effective as ibuprofen in the treatment of degenerative joint disease (2). Its role in the treatment of pain associated with inflammatory joint disease is less well defined. Intuitively, it would appear more reasonable to use an antiinflammatory drug in this setting.

The major limitation of acetaminophen is its flat dose-response curve. In single-dose studies, increasing the dose of acetaminophen beyond 1000 mg provides no additional analgesia. Daily doses greater than 4000 mg have been associated with hepatotoxicity (7). Patients who chronically abuse alcohol appear to be at greatest risk for the development of hepatic necrosis.

Acetaminophen can be used in combination with codeine or propoxyphene to provide short-term analgesia. The major problems with using analgesic combinations containing opiate derivatives are the development of tolerance and physical dependence. Addiction is a real but most likely overstated risk.

Salicylates

For many years, salicylates have been the favored drug for treating inflammatory joint disease. Salicylates have antiinflammatory, antipyretic, and analgesic properties. Although none of the newer NSAIDs have been shown to be superior to aspirin in the treatment of rheumatoid arthritis, the efficacy of aspirin for treating other inflammatory arthropathies is less clear. Aspirin may be less effective for treating patients with Reiter's syndrome or ankylosing spondylitis. The pain associated with gout and pseudogout also appears to respond better to NSAIDs than to salicylates.

Many formulations of salicylates are available (Table 36-1), yet aspirin remains the salicylate of choice in most instances. The major advantages of using nonaspirin salicylates are ease of administration, better patient tolerance, and fewer side effects. The major disadvantages are greater cost, less-flexible dosing schedules, and unpredictable absorption when administered orally.

TABLE 36-1. *Salicylates used in treatment of inflammatory joint disease*

Drug	Dose (mg)	Daily dose (mg)	Frequency
Aspirin	325	2500–5000	q.i.d.
Encaprin	325 500		b.i.d.
Easprin	975		q.i.d.
Cama	500		q.i.d.
Ascription	325		q.i.d.
Ecotrin	325		q.i.d.
Salts of salicylic acid			
Choline salicylate (Arthropan)	325	300–5000	q.i.d.
Choline magnesium trisalicylate (Trilisate)	500	3000	b.i.d.
Salicylsalicylic acid (Disalcid)	500, 750	3000	b.i.d.
Diflunisal (Dolobid)	500	1000	b.i.d.

Both the analgesic and the antiinflammatory effects of aspirin have flat dose-response curves. Analgesic doses of aspirin range from 650 to 1000 mg; antiinflammatory doses range from 3.5 to 5.0 g daily. A therapeutic blood level for antiinflammatory effects is between 15 and 20 mg/dl.

Data are lacking on the relationship between analgesia and salicylate blood levels in the absence of inflammation. Pain relief in inflammatory joint disease is probably due to the antiinflammatory rather than analgesic effects of salicylate. When treating pain with low doses of aspirin, it should be administered every 4 hours. As the dose is increased, the elimination half-life increases; hepatic enzymes become saturated. At higher doses, the aspirin can be administered as infrequently as every 8 to 12 hours (8). The exponential increase in salicylate blood levels seen with increasing dose means that small changes in doses can cause large changes in salicylate blood levels. Increasing the daily dose of aspirin by one or two tablets may result in toxicity. Tinnitus, although a useful marker for salicylate toxicity, may not be present in all cases. Therefore, salicylate blood levels should be measured in children and the elderly.

There are few data to support the use of salicylates and NSAIDs concurrently. It does not appear that combining aspirin with an NSAID will increase efficacy. The side effects may be greater when used in combination. The lack of synergism may be related to altered pharmacokinetics. The significance of these interactions is unknown; however, aspirin will decrease the absorption of fenoprofen and indomethacin.

The newer salicylates such as salicylate and choline magnesium trisalicylate have a better side-effect profile than aspirin but have not been shown to be more efficacious. They appear to cause less gastric mucosal damage than aspirin and not to adversely affect platelet function. They are most often used in patients who are intolerant of NSAIDs because of gastric irritation or ulcer.

Nonsteroidal Antiinflammatory Drugs

When treating rheumatoid arthritis, the choice between salicylates and NSAIDs is a matter of preference; none of the NSAIDs has been shown to be superior to aspirin in analgesic or antiinflammatory effects (9). This may not be true for other rheumatic diseases, however. For example, aspirin is not very effective in treating crystal-induced synovitis and appears to be less effective than NSAIDs in the treatment of spondyloarthropathies.

The role of newer NSAIDs such as ketorolac in the treatment of rheumatic pain is undefined. There are few data to support its use in either osteoarthritis or inflammatory joint disease. Its side-effect profile appears to be similar to that of other NSAIDs and therefore may add little to the treatment of pain associated with inflammatory joint disease.

A major limitation of NSAIDs is their flat dose-response curves; increasing the dose beyond the recommended level may not increase efficacy. This reflects the fact that they may act on only one component of the inflammatory response (i.e., inhibition of prostaglandin synthesis) (10).

NSAIDs appear to differ more in pharmacokinetics than in pharmacodynamics (Table 36-2). Drugs such as ibuprofen, fenoprofen, tolmetin, flurbiprofen, and meclofenamate have short elimination half-lives and must be administered every 6 to 8 hours. Sulindac, naproxen, and diclofenac have longer elimination half-lives and can be given twice a day. Piroxicam and nabumetone, having the longest elimination half-lifes, can be administered once daily.

Many of the side effects of treatment with NSAIDs relate to inhibition of prostaglandin synthesis (11). The side effect profiles of all NSAIDs are similar and are dose related. Nabumetone and meclofenamate may be exceptions. Nabumetone may have fewer gastrointestinal side effects because it is a prodrug whose active metabolite has no enterohepatic recirculation. Meclofenamate is unique in having a greater tendency to cause diarrhea.

All NSAIDs are potentially ulcerogenic. The risk of ulcer formation appears to be directly related to dose and duration of therapy. Phenylbutazone and indomethacin are thought to be more ulcerogenic than other NSAIDs, which may relate to their potency as inhibitors of mucosal cyclooxygenase. The risk of gastric ulcer appears to be less with salicylate and nabumetone.

All of the NSAIDs have the potential for causing bronchospasm in salicylate-sensitive asthmatics. Those who wheeze when taking aspirin will tend to wheeze when given other NSAIDs. This may relate to inhibition of prostaglandin E (PGE), which acts as a bronchodilator. Fortunately, only a small percentage of patients appear to be aspirin sensitive, and therefore NSAIDs can be used safely in many patients.

TABLE 36-2. *Pharmacokinetics of nonsteroidal antiinflammatory drugs*

Duration of action	Recommended daily dose (mg)
Short-acting	
Etodolac (Lodine)	300–1200
Fenoprofen (Nalfon)	1200–2400
Ketorolac (Zoradol)	40–60
Ketoprofen (Orudis)	150–300
Ibuprofen (Motrin, Rufen)	1200–3200
Indomethacin (Indocin)	75–200
Tolmetin (Tolectin)	800–1600
Meclofenamate (Meclomen)	200–400
Nabumetone (Relafen)	1000–2000
Intermediate-acting	
Diclofenac (Voltaren)	150–300
Naproxen (Naprosyn)	730–1000
Sulindac (Clinoril)	300–600
Long-acting	
Piroxicam (Feldene)	10–20
Phenylbutazone (Butazolidin)	300–400

As a group, all of the NSAIDs appear to adversely affect renal function by decreasing prostaglandin-dependent renal blood flow. Indomethacin may have a greater potential for decreasing renal blood flow than other NSAIDs. The question of sulindac having the least effect on renal blood is in dispute (12). Patients with compromised renal function from either volume contraction or intrinsic renal disease are at greatest risk for the development of azotemia. Diabetics may develop hyperkalemia as a consequence of hyporeninemic hypoaldosteronism caused by inhibition of PGE synthesis. Renal impairment due to hypersensitivity reactions is less predictable. Immune-mediated nephropathy can be caused by any of the NSAIDs but is more commonly seen in patients treated with fenoprofen. Patients who develop edema while taking aspirin will usually be intolerant of other NSAIDs. Phenylbutazone is unique in that it promotes fluid retention by two different mechanisms: inhibition of prostaglandin synthesis and an aldosterone-like effect on renal tubules.

Corticosteroids

Corticosteroids are potent antiinflammatory agents, but have no intrinsic analgesic properties. They are only useful for treating pain associated with inflammation. Corticosteroids do not appear to prevent joint destruction or alter disease progression. When treating rheumatoid arthritis, they are most often used in conjunction with remittent drugs. Their ability to relieve pain is well established but the appropriateness of their long-term use is still debated.

The major risks associated with chronic use of corticosteroids are osteoporosis, avascular necrosis of bone, hypertension, glucose intolerance, and cataract formation. There is no evidence that one class of corticosteroid is more efficacious or less toxic than another. Differences in side effects and efficacy relate more to differences in tissue half-life and potency than to mechanism of action (Table 36-3). Dexamethasone, the most potent corticosteroid, has the longest elimination half-life and therefore the longest duration of action.

TABLE 36-3. *Corticosteroids used in the treatment of inflammatory joint disease*

Relative Duration of action	Equivalent potency	doses (mg)
Short-acting		
Hydrocortisone	1	20
Prednisone	4	5
Methylprednisolone	4	4
Intermediate-acting		
Triamcinolone	5	4
Long-acting		
Betamethasone	25	0.6
Dexamethasone	30	0.75

Many physicians prefer using short-acting corticosteroids such as prednisone and prednisolone. Shorter acting corticosteroids are favored because they may have less risk of suppressing the hypothalamic-pituitary-adrenal (HPA) axis. The side effects of corticosteroids appear to be dose related. When using prednisone or its equivalent at doses less than doses of 7.5 to 10 mg/day, the side effects appear to be acceptable in most patients. There is also a relationship between side effects and duration of treatment. Alternate-day corticosteroid therapy may decrease the risk of side effects, but is usually less effective than daily corticosteroid administration in suppressing inflammation and pain.

The major factor determining suppression of the HPA axis is the duration of exposure to corticosteroids. For this reason, single daily dose or alternate-day regimens are preferred. Multiple daily doses are more effective in decreasing inflammation, but are also more likely to cause HPA axis suppression. The advantage of less HPA axis suppression with daily single-dose therapy is lost when doses of prednisone or its equivalent exceed 15 mg/day.

The role of corticosteroids in the treatment of inflammatory joint disease is controversial. The question is whether the benefits outweigh the potential risks. Low-dose corticosteroids appear to have a role in the treatment of rheumatoid arthritis (13). The role of corticosteroids in the treatment of crystal-induced arthropathies and spondyloarthropathies is less well defined, however. Corticosteroids are rarely administered systemically in acute gout because their use may prolong an attack. NSAIDs and colchicine are more efficacious, being less subject to rebound attacks after discontinuation of therapy.

Some physicians believe that corticosteroids have no place in the treatment of the spondyloarthropathies. This may relate to the need to justify the use of corticosteroids in diseases wherein the probability of remission is high and the risks of joint destruction are low. The use of corticosteroids potentially exposes patients to undue risks. Nevertheless, corticosteroids are frequently used to treat patients with Reiter's syndrome and ankylosing spondylitis who fail to respond to treatment with NSAIDs.

Systemic lupus erythematosus is one of the few rheumatic diseases in which there is little controversy over the appropriateness of corticosteroid therapy. Questions relate more to dosage regimens than to appropriateness of therapy. Corticosteroids may be more effective than NSAIDs in treating pain due to pleuritis, pericarditis, and abdominal serositis. Most patients with arthritis can be successfully treated with salicylates when used in high doses.

Intra-articular corticosteroids are useful in treating acute flares of synovitis involving one to several joints. Their use often leads to rapid relief of pain and swelling, but the duration of relief is highly variable. When used infrequently, the risks appear to be low. Chronic use may be associated with progressive joint deterioration. It appears that the risk of joint damage is related more to the frequency of administration than to the agent used. Therefore, they should be used only in patients who receive substantial prolonged relief of pain following injection.

There is little controversy regarding the effectiveness of intraarticular corticosteroids in the treatment of inflammatory joint disease. Their efficacy in treating patients with osteoarthritis is controversial, however (14). Most of the patients who respond to intraarticular corticosteroid injections will have effusions or a history of joint stiffness similar to those of patients with rheumatoid arthritis. Patients with osteoarthritis who have no evidence of synovitis tend to respond less well, having little relief of pain following intra-articular injections.

Perhaps the most successful use of depot corticosteroids is in treating patients with bursitis or tenosynovitis. These patients typically have rapid relief of symptoms following injection. The risks of single injections of corticosteroids appear to be small. The major complications following injection are infection and fat atrophy. As with other therapies, excessive use increases the risk of side effects. When used too frequently, patients may become cushingoid from systemic absorption of corticosteroids.

OSTEOARTHRITIS

Osteoarthritis is a chronic articular disease characterized by degeneration of cartilage, sclerosis of subchondral bone, and osteophyte formation. It is not a single disease but rather an expression of a final common pathway leading to joint destruction. Most oligoarticular disease probably arises from trauma or developmental abnormalities.

Osteoarthritis is divided into primary and secondary forms based on the presence or absence of an identifiable cause. It can also be subdivided into oligoarticular and polyarticular on the basis of the number of joints involved. Oligoarticular osteoarthritis involves weight-bearing joints such as the hips and knees. It rarely affects the shoulder or elbow in the absence of trauma. Generalized osteoarthritis typically involves distal and proximal interphalangeal joints as well as large weight-bearing joints such as the hips and knees.

Primary osteoarthritis can be further subdivided into primary generalized osteoarthritis and erosive osteoarthritis. Secondary osteoarthritis is defined by disease associations. It may be secondary to trauma, developmental abnormalities, or metabolic disease. Among the metabolic diseases associated with osteoarthritis are diabetes mellitus, ochronosis, acromegaly, hypothyroidism, and Wilson's disease.

Most patients with osteoarthritis complain of pain and stiffness in the involved joints. Their pain is characteristically aggravated by activity and relieved by rest. Patients with osteoarthritis may also complain of stiffness and aching following immobilization, however. Typically, their stiffness is relieved by movement. Most of their pain occurs late in the day as a consequence of excessive use. The joint examination typically shows bony overgrowth at articular margins, decreased range of motion with crepitus, and the absence of synovitis. Signs of systemic disease are typically lacking.

The pain of osteoarthritis arises in both articular and periarticular structures. The pain-sensitive structures within the joint are the joint capsule, articular fat pads, and subchondral bone (15). Extraarticular sources for pain include ligaments, tendons, and bursae. Pain arising from chronic repetitive mechanical stress in muscle may also contribute to discomfort.

Early osteoarthritis is typically painless because articular cartilage is aneural. Radiographic changes may precede symptoms. Pain may arise from microfractures in subchondral bone and synovium. Subclinical inflammation, commonly seen in specimens of synovial membrane, suggests that synovitis may be a source of pain. The possibility that rest pain in osteoarthritis is due to intraosseous venous engorgement has also been raised (16).

Treatment

Treatment of osteoarthritis is directed at symptoms rather than the underlying disease process. There are no known cures. Therapy must be individualized to meet the needs of the patient. Types of therapy include physical and occupational therapy, drugs, and surgery. Having an accurate diagnosis is a prerequisite for optimal care. The factors contributing to the pain behavior must be identified.

The goals of therapy are to relieve pain, to preserve function, and to prevent joint destruction. Pain can be treated with simple analgesics such as acetaminophen or NSAIDs. Physical therapy has an adjunctive role. Reconstructive surgery is reserved for the most intractable cases.

Patients should understand both the nature and the prognosis of their disease. Patient education will help dispel potentially unrealistic expectations and do much to improve patient compliance. An educated patient is less likely to abuse medications or seek care from nontraditional practitioners.

Drug Therapy

Salicylates and NSAIDs have been the mainstay of therapy because of their analgesic and antiinflammatory properties. In many cases, however, acetaminophen may be as effective as NSAIDs. Treatment is palliative; there is little evidence these drugs affect the underlying disease process.

Mild osteoarthritis is usually treated with simple analgesics such as acetaminophen or low-dose salicylates. Acetaminophen is administered orally in doses of 650 mg every 4 to 6 hours as needed. Aspirin is prescribed in analgesic doses of 2 to 3 g/day in divided doses. Patients with more-severe pain are often treated with aspirin or acetaminophen combined with either codeine or propoxyphene.

NSAIDs and high-dose salicylates are used for treating patients unresponsive to simple analgesics. They appear to be most effective in the presence of synovitis. Although there are few data suggesting that one NSAID is superior to another, indomethacin may be the exception. It may be more effective in treating the subset of patients with osteoarthritis who have coexistent crystal-induced synovitis. Patients having hydroxyapatite deposition disease or subclinical pyrophosphate arthropathy may respond better to indomethacin than to salicylates.

Intraarticular Corticosteroid Injections

Intraarticular corticosteroids are widely used for treating osteoarthritis; however, there is controversy over the appropriateness of their use. Data from controlled studies are contradictory; some studies show efficacy (17) whereas others show no benefit compared to placebo (18).

Questions regarding potential adverse effects on articular cartilage have also been raised (19). There are anecdotal reports of patients developing "Charcot-like" joints following repeated intraarticular injections of corticosteroids. Studies of the effects of corticosteroids on articular cartilage from animals are also contradictory. Intraarticular corticosteroids inhibit articular proteoglycan synthesis in rabbit, but not in primate cartilage. Taken together, these data indicate that intraarticular corticosteroids are useful in treating a subset of patients with osteoarthritis and that they have a significant potential for causing side effects when used inappropriately. Their use should be limited to patients who have not responded to either NSAIDs or high doses of salicylates. Intraarticular corticosteroids should not be administered more frequently than every 4 months and then only if the duration of benefit from the previous injection lasted more than 4 weeks. Short-term relief of pain does not justify the risks of repeated injections.

Physical Therapy

The major use of physical therapy is to correct postural abnormalities and to strengthen deconditioned muscles. Simple exercise programs such as walking can be helpful (20). Assistive devices such as canes, walkers, and crutches relieve pain by decreasing weight-bearing on symptomatic joints (21). Correction of structural abnormalities and weight reduction in the obese patient may be helpful. Application of heat and cold to symptomatic areas gives short-term relief, perhaps by decreasing muscle spasm.

RHEUMATOID ARTHRITIS

Rheumatoid arthritis, a chronic, polyarticular, multisystem disease, is distinguished from other rheumatic diseases by having symmetrical involvement of large and small joints of both upper and lower extremities. It is frequently associated with extraarticular manifestations such as subcutaneous nodules, serositis, pulmonary fibrosis, and vasculitis. Patients may be either seropositive or seronegative. Only 70 percent of patients have serum rheumatoid factor titers greater than 1:60. The prognosis is highly variable, and the course of individual patients is not predictable. The presence of subcutaneous nodules, high titers of rheumatoid factor, and the early appearance of joint erosion portend a poor prognosis and suggest the need for aggressive therapy.

The treatment of pain in rheumatoid arthritis is synonymous with suppression of inflammation; control of synovitis will result in control of pain. The pain of coexistent osteoarthritis is an exception. When pain is arising from nociceptors in subchondral bone, the pain will persist despite intensive use of antiinflammatory drugs.

Many patients with rheumatoid arthritis have a fibrositis-like syndrome as well as pain associated with synovitis. Successful management of myofascial pain requires muscle-stretching exercises, trigger-point injections, and at times the use of tricyclic antidepressants. Corticosteroids and NSAIDs are not effective in treating these noninflammatory pain syndromes.

Successful management of pain requires an accurate localization of the pain generators. Extraarticular pain syndromes such as bursitis, tenosynovitis, enthesopathy, and entrapment neuropathies may coexist with arthritis. Failure to identify these sources of pain will lead to suboptimal results. The symptoms of nonarticular rheumatic complaints are often poorly responsive to treatment with NSAIDs and salicylates. Using potentially remittent drugs to treat "burned-out" rheumatoid disease or nonarticular rheumatic complaints would be inappropriate.

Drug Treatment

When treating rheumatoid arthritis, one must understand the natural history of the disease untreated. Patients with definite rheumatoid arthritis (nodular erosive disease) have persistence of symptoms. In contrast, patients with "probable" rheumatoid arthritis have a more variable course. These patients may have either spontaneous remissions or persistence of symptoms without progression to joint destruction. At the outset, when the prognosis is in doubt, one should begin treatment with either salicylates or NSAIDs in maximally recommended doses. NSAIDs should be administered for at least 10 to 14 days before thinking of changing to another drug because it may take several weeks to obtain maximal effects. As a rule, if treatment with three consecutive NSAIDs does not provide adequate suppression of inflammation, it is unlikely that a fourth NSAID will be any more effective. Changing from one class of NSAIDs to another class of NSAIDs, although conceptually appealing, does not usually result in increased efficacy.

Before discontinuing treatment with an NSAID because of lack of benefit, one must confirm that the patient is taking the medication as prescribed. Compliance in taking medications is an important variable when assessing responses to treatment. One can confirm compliance by comparing the number of times a patient obtains refills of medication to the expected number of requests for refills.

When a patient has inadequate relief of pain or has had symptoms for more than 6 to 9 months, one should consider adding a remittent drug to the therapeutic regimen. One's choice of potentially remittent drug will vary depending on one's training and experience. Usually, either an antimalarial drug or chrysotherapy is considered as a first-line remittent agent. Auranofin, an oral gold compound, is often administered before treatment with parenteral gold or penicillamine because it is potentially less toxic (22). Remittent drugs are slow to act, requiring from 3 to 6 months before significant benefit is seen. The end point is having a decrease in inflammation, not just a decrease in pain.

Remittent drugs may have a significant placebo effect. Patients may claim improvement yet show no change in physical findings. Therefore, one needs to document a decrease in synovitis before committing a patient to a prolonged course of therapy. If no progress has been made after 3 months of therapy, one should change to another remittent drug.

Auranofin, a trialkylphosphine gold complex, can be administered orally. It has a lower frequency of mucocutaneous and renal toxicity than parenteral gold compounds. The major side effect of treatment is diarrhea. There is no correlation between auranofin blood levels and therapeutic efficacy (23). The usual dose is 3 mg given orally twice a day.

The use of gold compounds in the treatment of rheumatoid arthritis is controversial. Recent reports have questioned its value relative to toxicity. The issue is clouded by a lack of data from well-designed double-blind studies, however. Parenteral gold compounds include aurothioglucose and aurothiomalate (24). Both drugs have similar efficacy and potential toxicities. Aurothiomalate differs in causing a nitritoid reaction characterized by acute vasodilation and cutaneous flushing following intramuscular injection. The relationship between the dose of gold and efficacy is unclear. There is no difference in response when comparing the 10-mg weekly doses to the traditional 50-mg weekly dose. Doses higher than 50 mg/week appear to increase toxicity without conferring additional benefit. Parenteral gold is usually administered in doses of 25 to 50 mg weekly to a cumulative dose of 1,000 mg. Patients are then placed on long-term maintenance therapy because most patients will have an exacerbation of arthritis following discontinuation of treatment.

The major toxicities of parenteral gold are mucocutaneous and renal. Patients frequently develop stomatitis or dermatitis, requiring cessation of therapy. Renal toxicity presents as proteinuria; the major risk is the development of nephrotic syndrome. Renal biopsy findings have been variable, ranging from a focal proliferative glomerulonephritis to membranous nephropathy.

Penicillamine is also used for treating rheumatoid arthritis unresponsive to NSAIDs (25). It is usually administered orally in doses of 375 to 1000 mg/day. Treatment is begun at doses of 125 to 250 mg daily and increased by 125 mg every 2 to 4 weeks. By gradually increasing the dose, the frequency of intolerance is significantly decreased. Major side effects are rash and loss of taste. Proteinuria is a common complication with a potential for progressing to nephrotic syndrome. Thrombocytopenia is also seen. Anemia and leukopenia are less frequently noted. Blood studies should be done at least every 2 to 4 weeks during the first 6 months of therapy, and then at least every 4 to 6 weeks thereafter. Side effects such as myasthenia gravis, Goodpasture's syndrome, breast gigantism, and lupus-like syndrome should be anticipated.

Azathioprine can also be used but may not be the drug of next choice because of its oncogenic potential (26). Nevertheless, it has been approved for use in the treatment of rheumatoid arthritis. Patients who smoke cigarettes or have a strong family history of cancer may not be good candidates for treatment because of their having a greater risk of developing a neoplasm while taking an immunosuppressant drug. The possibility of azathioprine playing a permissive role by impairing immune surveillance cannot be discounted.

Methotrexate has become one of the most widely used drugs for treating rheumatoid arthritis (27). It has been shown to be both safe and efficacious, having a favorable benefit–side-effect profile. It is usually administered in doses ranging from 5 to 25 mg/week. The major side effects are stomatitis and gastrointestinal upset. Problems with abnormal liver function tests are common; however, the risk of hepatic fibrosis in this setting appears to be low. Patients with diabetes mellitus and alcoholics appear to have greater risks of liver toxicity following treatment with methotrexate. If there is a question about underlying liver disease, a percutaneous liver biopsy should be performed prior to beginning treatment. Patients having no risk factors may not need a liver biopsy at outset. The absence of abnormal liver function tests cannot be taken as evidence against the presence of hepatic damage. All patients should be biopsied after taking a cumulative dose of 2000 to 3000 mg, however.

Alkylating agents such as cyclophosphamide (28) and chlorambucil should be reserved for cases in which the indications for treatment are clear and incontrovertible. They are usually reserved for treating patients with life-threatening multisystem disease such as vasculitis.

There is no consensus on the use of corticosteroids in rheumatoid arthritis. They are usually given in low doses to treat patients who are candidates for remittent drugs, but not as first-line therapy. All patients taking corticosteroids should be placed on calcium supplements to prevent the development of osteoporosis; the exception is patients with absorptive hypercalcemia, who are at risk of nephrolithiasis.

Corticosteroids can be administered orally, parenterally, or intraarticularly. Prednisone, the most commonly used drug, is usually administered in doses of 5 to 7.5 mg daily. Split doses are more effective than single daily doses, but have a higher frequency of side effects. Depot corticosteroids are occasionally useful when one does not want to commit a patient to oral steroid therapy. Long-acting drugs such as triamcinolone acetonide can be used in doses of 30 to 60 mg intramuscularly. Long-term use is associated with the development of a cushingoid habitus with all the complications of chronic corticosteroid use.

Corticosteroids are injected intraarticularly to treat oligoarticular flares of synovitis. The risk of damage to articular cartilage is most likely overstated. The risks of articular damage are minimal when injections are given no more frequently than every 4 to 6 months. The incidence of septic arthritis, when using a sterile no-touch technique, is approximately 1:20 000 injections. The joint should be aspirated prior to injection. If the joint fluid is not removed, the corticosteroid crystals may be sequestered in synovial fluid and not reach the site of inflammation. It is important to avoid overdistending the joint during injection because excessive pressure will result in extravasation of drug into the subcutaneous tissue, increasing the risk of developing fat atrophy.

Antimalarials are useful in treating refractory synovitis (29). Controlled studies have confirmed their efficacy. Eye exams should be performed prior to beginning therapy and repeated every 4 to 6 months to identify subclinical retinopathy. Doses of chloroquine should not exceed 6 mg/kg/day; doses of hydroxychloroquine should not exceed 4 mg/kg/day. Doses should be decreased in patients with impaired renal function.

Physical Therapy

Physical therapy has a role in treating patients with rheumatoid arthritis (30). It provides short-term relief of symptoms both by promoting a sense of wellness and by helping to maintain function. There are few data to show that physical therapy has any effect on the progression of disease, however. Major problems with expense and poor patient compliance limit its use. Patients instructed by physical therapists seldom continue their exercises in an unsupervised setting. Nevertheless, the patient should be encouraged to see a therapist on a regular basis to prevent the development of contractures and damage to joints because of improper use.

"Step-Care" Approach

Rheumatoid arthritis is treated by a "step-care" approach whereby patients are given a series of potentially remittent drugs on a trial-and-error basis. Typically, patients will have taken a number of drugs to which there was an initial response but subsequent loss of efficacy. Drug-induced remissions may be lost following discontinuation of treatment; therefore, maintenance therapy is almost always indi-

cated. The exceptions are methotrexate and the cytotoxic drugs, because of their potential for cumulative toxicity. Methotrexate has a risk of causing hepatic fibrosis and possibly interstitial pulmonary disease. Cyclophosphamide has the potential for causing hemorrhagic cystitis and carcinoma of the bladder.

CRYSTAL-INDUCED ARTHRITIS

Crystal-induced arthritis, in contrast to other forms of arthritis, has well-defined causes. The major effector cells are neutrophils rather than mononuclear cells. Treatment is limited to antiinflammatory drugs and uric acid–lowering agents when appropriate. These arthritides lack systemic manifestations. There is no evidence that they respond to remittent drugs or benefit from immunosuppressive therapy.

Gout

Gout, perhaps the best understood of the crystal-induced diseases, arises as a consequence of hyperuricemia and crystal deposition. Monosodium urate crystals are the phlogistic agent. Treatment of acute attacks requires suppression of inflammation. Effective long-term treatment requires normalization of serum uric acid levels and depletion of the total body urate pools.

Pseudogout

Pseudogout, or calcium pyrophosphate deposition disease (CPPD), is caused by deposition of calcium pyrophosphate dihydrate in articular cartilage. Acute attacks of arthritis arise from shedding preformed crystals into joints, where they induce an inflammatory reaction similar to that seen with gout. Pseudogout can also present as pseudorheumatoid arthritis, pseudoosteoarthritis, pseudoneuropathic arthritis, and asymptomatic chondrocalcinosis. It can be idiopathic, familial, or associated with metabolic diseases such as hyperparathyroidism, hemochromatosis, hypothyroidism, ochronosis, or Wilson's disease. Treatment of calcium pyrophosphate deposition disease is palliative because there is no known cure.

Hydroxyapatite Deposition Disease

Hydroxyapatite deposition disease is also pleomorphic. It can present as an acute inflammatory arthritis, a chronic painful degenerative arthropathy, or periarthritis. Periarticular disease includes bursitis, tendinitis, and tenosynovitis. Hydroxyapatite crystals have been implicated in the "Milwaukee shoulder" syndrome, a chronic degenerative arthritis of the shoulders characterized by degeneration of the rotator cuff, joint space narrowing, and the presence of microspheres containing hydroxyapatite crystals. These crystals have also been implicated in both the periarthritis and the destructive arthropathy seen in patients on chronic hemodialysis.

Treatment

In most instances, crystal-induced arthritis responds to NSAIDs (31). Phenylbutazone and indomethacin are perhaps the most effective agents. Other NSAIDs have also been reported to be efficacious, however. Doses of NSAIDs used for treating acute attacks of gout are generally 25 percent higher than the doses used for treating rheumatoid arthritis. Pain associated with crystal-induced synovitis responds poorly to simple analgesics, salicylates, and opiates. Relief can only be obtained by suppression of inflammation.

Colchicine is effective in the treatment of both acute gout and pseudogout when administered intravenously (32). The usual dose is 2 mg in 20 ml of saline administered over 20 min. Additional 1-mg doses can be given every 3 to 6 hours if needed, to a maximum of 4 mg/24 hours. Colchicine can also be administered orally in doses of 0.6 mg every 1 to 2 hours until a maximum of 12 tablets is given or side effects occur (33). Most patients obtain relief after two or three doses. Oral colchicine is not usually effective in the treatment of pseudogout.

The choice between an NSAID and colchicine is arbitrary because both regimens are effective. Intravenous colchicine is preferred by many physicians for the treatment of acute gout, whereas an NSAID is preferred for the treatment of pseudogout. Colchicine can be used to treat patients with a history of peptic ulcer disease because it has no ulcerogenic potential. It should be avoided in patients with intercurrent diarrheal disease, chronic renal insufficiency, or bone marrow dysfunction. Colchicine is primarily excreted by the kidneys and therefore tends to be retained in patients with impaired renal function. Accumulation may lead to suppression of marrow function with resultant anemia or leukopenia.

NSAIDs are usually effective and well tolerated. Indomethacin and phenylbutazone are often given because of their efficacy and a long history of use. Phenylbutazone can never be considered a drug of first choice, however, because agents with less significant risks are available. Indomethacin may be the NSAID of choice in treating acute attacks of gout or pseudogout.

Oral corticosteroids have a limited role in the treatment of crystal-induced arthritis. Systemic corticosteroid therapy will suppress an acute attack, but often there is an exacerbation of the arthritis upon discontinuation of therapy. This is in contrast to intraarticular corticosteroid injections, which are useful in treating monarticular arthritis unresponsive to either colchicine or NSAIDs.

Acute attacks of gout should not be treated with agents that lower the serum uric acid because of their risk of exacerbating an attack. In general, one should not lower the serum uric acid until the attack has completely subsided; then either allopurinol or a uricosuric drug can be given along with colchicine or an NSAID. Colchicine is usually given in a dose of 0.6 mg three times a day for 3 to 6 months as prophylaxis to prevent an exacerbation of arthritis while lowering the serum uric acid level (34).

The treatment of chronic gout requires continuous therapy to lower the uric acid. The goal is to reduce the total urate pool to normal. This can be done by using either allopurinol (35) or a uricosuric agent. Allopurinol is usually administered at doses of 200 to 300 mg daily. Divided doses of allopurinol are not required because of the long elimination half-life of oxypurinol, its active metabolite. On occasion, doses of 600 to 800 mg/day must be given to maintain a uric acid level below 7 mg/dl. Patients who are taking high doses of allopurinol or taking thiazide diuretics concurrently are at risk for developing the Stevens-Johnson syndrome or hepatotoxicity. Patients with impaired renal function may tend to accumulate the drug because of decreased renal clearance.

In most cases the choice between allopurinol and a uricosuric agent is a matter of preference. The exceptions are patients with a history of nephrolithiasis and patients who are overexcreters (those who excrete more than 1000 mg of uric acid per day on a regular diet). These patients should be treated with allopurinol rather than a uricosuric agent. Drugs enhancing renal excretion of uric acid have a risk for causing nephrolithiasis.

Probenecid and sulfinpyrazone are the commonly used uricosuric agents. Like allopurinol, they should not be given during an acute attack of gout. Probenecid is given in an initial dose of 250 mg/day, with the dose being gradually increased to 1.0 to 1.5 g/day, over 7 to 10 days (36). It must be administered in divided doses because of it having a short elimination half-life. Sulfinpyrazone is given at doses of 50 mg twice daily and gradually increased to 200 to 800 mg in divided doses (37). The uricosuric effects of both probenecid and sulfinpyrazone are blocked by salicylates. Sulfinpyrazone also has an effect on platelet function and on the metabolism of both warfarin and tolbutamide. Appropriate dose adjustments for these drugs should be made.

SPONDYLOARTHROPATHIES

The spondyloarthropathies include ankylosing spondylitis, Reiter's syndrome, psoriatic arthritis, and enteropathic arthritis. The diseases classified as spondyloarthropathies share features of enthesopathy, sacroiliitis, iritis, seronegativity (i.e., they lack rheumatoid factors), and an association with the histocompatibility antigen HLA-B27.

Ankylosing Spondylitis

Ankylosing spondylitis is a chronic inflammatory disease that primarily involves the axial skeleton. It typically presents as back pain. The pain characteristically involves the low back or buttocks. The onset is often insidious without a history of antecedent trauma or a precipitating event. It is inflammatory in character, being associated with morning stiffness and improvement with activity. There may be an associated arthritis involving predominantly large joints such as the hips, shoulders, knees, and ankles. Involvement of the small joints of the hands and feet is less common. Small joint involvement is typically asymmetric. Enthesopathy is a characteristic feature of the disease. Patients may complain of chest pain due to involvement of costosternal and costochondral joints. Extraarticular manifestations such as iritis, conjunctivitis, and prostatitis are clues to the diagnosis. Late complications such as apical pulmonary fibrosis, aortic insufficiency, and cardiac conduction defects are uncommon.

Reiter's Syndrome

Reiter's syndrome is defined by the triad of arthritis, conjunctivitis, and urethritis. There may be associated stomatitis, balanitis, keratoderma, prostatitis, or diarrhea. The arthritis typically involves the large weight-bearing joints of the lower extremities. Tenosynovitis and enthesopathy are common features of the disease. The presence of Achilles tendinitis, plantar fasciitis, and costochondritis help distinguish incomplete Reiter's syndrome from rheumatoid arthritis. Extraarticular manifestations such as aortic insufficiency, pericarditis, and cardiac conduction defects are less commonly seen. Rarely one sees pleuritis or neurologic involvement with peripheral and cranial neuropathies.

Psoriatic Arthritis

Psoriatic arthritis is defined as a seronegative arthritis occurring in patients with psoriasis. Arthritis involving the distal interphalangeal joints and classic arthritis mutilans, although characteristic, is not the most common manifestation of the disease. Psoriatic arthritis typically presents as an asymmetric oligoarthritis. A small percentage of patients will have a rheumatoid arthritis–like pattern or will present with findings suggestive of ankylosing spondylitis. Extraarticular manifestations are uncommon. Conjunctivitis, iritis, and scleritis are seen in a minority of patients. Ocular involvement is strongly associated with sacroiliitis and the presence of the HLA-B27 histocompatibility antigen.

Enteropathic Arthritis

Arthritis, a major manifestation of inflammatory bowel disease, is typically seen with Crohn's disease and ulcerative colitis, but is also a feature of Whipple's disease, intestinal bypass arthropathy, and reactive arthritis following enteric infections. These diseases are typically nonerosive and nondeforming. Enteropathic arthritis usually presents as an acute oligoarthritis predominantly involving the joints of the lower extremities. Upper-extremity involvement does occur, but is less frequent. There is an association between the presence of arthritis and activity of the inflammatory

bowel disease. An association between spondylitis, iritis, and HLA-B27 is reported.

Treatment

As a group, the spondyloarthropathies are difficult to treat. With the exception of a subset of patients with psoriatic arthritis, there is no evidence that therapy with remittent drugs such as gold compounds is of any value. Therapy is limited to NSAIDs, physical therapy, and intraarticular corticosteroid injections. Remittent drugs such as antimalarials, gold compounds, and penicillamine have little value in treating patients with ankylosing spondylitis, Reiter's syndrome, or enteropathic arthritis. Physicians are less likely to treat these patients aggressively because the prognosis of the spondyloarthropathies is better than that of rheumatoid arthritis.

The choice of antiinflammatory drug is empiric. Patients with spondyloarthropathies may respond better to treatment with NSAIDs than to salicylates. Phenylbutazone, one of the most effective drugs for treating spondyloarthropathies, is seldom the drug of first choice because of the potential for causing agranulocytosis or aplastic anemia.

With the exception of psoriatic arthritis, corticosteroids are seldom appropriate for treating the spondyloarthropathies. In psoriatic arthritis they are often used for treating the skin manifestations. Because the prognosis of the spondyloarthropathies appears to be more favorable than the prognosis in rheumatoid arthritis, physicians are reluctant to treat these patients with corticosteroids. There is no evidence that corticosteroids will prevent ankylosis or alter the progression of disease.

Therapy is usually begun with either aspirin or an NSAID. When aspirin is used, it should be administered in maximally tolerated doses. Therapeutic blood levels should be documented to confirm compliance. Aspirin should be given with meals and antacids to decrease the development of gastric erosions. Patients with a history of peptic ulcer disease may be given H_2 blockers at bedtime to decrease HCl-induced gastric damage due to salicylates. If an NSAID is administered, it should be given in maximally recommended doses for at least 2 to 3 weeks before changing to another drug. The end point of therapy is suppression of inflammation as well as relief of pain.

Patients who may not respond to treatment with NSAIDs or salicylates may respond to treatment with cytotoxic drugs. Methotrexate and azathioprine are the most frequently used agents; however, data on their efficacy are lacking. There is no evidence that antibiotics have any role in the treatment of reactive arthritis due to venereal or enteropathic infection.

Some patients with psoriatic arthritis may respond to therapy with gold compounds. Others may be unresponsive, requiring treatment with cytotoxic agents. Methotrexate is the favored drug because it is effective in treating not only the arthritis, but the cutaneous manifestations as well. Only patients with chronic, potentially disabling disease should be considered for therapy.

Methotrexate is usually administered on a weekly rather than daily schedule. Doses range from 5 to 25 mg/week, with usual doses being from 5 to 7.5 mg/day. Methotrexate is absorbed well both orally and parenterally. The major factor determining toxicity is duration of exposure. Therefore, a single daily dose is to be preferred. Alternatively, the drug can be administered every 12 hours for three consecutive doses. Daily administration is associated with significant risk of toxicity. Patients with impaired renal function should not be given methotrexate because of the risk of accumulation. Patients taking aspirin are also at greater risk for toxicity. Potential drug interactions with probenecid and sulfonamides are important.

CONNECTIVE TISSUE DISEASES

The connective tissue diseases are a heterogeneous group that includes systemic lupus erythematosus, mixed connective tissue disease, progressive systemic sclerosis, and the systemic vasculitides. Pain most commonly arises from serositis and arthritis. Serositis manifests itself as pleuritis, pericarditis, and peritonitis. Patients complain of chest and abdominal pain.

Systemic lupus erythematosus (SLE) is a chronic, immunologically mediated multisystem disease characterized by the presence of multiple autoantibodies. It occurs most frequently in young women of childbearing age. Females are affected 7 to 10 times as often as males. The clinical manifestations of systemic lupus erythematosus are varied. Typically, patients will present with musculoskeletal complaints. They typically present with a polyarticular arthritis involving small joints of the hands, the wrists, and the knees. The arthritis is nonerosive but can be deforming, having an appearance similar to that of rheumatoid arthritis.

Patients may also have joint pain due to avascular necrosis of bone. This is usually seen in patients treated with corticosteroids. Patients complain of pain in the hips, knees, or shoulders. The pain of avascular necrosis generally does not respond to treatment with antiinflammatory drugs.

Cardiopulmonary complaints are very common. Pleuritic pain can occur with or without effusions. Pericarditis, a common cardiac manifestation, occurs in approximately one third of patients; patients complain of substernal chest pain that is typically aggravated by lying supine. Friction rubs are commonly heard, providing a clue to the diagnosis.

Patients with SLE may present with abdominal pain. The pain may be due to aseptic peritonitis or to mesenteric vasculitis. Ascites has been noted in up to 60% of patients who come to autopsy, suggesting that peritoneal involvement is more common than is clinically recognized. Mesenteric vasculitis with abdominal pain is uncommon, but may present as acute pancreatitis or ischemic bowel syndrome with perforation.

Sjögren's syndrome and mixed connective tissue disease have many features in common with systemic lupus erythematosus. Clinical manifestations are protean, involving almost every organ system. Patients may present with complaints of joint, chest, or abdominal pain.

The natural history of the connective tissue diseases is variable and unpredictable. The initial choice of therapy will depend on the severity of the illness and the organ system involvement. Pain arising from arthritis and serositis frequently responds to treatment with high-dose salicylates. The doses required to suppress articular inflammation range from 3.5 to 5.0 g daily. A few of these patients may develop salicylate-induced hepatitis, which usually subsides following discontinuation of the drug. In these cases, antimalarial drugs may be used to suppress the arthritis. Hydroxychloroquine is usually used in doses of 200 to 400 mg/day. The major risk is retinal damage with the potential for blindness. The risk of retinal damage is dose-related, and serious toxicity is rare if the patient is monitored appropriately.

Baseline eye exams should be done before beginning treatment and repeated every 4 to 6 months thereafter. NSAIDs drugs can also be used but are more likely than aspirin to cause side effects requiring discontinuation of therapy. Ibuprofen has been associated with central nervous system dysfunction and aseptic meningitis. NSAIDs have also been reported to cause significant impairment of renal function. This may range from a decrease in renal blood flow to acute renal failure due to interstitial nephritis.

Corticosteroids are indicated for the treatment of severe systemic manifestations of the disease. They are not usually needed for the treatment of either arthritis or serositis. If pain is unresponsive to treatment with either salicylates or NSAIDs, prednisone can be administered in doses of 5 to 10 mg/day as a single morning dose. Divided doses of corticosteroids, although potentially more effective, may suppress the HPA axis, causing obesity, hypertension, and glucose intolerance.

EXTRA-ARTICULAR PAIN SYNDROMES

Extra-articular pain syndromes can mimic arthritis. These include tendinitis, bursitis, and periarthritis. Recognition is imperative for optimal management. The periarthritis syndromes are characterized by enthesopathy. The character of the pain is variable but is generally described as aching, stabbing, or throbbing. The history, although suggestive, is often inconclusive. Diagnosis is made by physical examination and confirmed by infiltration block using local anesthetic. The local anesthetic should be infiltrated in the area of maximal tenderness. Assuming accurate placement, immediate relief of pain will confirm the diagnosis. Failure to relieve pain indicates either an incorrect diagnosis or improper injection technique. A depot corticosteroid can be mixed with the local anesthetic at the time of injection.

Rotator Cuff Tendinitis and Subacromial Bursitis

Rotator cuff tendinitis, a common cause of shoulder pain, can be acute, subacute, or chronic. Characteristically, patients complain of pain in the deltoid area rather than the shoulder. Exacerbation of pain at night is characteristic. A painful arc is typically noted between 60° and 100° of abduction; other motions may be painful as well. The diagnosis is easily confirmed by injection of local anesthetic into the subdeltoid area using a lateral approach (33). Relief of pain and improved range of motion are observed immediately following injection.

Bicipital Tendinitis

Patients with bicipital tendinitis frequently complain of pain in the area of the bicipital groove. The discomfort is reproduced by resisted supination of the hand with the elbow flexed. Marked tenderness is usually felt over the biceps tendon. Infiltration of the synovial sheath surrounding the biceps tendon with local anesthetic will result in immediate relief of pain (38). Many but not all patients respond to local injection of corticosteroid. Response to NSAIDs is less predictable.

Lateral Epicondylitis

Pain in lateral epicondylitis is localized to the dorsal aspect of the proximal forearm. Maximal tenderness is found over the insertion of the extensor muscles on the lateral epicondyle. Flexion and extension of the elbow is usually free and painless. Resisted extension of the wrist and resisted supination will exacerbate the pain. Patients are treated by splinting of the wrist, by local injections of corticosteroid, and less frequently by surgery. A small number of patients have entrapment of the deep radial nerve at the arcade of Frohse mimicking lateral epicondylitis. The differential diagnosis of entrapment neuropathy is confirmed by injection of local anesthetic, that is, conduction block of the deep radial nerve at the arcade of Frohse (39).

De Quervain's Tendinitis

In de Quervain's tendinitis there is tenderness over the radial styloid associated with inflammation of the abductor pollicis longus and extensor pollicis brevis tendons. The diagnosis is suggested by a positive Finkelstein's test (i.e., pain on lateral deviation of the wrist with the thumb adducted). It is often confused with superficial radial neuralgia and arthritis of the first carpal metacarpal joint. Patients are treated with NSAIDs, immobilization of the wrist and thumb, and local injection of corticosteroid.

Those who do not respond to conservative therapy should be considered for surgical treatment (40).

Anserine Bursitis

Anserine bursitis is characterized by knee pain associated with tenderness localized to the insertions of the medial collateral ligament and the sartorius muscle on the medial aspect of the proximal tibia. The pain, arising in the distribution of the infrapatellar branch of the saphenous nerve, is felt just distal to the medial joint line and proximal leg. Anserine bursitis is best treated by injecting a mixture of corticosteroid and local anesthetic at the point of maximal tenderness; it tends to respond poorly to treatment with NSAIDs (41). Anserine bursitis is most commonly seen in women with genu varum deformities of the knee and often coexists with osteoarthritis of the knees.

Achilles Tendinitis

Pain in the heel associated with erythema and tenderness is diagnostic of Achilles tendinitis or retrocalcaneobursitis. In most cases, inflammation is due to chronic trauma from ill-fitting shoes, but it can be a manifestation of an underlying spondyloarthropathy. Pain associated with trauma is usually short-lived and will respond to rest. Pain due to enthesopathy is persistent and usually requires treatment with NSAIDs or local injection of corticosteroid, however (42).

Polymyalgia Rheumatica

Polymyalgia rheumatica is a syndrome of diffuse proximal myalgias occurring in elderly patients (43). The onset can be acute or subacute. A subset of these patients will have giant cell arteritis. Another subset will have rheumatoid arthritis presenting with proximal joint involvement. The diagnosis of polymyalgia rheumatica is one of exclusion. Patients typically have a Westergren sedimentation rate of at least 50 mm/hour. Laboratory findings are nonspecific. The anemia of chronic disease, an elevated serum alkaline phosphatase level, and polyclonal hypergammaglobulinemia are frequently seen. Patients may have age-related antinuclear antibodies and rheumatoid factors but lack other serologic markers for autoimmune disease.

The diagnosis of giant cell arteritis is suggested by a patient having a history of headache, scalp tenderness, jaw claudication, or visual disturbance. In most cases the physical examination is normal. In a small percentage of patients, the temporal arteries will be tender and enlarged. The diagnosis is confirmed by temporal artery biopsy.

Treatment

The response to treatment with corticosteroids is also helpful diagnostically. Most patients with polymyalgia rheumatica will have a dramatic decrease in pain and stiffness within hours of beginning treatment with 7.5 to 10 mg of prednisone or its equivalent. Pseudopolymyalgia as seen in patients with rheumatoid arthritis will have a less impressive response to corticosteroids. Not having significant pain relief following treatment with low-dose prednisone should cause one to question the diagnosis of polymyalgia.

The term *polymyalgia rheumatica* is most likely a misnomer. There is little evidence that pain is of muscular origin. Muscle enzymes, electromyograms, and muscle biopsies are reported to be normal. Pain may arise from involvement of proximal joints such as shoulders and hips. The presence of synovitis is suggested by reports of increased uptake of radioisotopes in the shoulder region and by reports of an oligoarticular arthritis being present in many patients.

There is controversy over the need to use high doses of corticosteroid to treat patients with polymyalgia rheumatica who show no evidence of giant cell arteritis. Proponents of high-dose therapy argue that a negative biopsy does not rule out arteritis; therefore all patients should be treated as though they had the disease. Others argue that many patients with polymyalgia rheumatica do not have arteritis and that the use of high-dose corticosteroid therapy is unnecessary. Inappropriate use of corticosteroids in high doses will lead to increased morbidity and mortality from adverse effects of corticosteroids. In these cases, a negative temporal artery biopsy is reassuring.

The end point of treatment in polymyalgia rheumatica and giant cell arteritis is suppression of inflammation as evidenced by normalization of the erythrocyte sedimentation rate. These patients are usually given from 45 to 60 mg of prednisone daily for 1 month, followed by gradual tapering of the dose over 3 to 6 months while maintaining a normal erythrocyte sedimentation rate. Patients who have no evidence for arteritis can be treated symptomatically. In these cases, the end point of treatment is relief of pain. They are usually given from 7.5 to 10 mg of prednisone daily for control of symptoms, with tapering of the dose as tolerated. A small percentage of these patients will have subclinical arteritis; therefore, one should be prepared to increase the dose of corticosteroid when symptoms of vascular disease appear. Blindness is the major risk of inadequately treated giant cell arteritis. All patients should be given supplemental calcium to decrease the risk of corticosteroid-induced osteopenia. A minimum of 1,000 mg of elemental calcium should be administered daily. The question of using vitamin D or its analogues to prevent loss of bone is still debated.

REFERENCES

1. Capetola RJ, Rosenthale ME, Dubinsky B, McGuire JL. Peripheral antialgesics—a review. *J Clin Pharmacol* 1983;23:545–556.
2. Bradley JD, et al. Comparison of anti-inflammatory dose of ibuprofen and analgesic dose of ibuprofen and acetaminophen in the treatment of patients with osteoarthritis of the knee. *N Engl J Med* 1991; 325:87–91.
3. Rosenbaum JF. The drug treatment of anxiety. *N Engl J Med* 1982; 306:401–404.
4. Ward NG, Bloom VL, Friedel RD. The effectiveness of tricyclic antidepressants in the treatment of coexisting pain and depression. *Pain* 1979;7:331–341.
5. Beaver WT. Combination analgesics. *Am J Med* 1985;77:38–53.
6. Piletta P, et al. Central analgesic effect of acetaminophen but not of aspirin. *Clin Pharmacol Ther* 1991;49:350–354.
7. Bonkowsky HL, Mudge GH, McMurtry RJ. Chronic hepatic inflammation and fibrosis due to low dose paracetamol. *Lancet* 1978;1: 1016–1018.
8. Levy G, Tsuchiva T. Salicylate accumulation kinetics in man. *N Engl J Med* 1972;287:430–432.
9. Brooks PM, Day RO. Nonsteroidal anti-inflammatory drugs—differences and similarities. *N Eng J Med* 1991;324:1716–1725.
10. Ferreira SH. Peripheral analgesia: mechanisms of the analgesic action of aspirin-like drugs and opiate antagonists. *Br J Clin Pharmacol* 1980;10:2379–2455.
11. Blackshear JL, Napier JS, Davidman M, Stillman MI. Renal complications of nonsteroidal anti-inflammatory drugs: identification and monitoring of those at risk. *Semin Arthritis Rheum* 1985;14: 163–175.
12. Swainson CP, Griffiths P. Acute and chronic effects of sulindac on renal function in chronic renal disease. *Clin Pharmacol Ther* 1985;37: 298–300.
13. Byron MA, Mowat AG. Corticosteroid prescribing in rheumatoid arthritis—the fiction and the fact. *Br J Rheum* 1985;24:164–166.
14. Friedman DM, Moore MA. The efficacy of intraarticular corticosteroids for osteoarthritis of the knee. *Arthritis Rheum* 1978;21:556–559.
15. Wyke B. The neurology of joints in osteoarthritis. *Ann Rheum Dis* 19:257–261, 1981.
16. Arnold CC, Lemper RK, Linderholm H. Intraosseous hypertension and pain in the knee. *J Bone Joint Surg* 1975;57:360–363.
17. Hollander JL. Treatment of osteoarthritis of knee. *Arthritis Rheum* 1960;3:564–569.
18. Wright V, et al. Intraarticular therapy in osteoarthritis: comparison of hydrocortisone acetate and hydrocortisone tertiary butylacetate. *Ann Rheum Dis* 1960;19:257.
19. Butler M, et al. A new model of osteoarthritis in rabbits. III: Evaluation of antiarthrosic effects of selected drugs administered intraarticularly. *Arthritis Rheum* 1983;26:1380.
20. Kovar PA, et al. Supervised fitness walking in patients with osteoarthritis of the knees. A randomized controlled trial. *Ann Intern Med* 1992; 116:529–534.
21. Felson DT, et al. Weight loss reduces the risk of symptomatic knee osteoarthritis in women: the Framingham study. *Ann Intern Med* 1992; 116:535–539.
22. Davis P, Harth M (eds). Proceedings—therapeutic innovation in rheumatoid arthritis: worldwide auranofin symposium. *J Rheum* 1982; 90(Suppl 8):1–209.
23. Champion GD, et al. Auranofin in rheumatoid arthritis. *J Rheum* 1982;9(Suppl 8):137.
24. Cooperating Clinics Committee of the American Rheumatism Association. A controlled trial of gold salt therapy in rheumatoid arthritis. *Arthritis Rheum* 1973;16:353–358.
25. Dixon A St J, et al. Synthetic D(-) penicillamine in rheumatoid arthritis. Double blind controlled study of a high and low dose regimen. *Ann Rheum Dis* 1975;34:416–421.
26. Hunter T, et al. Azathioprine in rheumatoid arthritis: a long term follow up study. *Arthritis Rheum* 1975;18:15–20.
27. Kremer JM, Lee JK. The safety and efficacy of the use of methotrexate in long term therapy of rheumatoid arthritis. *Arthritis Rheum* 1986;29:822–831.
28. Cooperating Clinics Committee of the American Rheumatism Association. Controlled trial of cyclophosphamide in rheumatoid arthritis. *N Engl J Med* 1970;283:883–889.
29. Adams EM, et al. Hydroxychloroquine in the treatment of rheumatoid arthritis. *Am J Med* 1983;75:321–326.
30. Robinson HS, et al. Evaluation of a province-wide physical therapy monitoring service in an arthritis control program. *J Rheum* 1980; 7:387.

31. Kelly WN, Fox IH. Gout and related disorders of purine metabolism. In: Kelly WM, Harris E, Ruddy S, Sledge C, eds. *Textbook of rheumatology*, ed 2. Philadelphia: WB Saunders, 1985:1382–1388.
32. Wallace SL. The treatment of the acute attack of gout. *Clin Rheum Dis* 1977;3:133–143.
33. Wallace SL. Colchicine. *Semin Arthritis Rheum* 1974;3:369.
34. Yu TF, Gutman AB. Efficacy of colchicine prophylaxis in gout. *Ann Intern Med* 1961;35:179–192.
35. Brewis I. Single daily dose allopurinol. *Ann Rheum Dis* 1975;34:256–259.
36. Yu TF. Milestones in the treatment of gout. *Am J Med* 1974;56:676–685.
37. Emmerson BT. A comparison of uricosuric agents in gout with special reference to sulfinpyrazone. *Med J Aust* 1963;1:839–844.
38. Cogen L, et al. Medical management of the painful shoulder. *Bull Rheum Dis* 1982;32:88–92.
39. Goldie I. Epicondylitis lateralis humeroepicondyalgie or tennis elbow. *Acta Chir Scand Suppl* 1964;339:1.
40. Muckart RD. Stenosing tendovaginitis of abductor policis longus and extensor pollicis brevis at the radial styloid (de Quervain's disease). *Clin Orthop* 1964;33:201–207.
41. Larsson LG, Baum J. The syndrome of anserine bursitis. *Arthritis Rheum* 1985;28:1062–1065.
42. Sheon RP, Moscowitz RW, Goldberg VM. *Soft tissue rheumatic pain: recognition, management, prevention*. Philadelphia: Lea & Febiger, 1982:219–222.
43. Healy LA, et al. Polymyalgia rheumatica and giant cell arthritis. *Arthritis Rheum* 1971;14:138–141.

CHAPTER **37**

Evaluation and Management of Nonarticular Rheumatic Pain Disorders: Fibromyalgia Syndrome

Robert W. Simms

Fibromyalgia syndrome is the term employed to describe a musculoskeletal pain disorder characterized by the presence of chronic, widespread pain in muscles and joints, fatigue, sleep disturbance, and a variety of other somatic symptoms. It is among the most common rheumatologic conditions associated with chronic pain, second only to osteoarthritis in estimated prevalence in the general population. This condition was formerly called *fibrositis,* but this term is obsolete now that there is no evidence of muscle or joint inflammation. Fibromyalgia remains a controversial syndrome because of the lack of objective findings and the association with psychiatric conditions. It has also been linked to other controversial pain syndromes, including chronic fatigue syndrome, irritable bowel syndrome, and Gulf War syndrome. Much effort has been devoted to understanding the pathophysiology of the disorder, its clinical features, and management, and although significant progress has occurred, much remains unknown.

CLINICAL FEATURES AND DIAGNOSIS

Fibromyalgia syndrome is characterized by the presence of chronic, widespread musculoskeletal pain, generally associated with fatigue, disturbed sleep, and a variety and variable number of associated somatic complaint (1). The condition is approximately ten times more common in women than in men and has been described in virtually all age groups. There appears to be no clear socioeconomic risk factors, although epidemiological studies have been largely confined to industrial countries, and the prevalence of fibromyalgia in developing countries is currently unknown. It is often described in lay press and media reports as a relatively new

affliction of the latter portion of the twentieth century; however, medical reports that describe patients with symptoms of fibromyalgia date back as far as the eighteenth century (1). The term *fibrositis* was initially coined at the turn of the twentieth century with descriptions of muscle inflammation at the site of biopsies, but this term was abandoned approximately 15 years ago when it became certain that no inflammation could be found (2). Early attempts to define the syndrome were made by a number of investigators, all of whom developed their own *a priori* criteria. Common among these criteria was the observation of increased muscle tenderness, so-called trigger points, although the various criteria differed in the number of required trigger points and their location (3,4). In 1990, the American College of Rheumatology convened a committee of experts to devise classification criteria for the diagnosis of fibromyalgia syndrome (5). The committee employed an accepted methodology for the design of the study, i.e., patients with the syndrome were identified by the experts using *a priori* criteria. These patients, a set of normals and a disease control group (patients with symptoms that could be clinically confused with fibromyalgia syndrome), were then evaluated by a standardized assessment tool administered by a blinded observer. The factors that distinguished the patients from the controls were: (a) chronic widespread pain (defined as above and below the waist on both sides of the body) and (b) 9 of 11 bilateral tender locations or tender points (5). These criteria were shown to have high sensitivity and specificity and have now become the de facto standard for the diagnosis in clinical studies and in practice settings.

Early studies of fibromyalgia also identified several important clinical features, including the associated sleep disturbance and the association with psychiatric disorders. Most patients with fibromyalgia complain of poor sleep. This sleep disturbance consists of difficulty with getting to sleep, frequent awakenings, and early morning awakening. Formal sleep studies in patients with fibromyalgia identified a peculiar sleep electroencephalographic (EEG) pattern known as the alpha-delta sleep abnormality (6). This abnormality consisted of the normal awake EEG pattern, alpha wave sleep, superimposed on the deep sleep EEG pattern, delta waves (6). This pattern could be duplicated in normal controls by partially awakening them from deep sleep with a subliminal buzzer. This could also temporarily induce fibromyalgia-like symptoms the next morning in healthy controls (7). The alpha-delta pattern was identified in the majority of patients with fibromyalgia syndrome, initially suggesting that it might be important in the pathophysiology of the condition and might have diagnostic value. Subsequent studies found that the alpha-delta pattern was not specific to fibromyalgia and was found in a number of other conditions, including posttraumatic pain syndromes and depression (8).

A cardinal feature of fibromyalgia syndrome is the presence of increased tenderness at muscle and tendon insertion sites. Early criteria studies emphasized the significance of "tender points" and "control points" (4). "Control points" were anatomical locations, which were thought to be nontender in patients with fibromyalgia syndrome. These included the forehead, thumbnail, forearm, and dorsum of the foot (4). Tender points were also initially thought to have pathophysiologic significance because several biopsy studies suggested subtle abnormalities in muscle metabolism (see section on pathophysiology) (9). Subsequently, however, patients with fibromyalgia were found to be tender essentially all over, even at the *a priori* designated control sites, indicating that tenderness "all over" was the result of a lowered pain threshold (10). Additionally, carefully controlled studies of tender point locations failed to confirm metabolic abnormalities (2,9,11). The ACR classification criteria specify the location of these tender sites at the occiput, low cervical region, trapezius (midpoint), supraspinatus insertion, second rib, lateral epicondyle, upper gluteal insertion, greater trochanter, and medial knee (5). These anatomic locations function therefore as convenient sites to quickly elicit evidence of a low pain threshold.

Several studies have suggested that the number of tender points correlates with the degree of psychological distress (12,13). In one recent study, 289 subjects, who had demonstrated psychological distress (General Health Questionnaire score > or = 2), had a tender point examination and in-depth psychological evaluation (13). In addition, subjects were interviewed about a number of adverse childhood experiences. The 99 subjects with five or more tender points were compared with the remaining 190 subjects. A high tender point count (> or = 5) was associated with low levels of self-care (odds ratio [OR] 2.4, 95% confidence interval [95% CI] 1.1–5.0), reports of a greater number of

somatic symptoms (OR 2.2, 95% CI 1.0–4.9), high levels of fatigue (OR 3.3, 95% CI 1.7–6.3), and a pattern of illness behavior characterized by increased medical care usage (OR 4.2, 95% CI 2.1–8.4). Those with high tender point counts were substantially more likely to report adverse childhood experiences, including loss of parents (OR 2.1, 95% CI 1.1–3.9) and abuse (OR 6.9, 95% CI 2.0–24.6). The authors of this study suggested that these data add further weight to the hypothesis that tender points, as part of the fibromyalgia syndrome, are strongly associated with specific components of psychological distress, as well as characteristics of somatization and its antecedents (13).

ASSOCIATED DISORDERS

Many associated conditions have been described with fibromyalgia. One of the most important has been the myofascial pain syndromes. Myofascial pain syndromes comprise a group of regional chronic pain syndromes that share with fibromyalgia syndromes increased soft tissue tenderness and the absence of objective abnormalities by laboratory testing. They differ from fibromyalgia in the regional as opposed to generalized location of pain. Most frequently the myofascial pain syndromes involve the neck and shoulder girdle but may also involve the lower extremities and the face. Myofascial pain syndromes were initially thought to be accompanied by localized muscle tenderness that produce radiating symptoms or "trigger points," a local "twitch response," and palpable "taut bands" (14,15). These examination features were found to have no diagnostic sensitivity or specificity in a study involving blinded observers who evaluated preselected patients with fibromyalgia and myofascial pain syndrome (16). More importantly, myofascial pain syndromes were found to have symptoms common to patients with fibromyalgia syndrome, including fatigue, sleep disturbance, and depression (17). Both fibromyalgia syndrome and the more localized myofascial syndromes are frequently accompanied by numbness and tingling, although neurologic findings in both disorders are normal. Further underlining the similarity between these conditions is the observation that myofascial pain syndromes appear to frequently evolve into fibromyalgia syndrome (15).

Although fibromyalgia syndrome most frequently occurs independently of other musculoskeletal disorders, the ACR diagnostic criteria do not exclude other arthritis conditions in order to establish the diagnosis (5). Fibromyalgia may therefore occur concomitantly with conditions such as rheumatoid arthritis or systemic lupus erythematosus, which are also associated with chronic pain. In one study the prevalence of fibromyalgia syndrome, among a cohort of patients with systemic lupus, approached 40% (18). Furthermore, patients with fibromyalgia and lupus were more likely to be unemployed and receiving welfare or medical disability benefits compared to patients with lupus alone. The patients with lupus and fibromyalgia did not differ from their lupus counterparts without fibromyalgia with respect to measures of lupus activity such as the level of anti-DNA antibodies, serum complement levels, or levels of the erythrocyte sedimentation rate (18).

It appears that a variety of infectious conditions are associated with fibromyalgia syndrome. These infections include viral infections, such as Coxsackie's virus, parvovirus B19, human immunodeficiency virus, and hepatitis C (19–23). Lyme disease has also been linked to the development of fibromyalgia syndrome (24,25). The precise nature of the association between infectious conditions and fibromyalgia is uncertain. It does not appear that active infection is present at the time fibromyalgia is clinically apparent. Most of the studies reporting the association with fibromyalgia syndrome and infectious conditions are cross-sectional and detail old or prior infection rather than active infection. It is possible that viral infections may trigger fibromyalgia syndrome or, alternately, that both may share an associated feature. In the case of HIV infection, for example, the presence of depression, associated with HIV infection, is a strong risk factor for the development of fibromyalgia syndrome (21).

Fibromyalgia syndrome also shares many features with chronic fatigue syndrome, a disorder that early reports linked to chronic Epstein Barr virus infection (26,27). The association of chronic fatigue syndrome with EBV was later refuted, and no known virus has, to date, been conclusively associated with chronic fatigue syndrome. Fibromyalgia syndrome and chronic fatigue syndrome share many demographic and clinical features, including the predominance among females, the presence of debilitating fatigue, sleep disturbance, musculoskeletal pain, and self-reported impairment in concentration and short-term memory. Neither chronic fatigue syndrome nor fibromyalgia syndrome possess pathognomonic signs or diagnostic tests that have been validated in scientific studies (28–31). Furthermore, fibromyalgia and chronic fatigue syndrome have a similar prevalence of associated depression (29,30, 32). Studies that have examined the overlap between the two conditions indicate that a substantial proportion of patients with fibromyalgia meet proposed criteria for chronic fatigue syndrome and vice versa (28,33–36). At this time it appears logical to group these two conditions together.

EPIDEMIOLOGY

The development of classification criteria for the diagnosis of fibromyalgia facilitated subsequent epidemiological studies to identify the prevalence and demographic features of the syndrome. Furthermore, the advent of epidemiological studies facilitated studies of the factors involved in the development of the disorder. Early reports suggested that psychiatric disorders found in high prevalence among patients were the result of a selection bias: Patients who were seen in specialty clinics that reported the association were more likely to have a high prevalence of psychiatric disorders. For the first time, epidemiological studies could

explore the nature of this association to determine if the prevalence of psychiatric disease among the general population of patients with fibromyalgia had a similar prevalence to that reported in series of patients seen in specialty clinics. Later prospective studies could also explore the controversial question as to whether depression and other psychiatric diseases preceded the development of the condition or occurred subsequently: the key "chicken or egg" question, which fueled many years of debate.

Initial clinic-based studies estimated the prevalence of fibromyalgia to about 10% of general medical outpatients and up to 20% of rheumatology outpatients. Almost 90% were women between the ages of 35 and 55. The initial, large population-based telephone survey, to employ the ACR classification criteria, surveyed approximately 3000 adults in Wichita, Kansas, for the presence of chronic pain (37,38). Respondents were categorized into those who experienced no pain, regional pain, and widespread pain. Chronic widespread pain occurred in 10.6% of the sample. A subgroup of 391 individuals, including 193 with widespread pain, were examined and interviewed in detail. On the basis of this sample, the investigators estimated the prevalence of fibromyalgia in the general population to be 3.4% for women and 0.5% for men, with the age-specific prevalence in women increasing with age to a high of 7% among women aged 60–70. A cross-sectional postal survey of approximately 2000 adults in northern England found a prevalence of chronic widespread pain of 11.2%, although the age-specific prevalence among women was approximately evenly distributed (39). Both of these initial cross-sectional studies found strong correlations of widespread chronic pain with measures of depression and anxiety, indicating that referral bias was not likely to be an important explanatory factor in the association of fibromyalgia and psychiatric disorders and that depression specifically was probably a constitutive feature of the condition (37–39). Further support for the constitutive nature of depression came from another population-based, case-control survey of chronic widespread pain in 1953 subjects (40). Study subjects completed a questionnaire that included a pain assessment and the 12-item General Health Questionnaire (GHQ-12). Of 710 subjects scoring > 1 on the GHQ-12, 301 were assessed further using a structured psychiatric interview and detailed assessment of medical records to identify cases of mental disorder, in accordance with criteria of the tenth edition of the *International Classification of Diseases*. The association between chronic widespread pain and mental disorder was modeled using logistic regression, adjusting for possible confounders including age, sex, and nonresponders. The overall estimated population prevalence of mental illness was 11.9%. The odds of having a mental disorder for subjects with, versus those without, chronic widespread pain were 3.18 (95% confidence interval 1.97–5.11). Most subjects with mental disorders were diagnosed as having mood and anxiety disorders. Only three cases of somatoform disorders were identified, and all were associated with pain (40).

Several population-based studies have assessed the prevalence of tenderness in the general population (13,37). Both of the largest studies of chronic widespread pain in the general population found that tenderness was distributed as a continuum. In the Kansas study, tender point counts were distributed as a continuum in both men and women (38). In the English study there was a trend observed between the number of sites of pain and the number of tender points detected (13). Both studies suggest that fibromyalgia syndrome may not be a discrete entity but rather in some sense represents an arbitrary designation at one end of the continuum of pain and tenderness in the general population.

NATURAL HISTORY AND OUTCOME

The natural history of fibromyalgia syndrome is relatively unknown. There is limited data available on the natural history, and it is all derived from small studies. Most of these studies suggest that the majority of patients with fibromyalgia continue to have symptoms over time. Kennedy and colleagues performed a 10-year followup study of a small group of patients who were initially part of a therapeutic trial (41). Patients reported at the 10-year followup that their symptom severity was essentially unchanged but that overall they rated themselves as doing better. The authors interpreted this to mean that the patients were coping better with their symptoms (41). Two of 30 patients in this small study committed suicide, highlighting the importance of adequate identification and treatment of depression in this population of patients.

Disability associated with chronic pain syndromes without an objective diagnostic test or indication of severity remains a hotly contested issue (42–45). Several studies have attempted to assess the prevalence of work disability in fibromyalgia syndrome. In the largest population-based survey of fibromyalgia syndrome in the United States, high self-reported rates of disability were found (38). Among patients attending rheumatology clinics with an interest in fibromyalgia (and therefore likely biased in favor of more severely affected patients), almost 15% of patients were receiving Social Security disability payments compared to 2.2% of the general population (46). Because no independent measure of symptom severity exists in fibromyalgia, assessment of disabling symptoms is entirely dependent on patient's self-report. A number of authors have questioned the validity of self-reporting under these circumstances and raise the concern of exaggerated or even falsified symptom reporting (44–48). Others have suggested that concerns about exaggeration or malingering have been overblown and that the potential harm of denying justifiable disability is much greater (42). They point to the monetary disincentives for most workers to go on disability. Additionally, one small study found that monetary awards for disability associated with posttraumatic fibromyalgia did not result in improved symptoms following the monetary award.

PATHOPHYSIOLOGY

Muscle Studies

Because patients with fibromyalgia syndrome complain of pain in and around muscles, early interest in the syndrome focused on muscles. Early uncontrolled biopsy studies suggested that muscle ischemia could explain pain and tenderness that characterize the syndrome (9). These reports, in turn, fueled many studies that used a variety of methodologies to examine this possibility (1). A number of these reports found subtle changes in muscle metabolic parameters and suggested that fibromyalgia syndrome might be a type of metabolic muscle disease. The early studies, however, failed to control for the generally poor level of muscle conditioning that was found to occur in fibromyalgia syndrome patients. Because muscle deconditioning may produce reversible metabolic changes, the failure to control for this phenomenon was an important methodologic shortcoming. When muscle conditioning was adequately controlled for, no metabolic abnormalities could be detected (11).

Role of Disordered Sensory Processing

Allodynia is the abnormal experience of severe pain evoked by light touch (i.e., nonnociceptive pain or the perception of pain evoked by nonpainful stimulus) and occurs in a variety of disorders, including postherpetic neuralgia or phantom limb syndrome. There is increasing evidence that the phenomenon of allodynia may be relevant to the understanding of fibromyalgia. As indicated earlier, patients with fibromyalgia do not have focal areas of increased muscle tenderness but rather display a general lowering of pain threshold. This finding has led to the concept that perhaps a central abnormality in fibromyalgia is the result of disordered sensory processing. Several recent studies have documented abnormal pain processing in patients with fibromyalgia syndrome, perhaps indicating an abnormality in the normal inhibitory efferent spinal cord pathways that modulate pain perception. Somatosensory evoked potentials evaluate the electroencephalographic signals that can be measured in skull electrodes in response to peripheral sensory stimuli. Gibson and colleagues reported an increased late nociceptive evoked somatosensory response in 10 patients with fibromyalgia syndrome compared to 10 matched controls (50). Lorenz and colleagues found increased amplitude of evoked somatosensory potentials in patients with fibromyalgia syndrome compared to controls after laser stimulation of the skin (51). This finding occurred despite controlling for hypervigilance (the conditioned expectation response, which can confound these sort of studies) by using interspersed auditory stimuli. Interestingly, the somatosensory potentials evoked in response to these auditory stimuli were no different in patients with fibromyalgia syndrome than in control subjects (51).

The mechanism by which abnormal pain processing may occur in fibromyalgia syndrome remains unknown, but investigators have postulated that abnormally increased nociceptive transmission may occur, or perhaps decreased efferent inhibitory neuronal input may be to blame. Substance P, a putative, nociceptive transmitter, has been found to be increased in cerebrospinal fluid in patients with fibromyalgia syndrome, lending support to the former hypothesis (52,53). Curiously, one study did not find increased substance P in the cerebrospinal fluid of patients with chronic fatigue syndrome (54).

Neuroendocrine Studies (HPA)/Autonomic Nervous System

The lack of detectable abnormalities in muscle has led investigators, more recently, to pursue the central nervous system as the potential location of physiologic disturbance in fibromyalgia syndrome. Because the hypothalamic-pituitary-adrenal axis is thought to play an important role in the physiologic response to physical and emotional stress, investigators have studied this system in both fibromyalgia and chronic fatigue syndrome. Furthermore, hypothalamic corticotropin-releasing hormone (CRH), which stimulates the HPA axis, is also known to stimulate the central control nuclei of the sympathetic nervous system and inhibit ascending pain pathways.

In aggregate, the overall pattern of HPA axis function in both fibromyalgia and chronic fatigue syndrome appears similar in that basal urinary cortisol is low compared to healthy subjects, although there may be differences in adrenocorticotropin and cortisol responses to corticotropin-releasing hormone (27,55). In contrast to the HPA axis profile in fibromyalgia and chronic fatigue syndrome, the HPA axis of major depression appears to reflect hyperfunction. Nonmelancholic forms of depression, however, seem to have an HPA profile similar to that of fibromyalgia and chronic fatigue syndromes (56).

A number of reports recently have found evidence of autonomic nervous system dysfunction in fibromyalgia syndrome using a variety of techniques, including tilt table testing to assess neurally mediated hypotension and assessment of heart rate variability (57–61). One recent study has also potentially linked the HPA axis dysfunction to autonomic dysfunction in fibromyalgia (62). Interleukin-6 (IL-6), a cytokine capable of stimulating hypothalamic CRH release, was administered to fibromyalgia patients and controls. Compared to the controls, patients with fibromyalgia were found to have exaggerated norepinephrine responses, heart rate increases, and delayed corticotropin release, possibly consistent with a defect in hypothalamic CRH neural function, resulting in abnormal regulation of the sympathetic nervous system (62). These findings suggest what may be a lowered baseline tone of the HPA axis and autonomic nervous system in fibromyalgia. Whether these abnormalities represent cause or effect, however, remain unknown.

Cerebral Blood Flow Studies

Because it is known that regional alterations in cerebral blood flow occur in response to painful stimuli, it was logical for investigators to study regional blood flow in patients with fibromyalgia syndrome. Mountz and colleagues performed single photon emission computed tomography of the brain in 10 patients with fibromyalgia and 7 control subjects (63). Low regional blood flow was found in the caudate and hemithalamus in patients compared with control subjects and correlated with pain threshold but not with psychological status. This study points to possible disturbances in brain function in patients with fibromyalgia, although the possible confounding effects of medication, the influence of depression, sex differences in regional blood flow, and small numbers of study subjects warrant further study.

Studies of Psychological Disturbance

Fibromyalgia syndrome has been frequently associated with psychological disturbance, especially depression, although it has been hotly debated as to whether depression is a cause or effect of fibromyalgia. Initial studies that utilized psychiatric outcome measures such as the Minnesota Multiphasic Personality Inventory (MMPI) and showed a high rate of depression among patients with fibromyalgia were criticized because inherent symptoms of fibromyalgia, such as fatigue and unexplained widespread pain, automatically increased scores for depression and hypochondriasis (64). However, subsequent studies using more accepted methods, such as structured psychiatric interviews, also found high lifetime rates of major depression, ranging from 34% to 74% (30,65–67).

The high association of depression and fibromyalgia was initially thought to be the result of selection bias. Patients attending clinics specializing in fibromyalgia were thought to be more likely to possess high rates of psychiatric distress because of more severe symptoms (68). The finding of similar high levels of depression and psychiatric distress in a specialty clinic sample of patients and in patients from a population-based sample, however, agued that psychiatric distress is more inherent to the syndrome than a feature of health care-seeking behavior (38,39). Furthermore, individuals who meet criteria for fibromyalgia but who have never sought medical care for their symptoms ("nonpatients") have rates of depression that closely approximate those fibromyalgia patients who attend specialty clinics (69).

Several studies have suggested that depression precedes the development of fibromyalgia or widespread chronic pain (30,69,71). Silman and colleagues performed a prospective population-based study of chronic widespread pain among approximately 2000 adults (72). The strongest predictor of the development of widespread pain was the presence of high levels of psychological distress, including depression, suggesting an important causal relationship between psychological distress and fibromyalgia.

Additional evidence for the importance of depression in fibromyalgia syndrome comes from its association with other conditions that are, themselves, associated with depression. These conditions include migraine headaches, irritable bowel syndrome, and panic disorder. Hudson and Pope have postulated, on this basis, that fibromyalgia, migraine, irritable bowel syndrome, chronic fatigue syndrome, major depression, and panic disorder represent an "affective spectrum" of disorders that share a common physiologic, possibly hereditary, abnormality (73).

Barsky has applied the term *functional somatic syndromes* to multiple chemical sensitivity, the sick building syndrome, repetitive stress injury, the side effects of silicone breast implants, the Gulf War syndrome, chronic whiplash, chronic fatigue syndrome, irritable bowel syndrome, and fibromyalgia (33). Common among these disorders is the prominence of symptoms, suffering, disability, and the consistent lack of demonstrable tissue abnormality. Barsky has emphasized that patients with these functional somatic syndromes "have explicit and highly elaborated self-diagnoses, and their symptoms are often refractory to reassurance, explanation, and standard treatment of symptoms. They share similar phenomenologies, high rates of cooccurrence, similar epidemiological characteristics, and higher-than-expected prevalences of psychiatric comorbidity." Barsky has identified four psychosocial factors that propel this cycle of symptom amplification: the belief that one has a serious disease; the expectation that one's condition is likely to worsen; the "sick role," including the effects of litigation and compensation; and the alarming portrayal of the condition as catastrophic and disabling (33).

In summary, there is a diverse body of literature concerning the pathophysiology of fibromyalgia. Few studies have been able to discern cause versus effect. The preponderance of available evidence supports a central mechanism for the disorder, which is closely linked to psychiatric disorders, including depression.

MANAGEMENT

Role of Patient Education

Knowledge of fibromyalgia and its natural history appears to lessen anxiety and allow better coping strategies. Patients and their families should be instructed to view fibromyalgia syndrome as a disorder that is not crippling and to know that there is effective therapy, although there is no specific cure. When possible, patients should be encouraged to take an active, self-help–oriented approach, rather than a passive approach, to management of their condition.

Pharmacologic Agents

Controlled clinical trials have established the efficacy of several classes of antidepressants in the treatment of fibromyalgia (74). These include the tertiary amine tricyclics and the specific serotonin reuptake inhibitors (SSRIs). A recent metaanalysis of antidepressant therapy of fibromyalgia syndrome evaluated 21 controlled trials, of which 16 involved tricyclic agents (75). Effect sizes were determined for measures of physician and patient overall assessment, pain, stiffness, tenderness, fatigue, and sleep quality. Compared with placebo, tricyclic agents were associated with effect sizes that were significantly greater than zero for all measurements (75). The largest improvements were in measures of sleep quality, with the smallest improvements being in measures of stiffness and tenderness (75).

A combination approach employing both fluoxetine 20 mg daily with amitriptyline 10 mg at bedtime was shown to be more effective than placebo and either agent alone (76). Nonsteroidal antiinflammatory agents have been shown to be relatively ineffective in relieving symptoms but continue to be preferred by patients over acetaminophen (77). Corticosteroids have also been shown to be ineffective in one short-term controlled clinical trial (78).

Nontraditional Therapies

A number of nontraditional therapies, such as biofeedback, electroacupuncture, and hypnotherapy, have been evaluated in controlled settings in fibromyalgia, and they appear to be modestly beneficial in the short term (78).

A large number of uncontrolled therapies have been advocated for treatment of fibromyalgia, including local injection of tender points, transcutaneous electrical nerve stimulation, cognitive behavioral therapies, chiropractic manipulation, physical and massage therapy, and myofascial therapies. The role of these therapies and their cost effectiveness remain uncertain. Additionally, various vitamins, food supplements, herbal therapies, and other "alternative" remedies have been advocated. These latter approaches, in particular, should be viewed with cautious skepticism unless they are shown to be effective in controlled clinical trials.

Role of Exercise

Low-level aerobic exercise has been shown to provide therapeutic benefit in a number of, but not all, controlled studies (79–83). Unfortunately, many patients in clinical practice are unable to comply with long-term aerobic activity, and some patients will not participate at all because of immediate postexertion exacerbation of symptoms. Nevertheless, for patients who are able to participate in regular long-term aerobic exercise programs, many are able to successfully wean off other medications and become more functional. Those who do not improve function tend to develop a vicious cycle of worsening pain and muscle deconditioning. Although vigorous regular aerobic exercise may be the most beneficial, significant benefit is derived from low-level aerobic fitness that can be accomplished with simple activities such as a regular walking program.

Multidisciplinary Approaches

In some settings—for selected, especially more severely affected, patients—therapeutic approaches that employ combinations of several simultaneous disciplines under one roof (typically in outpatient settings), such as biofeedback, pharmacologic intervention, and exercise therapies, have been advocated and may be helpful.

Suggested Approach

The management of fibromyalgia should include an assessment of severity of symptoms and particularly their functional impact. For patients with mild symptoms and minimal functional impact, patient education and low-level aerobic exercise may be sufficient. For most patients, the use of antidepressant therapies forms the cornerstone of current effective treatment approaches. For these patients, initiating therapy with a low-dose tricyclic agent (e.g., 10–20 mg of amitriptyline or nortriptyline at bedtime) is reasonable. If there is no response to the initial dose, and side effects (usually transient dry mouth and/or excessive drowsiness) are minimal or tolerable, the dose should be increased in 10-mg increments weekly until there is benefit. In general, doses that exceed 50 mg daily seem to confer little additional benefit if there is no response to lower doses. For patients with more severe symptoms and for those with associated depression, an SSRI combined with low-dose tricyclic is most effective. For patients with more severe or agitated depression, psychiatric consultation may be required for optimal management. Additionally, for selected highly symptomatic patients with or without major depression, pain management or multidisciplinary approaches may be required.

REFERENCES

1. Simms RW. Fibromyalgia syndrome: current concepts in pathophysiology, clinical features, and management. *Arthritis Care & Research* 1996;9(4):315–328.
2. Simms RW. Fibromyalgia is not a muscle disorder. *Am J Med Sci* 1998;315:346–350.
3. Yunus MB, Masi AT, et al. Primary fibromyalgia (fibrositis): clinical study of 50 patients with matched normal controls. *Semin Arth Rheum* 1981;11:151–171.
4. Clark S, Campbell SM, et al. Clinical characteristics of fibrositis. II. A "blinded," controlled study using standard psychological tests. *Arth Rheum* 1985;28(2):132–137.
5. Wolfe F, Smythe HA, et al. The American College of Rheumatology 1990 Criteria for the Classification of Fibromyalgia. Report of the Multicenter Criteria Committee [see comments]. *Arth Rheum* 1990;33(2):160–172.
6. Moldofsky H, Scarisbrick P, et al. Musculoskeletal symptoms and non-REM sleep disturbance in patients with fibrositis syndrome and healthy subjects. *Psychom Med* 1975;37:341–351.
7. Moldofsky H, Scarisbrick P. Induction of neurasthenic musculoskeletal pain in non-articular rheumatism ("fibrositis syndrome"). *Pain* 1976;5:65–71.
8. Moldofsky H, Wong MT, et al. Litigation, sleep, symptoms and disabilities in post-accident pain (fibromyalgia) [see comments]. *J Rheum* 1993;20(11):1935–1940.
9. Simms RW. Is there muscle pathology in fibromyalgia syndrome? *Rheumatic Diseases Clinics of North America* 1996;22(2):245–266.
10. Simms RW, Goldenberg DL, et al. Tenderness in 75 anatomic sites. Distinguishing fibromyalgia patients from controls. *Arth Rheum* 1988;31(2):182–187.
11. Simms RW, Roy SH, et al. Lack of association between fibromyalgia syndrome and abnormalities in muscle energy metabolism [see comments]. *Arth Rheum* 1994;37(6):794–800.
12. Wolfe F. The relation between tender points and fibromyalgia symptom variables: evidence that fibromyalgia is not a discrete disorder in the clinic. *Annals of the Rheumatic Diseases* 1997;56(4):268–271.
13. McBeth J, Macfarlane GJ, et al. The association between tender points, psychological distress, and adverse childhood experiences: a community-based study. *Arth Rheum* 1999;42(7):1397–1404.
14. Simons DG. Fibrositis/fibromyalgia: a form of myofascial trigger points? *American Journal of Medicine* 1986;81(3A):93–98.
15. Smythe H. Links between fibromyalgia and myofascial pain. *J Rheum* 1992;19:842–843.
16. Wolfe F, Simons DG, et al. The fibromyalgia and myofascial pain syndromes: a preliminary study of tender points and trigger points in persons with fibromyalgia, myofascial pain syndrome and no disease. *J Rheum* 1992;19(6):944–951.
17. Goldenberg DL. Fibromyalgia, chronic fatigue syndrome, and myofascial pain syndrome. *Current Opinion in Rheumatology* 1997;9(2):135–143.
18. Middleton GD, McFarlin JE, et al. The prevalence and clinical impact of fibromyalgia in systemic lupus erythematosus [see comments]. *Arth Rheum* 1994;37(8):1181–1188.
19. Nash P, Chard M, et al. Chronic coxsackie B infection mimicking primary fibromyalgia. *J Rheum* 1989;16(11):1506–1508.
20. Leventhal LJ, Naides SJ, et al. Fibromyalgia and parvovirus infection. *Arth Rheum* 1991;34(10):1319–1324.
21. Simms RW, Zerbini CA, et al. Fibromyalgia syndrome in patients infected with human immunodeficiency virus. The Boston City Hospital Clinical AIDS Team. *American Journal of Medicine* 1992;92(4):368–374.
22. Berg AM, Naides SJ, et al. Established fibromyalgia syndrome and parvovirus B19 infection. *J Rheum* 1993;20(11):1941–1943.
23. Buskila D, Shnaider A, et al. Fibromyalgia in hepatitis C virus infection. Another infectious disease relationship. *Archives of Internal Medicine* 1997;157(21):2497–2500.
24. Dinerman H, Steere AC. Lyme disease associated with fibromyalgia. *Annals of Internal Medicine* 1992;117(4):281–285.
25. Sigal,LH, Patella SJ. Lyme arthritis as the incorrect diagnosis in pediatric and adolescent fibromyalgia. *Pediatrics* 1992;90(4):523–528.
26. Buchwald D, Goldenberg DL, et al. The "chronic, active Epstein-Barr virus infection" syndrome and primary fibromyalgia. *Arth Rheum* 1987;30(10):1132–1136.
27. Buchwald D. Fibromyalgia and chronic fatigue syndrome: similarities and differences. *Rheumatic Diseases Clinics of North America* 1996;22(2):219–243.
28. Goldenberg,DL, Simms RW, et al. High frequency of fibromyalgia in patients with chronic fatigue seen in a primary care practice. *Arth Rheum* 1990;33(3):381–387.
29. Lane TJ, Manu P, et al. Depression and somatization in the chronic fatigue syndrome. *Am J Med* 1991;91: 335-344.
30. Hudson, JI., DL. Goldenberg, et al. Comorbidity of fibromyalgia with medical and psychiatric disorders. *Am J Med* 1992;92(4):363–367.
31. Schaefer KM. Sleep disturbances and fatigue in women with fibromyalgia and chronic fatigue syndrome. *Journal of Obstetric, Gynecologic, & Neonatal Nursing* 1995;24(3):229–233.
32. Abbey SE, Garfinkel PE. Chronic fatigue syndrome and depression: cause, effect, or covariate. *Rev Infect Dis* 1991;13(Suppl 1):S73–83.
33. Barsky AJ, Borus JF. Functional somatic syndromes. *Annals of Internal Medicine* 1999;130(11):910–921.
34. Robertson TJ. Misunderstood illnesses: fibromyalgia and chronic fatigue syndrome. *Alta RN* 1999;55(3):6–7.
35. Aaron LA, Burke MM, et al. Overlapping conditions among patients with chronic fatigue syndrome, fibromyalgia, and temporomandibular disorder. *Archives of Internal Medicine* 2000;160(2):221–227.
36. White KP, Speechley M, et al. Co-existence of chronic fatigue syndrome with fibromyalgia syndrome in the general population. A controlled study. *Scand J Rheum* 2000;29(1):44–51.

37. Wolfe F, Ross K, et al. Aspects of fibromyalgia in the general population: sex, pain threshold, and fibromyalgia symptoms. *J Rheum* 1995;22(1):151–156.

38. Wolfe F, Ross K, et al. The prevalence and characteristics of fibromyalgia in the general population. *Arth Rheum* 1995;38(1):19–28.

39. Croft P, Rigby AS, et al. The prevalence of chronic widespread pain in the general population. *J Rheum* 1993;20(4):710–713.

40. Benjamin S, Morris S, et al. The association between chronic widespread pain and mental disorder: a population-based study. *Arth Rheum* 2000;43(3):561–567.

41. Kennedy MJ, Goldenberg DL, et al. A prospective long-term study of fibromyalgia syndrome. *Arth Rheum* 1995;38.

42. Bennett RM. Fibromyalgia and the disability dilemma. A new era in understanding a complex, multidimensional pain syndrome [see comments]. *Arth Rheum* 1996;39(10):1627–1634.

43. Turk DC, Okifuji A, et al. Pain, disability, and physical functioning in subgroups of patients with fibromyalgia. *J Rheum* 1996;23(7):1255–1262.

44. Wolfe F, Potter J. Fibromyalgia and work disability: is fibromyalgia a disabling disorder? *Rheumatic Diseases Clinics of North America* 1996;22(2):369–391.

45. Cohen ML, Quintner JL. Fibromyalgia syndrome and disability: a failed construct fails those in pain. *Medical Journal of Australia* 1998;168(8):402–404.

46. Wolfe F, Anderson J, et al. A prospective, longitudinal, multicenter study of service utilization and costs in fibromyalgia [see comments]. *Arth Rheum* 1997;40(9):1560–1570.

47. White KP, Harth M, et al. Work disability evaluation and the fibromyalgia syndrome. *Semin Arth Rheum* 1995;24:371–381.

48. Hadler NM. If you have to prove you are ill, you can't get well. The object lesson of fibromyalgia. *Spine* 1996;21(20):2397–2400.

49. Romano TJ. Clinical experiences with post-traumatic fibromyalgia syndrome. *West Virginia Medical Journal* 1990;86(5):198–202.

50. Gibson S, Littlejohn G, et al. Altered heat pain thresholds and cerebral event-related potentials following painful CO_2 laser stimulation in subjects with FM syndrome. *Pain* 1994;58:185–183.

51. Lorenz J, Grasedyck K, et al. Middle and long latency somatosensory evoked potentials after painful laser stimulation in patients with fibromyalgia syndrome. *Electroencephalogr Clin Neurophysiol* 1996;100:165–68.

52. Vaeroy H, Helle R, et al. Elevated CSF levels of substance P and high incidence of Raynaud's phenomenon in patients with fibromyalgia: new features for diagnosis. *Pain* 1988;32(1):21–26.

53. Russell IJ, Orr MD, et al. Elevated cerebrospinal fluid levels of substance P in patients with the fibromyalgia syndrome. *Arth Rheum* 1994;37(11):1593–1601.

54. Evengard B, Nilsson CG, et al. Chronic fatigue syndrome differs from fibromyalgia. No evidence for elevated substance P levels in cerebrospinal fluid of patients with chronic fatigue syndrome. *Pain* 1998;78(2):153–155.

55. Crofford LJ, Pillemer SR, et al. Hypothalamic-pituitary-adrenal axis perturbations in patients with fibromyalgia. *Arth Rheum* 1994;37(11):1583–1592.

56. Crofford LJ, Engleberg NC, et al. Neurohormonal perturbations in fibromyalgia. *Baillieres Clinical Rheumatology* 1996;10(2):365–378.

57. Bou-Holaigah I, Calkins H, et al. Provocation of hypotension and pain during upright tilt table testing in adults with fibromyalgia. *Clinical & Experimental Rheumatology* 1997;15(3):239–246.

58. Martinez-Lavin M, Hermosillo AG, et al. Circadian studies of autonomic nervous balance in patients with fibromyalgia: a heart rate variability analysis. *Arth Rheum* 1998;41(11):1966–1971.

59. Cohen H, Neumann L, et al. Autonomic dysfunction in patients with fibromyalgia: application of power spectral analysis of heart rate variability. *Seminars in Arth Rheum* 2000;29(4):217–227.

60. Raj SR, Brouillard D, et al. Dysautonomia among patients with fibromyalgia: a noninvasive assessment. *J Rheum* 2000;27(11):2660–2665.

61. Martinez-Lavin M, Hermosillo AG. Autonomic nervous system dysfunction may explain the multisystem features of fibromyalgia. *Semin Arth Rheum* 2000;29(4):197–199.

62. Torpy D, Papanicolaou D, et al. Responses of the sympathetic nervous system and the hypothalamic-pituitary-adrenal axis to interleukin-6: a pilot study in fibromyalgia. *Arth Rheum* 2000;43:872–880.

63. Mountz JM, Bradley LA, et al. Fibromyalgia in women. Abnormalities of regional cerebral blood flow in the thalamus and the caudate nucleus are associated with low pain threshold levels. *Arth Rheum* 1995;38(7):926–938.

64. Pincus T, Callahan LF, et al. Elevated MMPI scores for hypochondriasis, depression, and hysteria in patients with rheumatoid arthritis reflect disease rather than psychological status. *Arth Rheum* 1986;29:1456–1466.

65. Kirmayer LJ, Robbins JM, et al. Somatization and depression in fibromyalgia syndrome. *American Journal of Psychiatry* 1988;145(8):950–954.

66. Ahles TA, Khan SA, et al. Psychiatric status of patients with primary fibromyalgia, patients with rheumatoid arthritis, and subjects without pain: a blind comparison of DSM-III diagnoses. *American Journal of Psychiatry* 1991;148(12):1721–1726.

67. Yunus MB, Ahles TA, et al. Relationship of clinical features with psychological status in primary fibromyalgia. *Arth Rheum* 1991;34(1):15–21.

68. Bennett RM. Fibromyalgia and the facts. Sense or nonsense. *Rheumatic Diseases Clinics of North America* 1993;19(1):45–59.

69. Aaron LA, Bradley LA, et al. Peceived physical and emotional trauma as precipitating events in fibromyalgia. Associations with health care seeking and disability status but not pain severity [see comments] *Arth Rheum* 1997;40(3):453–460.

70. Hudson JI, Hudson MS, et al. Fibromyalgia and major affective disorder: a controlled phenomenology and family history study. *American Journal of Psychiatry* 1985;14(4):441–446.

71. Hudson JI, Pope HG Jr. The relationship between fibromyalgia and major depressive disorder. *Rheumatic Diseases Clinics of North America* 1996;22(2):285–303.

72. Silman AJ, McBeth J, et al. Features of somatization predict onset of chronic widespread pain: results from a large prospectie population study. *Arth Rheum* 1998;41:S358.

73. Hudson JI, Pope HG. The concept of affective spectrum disorde: relationship to fibromyalgia and other syndromes of chronic fatigue and chronic muslce pain. *Baillieres Clinical Rheumatology* 1994;8(4):839–856.

74. Simms RW. Controlled trials of therapy in fibromyalgia syndrome. *Baillieres Clinical Rheumatology* 1994;8(4)917–934.

75. Arnold LM, Keck PE Jr, et al. Antidepressant treatment of fibromyalgia. A meta-analysis and review. *Psychosomatics* 2000;41(2):104–113.

76. Goldenberg D, Mayskiy M, et al. A randomized, double-blind crossover trial of fluoxetine and amitriptyline in the treatment of fibromyalgia. *Arth Rheum* 1996;39(11):1852–1859.

77. Wolfe F, Zhao F, et al. Preference for nonsteroidal anti-inflammatory drugs over acetaminophen by rheumatic disease patients: a survey of 1,799 patients with osteoarthritis, rheumatoid arthritis, and fibromyalgia. *Arth Rheum* 2000;43(2):378–385.

78. Clark S, Tindall E, et al. A double blind crossover trial of prednisone versus placebo in the treatment of fibrositis. *J Rheum* 1985;12(5):980–983.

79. McCain GA. Role of physical fitness training in the fibrositis/fibromyalgia syndrome. *American Journal of Medicine* 1986;81(3A):73–77.

80. Mengshoel AM, Komnaes HB, et al. The effects of 20 weeks of physical fitness training in female patients with fibromyalgia. *Clinical & Experimental Rheumatology* 1992;10(4)345–349.

81. Wigers SH, Stiles TC, et al. Effects of aerobic exercise versus stress management treatment in fibromyalgia. A 4.5 year prospective study. *Scandinavian J Rheum* 1996;25(2):77–86.

82. Gowans SE, deHueck A, et al. A randomized, controlled trial of exercise and education for individuals with fibromyalgia. *Arthritis Care & Research* 1999;12(2):120–128.

83. Meiworm L, Jakob E, et al. Patients with fibromyalgia benefit from aerobic endurance exercise. *Clin Rheumatol* 2000;19(4):253–257.

CHAPTER 38

Myofascial Pain: Evaluation and Treatment Strategies

A Focus on Brachial Plexus Traction Injury (Neurogenic Thoracic Outlet Syndrome)

Robert L. Knobler

Acute pain is a survival mechanism that allows us to escape noxious stimuli that may prove harmful. As such, the reflex response to acute pain is integrally associated with the "fight or flight" response. There is much evidence to link the sensory components of the nervous system, and both the effector arms of the somatic neuromuscular system and the autonomic nervous system, which serve as the functional anatomical arms of this survival response. If we are to get away, we must be able to both sense and respond to a potentially harmful stimulus by moving away.

Emotional stress lowers the threshold of these responses, making us more sensitive to even the lightest touch. It is in this context that we recognize myofascial pain syndrome, which is a major contributing element in the production of localized spasm and muscle tightness, subjectively perceived in this disorder as painful. It is specifically this driving component, the focal tightness and spasm of muscles, which is made worse by strenuous, persistent, or repetitive physical activity, that plays a large role in the generation of common complaints that characterize myofascial pain disorders.

It has been estimated that more than 40 million people in the United States are affected by chronic and recurrent manifestations of myofascial pain syndrome, making this the second most common reason, after upper respiratory infections, for seeking medical attention and for missing days from work (1). Therefore, the recognition of myofascial pain syndromes is an important component in the eval-

uation and treatment of individuals who complain of these common and chronic pain syndromes.

A confounding factor in the assessment of people suffering from myofascial pain is the fact that it is frequently observed in the context of other problems as well and that its features may be confused with other pain syndromes for which the approach to treatment may be quite different (2). Therefore, this chapter differentiates myofascial pain syndrome (3,4) from other disorders such as fibromyalgia (5,6), autoimmune disorders, and metabolic endocrinopathies and focuses on its connection to such disorders as brachial plexus traction injuries, with secondary complex regional pain syndrome, type I (reflex sympathetic dystrophy), and complex regional pain syndrome type II (causalgia).

Myofascial pain syndrome is a distinct disorder from fibromyalgia (7,8). Myofascial pain syndrome is best described as a local and regional musculoskeletal pain syndrome and is best recognized in association with the limb girdles of the upper or lower extremities or as variations of either neck and shoulder or low back pain and may also include the spectrum of migraine headaches and temporomandibular joint dysfunction. The neck pain can also reflect other entities that must be ruled out, such as heart disease, ulcers, gallstones, tumors, and metastatic lesions.

In contrast, fibromyalgia is characterized by the American College of Rheumatology (ACR) criteria as a diffusely painful disorder (9), present for greater than 3 months, with associated muscle tenderness in all body quadrants (11 of

18 tender points that are painful on palpation). To further confuse matters, the diagnosis of fibromyalgia may coexist with other musculoskeletal conditions, such as myofascial pain syndrome.

Fibromyalgia has been recognized in 1% to 5% of those attending primary care clinics and in up to 20% of those attending rheumatology clinics. Fibromyalgia is much more common in women than in men. It is associated in particular with a variety of other symptoms such as fatigue, sleep disturbances (awakening unrefreshed), morning stiffness, irritable bladder, bowel syndromes, and diffuse headaches. The pain is described as aching, nagging, and radiating and often is associated with spasms.

There are no specific laboratory tests to diagnose fibromyalgia, although elevation of substance P in the spinal fluid has been reported (10). However, this is a non-specific finding, as are many of the other features of fibromyalgia. It is the constellation of these findings, and the absence of other conditions to explain them, that helps to establish the diagnosis of fibromyalgia (11).

The differential diagnosis of fibromyalgia includes autoimmune diseases such as systemic lupus erythematosus (SLE), looking for low-grade fever and a positive antinuclear antibody (ANA) test; rheumatoid arthritis (RA) (which has a positive rheumatoid factor and isolated joint tenderness and joint swelling); polymyositis and polymyalgia rheumatica (which often have an elevated erythrocyte sedimentation rate [ESR], diffuse proximal muscle weakness, and elevated muscle enzymes); degenerative cervical and lumbar spine disease (which have specific neurological radicular or myelopathic symptoms and radiographic findings); cardiac or pulmonary disease (which can cause chest pain and includes angina and pulmonary embolism); and various endocrinopathies affecting the pituitary, adrenal, thyroid, and parathyroid glands (causing measurably hyper- or hypoactive states, as well as deficiencies of ovarian or testicular function; may present with such clinical features as diffuse muscle pains and/or carpal tunnel syndrome).

BRACHIAL PLEXUS INJURIES

Brachial plexus traction injuries are addressed in greater detail later as a principal contributing cause of myofascial pain syndrome. In particular, the neurogenic form of thoracic outlet syndrome is characterized by a regional distribution of pain around the neck, radiating up into the head and down into the upper back between the shoulder blades, under the arm, and under the breast across the chest, as well as down the arm to the elbow or all the way down to all the fingers of the hand. In the vascular form of thoracic outlet syndrome, when Adson's maneuver is performed, there is a positive pulse response (with the patient seated establish the radial pulse; rotate head and elevate chin to side of pulse; if negative, rotate head and elevate chin to opposite side; a decrease in the radial pulse indicates com-

pression of the vascular component by the anterior scalene to same side or cervical rib to opposite side). In the neurogenic form of thoracic outlet syndrome, paresthesias will occur with this maneuver.

Brachial plexus traction injuries may often be accompanied by complex regional pain syndrome type I (reflex sympathetic dystrophy), where there is no clear-cut electrographic demonstration of a brachial plexopathy, or by complex regional pain syndrome type II (causalgia), where there is either electromyographic (EMG) or nerve conduction velocity (NCV) evidence of a partial injury to a component of the brachial plexus.

Muscle pain is always present in myofascial pain syndrome to some degree. However, a strained muscle may not develop pain for hours or days, whereas an unused muscle will be painful with virtually any activity. Therefore, it is important to know the genesis of the onset of the muscle pain.

In addition, some muscle pain tends to lessen with activity, albeit limited activity. Consequently, this type of pain is often worst after the individual has been relatively immobile for a while, such as in the morning after sleep, causing a complaint of pain on awakening, or from sitting or standing in a relatively fixed position for a prolonged period. Repetitive movement tends to worsen muscle pain due to excessive sustained contraction. Stress can perpetuate sustained muscle contraction and thus worsen muscle pain (12).

The hallmark of myofascial pain syndrome is the trigger point, which may vary in presentation with regard to acute or chronic overload of the particular muscle. Typically, the trigger points will be found in regions of trauma or repetitive strain injuries.

Trigger points may be latent or active. An active trigger point is very painful to touch and feels like a "taut band" on direct palpation and can produce a local twitch response when injected, reflecting contraction of the muscle fibers, with radiation from this site. The taut band is believed to represent a dysfunctional motor endplate, releasing sensitizing nociceptive substances during its sustained contraction.

A latent trigger point is not usually painful clinically but may present as a taut band, identified by palpation, and become painful when overloaded. A secondary trigger point reflects overload in an area that is compensating for an active trigger point. A satellite trigger point is one that is within the zone of radiation of the active trigger point.

These definitions are operational and anecdotal. Treatments have focused on injection of the trigger point, with the initial goal of its inactivation (13–15). Although this may provide immediate, albeit transient, relief, this does not address the cause of the problem. Without elimination of the conditions that have maintained the trigger point, the pain will likely recur (14). Overall, the elimination of the underlying cause of the trigger point is often more difficult to accomplish, requiring both recognition of the source of the trigger point (i.e., a brachial plexus traction injury) and then its specific treatment, which may mean the need for surgical repair and/or lifestyle modifications (less load bearing).

Manual techniques for trigger point inactivation include physical maneuvers such as deep tissue massage, trigger point compression, and local and regional stretching, sometimes using cold "spray and stretch" techniques (16,17). If these manual techniques fail, there has been fairly equal success of trigger point inactivation by injection, whether local anesthetic, steroid, or "dry needling" was used as the therapeutic modality (2,13–15).

Physical therapy following trigger point injection has merit. The taut band of the trigger point can lead to muscle shortening and interference with the normal mobility of the affected muscles. Injection of trigger points can permit the return of more normal body mechanics and range of motion.

In order to better understand the basis upon which the clinical diagnosis may be established, it is essential to explore the fundamental clinical presentation of myofascial pain disorders and how suggested treatment strategies may be employed to reduce symptoms and gain better control of the symptom complex of the patient. We will proceed with a general overview, then provide a specific discussion of brachial plexus traction injuries, and conclude with a case history of a specific patient in an effort to provide a more practical illustration of the points raised.

History and Physical Examination

This approach begins by detailing the history of chronic pain and the circumstances in which it arose. The mnemonic "**COLIC**" may be used to describe the **C**haracter of the pain, its **O**nset, **L**ocalization, **I**ntensity, and **C**omments on associated symptoms.

History: Chief complaint—What is the problem that led to medical attention?

History of Present Illness: COLIC mnemonic

Character of pain—aching, burning, shooting, squeezing, throbbing, viselike

Onset of pain—Was there a precipitating event?
  Trauma—whiplash, spinal cord injury, sprain, or strain
  Repetitive stress injury (work history)
  Medical illness—multiple sclerosis, orthopedic or arthritic condition, surgical procedure, casting or immobilization

Localization of pain—laterality
  Head, face, jaw; neck, shoulder, chest; trunk, upper back, lower back, buttock; arm, forearm, wrist, hand, fingers; hip, thigh, knee, lower leg, ankle, foot, toes

Intensity of pain—intermittent or constant
  Mild, moderate, severe, rating on a verbal scale of 1–10
  What worsens pain—cold, dependent posture, activity?
  What improves pain—heat, rest, immobility, exercise?

Comments on associated symptoms—depression, sleep, fatigue, ability to work

Medical History: Operations (scar formation, positioning during surgery, length of surgical procedure), illnesses (especially a pain history, such as migraines), accidents (any injuries, no matter how long ago)

Family History: Parents, siblings, children—operations, illnesses, accidents; any family members affected by similar disorders; when they occurred (anniversary reactions)

Social History: Education, habits (smoking, drinking), work and work schedule, living arrangements, hobbies (weight lifting, archery, riflery)

Physical Examination
  General examination of organ systems
  Inspect for overall mobility and tender points versus trigger points
  Head, face, jaw
  Neck (range of motion-rotation, flexion-extension, trapezius), shoulders (supraclavicular/infraclavicular fossa), chest (inhalation-expiration)
  Spine (deformity, mobility), trunk, upper back, lower back, buttocks
  Arm, forearm, wrist, hand, fingers (abduction, grip, index finger-thumb opposition)
  Hip, thigh, knee, lower leg, ankle, foot, toes
  Mental Status Examination
    Orientation to time, place, person
    Immediate recall; calculations
  Cranial Nerve Examination
    Smell, visual acuity, eye movements, pupil reactions, fundi
    Facial sensation, facial symmetry
    Hearing, swallowing, shoulder shrug, and tongue movements
  Motor Examination
    Strength, bulk (atrophy), tone
    Coordination, posture, movements, gait
    Upper and lower extremities
  Sensory Examination
    Light touch, position, temperature (warm, cold)
    Pressure, allodynia
    Upper and lower extremities
  Reflex Examination
    Biceps, brachioradialis, triceps
    Knee jerk, ankle jerk, Babinski

Diagnostic Review
  Evaluate chief complaint
  Is it localized or regional? versus Is it generalized?

What are the associated symptoms?
Localized headache versus diffuse headache?
Irritable bladder? Irritable bowel syndrome?
Sleep disturbance (falling asleep vs. staying asleep)?
Is the pain referred? Is the pain in multiple locations
on palpation?

Brachial Plexus Traction Injury

The assessment of neck pain requires a knowledge of the potential anatomical structures that may serve as the structural basis for the pain and what may be the source of dysfunction that has led to the pain. These include the vertebrae, ligaments, muscles, nerve roots, and blood vessels, among other structures.

A differential diagnosis is formulated, and the further evaluation of the patient is focused on distinguishing between potential causes of the neck pain (brachial plexus traction injuries, myofascial pain, tension headaches, and both carotid and vertebral artery dissection). At this point, it is also helpful to consider common occurrences that may also be present in the background, even if not the sole source of the pain, such as degenerative spine disease.

Throughout all, emphasis must be placed on taking a good history, performing a thorough examination, and carefully evaluating studies ordered, to be certain that important diagnostic considerations are not prematurely eliminated.

Pain-sensitive structures under consideration generally include the skin and subcutaneous tissues, including lymph nodes, muscles, blood vessels, bones and joints, nerve roots, and the spinal cord. We will focus primarily on brachial plexus traction injuries and their relationship to myofascial pain and tension headaches.

Most people over the age of 30 will already have some form of spondylosis in the cervical spine, most commonly at C-5–6, because back-and-forth movement of the cervical spine is typically greatest at this position. Therefore, it is not unexpected to find this pathoanatomical finding in the cervical spine following a whiplash injury because it is commonly observed in the general population. In contrast, straightening of the cervical spine, visible on either a plain x-ray or a cervical MRI, with loss of the normal lordotic curve, suggests the presence of paracervical muscle spasm and helps to corroborate the subjective complaint of neck pain following a whiplash injury.

Cervical spondylosis can complicate a whiplash injury further by tethering the nerve roots at the commonly spondylitic levels, such as C-5–6, and it is therefore not unusual to see a secondary problem of radiculopathy superimposed upon the whiplash injury. At its most extreme, this type of injury can involve trunks or divisions of the brachial plexus, with symptoms that involve not only the neck and head, but also the whole hand.

It should be noted that the mechanism of the injury varies a bit depending on the nature of the restraint placed on the patient at the time of the motor vehicle accident.

Lap belts alone will allow the body to move forward, while the inertia of the head will lead to an initial hyperextension and then hyperflexion. Even with a shoulder harness in place, these movements will occur, but hyperflexion may precede the hyperextension. In addition, there may be significant stresses on the cervical spine due to lateral movements of the head on the shoulders.

Slow motion movies of crash test dummies obtained through the Insurance Institute of Highway Safety provide highly informative demonstrations of the extent and force of movement elicited by even relatively low-speed collisions. There is a somewhat greater frequency of this type of injury in women, possibly reflecting a less muscular neck in women, with less tissue bulk to restrict the range of movements on impact.

The source of pain may derive from injured muscle and surrounding soft tissues initially, but this has the propensity to become a chronic problem and oftentimes with relatively few objective findings. It is for this reason, compounded by the potential for financial gain through insurance claims, that this has become a quite controversial clinical issue. Nevertheless, it has been observed that myofascial pain, possibly reflecting trauma to small nerve fibers from scar formation following the acute phase of injury with nociceptive pain reflecting the trauma to small blood vessels and surrounding tissues.

Myofascial pain is characterized by trigger points that are tender on direct palpation, radiate pain away from the maximum point of tenderness, and by a regional, rather than generalized, distribution. A myofascial trigger point is distinguished from a fibromyalgia tender point by its local twitch response on needling.

Although pain of cervical spine origin typically arises in the neck and radiates up the back of the head, it may also be projected into the shoulder and arm on the more affected side. It is also important to consider the potential contribution of referred pain, such as that from pressure on the diaphragm that radiates to the shoulder, when formulating a differential diagnosis. The cardinal feature of pain of cervical spine origin is that there are tenderness and limitation of motion of the cervical spine. MRI studies often reveal a pattern of stenosis at one or more neural foraminal levels, with corresponding changes in the related dermatomal patterns on EMG/NCV studies.

In contrast, pain arising in the region of the brachial plexus often radiates into the shoulder and is worsened by attempts to perform tasks that involve elevation of the arm, specifically if this involves elevation above shoulder level. Many focus attention on Adson's maneuver, obliteration of the radial pulse with rotation of the head, as the most meaningful test for this disorder. However, this test identifies only a vascular compromise, which may be present in some forms of thoracic outlet syndrome (vascular thoracic outlet syndrome).

Adson's maneuver does not always identify the neurogenic form of thoracic outlet syndrome. Specifically, it does not typically distinguish that form of thoracic outlet syndrome, which is due to trauma to the brachial plexus and in which a vascular component is not a significant element, yet in which numbness and tingling within the hand are important complaints signifying trauma to the neural component.

What are the principal findings in the neurogenic form of thoracic outlet syndrome? These include:

1. Numbness and tingling in the fingertips, radiating into all fingers of the ipsilaterally affected hand
2. Dropping objects from the ipsilateral hand without warning
3. Pain in the neck, radiating along the scapula and medial scapular border, between the shoulder blades, into the shoulder and down the arm, under the arm, under the breast, and into the chest
4. Difficulty in fully expanding the chest on inspiration and pain in the chest wall on coughing
5. Pain radiating down the arm and into the center of the chest, suggesting a heart attack or pulmonary embolism. These possibilities should be considered because they may be occurring concurrently along with neurogenic thoracic outlet syndrome.
6. Pain over the supraclavicular and/or infraclavicular fossa on the involved side on direct palpation, frequently eliciting a "jump" sign, with multiple trigger points identified around the neck
7. Pain worsened on the affected side when turning the head to the opposite side
8. Unilaterally predominant headache, ipsilateral to the side of brachial plexus involvement. Occasionally this pain will radiate into the eye on the affected side, having a "spike in the eye" character. This may be missed when there is a history of preexisting migraine or may be attributed to a later onset migraine.
9. A recent history of sinus disease due to secondary swelling in the sinus tissue of the affected side
10. Sudden drop attacks as the leg on the affected side gives way, leading to a history of frequent falls
11. Enlargement of the chest wall and the breast on the side of the thoracic outlet syndrome
12. Expression of reflex sympathetic dystrophy (complex regional pain syndrome type I) secondary to the neurogenic thoracic outlet syndrome. This can include burning or aching pain in the hand on the affected side, which may be the presenting symptom. On close inspection the hand is noted to swell, have increased sweating, altered color (flushed or blanched), altered temperature (increased or decreased), altered growth of the hair and nails (increased or decreased), and altered movement (difficulty in initiating movements, tremor, spasm, altered posture, brisk reflexes). If there is a partial, yet definite, peripheral nerve injury within the brachial plexus, demonstrable by EMG/NCV or a somatosensory evoked potential study, the correct diagnosis would be causalgia (complex regional pain syndrome type II).

Plain x-rays are appropriate to rule out structural lesions such as elongated lateral processes on one of the upper cervical vertebrae or a cervical rib. Other abnormalities include abnormal subclavian vessels and tumors or abscesses at the apex of the lung. The latter may require a chest x-ray or MRI/MRA to be identified. EMG/NCV studies and somatosensory evoked potential studies of the brachial plexus are often negative, which is attributed to the involvement of the smallest-diameter nerve fibers in this disorder, below the level of detection of such studies. Currently, there is no specific way to image muscle spasm, so the importance of its identification and localization can be determined only by the history and physical examination.

TREATMENT STRATEGIES

Treatment of myofascial pain involves physical measures to increase the range of motion of the affected muscles. This may include physical manipulation of the specific muscle areas that are most tender and painful through massage. Needle manipulations are the second method of treatment and can be accomplished with either a dry needle or the injection of some substance to temporarily manipulate the local environment and relieve the pain. Treatment of the underlying causative problem is the third and ultimate goal in order to prevent recurrence of myofascial pain. If this can be accomplished with any success, the entire disorder may resolve. However, if the condition is perpetuated, ongoing medical therapy may be needed for sufficient relief of symptoms.

Dry needling of the trigger point is separate from the injection of local anesthetics, steroids, or botulinum toxin. Local anesthetics may include short-acting agents like procaine or lidocaine (0.5% to 1%), which have far less muscle toxicity than the longer-acting bupivacaine. Corticosteroids have been injected as well, with the hope of reducing inflammation, but this has not been demonstrated to have any greater benefit than the other agents used alone. Saline injection may be used in the event of allergy to local anesthetics.

The greatest duration of action, for up to a period of months, may be accomplished through the use of botulinum toxin (both botulinum toxins A and B are now commercially available), but further studies are needed to better define the parameters of use, which remain empirical at present (18). Empirically, doses of 20 to 25 U per cc have been used for smaller muscles, and doses of 100 to 400 U per cc have been used for larger muscles.

Care is needed not to repeat these injections too frequently, generally at no more than a 3-month interval, to limit the chances of developing antibodies to the repeated dosing of the botulinum. Despite all of this information, at the present time there is no evidence to indicate the superiority of one agent over any other in trigger point inactivation (2,13–15).

Identification of the trigger point is dependent upon palpation. A taut band of increased resistance is noted.

The point of maximum tenderness is the ideal injection site. A local twitch response occurs upon penetration of this site within the muscle by the needle. A 25-gauge, 1.5-inch needle is preferred to either a potentially more effective, but more painful, larger-bore needle or a possibly less effective, but less painful, smaller-sized needle. There is no known relationship between acupuncture meridians and trigger points.

Complications of trigger point injections may include a failed trigger point injection, syncope, hematoma, infection, drug reaction, diffusion of the agent (botulinum toxin), nerve injury, vascular injury, penetration of an organ, or an inadvertent spinal nerve block. These can lead to circumstances in which the patient may require intubation and ventilatory support.

Successful management requires the combination of better sleep, improved posture, and movement and reduction of stress. Emphasis on exercise, gentle massage, physical therapy maneuvers, postural corrections, biofeedback, and counseling works toward stress reduction. Aquatic therapy is the least difficult to perform and consequently the most successful in restoring function. The aquatic environment provides support, limiting the risks from falls, and also simultaneously fosters exercise of all parts of the body.

Even simply walking in the water is adequate because displacement of each gallon of water is the equivalent of moving more than 8 pounds per gallon. Aquatic therapy also often provides a satisfactory alternative to social isolation and promotes both good posture and a sense of accomplishment at the end of each session, greatly reducing depression. Additional physical therapy maneuvers, such as wearing or using supportive devices, coupled with the application of ultrasound, have also been beneficial, including myofascial release.

Canes and crutches require special attention because their improper use can aggravate pain rather than aid the patient. These devices are meant to stabilize a patient and aid in ambulation. However, all too frequently, patients will place far too much of their weight onto the cane or crutches and thereby create a new source of neuromuscular pain in the brachial plexus.

A more perplexing issue is the associated problem of management of CRPS-I (RSD) dystrophy and headaches. It has been recognized that there is a broad but continuous spectrum between migraine and tension-type headaches (19). Therefore, agents once believed to be uniquely for migraine are now appreciated to also be effective in aborting severe and recurrent tension-type headaches.

There have been many advances in the treatment of headaches with the use of either low doses of the tricyclic antidepressant amitriptyline, up to 30 or 40 mg at bedtime, or long-acting propranolol, 60 mg to 120 mg twice daily, or the extended-release anticonvulsant valproate, 500 mg at bedtime for headache prophylaxis (20–22). In addition, the introduction and availability of the triptans as abortive therapy for migraines have greatly reduced the impact and the severity of headaches that do occur. Recent studies with sumatriptan have suggested that earlier treatment, with higher dosages of medication, can provide a pain-free response that is encouraging (22).

In contrast, the treatment of "reflex sympathetic dystrophy" has remained enigmatic. If identified early enough, "reflex sympathetic dystrophy" can be quieted by organized motor activity and regular movement of the affected extremity. Unfortunately, that is rarely the case, and this necessitates the use of rational polypharmacy in the management of the patient—the combination of multiple medications in an organized way. In this fashion, patients are asked to name the most bothersome problem from which they are suffering to provide a focal point of their treatment.

Whether it is their resting pain level or immobility, their inability to sleep, or movement-associated painful spasms (MAPS), this complaint is used as a focal point of all subsequent efforts as a benchmark for success of the agents and dosages chosen.

COMPLEX REGIONAL PAIN SYNDROME TYPE I

Reflex sympathetic dystrophy (RSD) is a form of neuropathic pain that may reflect disease in either the central nervous system or the peripheral nervous system. It is also known as complex regional pain syndrome type I, to contrast it to complex regional pain syndrome type II (causalgia), in which there is an identifiable, but partial, injury to a peripheral nerve. CRPS-I often follows a peripheral injury, such as a sprain or strain, and is characterized as pain out of proportion to the injury. There is usually a period of immobilization following the injury evident in the history.

The features of CRPS-I are complex and include burning or aching pain (worse distally), swelling, sweating, color changes, temperature changes, changes in the growth of the hair and nails as well as the skin, and abnormalities of movement. These features are made worse by activity, dependent posture, and cold ambient temperatures.

When confronted with this level of complexity of complaints, it is not unusual for patients to say they do not know where to begin if they are asked what bothers them the most. However, with a bit of effort, they almost always will indicate that it is the pain that occurs on movement that bothers them the most. This leads to a combination of medications and strategies to reduce their pain, including analgesics, anticonvulsants, antidepressants, antispasticity agents, antimigraine medications, and sleep-inducing agents.

First, an analgesic is used. This follows the guidelines of the WHO ladder, beginning with a simple nonsteroidal and escalating, depending on their need for pain relief, to various opioid compounds (23). The antiinflammatory component of a nonsteroidal has merit during the early injury because of inflammation associated with the initial injury. However, the analgesic level needed must be titrated to the patient.

Anticonvulsants are added for relief of the burning component, allodynia (the perception of light touch as pain), and shooting pains. Anticonvulsants have actions that empirically make some of them more suitable for some of these symptoms than for others. For example, gabapentin, tiagabine, and topiramate are more effective on the burning component and allodynia, whereas carbamazepine, oxcarbazepine, and zonisamide are more effective on the shooting component.

In the past low doses of tricyclic antidepressants had been used for these complaints, but their side effects make them less desirable choices. Selective serotonin reuptake inhibitor (SSRI) antidepressants have proven very effective in the treatment of depression. Because this is often an accompanying feature of ongoing long-term pain disorders, their use is growing. However, these agents do not have the same analgesic properties of the tricyclic antidepressants, so their use should be confined to the treatment of depression.

Caution must be exercised in combining the use of an SSRI with a triptan because of the possibility of serotonin syndrome due to the combination of increased serotonin availability from the SSRI and the selective serotonin agonist effect of the specific triptan. Finally, SSRI drugs should not be combined with monoamine oxidase inhibitors for similar reasons.

Of the antispasticity and antispasm agents available, baclofen and tizanidine get the most use, but some older agents serve multiple purposes. The latter include clonazepam and diazepam, which have merit because of their longer half-lives but have problems because of their potential for being habit forming. Adjustment of dosages must be made depending upon the needs of the patient.

The triptans have value as specific antimigraine agents, specifically when there is a history of a throbbing, pulsatile headache. Increasingly, it is being recognized that there is a broad continuum from tension-type headaches through migrainous headaches in which the triptans have demonstrated benefit.

Finally, sedative-hypnotic agents rarely are effective in the long term for individuals with chronic pain, other than for very brief periods. For this reason, other classes of medications are being explored. Of the latter, the atypical antipsychotic medications olanzepine and quetiapine have been quite helpful in achieving adequate rest on a regular basis. This is essential because lack of sleep worsens pain through stress mechanisms, unfavorable mood states, poor memory, increased frustration, and increasing fatigue.

With this background of information on the essential steps in eliciting the history and assessing the physical examination, it is best to review a specific case history to consolidate the essential features of the points that have been raised.

Case History: Neck and Shoulder Pain with Numbness and Tingling of the Hands

A 29-year-old left-handed woman was evaluated one year after being injured in a car accident. During the previous year she had been to multiple physicians who had attributed her complaints to a whiplash injury, which she was told should have been of limited duration. However, her pain in the neck and shoulders persisted, accompanied by tingling in all of the fingers on both hands. At the time of the accident, she was the driver of her vehicle and was stopped, holding the steering wheel with arms extended, waiting to make a left turn into her driveway. It was at this time that her vehicle was struck from behind by a car moving at about 50 mph.

What is the significance of her presenting complaint?

The differential diagnosis must address whether this pain is related to the trauma or independent of it. Some possible causes independent of the trauma would be an Arnold-Chiari malformation at the foramen magnum, a vascular malformation high in the cervical cord, an epidural abscess, blood or infection within the spinal cord and/or canal, multiple sclerosis, vitamin B12 deficiency with subacute combined degeneration, polyneuropathy, postsurgical changes, syringomyelia, or a neoplasm, such as a neurofibroma. The trauma may have led to direct damage to the spine, the cervical spinal cord, and/or nerve roots, or—more likely, with her arms extended at the time of impact—a traction injury to the brachial plexus from the whiplash motion of the head on the neck with or without the addition of an entrapment neuropathy of individual peripheral nerves.

She had a three-point restraint in place, but no air bags were present. After impact, she jumped out of her car and began directing traffic. She later went to the hospital and had x-rays of her neck performed because of pain in the neck and the nature of her injury. This showed straightening of the cervical spine. She was sent home with a prescription for ibuprofen.

What is the significance of the cervical spine straightening?

This indicates an abnormality in the posture of the cervical spine. There is normally a lordotic curve present where the lower end of the cervical spine is gently curved posteriorly, away from its position beneath the skull, toward the shoulder. Straightening of this portion of the spine generally indicates spasm of the muscles of the neck, if the bones and joints are not affected, altering the posture of the spine into a straight position. The clinical correlate of this change is pain in the neck, with imitation of the full range of movement, and appreciation of spasm and tenderness on direct palpation. Headache, radiating from the back or side of the neck, may also be associated with this finding.

The next day she developed a headache, with a left-sided preponderance, and could not spontaneously lift her head off the pillow without physically lifting her head using her hands. Her neck and upper back later bothered her, too, and this persisted over the ensuing months, although the headaches eventually decreased in intensity with physical therapy and medication with cyclobenzaprine. There were occasional pains in the left shoulder region but no burning sensations. There were no bladder or bowel complaints.

What is the significance of her headaches?

The headaches are localized, with a left-sided preponderance. This may indicate the presence of a chronic subdural hematoma as a consequence of the head trauma, but more commonly it indicates reflected muscle spasm, which is worse on one side of the neck and head. Other types of headaches to consider include those of migraine, cluster, aneurysm, arteriovenous malformation (AVM), or tumor. The history of the onset of this headache with trauma, the absence of changes in mental status, and the palpable tenderness and appreciable spasm in the neck on the side of the headache are clinical clues to the nature of this headache.

What is the significance of her shoulder pain?

The shoulder pain may reflect direct trauma to the shoulder, such as a torn rotator cuff. Alternatively, this may represent pain that is radiated from a herniated disc, affecting the C-5 nerve root, which supplies this anatomical region. In addition, brachial plexus traction lesions often are associated with radiation of pain and tenderness to the shoulder on the same side, pain that also radiates into the medial scapular border between the shoulder blades, under the arm and breast, and into the center of the chest, causing individuals to question whether they are having a heart attack. This latter pattern of radiation is quite characteristic of brachial plexus traction injuries, especially with increased exertion, but, of course, a high index of suspicion for cardiac causes should also be maintained, depending on the clinical context in which the pain occurs.

What is the significance of her absence of bowel/bladder complaints?

The normal bladder and bowel functions make it less likely that a cervical cord lesion has compromised the spinal cord. If that had happened, there probably would have been some manifestation of urinary urgency and frequency.

Medications: Aspirin, usually none, but up to six per day, depending on the intensity of her pain. Oxycodone with acetaminophen had also been used on occasion for very severe pain.

What other medications and/or treatments should be considered in her management?

Clinical management should progress from the simplest, most conservative, noninvasive methods to those that are more aggressively oriented forms of active intervention. Over-the-counter (OTC) medications are frequently used and specifically should be asked about. OTCs may give rise to rebound pain, just as certain prescription medications can do, and an awareness of the role of rebound in perpetuating the duration of the pain syndrome is needed before this issue can be addressed.

Allergies: None.

How might a history of seasonal allergies alter the evaluation of her complaints?

Focusing on the seasonal allergies, and the potential for a secondary sinusitis to develop, more attention would be given to the possibility of a sinus headache contributing to her overall picture. Unilaterally dominant sinus headaches are not uncommon, and caution must be exercised in not indicting a headache as due to sinus infection, thus missing the opportunity to treat the muscle or nerve injury basis of the posttraumatic headache.

Past Medical History: She had no prior history of medical illness, surgery, or trauma, although 12 years earlier she had been a passenger in the front seat of a car in another, but milder, accident. At the time she had hurt her right knee, which got better after a few years, requiring physical therapy for more than one year in duration.

What role does past trauma play in her present complaint?

The history of trauma in another car accident suggests the possibility of an earlier subclinical whiplash because neck and head complaints were not prominent at that time. However, cumulatively, the older injury can lower the threshold for soft tissue damage that later became clinically significant. Therefore, it is always important to address these issues.

Family History: Father, age 57, in good health. Mother, age 49, with a history of migraine headaches. A brother, age 25, with severe allergic rhinitis and asthma, otherwise in good health; and a sister, age 20, with a history of migraine headaches. She had no children.

Is there any correlation between her headaches and the family history of migraines noted?

There may be a correlation between family history of migraine and the subsequent development of migraine-like headaches in an individual. However, the history of intermittent headaches for some time prior to the precipitating trauma would have helped to secure this issue. Three possibilities exist. First, she has a migraine component reflecting her family history. Second, she has a migraine threshold that is lower than most, and the trauma provided a trigger to precipitate headaches. Third, regardless of the migraine family history, she had been essentially headache free until the trauma, which then resulted in a characteristic pattern of headache associated with muscle spasm at the site of the whiplash injury. These considerations clinically help to provide the optimum therapeutic choices.

Social History: Graduated from high school, then trade school in beautician work, which she no longer could do after the accident because of arm pain when she would lift her arms in styling hair. She had been dropping objects from her hands without warning, especially while working. In addition, after stopping her attempts at beautician work and after the more recent accident, she began attending college part-time, studying animal science with the hope of becoming a veterinarian. She also began working part-time as a veterinary assistant and was having problems lifting small animals as part of her job. She did not smoke and drinks on occasion, usually beer.

What is the significance of her difficulties in the use of her arms in her work history?

The limitations of arm movement, particularly those associated with elevating the arms and lifting following the type of trauma that she sustained, suggest injury to the brachial plexus. Other possible causes for her difficulties also exist but are in essence discounted by findings of a normal neurological examination and limited degenerative spine disease on the radiographic and other imaging studies. Rarely, seizures can be associated with dropping objects, but the time course of these events, the absence of specific movement abnormalities, and the lack of any alteration of consciousness mediate against this possibility.

On clinical examination, her major clinical findings were mild bilateral tenderness on direct palpation of the supraclavicular and infraclavicular fossa, which overlies the brachial plexus, with a slight left-sided preponderance and spasm of the paracervical spinal muscles. There were numbness and tingling throughout both hands, worse at the fingertips. There was a left Wartenberg reflex and slightly more brisk reflexes on the left side. This was consistent with her left-sided preponderance of the bilateral brachial plexus traction injuries.

What is the significance of the location of palpable tenderness and distribution of clinical symptoms?

Tenderness on palpation of the supraclavicular and infraclavicular fossa is indicative of either nerve root compression or bilateral brachial plexus traction injuries. The pattern of numbness and tingling in the whole hand suggests a diffuse rather than focal process, more consistent with involvement of the brachial plexus than a nerve root or entrapment of an individual peripheral nerve. The Wartenberg reflex indicates abnormal central nervous system function to some degree and represents the involuntary flexion of the extended thumb when there is effort to flex the four remaining fingers against resistance of the examiner's hand.

What can be done to objectively differentiate between these possibilities?

Plain x-rays of the cervical spine can be used to look for aberrant transverse spinal processes, a cervical rib, and a fractured clavicle, amongst other possibilities. In addition, an MRI of the cervical spine was performed to evaluate her to determine if there was either localized degenerative spine disease, a disc herniation, or spinal cord pathology such as a syrinx or compression.

My clinical impression was that of a bilateral brachial plexus traction injury secondary to her involvement in the more recent motor vehicle accident one year earlier. Furthermore, she had altered left-sided reflexes that were most consistent with her complaint of worse symptoms on the left side.

What can be done to confirm this impression?

An MRI examination of the cervical spine can be performed to be certain that there is neither nerve root nor spinal cord compression as a potential cause of her persistent symptoms. This was done and demonstrated a mild loss of the normal cervical lordotic curve. A nerve conduction study demonstrated slowing of conduction across the lateral cord component of the brachial plexus bilaterally. The latter test does not always reveal an abnormality because the problem frequently affects the smallest-diameter nerve fibers, which are characteristically below the level of detection using this test.

Regarding treatment, I suggested the use of cyclobenzaprine at bedtime for her pain due to muscle spasm. I also gave her a prescription for hydrocodone with acetaminophen 10/650 for severe pain if it should occur. However, she complained of feeling knocked out when taking either of these medications and did not use them. I then added the advice of using thick-soled shoes, with foam inserts and heavy socks, to absorb the shock of each step when walking. This lessened the impact of walking on her neck pain but did not provide needed analgesia to help her sleep through the night.

Propoxyphene had fewer cognitive effects than either the cyclobenzaprine or hydrocodone but also provided less pain relief than the hydrocodone/acetaminophen combination.

A trial with 1-mg (one quarter of a tablet) doses of tizanidine was then initiated to reduce muscle spasm and thus replaced the cyclobenzaprine. I had also made the suggestion of using the tizanidine as often as every 2 hours, if needed and tolerated, with the possibility of using even higher doses (up to one or two whole 4-mg tablets) at bedtime, to a maximum not to exceed 32 mg daily. In addition, 2 mg hydromorphone at bedtime provided better pain relief than did the hydrocodone-acetaminophen combination. Fluoxetine was added as an adjunct for the treatment of both pain and reactive depression, at a dosage of 20 to 40 mg daily.

Because of persistent symptoms and the requirement for continued dosing with analgesics and adjunctive medications, despite initial conservative intervention, surgical intervention was undertaken to decompress the brachial plexus bilaterally. This was done initially on the more severely affected left side and then 4 months later on the right.

She recovered with significant improvement in muscle strength and range of motion, using tizanidine occasionally at bedtime for control of persistent nighttime spasms. On this regimen, she has planned to resume her schooling but to pursue less physically demanding work.

REFERENCES

1. Fricton JR. Myofascial pain syndrome: characteristics and epidemiology. *Adv. Pain Res. Therapy* 1990;17:107–127.
2. Borg-Stein J, Stein J. Trigger points and tender points: one and the same? Does injection treatment help? *J Rheumatic Dis N Am* 1996;22:305–322.
3. Fischer AA. New approaches in the treatment of myofascial pain. *Phys Med Rehabil Clinics N Am* 1997;8:153–169.
4. Roth RS, Horowitz K, Bachman JE. Chronic myofascial pain: knowledge of diagnosis and satisfaction with treatment. *Arch Phys Med Rehabi* 1998;79:966–970.
5. Bennet R. Fibromyalgia, chronic fatigue syndrome and myofascial pain *Curr Opin Rheum* 1998;10:95–103.
6. Creamer P. Effective management of fibromyalgia. J. *Musculoskeletal Med* 1999;16:622–637.
7. Simons DG. Muscle pain syndromes - part I. *Am J Phys Med* 1975;54: 289–311.
8. Simons DG. Muscle pain syndromes - part II. *Am J Phys Med* 1975; 55:15–40.
9. Wolfe F, Smythe HA, Yunus MB, et al. The American College of Rheumatology 1990 criteria for the classification of fibromyalgia: report of the multicenter criteria committee. *Arth Rheum* 1990;33: 160–172.
10. Russell IJ, Orr MD, Littman B, et al. Elevated cerebrospinal fluid levels of substance P in patients with fibromyalgia syndrome. *Arth Rheum* 1994;37:1593–1601.
11. Burckhardt CS, Clark SR, Bennet RM. The fibromyalgia impact questionnaire—development and validation. *J Rheum* 1991;18: 728–733.
12. Sarno JE. Psychosomatic backache. *J Fam Pract* 1977;5:353–357.
13. Hong CZ. Myofascial trigger point injection. *Crit Rev Phys Med Rehab* 1993;5:203–217.
14. Hong CZ, Hsueh TC. Difference in pain relief after trigger point injections in myofascial pain patients with and without fibromyalgia. *Arch Phys Med Rehab* 1996;77:1161–1166.
15. Hopwood MB, Abram SE. Factors associated with failure of trigger point injections. *Clin J Pain* 1994;10:227–234.
16. Travell JG, Simons DG. *Myofascial pain and dysfunction: the trigger point manual.* Baltimore: Williams & Wilkins, 1983.
17. Travell JG, Simons DG. *Myofascial pain and dysfunction: the trigger point manual: the lower extremities* (Vol 2). Baltimore: Lippincott Williams & Wilkins, 1999.
18. Porta MA. Comparative trial of botulinum toxin type A and methylprednisolone for the treatment of myofascial pain syndrome and pain from chronic muscle spasm. *Pain* 2000;85:101–105.
19. Featherstone HJ. Migraine and muscle contraction headaches: a continuum. *Headache* 1985; 25:194–198.
20. Packard RC. Treatment of chronic daily posttraumatic headache with divalproex sodium. *Headache* 2000;40:736–739.
21. Peroutka SJ. Beyond monotherapy: rational polytherapy in migraine. *Headache* 1998;38:18–22.
22. Putnam GP, O'Quinn S, Bolden-Watson CP, et al. Migraine polypharmacy and the tolerability of sumatriptan: a large-scale, prospective study. *Cephalalgia* 1999;19:668–675.
23. Portenoy RK. Current pharmacotherapy of chronic pain. *J Pain Symptom Management* 2000;19(Suppl):S16–S20.

CHAPTER 39

The Somatizing Disorders: Diagnostic and Treatment Approaches for Pain Medicine

David A. Fishbain

The purpose of this chapter is to define, characterize, and suggest a treatment approach to a very difficult and common type of chronic pain patient (CPP): the one who has chronic pain complaints and associated functional dysfunction that are not proportional to the identified organic pathology or who has no organic pathology that can be identified to explain the chronic pain (CP). This chapter will describe the psychiatric syndromes thought to be associated with the preceding problems, difficulties with the diagnostic nomenclature of these syndromes, and, finally, a treatment approach to some of these syndromes. The key to understanding these syndromes is the concept of "somatization."

THE SOMATIZING DISORDERS

Although the term *somatization* is commonly used in the medical literature, there is no agreement about its definition (1). Recently *somatization* has been defined as "a tendency to experience and communicate somatic distress and symptoms that are unaccounted for by pathologic findings, to attribute them to physical illness, and to seek medical help for them" (2). Somatization is not a specific medical/psychiatric diagnosis. As such, it does not have operational criteria for arriving at this diagnosis. Somatization does not imply that the patient does not have a concurrent medical illness (3,4), nor does it imply that a psychiatric diagnosis is necessarily present (1).

Somatic symptoms are extremely common in the general population, and as such somatization is also common. About 60% to 80% of physically healthy people experience somatic symptoms in any given week (5). As such, somatic symptoms account for 30% to 40% of ambulatory medical visits, with only a small percentage of these having an identifiable organic etiology (6). As for somatization, it has been reported that of 260 000 patients in 325 hospitals, 5.2% or 13 520 patients were placed in the diagnostic category of "symptoms and ill-defined conditions" (7).

Patients with chronic pain (CP) have been reported to have multiple nonpain physical complaints, i.e., to have somatic symptoms or to somatasize. This problem has been studied in CPPs through a number of somatization questionnaire studies. Several of the studies do support this conclusion. A high percentage of CPPs demonstrate elevated hypochondriasis scores (8) and somatization scores (9) as measured by the Illness Behavior Questionnaire and the Modified Somatic Perceptions Questionnaire, respectively. In addition, when patients with various types of chronic pain are compared with appropriate controls on somatization measures, the CPPs are frequently demonstrated to have greater somatization scores. This finding has been demonstrated for CPPs with orofacial pain (10,11), migraines (12), noncardiac chest pain (13), chronic low back pain (14), and fibromyalgia (15). Finally, somatization scores appear to be predictors for treatment outcome in CPP with temporomandibular disorders (16) and low back pain (17). According to these questionnaire studies, somatization may be a significant problem in CPPs, and patients with this problem may be at risk for poor treatment outcome.

Somatization is commonly comorbidly associated with physical (3,4) and psychiatric illness (2,18). Somatizers often suffer from chronic illness and die early (19). Although it may simply be a reflection of medical problems (20) of aging, major depression has been shown to be associated with somatization (2,18).

It has been pointed out that a number of disorders described in the *Diagnostic and Statistical Manual of Mental Disorders, Fourth Edition (DSM-IV)* (21) encompass the concept of somatization (22) or abnormal illness behavior (23). These disorders are the following: the somatoform disorders (hypochondriasis, conversion disorder, somatization disorder, pain disorder, body dysmorphic disorder); factitious disorder with physical symptoms; and malingering (not officially a disorder). It has also been concluded (1) that there is a spectrum of severity for somatization from acute to chronic and that most somatization is transient. Thus, three types of somatization have been described (1): (a) related to acute situational stress; (b) comorbidly associated with acute psychiatric disorder or disorders; and (c) part of or related to a chronic psychiatric disorder (as in the preceding disorders). The relationship between these concepts is summarized in Table 39-1.

Key Points

Somatization is not a specific diagnosis.

Somatic symptoms are common in the general population and in CPPs.

Clinical Implications

The label of *somatization* or *somatic symptoms* should be avoided because it is imprecise.

Findings of somatic symptoms in CPPs should trigger a search for comorbidly associated problems, i.e., either primary or secondary somatization-associated disorders, as in Table 39-1.

THE PRIMARY SOMATIZING DISORDERS AND CHRONIC PAIN

A number of psychiatric researchers have reported on the alleged frequency of the primary somatizing disorders (Table 39-1) in CPPs. Their studies have usually utilized the *Diagnostic and Statistical Manual of Mental Disorders* system, which is the official nomenclature of the American Psychiatric Association (21). A summary of these studies is presented in Table 39-2. Although each of the disorders in Table 39-2 will be discussed in detail later, the following observations are evident from closer scrutiny of Table 39-2: (a) The reported frequency range for somatization disorder is 1.0% to 16.2%. It is likely less than 5%; (b) the reported frequency range for conversion disorder is 2% to 37.8%; (c) the reported frequency range for psychogenic pain/pain disorder is 0.3% to 97.0%; (d) the reported frequency range for hypochondriasis is 0.7% to 1.0%; (e) the reported frequency range for factitious disorder is 0.14% to 2.0%; (f) the reported frequency range for malingering is 0% to 22%; (g) no data are available for body dysmorphic disorder within CPPs.

TABLE 39-1. *Somatization: characteristics and associated syndromes*

	Primary somatizing disorders	Secondary somatizing disorders	
Related to:	Chronic psychiatric disorders	Acute situational stressor	Acute psychiatric disorder is comorbidly associated
Symptoms caused by:	Symptoms part of chronic psychiatric disorder: *Diagnoses* 1. Hypochondriasis 2. Pain disorder 3. Somatization disorder 4. Conversion disorder 5. Body dysmorphic disorder 6. Factitious disorder 7. Malingering (not a psychiatric disorder)	Stressful life events: *Diagnosis Example* Adjustment disorder	Symptoms part of acute psychiatric disorder, e.g., insomnia *Diagnosis Example* Major depression
Chronic problem (lasts lifetime, some degree of disability)	+++	No	+
Preoccupation with health and symptoms	+++	+	++
Fear or conviction of having a physical disease	+++	+	++
Likely to be persistent?	Yes	No	Dependent on the success of treatment for psychiatric disorder

(+ − +++), less likely to more likely.

TABLE 39-2. *Diagnostic frequency of somatizing disorders in chronic pain patients study*

	Fishbain et al. (24)	Reich et al. (25)	Katon et al. (26)	Large (27)	Fishbain et al. (28)	Fishbain et al. (29)	King* et al.	Polatin et al. (30)	Anooshian et al. (31)
Chronic pain patients (n)	283	43	37	50	Not available	2860	59	200	193
Diagnostic measure	DSM-III, 2-hour semi-structured interview	DSM-III, flow sheets	DSM-III DIS	DSM-III, Maudsley	DSM-III	DSM-III	DSM-IV	DSM-III-R SCID	DSM-IV
Diagnostic frequency									
Somatization disorder	3.9	5	16.2	8	—	—	—	1.0	—
Conversion disorder	37.8	2	—	8	—	—	—	—	—
Psychogenic pain/pain disorder	0.3	32	—	—	—	—	51.0	97.0	79% (with both psychological factors and medical condition) 9% (with psychological factors)
Hypochondriasis	0.7	—	—	—	—	—	—	1.0	—
Factitious disorders	—	2.0	—	—	—	0.14	—	—	—
Malingering	—	—	—	—	0.22	—	—	—	—

*King SA. Paper presented at the Eighth World Congress on Pain, Vancouver, 1996.
DIS, National Institutes of Mental Health Interview Schedule.
DSM-III, Diagnostic and Statistical Manual of Mental Disorders, 3rd ed.
DSM-III-R, Diagnostic and Statistical Manual of Mental Disorders, 3rd ed., revised.
DSM-IV, Diagnostic and Statistical Manual of Mental Disorders, 4th ed.
SCID—Structured Clinical Interview for DSM.

Key Point

There is little agreement between researchers on the prevalence percentages for the various primary somatization disorders within CPPs.

Clinical Implication

Reported prevalence percentages for these disorders cannot be utilized as clinical guides for decisions about presence/absence of these disorders in CPPs.

THE NONSPECIFIC PAIN PROBLEM

The common feature of the primary somatization disorders is the presence of physical symptoms that suggest a general medical condition but are not fully explained by a general medical condition. In the pain literature this problem has been called "nonspecific" pain. Nonspecific pain is the opposite of "specific pain," which is defined as pain where an underlying cause can be defined, such as infection, vertebral fracture, systemic disease, etc. (32). Currently, it is claimed that the vast majority of pain problems do not fit into the classical biomedical model that links symptomatology and disease process (33). As such, a definite somatic cause for the pain can be identified in no more than 10% to 20% of the cases (34). Thus, the "nonspecific" pain diagnosis is determined or defined by the process of excluding "specific" pain (34). As such, the pain physician's first task is to determine if a pain patient has "nonspecific" pain. If the pain physician is not convinced of this after the record review, history, and physical, he/she should proceed with further diagnostic procedures, including laboratory investigation (35). This is because patients with "nonspecific" pain become candidates for a diagnosis of one of the primary somatizing diagnoses. Do CPPs with nonspecific pain somatize more than CPPs without specific pain? There has been one study (36) that has addressed this issue. Here it was found that CPPs with nonspecific pain versus patients with specific pain *did not* exhibit more somatic complaints but were more distressed but not because of a greater tendency to somatize.

Key Point

Nonspecific pain is extremely common in CPPs and thus may be the rule rather than the exception.

Clinical Implication

Although every CPP with nonspecific pain will become a candidate for some primary or secondary somatizing diagnosis, the frequency of nonspecific pain would indicate that it is unlikely that all patients with nonspecific pain have a primary somatizing disorder.

THE FIBROMYALGIA SYNDROME AND MYOFASCIAL PAIN SYNDROME ISSUE

The second central question in the evaluation for the somatization disorders—after "specific" pain has been ruled out and "nonspecific pain" has been ruled in—relates to whether the CPP has physical findings indicative of fibromyalgia syndrome (FMS) or myofascial pain syndrome (MFPS). This is a group of soft tissue pain syndromes characterized by widespread pain and tender points in FMS (37) and regional pain and trigger points in MFPS (38). The important issue in reference to these syndromes is that they are commonly found in pain patients with intractable pain. For example, the proportion of new patients with FMS presenting in rheumatology clinics has been reported to be 10% to 20% (39). Even higher prevalence percentages for MFPS have been reported at pain facilities. Here, the numbers range from 30% to 100% (40,41). For example, in an early study, our group (42) had reported that of LBP patients with chronic intractable benign pain (CIBP), 96.7% had one or more trigger points. Of the neck patients with CIBP of the neck, 100% had one

or more trigger points (42). It was concluded that the vast majority CIBP patients demonstrate physical findings indicative of musculoskeletal diseases (42). Thus, it is unlikely that a significant number of pain patients presenting to a pain facility will have true "nonspecific" pain if an adequate soft tissue examination is performed (42).

The issue of whether the pain patient has "nonspecific" pain or actually suffers from a soft tissue syndrome such as FMS or MFPS is important not only diagnostically but also behaviorally. This is because the pain patient needs and awaits an explanation for the pain and feels that the pain needs to be legitimized (32). In addition, there may be legal and financial reasons why the pain patient requires a legitimate diagnosis. Indeed, Barkan et al. (43) demonstrated that pain patients considered "delegitimization," referring to the reputation of the patients' experience of pain and suffering, as one of the major perceived difficulties of the pain experience. In another study, addressing this issue in a different way, Diego and Diehl (44) demonstrated that LBP patient satisfaction with medical care was dependent on the pain patient receiving an adequate explanation for his/her problem. Those pain patients who perceived that they did not wanted more diagnostic tests, were less satisfied with their visit, and were less likely to want the same doctor again. Clearly, the "nonspecific" label does not provide an explanation, nor does it satisfy the patient's expectations of knowing the exact cause of the pain (32). Yet, there appear to be dangers in giving some pain patients a specific diagnosis. For example, Abenhaim et al. (45) showed that injured workers who received a specific diagnosis were significantly more likely to become chronic. Others have suggested that the FMS and MFPS diagnostic labels promote illness behavior (46). Thus, some authors (32) have suggested that pain explanations should put the patient's pain into a general context and avoid the "labeling effect." This author disagrees with this position. The patient with intractable pain needs to stop looking for a cure and thus stop doctor shopping. He/she needs to understand that he/she has a chronic condition that has no cure in most situations but can be managed. He/she then needs to learn to manage the pain. The process of learning how to manage the pain can begin only after the patient understands that his/her condition is chronic. Thus, pain patients labeled with FMS or MFPS should, in theory, decrease their health-care utilization. This is indeed the case: After the diagnosis is made, hospitalizations and health-care utilization do drop dramatically for FMS patients (47). There is, therefore, reason to believe that the labeling of pain patients with an FMS or MFPS diagnosis, if appropriate, can have positive behavioral consequences that can impact on pain treatment outcome. The diagnostic issue will be discussed later in reference to treatment of the somatizing disorders.

How does the preceding discussion in reference to FMS and MFPS relate to the issue of the primary somatizing disorders? If one understands the preceding logic, it becomes clear that a "nonspecific" pain diagnosis cannot and should not be assigned unless FMS and MFPS have been ruled out. It is the author's opinion, generally supported by the preceding literature, that if an adequate search is undertaken for FMS and MFPS in CPPs, few patients will be left in the "nonspecific pain" category. Thus, only a few patients will be left as candidates for a potential primary somatizing disorder diagnosis.

Key Point

FMS and MFPS are commonly found in CPPs. The presence of such a diagnosis in a CPP with alleged "nonspecific pain" generally precludes the CPP being assigned a primary somatizing disorder diagnosis.

Clinical Implication

Any CPP with alleged "nonspecific pain" should receive a careful soft tissue physical exam geared toward the diagnosis of FMS or MFPS.

NONORGANIC PHYSICAL FINDINGS

During the last 20 years Waddell et al. (48,49) standardized a group of low back pain (LBP) physical signs, which earlier in this century were identified as predominantly nonorganic (50–52). Earlier researchers thought that the presence of one or more of these signs indicated hysteria and/or malingering (50–52). Waddell et al. (49) described five types of physical signs (a total of eight signs). These are presented in Table 39-3. Waddell et al. (49) demonstrated that a large percentage of patients with chronic low back pain demonstrate these eight nonorganic physical signs. These signs

TABLE 39-3. *Waddell's nonorganic signs*

Tenderness
  Superficial skin tender to light touch
  Nonanatomical deep tenderness not localized to one area

Simulation
  Axial loading pressure on the skull of a standing patient induces low back pain
  Rotation: Rotating shoulders and pelvis in same plane induces pain

Distraction
  Difference in straight leg-raising in supine and sitting positions

Region
  Weakness: many muscle groups, "give-away weakness" (patient does not give full effort on minor muscle testing)
  Sensory: sensory loss in a stocking or glove distribution, nondermatomal
  Overreaction: disproportionate facial or verbal expression (i.e., pain behavior)

appear to be predictive of treatment outcome (49,53), and Waddell et al. (49) had suggested that their presence or absence should be used as a basis for surgical decisions. Most importantly, these signs correlate with a greater degree of pain behavior and, therefore, a more difficult treatment problem (54). Main and Waddell (54) have recently reappraised their position on these signs and have stated that these signs are not a test of credibility or faking but represent a "psychological yellow flag" indicating psychological factors need to be considered. This is an important restatement for the meaning of these signs, especially because recently the reliability of these signs, notably superficial tenderness and abnormal regional sensory or motor disturbance, has been questioned (55). It is clear that these signs are also influenced by subjective opinions of the examiners/raters. In addition, the author has demonstrated that one of these signs, nondermatomal sensory abnormalities, is not associated with any predominant psychiatric pathology as delineated by the *DSM-III* (56) and is directly related to the perception of pain in the affected extremity (52). The Somatic Amplification Rating Scale (57) has been developed as a method of quantifying nonorganic physical findings.

What is the significance of the presence of these signs of the primary somatizing disorders? According to the *DSM-IV* the presence of one or more of these signs makes the patient a candidate for a potential diagnosis of some somatizing disorder. Since Waddell's article (49), these signs have been utilized by clinicians to determine if CPPs have problems that "cause" the pain. As can be seen from the preceding discussion this is not a correct interpretation of these signs. The importance of these signs to the diagnostic process for the somatizing disorders will be outlined in a later section.

Key Points

Nonorganic physical findings are frequently found in CPPs.

Their presence indicates a more severe pain disorder, potential poor outcome, and a possibility for the presence of some somatizing disorder.

Their presence *does not* indicate that the pain has a psychiatric etiology or that the CPP is faking.

Clinical Implication

The presence of nonorganic physical findings indicates a need for a diagnostic psychiatric consultation in association with a special treatment plan developed for a potentially more difficult CPP.

PSYCHIATRIC COMORBIDITY AND "NONSPECIFIC PAIN"

Primary care studies (58) indicate that "unexplained symptoms are associated with comorbid mood or anxiety disorders." In addition, somatization has been demonstrated to be associated with current and past psychiatric illness and harm avoidance (59).

In reference to CPPs it has long been known that various psychiatric diseases such as depression are commonly associated with the presence of chronic pain (60). Yet, there are only a few studies on the association between chronic "nonspecific" pain and psychiatric comorbidity. These few studies, however, mirror the primary care studies. For example, Kouyanow et al. (61) recently reported that CPPs with "medically unexplained" pain demonstrated significant psychiatric comorbidity. Similarly, another recent study (62) indicated that CPPs with "medically unexplained" pain demonstrated a significantly greater comorbidity for anxiety disorders (phobia, harm avoidance) than controls. This brief discussion then indicates the importance of psychiatric comorbidity to chronic pain in general and to chronic "nonspecific" pain in particular.

Key Point

Patients with secondary somatizing disorders, primary somatizing disorders, chronic pain, and chronic "nonspecific" pain are all likely to demonstrate comorbid psychiatric disorders.

Clinical Implication

Because the comorbid psychiatric disorders are eminently treatable, CPPs with "nonspecific" pain should receive a psychiatric examination or psychological interview in order to identify a potentially treatable condition that could be making the patients' symptoms worse.

DO SOME OF THE SOMATIZING DISORDERS OVERLAP INTO THE OBSESSIVE-COMPULSIVE SPECTRUM?

Obsessive-compulsive spectrum disorders (OCSDs) are a group of disorders closely related to obsessive-compulsive disorder (OCD) (63,64). These disorders include the following: body dysmorphic disorder, anorexia nervosa, binge eating, hypochondriasis, sexual compulsions, pyromania, kleptomania, trichotillomania, compulsive buying, pathological gambling, and some self-injurious behaviors (63,64). It is to be noted that two of the somatizing disorders (hypochondriasis and body dysmorphic disorder) are included within this group but that pain disorder is not. The OCSD patients utilize the types of mechanisms and behaviors often noted in OCD. As such, these mechanisms and behaviors make the index disorder, e.g., gambling, worse and more difficult to treat. At issue then is whether these types of mechanisms operate in some other somatizing disorders such as pain disorder. The features of

OCSDs and OCD overlap in many respects, including demographics, repetitive intrusive thoughts or behaviors, comorbidity, and aetiology. Most important, it appears that this group of disorders responds preferentially to antiobsessional drugs such as clomipramine and the selective serotonin reuptake inhibitors (SSRIs), e.g., fluvoxamine (63,64). For example, body dysmorphic disorder, a somatizing disorder, is thought to be one of the OCSDs and has demonstrated a strong response to SSRIs (64). Recently (65) fluvoxamine was tried for some other somatizing disorders with encouraging results.

There have been no treatment studies utilizing the OCSD concept for pain disorder. However, a number of case reports have been published. The author has reported (66) on the positive response to antiobsessional agents in three cases of chronic atypical facial pain. Recently, there has also been a report of a positive response in two patients with schizophrenia and chronic pain to clomipramine (67). This limited evidence indicates that perhaps CPPs with "nonspecific" pain and prominent obsessive-compulsive components should be recruited into a treatment trial with antiobsessional agents.

Key Point

Some of the somatizing disorders such as BDD and pain disorder could have an OCD component, i.e., the patient could focus in on the symptom by OCD mechanisms.

Clinical Implication

Pain physicians should be aware of the OCSD concept and treat patients with a prominent OCD component accordingly.

THE SOMATIZING DISORDERS— INDIVIDUAL DESCRIPTIONS

Following is a brief description of each somatizing disorder of interest to this chapter.

Hypochondriasis

This disorder is characterized by a preoccupation of having a serious illness based on misinterpretation of bodily sensation. This preoccupation persists despite significant reassurance (21). It is a chronic disorder. There are discrepancies in its reported frequency. For example, some authorities (21) claim it is rare, whereas some authors (68) have reported a 4% to 6% prevalence in medical clinics. It is often comorbidly associated with other psychiatric disorders such as depression (69), anxiety (70), and somatization disorder (70,71). As seen in Table 39-2, the prevalence of hypochondriasis within CPPs appears to be small.

Key Point

Hypochondriasis is often comorbidly associated with other psychiatric disorders.

Clinical Implication

A diagnosis of hypochondriasis in a CPP should trigger a search for more treatable psychiatric diagnoses.

Somatization Disorder

The hallmark of somatization disorder is a history of many physical complaints occurring before age 30 that cannot be explained medically (21). The diagnostic criteria for this disorder are presented in Table 39-4. The prevalence for this disorder within the general population is claimed to be 1% (72), which is lower than that reported for CPPs (Table 39-2). Somatization disorder is usually comorbidly associated with other psychiatric disorders (22). These, in decreasing frequency, are major depression, dysthymia, panic disorder, generalized anxiety disorder, substance abuse, and personality disorders (73,74).

Key Point

Somatization disorder is frequently comorbidly associated with other psychiatric disorders.

Clinical Implication

A diagnosis of somatization disorder in a CPP should trigger a search for more treatable psychiatric diagnoses.

Body Dysmorphic Disorder

Body dysmorphic disorder (BDD) is a preoccupation with imagined or slight physical defects in appearance, such as

TABLE 39-4. *Diagnostic criteria for somatization disorder (21)*

History of many physical complaints beginning before age 30, occurring over many years, and resulting in treatment seeking or impairment.

Includes each of the following
1. Four pain symptoms
2. Two gastrointestinal tract symptoms
3. One sexual symptom
4. One pseudoneurologic symptom

Includes either of the following
1. Preceding symptoms cannot be explained.
2. Impairment exceeds that which would be warranted by physical findings.

---

hair or facial features (21). This preoccupation causes significant distress or impairment of social, occupational, or other functioning. Social anxiety with social avoidance is comorbidly associated with BDD. The prevalence of BDD is 1% to 2% in the U.S. population (75) and 11% to 12% in social anxiety disorder (75). Behaviors associated with BDD include mirror checking, physician visits, hair grooming, use of cosmetics, and social avoidance. Distress over BDD may lead these patients to undergo repeated cosmetic surgeries. Thus, BDD patients are seen with some regularity in plastic surgeons' and dermatologists' offices. There are no case reports for BDD within CPPs.

Key Point

BDD is often comorbidly associated with social anxiety disorder.

Clinical Implication

CPPs with social anxiety disorder should be evaluated for a possible diagnosis of BDD.

Conversion Disorder

The essential feature of conversion disorder is the presence of a conversion symptom(s) affecting voluntary or sensory function that suggests a medical problem (21). Conversion symptoms can be the following: (a) paralysis, (b) localized weakness, (c) impaired coordination or balance, (d) aphonia, (e) difficulty swallowing, (f) urinary retention, (g) loss of touch or pain sensation, (h) double vision, (i) blindness, (j) deafness, (k) hallucinations, and (l) seizures. There are two other criteria that are essential for the diagnosis of conversion disorder: The symptom cannot be fully explained by a medical condition, and psychological factors are judged to be associated with the symptom (21). The fact that psychological factors are usually ubiquitously present in relation to the general medical conditions (21) makes this diagnosis extremely imprecise. As a result, overreliance on the psychological criteria has caused frequent misdiagnoses with disastrous medicolegal consequences (76,77).

Conversion disorder has been reported to be present in 0.01% to 0.5% of the general population, 3% of outpatient referrals to mental health clinics, and 11% to 14% of general medical/surgical inpatients (21). Of patients admitted to a neurology service, 9% were found to have a conversion symptom. Of these, motor symptoms, including paralysis and paresis and gait disturbance, were found to be the most frequent, followed by dizziness, seizures, and sensory symptoms (anesthesia, analgesia) (78). In reference to CPPs the frequency of motor disturbance is unknown, although it has been reported (79) to be present. The frequency of nonanatomical sensory findings (anesthesia, analgesia, NDSA) is, however, extremely high: 37.8% (80). It is the opinion of this author that nondermatomal sensory abnormalities are the most frequent conversion symptom found in CPPs, followed by paralysis/paresis and then gait disturbance. It is to be noted that this author has investigated nonanatomical sensory findings in CPPs in two studies. In the first study (50) he was not able to demonstrate an association between other psychiatric diagnoses and NDSAs. In the second study (52) it was demonstrated that NDSAs do not occur in a random pattern, as would be expected if they were a conversion symptom, but occur in the extremity in which pain is present. In addition, this author has reviewed the literature on the conversion symptom of paralysis/paresis (79). It was found that in the vast majority of the reported cases of paralysis/paresis the paralysis/conversion occurred in the extremity where the pain was present. Finally, it is interesting to note that NDSA symptoms improve if the pain is treated and improves (80,81). Thus, the conversion symptoms of NDSA and paralysis/paresis may be a pain-related/associated phenomenon rather than causally related to some psychological problem. However, until more evidence is available to support the preceding hypothesis, CPPs with either of these two conversion symptoms become candidates for a diagnosis of conversion disorder.

Key Point

Conversion symptoms are commonly found in CPPs but may be pain-related phenomena.

Clinical Implication

Conversion symptoms should be treated as per the treatments outlined later but with the focus on pain treatment.

Pain Disorder

The pain disorder diagnosis is the result of renaming, reclassifying, and revising the criteria of two earlier diagnoses, the first being psychogenic pain and the second being somatoform pain disorder. These revisions became necessary because of problems of reliability and validity for the criteria of the two previous diagnostic entities (21). The concept behind the pain disorder diagnosis is that it should identify patients in whom psychological factors play or have played a significant part in the etiology of the pain. The criteria for pain disorder are as follows: (a) The pain must involve one or more anatomical sites and be the predominant focus of the clinical presentation; (b) the pain must cause clinically significant distress and impairment in social, occupational, or other important areas of functioning; and (c) psychological factors must play an important role in the onset, severity, exacerbation, or maintenance of the pain. In addition, this disorder has subtypes: pain disorder associated with psychological fac-

tors; pain disorder associated with a general medical condition only; or both. The subtype pain disorder associated with psychological factors applies when psychological factors appear to determine the onset, severity, exacerbation, or maintenance of the pain. The subtype pain disorder associated with both psychological factors and a general medical condition pertains when both psychological factors and a general medical condition appear to determine the onset, severity, exacerbation, or maintenance of the pain. The subtype pain disorder associated with a general medical condition is not a mental disorder; it is coded on Axis III and used for differential diagnosis only. Closer examination of the three criteria for this disorder reveals the following problems: (a) The vast majority of chronic pain patients have pain in one or more sites (e.g., low back plus neck, neck plus TMJ, hip plus leg, etc.). Thus, the vast majority of CPPs should fulfill criterion *(a)*, and the criterion, therefore, seems overinclusive. (b) Significant numbers of chronic pain patients are significantly distressed and impaired in social, occupational, or other important areas of functioning. Thus, criterion *(b)* is also overinclusive. (c) Criterion *(c)* requires a value judgment by the psychiatric examiner, and no guidelines exist to ensure validity. Taken together, these three criteria for the diagnosis of pain disorder should then have little diagnostic validity.

Two further problems with this revised diagnosis relate to the subtyping of pain disorder into (a) associated with psychological factors and (b) associated with a medical condition. In reference to psychological factors in the preamble to this diagnosis, the *DSM-IV* claims that psychological factors involved in this disorder "may consist of another Axis I or Axis II disorder or may be of a nature that does not reach the threshold for such a disorder (e.g., reactions to psychosocial stressors)." Most chronic pain patients are depressed (25), and whether this depression precedes, follows, and/or exacerbates chronic pain is at issue (82). Yet, in subtyping this disorder, the *DSM-IV* asks the psychiatric examiner to judge whether psychological factors have the major role in the onset, severity, exacerbation, or maintenance of the pain. Theoretically, then, a large percentage of chronic pain patients suffering from depression could become candidates for this subtype. Again, the issue of overinclusiveness surfaces. The final problem relates to the "associated with a medical condition" subtype. Here, if the pain is judged to be associated with a medical condition, it is not coded on Axis I but rather on Axis III and thus is not a mental disorder. However, as discussed under the section on fibromyalgia, few CPPs do not have physical findings of myofascial pain syndrome or fibromyalgia (42). As such, in a pain facility where such a diagnosis is made with regularity, no CPP would be a candidate for a pain disorder diagnosis on Axis I (a psychiatric disorder). In this case the criteria here lead to a situation of underinclusions.

Outside of the preceding problems with developing reliable and valid criteria for this diagnosis, there are general problems with the idea that the concept "psychological factors involved in the etiology of the pain" is a viable one. This is because a couple of studies have indicated that CPPs with a pain disorder diagnosis actually respond to pain medications as if they have real pain. In the first study, Chabal et al. (83) demonstrated that 91% of CPPs without objective physical findings responded to injections of intrathecal fentanyl as if the pain involved nociception. Similarly, results were obtained by Fishbain et al. (84) in a metaanalysis of antidepressant treatment for pain in somatoform pain disorder and psychogenic pain disorder. The results indicated that antidepressants are effective for the pain of somatoform pain disorder (84). Such studies certainly support the contention that we may not, as yet, understand the etiology of the pain in those patients with alleged somatoform pain disorder/psychogenic pain and raise questions regarding the validity of this diagnosis. However, until such time as we have further scientific evidence for the validity/nonvalidity of pain disorder, we should continue utilizing this diagnosis. However, as described earlier, the pain physician should keep the limitations of this diagnosis in a proper perspective.

Key Points

Pain disorder is a problematic diagnosis in terms of reliability and validity.
The concept behind this disorder may not be viable.

Clinical Implication

This diagnosis should be assigned with great care.

Factitious Disorder

The criteria for this disorder specify that physical or psychological symptoms are consciously feigned in order to assume the sick role (secondary gain) for which there is unconscious motivation (21). Factitious disorder is rare and is often comorbidly associated with personality disorders (borderline, antisocial) (85). It is difficult to make this diagnosis because the patient either has to admit to disease simulation or has to be caught in the act of disease simulation (29), e.g., injecting himself/herself with insulin in order to become hypoglycemic (in a nondiabetic patient). However, some characteristics of disease simulator patients, when present, can be utilized to raise the specter of suspicion for this diagnosis. These are presented in Table 39-5. A limited number (29,86) of CPPs have been identified as having this problem. The rarity of reports of this diagnosis from pain facilities speaks either to the problems in making this diagnosis or to the fact that it may indeed be rare in pain facilities.

TABLE 39-5. *Characteristics of disease simulation patients (29)*

Alienation from family	Drifter	Previous suicide ideation and/or attempts
Medical career	Spotty job history	Borderline personality characteristics
Disability status	Drug knowledge and interest	Staff dependency Hospital dependency
Complicated medical history	Drug dependence	Difficulties with patient at transfer or discharge from hospital
Great number of surgeries	Medical sophistication	Difficulties with detoxification
Multiple hospitalizations	Previous psychiatric treatment or hospitalization	Anger/hostility at transfer/discharge
Discrepancies in medical record		Suicidal ideation at transfer/discharge
Medical care all over United States	Family psychiatric history	Fear of vocational functioning
No permanent place of residence	Family history of alcohol or drug abuse	Pseudologica fantastica (Pathological lying intriguing to the listener)

Key Point

The diagnosis of factitious disorder should be entertained only on patient admission of disease simulation, i.e., pain simulation or observation of disease simulation.

Clinical Implication

Suspicion of factitious disorder should depend on whether the CPP has some characteristics previously described for this disorder.

Malingering

Malingering is not defined as a mental disorder, rather, it is an act and is therefore not an official psychiatric illness (21). *Malingering* is defined as the conscious and deliberate production, simulation, or exaggeration of a symptom for a conscious gain such as obtaining disability payments or avoiding military service (21). There are few studies of malingering; therefore, it is difficult to determine the prevalence of this condition. Fishbain et al. (28) have recently reviewed the literature on malingering as it relates to pain. They found that the range for reports on malingering in

CPPs is between 0% and 22%. This finding is in stark contrast to a report by the Institute of Medicine on pain and disability, which could not find any studies related to malingering and pain and concluded that malingering is rare in the chronic pain setting (87). Fishbain et al. (28), however, cautioned that their figures are likely to be incorrect and an overestimate due to the poor quality of the reviewed studies. In addition, Fishbain et al. (28) reported that there was no reliable and valid method of identifying the CPP malingerer yet available.

Key Point

Although some pain physicians believe that malingering is not rare within pain facilities, there is no reliable evidence to support this belief.

Clinical Implication

CPPs suspected of malingering should be treated like any other CPP until definitive evidence is available such as that provided by covert observation.

THE DIAGNOSTIC PROCESS FOR THE SOMATIZING DISORDERS

In this section all the information presented earlier will be integrated into an algorithm (Fig. 39-1) in order to generate a sequential process for the presented concepts. Referring to Fig. 39-1 the first question asked is whether the CPP has "nonspecific" pain. Absence of "nonspecific" pain or the presence of "specific" pain precludes any of the somatizing diagnoses in relationship to pain as a symptom. If the CPP is then found to have physical findings compatible with MFPS or FMS, he/she has "specific" pain and, therefore, also cannot have a somatizing diagnosis. In the next step the physician is asked to determine if the CPP has a nonorganic physical finding and/or a conversion symptom. Absence of both of these again precludes the CPP from being considered for a somatizing diagnosis. The CPP who is not eliminated by this process is then a candidate for a somatizing diagnosis and should now be referred for examination by a psychiatrist or psychologist. It is to be noted here that a somatizing diagnosis *cannot* be made through any kind of psychological testing, including the MMPI. Thus, if the CPP is referred to a psychologist, use of *DSM-IV* criteria should be expected. The psychiatrist or psychologist should examine the CPP utilizing *DSM-IV* criteria and first determine if the CPP has a secondary somatizing disorder. If so, the comorbid psychiatric disorder should be diagnosed and treated aggressively (maximum psychopharmacological doses indicated for that disorder). Such treatment, if successful, could improve or resolve the somatizing disorder. If the CPP is diagnosed as suffering from a chronic somatizing disorder (hypochondriasis, somatization disorder, BDD, conversion disorder, pain disorder, factitious disorder, malingering), then that psychiatrist or psychologist should decide if that CPP has some elements of obsessive-compulsive spectrum disorder. If so, aggressive treatment with antiobsessional agents should be instituted. Failure of this type of treatment is an indication to institute treatments specific to the type of somatizing disorder in question. In addition, as shown in Fig. 39-1, failure of aggressive treatment for the comorbid psychiatric disorder causing a secondary somatizing disorder is an indication for a search for obsessive-compulsive spectrum disorder features in that patient.

Key Point

As shown in Fig. 39-1, the diagnostic process for the somatizing disorders begins with an exclusionary process and focuses on identifying psychiatric comorbidity.

Clinical Implication

Failure to exclude treatable disorders such as MFPS or FMS or to identify comorbid psychiatric disorders may impact on the treatment outcome for CPPs with alleged somatizing disorders.

Specific Treatments for the Somatizing Disorders

Treatments for these disorders are summarized in Tables 39-6 and 39-7 and are broken down into two major categories: general treatment approach (Table 39-6) and specific treatment approaches (Table 39-7). The general treatment approach applies to the whole group of somatizing disorders and addresses the central issue in these disorders: the beliefs that the symptom experienced is a symptom of a serious disease and the expectation that he/she will get worse. It is to be noted that the suggested treatment here is acceptable explanation and reassurance. An incorrect approach is telling the patient that there is nothing wrong with him/her or that the symptom is in his/her head or that he/she has a psychiatric problem that causes the symptom. This general approach also addresses two other issues: the tendency to enter the sick role and the portrayal of the symptom as catastrophic. It is also important to address these two issues appropriately as in Table 39-6. This type of general approach has been embraced by pain facilities and has allowed whatever success is possible in the treatment of CPPs. Before the general acceptance and utilization of this approach, CPPs would simply go from doctor to doctor looking for someone who could give them an explanation for their nonspecific pain, thereby not engaging themselves in treatment.

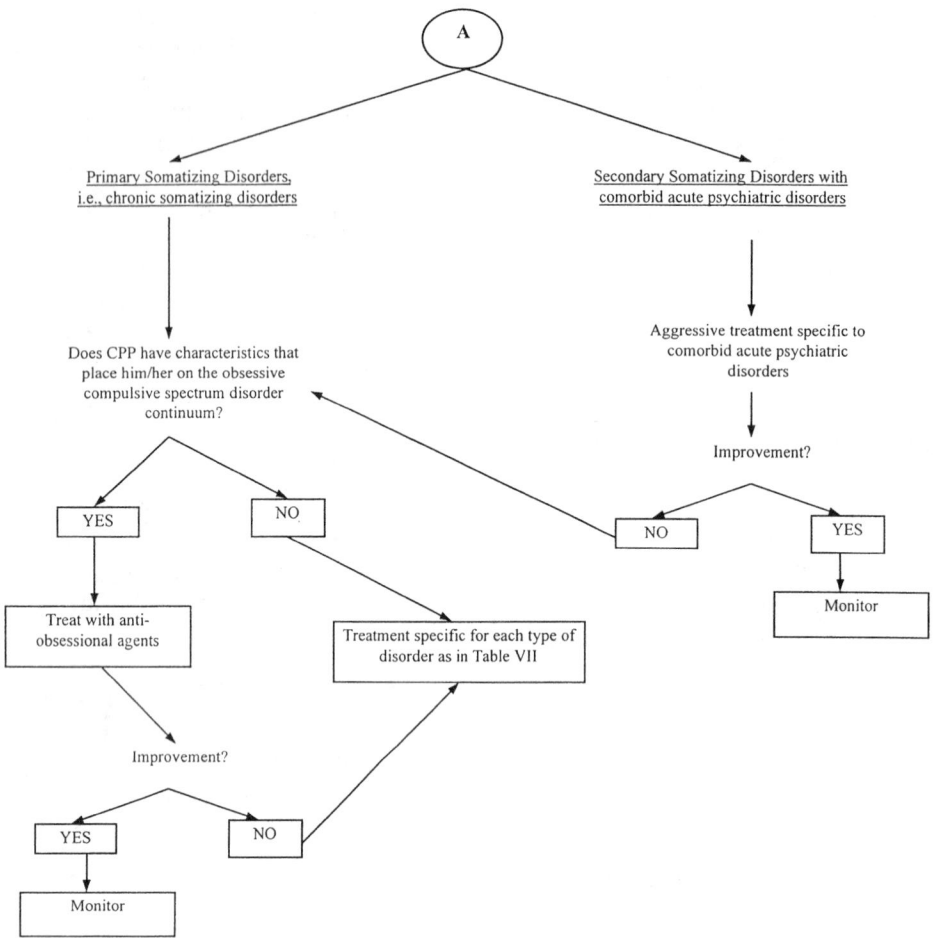

FIG. 39-1. Diagnostic process for the somatizing disorder.

Key Point

The general treatment approach to the somatizing disorders addresses the patients' belief system in reference to their symptom, e.g., pain, in an explanatory, reassuring fashion.

Clinical Implication

The somatizing disorders cannot be effectively treated without this general approach.

The specific treatments for the somatizing disorders are broken down by disorder in Table 39-7. For hypochondriasis three general types of treatments have been utilized with mixed success: psychotherapy utilizing the general treatment approach described earlier; behavioral-oriented psychotherapy; and antidepressant medications (Table 39-7). It is to be noted here that although many of these reported treatments were treatment studies, none of them

was placebo controlled. In reference to the reported success of antidepressants, it is unclear if the antidepressants are allegedly effective because of their antidepressant effect or because of their obsessive-compulsive spectrum disorder effect. In general, it appears that there is some limited success in the treatment of this somatizing disorder.

Somatization disorder is the next somatizing disorder to be considered. Here there are few treatment reports (Table 39-7 [II]) and limited treatment success. Again, these patients appear to respond best to a cognitive behavioral approach that stresses techniques in dealing with their physicians rather than approaches that advise them that their symptoms are not real. The best treatment efficacy studies with the somatizing disorders are for body dysmorphic disorder (Table 39-7 [III]). Here the studies break down into two groups: behavioral-oriented psychotherapy and medications. BDD patients appear to respond well to both types of treatments, with a particularly robust response to antidepressant antiobsessional agents (clomipramine, fluvoxamine). This type of response is in keeping with BDD, being one of the best-

TABLE 39-6. *General treatment approach to the somatizing disorders*

Issues that propel the cycle of symptom amplification (88)	Approach
1. Belief that one has serious disease (88)	1. Acceptable explanation for symptom (89)
	2. Serious illness not present (90)
2. Expectation that disease will get worse (88)	1. Suggest symptom will resolve over time (90)
3. The "sick role" (88)	1. Tell patient to return to normal activity (90)
4. Portrayal of condition as catastrophic or disabling (88)	1. Tell patient condition not catastrophic or disabling (90)

TABLE 39-7. *Various reported specific treatments for the somatizing disorders, with references*

	References
I. Hypochondriasis	
Cognitive behavior treatment	(97)
Explanatory therapy	(98)
Attention training	(99)
Exposure	(100)
Fluoxetine	(101)
Imipramine	(102)
Reassurance	(103)
II. Somatization disorder	
Cognitive behavioral group therapy	(104)
Electrosleep	(105)
III. BBD	
Fluvoxamine	(106)
Buspirone augmentation SSRI	(107)
Cognitive behavioral	(108)
Body image therapy	(109)
Behavioral treatment	(110)
Exposure with response prevention	(111)
Clomipramine	(112)
IV. Conversion disorder	
A. *Paralysis*	
Behavioral modification	(113,114)
Physical therapy	(113)
Suggestion hypnosis	(115)
Narcosuggestion	(113)
Functionally based rehab program	(113)
• EMG biofeedback	(79)
• Functional electrical stimulation	(91)
Combination treatment	(116)
Methamphetamine	(117)
B. *Nondermatomal sensory abnormalities*	
Blocks	(80,81)
C. *Gait abnormalities*	
Behavior modification	(118)
Psychotherapy	(119)
V. Pain disorder	
Antidepressants	(84)
Cognitive behavior therapy	(95)
Gabapentin	(96)
VI. Factitious disorder	
Psychotherapy	(120)
Pimozide	(121)
VII. Malingering	
No treatment reported	

characterized and best-studied obsessive-compulsive spectrum disorders.

As shown in Table 39-7, there are reports of treatments for three types of conversion disorders: paralysis, nondermatomal sensory abnormalities, and gait abnormalities. As pointed out earlier, these three types of conversion disorders are commonly seen in association with chronic pain, and thus the reported benefits of these treatments are of importance to the pain physician. It is important to emphasize that the evidence for the efficacy of these treatments for these three conversion disorders does not come from studies but rather from case report data. In reference to conversion paralysis, the reported treatments break down into the following general groups: hypnosis; behavioral modification, including EMG biofeedback, physical therapy, and drugs (methamphetamine); and functional electrical stimulation. It appears that the most successful treatments combine a behavior-modification regimen with activation and physical therapy. In our experience this type of combination is strengthened by the addition of functional electrical stimulation and/or EMG biofeedback (79,81). For details of how to perform functional electrical stimulation and/or EMG biofeedback in conversion paralysis patients, please refer to references (79) and (91). Medications have not been found to be particularly helpful here. Medications may, however, aid in a treatment combination rehabilitation program, especially if there is an obsessive component to the patient's psyche, although conversion paralysis is not an obsessive-compulsive spectrum disorder. As can be seen from Table 39-7 (IV B and C), there are few treatments reported to be successful for nondermatomal sensory abnormalities and for gait abnormalities. In the author's opinion, both of these conversion disorders are usually a function of pain and are best treated as part of a pain treatment program.

In reference to pain disorder, it needs to be noted that there is extensive chronic pain treatment outcome literature, including metaanalyses (92–94), that indicates that various

treatments, such as pain facility treatment, antidepressants, cognitive behavioral, etc., are effective for the treatment of chronic pain. However, these data do not address pain disorder that forms a subcategory within the chronic pain population. Because of the difficulties with the diagnostic nomenclature of pain disorder (described earlier) there are few treatment studies for this disorder. The available information on the treatment for this disorder is presented in Table 39-7 (V). There is actually good evidence on the efficacy of antidepressants for this disorder. This information has been compiled into a metaanalysis (84) that indicated that antidepressants are effective for *the pain of pain disorder*. If the pain of pain disorder was a behavior phenomenon, response to antidepressants should be no greater than to placebo. Such is not the case. As such, these drugs appear to treat "real" perceived pain. In addition to antidepressants there has been one reported study of cognitive behavior therapy being effective (95). Finally, gabapentin, an anticonvulsant, has also been reported to be effective in one study (96).

Patients with factitious disorder on discovery usually leave the hospital or facility Against Medical Advice (AMA). Thus, there are few treatment reports for this condition. Currently there are only two case reports in the literature reporting on the use of psychotherapy and pimozide (Table 39-7 [VI]). Pimozide is a neuroleptic that has had some success in the treatment of delusional disorders with a somatic delusion such as being infected with AIDS.

Malingering is the final somatizing disorder to be discussed in terms of treatment. There are no reports in the literature of treatment for malingering. This is because of the difficulty of arriving at a malingering diagnosis and the usual reaction (anger) of the patient at such an accusation. Usually after the accusation, treatment is terminated by the patient.

CONCLUSION

Overall, there is little information on the treatment of the somatizing disorders. The best scientific evidence for treatment efficacy exists for the best-characterized and most diagnostically sound disorders, such as BDD and hypochondriasis. This area awaits further improved research.

Key Point

There are limited data on specific treatment for the somatizing disorders.

Clinical Implication

Pain physicians will need to be creative in their decisions about treatment for this group of disorders, utilizing the previously reviewed literature as much as possible.

REFERENCES

1. Sullivan M, Katon W. The path between distress and somatic symptoms. *Am Pain Soc J* 1993;2:141–149.
2. Lipowski ZJ. Somatization and depression. *Psychosomatics* 1990;31:13–21.
3. Bridges RN, Goldberg DP. Somatic presentation of DSM-III psychiatric disorders in primary care. *J Psychosom Res* 1985;29:563–569.
4. Ford CV. The somatizing disorders. *Psychosom* 1986;27:327–337.
5. Kellner R, Sheffield BR. The one-week prevalence of symptoms in neurotic patients and normals. *Am J Psych* 1973;130:102–105.
6. Kroenke K, Mangelsdorff A. Common symptoms in ambulatory care: incidence, evaluation, therapy, and outcome. *Am J Med* 1989;86:262–266.
7. Wallen J, Pincus HA, Goldman HH. Psychiatric consultations in shorts-term general hospitals. *Arch Gen Psych* 1987;44:163–168.
8. Pilowsky I, Spence ND. Patterns of illness behaviour in patients with intractable pain. *Psychosom Res* 1975;19:279–287.
9. Sikorski JM, Stampfer HG, Cole RM. Psychological aspects of chronic low back pain. *Aust N Z J Surg* 1996;66:294–297.
10. Zach GA, Andreasen K. Evaluation of the psychological profiles of patients with signs and symptoms of temporomandibular disorders. *J Prosthet Den* 1991;66:810–812.
11. McGregor NR, Butt HL, Zerebes M, et al. Assessment of pain (distribution and onset), symptoms, SCL-90-R inventory responses, and the association with infectious events in patients with chronic orofacial pain. *J Orofac Pain* 1996;10:339–350.
12. Merkangas KR, Stevens DE, Angst J. Headache and personality: results of a community sample of young adults. *J Psych Res* 1993;27:187–196.
13. Serlie AW, Duivenvoorden HJ, Passchier J, et al. Empirical psychological modeling of chests pain: a comparative study. *J Psych Res* 1996;40:625–635.
14. Bacon NM, Bacon SF, Atkinson JH, et al. Somatization symptoms in chronic low back pain patients. *Psychosom Med* 1994;56:118–127.
15. Ahles TA, Khan SA, Yunus MB, et al. Psychiatric status of patients with primary fibromyalgia, patients with rheumatoid arthritis, and subjects without pain: a blind comparison of DSM-III diagnoses. *Am J Psych* 1991;148:1721–1726.
16. Vassend O, Krogstad BS, Dahl BL. Negative affectivity, somatic complaints, and symptoms of temporomandibular disorders. *J Psychosom Res* 1995;39:889–899.
17. Dionne CE, Koepsell BS, Dahl BL. Predicting long-term functional limitations among back pain patients in primary care settings. *J Clin Epidemiol* 1997;50:31–43.
18. Katon W, Kleinman A, Rosen G. Depression and somatization: a review Part I. *Am J Med* 1982;72:127–135.
19. McFarland BH, Freeborn DK, Mullooly JP. Utilization patterns among long-term enrollees in a prepaid group practice health maintenance organization. *Med Care* 1985;23:1221–1233.
20. Chandler JD, Gerndt J. Somatization, depression and medical illness in psychiatric inpatients. *Acta Psychiatr Scand* 1988;77:67–73.
21. American Psychiatric Association. *Diagnostic and Statistical Manual of Mental Disorders*, 4th ed. Washington, DC: American Press 1994.
22. Ford CV. Dimensions of somatization and hypochondriasis. *Neurologic Clin* 1995;13:241–253.
23. Pilowsky I. The concept of abnormal illness behavior. *Psychosomatics* 1990;31(2):207–213.
24. Fishbain DA, Goldberg M, Meagher BR, et al. Male and female chronic pain patients categorized by DSM-III psychiatric diagnostic criteria. *Pain* 1986;26:181–197.
25. Reich J, Rosenblatt RM, Tupen J. DSM-III: a new nomenclature for classifying patients with chronic pain. *Pain* 1983;16:201–206.
26. Katon W, Egan K, Millder D. Chronic pain: lifetime psychiatric diagnoses and family history. *Am J Psych* 1985;142:1156–1160.
27. Large RG. DSM-III diagnosis in chronic pain—confusion or clarity? *J Nerv Ment Dis* 1986;174:295–302.
28. Fishbain DA, Cutler R, Rosomoff HL, et al. Chronic pain disability exaggeration/malingering research and submaximal effort research. *Clin J Pain* 1999;15(4)244–274.
29. Fishbain DA, Goldberg M, Steele-Rosomoff et al. More munchausen with chronic pain. *Clin J Pain* 1991;7:237–244.
30. Polatin PB, Kinney RK, Gatachel RJ, et al. Psychiatric illness and chronic low back pain. *Spine* 1993;18:66–71.
31. Anooshian J, Streltzer J, Goebert D. Effectiveness of a psychiatric pain clinic. *Psychosomatics* 1999;40:226–232.
32. Cedraschi C, Nordin M, Nachemson AL, Vischer TL. Health care providers should use a common language in relation to low back pain patients. *Bailliere's Clin Rheumatology* 1998;12(1):1–13.
33. Haldeman S. Failure of the pathology model to predict back pain. *Spine* 1990;15:718–724.
34. Deyo RA, Fihillips WR. Low back pain. A primary care challenge. *Spine* 1996;21:2826–2832.
35. Kennedy LD. Laboratory Investigation. Chapter 5, In: Raj PP, ed. *Pain medicine, a comprehensive review*. St. Louis, MO: Mosby, 1996:47–54.

36. Peyrot M, Moody PM, Wiese HJ. Biogenic, psychogenic, and sociogenic models of adjustment to chronic pain: an exploratory study. *Int J Psych Med* 1993;23(1):63–80.
37. Wolfe F, Smythe HA, Yunus MB. The American College of Rheumatology 1990 criteria for the classification of fibromyalgia: report of the Multicenter Criteria Committee. *Arth Rheum* 1990;33:160–172.
38. Simons DG. Referred phenomena of myofascial trigger points. In: Vechiet L, Albe-Fessard D, Lindblom U, eds. *New trends in referred pain and hyperalgesia.* Amsterdam: Elsevier 1993;341.
39. Wolfe F, Ross K, Anderson J, et al. The prevalence and characteristics of fibromyalgia in the general population. *Arth Rheum* 1995;38:19–28.
40. Han SC, Harrison P. Myofascial pain syndrome and trigger point management. *Reg Anesth* 1997;22:89–101.
41. Hubbard DR. Chronic and recurrent muscle pain: pathophysiology and treatment and review of pharmacologic studies. *J Musculoskeletal Pain* 1996;4:123–143.
42. Rosomoff HL, Fishbain DA, Goldberg M, et al. Physical findings in patients with chronic intractable benign pain of the neck and/or back. *Pain* 1989;37:279–287.
43. Borkan JM, Reius S. Hermoni D, Biderman A. Talking about the pain: a patient-centered study of low back pain in primary care. *Social Sci Med* 1995;40:977–988.
44. Deyo RA, Diehl AK. Patient satisfaction with medical care for low-back pain. *Spine* 1986;11:28–30.
45. Abenhaim L, Rossignol M, Gobeille D. The prognostic consequences in the making of the initial medical diagnosis of work-related injuries. *Spine* 1995;20:791–795.
46. Bohr T. Problems with myofascial pain syndrome and fibromyalgia. *Neurology* 1996;46:593–597.
47. Cathey MA, Wolfe K, Dleinhekss SM, Hawley DJ. Socioeconomic impact of fibrositis: a study of 81 patients with primary fibrositis. *Am J Med* 1986;81:78–84.
48. Waddell G. A new clinical model for the treatment of low-back pain. *Spine* 1987;12:632–670.
49. Waddell G, McCulfoch JA, Kimmel E, Verner RM. Non-organic physical signs in low back pain. *Spine* 1980;5:117–125.
50. Kiesler PD, Duke AD. Is it malingering or is it real? Eight signs that point to non-organic back pain. *Post Grad Med* 1999;106(7):1–8.
51. Sculzitti DA. Screening for psychological factors in patients with low back problems: Waddell's non-organic signs. *Physical Therapy* 1997;77(3):306–311.
52. Fishbain DA, Goldberg M, Ferretti T, et al. The non-dermatomal sensory abnormality (NDSA) and pain perception. *Pain* 1990;(suppl S5):S332.
53. Lehmann TR, Russell DW, Spratt KF. The impact of patients with non-organic physical findings on a controlled trial of transcutaneous electrical nerve stimulation. *Spine* 1983;8:625–634.
54. Main CJ, Waddell G. A reappraisal of the interpretation of "nonorganic signs." *Spine* 1998;23(21):2367–2371.
55. McCombe PF, Fairbank JCT, Cockersole BC, Pysent PB. Reproducibility of physical signs in low back pain. *Spine* 1989;14:908–917.
56. Fishbain DA, Goldberg M, Steele-Rosomoff R, Rosomoff HL. Chronic pain patients and the non-organic physical sign of non-dermatomal sensory abnormalities (NDSA). *Psychosomatics* 1991;32:294–303.
57. Korbon GA, DeGood DE, Schroeder ME. The development of a somatic amplification rating scale for low back pain. *Spine* 1987;12(8):787–791.
58. Kroenke K, Spitzer RL, Williams JBW, et al. Physical symptoms in primary care. Predictors of psychiatric disorders and functional impairment. *Arch Fam Med* 1994;3:774–779.
59. Russo J, Katon W, Sullivan M, et al. Severity of somatization and its relationship to psychiatric disorders and personality. *Psychosomatics* 1994;35:546–556.
60. Fishbain DA, Cutler BR, Rosomoff H, Steele Rosomoff R. Comorbidity between psychiatric disorders and chronic pain. *Curr Rev of Pain* 1998;2:1–10.
61. Kouyanou K, Pither CE, Rabe-Hesketh S, Wessely S. A comparative study of iatrogenesis, medication abuse, and psychiatric morbidity in chronic pain patients with and without medically explained symptoms. *Pain* 1998;76:417–426.
62. Asmundson GJG, Rorton GR, Jacobson SJ. Social, blood/injury, and agoraphobic fears in patients with physically unexplained chronic pain: are they clinically significant? *Anxiety* 1996;2:28–33.
63. McElroy SL, Phillips KA, Keck PE Jr. Obsessive compulsive spectrum disorder. *J Clin Psych* 1994;55(Suppl):33–53.
64. Hollander E. Treatment of obsessive-compulsive spectrum disorders with SSRIs. *Brit J Psych* 1998;35(S):7–12.
65. Noyes R Jr, Happel RL, Muller BA, et al. Fluvoxamine for somatoform disorders: an open trial. *Gen Hosp Psych* 1998;20(6):339–344.
66. Fishbain DA, Trescott J, Cutler B, et al. Do some chronic pain patients with atypical facial pain overvalue and obsess about their pain? *Psychosomatics* 1993;34(4):355–359.
67. Kurokawa K, Tanino R. Effectiveness of clomipramine for obsessive-compulsive symptoms and chronic pain in two patients with schizophrenia. *J Clin Psychopharm* 1997;17(4):329–330.
68. Barsky AJ, Wyashak GL. The prevalence of hypochondriasis in medical outpatients. *Soc Psych Epidemiol* 1990;25:89–94.
69. Fischer-Homberger E. Hypochondriasis of the eighteenth century—neurosis of the present century. *Bull Hist Med* 1972;46:391–401.
70. Barsky AJ, Wyshak G, Klerman GL. Psychiatric comorbidity in DSM-III-R hypochondriasis. *Arch Gen Psych* 1992;49:101–108.
71. Noyes R Jr., Holt CS, Happel RL, et al. A family study of hypochondriasis. *J Nerv Ment Dis* 1997;185:223–232.
72. Liskow B, Othmer E, Penick EC. Is Briquet's syndrome a heterogenous disorder? *AM J Psychiatry* 1986;143:626–629.
73. Brown FW, Golding JM, Smith GR Jr. Psychiatric comorbidity in primary care somatization disorder. *Psych Med* 1990;52(4):445–551.
74. Rost KM, Akins RN, Brown FW. The comorbidity of DSM-III-R personality disorders in somatization disorder. *Gen Hosp Psychiatry* 1992;14:322–326.
75. Hollander E, Aronowitz BR. Comorbid social anxiety and body sysmorphic disorder: managing the complicated patient. *J Clin Psych* 1999;60(9):27–31.
76. Fishbain DA, Goldberg M. The misdiagnosis of conversion disorder in a psychiatric emergency service. *General Hospital Psych* 1991;13:177–181.
77. Fishbain D. Response to "the misdiagnosis of conversion disorder in a psychiatric emergency service." *Gen Hosp Psych* 1992;14(2):146–148.
78. Lempert T, Dieterich M, Huppert D, Brandt T. Psychogenic disorders in neurology: frequency and clinical spectrum. *Acta Neuro Scand* 1990;82(5):335–340.
79. Fishbain DA, Goldberg M, Khalil TM, et al. The utility of electromyographic biofeedback in the treatment of conversion paralysis. *Am J Psych* 1988;145(12):1572–1575.
80. Verdugo RJ, Ochoa JL. Reversal of hypesthesia by nerve block, or placebo: a psychologically mediated sign in chronic pseudoneuropathic pain patients. *J Neurology, Neurosurg & Psych* 1998;65(2):196–203.
81. Moriwaki K, Yugae O, Nishioka K, et al. Reduction in the size of tactile hypesthesia and allodynia closely associated with pain relief in patients with chronic pain. *Progress Pain Research Management* 1994;2:819–830.
82. Fishbain DA, Cutler R, Rosomoff HL, Steele Rosomoff R. Chronic pain-associated depression: antecedent or consequence of chronic pain? a review. *Clin J Pain* 1997;13:116–137.
83. Jacobson L, Chabal C, Mariano AJ, Chaney EF. Persistent low-back pain is real. However, diagnostic spinal injections are not helpful in its evaluation. *Clin J Pain* 1992;8:237–241.
84. Fishbain DA, Cutler RB, Rosomoff HL, Rosomoff RS. Do antidepressants have an analgesic effect in psychogenic pain and somatoform pain disorder? A meta-analysis. *Psychosom Med* 1998;60(4):503–509.
85. Nadelson T. False patients/real patients: a spectrum of disease presentation. *Psychother Psychosomatics* 1985;44:175–184.
86. Wemyss-Gorman PB. Munchausen's syndrome and chronic pain. *Hosp Med* 1998;59(9):738.
87. Institute of medicine. Pain and disability, clinical, behavioral, and public policy perspectives. Edited by Osterweis M, Kleinman A, Mechanic D. Washington, DC. National Academy Press, 1987.
88. Barsky AJ, Borus JF. Functional somatic syndromes. *Ann Intern Med* 1999;130(11):910–921.
89. Servan-Schreiber D, Kolb R, Tabas G. The somatizing patient. *Prim Care; Clinics in Office Practice* 1999;26(2):225–242.
90. Kathol RG. Reassurance therapy: what to say to symptomatic patients with benign or non-existent medical disease. *Int J Psych Med* 1997;27(2):173–180.

91. Abdel-Moty E, Fishbain DA, Goldberg M, et al. Functional electrical stimulation treatment of postradiculopathy associated muscle weakness. *Arch Phys Med Rehabil* 1994;75:680–686.

92. Fishbain DA. Non-surgical chronic pain treatment outcome: a review. *Int Rev Psych* 2000;12:170–180.

93. Fishbain DA, Cutler R, Rosomoff HL, Steele Rosomoff R. What is the quality of the implemented meta-analytic procedures in chronic pain treatment meta-analyses? *Clin J Pain* 1999;16:73–85.

94. Fishbain DA, Rosomoff HL, Steele Rosomoff R, Cutler BR. Types of pain treatment facilities and referral selection criteria: a review. *Arch Fam Med* 1995;4:58–66.

95. Mayou RA, Bryant BM, Sanders D, et al. A controlled trial of cognitive behavioural therapy for non-cardiac chest pain. *Psych Med* 1997;27(5):1021–1031.

96. Maurer I, Volz HP, Sauer H. Gabapentin leads to remission of somatoform pain disorder with major depression. *Pharmacopsych* 1999;32(6):255–257.

97. Clark DM, Salkovskis PM, Hackmann A, et al. Two psychological treatments for hypochondriasis. a randomized controlled trial. *Brit J Psych* 1998;173:218–225.

98. Fava GA, Grandi S, Rafanelli C, et al. Explanatory therapy in hypochondriasis. *J Clin Psych* 2000;61(4):317–322.

99. Papageorgiou C, Wells A. Effects of attention training on hypochondriasis: a brief case series. *Psychological Med* 1998;28(1):193–200.

100. Tearnan BH, Goetsch V, Adams HE. Modification of disease phobia using a multifaceted exposure program. *J Behav Ther & Exper Psych* 1985;16(1):57–61.

101. Fallon BA, Liebowitz MR, Salman E, et al. Fluoxetine for hypochondriacal patients without major depression. *J Clin Psychopharm* 1993;13(6):438–441.

102. Wesner RB, Noyes R Jr. Imipramine an effective treatment for illness phobia. *J Affective Disorders* 1991;22(1-2):43–48.

103. Starcevic V. Reassurance and treatment of hypochondriasis. *Gen Hospital Psych* 1991;13(2):122-127.

104. Lidbeck J. Group therapy for somatization disorders in general practice: effectiveness of a short cognitive-behavioural treatment model. *Acta Psych Scand* 1997;96(1):14–24.

105. Scallet A, Cloninger R, Othmer E. The management of chronic hysteria: a review and double-blind trial of electrosleep and other relaxation methods. *Dis Nerv System* 1976;91:347–353.

106. Phillips KA, Dwight MM, McElroy SL. Efficacy and safety of fluvoxamine in body dysmorphic disorder. *J Clin Psych* 1998;59(4):165–171.

107. Phillips KA. An open study of buspirone augmentation of serotonin-reuptake inhibitors in body dysmorphic disorder. *Psychopharm Bull* 1996;32(1):175–180.

108. Wilhelm S, Otto MW, Lohr B, Deckersbach T. Cognitive behavior group therapy for body dysmorphic disorder: a case series. *Behav Res & Ther* 1999;37(1):71–75.

109. Rosen JC, Reiter J, Orosan P. Cognitive-behavioral body image therapy for body dysmorphic disorder. *J Consult & Clin Psychol* 1995; 63(2):263–269.

110. McKay D. Two-year follow-up of behavioral treatment and maintenance for body dysmorphic disorder. *Behav Mod* 1999;23(4): 620–629.

111. McKay D, Todaro J, Neziroglu K, et al. Body dysmorphic disorder: a preliminary evaluation of treatment and maintenance using exposure with response prevention. *Behav Res & Ther* 1997;35(1):67–70.

112. Hollander E, Allen A, Kwon J, et al. Clomipramine vs desipramine crossover trail in body dysmorphic disorder: selective efficacy of a serotonin reuptake inhibitor in imagined ugliness. *Arch Gen Psych* 1999;56(11):1041–1042.

113. Watanabe TK, O'Dell MW, Togliatti TJ. Diagnosis and rehabilitation strategies for patients with hysterical hemiparesis: a report of four cases. *Arch Phys Med Rehabil* 1998;79(6):709–714.

114. Campo JV, Negrini BJ. Case study: negative reinforcement and behavioral management of conversion disorder. *J Am Acad Child & Adolescent Psychiatry* 2000;39(6):787–790.

115. Moene FC, Hoogduin KA, Van Dyck R. The inpatient treatment of patients suffering from (motor) conversion symptoms: a description of eight cases. *J Clin & Exper Hypnosis* 1998;46(2):171–190.

116. Speed J. Behavioral management of conversion disorder: retrospective study. *Arch Phys Med & Rehab* 1996;77(2):147–154.

117. Hafeiz HB. Hysterical conversion: a prognostic study. *Brit J Psych* 1980;136:548–551.

118. Teasell RW, Shapiro AP. Strategic-behavioral intervention in the treatment of chronic nonorganic motor disorders. *Am J Phys Med & Rehab* 1994;73(1):44–50.

119. Sinel M, Eisenberg MS. Two unusual gait disturbances: astasia abasia and camptocormia. *Arch Phys Med & Rehab* 1990;71(13):1078–1080.

120. Plassmann R. Inpatient and outpatient long-term psychotherapy of patients suffering from factitious disorders. *Psychother & Psychosom* 1994;62(1–2):96–107.

121. Prior TI, Gordon A. Treatment of factitious disorder with pimozide. *Can J Psych* 1997;42(5):532.

Cancer Pain

CHAPTER **40**

Cancer Pain Management

Richard B. Patt

SYMPTOM CONTROL: AN ESSENTIAL COMPONENT OF COMPREHENSIVE CANCER CARE

Until recently, curative and even palliative treatments for patients with neoplastic disease have focused on survival, whereas supportive care was more likely to be regarded as a secondary consideration, pertaining uniquely to the end of life (1,2). Recent initiatives, emphasizing the concept of comprehensive cancer care, mandate that attention to symptom control and psychosocial concerns be applied in an integrated fashion throughout the course of a cancer diagnosis (3,4). Contemporary approaches to managing pain and other symptoms emphasize earlier and more liberal use of opioids, recognizing their low addiction potential and overall favorable risk/benefit ratio (5,6,7,8). A second important concept, which has only recently become well established, relates to the use of the less traditional adjuvant analgesics (e.g., selected antidepressants, anticonvulsants) for specific types of pain (9). A corollary principle of critical importance is that these agents be integrated into the therapeutic matrix as adjuvants ("helpers") rather than as *substitutes* for the more reliable but more stigmatized traditional opioid analgesics (10). The role of invasive pain therapies, although critical, remains less well defined (11–13). Although the principles of contemporary pain management more than ever comprise a fundamental area of knowledge for providers of cancer care, unfortunately they remain underutilized despite unparalleled ongoing initiatives.

The prospect of suffering from unrelieved pain is one of the most feared aspects of a cancer diagnosis for most patients and their families (14). Optimal management parallels that of cancer treatment and involves careful assessment, individualization of therapy, close followup, and a proactive approach. Adequate control of pain can be achieved in the vast majority of patients with the rigorous and aggressive application of measures that are ultimately quite straightforward. Patients are reassured and symptoms are easier to control when it is communicated that pain is treatable and that symptom control is one of the treatment team's priorities. Optimal control of pain and related symptoms facilitates cancer treatment and promotes an enhanced quality of life, improved functioning, better compliance, and a means for patients to focus on those things that give meaning to life.

PUBLIC HEALTH ASPECTS: OPIOPHOBIA AND THE UNDERTREATMENT OF CANCER AND CHRONIC PAIN

Cancer pain is a significant public health problem that has, especially recently, galvanized the attention of health-care providers, professional societies, governmental agencies, and the general public (15,16). Cultural, philosophic, and especially logistic responses to the management of pain and suffering viewed against the backdrop of suggestions of a stalemate in the "war on cancer" (17) are an especially visible and compelling focus in the context of contemporary society's uniquely burgeoning interest in end-of-life issues (18–20). The synchronicity of a widespread recognition of ongoing undertreatment of cancer pain despite the availability of adequate resources and a heightened interest and advocacy of physician-assisted suicide and euthanasia can reasonably be interpreted as evidence for the failure of our health-care delivery systems to reflect societal values.

Another highly significant aspect of the status of our progress in addressing the symptomatic needs of cancer patients is its relationship and influence on the approaches applied to the management of chronic symptoms in nononcologic patients with refractory medical disorders (21). Despite the appearance of recent improvements in palliative care, epidemic historic undertreatment of cancer pain suggests inestimably far greater unmet needs in chronic pain patients who possess greater potential life expectancy and productivity but lack the compelling stigmata of cancer. Although a perplexingly new field, cancer pain management can in a very real and ethically sound sense be viewed as representing a "proving ground" for therapies that, although apparently safe, have been traditionally withheld for more obscure cultural reasons. After safety, efficacy, and familiarity are established in the more temporally desperate setting of cancer, many of the same therapies are finally considered more liberally in the setting of chronic pain due, for example, to sickle cell disease, HIV infection, and degenerative disorders (22–26).

OUTCOME DATA

Despite a legacy of undertreatment, contemporary experience has demonstrated that when evidence-based guidelines are applied in a systematic but individualized manner, favorable outcomes that are reproducible and cost effective can be achieved in most patients (27). Although significant pain is ultimately present in about two thirds of cancer patients, despite the dynamic nature of cancer and its attendant pain, durable relief can be obtained in 70% to 90% of patients with the application of straightforward "low tech" (noninvasive) pharmacologic approaches (e.g., oral, transdermal, and transmucosal medications) (28) that can be effectively delivered by primary-care providers (29). Most remaining patients can achieve satisfactory pain control with the judicious application of moderately invasive pharmacologic techniques (e.g., subcutaneous and intravenous infusions) (30,31) and, when appropriate, more highly invasive anesthetic and neurosurgical interventions carefully provided by specially trained consultants (32,33). Although the principles of pain management in cancer patients are ultimately straightforward, optimal delivery is time intensive, requires considerable attention to detail, and is best accomplished in an interdisciplinary context. Poorly controlled pain not only is demoralizing to patients, their relations, and health-care providers, but also can interfere with the delivery of timely antineoplastic therapy and may influence survival (34,35).

UNDERTREATMENT

Despite vast improvements in our understanding of pain and its management over the last decade, it is curious and, indeed, tragic that despite the availability of straightforward cost-effective therapies, cancer pain remains undertreated even in developed nations (36–38). The factors contributing to undertreatment are complex but well documented. Undertreatment is usually conceived of as relating to knowledge deficits, beliefs, and attitudes maintained by (a) health-care providers, (b) patients and family members, and (c) regulators and health-care delivery systems (39). Representative barriers are listed in Table 40-1. The most prevalent underlying issues relate to an inadequate understanding of the pharmacology of the opioid drugs and exaggerated fears of addiction. Thus, workable solutions relate less to developing new drugs or technology and instead involve improving the utilization of currently available techniques.

EPIDEMIOLOGY

Pain is among the most common symptoms associated with cancer, affecting about two thirds of patients overall (40,41). A considerable proportion of patients (15% to 25%) experience significant pain in association with early, localized, even curable disease (42). If pain is poorly controlled in this setting, then its effects may reduce the patient's compliance with plans for demanding cytotoxic therapies and, by influencing performance status, may exclude patients from entering protocols for investigational therapies. With the development of metastases, the incidence of pain increases to 40% to 60%, and in far advanced disease, 60% to 90% of patients report significant pain (43–47). As curative options become exhausted, the focus of care shifts, and symptom control assumes paramount importance.

CONTEMPORARY THEMES

Recent initiatives emphasizing the concept of comprehensive cancer care mandate that attention to symptom control and psychosocial concerns be applied in an integrated fashion throughout the course of a cancer diagnosis (48). Contemporary approaches to managing cancer pain can be viewed in the context of a number of themes and principles that underpin successful outcomes (Tables 40-2–40-4). The most prominent of these include (a) the need to individualize doses based on therapeutic response, (b) the use of adjuvant analgesics for neuropathic pain syndromes, (c) the time-contingent use of long-acting analgesics, and (d) the need for aggressive management of the temporary flares in pain that have come to be known as breakthrough pain (49,50).

ASSESSMENT

Assessment is the cornerstone for developing a diagnosis and effective treatment plan and should be explicitly performed in all cancer patients (Tables 40-2 and 40-3). The experience of pain varies according to many factors, including the meaning it imparts to the patient, and, as a result, the initial encounter should be broad based. In addition to focusing the inquiry on the pain syndrome *per se* (Table 40-5), the process should encompass evaluation of the person, his/her feelings and attitudes about pain and disease, and family concerns.

TABLE 40-1. *Barriers to effective cancer pain management*

I. Health-care provider–related barriers
  A. Lack of education and knowledge
    1. Re. assessment and management of pain, e.g., pharmacology of chronically administered opioids, management of opioid-mediated side effects
    2. Re. assessment and management of refractory pain, especially use of alternative treatments, e.g., adjuvant analgesics (antidepressants, anticonvulsants, etc.), parenteral routes, other treatment modalities
    3. Re. risks of analgesic therapy, e.g., addiction versus physical dependence versus tolerance, respiratory depression
  B. Outdated beliefs
    1. Pain is an unmanageable and inevitable feature of advanced cancer
    2. Use of opioids at effective doses is equivalent to euthanasia
    3. Opioids should be reserved for the dying patient
    4. Patient reports of pain are unreliable
  C. Reluctance to use triplicate prescriptions
    1. Added cost and effort
    2. Fear of reprisal from regulatory agencies
    3. Restrictions due to limits on quantities prescribed and telephone refills
  D. Practice management
    1. Lack of time, energy, motivation to make the frequent changes necessary to maintain pain control
    2. Inability to recognize patients' reluctance to discuss pain

II. Cultural or health-care system–related barriers
  A. War on drugs
    1. Failure to distinguish between illicit and medicinal uses
    2. Restrictive limits on prescribing
    3. Failure of pharmacies to stock strong opioids
  B. Medical education
    1. Medical school curricula and residency training programs do not provide information or adequate reference material on management of chronic pain
    2. Do not recognize pain management or palliative care as legitimate subspecialty
    3. Texts fail to distinguish between acute and chronic pains
  C. Health care
    1. Acute disease-oriented health-care model leads to lack of accountability for control of chronic symptoms, failure to coordinate as patient moves between care settings (e.g., hospital, home, nursing home, etc.)
    2. Inadequate resources for procedurally based pain management
    3. Fragmentation of care due to multiple specialists
    4. Resultant failure of some insurers to provide hospice care or to consider reimbursement for treatment aimed at comfort

III. Patient and family-related barriers
  A. Beliefs
    1. Pain inevitably accompanies cancer and is unmanageable
    2. Painkillers must be withheld until late in the disease process, or else they won't be effective
    3. Opioids have serious side effects, making people incoherent and high and leading to addiction
    4. Reluctance to take opioids due to their association with serious illness: may hasten death or signify the disease is incurable
  B. War on drugs
    1. Pressure (family, media, government) *never* to take opioids under any circumstances
    2. Reluctance to discuss pain with health-care provider
    3. Desire to be seen as a "good" patient
    4. Complaints may be regarded as weak character or an insult to the providers
    5. Reluctance to "use up" doctor's time
    6. Fear of an acknowledgment that the cancer has returned or is progressing

Published guidelines recommend that pain be assessed initially and then reassessed at regular intervals, at each new report of pain, and at suitable times following new interventions (e.g., 15 to 30 minutes after parenteral therapy and one hour after oral therapy) (51).

The assessment process may also serve to educate patient, family members, and referring physicians regarding the usually favorable prognosis for controlling pain. A compassionate, but objective, approach to assessment establishes a therapeutic alliance and serves to instill

TABLE 40-2. *General principles of pain management in the cancer patient: assessment*

- Assess the patient carefully prior to initiating treatment. A careful history and directed physical examination (especially of the painful region and neurologic and musculoskeletal systems) are essential.
- Assess pain in a global context. Elicit medical history, oncologic and social history, and presence of other distressing symptoms. Seek history of alcohol or drug abuse.
- Listen to and believe the patient's reports of pain and other symptoms, as well as the observations of the patient's relations.
- Ask explicitly about the presence and nature of pain and other symptoms. Pertinent information is often not otherwise volunteered.
- Seek the presence of multiple complaints of pain. When multiple complaints exist, they should each be evaluated as discrete, independent entities, as well as in their wider context. When appropriate, prioritize complaints based on how distressing they are, as well as their treatability.
- Assess the characteristics of each pain complaint: chronicity, location and referral or radiation, severity (best, worst, average, current), quality, temporal features, associated symptoms, aggravating and relieving factors.
- Assess pain complaints globally: in addition to pertinent physical aspects, assessment and ultimately management should address emotional, psychological, environmental, and spiritual factors that influence pain and well-being.

- Determine beneficial and adverse effects for each analgesic in current use, as well as those taken in the past. Determine to what degree trials of other agents have been adequate and thorough.
- Determine to what degree pain and other symptoms are distressing and interfere with activities that are important to the patient.
- Consider the use of a simple validated written instrument that can be rapidly completed to document self-report (e.g., Brief Pain Inventory or Memorial Pain Assessment Card).
- Teach and encourage the consistent use of a simple verbal tool to monitor pain intensity (e.g., 0 to 10, none–slight–moderate–severe).
- Develop a problem list based on data obtained during assessment.
- Based on the initial evaluation, develop a provisional diagnosis for the cause and type of each pain.
- Formulate a treatment plan that includes primary recommendations for each targeted symptom, with contingencies for titration or alternate interventions.
- Obtain and personally review needed diagnostic tests.
- Document findings and recommendations in medical record, and communicate with the patient and family and the referring and other treating physicians.

---

confidence in the patient and family that will be of value throughout treatment.

PAIN CHARACTERISTICS

Various schemata for classifying cancer pain have been suggested that, especially when applied together, have potential utility to aid in diagnosis and management (Table 40-6) (52). Although efforts at classification help guide treatment, pain in the cancer patient is ultimately an individual phenomenon, and optimal treatment requires careful assessment and management tailored to meet the unique needs of the individual patient.

Etiology and Pathophysiology

Given the variety of clinically relevant methods for classifying cancer pain, classification is best approached by considering general schema first. Foremost in this context is a broad etiologic classification that distinguishes among the general causes of pain in patients with cancer (Table 40-7). Tumor invasion accounts for two thirds to three quarters of significant pain in cancer patients, with most of the remainder of cases comprised of sequelae of cancer therapy and, to a lesser extent, diagnostic procedures. A smaller proportion of pain problems results from general debility, chronic illness, and chronic disorders that predate, and are not directly related to, the diagnosis of cancer, such as

---

TABLE 40-3. *General principles of pain management in the cancer patient: reassessment*

- Reassess at appropriate, individualized intervals: gauge response to interventions; monitor for disease progression; development of new symptoms.
- Reassess at frequent intervals after initial evaluation, commencing new drugs, performing an intervention (e.g., nerve block.).
- Use established verbal tools to assess pain intensity longitudinally (e.g., 0 to 10, none–slight–moderate–severe).
- When reassessing, ask about efficacy and side effects of current treatment regimen.
- When reassessing, routinely inquire about bowel habit, nausea, and alertness.

- Be alert to findings consistent with epidural spinal cord compression and other neurologic syndromes. Pertinent information is often not otherwise volunteered.
- Review problem list and progress made in treating each distressing symptom.
- Encourage patients to focus on whether symptoms have improved rather than on whether they've been eliminated.
- Determine overall satisfaction with treatment.
- Document findings and recommendations in medical record, and communicate changes in condition and modifications in treatment regimen with referring and other treating physicians.

TABLE 40-4. *General principles of pain management in the cancer patient: management*

- Develop and apply an algorithmic approach to each pain problem, always being prepared to modify care plans based on individual features of a patient's presentation and response.
- When feasible, treat pain by attempting to modify its cause, usually with antineoplastic therapy. Institute concurrent symptomatic treatment with analgesics while awaiting therapeutic response, which may be delayed.
- Select specific drugs for specific reasons.
- Keep the treatment regimen simple whenever possible. Avoid polypharmacy unless indicated for specific reasons. Review drug regimen regularly, and consider discontinuing agents that are of questionable value. They can always be restarted.
- Maintain exquisite familiarity with a core group of drugs that is frequently used. Ensure ready access to reliable information on less frequently prescribed drugs.
- Be knowledgeable about the range of side effects associated with prescribed drugs. When considering drugs with similar primary effects, be aware of the opportunity to exploit "side effects" (secondary effects) that may be beneficial in a given patient (e.g., nighttime use of a sedating antidepressant for neuropathic pain in a patient with concomitant insomnia).
- Start new drugs in low doses, and be prepared to titrate dose upward rapidly after a therapeutic response and the presence or absence of side effects have been established.
- Avoid starting multiple drugs simultaneously, both to minimize the risk of drug interactions and to avoid uncertainty about which agent is responsible for changes.
- Always express a generic willingness to help the patient and family. Ask explicitly what they want or need. Be aware that it may not be a prescription, but rather advice or just an empathetic listener. Never say or imply that "nothing more can be done."
- Consider nonpharmacologic therapies, both invasive (antineoplastic, anesthetic, neurosurgical, orthopedic) and noninvasive (behavioral, counseling, physiatric), when appropriate.
- Discuss treatment decisions with patient and family members. When appropriate, present options in the context of their alternatives and relative risk and benefit. Always try to provide clear recommendations based on your knowledge of the patient and the merits of each treatment option.
- Provide education to the patient and family or significant others regarding all aspects of treatment. When appropriate, involve the family in establishing realistic goals. Seek their help in maintaining compliance with treatment recommendations. Interact with family members in a supportive manner that communicates concern about their well-being and a willingness to ease their distress.
- Encourage patients to understand their illness and the treatments they are receiving and to maintain and carry with them a list of medications they take. When appropriate, provide instructions on the use of pain dairies.
- Discuss advanced directives when appropriate.

degenerative joint disease or disc protrusion (premorbid chronic pain).

In addition to its etiology, cancer pain can be considered as emanating from a variety of pathophysiologic processes. Tumor-mediated pain may emanate from mechanisms that include inflammation, edema, or necrosis of pain-sensitive tissues or impingement on neighboring structures. Specific mechanisms include invasion of bone or soft tissues, obstruction of lymphatic and vascular channels, mesenteric torsion, distension of a hollow viscus, capsular stretch of a solid viscus, and involvement of nervous system structures. The underlying pathologic processes and events that appear to initiate and maintain pain (Tables 40-8 and 40-9) are typically inferred by the patient's clinical presentation and the results of diagnostic imaging studies. Although it is often the case that more than one mechanism is operant, it remains useful to determine the predominant mechanism in order to plan treatment directed at the source of pain.

Tumor-Mediated versus Treatment-Related Pain

The incidence of pain due to cancer therapy is naturally greater in communities where antineoplastic therapy is administered aggressively, and, conversely, the incidence of pain due to tumor progression is typically greater in rural or less developed regions where cancer treatment is prescribed less intensively, either because patients initially present with advanced disease that is beyond treatment or because limited resources preclude comprehensive treatment. Pain that is progressively severe or that spreads, especially to anatomically unrelated areas, is more likely to be directly related to tumoral activity than to cancer treatment.

Pain related to cancer treatment typically has mixed neuropathic and musculoskeletal features, is more likely to remain localized to the same region, and, although it may wax and wane, has severity that is less likely to steadily mount than when symptoms are due to tumor progression. Because evidence of tissue damage may be absent, treatment-related pain is often poorly understood and is more likely to be undertreated, especially in the cancer survivor who is in remission. Despite survivorship, significant pain may persist indefinitely, particularly with tumors associated with intensive treatment (e.g., head and neck) but also after more apparently innocuous therapies like mastectomy (53) or chemotherapy (54,55). Various pain syndromes (see following) have been described both for tumor-mediated (56) and treatment-related pain (57,58) (Table 40-5) that are unique to the cancer population and are characterized by more discrete clinical features.

TABLE 40-5. *Examples of cancer pain syndromes*

Bone invasion	Presentation is variable; usually constant, often greatest at night and with movement or weight bearing; often a dull ache or deep, intense pain; may be associated with referred pain and muscle spasm or, when there is nerve compression, paroxysms of stabbing pain.
Vertebral body invasion	Often presents as severe, localized, dull, steady, aching pain; often exacerbated by recumbency, sitting, movement, and local pressure; may be relieved by standing; localized midline tenderness may be present; associated nerve compression may produce radiating dermatomal pain and corresponding neurologic changes; may be associated with epidural spinal cord compression.
Base of skull metastases	Numerous specific syndromes described (middle fossa syndrome, jugular foramen syndrome, clivus metastases, orbital metastases, parasellar metastases, sphenoid sinus metastases, occipital condyle invasion, odontoid fractures); usually present with headache and a spectrum of neurologic findings, especially involving cranial nerves; usually a late finding; may be difficult to diagnose radiographically.
Nerve invasion	Typically a constant, burning dysesthetic pain, often with an intermittent lancinating, electrical component; may be associated with neurologic deficit or diffuse hyperesthesia and localized paresthesia; muscle weakness and atrophy may be present in mixed or motor nerve syndromes.
Leptomeningeal metastases, meningeal carcinomatosis	Most common with primary malignancies of breast and lung, lymphoma, and leukemia; headache is most common presenting complaint; characteristically unrelenting, may be associated with nausea, vomiting, nuchal rigidity, and mental status changes; associated neurologic abnormalities may include seizures, cranial nerve deficits, papilledema, hemiparesis, ataxia, and cauda equina syndrome; diagnosis confirmed with lumbar puncture.
Spinal cord compression	Pain almost always precedes neurologic changes; urgent radiologic workup required for rapid progression of neurologic deficit, particularly motor weakness or incontinence; early treatment may limit neurologic morbidity.
Cervical plexopathy	May result from local invasion by head and neck cancers or pressure from enlarged nodes; symptoms primarily sensory, experienced as aching preauricular, postauricular, or neck pain.
Brachial plexopathy	Most commonly due to upper lobe lung cancer (Pancoast's syndrome), breast cancer, or lymphoma; pain is an early symptom, usually preceding neurologic findings; usually diffuse aching in shoulder girdle, radiating down arm, often to the elbow and medial (ulnar) aspect of the hand; Horner's syndrome, dysesthesias, progressive atrophy, and neurologic impairment (weakness and numbness) may occur; must differentiate from radiation fibrosis, which characteristically is less severe, less often associated with motor changes, tends to involve the upper trunks, and may be associated with lymphedema.
Lumbosacral plexopathy	May be due to local soft tissue invasion or compression; pain is usually presenting sign; may be referred to low back, abdomen, buttock, or lower extremity.
Celiac plexopathy	Usually relentless, boring, midepigastric aching pain radiating to midback; often relieved by fetal position and worsened by recumbency.
Chemotherapy-induced polyneuropathy	Most common with vincristine, vinblastine, and cis-platinum; may include jaw pain, claudication, and dysesthetic pain in the hands or feet.
Postsurgical syndromes	Most common after mastectomy, thoracotomy, radical neck dissection, nephrectomy, and amputation; usually aching, shooting, or tingling in distribution of peripheral nerves (intercostal brachial, intercostal, cervical plexus, etc.) with or without skin hypersensitivity.

Pain Due to Diagnostic Procedures

Whereas pain due to cancer or its treatment is typically chronic and ongoing, pain related to diagnostic procedures is acute and transient in nature. Pain due to diagnostic procedures is an especially important consideration in children because "routine" procedures (e.g., venipuncture, lumbar puncture, bone marrow aspiration, biopsy) that are often viewed as innocuous by adults are a major source of distress in children (59). Distress and pain produce similar behavioral responses in children and thus may be difficult to distinguish (60). Unfortunately, the significance and even the existence of procedure-related pain are often not considered due to busy hospital routines, outmoded beliefs that children do not appreciate or remember pain, and insufficient resources. Treatment with standard pharmacologic and behavioral approaches, especially using parents as coaches, is usually effective but requires proactive, systematic application, usually in a programmatic context (61). Effective management is especially important from the start to avoid anticipatory distress in children and when repeated painful diagnostic procedures are planned.

TABLE 40-6. *Methods of classifying cancer pain*

Method	Example	Clinical significance
General etiology	Tumor-related pain Treatment-related pain Procedure-related pain Debility and chronic illness Premorbid chronic pain	Broadest of all classification schema. Determination of general etiology aids the clinician in formulating a rational treatment plan that takes into account the patient's prognosis for survival and the natural longitudinal course of the painful condition. Recognition of the broad underlying cause of pain is useful in determining what resources are best applied for management.
Chronicity	Acute Chronic	Relative acuity/chronicity helps determine the degree to which pain should be regarded as a diagnostic sign that may signal new underlying pathology. Acute pain may be more likely to respond to treatment directed at its source. Patients with chronic pain may require additional interdisciplinary resources to help manage depression and suffering and to facilitate rehabilitation.
Severity or intensity	Mild, moderate, severe Visual Analog Scale faces 0–10 numerical score	Usual determinant of the potency of prescribed analgesic (NSAID for mild pain, "weak" opioid for moderate pain, "strong" opioid for severe pain). Regular measurement is required to gauge treatment outcome.
Pathophysiology	Somatic nociceptive Visceral nociceptive Neuropathic	By helping target the source of pain, more specific treatment may be offered (e.g., sympathetic block for visceral nociceptive pain). The presence of neuropathic pain, which is typically less opioid responsive than nociceptive pain, is an important feature because adjuvant analgesics (antidepressants, anticonvulsants, oral local anesthetics) may play a relatively more important role.
Syndromal presentation	Plexopathy Cord compression Postsurgical syndromes, etc.	Recognition may provide valuable information about etiology, prognosis, and optimal treatment.
Disease stage	Newly diagnosed or recurrent disease Curable versus terminal disease, etc.	May suggest specific treatment options and may predict response to therapy, e.g., patients in active treatment may exhibit high pain thresholds and may be reluctant to report pain, whereas pain control is usually a high priority for patients with terminal disease.
Patient characteristic	Anxiety, distant/recent history of alcohol or drug use, etc.	Special features may help determine need for multimodal therapy.
Temporal features	Constant, intermittent, mixed, breakthrough pain	This helps determine optimal schedule for prescribing analgesic drugs (PRN vs. around-the-clock vs. around-the-clock + PRN).
Responsivity	Highly opioid responsive, moderately opioid responsive, poorly opioid responsive	Empiric responsivity to opioids, adjuvants, and other modalities helps determine best treatment strategy in a given patient.

Premorbid Chronic Pain

Patients with preexisting chronic pain due to traumatic, degenerative, or idiopathic causes comprise a smaller proportion of consultations for pain control. Assessment and management of these patients may be more complex because of the presence of psychological adaptation and established pain behaviors (62).

Chronicity of Pain: Acute versus Chronic Pain

Acute pain is frequently associated with signs of sympathetic hyperactivity and heightened distress. It often is manifest at the onset of disease, and, although analgesics may be required on a transient basis, symptoms may resolve as antitumor therapy progresses (63). In contrast, assessment and management of patients with chronic pain tend to be more complex. With time, biologic and behavioral adjustment to symptoms occurs, and associated signs of tachycardia, hypertension, and diaphoresis are often absent. Various pain behaviors (alterations in facial expression, gait, posture, and mood) may be observed and may persist throughout treatment. Premorbid chronic nonmalignant pain that precedes the diagnosis of cancer can complicate management. Pain due to cancer *per se* usually signals tumor progression with actual injury to tissue, and, as a result, response to intervention is relatively predictable. In contrast, chronic nonmalignant pain, even in the cancer patient, is more often an ingrained behavior and personality feature that may be associated with drug-seeking behavior, symptom magnification, and pain on the basis of depression, and thus symptoms may persist despite intervention (64,65). Alternatively, a proportion of patients are pleasantly surprised to find that relief of their chronic pain

TABLE 40-7. *Classification of cancer pain by general etiology*

Pain due to direct effects of tumor progression
  e.g., compression or ischemia of pain-sensitive structures

Pain due to cancer treatment
  e.g., osteoradionecrosis, chemotherapy-induced neuropathy, postmastectomy syndrome

Pain due to diagnostic procedures
  e.g., venipuncture, lumbar puncture, bone marrow biopsy

Pain due to chronic illness and debility
  e.g., muscle spasm from prolonged bedrest, decubitus ulcers

Premorbid chronic pain
  e.g., chronic radiculitis, osteoarthritis

TABLE 40-8. *Classification of cancer pain by its underlying pathophysiology*

Tumor invasion or compression of pain-sensitive structures (e.g., periosteum, nerve, muscle)
Reflex neural activity arising from nerve invasion or compression (neuropathic pain with windup)
Pressure and obstruction of lymphatics and vessels
Localized edema and inflammation
Distention, stretch, or abnormal contraction (reflex spasm) of hollow viscera
Stretch of the capsule surrounding solid viscera
Ischemia or necrosis of smooth muscle of hollow viscera
Chemical irritation of the serosal or mucosal surfaces of hollow viscera
Distention, traction, or torsion of mesenteric and vascular attachments of viscera

can be readily achieved after medications are prescribed more liberally based on their status as a cancer patient.

Mechanism

A mechanistic classification based on inferred pathophysiology of pain that distinguishes among nociceptive (somatic and visceral) and neuropathic pain has become increasingly well accepted (Table 40-9) (66). Common clinical characteristics and shared responsivity to various therapeutic interventions have been observed for each type of pain, and, hence, consideration of this classification is useful when formulating an initial treatment approach. Cancer pain, especially when advanced, usually involves multiple sensory pathophysiologic mechanisms ("mixed pain") that interact with related characterologic and environmental components (affective, cognitive, and behavioral), the sum of which contributes to a complex experience that defies simple categorization or management per a simple algorithm.

NOCICEPTIVE PAIN

Nociceptive and *neuropathic pain* refer to broad categories of painful conditions, distinguished from each other based on their inferred mechanisms. Nociceptive pain is further comprised of somatic nociceptive pain and visceral nociceptive pain. Each type of pain is characteristically described by patients in similar terms and tends to respond similarly to various therapeutic interventions (67).

Nociceptive pain results from an injury or insult to nonneurologic structures and occurs in the presence of a fundamentally intact nervous system, i.e., under conditions of normal peripheral and central nervous system function. Characteristically, pain appears to be proportional and commensurate with the underlying tissue injury.

TABLE 40-9. *Classification of pain by its underlying mechanism*

Type of pain	Common clinical features	Responsivity to opioids and NSAIDs, adjuvants, neural blockade
Somatic nociceptive	Constant, well localized; dull, sharp, aching, throbbing, gnawing. Examples: bone metastases, skin infiltration, muscle spasm	(+++)(-)(++)
Visceral nociceptive	Constant or paroxysmal; vague in distribution and quality; deep, dull, aching, dragging, squeezing, or pressure-like; acute: may be colicky; associated with nausea, vomiting, diaphoresis, and alterations in vital signs. Examples: liver metastases, bowel or ureteral obstruction, pancreatic cancer	(++)(-)(++)
Neuropathic	When constant: burning, tingling, numbing, pressing, squeezing, and/or itching; when paroxysmal: shooting, stabbing, lancinating, electrical, jolting, shocklike. Examples: herpes zoster, postmastectomy or thoracotomy pain, brachial or lumbosacral plexopathy, phantom limb pain, spinal cord injury, diabetic neuropathy, leptomeningeal metastases	(+)(++)(+)
Mixed	Various features from preceding, depending on predominant mechanism(s)	Variable

Noxious stimuli result in transmission of impulses along classical pain pathways. Symptoms consist of sensations to which most people have a familiar frame of reference from prior painful experiences (e.g., trauma, surgery, and childbirth) and are characteristically described with adjectives or descriptors that are traditionally associated with pain. Nociceptive pain typically responds favorably and predictably to treatment with NSAIDs (nonsteroidal anti-inflammatory drugs) and the opioids in a graded fashion that is relatively proportional to dose, and favorable responses to treatment with adjuvant analgesics are unlikely (Table 40-9). When appropriate, nociceptive pain is often amenable to relief by interruption of proximal pathways by neural blockade or surgery, at least temporarily.

Somatic Nociceptive Pain

Nociceptive pain can be further subdivided into somatic nociceptive pain and visceral nociceptive pain. Somatic nociceptive pain occurs as a result of ongoing activation of cutaneous and deep nociceptors in somatic tissues (skin, muscle, bone, joint, tendon, and other connective tissues). These nociceptors are activated by mechanical, thermal, and chemical stimuli (68,69). Pain may be acute or chronic in nature, is typically well localized, and is often characterized as aching, dull, sharp, or gnawing (Table 40-9).

Visceral Nociceptive Pain

Visceral nociceptive pain arises from injury to internal organs (thorax, abdomen, pelvis). Although insensitive to simple manipulation, cutting, and burning, visceral pain is elicited as a result of distention, stretch, abnormal contraction, or reflex spasm, ischemia, or necrosis of smooth muscle, chemical irritation of serosal or mucosal surfaces of hollow viscera, stretch of the capsular investment of solid viscera and distention, and traction or torsion of mesenteric and vascular attachments (70–72). Visceral injury often produces referred pain, defined as pain and hyperalgesia (hypersensitivity) that is localized to superficial and/or deep tissues often distant to the source of pathology (e.g., back pain secondary to pancreas cancer, right shoulder pain secondary to diaphragmatic irritation). In contrast to somatically mediated pain, visceral pain is characteristically described as vague in distribution and quality and is often deep, dull, aching, dragging, squeezing, or pressure-like. When acute, it may be paroxysmal and colicky and can be associated with nausea, vomiting, diaphoresis, and alterations in blood pressure and heart rate.

NEUROPATHIC PAIN

In contrast to nociceptive pain, neuropathic pain occurs as a consequence of neural injury and abnormal/pathologic transmission, processing, and integration. Peripheral or central nervous system injury results in aberrant somatosensory processing, and the resulting pain appears to be self-sustaining and poorly correlated with the degree of apparent tissue injury (66,67). Neuropathic pain is often associated with objective neurologic signs or subjective reports of altered sensation and especially alterations in sensory threshold, including anesthesia and allodynia (pain in response to a stimulus that usually does not provoke pain, e.g., light stroke). Patients report experiences that are distinct from ordinary, familiar sensations of pain (e.g., burning, tingling, itching, numbness), considered together under the rubric "*dysesthesias*" (Latin for "bad feeling"). Pain is often diffuse and may be accompanied by exaggerated skeletal muscle and autonomic responses.

Neuropathic pain may be relatively constant and unrelenting (so-called tonic pain) or predominantly intermittent, spontaneous, and shocklike or lancinating or commonly a mix of tonic dysesthesia with superimposed electrical spikes. As a rule, neuropathic pain is more difficult to treat than nociceptive pain because it tends to be less responsive than nociceptive pain to opioids administered in "routine" doses and typically requires the addition of adjuvant analgesics, including antidepressants and anticonvulsants (Table 40-9). Examples of neuropathic pain include phantom limb pain, spinal cord injury, postherpetic neuralgia, and neuropathy due to chemotherapy or diabetes.

IDIOPATHIC OR "PSYCHOGENIC" PAIN

Great controversy surrounds labeling a pain syndrome as wholly psychogenic in origin. The fact that patients' psychologic states contribute significantly to complaints of pain and suffering is fundamental to the subjective nature of pain and is now well accepted (64,65). The presence of psychological influences on pain report or evidence for a placebo response should in no way be regarded as detracting from the authenticity of a complaint of pain. It is often difficult to ascertain the degree to which psychological disturbances are sequelae of chronic pain or constitute a more primary disorder that is expressed as pain. Regardless, symptoms and their associated distress are real to the patient, independent of the degree to which psychological factors are involved in their maintenance, and thus should always be taken seriously. Although it is essential that the clinician maintain a willingness to believe the patient's report of pain and investigate its cause, the presence of anxiety or depression should be carefully assessed in order that appropriate supportive care and/or pharmacotherapy can be instituted.

PAIN INTENSITY AND SELF-REPORT

Classification of cancer pain based on its intensity has considerable practical relevance (41). Because self-report remains the gold standard for assessing pain intensity, providing patients with the tools for assessing and reporting changes in pain intensity is a key patient education goal. Patients should be familiarized with a suitable measure of pain intensity on their first encounter, which should then be applied consistently from visit to visit. The use of a simple self-report scale empowers patients by providing a simple means for them to rapidly communicate volumes about a complex personal experience that is not otherwise readily accessible to an observer. In the absence of a shared language or tool for communicating changes in subjective symptoms, it is unreasonable for the clinician to expect to otherwise gauge outcome and the need to appropriately modify ongoing therapy.

Especially for unstable pain, patients may be instructed in the use of a pain diary to document changes in pain intensity between visits. The consistent use of a single schema for measuring pain intensity aids in the reliable assessment of patients' progress and serves as a basis for interpatient comparison when data are being gathered for research purposes.

Any inclination to rely on measures other than self-report (observation, reports of family members and nurses, changes in vital signs or radiographs) except as adjunctive tools should be rejected because numerous studies have demonstrated the superiority of self-report (73,74). The particular tool utilized to glean self-report appears to be less important than the use of an appropriate method consistently in a given patient. Most clinics use a 0–10 scale (0 = no pain, 10 = the worst pain the patient can imagine), administered either verbally or with pen and paper. Patients are ideally asked for a numeric rating of their pain at present and over the prior week, with a best, worst, and on average (75). The visual analog scale, a pen-and-paper method, although somewhat abstract and potentially confusing, is the standard against which other scales are measured. The prevailing convention involves the use of an uncalibrated 10-cm horizontal line that is anchored at its extremes with descriptors indicating "no pain" and "the most severe pain imaginable."

Numeric ratings rely on a somewhat abstract concept, and difficulties may arise particularly in the very young, very old, unschooled, or impatient patient, as well as in the presence of factors that impair concentration such as severe pain or distress, debility due to chronic illness, and the effects of anesthetic or analgesic drugs. Novel tools have been developed for special indications, especially as age-specific techniques used in pediatric populations. These include pain thermometers, color scales, and sketches of faces that depict a continuum of changing expressions (76).

CLINICAL SIGNIFICANCE OF PAIN INTENSITY RATINGS

Classification of cancer pain based on its intensity determines where the patient is likely to fall along the WHO-endorsed "analgesic ladder" (41), an effective but almost deceptively simple schema that has been incorporated into guidelines adopted by other expert bodies (5–8). The ladder employs a primary strategy of matching analgesic potency with pain intensity (NSAIDs for mild pain and various opioids for moderate to severe pain) and, secondarily, recommends selecting drugs based on the presumed mechanisms of pain (NSAIDs and opioids for nociceptive pain and adjuvants for neuropathic pain). Pain severity serves as the main determinant for determining the level at which the ladder is accessed and thus whether treatment is rendered with a nonopioid analgesic, a so-called weak opioid, or a so-called strong/potent opioid. Recently, the terms "opioid conventionally used to treat moderate pain" and "opioid conventionally used to treat severe pain" have been advocated in preference to "weak" and "strong" opioid (77).

Consistently high pain scores should obviously alert the clinician to the urgent need for aggressive intervention. Because, with the exception of the adjuvant analgesics, the dose-response relationship of drugs used in the ladder is tightly linked, when necessary, patients should be moved briskly through its tiers to avoid unnecessary delays in achieving pain relief. A determination of whether a drug of adequate potency and dose has been initially prescribed can usually be made with the administration of just a few doses or at most after a few days. The WHO treatment hierarchy can be accessed at any level: Patients presenting initially with severe pain can be managed from the start with low doses of potent opioids (41).

TEMPORAL PATTERN OF PAIN

Pain may be constant and unremitting, in which case it is most amenable to an around-the-clock dosing schedule, contingent on time rather than symptoms. This approach to management endeavors to prevent pain rather than treat it retroactively and is best accomplished by the optimal use of long-acting oral or transdermal analgesics or, when indicated, a continuous parenteral infusion.

Despite establishing an effective preventative schedule, breakthrough pain is still a common phenomenon that must be anticipated and addressed. *Breakthrough pain* (49,50) refers to intermittent exacerbations of pain that can occur spontaneously or in relation to specific activity against a background of chronic unremitting pain. Breakthrough pain that is related to a specific activity, such as eating, bowel movements, socializing, or walking is referred to as *incident pain* (49). Breakthrough pain may also be idiopathic or related to the around-the-clock (ATC) dosing regimen (end-of-dose failure), in which case it usually occurs predictably near the end of a dosing interval, has a more gradual onset, and is more likely to be persistent. The incidence and severity of end-of-dose failure usually correlate with the adequacy of ATC dosing regimens prescribed for the management of basal pain, and this type of breakthrough pain is best countered by modifying the dose or schedule of long-acting ATC opioids. Idiopathic and incident types of breakthrough pain are best managed by supplementing the preventative regimen with analgesics characterized by rapid onset and short duration. After a pattern of incident pain is established, breakthrough doses, rescue doses, or escape doses of analgesics can be administered in anticipation of the pain-provoking activity. When treatment with an infusion (subcutaneous, intravenous, epidural) has been elected, the addition of patient-controlled analgesia (PCA), which permits patients to administer a preset amount of narcotic at preset intervals, is an effective means to manage breakthrough and incident pain (31).

Pain that is intermittent and unpredictable in onset represents a further challenge to management. Around-the-clock dosing is likely to be unsatisfactory because analgesia is often inadequate during painful episodes, and sedation usually supervenes during pain-free intervals. Pain that occurs intermittently is usually best managed by the *pro re nata* (PRN) administration of an appropriately potent analgesic of rapid onset and short duration (e.g., morphine, hydromorphone, oxycodone, oral transmucosal fentanyl citrate). When intermittent pain is well localized there may be a role for nerve blocks as well (13).

PATIENT AND DISEASE CHARACTERISTICS

The concept that assessment should include attention to disease-specific and person-specific factors that contribute to the meaning of pain is well accepted (Table 40-10), although formal schemata have not been detailed or validated. Neither assessment nor treatment should be strictly limited to a disease-specific focus. Optimally, the clinician's focus is on a human being who, in addition to cancer and pain, has thoughts, feelings, prior experiences, and memories that influence report and response. For example, the optimal approach needed to provide treatment for a patient who has observed a loved one die with unrelieved pain will necessarily differ from that needed in a patient who has observed family members' experiences with drug abuse. A classification scheme based on stage of disease and patient characteristics that may help predict patients' response to pain is summarized in Table 40-10 (63).

Syndromal Presentation

The importance of classifying cancer pain based on its syndromal presentation has become increasingly appreciated (56). The clinical recognition of cancer pain syndromes is based on the clinician's knowledge of their

TABLE 40-10. *Classification of cancer pain by disease stage and patient characteristics*

Acute cancer-related pain	Biologic "red flag" signifying need to simultaneously investigate cause and rapidly institute treatment
Related to diagnosis or treatment	Patients tend to be hopeful; may readily endure pain, often without seeking treatment
Recurrent pain	Identification with recrudescence of disease, psychological effects potentially devastating
Chronic cancer-related pain	Behavioral adaptation/maladaptation, pharmacologic tolerance, and physical dependence may be established
Associated with treatment	Overriding concern is reestablishment of functional lifestyle
Associated with progression	Hopelessness, helplessness often predominate
Preexisting chronic pain	Pain behavior established; may require intensive intervention and support; accurate diagnosis essential
Dying patients	Adequacy of treatment has great impact on patient and family; assure comfort at all reasonable costs
History of drug abuse	Evaluation and management are often complicated by legitimate concerns that pain treatment may result in maintenance or recrudescence of aberrant drug use; by the same token, a significant risk of undertreatment of pain exists as a consequence of such concerns
Distant history of abuse	Patient may be reluctant to use opioids due to fear of readdiction and criticism of peers and family
Ongoing methadone maintenance	May complicate pharmacologic management; requires coordination
Active drug abuse	Most challenging; interdisciplinary/multimodal management helpful; coordinate support services (e.g., rehabilitation, social work)
Pediatrics	Pain, anxiety, and distress evoke equivalent responses
Preverbal children	Pain expressed by crying, grimacing, facial expressions
Toddlers	Tend to regress
Adolescents	Tend to withdraw

clinical presentation and a careful history, physical examination, and review of diagnostic studies. Although an exhaustive description of known cancer pain syndromes is beyond the scope of this text, brief descriptions follow.

Bone Metastases

Skeletal metastases are clinically evident in one third of cancer patients and are present in two thirds of cancer patients at autopsy (78), and thus it is not surprising that infiltration of bone is the most common cause of cancer pain. Neoplasms with the greatest propensity to metastasize to bone include multiple myeloma, breast cancer, prostate cancer, and lung cancer.

Because up to 50% decalcification must be present before osseous lesions are visible on plain roentgenograms, scintigraphy (radioisotope scanning) is the diagnostic imaging technique of choice except in the case of primary bone tumors, thyroid cancer, and multiple myeloma. Although ordinarily more sensitive than plain films, scintigrams are not highly specific; therefore, findings must be interpreted in the context of clinical findings and other studies. A biochemical mechanism has been advocated to explain much of the pain associated with osseous invasion, which would help explain why 20% to 25% of patients with even very large bone metastases are asymptomatic, whereas sometimes even very small lesions produce severe pain. Osseous metastases elaborate prostaglandin E2 (PGE2), which, it is hypothesized, contributes to pain by sensitization of peripheral nociceptors. Nonsteroidal anti-inflammatory agents and steroids are postulated to be effective in the treatment of painful bony metastases on the basis of their activity to inhibit the cyclooxygenase pathway of arachidonic acid breakdown, thus decreasing the formation of PGE2. As deposits enlarge, stretching of the periosteum, pathologic fracture, and perineural invasion contribute to pain, and requirements for more potent analgesics increase. It has also been suggested that pain is more closely correlated with the rate of expansion of bony lesions rather than their absolute size *per se* (79). External beam radiotherapy has long been successfully employed to relieve pain emanating from bony metastases. More recently, radionuclides (e.g., strontium-89, samarium) have been used to treat pain in specific settings (after conventional radiotherapy has been maximized), especially in the presence of diffuse metastases and in patients with hormonal-dependent cancers (i.e., breast and prostate cancer) (80). Hormonal therapy (e.g., chemotherapy, orchiectomy, hypophysectomy) is also often effective in reducing bony pain in patients with hormonal-dependent disease, although the estrogen agent, tamoxifen, may increase pain transiently before it is relieved in a proportion of patients (tamoxifen flare) (81). Metastases to the skull, sternum, and upper limb tend not to be painful. When investigating pain that is thought to emanate from bony deposits, the clinician should consider imaging adjacent structures to exclude referred pain, as in the case of knee pain associated with metastatic involvement of the hip.

Epidural Spinal Cord Compression

Epidural spinal cord compression is a critically important clinical entity that all practitioners should be capable of recognizing. Onset is almost always heralded by pain, usually well in advance of discrete neurologic findings, and, therefore, a diagnosis should be considered in all at-risk patients who present with new onset or rapidly changing back pain (82,83). Early recognition and intervention may limit neurologic morbidity. Pain may be localized to the midline of the spine or associated with a radicular pattern of weakness and tingling. It tends to be dull, steady, and aching, increasing gradually over time, and often is exacerbated with recumbency or straining. Rapid progression of neurologic deficit, particularly of motor weakness or incontinence, signals progressive epidural spinal cord compression and warrants urgent intervention. MRI (magnetic resonance imaging) has all but replaced CT (computed tomography) as the study of first choice, and treatment planning often involves collaboration of a neurosurgeon, radiologist, and radiation oncologist (84,85).

Neural Invasion

Invasion or compression of somatic nerves by tumor is generally associated with constant, burning dysesthetic pain, often with a superimposed intermittent stabbing component. Diffuse hyperesthesia and localized paresthesia are common, and muscle weakness and atrophy may be present if a mixed or motor nerve is involved in the affected structure. Pain attributable to nerve compression by tumor was diagnosed in 34%, 40%, 20%, and 31% of patients referred to an anesthesiology-pain service, tertiary care center, neurology service, and hospice, respectively (86–88).

Brachial and Lumbosacral Plexopathy

Brachial plexus invasion (Pancoast's or superior sulcus syndrome) is associated most commonly with carcinoma of the lung (primary or metastatic) or breast and lymphoma (89). Differentiating brachial plexus abnormalities due to radiation fibrosis versus tumor invasion can be difficult because clinical findings are similar. Horner's syndrome and severe pain and weakness in the C-8–T-1 (lower plexus) distribution are more commonly associated with tumor invasion, whereas lymphadenopathy and weakness of shoulder abduction and arm flexor (upper plexus) are more commonly encountered after radiation injury (56). Workup of suspected brachial plexopathy includes MRI, nerve conduction studies, and, if epidural extension is suspected, consideration of spinal studies.

Lumbosacral plexopathy, due to invasion of local soft tissue by tumor, lymphadenopathy, or compression from bony metastases, occurs most commonly in association with tumors of the rectum, cervix, breast, sarcoma, and lymphoma. Involvement of the lumbar plexus characteristically produces radicular lower extremity pain that is usually described as aching or pressure-like. Pain is the presenting symptom in most patients, about half of whom will go on to develop significant weakness and numbness within weeks or months of the initial appearance of pain (90). Reflex asymmetry and mild sensory and motor changes are relatively early findings, whereas impotence and incontinence are infrequent findings. Suspected plexopathy must be differentiated from cord compression, cauda equina, and leptomeningeal metastases. CT investigations of the pelvis and lumbar spine and diagnostic nerve blocks are helpful to corroborate clinical findings.

Invasion of the sacral plexus is most often associated with severe constant lower backache, often progressing to perineal sensory loss and bowel or bladder dysfunction. Plain films, tomography, and scintigrams frequently demonstrate bony invasion of the sacral plates. Symptom control is most important in these settings because constant pain will likely lead patients to become immobilized, depressed, and subject to increased risks of venous thrombosis, decubiti, and infection.

Cranial Neuralgias and Associated Orofacial Pain

Although the responsivity of pain from head and neck tumors to routine analgesics is a subject of some controversy (91,92), pain in this setting can be extremely challenging for many reasons, not the least of which relates to the depression and impairment that often accompany treatment of these tumors (93). New pain or an exacerbation after a long interval of stable symptoms should always raise the suspicion of recurrence, even when not clinically apparent (94).

The head and neck are richly innervated by contributions from cranial nerves V, VII, IX, X, and the upper cervical nerves. Pain commonly emanates from bony and soft tissue growths that may impinge on cranial nerves and their branches. Specific etiologies for pain include soft tissue ulceration, infection, compression from adenopathy or tumor, mucositis, bony erosion, and nerve invasion. Analgesia may be difficult to achieve due to the erosive character of many tumors and the ineffectiveness of physiologic splinting; the latter is an ordinarily protective reflex that is overridden by the pain that accompanies the relatively involuntary motion produced by swallowing, eating, coughing, talking, and other movements of the head. When cranial nerves and their branches are involved, symptoms may mimic trigeminal or glossopharyngeal neuralgia, with baseline dysesthetic pain and superimposed sudden, severe shocklike lancinating pain radiating to the receptive field of the affected division(s). Glossopharyngeal and intermedium neuralgias produce similar symptoms but with pain more localized to the throat and ear, respectively.

If the tumor is unresectable, then early consideration should be given to palliative radiotherapy. Depending on its underlying mechanism, pain may be responsive to treatment with steroids, NSAIDs, opioids, and anticonvulsants or antidepressants. Refractory pain may warrant empiric treatment with antibiotics because infection may be masked by bone marrow failure or sequestration (95). Neurolytic blocks, neurosurgery, and intraventricular opioids are often successful for pain that is otherwise intractable (96).

Leptomeningeal Metastases/Meningeal Carcinomatosis

Diffuse infiltration of the meninges by tumor has the potential to produce protean signs and symptoms, and, as a result, a high index of suspicion is required to make an accurate diagnosis (97,98). This condition is most common in patients with primary malignancies of the breast and lung, lymphoma, and leukemia. About 40% of patients have headache or back pain due to traction on pain-sensitive structures (meninges, cranial spinal nerves) and/or raised intracranial pressure. The most common presenting complaint is headache, which is characteristically unrelenting and may be associated with nausea, vomiting, nuchal rigidity, and mental status changes. Other neurologic abnormalities that may develop include seizures, cranial nerve palsies, papilledema, hemiparesis, ataxia, and cauda equina syndrome. Diagnosis is confirmed by lumbar puncture (LP) and cerebrospinal fluid (CSF) analysis, which will identify malignant cells and may also be remarkable for an increased opening pressure, raised protein, and decreased glucose. Computerized tomography, MRI with contrast, and myelograms are helpful to evaluate the extent of disease. The natural history of patients with clinically evident leptomeningeal metastases is gradual decline and death over 4 to 8 weeks, although survival may be extended to 6 months or more when treatment with radiotherapy and/or intrathecal methotrexate is instituted. Steroids may be useful in the management of associated headache (99).

Headache

Headache is a major, but not invariable, symptom of intracranial neoplasm (71), present in 60% of patients in one survey, half of whom classified headache as their primary complaint (72). Its pattern is indistinctive (100). Patients typically describe pain that is steady, deep, dull, and aching and is rarely rhythmic or throbbing. It is usually intermittent and may be worse in the morning, with coughing or straining. Characteristically, the intensity of pain is only moderate, rarely awakening patients from sleep and generally less than that which is typically described in so-called benign headache syndromes. Symptoms often respond to simple measures, including recumbency, the administration of aspirin or steroids (101), and the application of cold packs. Symptoms often improve when whole brain irradiation is applied to treat multiple metastases (102), whereas the gamma knife is being used with increased frequency for discrete and usually solitary lesions (103).

Cerebral tissue *per se* is insensitive to noxious stimuli, and, thus, headache is mediated by indirect mechanisms, with pain referred from adjacent pain-sensitive structures such as the venous sinuses and their tributaries, dural and cerebral arteries, the dura (especially at the base of the brain), cranial nerves V, IX, X, and the upper three cervical nerves. Mechanisms include traction, displacement and dilation of veins and arteries, inflammation near pain-sensitive structures, and direct pressure on cranial and cervical nerves. Reflex contraction of the cervical muscles is a common finding with headache in general and accompanies headache of neoplastic origin in a high proportion of cases. Although an important diagnostic sign of raised intracranial pressure (along with nausea, vomiting, mental status changes, and papilledema), headache may be absent, particularly when elevations in pressure are gradual or chronic.

CANCER PAIN TREATMENT

Antineoplastic Treatment

Ideally, cancer pain is managed by direct treatment of its underlying cause. After it has been elucidated, the pathologic process responsible for pain can often be altered with surgical extirpation, external beam radiotherapy (targeted fractionated or single-dose therapy, hemibody or total body irradiation) (104–106), radionuclides (e.g., strontium-89, samarium) (107,108), hormonal treatment (109,110), chemotherapy, and even hyperthermia (111,112). Many patients are pleased to realize prompt and significant pain relief when their cancer responds to antitumor therapy. This is especially true for lymphoma treated with various chemotherapies and painful bone metastases that often respond promptly and dramatically to local irradiation, which, in some settings, can be administered in a single, nonfractionated dose (113). Nevertheless, the majority of patients will require some form of primary analgesic therapy while awaiting a tumorocidal response or because antitumor therapy has been maximized or is no longer applicable. Even when the goal of cancer cure has been abandoned, further antitumor therapy should be considered when new symptoms arise or a change in the pain treatment strategy is planned. For rapid palliation of symptoms, as opposed to cure, radiotherapy is generally the most applicable of these modalities. It is important to recognize, however, that palliative antitumor measures have definite limitations with regard to efficacy, patient acceptance, and adverse effects, especially in patients with advanced disease. Interestingly, although the use of analgesics has been alleged to be associated with shortening

patients' lives, the ill-advised continuation of "palliative" chemotherapy in the setting of refractory malignancy is more likely to be associated with premature mortality. Finally, the decision to pursue antitumor therapy does not imply that analgesic drugs and other supportive therapy should be discontinued and indeed argues that they occupy a more central therapeutic role.

Pharmacologic Management

Pain management was regarded and provided very differently in the eras that predated contemporary medicine's emphasis on evidence-based practice. Up until the last decade, rather than reliance on a formal curricula or controlled trials (which were nonexistent), prescribing practices emanated largely from trainee-modeling of the unconscious behaviors of generations of physicians troubled by exaggerated concerns regarding addiction and legitimate concerns about regulatory sanctions. Further influenced by the transmission of misinformation and a legacy of clinical lore that arose in the context of a tradition of undertreatment and unscientific prescribing, massive efforts to institutionalize and imbue current practices with science are only now beginning to bear fruit.

Most knowledge gleaned about opioid pharmacology was, until recently, derived from single- or limited-dose studies conducted in the presence of either experimentally induced or acute pain. In a construct that recognizes chronic and acute pain as distinct disorders, there is limited justification for applying knowledge gained from one setting to the other uncritically. The inadequate scientific basis for prescribing practices is compounded by firmly held beliefs regarding the dangers of opioid therapy (114). Such beliefs are now widely understood to be based more on cultural bias than medical considerations (115–118). Recognition of these deficiencies has engendered an almost unparalleled scientific activism to dispel myths surrounding the treatment of pain with drugs and improve the plight of symptomatic cancer patients. Guidelines released by the World Health Organization (41,77), American Pain Society (6), American Society of Clinical Oncology (7), American Society of Anesthesiologists (8), and the U.S. government's Agency for Health Care Policy Research (5) stress the importance of opioid therapy and articulate the need to overcome exaggerated concerns about its risks.

Oral analgesics are the mainstay of therapy for patients with cancer pain (Tables 40-11–40-13). An estimated 70% to 90% of patients can be rendered relatively free of pain when straightforward guideline-based principles of pharmacologic management are applied in a thorough, careful manner (5,7,27,41). Treatment is effective in adults and children across different cultures and in patients who are ambulatory or debilitated. The analgesia that is associated with systemically administered medications is titratable and suitable for pain that is multifocal and/or progressive.

TABLE 40-11. *Opioid agonists conventionally used to manage mild-moderate cancer pain (weak opioids)*

Most "weak" opioids are weak only insofar as the inclusion of aspirin or acetaminophen imposes a ceiling dose above which further increases promote risks of toxicity.

With increasing recognition that the distinction between so-called weak and potent opioids is more cultural and ideologic than medical in nature, "potent" opioids are being prescribed earlier, albeit in low doses.

The recent availability of oxycodone as a single-entity agent (without acetaminophen or aspirin) has demonstrated that increasing doses of a "weak" analgesic may provide clinical analgesia that is equipotent with that of morphine.

Although 100 times more potent than morphine, fentanyl is now widely used in the microgram range.

Although not a meaningful therapeutic advantage, these agents have the *perceived* advantage of being less highly regulated (with the exception of oxycodone, which requires a multiple copy prescription in most states).

Despite a trend toward skipping this analgesic "step" in favor of earlier use of "potent" opioids in patients with pain that is expected to be chronic and progressive, the "weak" opioids are often prescribed beyond their utility or in potentially toxic doses in ill-advised attempts to avoid dispensing more highly regulated drugs due to exaggerated fears of regulatory reprisal and addiction liability.

Opioid	Examples (proprietary names)	Coanalgesic
Propoxyphene hydrochloride (32–65 mg); napsylate (50–100 mg)	Darvon, Darvon Compound, Darvocet, Wygesic	Usually 325–650 mg acetaminophen or 325–389 mg aspirin
Codeine (7.5–60 mg)	Tylenol with codeine #2, #3, #4; Empirin and Empracet with codeine #2, #3, #4; Phenaphen with codeine #2, #3, #4	Usually 325 mg aspirin or 300–650 mg acetaminophen
Hydrocodone (2.5–10 mg)	Lortab, Lorcet, Lortab elixir, Vicodin, Vicodin ES, Hydrogesic, Hydrocet, Hy-Phen, Co-gesic	Usually 500 mg aspirin or 500–750 mg acetaminophen
Dihydrocodeine (16 mg)	Synalgos DC	Usually 356.4 mg acetaminophen and 30 mg caffeine
Oxycodone (2.25–5 mg)	Roxicet, Percocet, Percodan, Percodan-demi, Tylox	325–500 mg acetaminophen or 325 mg aspirin

Effects and side effects are reversible, and widespread implementation does not depend on sophisticated technology or scarce resources (119). The World Health Organization has developed a three-step "ladder" approach to cancer pain management that relies exclusively on the administration of oral agents, and this approach is usually effective (41,77). For example, in a prospective evaluation of the WHO method, Zech et al. observed good results in 76% of 2118 cancer patients treated over a 10-year interval (27).

Although pain can be managed in most patients with oral agents alone, even through the terminal stages of illness, a small but important proportion of patients require alternative forms of therapy (120). The role of more interventional forms of analgesia, ranging from parenteral analgesics to neural blockade and CNS opioid therapy, remains poorly defined, although it is widely recognized that the judicious application of such approaches is essential when more conservative therapies produce inadequate results.

Noninvasive routes (e.g., oral, transdermal, transmucosal) should be maintained as long as possible for reasons that include simplicity, maintenance of independence and mobility, convenience, and cost. Treatment has been markedly simplified by the introduction of controlled-release preparations of oral opioids (e.g., MS Contin, Oramorph, Kadian, Oxycontin), novel noninvasive approaches (e.g., transdermal fentanyl, oral transmucosal fentanyl citrate), and most importantly, the widespread acceptance of guideline-based therapies.

NONSTEROIDAL ANTIINFLAMMATORY DRUGS (NSAIDS)

Despite their ubiquitous role in chronic pain management and their designation as the primary treatment for mild cancer pain (Table 40-14), NSAID use is limited in ongoing cancer pain primarily by their toxicities, which are significant in medically ill populations (121). When tolerated, however, regular NSAID use is especially warranted for cancer pain of musculoskeletal, bony metastatic, and inflammatory origin by virtue of their ability to impede the production of prostaglandins, which are intimately involved in the pathogenesis of each of these conditions.

Thus, regular (around-the-clock) administration of an NSAID is an appropriate starting point as the sole treatment for mild pain, and an NSAID combined with an opioid analgesic may be considered for moderate to severe

TABLE 40-12. *Comparison of opioid agonists conventionally used in cancer pain management (potent opioids)*

Generic name	Proprietary name	Route	Equivalent dose	Schedule	Formulations
Morphine (parenteral)	various	oral	10 mg	q3–4 hr	various
Comments: 10 mg IM morphine is the standard against which other opioids are compared; used for PCA (acute: postop and pain crisis; chronic by SC route)					
Controlled Release (CR)	MS Contin, Oramorph	oral	30 mg	q12–8 hr	15, 30, 60, 100, 200 mg
Comments: intended for around-the-clock (ATC) use; do not break, crush or chew; usually effective q 12 hour; MS Contin has been reported to be effective rectally					
Immediate Release	MSIR, Roxanol, various	oral	30-20 mg	q3–4 hr	10, 15, 30 mg
Comments: consider an alternate opioid if refractory nausea or sedation arise; a metabolite M6G may accumulate, especially if renal function is impaired					
Hydromorphone	Dilaudid	IV, IM, SC	1.5 mg	q3–4 hr	—
Hydromorphone	Dilaudid	oral	7.5 mg	q3–4 hr	2 mg, 4 mg, 8 mg
Comments: despite reputation for street abuse is an excellent alternative to MS; main use is for intermittent pain or as a supplement to ATC meds for breakthrough pain					
Oxycodone	Roxicodone	oral	20-30 mg	q3–4 hr	5 mg
Comments: long available combined w/aspirin and acetaminophen as Percodan and Percocet; single entity drug reduces concerns regarding toxicity					
CR Oxycodone	Oxycontin	oral	20-30 mg	q12–8 hr	10, 20, 40, 80 mg
Comments: for ATC use, usually every 12 hr; do not break, crush or chew					
Fentanyl	Duragesic	TD		q72–48 hr	25, 50, 75, 100 ug/hr
Comments: patches may be combined for optimal dose; ATC use for stable pain, usually q72 hr; lag time w/initial application & after stopping; probably less constipation					
Fentanyl	Sublimaze	IV	100 ug	q30 min	50 ug/ml
Comments: once used only for anesthesia; excellent morphine alternative; no active metabolites					
Methadone	Dolophine	oral	20 mg	q4–12 hr	5 and 10 mg
Methadone	Dolophine	IV, IM	10 mg	q4–12 hr	—
Comments: although inexpensive, first-line use is not recommended due to potential for accumulation second to long, variable life, especially with advanced age and renal impairment; action at NMDA receptor may promote added efficacy; ideal interval between doses is variable, so start prn until optimal schedule established; more potent than suggested by tables, esp. at higher doses.					
Levorphanol	Levodromoran	oral	4 mg	q4–8 hr	—
Levorphanol	Levodromoran	IM/IV	2 mg	q4–8 hr	2 mg
Comments: pharmacokinetics similar to methadone, with similar need to monitor for toxicity as a consequence of accumulation, especially with advanced age and renal impairment					
Oxymorphone	Numorphan	IM./IV / rectal	1 mg / 10 mg	q4–6 hr	10 mg suppository
Comments: no longer available in oral formulation; relatively long acting					

pain (122). Potential benefits need to be balanced against potential toxicity (e.g., GI, GU, CNS, hematologic toxicities, and masking of fever)—considerations that are especially pertinent in the context of recent antitumor therapy and advanced age. Consider avoiding NSAIDs altogether or instituting prophylaxis in patients with bone marrow depression or those who are predisposed to developing gastropathy. If prophylaxis is indicated, then misoprostol appears to be the most effective protective regimen (123).

The nonacetylated salicylates (sodium salicylate, choline magnesium trisalicylate) are associated with a favorable toxicity profile in that they fail to interfere with platelet aggregation, are rarely associated with GI bleeding, and are well tolerated in asthmatic patients (124,125).

A parenteral formulation of ketorolac has been shown to be equianalgesic to low doses of morphine in some settings but is associated with the same range of potential side effects as oral NSAIDs (126).

The recent discovery of subtypes of prostaglandin receptors and the release of more highly selective COX-2 selective prostaglandin inhibitors are predicted to open the door to a new era of more safe and effective antiinflammatory use (127). COX-2 selective NSAIDs appear to provide similar analgesic and antiinflammatory activity as previously available less selective agents but do so at the expense of modest or absent toxicity (128). Although the studies leading to drug approval are extremely encouraging, the true incidence of toxicity will become completely apparent

TABLE 40-13. *Dosage equivalency for transdermal fentanyl*(hourly dose based on 24-hour morphine equivalents*)*

Oral morphine* ** (mg/24 hours)	IM morphine* *** (mg/24 hours)	Transdermal fentanyl (µg/hours)
45–134	8–22	25
135–224	23–37	50
225–314	38–52	75
315–404	53–67	100
405–494	68–82	125
495–584	83–97	150
585–674	98–112	175
675–764	113–127	200
765–854	128–142	225
855–944	143–157	250
945–1034	158–172	275
1035–1124	173–187	300

Courtesy: Janssen Pharmaceutica (modified by author).

*These recommendations originate from the product's package insert.

**Conversion from oral morphine: Based on a *conservative* analgesic activity ratio of 60 mg oral morphine:10 mg IM morphine (6:1 oral:parenteral conversion ratio rather than the widely accepted 3:1 ratio). As a result, converting from oral morphine to transdermal fentanyl using this chart, although generally quite safe, may result in *underdosing* of up to half of patients, who will then require rapid upward titration to achieve analgesia.

***Conversion from IV or IM morphine: An analgesic activity ratio of 10 mg IM morphine:100 ug IV fentanyl was used to derive the equivalence of parenteral morphine to transdermal fentanyl. *These recommendations tend to be reliable.*

only with more widespread use. The new more selective NSAIDs are indicated as treatment for mild to moderate pain because they still have a "ceiling effect" above which further titration is not associated with additional analgesia. Their direct costs are typically greater than those of classic agents, although when considered globally, fewer complications and side effects may result in a lower overall cost. Currently available agents include celecoxib (Celebrex) (usually 100 to 200 mg orally, twice daily) and rofecoxib (Vioxx) (12.5 to 50 mg orally, once daily), which have been variously approved for acute pain, osteoarthritis, and primary dysmenorrhea and which are especially sensible choices in patients with oncologic disease who are especially vulnerable to the side effects of the "classic" less selective NSAIDs.

In contrast to the opioid analgesics, NSAIDs are associated with a ceiling effect, above which dose escalations produce toxicity but no greater analgesia. However, the ceiling dose for a given drug differs from patient to patient, allowing some potential for dose titration. Regular (as opposed to intermittent) use promotes both antiinflammatory as well as analgesic effects. Despite their apparent heterogeneity, the NSAIDs are, in most respects, clinically indistinguishable. Selection is based on the patient's prior experience, minor differences in toxicity, clinician experience, schedule, and cost. When efficacy is poor, the clinician may consider rotating to another NSAID, usually from a distinct biochemical class.

TABLE 40-14. *NSAID use in the management of cancer pain*

Mechanism: Tumor growth produces inflammatory and mechanical effects in adjacent tissues that can trigger the release of prostaglandins (PG), bradykinin, and serotonin, which may precipitate or exacerbate pain in the surrounding tissues. A biochemical, PG-mediated effect is particularly attractive to explain metastatic bone pain because even small lesions may be painful. By inhibiting PG-synthetase (cyclooxygenase), an enzyme involved in the conversion of arachidonic acid to PG.

NSAIDs are considered a first-line drug for mild to moderate cancer pain. Because their mechanism of analgesia is distinct from that of opioids, when they are used together, effects may be additive or even synergistic. Thus, when appropriate, NSAIDs may be used longitudinally throughout the course of management of chronic cancer pain.

In the absence of contraindications, NSAIDs are especially indicated for:
- low-grade, mild pain
- pain due to bone metastases
- bladder spasm
- pain in patients sensitive to opioids
- intermittent pain
- pain associated with inflammation or infection
- pain associated with cutaneous ulcerations
- other musculoskeletal aches and pains

Despite the extensive variety of NSAIDs available, few generalizable, clinically important differences appear to exist among NSAIDs. However, as with opioids, patients may respond more favorably to one than another, with respect to both analgesic efficacy and side-effect profile. Factors influencing the choice of NSAIDs include:
- prior positive and negative experiences
- cost
- schedule
- differences in toxicity

Cancer patients, especially those who are ill, have received chemotherapy, or are in the geriatric age range, are vulnerable to NSAID side effects, which often preclude their use, and, thus, despite WHO guidelines, many clinicians avoid routine NSAID use because their mild opioid-sparing effect may be overshadowed by the potential for side effects and drug interactions.

"WEAK" OPIOIDS (OPIOIDS CONVENTIONALLY USED TO TREAT MODERATE PAIN)

Opioids continue to constitute the mainstay of treatment for cancer pain, especially when it is progressive and related to tumor infiltration. When NSAIDs provide insufficient relief, are contraindicated or poorly tolerated or when pain is severe at presentation, the addition or substitution of a so-called weak opioid (i.e., codeine, hydrocodone, dihydrocodeine, oxycodone preparations) is recommended as an analgesic of intermediate potency (Table 40-11) (16). Usually formulated as combination products, these agents are "weak" only insofar as the inclusion of aspirin, acetaminophen, or ibuprofen results in a ceiling dose above which the incidence of toxicity increases (129). The term "opioids conventionally used to treat moderate pain" is now endorsed in preference to "weak opioids" in recognition of the fact that, when equianalgesic dosing is applied, the potency of the opioid *per se* is not a clinically important distinguishing feature of this class of drugs. For example, a sole entity preparation of oxycodone is now available that, when prescribed in sufficient doses, is effective for even severe pain (130,131) because the ceiling effect imposed by the aspirin/acetaminophen is absent. Likewise, fentanyl, although up to 100 times more potent than parenteral morphine, is rendered clinically useful by utilizing a dosing schedule in a microgram rather than milligram range.

Although the "weak opioids" are appropriate for mild or intermittent pain, practitioners often rely excessively on these agents, frequently continuing their use after they are no longer effective in an ill-advised attempt to avoid prescribing more potent opioids that are also more highly regulated (115). Although propoxyphene has generally been considered inappropriate for the management of cancer pain because of its low potency (132), new studies suggest that it may be more effective than previous, largely single-dose trials have suggested, based on its potential to antagonize NMDA receptors (133). Codeine is considerably emetogenic and constipating relative to its analgesic potency (134) but because of familiarity remains commonly prescribed. Oxycodone, now available not only as a combination product (e.g., Percocet, Percodan) but also as a sole entity preparation (e.g., Roxycodone, Oxy-IR, Oxy-Alone) and in a slow-release formulation (Oxycontin) (135), is considerably more potent than codeine and may be the most useful drug in this class. The potency of hydrocodone and dihydrocodeine preparations (e.g., Lortab, Vicodin) is between that of codeine and oxycodone (136). These agents have the perceived advantage of not requiring triplicate prescriptions (DEA Class C-III vs. C-II), although the clinician must be cautious not to exceed the usual recommended dose of acetaminophen (4 gm/day) as opioid requirements increase.

"POTENT" OPIOIDS (OPIOIDS CONVENTIONALLY USED TO TREAT SEVERE PAIN)

When combinations of codeine-like drugs and NSAIDs provide insufficient analgesia, or when pain is severe at presentation, therapy should progress to include more potent opioid analgesics in a "ladder" fashion (Tables 40-12 and 40-13) (41,77). Morphine, hydromorphone, transdermal fentanyl, and oxycodone are appropriate first-line agents for the institution of basal analgesia, whereas methadone and levorphanol are generally considered second-line agents (see following). Less potent analgesics should not be summarily excluded because NSAIDs may provide additive or synergistic analgesia, and codeine-like preparations may be useful for breakthrough or incident pain. Opioids should initially be introduced in low doses because the early development of side effects will negatively influence compliance but should be rapidly titrated to effect. Pretreatment counseling is important to convert the common but unrealistic expectation that pain be eliminated to one of achieving the best balance possible between comfort and adverse effects.

Morphine

Morphine remains the standard of reference to which other analgesics are compared. Despite widespread use and extensive research, misconceptions about the use of morphine for chronic pain management continue to interfere with its optimal use (115,116).

Morphine is readily absorbed from the gastrointestinal tract and is metabolized in the liver. With chronic use, about one third of the orally administered dose ultimately exerts an analgesic effect (oral bioavailability of 3:1). This is in contrast to the 6:1 parenteral:oral ratio determined from single-dose studies for acute pain. Because parenterally administered drug is not subject to this first-pass effect, clinicians may incorrectly perceive parenterally administered opioids as more effective than orally administered opioids. Recent research has focused on the role of morphine metabolites, once thought to be inactive. Morphine-3-glucuronide has been postulated to antagonize opioid analgesia, whereas morphine-6-glucuronide appears to possess potent analgesic properties and may induce persistent nausea and sedation, especially in the presence of altered renal function (137,138). Although the clinical relevance of these metabolites is currently uncertain, persistent nausea or sedation during morphine therapy should warrant consideration of switching to an alternate opioid.

Morphine is available in a variety of formulations and is appropriate for administration by a variety of routes. The most important distinctions are between (a) so-called immediate-release preparations (e.g., Roxanol), which have a short latency to effect (about 30 minutes) and a short duration (2 to 4 hours) and are usually administered every 3 to 4 hours, and (b) "controlled-release preparations" (e.g., MS Contin, Oramorph), which have a longer latency to effect and duration and, as a result, are usually administered every 12 or sometimes 8 hours (139). New controlled-release preparations include a capsular form that may be suitable for once-daily administration and a q12-hour rectal suppository (140,141).

Alternative Potent Opioids

Hydromorphone (Dilaudid) is available in a variety of formulations and can be administered by the oral, rectal, subcutaneous, and intravenous routes. It is seven to eight times more potent than morphine when administered parenterally and, enterally, is about four times more potent than oral morphine (parenteral to oral dose ratio of about 5:1). Administered by either route, its latency to effect and duration are relatively short (about 30 minutes and 2 to 4 hours, respectively). The main uses of hydromorphone are for subcutaneous infusions (in view of its solubility of up to 200 mg/mL), for oral breakthrough dosing, and for patients who are intolerant to morphine. Despite an unfortunate reputation for street abuse, hydromorphone represents an excellent alternative to morphine in most settings. Because of its high solubility, large doses of hydromorphone can be concentrated in small volumes, making it the usual drug of choice for chronic subcutaneous administration, which is the preferred route of parenteral administration in hospice care because intravenous lines do not need to be maintained. Heroin has the same solubility advantages and is used in the United Kingdom for similar indications but is not available in the United States for routine medical treatment.

Methadone and, to a lesser extent, levorphanol are usually reserved for refractory pain because their half-lives are long and unpredictable, introducing the potential for accumulation, especially in the presence of advanced age and altered renal function (142–144). Most charts describe methadone as equipotent with morphine when administered intramuscularly and slightly more potent when administered orally, although newer data suggest that potency may be significantly greater over time as a result of accumulation. Although it is extremely inexpensive, this advantage is offset by a long and variable half-life (13 to 51 hours in most studies, and even up to 100 hours in others) that may lead to drug accumulation, especially in patients who are elderly or who have renal failure. Treatment may best be initiated by parenteral (PRN) administration until a steady state is achieved, following which the interval between ATC administration may still vary between 4 hours and 12 hours. Levorphanol (145) (Levodromoran) resembles methadone in that, due to its relatively long half-life (11 hours), accumulation may occur. Dosing intervals may vary from 4 to 8 or even 12 hours, and, as a

result, the same precautions described for methadone apply to its use. A parenteral dose of 2 mg and oral dose of 4 mg of levorphanol are usually equianalgesic to 10 mg of parenteral morphine.

Pragmatic and Operational Use of Oral Opioids

Schedule

Most patients will require simultaneous treatment with two different formulations of an opioid: a long-acting (basal) analgesic administered around-the-clock (ATC) and a short-acting analgesic administered as-needed (PRN). This schema is analogous to the treatment of diabetes mellitus with long-acting (NPH) and short-acting (regular) formulations of insulin concurrently. A predominantly time-contingent (around-the-clock) schedule for the administration of analgesics is generally preferred to symptom-contingent (PRN) administration. With prolonged PRN administration, patterns of anticipation and memory of pain become established and may contribute to suffering, even during periods of adequate analgesia.

Basal (Around-the-Clock) Analgesia

Compliance and overall quality of analgesia are enhanced by the regular administration of a long-acting opioid analgesic for basal pain control, supplemented by a short-acting opioid analgesic administered PRN ("escape doses" or "rescue doses") for breakthrough and incident pain. This strategy promotes consistent therapeutic plasma levels and avoids "roller coaster" or sine wave kinetics and dynamics characterized by alternating bouts of pain and toxicity. If analgesics are withheld until pain becomes severe, sympathetic arousal occurs, and even potent analgesics may be ineffective. Prolonged PRN administration may lead to the establishment of a pattern of anticipation and memory of pain that predisposes to persistent suffering even after a more regular administration of analgesics has been instituted (146–148). Preferred basal analgesics include controlled-release morphine and oxycodone preparations that are available in a wide range of doses (but cannot be broken, crushed, or chewed) and transdermal fentanyl (149,150). Transdermal fentanyl is best reserved for the management of relatively stable basal pain. When these agents are poorly tolerated, methadone or levorphanol may be prescribed with careful monitoring, particularly in the presence of altered renal function and advanced age, to avoid accumulation and overdose, risks that are greatest during the initiation of treatment (142).

Supplemental (PRN) Analgesia with Escape or Rescue Doses

In addition to the preceding regimen, potent short-acting opioids with minimal potential for accumulation (immediate-release morphine, hydromorphone, oxycodone) are generally made available on an as-needed basis, usually at intervals of 2 to 4 hours for exacerbations of pain (breakthrough pain) (50). The dose of PRN analgesic is usually empirically derived by giving the equivalent of 10% of the sum of long-acting analgesics administered over 24 hours. For example, the patient taking 100-mg controlled-release morphine q12h should be started at about 20-mg immediate-release morphine sulfate every 3 to 4 hours, after which the ideal dose is found through titration. Rescue doses are often prescribed in a range (i.e., 1 to 3 tablets q 3 to 4 hours), depending on the severity of each episode of breakthrough pain. Patients should be instructed to maintain careful records that accurately reflect their analgesic use. When rescue doses are consistently needed more than 2 to 3 times over a 12-hour period, the dose of the basal, long-acting analgesic should be increased. Breakthrough pain that is predictably triggered by a specific event or activity is referred to as incident pain, which, if prevalent, is a signal that patients should be instructed to take their PRN (rescue) dose in anticipation of the pain-provoking activity (151).

A formulation of oral transmucosal fentanyl citrate (Actiq) has been introduced that produces meaningful relief of breakthrough pain within 5 minutes of initiating consumption, an onset that mimics IV administration, despite its noninvasive character (152,153). About half of the delivered dose is ultimately swallowed and is subject to hepatic first-pass metabolism, resulting in a usual duration of effect of 4 hours. About 15 minutes is usually required for complete consumption, and for maximum effectiveness lozenges should not be chewed. Patient education about child safety is mandatory.

Initiating Opioid Therapy

Because dose response and side effects vary widely based on a number of physiologic and behavioral factors (e.g., age, drug history, extent of disease, etc.), therapy should be individualized to suit the patient's needs. Effective doses often dramatically exceed guidelines recommended in standard texts (morphine 10 mg IM, 30 mg PO), which for the most part are derived from experience with acute or postoperative pain in opioid naive patients.

Treatment with oral morphine can be started several ways. In cases of severe pain, it may be desirable to initiate therapy with parenteral morphine that can later be converted to an oral drug regimen using a 3:1 ratio. More commonly, immediate-release oral morphine is administered every 3 to 4 hours to determine opioid requirements, following which the sum of the daily dose is halved and administered as a controlled-release preparation and supplemented by rescue doses of immediate-release morphine, each aliquot of which should equal 5% to 15% of the 24-hour dose of long-acting opioid. Alternatively, treatment can be initiated with an empirically selected dose of controlled-release morphine, supplemented by appropriate doses of immediate-release morphine. Regardless of the regimen that is selected, low starting doses with rapid upward titration are preferred to limit the frequency of side effects and enhance compliance.

Dose Titration

The correct dose of morphine (or a morphine-like drug) for the management of cancer pain is the dose that effectively relieves the pain without inducing intolerable side effects. Daily doses of morphine required to adequately relieve cancer pain may vary from 30 mg to several grams in divided doses. There is no ceiling effect for morphine; that is, an increase in the dose will always produce a concomitant increase in pain relief. The starting dose is gradually and steadily titrated upward until either pain control is achieved or side effects occur. If dose increases result in worsening side effects and only small increments in analgesia, then the pain syndrome may be relatively opioid resistant (e.g., neuropathic pain or movement-related incident pain) (154). Relatively opioid-resistant pain may require alterative therapeutic approaches.

Individualization

Pharmacologic therapy should be individualized in light of the specific characteristics and needs of each patient (155). Dose response and side effects vary widely based on various physiologic and behavioral factors (e.g., age, drug history, extent of disease, etc.) (156). As noted, effective doses of an analgesic in the presence of chronic pain often dramatically exceed those utilized for treating acute or postoperative pain in opioid naive individuals.

Guidelines for Dosing

The aphorism that the correct dose of an opioid for the management of cancer pain is ultimately that which effectively relieves pain without resulting in unacceptable side effects is indeed well founded (5,7,154). Ideally, the starting dose is gradually and steadily titrated upward until either pain control is achieved or side effects occur. If the latter ensues before adequate comfort is established, then side effects are treated aggressively in an algorithmic fashion (e.g., palliative measures, adjuvant analgesics, opioid rotation, anesthetic interventions).

Adverse Effects

Treatment with the opioids may be associated with side effects, although, in many cases, these are transient and, in most cases, manageable. Prompt identification, assessment, and management of side effects are a cornerstone of treatment. Adverse effects are often perceived of as barriers to the utilization of analgesics in doses required to relieve pain effectively (dose-limiting side effects). Most drug-related side effects can be effectively relieved with careful management, but the same attention and skill required to tailor a pain management program need to be applied to selecting and titrating drugs to minimize the impact of side effects. Patient education is essential to ensure the best outcome and to avoid confusion between manageable side effects and allergy (157). Patients should be encouraged to report problems as they occur.

Constipation

Opioid-induced constipation is sufficiently common that it should almost universally be treated prophylactically. Usually a combined mild stimulant and softener is prescribed when opioid therapy commences, along with instructions for a "sliding scale" regimen that provides progressively stronger cathartics until a regular bowel habit ensues (158,159). An osmotic agent (e.g., lactulose) is the usual second-line agent of choice for refractory constipation. Although their acceptance will vary with the patient's age, sex, and cultural and ethnic background, enemata are often useful to help resolve an established dilemma, but their routine use should be avoided. Although no support from the literature is available, in the context of a major cancer hospital, the author has encountered countless excellent outcomes and acceptance using a preparation of milk and molasses (8 oz warm water, 3 oz powdered milk, 4.5 oz molasses), delivered high by means of soft tubing passed gently 12 inches beyond the sphincter. Although specific commercial preparations are not yet available, based on its presumed action at opioid receptors in the gut wall, oral naloxone has been shown to be an effective cathartic for constipation that is specifically mediated by opioids (160,161). Although relatively high doses are required (about 5 to 15 mg/day), results appear to be reliable and dramatic. Because naloxone does not readily cross the gut wall, treatment is associated with only a modest, but still significant, risk of reversing analgesia, inducing withdrawal and cramping. Whenever encountering refractory constipation, the evaluating clinician should remain alert for the presence of bowel obstruction, as well as fecal impaction, which may present as spurious diarrhea due to the leakage of liquid stool around a distal fecal plug. Impaction is confirmed by manual rectal examination, and its occurrence leaves no other alternative than manual disimpaction, which is time consuming, unpleasant, and usually requires strong analgesics. Finally, unrecognized constipation can contribute to nausea and vomiting.

Nausea and Vomiting

Opioid-mediated nausea and vomiting occur in up to half of patients first exposed to an opioid and after a dose increase (162). These symptoms usually resolve spontaneously with continued opioid use, and thus patients should be reassured and encouraged to adhere to their prescribed regimen of analgesics. Patients who are not routinely apprized of these features will mistake side effects for allergy. For nausea and/or vomiting, a major tranquilizer (e.g., prochlorperazine, chlorpromazine) administered orally or rectally is the usual first-line agent of choice, especially when cost is a consideration (163). A properistaltic agent (e.g., metoclopramide) is appropriate when gastric stasis is suggested by nausea, bloating, and early satiety (164). Scopolamine is particularly useful for nausea that is vertiginous in nature (i.e., amplified by ambulation) (165). In addition to their potential to reduce peritumoral edema and pain, stimulate weight gain and appetite, and enhance mood, corticosteroids are among the most reliable of antiemetics, although the advisability of chronic use is a complex medical decision. Commonly used as an adjunct to emetic chemotherapies, ondansetron (Zofran) and similar agents can be considered for refractory nausea but are usually avoided due to their excessive cost (166). In addition to its new indication as an antianorectic agent (167), Dronabinol, an oral agent containing active elements of marijuana and corticosteroids, is another alternative for refractory nausea (168) and, interestingly, appears not to be regarded as having significant "street value" as a drug of abuse (169). Finally, as is the case with the palliation of other symptoms, the combination of agents that acts by distinct mechanisms may be more effective than the administration of a single agent alone.

Somnolence and Cognitive Impairment

As with nausea, central nervous system side effects occur commonly when opioid therapy is commenced or escalated, but they usually resolve spontaneously with uninterrupted use. Cognitive dysfunction is best regarded as a spectrum of phenomena ranging from drowsiness to confusion and hallucinations. When these occur immediately after treatment is instituted for persistent severe pain, they should be distinguished from "catch-up sleep." When persistent, these effects may reflect interactions between symptom management and comorbidities that can include preexisting dementia, brain or leptomeningeal metastases, whole brain irradiation, and indirect effects due to anorexia, cachexia, and malnutrition, chemotherapy, humoral substances elaborated by certain tumors and paraneoplastic syndromes, and metabolic abnormalities such as dehydration, hypercalcemia, hyponatremia, and sepsis. Of the drugs with the potential to produce adverse CNS effects, used in steady doses, the opioids are actually among those that are the least offensive, especially compared to the benzodiazepines, other sedatives, and polypharmacy in general. The consultant should be aware, however, that as a highly stigmatized therapeutic class of drugs, the opioids are nevertheless most commonly implicated by patients, family members, and even other physicians, especially in the setting of the emergency room. Family members typically find it easier to indict a therapeutic intervention than to acknowledge the progression of a loved one's underlying malignancy. An especially useful "clinical pearl" is the recognition that the sudden onset of delirium is almost never due predominantly to opioids if their dose has remained stable over the preceding weeks or even days. As a result, except in the presence of profound respiratory depression, the reflex administration of naloxone, especially in large bolus doses, should be avoided, lest the patient's new, undiagnosed confusional state be unnecessarily compounded by the sudden reemergence of pain and symptoms of withdrawal.

Opioid-mediated sedation that has not responded to a rotation of agents, trials of "opioid-sparing" adjuvant analgesics, or the passage of time can often be managed surprisingly effectively with titrated doses of a psychostimulant such as methylphenidate or dextroamphetamine (170–172). Methylphenidate is usually started in doses of 10 mg on awakening and 5 mg at noon but may require titration, especially over time. The stimulants appear to enhance analgesia (172) and are also associated with potent antidepressant actions that, in contrast to classic antidepressants, are usually evident almost immediately. Other than jitteriness, side effects are infrequent, although caution should be exercised in the presence of brain metastasis, psychotic disorders, hyperactive delirium, and tachyarrhythmias. Anorexia appears not to be a practical problem, and, in fact, patients have anecdotally been observed to experience paradoxic weight gain, presumably as a result of increased wakefulness and arousal. Both methylphenidate and dextroamphetamine have relatively short half-lives, so sleep is typically not disturbed, and, should it be necessary, both agents are available in extended-release formulations. The judicious use of psychostimulants in patients with significant symptom burdens may reduce the need for more inherently risky anesthetic interventions, and by restoring or maintaining lucidity such use is often met with extraordinary gratitude and thus should be considered more routinely.

Refractory Side Effects

When side effects are refractory to pharmacoreversal, consideration should be given to a trial of a similar, alternative opioid because side effects are often idiosyncratic and may not be triggered by agents that are in other respects similar (173). If indicated, the addition of a nonopioid adjuvant analgesic can be considered, which, if successful, may serve to reduce side effects by an opioid-sparing effect (174). Finally, in patients with amenable pain syndromes, the presence of refractory side effects is an indication to consider other more invasive therapeutic modalities, such as nerve blocks or spinal opioid therapy (13).

Reassessment

After an acceptable drug regimen has been established, adequacy should be periodically reassessed (Table 40-3). Patients are often reluctant to spontaneously request more potent analgesics because of fear of addiction and other factors that, regrettably, often include barriers unconsciously erected by the treatment team or the health-care delivery system. In the setting of an established malignancy, increased drug requirements should be anticipated as a consequence of disease progression and its attendant pain, as well as the development of tolerance. Although tolerance is now viewed as a less vexing problem than in the past, when it occurs, it is most frequently manifested by decreased duration of analgesic effect.

EDUCATION AND ADDICTION POTENTIAL

Patient and family education is an essential precursor to effective symptom control and is ideally accomplished through the combined efforts of physicians, nurses, pharmacists, and other providers. Patients commonly maintain deeply rooted fears of addiction that are culturally reinforced, regrettably often by their physicians. Distinctions among addiction (psychological dependence), physical dependence, and tolerance should be explained preemptively (175). Tolerance (the need for increasing dosages to maintain a desired drug effect) and physical dependence (drug use that is sufficiently established that characteristic withdrawal symptoms occur when treatment is stopped precipitously or a specific antagonist is administered) are biophysiologic phenomena that inevitably accompany chronic opioid use and that thus are best regarded as pharmacologic effects that are unrelated to addiction and that, when recognized, need not impede successful analgesic therapy. Because tolerance also develops rapidly to most opioid side effects (except constipation, miosis, and myoclonus), doses can usually be simply increased to recapture analgesia. Likewise, physical dependence is rarely problematic because, should opioid therapy become unnecessary, patients are generally able to readily discontinue drug use when a gradual tapering schedule is instituted (173).

Tolerance, physical dependence, and psychological dependence (addiction), once considered uncritically as part of a single syndrome, are increasingly recognized as distinct phenomena. In contemporary parlance, addiction is regarded as a psychobehavioral phenomenon with possible genetic influences characterized by (a) overwhelming drug use and loss of control over drug use, (b) nonmedical drug use, and (c) continued use despite the presence or threat of physiological, psychological, or environmentally harmful consequences. In contrast to tolerance and physical dependence—which are, to varying degrees, inevitable with chronic use—addiction is an infrequent outcome of medical treatment with opioids, except in patients with histories of drug or alcohol abuse who are at increased risks of both developing aberrant drug use and of being subjected to undertreatment as a consequence of prescribers' fears of rekindling addiction (176). Rather than positing addiction as a substance-specific phenomenon, arising from simple exposure to an offensive agent, current thinking recognizes the importance of the context of drug use.

ADJUVANT ANALGESICS

As opposed to opioids, whose effects are relatively reliable in virtually all settings, the so-called adjuvant analgesics (see following) are mechanism specific and thus should be utilized based on specific indications, such as neuropathic pain (selected antidepressants and anticonvulsants), bone pain (NSAIDs), or pain due to raised intracranial pressure (corticosteroids). In patients with amenable pain syndromes, successful treatment with agents from among this heterogeneous classification is heralded by an opioid-sparing effect, often with reduced toxicity.

ROUTES OF OPIOID ADMINISTRATION (TABLE 40-15)

Oral Administration

When possible, analgesics should be administered orally or by a similarly noninvasive route (transdermal, rectal, oral transmucosal) to promote independence and mobility and to provide ease of titration (5,41). In the presence of a functional, intact GI system, after dose is adjusted to account for hepatic first-pass effect, oral administration provides analgesia that is as effective as parenteral (but usually not spinal) administration. Other than transdermal administration, which has attributes similar to oral therapies, alternate routes should otherwise be generally considered only for specific indications. When patients are followed longitudinally through the end of life, however, ultimately it appears that at least one third to two thirds of patients will benefit from at least the transient use of an alternate route, usually subcutaneous or intravenous administration (30,120,177).

Transdermal Administration

Transdermal fentanyl is associated with advantages similar to those cited for oral administration except that, due to its pharmacokinetics, it is best reserved for patients with stable pain and should not be relied on in the presence of rapidly changing dose requirements (178–180). Although its use can be maintained in the presence of alimentary tract dysfunction, it need not be reserved specifically for this setting. It is particularly useful in patients with otherwise poor compliance, is generally associated with high levels of patient acceptance, and may produce less constipation than oral opioids (181).

After treatment is established, steady plasma levels of fentanyl are maintained for 72 hours following a single

application of a 25-, 50-, 75-, or 100-mcg/hour patch (182). The surface area of the patch is directly proportional to the administered dose of fentanyl, and patches can be combined to arrive at the desired dose. The system's rate-controlling membrane regulates drug release at a slower rate than average skin flux, thus ensuring that the delivery system, rather than the skin, is the main determinant of absorption. Of factors with the potential to influence the rate of absorption through the skin, temperature is most important, and, as a result, patients should be warned against applying heating pads, etc. (183). Although low levels of fentanyl can be detected in the bloodstream just one hour after administration, because of the relative impermeability of the epidermis, a consistent, near-peak (pseudosteady state) level is not obtained for a period of 12–18 hours after treatment is initiated or the dose is increased. Patients need to be cautioned that pain relief will accrue over the first day of treatment and should be provided with rescue doses of short-acting analgesics during this interval. In addition, as a result of the formation of a subcutaneous depot of drug, effects persist for 12–18 hours following removal of the patch, so that adverse effects may require prolonged treatment. Although the transdermal fentanyl system was originally studied predominantly in the perioperative setting, its ultimate approval was limited to the management of chronic pain. Conversion schemes are conservative, so that up to half of patients dosed according to the product's package insert will require rapid upward titration. Because of the lag between dose and response, transdermal fentanyl analgesia is best suited for patients with relatively stable dose requirements and is particularly useful when the oral route is contraindicated but is considered any time a patient requires chronic opioid therapy.

Rectal Administration

When the oral and transdermal routes are inappropriate, rectal administration is reliable for short-term use (184,185) except in the presence of diarrhea, fistulas, or other anatomic abnormalities. Rectal administration is usually avoided in older children and in the presence of conditions that increase pain when patients are positioned for suppository insertion. Morphine and hydromorphone are available in rectal preparations, and oxymorphone hydrochloride (Numorphan) rectal suppositories provide 4 to 6 hours of potent analgesia. Rectal methadone has been shown to be safe and effective but must be compounded by a manufacturing pharmacist (186).

Parenteral Administration

With the growth of the hospice and home care movement, there has been increasing acceptance of chronic parenteral opioid administration by means of continuous subcutaneous or intravenous infusions administered by a portable

TABLE 40-15. *Comparison of routes of drug administration*

Route	Comments	Available drugs
Oral (PO)	Generally the preferred route of administration (see transdermal); after adjustment in dose to account for hepatic first pass effect, oral and systemic (IV, SC, IM) analgesics are equipotent; reliance on oral (and transdermal) route enhances independence	Acetaminophen, NSAIDS, codeine, propoxyphene, morphine, hydromorphone, levorphanol, methadone, oxycodone
Rectal (PR)	Useful for short intervals when oral route is compromised; limitations: colostomy, resection, anorectal tumor, radiation fibrosis, scarring, embarrassment (esp. in adolescents), diarrhea, impaction, hemorrhoids, pain on positioning (esp w/bone metastases), etc.; potency ratio is variable, usually considered 1:1; often impractical due to limited available formulations; custom made suppositories can be prepared by compounding pharmacist; anecdotal experience suggests efficacy for MS Contin	Morphine, hydromorphone, oxymorphone
Intramuscular (IM)	Not recommended; unnecessarily painful, especially for children; no pharmacokinetic advantage; risk of sterile abscess	Morphine, hydromorphone, levorphanol, methadone, oxymorphone
Transdermal (TD)	Associated with most of same benefits as oral route; appropriate as basal analgesic for pts with stable pain; slow onset of action after first application and dose increases due to epidermal barrier; slow offset after removal due to SC skin depot; almost always effective for 72 hours, occasionally only 60 or 48 hours; especially advantageous when oral route is compromised and for noncompliants; inappropriate for unstable pain	Fentanyl
Intravenous (IV)	Standard against which other routes are compared; commonly used postop; since potency is no greater than oral administration (after adjustments for hepatic first pass effect), reserve for unstable pain (rapidly changing dose requirements) and pain emergencies, or for when oral route is compromised (xerostomia, dysphagia, obstruction, nausea and vomiting, malabsorption, coma). When feasible, continuous infusion is supplemented with PCA	Morphine, hydromorphone, fentanyl, methadone, levorphanol, oxymorphone
Subcutaneous (SQ or SC)	When chronic parenteral analgesia is required due to alimentary tract failure (see IV, above), especially at home or in hospice, this is the route of choice unless a durable IV catheter is already in place; pharmacokinetics are essentially the same as for IV and, administered with a portable pump and through a butterfly needle, nursing requirements are less than for IV; when drug is concentrated to deliver required dose at under 1–2 mL/hour, site usually needs to be rotated only 1X/week; analgesics may be combined with antiemetics, steroids and, with hyaluronidase can use fluid for hydration	Morphine, hydromorphone, fentanyl
Epidural and intrathecal	Because drug is administered close to receptors, low doses usually result in profound analgesia with few side effects; institution requires specialized skills, good home care and a committed family; requires maintenance of catheter and pump; careful decision making is required to ensure cost effectiveness; especially useful for lower extremity pain, diffuse pain and pelvic, rectal or gynecologic pain	Morphine, hydromorphone fentanyl, sufentanil, dilute local anesthetic (bupivacaine) admixtures, clonidine
Oral transmucosal (OT) Sublingual (SL)	Avoids first pass metabolism; FDA approval for oral transmucosal fentanyl citrate (OTFC), a rapid acting drug for treating breakthrough pain is pending; although commonly used in hospice, efficacy of SL morphine is marginal	Fentanyl, morphine

pump, with or without a patient-controlled analgesia feature. When equianalgesic conversion is accounted for, there is no evidence that parenteral administration is associated with superior analgesia, and, as a result, conversion should be reserved for specific indications, such as titration for a pain emergency or alimentary tract failure (xerostomia, dysphagia, malabsorption, obstruction, vomiting, coma) (187,188).

Continuous Subcutaneous and Intravenous Opioid Infusions

Due to reduced nursing requirements, the continuous subcutaneous infusion (CSCI) of opioids currently represents the route of choice for chronic home-based administration, unless permanent IV access has already been established (31,189). A variety of commercially available infusion pumps are available that are portable, battery-driven, inexpensively leased, and equipped with alarm systems.

To initiate a CSCI, the 24-hour dose of parenteral drug is summed. If the patient's drug regimen includes oral analgesics, then conversion tables are utilized (Tables 40-12 and 40-13) to calculate the equianalgesic parenteral dose of opioid (usually morphine or hydromorphone). The total daily dose of parenteral drug is divided by 24, and the pump is set accordingly. Tissue irritation is minimized when volumes under 1 to 2 mL are delivered, which is facilitated by ordering an appropriately concentrated formulation of the opioid. The pump's tubing is primed with drug, and it is attached to a 27-gauge pediatric butterfly needle, which is inserted subcutaneously and taped flush to the patient's skin. Any subcutaneous site can be utilized, although the infraclavicular fossa and chest wall are frequently selected to facilitate ambulation. The infusion site is ideally checked twice daily for signs of irritation and is changed weekly, or as needed (190).

Absorption of subcutaneously administered opioids is rapid, and steady-state plasma levels are generally approached within one hour (191). Most parenteral opioids are suitable for CSCI, although morphine and hydromorphone are used most commonly, and meperidine, methadone, and pentazocine are best avoided due to the potential for tissue irritation. Physician orders should provide for rescue doses of drug adequate to counter incomplete analgesia (usually a subcutaneous bolus injection equal to the hourly dose administered every 30 to 60 minutes PRN), and, at the end of 24 hours, the basal infusion can be increased by the sum of the recorded rescue doses. If analgesia is adequate, but side effects are prominent (usually oversedation), the infusion rate may be halved and titrated upward, as needed, or opioid rotation can be considered. In the United States, hydromorphone is the usual subcutaneous drug of choice because large doses can be concentrated into small volumes due to its high solubility. In the United Kingdom, where parenteral hydromorphone is not routinely used, diamorphine (heroin) is utilized preferentially for the same reasons.

More sophisticated hospice programs routinely infuse combinations of opioids, antiemetics, and steroids simultaneously without side effects or difficulties. Novel subcutaneous applications include continuous infusions of ketamine (193) and lidocaine (194) for refractory neuropathic cancer pain syndromes and the development of a hydromorphone pellet that, when implanted, provides continuous pain relief for periods of up to 4 weeks (195).

Alternate Opioid Analgesics, Including Tramadol

Clinicians should maintain familiarity with the pharmacologic profiles of a variety of opioids (Tables 40-11–40-14) and should consider drug rotation when a favorable bal-

ance between comfort and side effects cannot be achieved with a given regimen (155). When converting between drugs or routes, one half to two thirds the calculated equianalgesic dose of the new drug is usually recommended as a starting dose (5,6), which is then titrated rapidly, as needed.

Despite a unique mechanism that involves weak mu-agonist activity, as well as inhibition of norepinephrine and serotonin reuptake, the synthetic codeine analog tramadol has, at best, a moderate role in the management of cancer pain. Although it may be used as an alternative to codeine or hydrocodone, it is unclear whether tramadol possesses any particular advantages, and it appears to be less satisfactory than morphine for the management of severe pain. Higher doses are associated with a ceiling effect and side effects that include dizziness, nausea, dry mouth, and sedation. However, abuse potential may be lower than that of classic pure agonist opioid analgesics.

Opioid Analgesics Best Avoided (Table 40-16)

The chronic administration of meperidine, especially by the oral route, is contraindicated (5,6,41). Administered chronically, all opioids may produce some degree of myoclonus, but the accumulation of normeperidine, a metabolite, may lead to frank seizure activity, especially with oral use, when renal function is impaired and when the patient is elderly (196,197).

Agonist-antagonist and partial agonist opioids should generally be avoided for a variety of reasons, the most important of which is the presence of a ceiling effect for analgesia (198). With the usual exception of buprenorphine, these agents may precipitate withdrawal, and their administration complicates the eventual, usually inevitable, transition to pure agonist agents. Pentazocine (Talwin), the only one of these agents widely available orally, is associated with a high incidence of hallucinations and confusion, and buprenorphine is not easily or reliably reversed by naloxone.

Brompton's cocktail, one of the first preparations of an oral opioid to gain clinical acceptance, is now used only infrequently. Developed at Brompton's Chest Hospital in the United Kingdom, it consisted of a mixture of morphine hydrochloride (or heroin), cocaine hydrochloride, alcohol, syrup, and chloroform water. In blinded trials it has not been shown to produce analgesia that is superior to that of an oral opioid administered alone (199), and its use should be discouraged because of the problems associated with titrating fixed-dose combinations. Likewise, no advantage has been demonstrated for treatment with heroin (200), although it is still sometimes used in the United Kingdom and Canada, predominantly for subcutaneous infusions by virtue of its high solubility.

TABLE 40-16. *Drugs to avoid for management of chronic cancer pain*

Generic name	Proprietary name	Comments
Meperidine	Demerol, Pethedine	Accumulation of a toxic metabolite, normeperidine, may result in CNS excitation leading to seizures, sequelae that are not naloxone reversible; also short duration and low potency do not favor its use
Heroin	Diamorphine	Available in United Kingdom; rapidly deacetylated into morphine; analgesic efficacy is no greater than that of morphine; high abuse potential
Brompton's Cocktail	Heroin or morphine + cocaine, alcohol, and phenothiazine	Used in UK; avoid fixed combination products when possible; efficacy is no greater than that of morphine
Pentazocine Nalbuphine Butorphanol	Talwin Nubain Stadol	Mixed agonist-antagonist; associated with ceiling dose; may cause dysphoria; pentazocine is the only agent available in oral formulation
Buprenorphine Dezocine	Buprenex Dalgan	Partial agonist; associated with ceiling dose; may cause dysphoria; buprenorphine available as sublingual preparation outside United States

Note: Although benzodiazepines and major tranquilizers may have important roles for the management of other symptoms (e.g., nausea, agitation, anxiety), they are not substitutes for true analgesics.

Adjuvant (Nonopioid) Analgesics

The term *adjuvant analgesic* is used to refer to a heterogeneous group of medications originally developed for purposes other than relief of pain that has been observed to promote analgesia in specific clinical settings. Although a large variety of drugs are purported to possess adjuvant properties, only a limited number have been shown to reliably relieve pain in controlled or partially controlled trials. Patients with cancer pain may benefit, usually from the addition of (a) corticosteroids, (b) selected, usually tricyclic, antidepressants, (c) anticonvulsants, (d) amphetamines and, more rarely, (e) N-methyl D-aspartate antagonists, (f) alpha-adrenergic antagonists, (g) antihistamines, and (h) phenothiazines. Interestingly, not every agent belonging to each class appears to possess analgesic properties, and even those agents with confirmed analgesic properties are applicable only for specific types of pain, and even then, pain relief does not accrue in all potential candidates.

The adjuvant analgesics differ from opioid analgesics in important general ways. Opioids are "all purpose" analgesics in that, independent of the clinical condition being treated, if administered in an adequate dose, they always elicit some degree of pain relief. Although, admittedly, some conditions appear to be less opioid responsive than others, the clinician can still count on achieving some degree of analgesia if an opioid is administered in a sufficient dose. Regrettably, in less opioid responsive conditions, escalating side effects may eclipse the utility of analgesia, rendering therapy unacceptable. In contrast, responses to adjuvant analgesics are more binary in nature in that, depending on the nature of the clinical condition being treated (and perhaps other more obscure variables), treatment may or may not elicit pain relief. It happens that most currently recognized adjuvants are most likely to be effective for various types of neuropathic pain. A second fundamental difference relates to the dose-response relationship. Even in conditions in which adjuvants are clearly effective, the nature of the dose-response relationship is fundamentally different from that of the opioids. The relationship between dose and response is usually relatively linear for opioids, even though, depending on the responsivity of the pain, the slope of the line describing the dose-response relationship may be shallow or steep. In contrast, even should an adjuvant produce a desirable effect, there is no certainty that raising the dose will enhance analgesia or that if a positive response occurs, it will be proportionate or replicable. These features of the adjuvants dictate the development of novel study methodologies (201).

Antidepressants

The efficacy of selected antidepressants as analgesics, independent of their effects on mood and nighttime sleep, has been demonstrated initially in noncancer models (202–204) and, more recently, in cancer patients as well (205–206). Because analgesia is characteristically induced with doses generally considered insufficient to relieve depression, there is an argument for a direct, independent underlying mechanism of effect. In addition, although onset is not immediate, analgesia is generally established more rapidly than are antidepressant effects (typically 3 to 7 days vs. 14 to 21 days). The operant mechanism for antidepressant-mediated analgesia presumably relates to increased circulating pools of norepinephrine and serotonin induced by reductions in the postsynaptic uptake of these neurotransmitters. The most compelling indication for tricyclic antidepressant (TCA) therapy remains variants of neuropathic pain (e.g., postherpetic neuralgia, central pain, diabetic neuropathy), although more recent trials have demonstrated efficacy for disorders that include headache, arthritis, chronic low back pain, and "psychogenic" pain.

Amitriptyline and, to a lesser extent, imipramine remain the most extensively studied of these agents and, as a result, are the usual first choices of academically based pain specialists. Although usually relatively innocuous, side effects are especially prominent with these agents. Because amitriptyline and imipramine are, respectively, metabolized to nortriptyline and desipramine—agents with superior side-effect profiles—many authorities, especially in private practice, advocate the latter two agents as drugs of first choice. Data from controlled clinical trials support the use of amitriptyline, nortriptyline, desipramine, imipramine, doxepin, maprotiline, and clomipramine. Trazodone, although sedating and, thus, potentially helpful for sleep disturbances, appears to be of limited value as an analgesic. Interestingly, despite their efficacy for depression and generally favorable side-effect profiles, the newer selective serotonin reuptake inhibitors (SSRIs), such as fluoxetine (Prozac), paroxetine (Paxil), and sertraline (Zoloft), appear to be less effective for treating pain than are the heterocyclic antidepressants. Obviously, in cases where pain is a secondary manifestation of depression, the SSRIs and other antidepressants, administered in therapeutic doses, may be beneficial.

The main indication for treatment with the heterocyclic antidepressants is neuropathic pain that is relatively constant and unrelenting and is not predominantly intermittent, lancinating, jabbing, or shocklike. Neuropathic pain of the latter (paroxysmal) type may also be treated effectively with TCAs but is often first treated with an anticonvulsant. As noted, TCAs have also been used successfully in headache and other syndromes, and thus a trial in nearly any cancer pain syndrome that has not responded favorably to primary analgesics is justified.

Usually, amitriptyline, nortriptyline, or desipramine are started in doses of 10 to 25 mg nightly and are gradually titrated upward, usually to a range of 50 to 125 mg and occasionally higher, until toxicity occurs or analgesia is established. Dry mouth, constipation, drowsiness, and dysphoria are the most prominent of a wide range of potential side effects, although more serious, usually anticholinergic, side effects may occur (e.g., urinary retention, cardiac dysrhythmias). Unlike the side effects of opioid therapy, the development of tolerance is less robust, and side effects are less readily reversible; as a result, if side effects are more prominent than analgesia, then the offending agent is usually discontinued, and a pharmacologic analog or a drug from another class is usually started. Although not as reliably analgesic as the TCAs, the newer SSRIs may be preferred for (a) the fragile elderly, (b) patients predisposed to developing serious anticholinergic side effects, (c) patients who have failed

multiple trials of tricyclics due to side effects, and (d) patients in whom depression is a prominent comorbidity. Usual starting doses of the SSRIs are the same as are suggested for the management of depression (fluoxetine 20 mg, paroxetine 20 mg, sertraline 50 mg), administered as a single morning dose to take advantage of their propensity to mildly stimulate activity. Interestingly, although these agents are not considered as reliable for analgesia as the heterocyclic antidepressants, paroxetine has been reported to be effective for refractory pruritus in patients with advanced cancer (208).

Anticonvulsants and Baclofen

Based on ample, but predominantly anecdotal, reports on the efficacy of carbamazepine for the nonsurgical treatment of trigeminal neuralgia (tic douloureux) (209), carbamazepine, phenytoin, valproate, clonazepam, and, most recently, gabapentin—alone or in combination with the TCAs—have been used successfully to treat pain of neuropathic origin (210–212). Most authorities consider them as drugs of first choice for neuropathic pain that resembles classic trigeminal neuralgia (i.e., predominantly paroxysmal, jabbing, shocklike pain). Anticonvulsants are also usually considered a second-line therapy for relatively steady, constant neuropathic pain when TCAs are poorly tolerated or have been ineffective or only partially effective (5). Anticonvulsants relieve pain in these settings as a result of their ability to dampen ectopic foci of electrical activity and spontaneous discharge from injured nerves, in a manner analogous to their salutary effects in seizure disorders.

Carbamazepine therapy has been most thoroughly documented, and, thus, in the absence of contraindications, it is usually considered the drug of first choice. The most toxic of the anticonvulsants used to treat pain, carbamazepine is associated with idiosyncratic hepatotoxicity (rare) and bone marrow depression (incidence of up to 2%), and thus is avoided in patients with liver metastases or bone marrow depletion or those receiving cytotoxic therapy. Used chronically, carbamazepine therapy requires monitoring of CBC and liver function tests every 2 to 3 months. Ataxia, confusion, dizziness, and nausea are relatively common with upward dose titration, and therefore carbamazepine is also best avoided in the fragile elderly, especially combined with other psychotropic agents. Clonazepam, in doses of 0.5 mg b.i.d., is often well tolerated in patients who have experienced or are at risk for side effects with carbamazepine, phenytoin, and valproate. Carbamazepine is usually started at 100 mg b.i.d. and titrated upward toward 300 to 400 mg q.i.d. while awaiting an analgesic response or toxicity.

Failure of one anticonvulsant does not appear to predict outcome for trials of an alternate agent. Gabapentin (213) is a new anticonvulsant that, according to anecdote, may be highly efficacious for neuropathic pain, especially when lancinating, although controlled trials have not yet been reported. Trials of gabapentin for neuropathic pain, in doses commencing at 100 mg t.i.d. and ranging to 300 q.i.d., have become almost ubiquitous largely because serious side effects are infrequent. Although felbamate, another new anticonvulsant, is known to interact with the NMDA receptor, its use is probably only rarely warranted due to concerns regarding the development of aplastic anemia (214).

Although it is a GABA agonist and not an anticonvulsant, baclofen, with or without carbamazepine, has been reported to be effective for lancinating, ticlike neuropathic pain. Baclofen is usually started at a dose of 5 mg b.i.d. or t.i.d. and may be titrated up to 30 to 90 mg/day, as tolerated. The other main role for baclofen in pain management is as an intrathecal infusion for spasticity, due especially to spinal cord injury and multiple sclerosis (215).

Oral Local Anesthetics

Based on historic accounts of transient relief of pain after IV infusions of local anesthetics, oral (and rectal) analogs already in use as antiarrhythmics have been exploited for relief of neuropathic pain (216,217). The agent of choice from this group is mexiletine, which is usually regarded as a second- or third-line agent for continuous or intermittent neuropathic pain disorders. The oral local anesthetics block sodium channels and relieve pain by mechanisms similar to those at work in anticonvulsant-mediated analgesia. Mexiletine is usually started in doses of 150 mg/day and is titrated upward to a maximum dose of 300 mg t.i.d. Up to 40% of patients may discontinue therapy due to side effects, the most common of which are nausea and vomiting.

Psychostimulants: Amphetamines

The most accepted use for amphetamines in palliative care is as a means to reverse opioid-mediated sedation (172). A recent report even suggests durable improvements in cognitive function in cancer patients receiving opioids (218). In addition to these primary effects, research suggests that dextroamphetamine and methylphenidate (Ritalin) possess analgesic properties (170) and are excellent antidepressants. Unlike classic antidepressants, their effect on mood is usually apparent with the first dose. Further, prior to the introduction of SSRIs, methylphenidate had developed an excellent record of safety in geriatric patients with refractory depression, and their safe use has recently been reported in adolescent cancer patients on opioid therapy (219). Arrhythmias are almost nonexistent, and, instead of inducing anorexia, these agents typically have a paradoxic effect of increasing appetite by enhancing alertness. Nervousness and agitation are the most common adverse effects and usually respond to dose reductions. Agitated delirium may occur in patients with coexisting psychiatric disorders, brain metastases, or metabolic disturbances, all of which are relative contraindications to use. Methylphenidate is typically started in doses of 10 mg on awakening and 5 mg with the noontime meal, after which titration to effect is instituted. Because of its short half-life, patients are usually able to sleep well at night (220), especially if they have become more active as a result of increased alertness. Dextroamphetamine can be administered on a similar schedule, and extended-release formulations are available for both agents.

Corticosteroids

The efficacy of corticosteroids as treatment for acute pain resulting from raised intracranial pressure (ICP) and spinal cord compression is well established. In addition, these agents have been administered empirically for a variety of cancer pain syndromes with good results (221,222). Pain relief is presumably related to reduced peritumoral edema and inflammation, with consequent relief of pressure and traction on nerves and other pain-sensitive structures, although beneficial effects on mood, appetite, and weight also may indirectly contribute to improved subjective pain reports. Improvements in pain are often rapid and dramatic but usually depend on continued administration. Although results may be maintained in a proportion of patients, benefits are often short lived, plateauing in a few weeks, presumably due to the replacement of edema by tumor growth in patients with aggressive disease. A trial of oral steroids may be beneficial in any patient with pain that appears to be predominantly due to spread of bulky tumor (e.g., selected patients with pelvic, rectal, esophageal, or hepatic tumor deposits or invasion of the brachial and lumbosacral plexus).

Dexamethasone is the usual drug of choice because it possesses less potent mineralocorticoid effects. Although a variety of side effects and complications can occur as a result of even acute steroid administration (e.g., diabetes mellitus, psychosis), serious problems usually arise only from chronic use. As a result, when a trial produces beneficial results, it is reasonable to maintain use, without tapering, in the presence of progressive cancer (223). Although most patients note improvements in mood when steroid therapy is commenced, a small proportion experience dysphoria and even florid psychosis. Interestingly, the occurrence of such an episode does not appear to predict similar reactions on reexposure. The optimal dose of steroids, both for oncologic emergencies (e.g., raised ICP, cord compression) and chronic pain, is not known. For the former, 100 mg IV dexamethasone is administered initially in some institutions, followed by IV maintenance. The large bolus dose produces severe, but transient, perineal burning ("like ants in my pants") due to an unknown mechanism. For the management of nonemergent pain, an oral dose of 2 to 6 mg dexamethasone q.i.d. or t.i.d. is common.

N-Methyl D-Aspartate (NMDA) Antagonists

The NMDA receptor has recently been described and implicated in the transmission of pain (224). Although research on various agents with antagonist activity at the NMDA receptor is underway, ketamine, a partial NMDA antagonist, is the only agent currently available that appears to mediate pain by this nonopioid mechanism (225). Long used as an IV anesthetic agent, subanesthetic doses have been administered for prolonged periods with fair success in a small number of patients with refractory neuropathic cancer pain (193,226). Due to side effects and the risk of complications, ketamine infusion should be regarded as a treatment of desperation, reserved for rare use, until additional experience has been reported.

Alpha-2 Adrenergic Antagonists

The centrally acting antihypertensive clonidine has been observed to promote analgesia for neuropathic pain when administered near the neuroaxis. Epidural administration has recently received FDA approval, and trials of intrathecal clonidine are underway. In a prospective randomized study of 38 patients with severe cancer pain that had persisted despite large doses of spinal opioids, the addition of epidural clonidine was associated with significant improvement in 45% of patients overall and in 56% of patients with neuropathic pain (227). Hypotension during the initiation of treatment and rebound hypertension during withdrawal are the main potential risks of treatment.

Bisphosphonates

Although the primary indication for the bisphosphonates remains the management of symptomatic hypercalcemia, important roles for these agents are emerging for the prevention of skeletal complications of cancer. Nearly all of the bisphosphonates have been implicated in the reduction of phenomena that include osseous metastases, pain emanating from established bone metastases, osteoporosis, pathologic fracture, and immobility. Most studies demonstrating efficacy have been conducted in patients with multiple myeloma and metastatic breast and prostate cancer. Etidronate appears to be relatively ineffective for treating pain, whereas monthly IV injections of pamidronate appear to be the most reliable approach to inducing analgesia (228,229). The utility of oral pamidronate is unfortunately hampered by poor bioavailability and adverse effects, including GI toxicity, renal impairment, anemia, and electrolyte abnormalities. In one report, a series of five daily IV injections of olpadronate was observed to dramatically reduce bone pain for a period of 4 to 6 weeks, beyond which analgesia persisted only in patients maintained on oral therapy (230). A trial of clodronate, administered as 600 to 1500 mg IV in 500-mL normal saline over 3 hours q 1 to 2 weeks, is an alternate regimen that has been shown to be effective for the management of painful bone metastases.

Other Purported Adjuvants

Despite an absence of data from controlled trials, antihistamines, benzodiazepines, and antipsychotics have been used, mostly historically, in efforts to enhance analgesia. Although these agents have clear roles for primary indications other than pain (e.g., anxiolysis, antiemesis, etc.), with few exceptions they are not reliably associated with analgesia (231,232) and thus should not be relied on as substitutes for opioid analgesics.

In contrast to other neuroleptics, methotrimeprazine reliably produces dose-related analgesia that is comparable to that of opioid-mediated analgesia (233) but has recently become difficult to obtain in the U.S. marketplace. Although clinical lore has perpetuated the hypothesis that the butyrophenones have utility as primary or adjuvant analgesics, this lore has been confirmed neither by controlled trials nor survey data. Proponents advocate trials for rectal tenesmus, bladder tenesmus, and neuropathic pain and for prominent suffering or psychological distress.

A careful review of the literature reveals insufficient evidence to support the contention that the benzodiazepines have meaningful analgesic properties in most clinical circumstances (231). Although treatment with the benzodiazepines may reduce complaints of pain, this appears to be an indirect effect related to their psychotropic properties, rather than true analgesia. Thus, the use of benzodiazepines should be discouraged except in extremely specific settings. Clinical experience suggests a potential role for short-term use for acute muscle spasm, for anxiolytic use when stress appears to influence reports of pain, and for lancinating neuropathic pain as a part of sequential trials, in which case clonazepam and alprazolam are the agents of choice. They should probably not be considered as first-line choices even for the preceding indications because potential benefits are often eclipsed by the potential for the development of cognitive impairment, physical and psychological dependence, worsening depression, the risk of overdose, and other side effects.

Adequate pain relief cannot always be achieved through pharmacologic means alone. Initial screening should identify patients in whom behavioral or psychological modalities may be employed successfully. When careful trials of pharmacologic therapy have failed, consideration should be given to alternative modalities, including additional antitumor therapy, neural blockade, CNS opioids, neurosurgical options, and, rarely, electrical stimulation.

NONPHARMACOLOGIC INTERVENTIONAL THERAPIES FOR CANCER PAIN

Historically, a variety of alternatives to systemic analgesics for controlling cancer pain have been advocated with varying enthusiasm (11). Prior to the widespread availability of safe analgesics, interventional therapies were in greater vogue, a trend that persisted through the recent past,

TABLE 40-17. *Early consideration of neurolysis**

Indication	Procedure
Visceral pain in the abdomen and back	Celiac plexus neurolysis
Visceral pelvic or rectal pain	Superior hypogastric plexus neurolysis
Visceral pain of anus or genitalia	Ganglion impar neurolysis
Perineal pain with urinary diversion	Phenol saddleblock
Focal chest wall pain	Thoracic subarachnoid neurolysis
Focal chest wall pain	Intercostal neurolysis
Unilateral leg pain in bedbound patient	Lumbar subarachnoid neurolysis
Unilateral pain below midtrunk	Percutaneous cordotomy

*The risk-benefit ratio of these procedures in the specified settings is sufficiently favorable and well established to warrant early consideration.

mostly as a consequence of exaggerated concerns about iatrogenic addiction and fear of regulatory reprisal. With more widespread dissemination and acceptance of contemporary pharmacotherapeutic strategies and guidelines (5), interventional techniques are now generally considered as being best reserved for discrete settings characterized by refractory pain or unremitting medication-mediated side effects (12).

The more circumscribed role of interventional therapies in contemporary practice has evolved out of a recognition that (a) indications are more discrete, (b) implementation is associated with greater acute risk, and (c) both treatment and maintenance are usually more demanding of institutional and family resources. Generally provided by anesthesiologists and neurosurgeons, these therapies are most commonly considered after advanced, irreversible disease has been established, but in specific settings they are occasionally considered relatively early in the course of a painful neoplastic disorder (Table 40-17).

Although the applications for interventional approaches for cancer pain are more limited, they remain essential in a small proportion of patients (11). Even when indicated, however, they are rarely a panacea, especially when instituted in isolation. Interventional techniques are best regarded as a component of a therapeutic matrix that includes antitumor therapy, various pharmacologic strategies, and behavioral and psychiatric approaches (13). A comprehensive multimodal approach is preferred due to the heterogeneous and often progressive nature of cancer pain and in recognition of the fact that pain may comprise just one component of a broader symptom complex in patients with advanced medical illness.

Classification: Neuroablation versus Neuromodulation

Interventional therapies for managing cancer pain are of two fundamental types. Neuroablative (neurolytic, neurodestructive) techniques involve intentional injury to elements of the nervous system implicated in the transmission of pain (234). Lesions are produced by surgical, chemical, thermal, or cryogenic means. Neuroaugmentative techniques rely on modulating the endogenous regulation of pain and include local anesthetic blockade, regional infusions of drugs at epidural, intrathecal, intraventricular, or perineural sites, and electrical stimulation.

Neuroablative Interventions

Chemical neurolysis is generally performed with either 100% (absolute or dehydrated) ethyl alcohol or phenol compounded with contrast medium, water, or, for intrathecal use, glycerin. Ammonium salts (pitcher plant distillate) and chlorocresol are rarely used in contemporary practice, and the use of glycerol is confined almost exclusively to the treatment of trigeminal neuralgia of nonmalignant origin. Radiofrequency thermocoagulation, initially used almost exclusively by neurosurgeons for percutaneous cordotomy, is now more often considered whenever long-lasting block of a discrete neural target is desired (235). Although equipment is costly and the technique more complex, thermoablation may lower the risk of undesired deficits by producing a more controllable lesion both because circuitry for electrical stimulation makes localization more certain and because untoward spread after injection is eliminated. Chemical neurolysis is still preferred for interventions that depend on disrupting a more diffuse neural network, as in the case of celiac plexus block. Cryoanalgesia is less commonly employed due to impressions that durable analgesia is more difficult to achieve, but it may be preferred for patients with longer life expectancies because preservation of the underlying neural architecture may reduce the risk of postablative dysesthesias (236).

Specific Neuroablative Procedures

These procedures are generally undertaken only after careful consideration due to their hazards (Table 40-18), which may persist indefinitely. Risks include undesired deficit from untoward lesion extension or placement, physical trauma from needle or probe insertion, and new pain due to denervation and neuroma formation. With good patient selection (Table 40-19) and expertise, however, complications are infrequent. Regrettably, pain relief is rarely permanent as a consequence of central nervous system

TABLE 40-18. *Potential hazards of neuroablation*

- Development of new dysesthetic pain due to deafferentation or neuroma formation
- Accidental damage to nontargeted nonneurologic tissue (e.g., pneumothorax)
- Accidental damage to nontargeted neurologic tissue (e.g., paraplegia)
- Impermanence due to axonal regrowth, plasticity, or disease progression
- Incomplete pain relief due to incomplete ablation, overlapping distribution of neighboring nerves, or faulty diagnosis

plasticity, axonal regrowth, and progressive tumor growth. Nevertheless, when a neuroablative procedure can be performed with relative safety and a good likelihood of a successful outcome, drug burden can be significantly reduced, and the more extensive needs for the supportive care associated with regional infusion therapy are absent.

Ablation of peripheral nerves is conducted infrequently because of a relatively higher incidence of neuritis, which is said to be more common with alcohol than phenol. Intercostal blockade can be conducted with a low incidence of pneumothorax (237), although neighboring nerves must be destroyed to account for overlapping innervation, and many experts prefer subarachnoid neurolysis. Alcohol, phenol, or radiofrequency ablation of the fifth and occasionally ninth and tenth cranial nerves may be appropriate for orofacial pain that is unresponsive to radiotherapy. Although it is available only in select centers, preliminary evidence suggests that gamma knife irradiation is an additional option, although immediate relief is not typically forthcoming (238).

Sympathetic neuroablation for refractory visceral pain is typically approached somewhat more liberally because successful treatment is associated with a very low incidence of new pain and no numbness or motor weakness. Celiac plexus or splanchnic nerve block is often considered early for abdominal and back pain secondary to visceral or

TABLE 40-19. *Relative indications for neuroablative procedures*

Patient characteristics
- Limited life expectancy (up to about 12 months)
- Tolerance of effects achieved with prognostic block (when appropriate)
- Valid informed consent

Pain characteristics
- Pain is severe
- Pain is expected to persist
- Pain cannot be modified by less invasive measures
- Pain is well localized and characterized in a consistent fashion
- Pain is relieved with local anesthetic block (when appropriate)
- Relief is most likely with somatic and visceral pain

retroperitoneal disease and can be accomplished by a variety of approaches (239). Although usually performed percutaneously by an anesthesiologist, injections can be performed at the time of surgery, and splanchnic nerves can be sectioned via thoracoscopy (240). Although partially controlled trials suggest that pancreatic cancer pain may not vary significantly with pharmacotherapy versus neural blockade, better performance status and fewer side effects, presumably as a consequence of reduced opioid burden, are common (241,242). One recent double-blinded placebo-controlled trial of celiac block serendipitously suggested a significant survival benefit in treated patients, a portentous finding that requires confirmation (243). The more recent introduction of superior hypogastric plexus block targets the sympathetic system near the sacral promontory bilaterally and is effective for visceral pelvic pain with no reported complications (244). Surprisingly, reflex sympathetic dystrophy (complex regional pain syndrome) infrequently accompanies a diagnosis of cancer, so stellate ganglion ablation, which is associated with risks of brachial plexus injury, is rarely required. Likewise, most lower extremity oncologic pain is somatically mediated, creating little role for lumbar sympatholysis.

Intrathecal neurolysis is a time-tested intervention that, although infrequently performed in contemporary practice, is in many respects straightforward (245). When coupled with scrupulous decision making and technique treatment, it is associated with highly rewarding outcomes, especially for chest wall pain, because targeted fibers are so distant from the outflow to the extremities and sphincters. Although serial epidural neurolysis has a few proponents, intrathecal injections of absolute alcohol or phenol and glycerin are usually preferred because their respective hypobaricity and hyperbaricity confer much more exquisite control over drug spread.

Neuromodulation

With Wall and Melzack's introduction of the gate control theory of pain (246) and reluctant abandonment of the linear Cartesian theory of pain transmission it has come to be recognized that all interventions constitute some form of modulation. Nevertheless, the term *neuromodulation* has come to be equated with techniques that up- or down-regulate the substrates that appear to be involved in pain generation and is especially used to refer to electrical stimulation and regional infusion therapy.

Local Anesthetic Blockade

Because results are typically transient, local anesthetic blocks play a relatively limited role in the management of well-established cancer pain (247). Local anesthetic neural blockade may be performed for diagnostic, prognostic, or therapeutic purposes. Diagnostic and prognostic nerve blocks help characterize the underlying mechanism of pain (somatic, visceral, sympathetic, neuropathic, psychogenic) and may be predictive of the potential for a subsequent neuroablative procedure to relieve pain or produce side effects.

Local anesthetic injections with or without the addition of corticosteroids may provide lasting relief in specific settings such as muscle spasm, postsurgical nerve impingement, herpes zoster, sympathetic dystrophy, and premorbid chronic low back pain. Therapeutic local anesthetic injections are associated with relatively low risks, can often be performed at the bedside, and under selected circumstances may be rendered by physicians with a variety of backgrounds.

Electrical Stimulation

Despite anecdotal and investigational reports, these techniques are infrequently applied to treat cancer pain in routine clinical practice. Contemporary interest is more focused on their role in the management of nonmalignant pain. Although all modalities involve attempts to relieve pain by the application of electrical current, each has distinct indications that are only briefly considered here.

Although still widely used as an adjunct for the ambulatory management of chronic nonmalignant pain, TENS is usually restricted in the oncologic setting to physical therapy and the rehabilitative treatment of survivors. Despite the advantage of empowering patients by allowing them control over some treatment parameters, efficacy is minimal for severe pain, and results are uneven and often deteriorate rapidly after commencing treatment, suggesting a high rate of placebo response, especially for cancer pain (248).

Despite increasing use for the management of nonmalignant pain, spinal cord stimulation is rarely considered appropriate for treating cancer pain (249). Pain from active cancer is generally too severe, fluctuating, or mixed in etiology to warrant the expense of establishing and maintaining treatment. Other considerations weighing against its consideration in the setting of active cancer include concerns about epidural tumor spread, the risk of infection due to depressed immune function, and the frequent need for reoperation to maintain appropriate anatamo-topographic coverage.

Despite a dearth of published reports, spinal cord stimulation is a logical alternative for cancer survivors with stable patterns of refractory pain. Best candidates are those with well-localized neuropathic pain associated with cancer treatment, particularly pain after mastectomy or thoracotomy, postherpetic neuralgia, and radiation-induced brachial plexopathy.

Despite convincing early data and the use of minimally invasive (stereotactic) surgery, deep brain stimulation analgesia is used infrequently in contemporary practice. Impressive results have been obtained in cancer pain patients when miniaturized electrodes are implanted in areas rich in opioid receptors (e.g., periventricular and periaqueductal regions) (250). Analgesia appears to be related to the release of endogenous opioid-like substances, and effects are diffuse and bilateral rather than restricted to an area subserved by a single nerve (251). In contrast, thalamic stimulation produces contralateral, position-specific effects limited to a discrete topographic region. The effects of thalamic stimulation are not naloxone reversible, and efficacy has been demonstrated mostly for neuropathic pain, especially of central origin, making treatment more appropriate for chronic rather than cancer pain (252).

Regional Drug Infusions

The recognition that opioids produce their protean effects by activating stereospecific receptors laid the groundwork for the administration of these and other substances discretely near the central nervous system's targets where they are believed to have their primary effects. A variety of devices have been pioneered to permit highly regulated infusions for the management of refractory chronic pain.

Although parenteral drug administration has an important role when the alimentary tract is compromised by disease (e.g., xerostomia, dysphagia, malabsorption, obstruction, vomiting, coma), other than rapidity of onset, there appear to be no specific advantages to intravenous (253) or subcutaneous (254) drug administration. The recent availability of an oral transmucosal preparation of fentanyl citrate constitutes a novel means to administer a strong opioid in such settings as well (255).

In contrast to systemically administered parenteral drugs, the deposition of opioids and other novel substances in close proximity to central nervous system receptors may provide more potent analgesia with fewer side effects. Various delivery systems have been developed to facilitate treatment, although none is without some drawbacks.

The epidural administration of opioids, although in many respects ideal for the management of acute pain, has some limitations for the treatment of chronic cancer pain. Despite the development of improved external pumps, biocompatible Silastic catheters, and increased experience with their surgical placement, concerns include dislodgement, infection, fibrin deposition, cord compression, and the fear that with chronicity, near-systemic doses may be required with attendant side effects. The main advantage of the epidural route is that a dilute admixture of local anesthetic can be gradually added to achieve a degree of dermatomal numbness that is sometimes needed for pain associated with severe tissue damage or neuropathy (256).

Intrathecal administration of opioids is associated with even lower doses than the epidural route, and fully implantable systems are now widely available that enhance patient independence and reduce the risk of infection (257). Although access to a specialized laptop computer is required for Medtronic's most sophisticated SynchroMed system, ultimately the need for supportive care in the form of nursing visits, pharmacy services, and pump maintenance is dramatically reduced (258). High initial equipment and professional costs prohibit the use of fully implantable systems in patients unless at least a 3- to 6-month survival is predicted, in which case costs may ultimately be much less than for epidural and subcutaneous infusions. Although the SynchroMed system is reliable over a breadth of infusion rates that can be preprogrammed for circadian variations in pain, systems still lack a patient-activated feature. Less expensive patient-activated devices are currently available outside of the United States and are anticipated to find an important niche in more preterminal patients. Although admixtures of local anesthetic and opioids may somewhat enhance intrathecal analgesia, unlike epidural treatment, discrete dermatomal numbness cannot be achieved.

Epidural and intrathecal clonidine (259) may enhance regional analgesia, and the future is undoubtedly ripe for the development of more selective opioid compounds and other novel analgesic substances, although it is essential that neurotoxicity be scrupulously evaluated before embarking on the imprudent use of otherwise-promising therapies (260).

CONCLUSION

Cancer pain can now be effectively managed in a satisfying majority of patients with rigorously applied pharmacotherapies applied by motivated and compassionate professionals, especially with an increased public health mandate and better availability of institutional support. Although pharmacotherapy is in many respects straightforward, careful interdisciplinary communication and frequent adjustments are required, making optimal symptom control a time-intensive, though characteristically satisfying, endeavor. Arising from fundamental, straightforward, easily reproducible guidelines, drug therapy has been enriched by an increasing plethora of new drugs and means of administration that, although potentially confounding to decision making and expensive, ultimately enrich treatment options tremendously. Whereas relatively "low-tech" approaches are adequate for most patients, "medium-tech" interventions in the form of systemic parenteral (intravenous and subcutaneous) infusions are increasingly accepted in preterminal patients with poor alimentary function, although the ensuing results tend to be more convenient than effective (253,254).

Even with the most facile use of noninterventional pharmacotherapies, rehabilitative approaches, and behavioral management, an important 10% to 30% of cancer pain patients will benefit from more invasive therapies, which, regrettably, are not routinely available. More importantly, in contrast to pharmacotherapies, the scientific literature's relative dearth of controlled trials of interventional therapies makes evidence-based decision making difficult and sometimes apparently idiosyncratic (233). An emerging literature suggests that a tendency to pain that is refractory to conventional therapies may be prospectively identified based on the presence of various clinical features, the most prominent of which appears to be movement-related pain but which also may include neuropathic pain, cutaneous ulcerative pain, massive tissue distortion, recent tolerance to analgesics, a history of alcohol or drug abuse, and the presence of severe psychological distress.

An immense range of invasive techniques for managing intractable cancer pain has been advocated (11,13,234). Approaches involving intended injury or destruction of the neural components involved in pain transmission, predominantly by injecting alcohol or phenol near nerve trunks, were once quite popular. More liberal and facile use of oral and parenterally administered opioids and the advent of perispinal analgesic therapy have largely, but by no means entirely, supplanted neurodestructive (neurolytic) techniques. Relative to "highly" invasive destructive techniques, "moderately" invasive (parenteral or regional) drug infusion therapies are often preferred by contemporary pain management experts because of their reversibility and a risk-benefit ratio that is usually, but not always, more favorable. Nevertheless, a proportion of patients exposed to even state-of-the-art infusion therapies continue to experience inadequate control of pain or refractory drug-related side effects. As a result of near-universal acceptance of the construct that the correct dose of analgesic is dynamic and not fixed and thus consists of that which is effective (i.e., that which relieves pain adequately without unacceptable side effects), dose-limiting side effects ultimately constitute the primary indication for more invasive pain therapies. Interestingly, an emerging literature (233) suggests that such patients may be prospectively identified based on the presence of clinical factors, the most prominent of which appears to be movement-related pain but which also may include neuropathic pain, cutaneous ulcerative pain, massive tissue distortion, recent tolerance to analgesics, a history of alcohol or drug abuse, and the presence of severe psychological distress.

Although an immense range of invasive techniques for managing intractable cancer pain has been advocated, conceptual and scientific breakthroughs coupled with ongoing attitudinal shifts have reduced the role of interventional therapies considerably, a trend that in reality heightens rather than reduces their importance in the correct setting. A regrettable consequence of the current emphasis on less invasive approaches that are well within the purview of the motivated generalist is that more invasive alternative therapies will be taught less often and less effectively. Thus, despite their critical role, the use of invasive therapies in just a small proportion of patients dictates that adequate clinical exposure may occur only in centers caring for large volumes of patients with oncologic pain or in the presence of carefully established referral patterns. Although understandable, evolving educational deficits position these interventions tragically at risk of achieving the status of a "lost art," introducing risks both that appropriate techniques will be overlooked despite important indications and that hazardous therapies may be applied injudiciously. Although technical expertise is an obvious predictor of outcome, optimal clinical decision making is an even more evasive and ethereal entity that is difficult to impart to the most motivated acolyte, even when adequate clinical material and expertise are available. Detailed algorithm, clinical pathways, and hierarchies of interventions have been proposed, but ultimately they are inadequate substitutes for highly individualized decision making. This is especially frustrating because other than the need for exquisite attention to detail, many invasive techniques are neither excessively technically demanding nor hazardous when scrupulous patient selection is exercised (11,13,234).

Even exploiting the full range of uses for more conventional therapies, interventional approaches by no means constitute a panacea and are ideally integrated within a broad interdisciplinary matrix. Of note is that, in addition to the capacity for well-selected interventional therapies to control pain, by lowering drug burden other symptoms are often ameliorated and performance status improved—features that may influence not only quality of life but also length of survival.

Of these approaches, there remains an important, though circumscribed, role for neuroablative or neurolytic procedures that involve intentional damage to elements of the nervous system. Although potentially hazardous, especially due to their irreversibility, these therapies require lower chronic maintenance and are especially ideal when pain is well localized and when support systems are inadequate, as in the case of rural settings. Many of these techniques are surprisingly straightforward and, when coupled with careful decision making, are associated with highly rewarding outcomes.

In addition to the more liberal, facile, and generalized use of oral and parenterally administered opioids, akin to a democratization of techniques previously reserved for the privileged or agonal, the development of techniques for regional drug infusions and the dissemination of specialized delivery systems has largely, but by no means entirely, supplanted neurodestructive techniques. Relative to "highly" invasive destructive techniques, "moderately" invasive (parenteral or regional) drug infusion therapies are often preferred by contemporary pain management experts because of their reversibility and a risk-benefit ratio that is usually, but not always, more favorable. Although more demanding of patients and their support systems than conventional therapies, regional analgesic infusions share most of their same favorable aspects, including generalizability among disparate patient populations (e.g., regardless of fitness, fragility, age, and culture), a wide range of topographic and mechanistic predecessors (e.g., pain that is neuropathic, nociceptive, and mixed and

multifocal, disseminated, and bilateral), and especially reversibility and titratability—cardinal features for a target disease as unpredictable and potentially progressive as cancer (257).

Finally, although no single technique is a panacea, the motivated clinician or team possessing the background and skills—or at least access to interventional therapies that, although increasingly arcane, are better understood—can evoke a highly satisfying treatment response despite the diversity and challenges of neoplastic disorders. Ultimately, cancer pain has been and will continue to serve as a stimulating proving ground for techniques that, with careful retrospective and prospective analysis, benefit the larger and more highly underserved population of patients with chronic painful medical disorders of nononcologic origin.

Regrettably, chronic pain and acute pain occur in a high frequency of cancer patients. If inadequately addressed by the clinician, pain and other distressing symptoms may interfere with primary antitumor therapy and will markedly detract from the quality of life of patients, family members, and care providers. Although a strong focus on pain control is important, independent of disease stage, it is a special priority in patients with advanced disease who are no longer candidates for potentially curative therapy.

Although rarely eliminated altogether, pain can be controlled in the vast majority of patients, usually with the careful application of straightforward pharmacologic measures, combined with diagnostic acumen and conscientious followup. In the small, but significant, proportion of patients whose pain is not readily controlled with noninvasive analgesics, a variety of alternative measures are available that, when selected carefully, are also associated with a high degree of success. An increasingly large cadre of clinicians has come to recognize that, far from an exercise in futility, caring for patients with advanced, irreversible illness can represent a highly satisfying endeavor that is usually met with considerable success. Thus, no patient should ever wish for death as a result of inadequate control of pain or other symptoms, and clinicians need never communicate overtly or indirectly that "there is nothing more that can be done." Comprehensive cancer care is best regarded as a continuum that commences with prevention and early detection, focuses intensely on curative therapy, and is ideally rendered complete by a seamless transition to palliation and attention to quality of life.

REFERENCES

1. Pickett M, Cooley ME, Gordon DB. Palliative care: past, present, and future perspectives. *Semin Oncol Nurs* 1998;14:86.
2. Burge F. The epidemiology of palliative care in cancer. *J Pall Care* 1992;8:18.
3. Brescia FJ. Pain management issues as part of the comprehensive care of the cancer patient. *Sem Oncol* 1993;20(suppl A):48.
4. MacDonald N. Cancer centres: their role in palliative care. *J Pall Care* 1992;8:38.

5. Management of Cancer Pain Guideline Panel. *Management of cancer pain: clinical practice guideline no 9*. Rockville, MD: AHCPR Publication No. 94–0592; March 1994.

6. American Pain Society. *Principles of analgesic use in the treatment of acute pain and chronic cancer pain*, 3rd ed. Skokie, IL: American Pain Society, 1992.

7. Cancer pain assessment and treatment curriculum guidelines. *J Clin Oncol* 1992;10:1976.

8. Ferrante, Patt RB, et al. Practice guidelines for cancer pain management: a report by the ASA Task Force on Pain Management, Cancer Pain Section. *Anesthesiology* 1996;84:1243–1257.

9. Breitbart W. Psychotropic adjuvant analgesics for pain in cancer and AIDS. *Psychooncology* 1998 7:333–345.

10. Caraceni A, Zecca E, Martini C, De Conno F. Gabapentin as an adjuvant to opioid analgesia for neuropathic cancer pain. *J Pain Symptom Manage* 1999 17:441–445.

11. Patt RB. Anesthetic procedures for the control of cancer pain. In: Arbit E, ed. *Management of cancer related pain*. Mount Kisco, NY: Futura, 1993:381.

12. Patt RB, Jain S, et al. The outcomes movement and neurolytic blockade for cancer pain management. *Pain Digest* 1995;5:268.

13. Patt RB, Jain S. Therapeutic decision making for invasive procedures. In: Patt RB, ed. *Cancer pain*. Philadelphia, PA: Lippincott, 1993:275.

14. Zimmerman L, Story KT, Gaston-Johansson F, Rowles JR. Psychological variables and cancer pain. *Cancer Nurs* 1996 19:44–53.

15. Melzack R. The tragedy of needless pain. *Scientific American* 1990; 262:27–33.

16. Levy MH. Pharmacologic treatment of cancer pain. *N Engl J Med* 1996;335:1124–1132.

17. Witte MH, Witte CL. Epilogue: what we don't know about cancer. *Anticancer Res* 1999;19(6A):4919–4933.

18. Emanuel EJ, Fairclough D, Clarridge BC, et al. Attitudes and practices of U.S. oncologists regarding euthanasia and physician-assisted suicide. *Ann Intern Med* 2000;133:527–532.

19. Wilson KG, Scott JF, Graham ID, et al. Attitudes of terminally ill patients toward euthanasia and physician-assisted suicide. *Arch Intern Med* 2000;60:2454–2460.

20. Rosenfeld B, Breitbart W, Galietta M, et al. The schedule of attitudes toward hastened death: measuring desire for death in terminally ill cancer patients. *Cancer* 2000 88:2868–2875.

21. Passik SD, Weinreb HJ. Managing chronic nonmalignant pain: overcoming obstacles to the use of opioids. *Adv Ther* 2000;17:70–83.

22. Brookoff D, Polomano R. Treating sickle cell pain like cancer pain. *Ann Intern Med* 1992;116:364–368.

23. Belgrade MJ. Opioids for chronic nonmalignant pain. Choosing suitable candidates for long-term therapy. *Postgrad Med* 1999;106:115–116.

24. Anderson VC, Burchiel KJ. A prospective study of long-term intrathecal morphine in the management of chronic nonmalignant pain. *Neurosurgery* 1999;44:289–300.

25. Zenz M, Strumpf M, Tryba M. Long-term oral opioid therapy in patients with chronic nonmalignant pain. *J Pain Symptom Manage* 1992;7:69.

26. Roth SH, Fleischmann RM, Burch FX, et al. Around-the-clock, controlled-release oxycodone therapy for osteoarthritis-related pain: placebo-controlled trial and long-term evaluation. *Arch Intern Med* 2000;60:853–860.

27. Zech DFJ, Grong S, Lynch J, et al. Validation of the world health organization guidelines for cancer pain relief: a 10-year prospective study. *Pain* 1996;63:65–76.

28. Grond S, Zech D, Diefenbach C, Bischoff A. Prevalence and pattern of symptoms in patients with cancer pain: a prospective evaluation of 1635 cancer patients referred to a pain clinic. *J Pain Symptom Manage* 1994; 9:372–382.

29. Zech DFJ, Grond S, Lynch J, et al. Validation of world health organization guidelines for cancer pain relief: a 10-year prospective study. *Pain* 1995;63:65–76.

30. Moulin DE, Johnson NG, Murray-Parsons N, et al. Subcutaneous narcotic infusions for cancer pain: treatment outcome and guidelines for use. *CMAJ* 1992;146:891–897.

31. Moulin DE, Kreeft JH, Murray-Parsons N, Bouquillon AI. Comparison of continuous subcutaneous and intravenous hydromorphone infusions for management of cancer pain. *Lancet* 1991;337:465–468.

32. Ferrante FM, Bedder M, Caplan RA, et al. Practice guidelines for cancer pain management: A report by the American Society of Anesthesiologists Task Force on Pain Management, Cancer Pain Section. *Anesthesiology* 1996; 84:1243–1257.

33. Patt RB. The current status of anesthetic approaches to cancer pain management. In: Payne R, Patt RB, Hill CS Jr, eds. *Assessment and treatment of cancer pain: progress in pain research and management*, Vol 12. Seattle: IASP Press, 1998.

34. Liebeskind JC. Pain can kill. *Pain* 1991;44:3–4.

35. Lillemoe KD, Cameron JL, Kaufman HS, et al. Chemical splanchnicectomy in patients with unresectable pancreatic cancer. *Annals of Surgery* 1993;217:447–457.

36. Cleeland CS, Gonin R, Hatfield AK, et al. Pain and its treatment in outpatients with metastatic cancer. *New Engl J Med* 1994;330:592.

37. Jadad AR, Browman GP. The WHO analgesic ladder for cancer pain management: stepping up the quality of its evaluation. *JAMA* 1995;274:1870.

38. Ventafridda V, De Conno FD. Status of cancer pain and palliative care worldwide. *J Pain Symptom Manage* 1996;12:79.

39. Cleeland CS. Barriers to the management of cancer pain. *Oncology* 1987;12(Suppl):19.

40. Daut RL, Cleeland CS. The prevalence and severity of pain in cancer. *Cancer* 1982:50;1913.

41. World Health Organization. *Cancer pain relief*. Geneva: WHO, 1986.

42. Vuorinen E. Pain as an early symptom in cancer. *Clin J Pain* Dec 1993;9(4):272–278.

43. Wagner G. Frequency of pain in patients with cancer. Recent results. *Cancer Res* 1984;89:64–71.

44. Franks PJ, Salisbury C, Bosanquet N, et al. The level of need for palliative care: a systematic review of the literature. *Palliat Med* 2000; 14:93–104.

45. Petzke F, Radbruch L, Zech D, et al. Temporal presentation of chronic cancer pain: transitory pains on admission to a multidisciplinary pain clinic *J Pain Symptom Manage* 1999;17:391–401.

46. Caraceni A, Portenoy RK. An international survey of cancer pain characteristics and syndromes. IASP Task Force on Cancer Pain. *Pain* 1999;82:263–274.

47. Banning A, Sjogren P, Henriksen H. Pain causes in 200 patients referred to a multidisciplinary cancer pain clinic. *Pain* 1991;45:45–48.

48. Brescia FJ. Pain management issues as part of the comprehensive care of the cancer patient. *Sem Oncol* 1993;20(suppl A):48–52.

49. Portenoy RK, Payne D, Jacobsen P. Breakthrough pain: characteristics and impact in patients with cancer pain. *Pain*1999 81:129–134.

50. Patt RB, Ellison NM. Breakthrough pain in cancer patients: characteristics, prevalence, and treatment. *Oncology* 1998;12:1035–1046.

51. Jacox A, Carr DB, Payne R, et al. Management of cancer pain. *Clinical practice guideline no 9*. Rockville, MD: AHCPR Publication No. 94-0592; March 1994.

52. Rowlingson J, Hammill RJ, Patt RB. Assessment of the patient with oncologic pain. In: Patt R, ed. *Cancer pain*. Philadelphia, PA: Lippincott, 1993:23.

53. Tasmuth T, Kataja M, Blomqvist C, et al. Treatment-related factors predisposing to chronic pain in patients with breast cancer—a multivariate approach. *Acta Oncol* 1997;36:625.

54. Uhm JH, Yung WK. Neurologic complications of cancer therapy. *Curr Treat Options Neurol* 1999;1:428–437.

55. McCarthy GM, Skillings JR. Jaw and other orofacial pain in patients receiving vincristine for the treatment of cancer. *Oral Surg Oral Med Oral Pathol* 1992;74:299.

56. Patt RB. Cancer pain syndromes. In: Patt RB, ed. *Cancer pain*. Philadelphia, PA: Lippincott, 1993:3.

57. Campa JA, Payne R. Pain syndromes due to cancer. In: Patt RB, ed. *Cancer pain*. Philadelphia, PA: Lippincott, 1993:41.

58. Ross EL. The evolving role of antiepileptic drugs in treating neuropathic pain. *Neurology* 2000;55:S41–S46.

59. Harris CV, Bradlyn AS, Ritchey AK, et al. Individual differences in pediatric cancer patients' reactions to invasive medical procedures: a repeated measures analysis. *Pediatr Hematol Oncol* 1994;11:293.

60. Broome ME, Rehwaldt M, Fogg L. Relationships between cognitive behavioral techniques, temperament, observed distress, and pain reports in children and adolescents during lumbar puncture. *J Pediatr Nurs* 1998;13:48.

61. McCarthy AM, Cool VA, Petersen M, et al. Cognitive behavioral pain and anxiety interventions in pediatric oncology centers and bone marrow transplant units. *J Pediatr Oncol Nurs* 1996;13:3.

62. Reddy SK, Weinstein SM. Medical decision-making in a patient with a history of cancer and chronic non-malignant pain. *Clin J Pain* 1995; 11:242.

63. Foley KM. Treatment of cancer pain. *N Engl J Med* 1985;313:84.

64. Gamsa A. The role of psychological factors in chronic pain. I. A half century of study. *Pain* 1994;57:5.

65. Gamsa A. The role of psychological factors in chronic pain. II. A critical appraisal. *Pain* 1994;57:17.

66. Martin LA, Hagen NA. Neuropathic pain in cancer patients: mechanisms, syndromes, and clinical controversies. *J Pain Symptom Manage* 1997;14:99–117.

67. Portenoy RK, Kanner RM. Nonopioid and adjuvant analgesics. In: Portenoy RK, Kanner RM, eds. *Pain management: theory and practice.* Philadelphia, PA: F. A. Davis, 1996:219.

68. Raja SN, Meyer RA, Campbell JN. Peripheral mechanisms of somatic pain. *Anesthesiology.* 1988;68:571–590.

69. Bennett GJ. Update on the neurophysiology of pain transmission and modulation: focus on the NMDA-receptor. *J Pain Symptom Manage* 2000;19(Suppl 1):S2–S6.

70. Joshi SK, Gebhart GF. Visceral pain. *Curr Rev Pain* 2000;4:499–506.

71. Gebhart GF. J.J. Bonica lecture-2000: Physiology, pathophysiology, and pharmacology of visceral pain. *Reg Anesth Pain Med* 2000;25: 632–638.

72. Rigor BM SR. Pelvic cancer pain. *J Surg Oncol* Dec 2000;75(4): 280–300.

73. Grossman SA, Sheidler VR, Swedeen K, et al. Correlation of patient and caregiver ratings of cancer pain. *J Pain Symptom Manage* 1991; 6:53.

74. O'Brien J, Francis A. The use of next-of-kin to estimate pain in cancer patients. *Pain* 1988;35:171.

75. Cleeland CS, Nakamura Y, Mendoza TR, et al. Dimensions of the impact of cancer pain in a four country sample: new information from multidimensional scaling. *Pain* 1996;67:267–273.

76. Beyer JE, Wells N. Assessment of cancer pain in children. In: Patt RB, ed. *Cancer pain.* Philadelphia, PA: Lippincott Co, 1993:57.

77. WHO Expert Committee. *Cancer pain relief and palliative care.* Geneva: WHO, 1990.

78. Enneking WF, Conrad EU III. Common bone tumors. *Clin Symp* 1989;41:1.

79. Akakura K, Akimoto S, Shimazaki J. Pain caused by bone metastasis in endocrine-therapy-refractory prostate cancer. *J Cancer Res Clin Oncol* 1996;122:633.

80. Papatheofanis FJ. Variation in oncologic opinion regarding management of metastatic bone pain with systemic radionuclide therapy *J Nucl Med* 1999;40:1420–1423.

81. DeVita VT Jr, Hellman S, Rosenberg SA, eds. *Cancer: principles and practice of oncology,* 5th ed. Philadelphia, PA: Lippincott, 1997: 1604.

82. Bryne TN. Spinal cord compression from epidural metastases. *N Engl J Med* 1992;327:614.

83. Sorensen S, Borgesen SE, Rohde K, et al. Metastatic epidural spinal cord compression. *Cancer* 1990;65:1502.

84. Ingham J, Beveridge A, Cooney NJ. The management of spinal cord compression in patients with advanced malignancy. *J Pain Symptom Manage* 1993;8:1.

85. Maranzano E, Latini P, Checcaglini F, et al. Radiation therapy of spinal cord compression caused by breast cancer: report of a prospective trial. *Int J Radiat Oncol Biol Phys* 1992;24:301.

86. Grond S, Zech D, Diefenbach C, et al. Assessment of cancer pain: a prospective evaluation in 2266 cancer pain patients referred to a pain service. *Pain* 1996;64:107.

87. Patchell RA, Posner JB. Neurologic complications of systemic cancer. *Neurol Clin* 1985;3:729.

88. Gilbert MR, Grossman SA. Incidence and nature of neurologic problems in patients with solid tumors. *Am J Med* 1986;81:951.

89. Kori SH, Foley KM, Posner JB. Brachial plexus lesions in patients with cancer: 100 cases. *Neurology* 1981;31:45.

90. Jaekle KA, Young DF, Foley KM. The natural history of lumbosacral plexopathy in cancer. *Neurology* 1985;35:8.

91. Vecht CJ, Hoff AM, Kansen PJ, et al. Types and causes of pain in cancer of the head and neck. *Cancer* 1992;70:178.

92. Grond S, Zech D, Lynch J, et al. Validation of World Health Organization guidelines for pain relief in head and neck cancer. A prospective study. *Ann Otol Rhinol Laryngol* 1993;102:342.

93. Bjordal K, Kaasa S. Psychological distress in head and neck cancer patients 7–11 years after curative treatment. *Br J Cancer* 1995; 71:592.

94. Wong JK, Wood RE, McLean M. Pain preceding recurrent head and neck cancer. *J Orofac Pain* 1998;12:52.

95. Bruera E, MacDonald RN. Intractable pain in patients with advanced head and neck tumors: a possible role for local infection. *Cancer Treat Rep* 1986;70:691.

96. Patt RB, Jain S. Management of a patient with osteoradionecrosis of the mandible with nerve blocks. *J Pain Symptom Manage* 1990; 5:59.

97. Wasserstrom WR, Glass JP, Posner JB. Diagnosis and treatment of leptomeningeal metastases from solid tumor: experience with 90 patients. *Cancer* 1982;49:759.

98. Glass JP, Foley KM. Carcinomatous meningitis. In: Harris JR, Hellman S, Henderson IC, et al, eds. *Breast diseases,* 2nd ed. Philadelphia, PA: Lippincott, 1987:700.

99. Elliot K, Foley KM. Neurologic pain syndromes in patients with cancer. *Crit Care Clin* 1990;6:393.

100. Zimm S, Wampler GL, Stablein D, et al. Intracerebral metastases in solid tumor patients: Natural history and results of treatment. *Cancer* 1981;48:384.

101. Gutin PH. Corticosteroid therapy in patients with brain tumors. *Natl Cancer Inst Monograph* 1977; 46:151–156.

102. Armstrong TS, Gilbert MR. Metastatic brain tumors: diagnosis, treatment, and nursing interventions. *Clin J Oncol Nurs.* 2000;4: 217–225.

103. Nakagawa K, Tago M, Terahara A, et al. A single institutional outcome analysis of Gamma Knife radiosurgery for single or multiple brain metastases. *Clin Neurol Neurosurg* 2001;102(1):227–232.

104. Hoskin PJ. Radiotherapy in the management of bone pain. *Clin Orthop* 1995;312:105.

105. Salazar OM, Da Motta NW, Bridgman SM, et al. Fractionated half-body irradiation for pain palliation in widely metastatic cancers: comparison with single dose. *Int J Radiation Oncology Biol Phys* 1996;36:49.

106. Needham PR, Mithal NP, Hoskin PJ. Radiotherapy for bone pain. *J R Soc Med* 1994;87:503.

107. Baziotis N, Yakoumakis E, Zissimopoulos A, et al. Strontium-89 chloride in the treatment of bone metastases from breast cancer. *Oncology* 1998;55:377.

108. Serafini AN, Houston SJ, Resche I, et al. Palliation of pain associated with metastatic bone cancer using samarium-153 lexidronam: a double-blind placebo-controlled clinical trial. *J Clin Oncol* 1998; 16:1574.

109. Mellette SJ. Management of malignant disease metastatic to the bone by hormonal alterations. *Clin Ortho* 1970;73:73.

110. Takeda F, Uki J, Fuse Y, et al. The pituitary as a target of antalgic treatment of chronic cancer pain: a possible mechanism of pain relief through pituitary neuroadenolysis. *Neurol Res* 1986;8:194–200.

111. Estes NC, Morphis JG, Hornback NB, et al. Intraarterial chemotherapy and hyperthermia for for pain control in patients with recurrent rectal cancer. *Am J Surg* 1986;152:597.

112. Petrovich Z, Langholz B, Gibbs FA, et al Regional hyperthermia for advanced tumors: a clinical study of 353 patients. *Int J Radiat Oncol Biol Phys* 1989;16:601–607.

113. Price P, Hoskin PJ, Easton D, et al. Prospective randomized trial of single and multifraction radiotherapy schedules in the treatment of painful bone metastasis. *Clin Oncol* 1989;1:56.

114. Cleeland CS. Documenting barriers to cancer pain management. In: Chapman CR, Foley KM, eds. *Current and emerging issues in cancer pain: research and practice.* New York: Raven Press, 1993:321.

115. Hill CS. Oral opioid analgesics. InL Patt RB, ed. *Cancer pain.* Philadelphia, PA: Lippincott, 1993:129.

116. Portenoy RK. Inadequate outcome of opioid therapy for cancer pain: influences on practitioners and patients. In: Patt RB, ed. *Cancer pain.* Philadelphia, PA: Lippincott, 1993:119.

117. Hill CS, Jr.. Relationship among cultural, educational, and regulatory agency influences on optimum cancer pain treatment. *J Pain Symptom Manage* 1990;5(Suppl):S37.

118. Joranson DE, Gilson AM. Regulatory barriers to pain management. *Semin Oncol Nurs* 1998;14:158–163.

119. Ventafridda V, De Conno FD. Status of cancer pain and palliative care worldwide. *J Pain Symptom Manage* 1996;12:79.

120. Coyle N, Adelhardt J, Foley KM, et al. Character of terminal illness in the advanced cancer patient: pain and other symptoms during the last four weeks of life. *J Pain Symptom Manage* 1990;5:83.

121. Mercadante S, Maddaloni S, Roccella S, Salvaggio L. Predictive factors in advanced cancer pain treated only by analgesics. *Pain* 1992;50:151–155.

122. Eisenberg E, Berkey CS, Carr DB, et al. Efficacy and safety of nonsteroidal anti-inflammatory drugs for cancer pain: a meta-analysis. *J Clin Oncol* 1994;12:2756–2765.

123. Valentini M, Cannizzaro R, Poletti M, et al. Nonsteroidal antiinflammatory drugs for cancer pain: comparison between misoprostol and ranitidine in prevention of upper gastrointestinal damage. *J Clin Oncol* 1995;13:2637.

124. Rothwell KG. Efficacy and safety of a non-acetylated salicylate, choline magnesium trisalicylate in the treatment of rheumatoid arthritis. *J Int Med Res* 1983;11:343.

125. Johnson JR, Miller AJ. The efficacy of choline magnesium trisalicylate (CMT) in the management of metastatic bone pain: a pilot study. *Palliat Med* 1994;8:129–135.

126. Buckley MMT, Brogden RN. Ketorolac: a review of its pharmacodynamic and pharmacokinetic properties and therapeutic potential. *Drugs* 1990;39:86.

127. Everts B, Wahrborg P, Hedner T. COX-2-Specific inhibitors—the emergence of a new class of analgesic and anti-inflammatory drugs. *Clin Rheumatol* 2000;19:331–343.

128. Jackson LM, Hawkey CJ. COX-2 selective nonsteroidal anti-inflammatory drugs: do they really offer any advantages? *Drugs* 2000;59:1207–1216.

129. Dhaliwal HS, Sloan P, Arkinstall WW, et al. Randomized evaluation of controlled-release codeine and placebo in chronic cancer pain. *J Pain Symptom Manage* 1995;10:612.

130. Kalso E, Vainio A. Morphine and oxycodone hydrochloride in the management of cancer pain. *Clin Pharm and Ther* 1990;47:639.

131. Glare PA, Walsh TD. Dose-ranging study of oxycodone for chronic pain in advanced cancer. *J Clin Oncol* 1993;11:973.

132. Li Wan Po A, Zhang WY. Systematic overview of co-proxamol to assess analgesic effects of addition of dextropropoxyphene to paracetamol. *Br Med J* 1997;315:1565.

133. Ebert B, Andersen S, Hjeds H, Dickenson AH Dextropropoxyphene acts as a noncompetitive N-methyl-D-aspartate antagonist. *J Pain Symptom Manage* 1998;15:269–274.

134. Minotti V, De Angelis V, Righetti E, et al. Double-blind evaluation of short-term analgesic efficacy of orally administered diclofenac, diclofenac plus codeine, and diclofenac plus imipramine in chronic cancer pain. *Pain* 1998;74:133.

135. Heiskanen T, Kalso E. Controlled-release oxycodone and morphine in cancer related pain. *Pain* 1997;73:37.

136. Hopkinson JH III. Vicodin: a new analgesic: clinical evaluation of efficacy and safety of repeated doses. *Curr Ther Res* 1978;24:633.

137. Portenoy RK, Foley KM, Stulman J, et al. Plasma morphine and morphine-6-glucuronide during chronic morphine therapy for cancer pain: plasma profiles, steady-state concentrations and the consequences of renal failure. *Pain* 1991;47:13.

138. Portenoy RK, Thaler HT, Inturrisi CE, et al. The metabolite morphine-6-glucuronide contributes to the analgesia produced by morphine infusion in patients with pain and normal renal function. *Clin Pharmacol Ther* 1992;51:422.

139. Warfield CA. Controlled-release morphine tablets in patients with chronic cancer pain: a narrative review of controlled clinical trials. *Cancer* 1998;82:2299.

140. Broomhead A, Kerr R, Tester W, et al. Comparison of a once-a-day sustained-release morphine formulation with standard oral morphine treatment for cancer pain. *J Pain Symptom Manage* 1997;14:63.

141. Bruera E, Fainsinger R, Spachynski K, et al. Clinical efficacy and safety of a novel controlled-release morphine suppository and subcutaneous morphine in cancer pain: a randomized evaluation. *J Clin Oncol* 1995;13:1520.

142. Ettinger DS, Vitale PJ, Trump DL. Important clinical pharmacologic considerations in the use of methadone in cancer patients. *Cancer Treat Rep* 1979;63:457.

143. Ripamonti C, De Conno F, Groff L, et al. Equianalgesic dose/ratio between methadone and other opioid agonists in cancer pain: comparison of two clinical experiences. *Ann Oncol* 1998;9:79.

144. Lawlor PG, Turner KS, Hanson J, et al. Dose ratio between morphine and methadone in patients with cancer pain: a retrospective study. *Cancer* 1998;82:1167.

145. Dixon R. Pharmacokinetics of levorphanol. *Adv Pain Res Ther* 1986;8:217.

146. Paalzow LK. Pharmacokinetic aspects of optimal pain treatment. *Acta Anaesthesiol Scand* 1982;74(Suppl):37.

147. Ferrell BR, Dean G. The meaning of cancer pain. *Semin Oncol Nurs* 1995;11:17.

148. Ersek M, Ferrell BR. Providing relief from cancer pain by assisting in the search for meaning. *J Palliat Care* 1994;10:15.

149. Sloan PA, Moulin DE, Hays H. A clinical evaluation of transdermal therapeutic system fentanyl for the treatment of cancer pain. *J Pain Symptom Manage* 1998;16:102.

150. Jeal W, Benfield P. Transdermal fentanyl. A review of its pharmacological properties and therapeutic efficacy in pain control. *Drugs* 1997;53:109.

151. Rogers AG. How to manage incident pain. *J Pain Symptom Manage* 1987;2:99.

152. Farrar JT, Cleary J, Rauck R, et al. Oral transmucosal fentanyl citrate: randomized, double-blinded, placebo-controlled trial for treatment of breakthrough pain in cancer patients. *J Natl Cancer Inst* 1998;90:611.

153. Christie JM, Simmonds M, Patt R, et al. Dose titration, multicenter study of oral transmucosal fentanyl citrate for the treatment of breakthrough pain in cancer patients using transdermal fentanyl for persistent pain. *J Clin Oncol* 1998;16:2238.

154. McQuay HJ. Pharmacological treatment of neuralgic and neuropathic pain. *Cancer Surv* 1988;7:141.

155. Galer BS, Coyle N, Pasternak GW, et al. Individual variability in the response to different opioids: report of five cases. *Pain* 1992;49:87.

156. Kaiko RF, Wallenstein SL, Rogers AG, et al. Sources of variation in analgesic responses in cancer patients with chronic pain receiving morphine. *Pain* 1983;15:191.

157. Ellison NM. Opioid analgesics: toxicities and their treatment. In: Patt RB, ed. *Cancer pain*. Philadelphia, PA: Lippincott, 1993:185.

158. Cameron JC. Constipation related to narcotic therapy. A protocol for nurses and patients. *Cancer Nurs* 1992;15:372.

159. Glare P, Lickiss JN. Unrecognized constipation in patients with advanced cancer: a recipe for therapeutic disaster. *J Pain Symptom Manage* 1992;7:369.

160. Sykes NP. An investigation of the ability of oral naloxone to correct opioid-related constipation in patients with advanced cancer. *Palliat Med* 1996;10:135–144.

161. Latasch L, Zimmermann M, Eberhardt B, Jurna I. Treament of morphine-induced constipation with oral naloxone. *Anaesthesist* 1997;46:191–194.

162. Baines M. Nausea and vomiting in the patient with advanced cancer. *J Pain Symptom Manage* 1988;3:81.

163. Frytak S, Moertel CG. Management of nausea and vomiting in the cancer patient. *JAMA* 1981;245:393.

164. Bruera E, Seifert L, Watanabe S, et al. Chronic nausea in advanced cancer patients: a retrospective assessment of a metoclopramide-based antiemetic regimen. *J Pain Symptom Manage* 1996;11:147.

165. Ferris FD, Kerr IG, Sone M, et al. Transdermal scopolamine use in the control of narcotic-induced nausea. *J Pain Symptom Manage* 1991;6:389.

166. Cubeddu LX, Pendergrass K, Ryan T, et al. Efficacy of oral ondansetron, a selective antagonist of 5-HT3 receptors, in the treatment of nausea and vomiting associated with cyclophosphamide-based chemotherapies. Ondansetron Study Group. *Am J Clin Oncol* 1994;17:137.

167. Beal JE, Olson R, Laubenstein L, et al. Dronabinol as a treatment for anorexia associated with weight loss in patients with AIDS. *J Pain Symptom Manage* 1995;10:89–97.

168. Gilbert CJ, Ohly KV, Rosner G, Peters WP. Randomized, double-blind comparison of a prochlorperazine-based versus a metoclopramide-based antiemetic regimen in patients undergoing autologous bone marrow transplantation. *Cancer* 1995;76:2330–2337.

169. Calhoun SR, Galloway GP, Smith DE. Abuse potential of dronabinol (Marinol). *J Psychoactive Drugs* 1998;30:187–196.

170. Bruera E, Chadwick S, Brenneis C, et al. Methylphenidate associated with narcotics for the treatment of cancer pain. *Cancer Treat Rep* 1987;71:67.

171. Bruera E, Miller MJ, Macmillan K, Kuehn N. Neuropsychological effects of methylphenidate in patients receiving a continuous infusion of narcotics for cancer pain. *Pain* 1992;48:163–166.

172. Forrest WH Jr, Brown BM Jr, Brown CR. Dextroamphetamine with morphine for the treatment of postoperative pain. *N Engl J Med* 1977;13:712.

173. Zenz M, Strumpf M, Tryba M. Long-term oral opioid therapy in patients with chronic nonmalignant pain. *J Pain Symptom Manage* 1992;7:69.

174. Bryson HM, Wilde MI. Amitriptyline. A review of its pharmacological properties and therapeutic use in chronic pain states. *Drugs Aging* 1996;8:459.

175. Portenoy RK. Opioid therapy for chronic nonmalignant pain: a review of the critical issues. *J Pain Symptom Manage* 1996;11:203.

176. Porter J, Jick H. Addiction rare in patients treated with narcotics. *N Engl J Med* 1980;302:123.

177. Moulin DE, Kreeft JH, Murray-Parsons N, Bouquillon AI. Comparison of continuous subcutaneous and intravenous hydromorphone infusions for management of cancer pain. *Lancet* 1991; 337:465–468.

178. Sloan PA, Moulin DE, Hays H. A clinical evaluation of transdermal therapeutic system fentanyl for the treatment of cancer pain. *J Pain Symptom Manage* 1998;16:102.

179. Jeal W, Benfield P. Transdermal fentanyl. A review of its pharmacological properties and therapeutic efficacy in pain control. *Drugs* 1997;53:109.

180. Korte W, de Stoutz N, Morant R. Day-to-day titration to initiate transdermal fentanyl in patients with cancer pain: short- and long-term experiences in a prospective study of 39 patients. *J Pain Symptom Manage* 1996;11:139–146.

181. Ahmedzai S, Brooks D. Transdermal fentanyl versus sustained-release oral morphine in cancer pain: preference, efficacy, and quality of life. The TTS-Fentanyl Comparative Trial Group. *J Pain Symptom Manage* 1997;13:254–261.

182. Portenoy RK, Southam MA, Gupta SK, et al. Transdermal fentanyl for cancer pain. Repeated dose pharmacokinetics. *Anesthesiol* 1993;78:36.

183. Rose PG, Macfee MS, Boswell MV. Fentanyl transdermal system overdose secondary to cutaneous hyperthermia. *Anesth Analg* 1993;77:390.

184. Cole L, Hanning CD. Review of the rectal use of opioids. *J Pain Symptom Manage* 1990;5:118.

185. De Conno F, Ripamonti C, Saita L, et al. Role of rectal route in treating cancer pain: a randomized crossover clinical trial of oral versus rectal morphine administration in opioid-naive cancer patients with pain. *J Clin Oncol* 1995;13:1004.

186. Ripamonti C, Zecca E, Brunelli C, et al. Rectal methadone in cancer patients with pain. A preliminary clinical and pharmacokinetic study. *Ann Oncol* 1995;6:841.

187. Bruera E, Ripamonti C. Alternate routes of administration of narcotics. In: Patt RB, ed. *Cancer pain*. Philadelphia, PA: Lippincott, 1993:16.

188. Stevens RA, Ghazi SM. Routes of opioid analgesic therapy in the management of cancer pain. *Cancer Control* 2000;1:132–141.

189. Nelson KA, Glare PA, Walsh D, et al. A prospective, within-patient, crossover study of continuous intravenous and subcutaneous morphine for chronic cancer pain. *J Pain Symptom Manage* 1997;13:262.

190. Bruera E, MacEachern T, MacMillan K, et al. Local tolerance to subcutaneous infusions of high concentrations of hydromorphone: a prospective study. *J Pain Symptom Manage* 1993;8:201.

191. Nahata MC, Miser AW, Miser JS, et al. Analgesic plasma concentrations of morphine in children with terminal malignancy receiving a continuous subcutaneous infusion of morphine sulfate to control severe pain. *Pain* 1987;18:109.

192. Reference deleted in text.

193. Mercadante S, Lodi F, Sapio M, et al. Long-term ketamine subcutaneous continuous infusion in neuropathic cancer pain. *J Pain Symptom Manage* 1995;10:564.

194. Devulder JE, Ghys L, Dhondt W, et al. Neuropathic pain in a cancer patient responding to subcutaneously administered lignocaine. *Clin J Pain* 1993;9:220.

195. Lesser GJ, Grossman SA, Leong KW, et al. In vitro and in vivo studies of subcutaneous hydromorphone implants designed for the treatment of cancer pain. *Pain* 1996;65:265.

196. Kaiko RF, Foley KM, Grabinski PY, et al. Central nervous system excitatory effects of meperidine in cancer patients. *Ann Neurol* 1983; 13:180.

197. Szeto HH, Inturrusi CE, Houde R, et al. Accumulation of normeperidine, an active metabolite of meperidine, in patients with renal failure or cancer. *Ann Int Med* 1977;86:738.

198. Bono AV, Cuffari S. Effectiveness and tolerance of tramadol in cancer pain. A comparative study with respect to buprenorphine. *Drugs* 1997;53(Suppl 2):40.

199. Twycross RG. The brompton cocktail. *Adv Pain Res Ther* 1979; 2:291.

200. Twycross RG. The measurement of pain in terminal carcinoma. *J Int Med Res* 1976;4:58.

201. Byas-Smith MG, Max MB, Muir J, et al. Transdermal clonidine compared to placebo in painful diabetic neuropathy using a two-stage 'enriched enrollment' design. *Pain* 1995;60:267.

202. Kishore-Kumar R, Max MB, Schafer SC, et al. Desipramine relieves post-herpetic neuralgia. *Clin Pharmacol Ther* 1990;47:305–372.

203. Panerai AE, Monza G, Mouilia P et al. A randomized, within-patient, crossover, placebo-controlled trial on the efficacy and tolerability of the tricyclic antidepressants chlorimipramine and nortriptyline in central pain. *Acta Neurol Scand* 1990;82:(Suppl)34–38.

204. Sindrup SH, Gram LF, Skjold T, et al. Clomipramine vs desipramine vs placebo in the treatment of diabetic neuropathy symptoms. A double-blind cross-over study. *Br J Clin Pharmac* 1990; 30:683–691.

205. Eija K, Tiina T, Pertti NJ. Amitriptyline effectively relieves neuropathic pain following treatment of breast cancer. *Pain* 1996;64:293.

206. Holland JC, Romano SJ, Heiligenstein JH, et al. A controlled trial of fluoxetinendesipramine in depressed women with advanced cancer. *Psychooncol* 1998;7:291.

207. Reference deleted in text.

208. Zylicz Z, Smits C, Krajnik M. Paroxetine for pruritus in advanced cancer. *J Pain Symptom Manage* 1998;16:121.

209. Sweet WH. Treatment of trigeminal neuralgia (tic douloureux). *N Engl Jed* 1986;315:174.

210. McQuay H, Carroll D, Jadad AR, et al. Anticonvulsant drugs for management of pain: a systematic review. *Br Med J* 1995;311:1047.

211. Yajnik S, Singh GP, Singh G, et al. Kumar M: Phenytoin as a coanalgesic in cancerain. *J Pain Symptom Manage* 1992;7:209.

212. Chang VT. Intravenous phenytoin in the management of crescendo pelvic cancer- related pain. *J Pain Symptom Manage* 1997;13:238.

213. Rosner H, Rubin L. Gabapentin adjunctive therapy in neuropathic pain states. *Clin J Pain* 1996;12:56.

214. Rho JM, Donevan SD, Rogawski MA. Mechanisms of the anticonvulsant felbamate: opposing effects on N-methyl-D-aspartate and gamma aminobutyric acid-A receptors. *Ann Neurol* 1994;35:229.

215. Ordia JI, Fischer E, Adamski E, et al. Chronic intrathecal delivery of baclofen by programmable pump for the treatment of severe spasticity. *J Neurosurg* 1996;85:452.

216. Dejgard A, Petersen P, Kastrup J. Mexiletine for treatment of chronic painful diabetic neuropathy. *Lancet* 1988;9.

217. Lindstrom P, Lindblom U. The analgesic effect of tocainide in trigeminal neuralgia. *Pain* 1987;28:45.

218. Bruera E, Miller MJ, MacMillan K, et al. Neuropsychological effects of methylphenidate in patients receiving a continuous infusion of narcotics for cancer pain. *Pain* 1992;48:163.

219. Yee JD, Berde CB. Dextroamphetamine or methylphenidate as adjuvants topioidnalgesia for adolescents with cancer. *J Pain Symptom Manage* 1994;9:122.

220. Wilwerding MB, Loprinzi CL, Mailliard JA, et al. A randomized, crossover evaluation of methylphenidate in cancer patients receiving strong narcotics. *Support Care Cancer* 1995;3:135.

221. Watanabe S, Bruera E. Corticosteroids as adjuvant analgesics. *J Pain Symptom Manage* 1994;9:442.

222. Twycross R. The risks and benefits of corticosteroids in advanced cancer. *Drug Saf* 1994;11:163.

223. Bruera E, Roca E, Cedaro L, et al. Action of oral methylprednisolone in terminal cancer patients: A prospective randomized double-blind study. *Cancer Treat Rep* 1985;69:751.

224. Pud D, Eisenberg E, Spitzer A, et al. The NMDA receptor antagonist amantadine reduces surgical neuropathic pain in cancer patients: a double blind, randomized, placebo controlled trial. *Pain* 1998;75:349.

225. Mercadante S. Ketamine in cancer pain: an update. *Palliat Med* 1996;10:225.
226. Yang CY, Wong CS, Chang JY, et al. Intrathecal ketamine reduces morphine requirements in patients with terminal cancer pain. *Can J Anaesth* 1996;43:379.
227. Eisenach JC, DuPen S, Dubois M, et al. Epidural clonidine analgesia for intractableancer pain. *Pain* 1995;61:391.
228. Harvey HA, Lipton A. The role of bisphosphonates in the treatment of bone metastases—the U.S. experience. *Support Care Cancer* 1996;4:213.
229. Diener KM. Bisphosphonates for controlling pain from metastatic bone disease. *Am J Health Syst Pharm* 1996;53:1917.
230. Pelger RC, Hamdy NA, Zwinderman AH, et al. Effects of the bisphosphonate olpadronate in patients with carcinoma of the prostate metastatic to the skeleton. *Bone* 1998;22:403.
231. Patt RB, Reddy S. The benzodiazepines as adjuvant analgesics. *J Pain Symptom Manage* 1994;9:510.
232. Patt RB, Proper G, Reddy S. The neuroleptics as adjuvant analgesics. *J Pain Symptom Manage* 1994;9:446.
233. Lasagna L, DeKornfeld TJ. Methotrimeprazine: a new phenothiazine derivative with analgesic properties. *JAMA* 1961;178:887–890.
234. Patt RB, Cousins MJ. Neurolytic blockade techniques for chronic and cancer pain. In: Cousins MJ, Bridenbaugh PO, eds. *Neural blockade*, 3rd ed, Philadelphia, PA: JB Lippincott, 1007–1061.
235. Cheng TM, Cascino TL, Onofrio BM. Comprehensive study of diagnosis and treatment of trigeminal neuralgia secondary to tumors. *Neurology* 1993;43:2298–2302.
236. Ramamurhty S, Walsh NE, Schoenfeld LS, Hoffman J. Evaluation of neurolytic blocks using phenol and cryogenic block in the management of chronic pain. *Pain Symptom Manage* 1989;4:72–75.
237. Moore D, Bridenbaugh DL. Intercostal nerve block in 4333 patients: Indications, techniques, complications. *Anesth Analg* 1962;41:1.
238. Young RF, Vermeulen SS, Grimm P, et al. Gamma Knife radiosurgery for treatment of trigeminal neuralgia: idiopathic and tumor related. *Neurology* 1997;48:608–614.
239. Eisenberg E, Carr, DB, Chalmers TC. Neurolytic celiac plexus block for treatment of cancer pain: a meta-analysis. *Anesth Analg* 1995;80:290–295.
240. Olak J, Gore D. Thoracoscopic splanchnicectomy: technique and case report. *Surg Laparoscop Endosc* 1996;6:228–230.
241. Mercadante S. Celiac plexus block versus analgesics in pancreatic cancer pain. *Pain* 1993;52:187–192.
242. Kawamata M, Ishitani K, Ishikawa K, et al. Comparison between celiac plexus block and morphine treatment on quality of life in patients with pancreatic cancer pain. *Pain* 1996;64:597–602.
243. Lillemoe KD, Cameron JL, Kaufman HS, et al. Chemical splanchnicectomy in patients with unresectable pancreatic cancer. *Annals of Surgery* 1993;217:447–457.
244. Plancarte R, Amescua C, Patt R, Aldrete A. Superior hypogastric plexus block for pelvic cancer pain. *Anesthesiology* 1990;73:236.
245. Patt RB, Reddy S. Spinal neurolysis for cancer pain: indications and recent results. *Annals Academy Medicine Singapore* 1994;23:216–220.
246. Melzack R. Gate control theory: on the evolution of pain concepts. *Pain Forum* 1996;5:128–138.
247. Abrams SE. The role of non-neurolytic blocks in the management of cancer pain. In: Abrams SE, ed. *Cancer pain*. Boston: Kluwer Academic, 1989:67–75.
248. Ventafridda V, Sganzerla EP, Fochi C, et al. Transcutaneous nerve stimulation in cancer pain. *Adv Pain Res Ther* 1979;2:509–515.
249. Loeser JD. Dorsal column and peripheral nerve stimulation for relief of cancer pain. *Adv Pain Res Ther* 1979;2:499–507.
250. Young RF, Brechner T. Electrical stimulation of the brain for relief of intractable pain due to cancer. *Cancer* 1986;57:1266–1272.
251. Akil H, Richardson DE, Hughes J, et al. Elevations in levels of enkephalin-like materials in the ventricular CSF of pain patients upon analgetic focal stimulation. *Science* 1979;201:463–465.
252. Hosobuchi Y. Subcortical electrical stimulation control of intractable pain. Report of 122 cases. *J Neurosurg* 1986;64:543–553.
253. Cohen MH, Johnston-Anderson A, Krasnow SH, Wadleigh RG. Continuous intravenous narcotic infusions for cancer pain. *Cancer Invest* 1993;11:169–173.
254. Coyle N, Cherny NI, Portenoy RK. Subcutaneous opioid infusions at home. *Oncology* 1994;8:21–27.
255. Christie JM, Simmonds M, Patt R, et al. Dose titration, multicenter study of oral transmucosal fentanyl citrate for the treatment of breakthrough pain in cancer patients using transdermal fentanyl for persistent pain. *J Clinical Oncology* 1998;16:2238–2246.
256. Du Pen SL, Williams AR. Management of patients receiving combined epidural morphine and bupivacaine for the treatment of cancer pain. *J Pain Symptom Manage* 1992;7:125–127.
257. DuPen SL, Williams AR. Spinal and peripheral drug-delivery systems. *Pain Digest* 1995;5:307–317.
258. Hassenbusch SJ, Paice JA, Patt RB, et al. Clinical realities and economic considerations: economics of intrathecal therapy *J Pain Symptom Manage* 1997;14:S36–S48.
259. Eisenach JC, DuPen S, Dubois M, et al. Epidural clonidine analgesia for intractable cancer pain: The Epidural Clonidine Study Group. *Pain* June 1995;61:391–399.
260. Malinovsky JM, Cozian A, Lepage JY, Mussini JM, Pinaud M, Souron R. Ketamine and midazolam neurotoxicity in the rabbit. *Anesthesiology* 1991;75:91–97.

CHAPTER 41

Management of Cancer Pain Utilizing Radiation Therapy

Tony Y. Eng, Charles R. Thomas, Jr. and Richard H. Fitzgerald, Jr.

Management of cancer pain is one of the major challenges in the clinical practice of oncology. Approximately 30% of all cancer patients and as many as 70% to 90% of those with advanced cancer will experience some pain in the course of their disease (1–3). Radiation therapy is one of the most common and effective treatments in cancer pain control. There are now few communities without access, yet, it is often forgotten or left as a last resort. The majority of patients will experience an improvement in symptoms after appropriate irradiation. This is in large part independent of the histology of the malignancy being treated (4–7). There are still many who fear radiation treatment because of ignorance of its capability. Radiation therapy is an integral part of the cancer management team. Radiation therapy does cure many cancers. Where cure is not possible, radiation can reduce or stabilize a malignancy, stop active bleeding, lessen obstruction, restore luminal patency, preserve skeletal or organ integrity, and relieve cancer pain or other cancer-related symptoms. The goal of radiation therapy palliation is to improve the quality of life by reducing pain and suffering during whatever period of life remains.

Scope of the Problem

The American Cancer Society estimates project that over 10 million Americans alive today have a history of cancer. More than one million new invasive cancer cases will be diagnosed in the year 2000, and one half million will die of malignancy (8). Many of those with advanced disease require some forms of palliative therapy for comfort. A reasonable approximation for health-care economic planning is that 50% of cancer patients will receive radiation treatment at some time during their illness, either alone or in combination with surgery, chemotherapy, or other bio-

logic therapies. Cancers have a high propensity to metastasize to bone. Bone metastases can be quite painful and are addressed by analgesics, orthotics, and irradiation. Palliative radiation therapy is often underused and may be withheld except as a "last resort" (9). Because people do not understand that radiation therapy palliates and often completely relieves cancer-related pain and discomforting symptoms, appropriate referral may be delayed or omitted. Some treatises on cancer pain address radiation therapy only to accentuate the very uncommon and even rare neurologic complications (10). This is regrettable because radiation palliation is often very long-lasting and contributes to the comfort of hundreds of thousands of patients each year (11). There is no nonpharmacologic technique, technology, or agent that benefits the pain management of as many patients with malignancy as does radiation therapy. This chapter is intended for clinicians and other health professionals who interact with cancer patients in the hope of imparting a better understanding of the value of palliative radiation therapy in cancer pain management.

BRIEF PATHOPHYSIOLOGY OF CANCER PAIN

Cancer pain most often is due to tumor infiltration of local structures. It may also be referred or related to cancer therapy (12). Knowledge of the causes of cancer pain is essential to a proper pain evaluation and assessment that subsequently lead to optimal pain management. Cancer pain can be categorized as somatic, visceral, or neuropathic, which differ in causation, symptoms, characteristics, and response to palliative radiation therapy and analgesics (13,14). Psychogenic pain is also important in the overall impairment and quality of life and requires skill in appreciation and management. It is beyond the scope of this chapter. In general, somatic pain, e.g., bone pain and neuropathic pain caused by nerve compression or infiltration, can be more effectively diminished by irradiation; visceral pain is better managed by pharmacologic and interventional anesthesia techniques (13,15). However, it may be difficult to determine the relative contributions of the somatic and visceral systems to a particular patient's pain because of associated autonomic components (16).

Somatic Cancer Pain

Somatic cancer pain is due to direct tumor invasion or impingement of pain-sensitive structures, including bone, joint, muscle, or connective tissue. The invasion process induces an inflammatory response and stimulates local production of chemical mediators, such as prostaglandin, bradykinin, and cellular release of potassium. These, along with mechanical stimulation by the tumor mass, can sensitize and activate the nociceptor, a pain receptor located at the terminal peripheral branches of sensory nerve fibers and sensitive to noxious stimuli (13). Bone pain is the most prevalent cancer-induced somatic pain, either due to direct tumor invasion, nerve compression, or local release of algesic substances (e.g., substance P) from the bone marrow (17). The periosteum contains a high concentration of nociceptive afferents, which become distorted and stretched by the increasing intraosseal pressure. Local pain of varying intensity develops and is exacerbated by movement or weight bearing.

Visceral Cancer Pain

Visceral organs, such as lung, liver, and kidney, have sensory afferents that project to the spinal cord along sympathetic fibers. Visceral pain can arise from direct stimulation of these afferent fibers due to secondary distention or actual infiltration of organs or their covering capsule or adjacent structures. Visceral pain tends to be diffuse and poorly localized. It may be referred to a remote dermatome, making the source of pain difficult to elucidate. For example, pancreatic malignancy may be associated with referred pain to the shoulder or upper back. Liver metastases, capsular distention by the liver masses, biliary obstruction, bowel or ureteral obstruction, and soft tissue distention from an expanding tumor are other examples of visceral pain. Anesthetizing the appropriate sympathetic fiber or ganglia may ameliorate visceral pain. For example, epigastric and upper abdominal visceral pain may sometimes be relieved by local anesthetic blockade of the sympathetic and accompanying visceral afferent fibers at the celiac plexus or splanchnic nerves, whereas visceral pain originating from the lower abdomen and pelvic organs may sometimes be successfully relieved by neurolytic block at the superior hypogastric plexus (13). This does not address the cause of the pain but may relieve symptoms.

Neuropathic Cancer Pain

Neuropathic (or neurogenic) pain occurs when a peripheral nerve or nerve plexus is injured or impinged upon by cancer. Damage to the dorsal root ganglia, dorsal roots, spinal cord, brainstem, thalamus, or cerebral cortex may cause central neuropathic pain. A sharp, stabbing, burning, or shooting pain, often associated with alteration in sensation, such as hyperalgesia or paresthesia, is experienced. As with visceral pain, neuropathic pain sometimes has a sympathetic component associated, such as CRPS-II (causalgia) and CRPS-I (reflex sympathetic dystrophy) (16).

ASSESSMENT OF CANCER PAIN

Patient Assessment

Proper management of cancer pain requires a comprehensive and accurate assessment of its pathogenesis and the effect on the individual patient's quality of life and a knowledge of analgesic pharmacology, orthotics, chemotherapy and hormonal efficacy, the impact of comorbid conditions, and, at times, economics. A recent Radiation Therapy Oncology Group (RTOG) survey concluded that an adequate pain assessment remains a barrier to effective cancer pain management. Seventy-seven percent of physicians rated poor pain assessment as a major barrier to good pain management (18). Pain can be assessed objectively or subjectively. The proper assessment of pain involves performing a detailed history and physical examination to formulate the characteristics and etiology of the pain. The location, pattern of radiation, character, intensity, correlated factors, timing, and duration of prior or current therapies all may provide valuable insight (19) and help to predict the analgesic efficacy of any intervention, including irradiation (20). The patient's description of pain is important. Pain described as hot or burning or scalding or paroxysmal or shocklike predicts the presence of neuropathic pain (21). Pain described as constant, aching, or gnawing may suggest somatic pain, which may be well localized. Visceral pain is frequently a more diffuse aching and may be accompanied by nausea (22). Laboratory data and appropriate imaging studies are crucial in evaluating and planning a therapeutic approach. Subjective pain rating is a useful measure of a patient's pain and may be employed to help in the selection of therapy and monitoring of its results. Some of the commonly used assessment tools are the Wisconsin Brief Pain Inventory (23), Memorial Pain Assessment Card (24), and the Hopkins Pain Rating Index (25). Because cancer patients may have other symptoms, multisymptom scales, such as the Anderson Symptom Inventory, can be used (26). These assessment tools use a numerical scale to record patient descriptions to attempt some precision and consistency. The reproducibility of these scales allows a more accurate assessment of the patient's perception of pain. Recent attempts to employ technology and allow for a relaxed, patient-friendly system are evaluating pain assessment using a software program at bedside on a laptop computer (27).

Radiographic Assessment

X-rays

Plain radiographs are extremely useful in detailing bony metastases and impending pathologic fractures. Conventional radiographs are most cost effective and readily available in all cancer treatment facilities. They may be obtained and interpreted quickly. Their noninvasive nature and short exposure times make them acceptable and practical to most patients. To be recognized as abnormal, changes in density and trabecular bone pattern need to be recognized. Most bone metastases exhibit osteolytic change, which may be described as a moth eaten or diffusely infiltrated or expansile pattern. Fracture through a bone defect caused by malignancy is called a pathologic fracture. The risk of pathologic fracture is correlated with the degree of cortical bone destruction (28). When there is cortical bone loss exceeding 40% to 50% in a weight-bearing bone, impending fracture is suggested, and surgery should be considered to provide stabilization prior to palliative radiation therapy. Whether surgery is done or not depends on the activity of the patient, the patient's overall condition and prognosis, and other factors associated with morbidity and economics. Osteoblastic lesions are less common. They may be seen as well circumscribed, round, or discrete, or they may be mottled with irregular areas of varying sclerosis. Some metastases manifest a "mixed" pattern, containing both lytic and blastic characteristics.

Bone Scintigraphy (Scan)

A radionuclide bone scan is a cost-effective study to survey the skeleton in symptomatic or asymptomatic patients. It will often detect metastatic lesions before they can be seen on plain radiograph. It is more sensitive than plain x-rays in identifying metastasis because it detects functional rather than structural changes, that is, the functional physiology of active bone formation. A small and localized area of increased activity can be detected by bone scan, whereas a minimum of 40% to 50% trabecular bone destruction is required for plain x-ray detection (29). Radiographs and bone scanning are often complementary studies in the evaluation of skeletal pain. An x-ray skeletal survey is more useful than bone scan in detecting an area of pure bone destruction, that is, with no area of new bone formation. Such osteolytic photopenic lesions are seen in patients with multiple myeloma and some rapidly growing solid tumors.

Computed Tomography

Computed tomography (CT) allows reconstructed images of bone and soft tissue. Defects and mass lesions not

detected by plain x-rays or scans thus are revealed. It is more expensive than plain x-rays or scans. It is more widely available than magnetic resonance imaging (MRI). CT scans can evaluate both soft tissue and bone metastasis. CT can be especially useful in evaluating equivocal lesions that may be located in the spine or other areas difficult to evaluate by conventional radiographs. The cross-sectional reconstructed images provide a good assessment of the spinal cord and spinal canal. Many thoracic and abdominal processes are imaged by CT. Discrimination of vascular images from abnormal lymph nodes or masses and visualization of urologic and gastrointestinal tissues are enhanced by intravenous contrast for opacification of the urinary tract and vascular structures and by oral contrast for clarification of gastrointestinal tract volume.

Magnetic Resonance Imaging

Magnetic resonance imaging (MRI) is more expensive than CT scanning. It requires a longer examination time, and more patients have a sense of claustrophobia because of the configuration of the imaging device. MR signals are based on magnetic relaxation times and tissue characteristics other than electron density. Normal bone marrow has a high fat content that appears bright; whereas tumors often have increased cellularity and high water content and appear darker on the same image reconstructions. MRI can image lytic bone lesions not detected by bone scan. In one prospective study, 30 patients with multiple myeloma were evaluated by a battery of studies. Abnormalities on any study were confirmed by needle aspiration biopsy. The specificity in determining malignant lesions was 67% for plain x-rays, 20% for bone scan, 37% for CT scan, and 100% for MRI scan (30). With MRI, there is excellent soft tissue contrast and multiplanar imaging capability. MRI provides good visualization of the entire spine and evaluation of the spinal cord and nerve roots. It is easier to tolerate for patients with spinal instability (31).

Laboratory Assessment

There is no serum marker that indicates the presence or absence of bone metastasis in all patients. The majority of prostate patients with bone involvement have an elevated PSA; but this is nonspecific for bone metastasis. At times, alkaline phosphatase, acid phosphatase, lactate dehydrogenase (LDH), PSA, CEA, and other tumor markers are of benefit. The knowledge of blood chemistries, especially liver and renal chemistries, may help in the anticipation of metabolism of analgesics.

PALLIATIVE RADIATION THERAPY

Historical Aspect of Radiation Therapy (32)

Empiric therapeutic use of Roentgen's x-rays evolved in parallel with clinical radiobiological experimentation.

Before the end of the nineteenth century, many observations of skin and tissue reaction were made. In the early twentieth century, radiosensitivity of tissue was found to be in close relationship with cellular proliferation as determined by a "mitotic index" of cells in active division. Later studies identified an association of sensitivity with oxygenation. Becquerel discovered radioactivity in 1898. He left a container of radium in his vest pocket and made an important observation of skin erythema several weeks thereafter. Some early experiments in "fractionation," i.e., smaller, multiple dosing, were performed in Paris in the 1920s. After irradiating ram scrota, it was observed that severe skin reactions occurred if a single dose of x-rays was given to sterilize the testes, whereas if smaller doses were given, over a longer period of time to provide the same end result of sterility, the scrotal skin was less irritated. Thus arose a concept of "therapeutic gain" by fractionation. In that example, the testes represent fast-growing tumor cells, and the skin of the scrotum represents normal, more slowly growing tissue. Later in the twentieth century, Withers proposed principles commonly called the four *R*s of radiobiology, which are *repair, reassortment, repopulation,* and *reoxygenation*. These will be discussed later. Contemporary radiobiology considers factors that include the total dose, number of fractions, fraction size, total time of exposure, total time to provide the summated dose, and other treatment parameters. Innovations allowed concentrated isotope machines and linear accelerator technology, which provided for greater accuracy and enhanced sparing of normal tissues. Advances continue today, integrated with oncologic specialties and molecular biology. We now have a better understanding of tumor biology, radiobiological principles, surgery, and medical oncology. We have more energetic treatment delivery machines that can shape treatment fields in three dimensions (conformal therapy), optimize dose distribution, calculate dose delivered to complex fields, and provide for greater homogeneity of dose in the treated volume of interest.

Basic Radiation Biology (32)

Tissue Interaction

When ionizing radiation interacts with matter, it incites ionization or excitation. Ionization is a process whereby one or more bound orbital electrons are ejected from the parent or constituent atom. Excitation requires less energy and raises the energy state of a bound orbital electron to a higher or more excited energy state. It has little or no radiobiologic significance but consumes some energy of the incident x-rays. The Compton scatter process is the most important mechanism of ionizing radiation absorption in clinical radiation therapy. It involves the ejection of a loosely bound outer orbital electron by the incident radiation. Compton scatter is independent of the atomic number of the medium or tissue in which radiation is absorbed.

Very similar energy is absorbed in soft tissue or bone. This separates contemporary radiation from that of an earlier era wherein higher density structures, most notably bone, experienced a higher energy deposition than soft tissue.

Direct and Indirect Effects

Ionization results in charged atoms or molecules, which may have direct biological effects on the stability of adjacent molecules leading to radiochemical lesions in critical cellular targets. However, indirect action mediated by highly reactive "free radicals" is believed causative for the greater proportion of cellular damage produced by radiation. Mammalian cells are mostly water, which interacts with ionizing radiation to form free radicals. These are quite short-lived and highly reactive chemically. They produce cellular damage. The critical cellular targets are thought to include deoxyribonucleic acid (DNA) residing in chromosomes or mitochondria. The direct and indirect effects of ionizing radiation lead to molecular damage, which interferes with cellular reproductive integrity, that is, cell death or the loss of ability to undergo multiple cell divisions.

Oxygen Effect

Water will form free radicals. In the presence of molecular oxygen, more free radicals are produced, resulting in greater cell damage. This is the basis for an "oxygen enhancement effect" or oxygen enhancement ratio (OER). This is the ratio of radiation required to produce a similar percentage of cell death in a hypoxic medium as opposed to that dose of radiation required in a well-oxygenated medium. This ratio is typically between 2 and 3.

There is more preferential tumor cell death in those areas with higher oxygen concentration. In tissue that has a compromised vascular supply or necrosis, the oxygenated portion of the tumor shrinks preferentially, allowing the hypoxic cells to become oxygenated again. This reoxygenation allows sensitization to subsequent doses of radiation with an improved oxygen enhancement ratio. The extent and rapidity of reoxygenation are variable. Clinical exploitation of oxygenation in human tumors has been difficult. Hemoglobin concentration has shown correlation with response in curative series.

Cell Cycle Sensitivity and Reassortment

Radiosensitivity varies during the cellular mitotic cycle. In general, cells that are actually dividing are more sensitive to radiation; more specifically, late G2 and M-phases are more radiosensitive than late S-phase. These differences appear to reflect cyclic variation in sulfhydryl (-SH) content, especially glutathione, which is known to be more prevalent in late S-phase. Sulfhydryl radicals function as free radical scavengers, which reduce the radiobiological impact of a given radiation dose.

In a general tumor cell population, after exposure to a single large dose of radiation, most survivors will be in those resistant phases of the cell cycle. Because those more sensitive will have been killed, there will be a partial synchronization of cells more resistant. These cells then reassort themselves and again become asynchronous, with a portion moving from resistant into sensitive phases of the cell cycle. A second dose of irradiation, therefore, will render cells newly recruited into the sensitive phase killed. The degree of tissue differentiation and mitotic activity can affect radiosensitivity. For most tissues, as mitotic activity increases or cellular differentiation decreases, radiosensitivity increases. This has been termed the Law of Bergonié and Tribondeau (33). A poorly differentiated tumor with a high mitotic activity is theoretically quite sensitive and will, in theory, require a lower dose of irradiation for eradication when compared to a well-differentiated tumor with a low mitotic activity.

Cell Repair and Repopulation

The extent of cellular repair of damage that is not lethal varies widely among different cells and tissues. Types of cellular repair have been categorized as sublethal damage repair (SLDR) and potentially lethal damage repair (PLDR). SLDR is observed when there are fewer cells killed following a dose of radiation given in fractions instead of a single dose. The prolonged time between fractions allows the cells to undergo SLDR, whereby enzymatic and reparative mechanisms are restored. This has been demonstrated in cell cultures, transplanted tumor systems, and normal tissue assays. PLDR occurs when more cells survive following irradiation if the postirradiated cell environment is manipulated to prevent cell division. This is a contrived and experimental observation, but it suggests that, given time, cells can repair potential lethal damage by radiation if they are not allowed to proceed directly with mitosis and subsequent division but have time and nutrients for resynthesis and repair. PLDR has been observed in cells from both normal and malignant lines in vitro. Clinically, high doses of radiation can kill growing normal and malignant cells. However, theoretically, cancer cells are growing more rapidly and lack the ability to repair radiation damage as efficiently as normal cells. They are, therefore, killed by radiation more so than normal cells are.

Basic Radiation Physics (34)

X-rays and Gamma Rays

Ionizing radiation has a higher frequency and shorter wavelength than visible light and is in the form of either gamma or x-rays. Therapeutic x-rays are generated electrically, whereas gamma rays are a product of disintegration of a nucleus of a radioactive atom. X-rays and gamma rays are physically identical and are referred to as photons.

Higher energy radiation machinery allows superficial tissues to be spared by depositing the maximal dose below the skin surface. In addition, sharper beam edges and less side scatter provide for less normal tissue reaction. Megavoltage x-ray machines, capable of producing electron beams, are replacing lower energy superficial and orthovoltage machines in the treatment of superficial malignancies. Whereas the maximum dose of a superficial or orthovoltage machine is on the surface of the skin with little tissue penetration, high energy photons in the range of 4 to 20 million electron volts are commonly used today, providing maximum dose buildup at 1.5 to 3.5 cm with a skin dose a fraction of the maximum dose.

Particulate Radiation

Particulate radiation is the use of particles that combine with matter to induce x-rays, which then interact to produce free radicals and ionization. Electron beam is the most common form of particulate radiation in use. The main advantage of electron beam is the ability to control the depth of penetration by varying the energy of the electron beam. It is ideal for treating superficial cancers while avoiding radiation to underlying normal tissues. Unlike photon beams, where the percent surface dose decreases as energy increases, with electron beam, the percent surface dose increases with higher electron beam energy. In clinical practice, treatment planning for the use of radiation takes into account air cavity, bones, and other inhomogeneities that can affect electron dose absorption.

There are other particle types that are used experimentally or in selective clinical circumstances in a few institutions. These include protons, neutrons, and negative pi-mesons. The main advantage of these types of particles is the presence of the "Bragg peak." There is a finite depth of penetration of the particle, and the biological effectiveness increases as the particle beam slows at the end of its trajectory. By using devices to modify the peak, the therapeutic ratio can be significantly improved. These particle beams require more complex and expensive equipment to accelerate them. They are very expensive and are associated with research facilities.

External Beam Radiation Therapy

The exact mechanism by which radiation relieves cancer pain is not understood. Although mechanical pressure does have a major role in the pathogenesis of cancer-related pain, relief can be achieved prior to or in the absence of shrinkage after palliative radiation therapy. It has been postulated that an inhibition of pain mediators may be responsible for the palliative effect (35). Nevertheless, palliative external beam radiation therapy is one of the most cost-effective treatments for cancer pain and has a different side-effect profile compared with narcotic analgesics (36). In the majority of cases, radiation therapy can achieve meaningful pain relief. It is estimated that 60% to 90% of patients with cancer-related bone pain may benefit from palliative radiation therapy, using low doses of radiation, in the range of 2000 to 3000 cGy to the painful site (37,38).

The process of radiation therapy involves initial consultation, which includes a history and physical examination. The recommendation for radiation therapy is discussed relative to logistical and individual concerns. The patient returns for a simulated treatment, which allows for taking measurements and definition of treatment portals and documenting radiographs using machinery of similar geometry with actual treatment machines. This process often takes 30 to 60 minutes. Treatment begins after adequate time for planning and completion of dosimetry and formulation or fabrication of delineating heavy metal blocks. Radiation therapy is typically given 5 days a week for 5 to 7 weeks if cure is intended. Palliative care may be given for a substantially shorter time, ranging from 1 to 4 weeks. Radiation therapy may be provided as external beam (teletherapy) utilizing x-ray photons or electron beam. It may be provided internally, either by pellets or needle implantation (brachytherapy), intraoperative radiation therapy (IORT), or by injection of systemic radionuclides. External beam radiation therapy itself is painless, similar to having a chest radiograph. The patient does not become radioactive or a health hazard after external beam radiation therapy.

Localized Irradiation

Local fields can adequately encompass most symptomatic lesions. Typically a margin is provided around the area of metastasis (Fig. 41-1). During simulation, a marker may sometimes be used to minimize fluoroscopic time and radiographic exposure and allow for greater simulation time efficiency. The final field size is limited by the characteristics of the metastasis, potential side effects, normal tissue tolerance, surrounding critical organs, and prior treatments. Therefore, one must recognize that, as with the use of analgesic drugs for cancer pain (39), the fundamental dictum of use of palliative irradiation is individualization without rigidity.

Energy of Irradiation

Most superficial lesions of the skin can be treated with low energy (100 to 500KVP) machines or with electron beams from linear accelerators. The need is for radiation energy to be deposited in the first few millimeters of tissue. Different energies of electrons may be selected to treat lesions at different depths. Similarly, when available, higher energy photons are chosen, which best suit the depth of interest.

Radiation Dose and Fractionation

There is no known best radiation therapy regimen established for palliation of cancer pain. Traditionally, in the

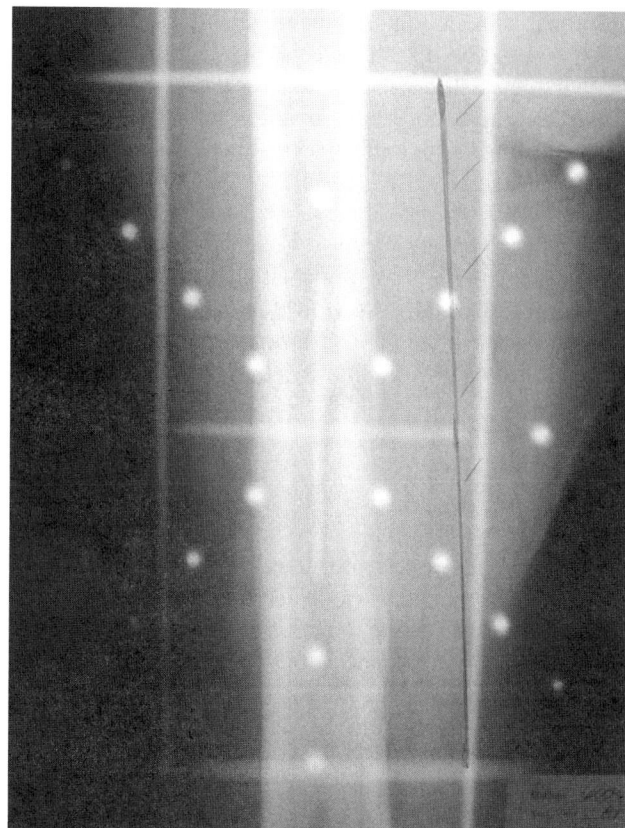

FIG. 41-1. Radiation treatment port for metastasis to the right midfemur. (Courtesy of Dr. Keith E. Eyre)

United States, the most common dose regimen has been 3000 cGy delivered in 10 daily fractions to sites of metastatic cancer, regardless of origin, unless limited by surrounding normal tissue. This 3000 cGy regimen takes approximately 2 weeks to deliver and provides a relatively durable response of 80% to 90% pain relief at a median of 4 to 6 months (38,40). In a large, multicenter RTOG study that accrued 1016 patients from 39 institutions over 6 years, there was no statistically significant relationship concluded between the total dose or fraction number and the probability of complete pain relief (38). A reanalysis of that pain study used different endpoints, including the need for retreatment and analgesics, and showed a stepwise association between higher doses with greater fractionation and complete pain relief. That is, higher doses given over a longer period of time produced a more durable benefit (41). Other large randomized studies have demonstrated that various dose fractionation schemes may be equally effective, at least over a short time period (35,40,42–46). Currently, there are still insufficient data to support a clear consensus concerning a dose-response relationship (47–50). More recent analyses have looked at cost-effectiveness and quality-of-life issues (46,51).

An "expert panel for the radiation oncology bone metastasis work group" concluded that 2000 cGy in five fractions, 3000 cGy in 10 fractions, and 3500 cGy in 14 fractions are appropriate schemes for the initial treatment of bone metastases (52). Because many patients with metastases have uncertain prognosis, it is important to deliver an appropriate effective treatment so that quality of life is not compromised. In such cases, shorter treatment might be considered. Patients with an otherwise good prognosis might be treated to a higher dose over a more protracted time for an anticipated more effective and durable response (50). An individualized approach, mindful of clinical, biologic, and economic considerations, is required (53).

Specific Palliation

Bone Pain

Mature bone has nociceptor fibers in the endosteum and periosteum, supporting vascular structures and ligamentous and muscular attachments. Bone metastases occur in as many as 84% of patients with advanced or terminal disease, the percentage depending somewhat on the site of the primary malignancy and the intensity of investigation (38). Bone pain is usually aching and often worsened with movement or weight bearing (54). Pain may be the result of chemical mediators produced by the malignancy. A prostaglandin or other kinin is thought to be associated and may explain the pain relief seen with some analgesics and the rapid onset of pain relief seen in some patients following the initiation of irradiation (10,55). The observation of a brisk response allows the conclusion that less chemical mediator is being produced by disruption of the metabolism of the irradiated tumor cell and its environment. More often, however, pain relief is delayed for 1 to 4 weeks and may then be due to a reduction in the bulk of tumor deposits and a release of pressure on compressed or entrapped nerves or surrounding sensitive structures (55). Repeatedly, it has been demonstrated that 80% of patients treated with radiation for cancer-related bone pain will achieve either complete or substantial partial relief of pain (35). Furthermore, more than two thirds of those patients will remain pain free in the area irradiated for the remainder of their life (38,56). Some patients with metastatic bone disease will live for many years (11,57). Patients with symptomatic bone metastasis who are palliated by irradiation can expect less obtundation and constipation from analgesics, improved mobility, and less attendant depression and anxiety.

Neuropathic Pain

The origin and course of the brachial and lumbosacral plexi are intimately associated with bone and soft tissue. Direct invasion or compression of these structures results in severe and complex pain patterns. The violation of nerve trunks by malignancy causes a pain more akin to causalgia. When nerves are actually invaded or infiltrated and disrupted, irradiation-associated palliation is usually less than complete and may be minimal. At times, however, treatment can be very gratifying, and irradiation should not be withheld only because of the anatomic location of the disease. Some malignancies are more quickly responsive to irradiation. These would include lymphomas and small-cell carcinoma of the lung.

Pathologic Fracture

Most bone metastases occur in the area of active blood-producing red marrow with its associated rich vascular supply. The weight-bearing areas of the femur and acetabulum, which make up the functioning ball and socket joint of the hip, are often involved. Radiographic demonstration of lytic defects in those bones may herald a pathologic fracture (35). Those at higher risk have cortical defects greater than 2.5 cm or have lost more than 50% of the bone cortex (35). By recognizing that full function and stability may never be returned to those bones, delivering appropriate radiation therapy, and counseling the patient to modify activity in spite of pain improvement, it may be possible to avoid pathologic fracture (35). The personal drain of being bedfast, the loss of economic productivity, and the cost of surgical repair of a pathologic fracture are better avoided. Bone healing and remodeling can occur after irradiation, but extreme loss may require surgical stabilization (58). The irradiation may follow surgical stabilization to minimize regrowth of the metastasis and assist in the stability of the bone and any surgically placed prosthesis. The American College of Radiology consensus panel on the radiation of bone metastasis recommends surgical intervention for lytic lesions greater than 3.0 cm and involvement of more than one third of the cortex (59). Based on clinical judgment, palliative radiation treatment can be initiated after demonstration of primary healing of the incision. Pathologic fractures are associated with pain and are a special concern in vertebrae because of spinal cord compression.

Spinal Cord Compression and Back Pain

The spinal cord is encased in a rigid bony canal with little room for extraneous tissue. It is quite sensitive to injury that alters blood supply. Compression obstructs the nutrient spinal artery of the spinal cord. Ischemia results in the death of the spinal cord below the site of damage. There are two common patterns of compression: First, there is direct extension of a malignant mass from the involved vertebral bone. Second, spinal cord compression is by direct extension of soft tissue disease through an intervertebral foramen. Direct metastasis to the epidural space or spinal cord is rare (60). A limited vascular supply and rigid envelope of bone contribute to the sensitivity of the cord to ischemia (61,62). Early recognition and intervention are critical to restore neural function. Treatment can be by surgery or by means of radiation therapy, depending on the availability of technology, the rapidity of change of neurologic function, and the site of primary malignancy (63). Findlay reviewed 1816 patients with spinal cord compression, of which 25% were referred for treatment when still able to walk, that is, with function preserved well enough to stand and move. Among that group, of those treated with surgery, 48% remained ambulatory following decompression. Of those patients who received surgery followed by irradiation, 67% remained ambulatory. Of those patients treated with radiation therapy only, 79% remained able to walk (35,64). Posterior decompression of the spinal laminae will decompress the spinal cord in the area of bone resection. It cannot address the bulk and distortion arising from the vertebra in the anterior aspect of the spinal canal ventral to the spinal cord. Anterior approaches to the spinal canal through the neck or thorax are more demanding on the patient and the surgeon and often require stabilization by means of a prosthesis to strut the surgical or neoplastic defect. After any surgical decompression, irradiation is appropriate to further safeguard the spinal cord by treating the encroaching malignancy.

Almost all spinal cord compression by malignancy can be appropriately treated with radiation. Over 90% of patients who present with symptoms of early spinal cord compression and are still ambulatory before treatment will remain ambulatory after prompt immediate radiation therapy (65,66). As with surgery, poor results are obtained in patients who have manifest paraplegia and bladder dysfunction. Some nonambulatory patients may regain lower extremity function; but the majority experience little or no improvement after irradiation. When spinal cord compression occurs in an area previously irradiated, surgical intervention may be most appropriate. Situations where a surgical approach should be considered prior to irradiation for spinal cord compression include: a lack of tissue diagnosis, instability of vertebral bodies, compression due to a large paravertebral mass, a known radio-resistant tumor, and, perhaps, the rapid progression of neurologic symptoms.

All tissues have an innate tolerance to irradiation. Spinal cord tolerance exceeds the dose most often needed to relieve bone pain. However, if symptoms return or symptoms of compression and neurologic deficit become evident again, retreatment poses a complex problem. Additional doses may cumulatively approach or exceed spinal cord tolerance. Fundamentally, it should be remembered that spinal cord injury and death by malignancy are more problematic and common than irradiation-induced damage. Injury to any tissue during a therapeutic endeavor is to be avoided whenever possible. An occasional patient will be seen who has severe vertebral pain or impending spinal cord compression in an area already irradiated. The therapeutic dilemma then arises of whether to treat further with the goal of improving mobility and decreasing pain by reducing tumor volume or only to address the pain with greater doses of analgesics, anticipating worsening of paresis. These circumstances call for philosophic, practical, and prudent analyses of the patient's individual prognosis and desires. This is the crux of why palliative treatment is demanding on the caregiver.

Headaches and Brain Metastasis

Brain metastases are the most common brain tumor in adults. The brain is within the rigid bony calvarium, which does not allow the brain to expand after insult or injury. Metastasis to the cerebral cortex can produce a mass or edema, with an increase in intracranial pressure leading to headache, focal weakness, mental status changes, gait disturbances, seizures, etc. (67). The effect of these symptoms on the quality of life can be profound and contribute to morbidity and mortality. Radiation therapy has been the mainstay of palliation of brain metastases for decades. By decreasing the bulk of the metastasis by irradiation, and by decreasing any attendant edema by corticosteroids, headache pain and neurologic loss can often be alleviated. Surgery may be considered for a dominant, superficial lesion in a nonelegant area of the brain.

Various dose and fractionation schemes have been used. Most commonly in the United States, the brain receives 3000 cGy in 2 weeks (68). Some patients are better served by a more protracted course of radiation therapy (69). Intensely focused irradiation, by means of stereotactic technology, using linear accelerator or Gamma Knife radiosurgery, is of benefit in selected patients. In those patients who are treated with surgery or radiosurgery, external beam subsequently increases the degree and duration of improvement (70–74).

Superior Vena Cava Syndrome (SVCS)

Venous drainage from the upper extremities and head is afforded by a large vein just proximal to the heart, the superior vena cava. Central mediastinal masses that compress the superior vena cava result in a syndrome of edema of the arms, neck, and face, accompanied by a throbbing headache, presumably due to edema of the brain and meninges. Irradiation of mediastinal masses with resultant decrease in the obstruction can relieve headache and improve the comfort of patients with superior vena cava syndrome (75). Less commonly are other thin-walled, low-pressure venous structures compressed (e.g., the axillary vein or inferior vena cava). Minimal change in the radius of the lumen of a vessel can result in substantial improvement in blood flow and comfort. The same principle pertains to those obstructed bronchial lumens, which are discussed later. Irradiation to the mediastinum will ameliorate superior vena cava syndrome symptoms in the majority of patients. In a study of 34 patients with lung cancer and associated SVC not responsive to chemotherapy, 76% with nonsmall-cell lung carcinoma and 94% with small-cell carcinoma showed response as measured in relief of symptoms. Some patients were improved within 3 days after initiating palliative radiation therapy (76). Diagnostic procedures are most often performed prior to irradiation if superior vena cava syndrome is the first presentation of malignancy. This is done to formulate an overall treatment approach. Lymphoproliferative disorders may be treated differently than epithelial malignancies.

Bronchial Obstruction

External beam radiation therapy is often quite effective in palliating bronchial obstruction. The symptoms of breathlessness, cough, hemoptysis, and chest pain may be well palliated (77,78). The goal is complete reaeration and reexpansion of an atelectatic lung (79). Intraluminal endobronchial radiation therapy is sometimes used with or without rigid stenting. In one analysis of endobronchial treatment, among 52 patients with malignant airway occlusion, radiographic reaeration was seen in 73% (80).

The symptoms mentioned earlier are also seen in patients at initial presentation who are treated with curative intent. The symptoms alone do not relegate the patient to palliative status only. To rephrase this statement, in oncology, palliation of symptoms is often an important milestone on the pathway to cure.

Uncontrolled Bleeding

Acute bleeding from advanced neoplasms is a challenge. Patients with advanced cervical cancer can develop bleeding severe enough to require transfusion. Radiotherapy can slow down or completely stop bleeding. In a study of 35 patients with massive bleeding from cervical carcinoma, all but one responded with the cessation of bleeding with no treatment-related complications (81).

Visceral Organs

Pleuritic pain may be improved by irradiation of the area of concern. Often it is difficult to distinguish between pleural-based or rib-associated pain. The capsule of the liver may be infiltrated or stretched by neoplastic enlargement of the liver. The pain is deep and may limit the depth of inspiration. Treatment of the liver capsule can provide greater comfort with a decrease in the need for narcotics and improvement in sensorium and function (82,83). The spleen may be enlarged by infiltration of lymphoma or leukemia. Splenomegaly can be uncomfortable and associated with dyspnea. Irradiation of the spleen in this circumstance is indicated to provide comfort.

Occasionally, the bowel or mesentery will be involved with lymphoma. Irradiation of that section of the bowel or the entire abdominal or pelvic cavity may result in improvement in comfort and well-being. Ovarian and colonic carcinoma can also widely involve the abdomen; but these conditions are much less subject to manipulation by irradiation.

Organs high in the abdomen, especially the pancreas, can directly invade and infiltrate the prevertebral soft tissue and splanchnic nerve plexus. This results in a severe, deep, and boring pain that is quite debilitating and often the dominant site of concern. Irradiation may improve the comfort of these patients. If the pain is not severe, it may be more indicative of mass effect than of nerve infiltration. Treatment may obviate the occurrence of severe pain throughout the course of the patient's life (75).

Soft Tissue Masses

Direct, contiguous extension of disease into soft tissue, or metastasis to tight compartments or areas associated with muscular activity, is painful and debilitating. Low pelvic and perineal involvement by malignancy may make it difficult to sit. Metastasis to nodes in the groin or axilla allows for maceration of the overlying skin, which may become tight and thin and be associated with compression of vascular and neural structures with attendant morbidity. Irradiation of these soft tissue masses can be very gratifying and result in a decrease of the mass and release of associated pressure.

Hemibody Irradiation

When patients develop multiple symptomatic lesions, localized treatment may be impractical and time consuming and require overlapping of treatment fields. If possible, that is to be avoided to minimize excessive toxicity. With multiple symptomatic lesions, patients may be treated with upper or lower hemibody irradiation. Because of the large volume of the body treated and the use of larger doses with each fraction, there is a greater morbidity to gastrointestinal and hematologic toxicity (84,85). Because multiple organs are irradiated, the patients may require hospital admission, hydration, and premedication to decrease potential side effects of nausea, vomiting, diarrhea, and hypotension. Individual customized metal blocks are fabricated to spare areas that might be excluded. Typically, areas such as the salivary glands or the entire head may be spared. Upper hemibody irradiation can occasionally cause radiation pneumonitis. Lower hemibody irradiation may lead to potential severe bone marrow toxicity that may preclude the use of systemic chemotherapy. For these reasons, hemibody irradiation is not often used. Fractionated hemibody irradiation may be more tolerable (86).

Reirradiation

Reirradiation is not uncommon in oncologic practice (87). As supportive care is improved, many patients survive longer. Reirradiation may be done for palliation of mucosal malignancies of the pharynx (88,89), brain lesions, lung carcinoma with compression symptoms, and breast and chest wall malignancies, to mention only a few (87,90,91). Likewise, recurrent symptomatic bone metastasis may respond to retreatment with radiation (87,92). As with primary treatment, tissue tolerance limits repeat irradiation (93). Therefore, a lower than initial benefit may be expected. The reported response rates for reirradiation vary widely, ranging from 15% to 90%, depending on the site of recurrence, patient selection, and dose administered at retreatment (87).

Brachytherapy

Low Dose Rate (LDR)

Brachytherapy means radiation treatment done at short distance by placing radioactive sources next to or on the tissue target. It is sometimes used with palliative intent when the patient has already received previous external beam therapy and reirradiation poses unacceptable risk to surrounding tissues. Brachytherapy provides a relatively high dose of radiation to the target while minimizing the dose to surrounding tissues (94–96). The basic principles, indications, patient selection, techniques, and radionuclides used for palliative brachytherapy have recently been reviewed by Shasha and Harrison (97).

High Dose Rate (HDR)

High dose rate therapy utilizes a more concentrated source of radioactivity. It allows for shorter treatment time and often avoids hospitalization. No general anesthesia is used. There may be less patient motion because of shorter treatment time requirements. There is often patient preference because of outpatient possibility and improved personnel safety. Optimal dose and fractionation schedules are being evaluated (97–103). Reirradiation utilizing high dose rate brachytherapy should be done with caution. Severe complications are potential, and skill and judgment are paramount (104,105).

Systemic Radiation Therapy

Radiation therapy using bone-seeking radionuclides is considered when multiple bony sites are involved (106). Unlike hemibody irradiation, as mentioned, systemic radionuclides are less cumbersome to administer, provide less acute radiation toxicity, and simultaneously treat the entire bony skeleton. Approximately 60% to 80% of patients treated with systemic nuclides experience pain reduction or complete pain relief (107). Hematologic toxicity limits its use to selected patients who have acceptable marrow and renal function. Treatment planning for systemic administration of radioisotopes includes the documentation of some element of osteoblastic activity (108).

If treatment is administered to patients with purely lytic or no osteoblastic abnormality at the painful site, there is less likely a preferential accumulation of radioisotope, and pain is less likely to be relieved.

Although iodine-131 is used specifically and extensively to treat appropriate thyroid carcinomas, for nonthyroid malignancy with symptomatic bone metastasis, phosphorus-32 (P-32), strontium-89 (Sr-89), and samarium-153 (Sm-153 EDTMP) have been approved by the United States Food and Drug Administration (108–110). The most appropriate dosing and scheduling have not been adequately established. Overall response rates are anticipated to vary between 75% and 80% (111). When compared with the use of local external beam therapy, it was concluded that both treatments are similarly effective in pain relief; but patients treated with radionuclide may show less likelihood to develop new sites of pain (112). When radionuclide and external beam are used together, there may be an improvement in overall pain control and decreased analgesic requirement with further delay in disease progression.

As might be anticipated, hematologic toxicity is the limiting aspect of widespread clinical use of strontium or samarium (113,114). This is a promising area, and other radioisotopes are being evaluated (107,108,115).

Radioimmunotherapy

Radioimmunotherapy uses antibodies or antibody-derived constructs as direct carriers for radionuclide. These circulating radio-labeled monoclonal antibodies specifically bind to antigens on tumor cells and deliver systemically targeted radiation to the tumor with relative sparing of surrounding normal tissues. Results from clinical trials have been promising, especially for lymphomatous malignancies (116,117). However, the antibody may itself induce an allergic reaction. This therapeutic modality remains investigational.

Radiation Toxicity and Tissue Tolerance

Radiation therapy morbidity is complex and is dependent on many factors. Palliative, low dose irradiation to an extremity, for example, produces almost no side effects or complications, whereas a similar dose to the upper abdomen may be associated with nausea and vomiting. Each organ, system, and body area has a different radiation tolerance, side-effect profile, and complication possibility. Table 41-1 is a listing of selected tissue tolerances to radiation (118). Side effects are dependent on the region of the body, the organ system, the volume of the organ treated, the dose delivered in each treatment session, somewhat on the characteristic of the x-ray, and dose rate. There is a less predictable toxicity, depending on the general state of health or debility of the patient, the patient's nutritional status, other medical illnesses, concurrent medications,

TABLE 41-1. *Selected normal tissue tolerance to therapeutic radiation (modified from Emami et al.) (118)*

Organ	TD 5/5* Volume 1/3	2/3	3/3	Selected endpoint
Brain	6000	5000	4500	Necrosis infarction
Optic nerve	No partial volume		5000	Blindness
Optic chiasm	No partial volume		5000	Blindness
Eye lens	No partial volume		1000	Cataract requiring intervention
Retina	No partial volume		4500	Blindness
Ear mid/external	3000	5500	3000	Acute serous otitis
	5500	3000	5500	Chronic serous otitis
TMJ mandible	6500	6000	6000	Marked limitation of joint function
Parotid	—	3200	3200	Xerostomia
Larynx	7900	7000	7000	Cartilage necrosis
Spinal cord	5 cm/5000	10 cm/5000	20 cm/4700	Myelitis necrosis
Rib cage	5000	—	—	Pathologic fracture
Lung	4500	3000	1750	Pneumonitis
Heart	6000	4500	4000	Pericarditis
Esophagus	6000	5800	5500	Clinical stricture/perforation
Stomach	6000	5500	5000	Ulceration perforation
Liver	5000	3500	3000	Liver failure
Colon	5500		4500	Ulceration perforation
Kidney	5000	3000	2300	Clinical nephritis
Bladder	N/A	8000	6500	Symptomatic bladder contracture and volume loss
Femoral head	—	—	5200	Necrosis
Skin	—	—	100 cm²/5000	Telangiectasia

*Tolerance dose, 5% incidence in 5 years.

and prior surgical or radiation procedures. Table 41-2 lists a comprehensive schema of the potential side effects of radiation as considered and compiled by the largest cooperative clinical radiation research organization, the Radiation Therapy Oncology Group (119). Please note that this is a broad compendium and is presented for the elucidation of the reader. Just as medication has potential adverse effects, and surgery has attendant morbidity, irradiation sometimes can be associated with acute and chronic sequelae. It is the judicious use of any therapy that identifies the expert. Recognizing that all forms of therapeutic endeavor have some attendant cost and potential detriment, the goal in palliating cancer pain is to minimize cost and treatment-related morbidity while maximizing the degree and duration of improvement. In Table 41-2, acute toxicity is considered. Morbidity scores 4 and 5 are exceptionally unusual. In clinical practice, one structures a treatment regimen with all attempts to minimize acute and late adverse effects. Toxicity scores of 0 to 2 are most often the extent of adverse acute effects, whereas a 0 morbidity for chronic effects is the ideal (Table 41-3) (119). The side effects and toxicities noted earlier are much less likely to be observed or experienced with doses most often employed in palliative circumstances. The radiation oncologist chooses his treatment mindful of the particular problem to be addressed and the goal of therapy in the individual patient.

TABLE 41-2. *Acute radiation morbidity scoring criteria (RTOG) (119)*

Organ/tissue	0	Grade 1	Grade 2	Grade 3	Grade 4
Skin	No change over baseline	Follicular, faint, or dull erythema, epilation, dry desquamation, decreased sweating	Tender or bright erythema, patchy moist desquamation, moderate edema	Confluent, moist desquamation other than skin folds, pitting edema	Ulceration, hemorrhage, necrosis
Mucous membrane	No change over baseline	Injection, may experience mild pain not requiring analgesic	Patchy mucositis that may produce an inflammatory sero-sanguinous discharge, may experience moderate pain requiring analgesic	Confluent fibrinous mucositis; may include severe pain requiring narcotic	Ulceration, hemorrhage, necrosis

TABLE 41-2. *Continued*

Organ/tissue	0	Grade 1	Grade 2	Grade 3	Grade 4
Eye	No change	Mild conjunctivitis with or without scleral injection, increased tearing	Moderate conjunctivitis with or without keratitis requiring steroids or antibiotics, dry eye requiring artificial tears, iritis with photophobia	Severe keratitis with corneal ulceration, objective decrease in visual acuity or in visual fields, acute glaucoma, panophthalmitis	Loss of vision (unilateral or bilateral)
Ear	No change over baseline	Mild external otitis with erythema, pruritus, secondary to dry desquamation not requiring medication. Audiogram unchanged from baseline	Moderate external otitis requiring topical medication, serous otitis medius, hypoacusis on testing only	Severe external otitis with discharge or moist desquamation, symptomatic hypoacusis, tinnitus, not drug related	Deafness
Salivary gland	No change over baseline	Mild mouth dryness; slightly thickened saliva; may have slightly altered taste such as metallic; these changes not reflected in alteration in baseline feeding behavior, such as increased use of liquids with meals	Moderate to complete dryness; thick, sticky saliva, markedly altered taste	—	Acute salivary gland necrosis
Pharynx and esophagus	No change over baseline	Mild dysphagia or odynophagia; may require topical anesthetic or nonnarcotic analgesics; may require soft diet	Moderate dysphagia or odynophagia; may require narcotic analgesics; may require purge or liquid diet	Severe dysphagia or odynophagia with dehydration or weight loss (>15% from pretreatment baseline) requiring NG feeding tube, IV fluids, or hyperalimentation	Complete obstruction, ulceration, perforation, fistula
Larynx	No change over baseline	Mild or intermittent hoarseness; cough not requiring antitussive; erythema of mucosa	Persistent hoarseness but able to vocalize; referred ear pain, sore throat, patchy fibrinous exudate or mild arytenoid edema not requiring narcotic; cough requiring antitussive	Whisper speech, throat pain or referred ear pain requiring narcotic; confluent fibrinous exudates, marked arytenoids edema	Marked dyspnea; stridor or hemoptysis with tracheostomy or intubation necessary
Upper GI	No change	Anorexia with <5% weight loss from pretreatment baseline; nausea not requiring antiemetics; abdominal discomfort not requiring parasympatholytic drugs or analgesics	Anorexia with <15% weight loss from pretreatment baseline; nausea or vomiting requiring antiemetics; abdominal pain requiring analgesics	Anorexia with >15% weight loss from pretreatment baseline or requiring NG tube or parenteral support; nausea or vomiting requiring NG tube or parenteral support; abdominal pain, severe despite medication; hematemesis or melena; abdominal distention (flat plate radiograph demonstrates distended bowel loops)	Ileus, subacute or acute obstruction, perforation, GI bleeding requiring transfusion; abdominal pain requiring tube decompression or bowel diversion

Continued

TABLE 41-2. *Continued*

Organ/tissue	0	Grade 1	Grade 2	Grade 3	Grade 4
Lower GI including pelvis	No change	Increased frequency or change in quality of bowel habits not requiring medication; rectal discomfort not requiring analgesics	Diarrhea requiring parasympatholytic drugs (e.g., diphenoxylate); mucous discharge not necessitating sanitary pads; rectal or abdominal pain requiring analgesics	Diarrhea requiring parenteral support; severe mucous or blood discharge necessitating sanitary pads; abdominal distention (flat plate radiograph demonstrates distended bowel loops)	Acute or subacute obstruction, fistula, or perforation, GI bleeding requiring transfusion, abdominal pain or tenesmus requiring tube decompression or bowel diversion
Lung	No change	Mild symptoms of dry cough or dyspnea on exertion	Persistent cough requiring narcotic, antitussive agents; dyspnea with minimal effort but not at rest	Severe cough unresponsive to narcotic antitussive agent or dyspnea at rest; clinical or radiologic evidence of acute pneumonitis; intermittent oxygen or steroids may be required	Severe respiratory insufficiency; continuous oxygen or assisted ventilation
Genitourinary	No change	Frequency of urination or nocturia twice pretreatment habit; dysuria, urgency not requiring medication	Frequency of urination or nocturia less frequent than every hour; dysuria, urgency, bladder spasm requiring local anesthetic (e.g., phenazopyridine)	Frequency with urgency and nocturia hourly or more frequently; dysuria, pelvic pain, or bladder spasm requiring regular, frequent narcotic; gross hematuria with or without clot passage	Hematuria requiring transfusion; acute bladder obstruction not secondary to clot passage, ulceration, or necrosis
Heart	No change over baseline	Asymptomatic but objective evidence of EKG changes or pericardial abnormalities without evidence of other heart disease	Symptomatic with EKG changes and radiologic findings of congestive heart failure or pericardial disease; no specific treatment required	Congestive heart failure, angina pectoris, pericardial disease responding to therapy	Congestive heart failure, angina pectoris, pericardial disease, arrhythmias not responsive to nonsurgical measures
CNS	No change	Fully functional status (able to work) with minor neurologic findings; no medication needed	Neurologic findings sufficient to require home care; nursing assistance may be required; medication including steroids; antiseizure agents may be required	Neurologic findings requiring hospitalization for initial management	Serious neurologic impairment that includes paralysis coma, or seizures >3 per week despite medication; hospitalization required

TABLE 41-2. *Continued*

Organ/tissue	0	Grade 1	Grade 2	Grade 3	Grade 4
Hematologic WBC (×1000)	−4.0	3.0– < 4.0	2.0– < 3.0	1.0– < 2.0	< 1.0
Platelets (×1000)	> 100	75– < 100	50– <75	25– < 50	< 25 or spontaneous bleeding
Neutrophils (×1000)	−1.9	1.5– < 1.9	1.0– < 1.5	0.5– < 1.0	< 0.5 or sepsis
Hemoglobin (GM %)	> 11	11–9.5	< 9.5–7.5	< 7.5–5.0	—
Hematocrit (%)	−32	20– < 32	20	Packed cell transfusion required	—

Guidelines: The acute morbidity criteria are used to score/grade toxicity from radiation therapy. The criteria are relevant from day 1, the commencement of therapy, through day 90. Thereafter, the EORTC/RTOG Criteria for Late Effects are to be utilized. The evaluator must attempt to discriminate between disease and treatment-related signs and symptoms. An accurate baseline evaluation prior to commencement of therapy is necessary. All toxicities of grade 3, 4, or 5 must be verified by the principal investigator (any toxicity that caused death is graded 5).

TABLE 41-3. *Late radiation morbidity scoring scheme (RTOG, EORTC) (119)*

Organ/tissue	0	Grade 1	Grade 2	Grade 3	Grade 4	Grade 5
Skin	None	Slight atrophy pigmentation change, some hair loss	Patchy atrophy, moderate telangiectasia, total hair loss	Marked atrophy, gross telangiectasia	Ulceration	Death directly related to radiation late effect
Subcutaneous tissue	None	Slight induration (fibrosis) and loss of subcutaneous fat	Moderate fibrosis but asymptomatic, slight field contracture; < 10% linear reduction	Severe induration and loss of subcutaneous tissue; field contracture > 1016 linear measurement	Necrosis	
Mucous membrane	None	Slight atrophy and dryness	Moderate atrophy and telangiectasia, little mucus	Marked atrophy with complete dryness, severe telangiectasia	Ulceration	
Salivary glands	None	Slight dryness of mouth, good response on stimulation	Moderate dryness of mouth, poor response on stimulation	Complete dryness of mouth, no response on stimulation	Fibrosis	
Spinal cord	None	Mild Lhermitte's sign	Severe Lhermitte's sign	Objective neurologic findings at or below cord level treated	Mono-, para-quadriplegia	
Brain	None	Mild headache, slight lethargy	Moderate headache, great lethargy	Severe headache, severe CNS dysfunction (partial loss of power or dyskinesia)	Seizures or paralysis, coma	
Eye	None	Asymptomatic cataract, minor corneal ulceration or keratitis	Symptomatic cataract, moderate corneal ulceration, minor retinopathy or glaucoma	Severe keratitis, severe retinopathy or detachment, severe glaucoma	Panophthalmitis, blindness	
Larynx	None	Hoarseness, slight arytenoid edema	Moderate arytenoid edema, chondritis	Severe edema, severe chondritis	Necrosis	

Continued

TABLE 41-3. *Continued*

Organ/tissue	0	Grade 1	Grade 2	Grade 3	Grade 4	Grade 5
Lung	None	Asymptomatic or mild symptoms (dry cough), slight radiographic appearances	Moderate symptomatic fibrosis or pneumonitis (severe cough); low-grade fever, patchy radiographic appearances	Severe symptomatic fibrosis or pneumonitis, dense radiographic changes	Severe respiratory insufficiency, continuous O$_2$, assisted ventilation	
Heart	None	Asymptomatic or mild symptoms, transient T-wave inversion and ST changes, sinus tachycardia >110 (at rest)	Moderate angina on effort, mild pericarditis, normal heart size, persistent abnormality T-wave and ST changes, low ORS	Severe angina, pericardial effusion, constrictive pericarditis, moderate heart failure, cardiac enlargement, EKG abnormalities	Tamponade, severe heart failure, severe constrictive pericarditis	
Esophagus	None	Mild fibrosis, slight difficulty in swallowing solids, no pain on swallowing	Unable to take solid food normally, swallowing semisolid food, dilatation may be indicated	Severe fibrosis, able to swallow only liquids, may have pain on swallowing; dilatation required	Necrosis, perforation, fistula	
Small/large intestine	None	Mild diarrhea, mild cramping, bowel movement 5 times daily, slight rectal discharge or bleeding	Moderate diarrhea and colic, bowel movement > 5 times daily excessive rectal mucus or intermittent bleeding	Obstruction or bleeding requiring surgery	Necrosis, perforation, fistula	
Liver	None	Mild lassitude, nausea, dyspepsia, slightly abnormal liver function	Moderate symptoms, some abnormal liver function tests, serum albumin normal	Disabling hepatitis insufficiency; liver function tests grossly abnormal, low albumin, edema, or ascites	Necrosis, hepatic coma or encephalopathy	
Kidney	None	Transient albuminuria, no hypertension, mild impairment renal function, urea 25 to 35 mg %, creatinine 1.5 to 2.0 mg %, creatinine clearance >75%	Persistent moderate albuminuria (2+); mild hypertension, no related anemia, moderate impairment renal function; urea >36 to 60 mg %, creatinine clearance (50 to 74%)	Severe albuminuria, severe hypertension, persistent anemia (< 100%), severe renal failure, urea >60 mg%, creatinine >4.0 mg %, creatinine clearance < 50%	Malignant hypertension, uremic coma; urea >100%	
Bladder	None	Slight epithelial atrophy; mild telangiectasia (microscopic hematuria)	Moderate frequency, generalized telangiectasia, intermittent macroscopic hematuria	Severe frequency and dysuria, severe generalized telangiectasia (often with petechiae), frequent hematuria reduction in bladder capacity (<150 mL)	Necrosis, contracted bladder (capacity < 100 mL), severe hemorrhagic cystitis	
Bone	None	Asymptomatic, no growth retardation, reduced bone density	Moderate pain or tenderness, growth retardation, irregular bone sclerosis	Severe pain or tenderness, complete arrest of bone growth, dense bone sclerosis	Necrosis, spontaneous fracture	
Joint	None	Mild joint stiffness, slight limitation of movement	Moderate stiffness, intermittent or moderate joint pain, moderate limitation of movement	Severe joint stiffness, pain with severe limitation of movement	Necrosis, complete fixation	

CONCLUSION

Radiation therapy is an effective treatment in the management of cancer pain. It is a preferred treatment for cancer pain relief in cases of bone metastasis, soft tissue masses, lumen compromise, and bleeding. Until mechanisms that will prevent the development of malignancy are established, major lifestyle changes regarding cigarettes and diet are implemented, and mechanisms for earlier diagnoses are developed, palliation of patients with advanced malignancy will remain a problem of great magnitude. Radiation therapy is one tool in the armamentarium of caregivers who have chosen to relieve the chronic pain and suffering of patients with malignancy. The aggressive and appropriate use of radiation oncology consultation and therapy may provide more effective and less costly care and minimize the burden to patients and caregivers (120).

REFERENCES

1. Cleeland CS, Gonin R, Hatfield AK, et al. Pain and its treatment in outpatients with metastatic disease. *N Engl J Med* 1994;330:592–596.
2. Bonica JJ. Treatment of cancer pain: current status and future needs. In: Fields EL, Dubner R, Cervero F, eds. *Advances in pain research and therapy*, Vol 9. New York: Raven, 1985:589–616.
3. Portenoy RK, Thaler HT, Kornblith AB, et al. Symptom prevalence, characteristics and distress in a cancer population. *Qual Life Res* 1994;3:183–189.
4. Ciezki J, Macklis RM. The palliative role of radiotherapy in the management of the cancer patient. *Sem in Oncol* 1995;22(2)(Suppl3):82–90.
5. Hoskin, PJ. Radiotherapy in the management of bone pain. *Clin Ortho Rel Res* 1995;312:105–119.
6. Macklis RM, Cornelli H, Lasher J. Brief course of palliative radiotherapy for metastatic bone pain: a pilot cost-minimization comparison with narcotic analgesics. *Am J Clin Oncol* 1998;21(6):617–622.
7. Gilbert HA, Kagan AR, Nussbaum H, et al. Evaluation of radiation therapy for bone metastases: pain relief and quality of life. *Am J Roentgenol* 1977;129:1095–1096.
8. Greenlee RT, Murray T, Bolden S, Wingo PA. Cancer Statistics, 2000. *Ca J Clin* 2000;50(1):7–34.
9. Skolnick AA. New study suggests radiation often underused for palliation. *JAMA* 1998;279(5):343–4.
10. Foley KM. Diagnosis and treatment of cancer pain. In: Holleb A, Fink D, Murphy G, eds. *American Cancer Society textbook of clinical oncology*. Atlanta, GA: American Cancer Society, 1991:555–575.
11. Schocker JD, Brady LW. Radiation therapy for bone metastasis. *Clin Orthop Rel Res* 1982;169:38–43.
12. Lesage P, Portenoy RK. Trends in cancer pain management. *Cancer Control* 1999;6(2):136–145.
13. Regan JM, Peng P. Neurophysiology of cancer pain. *Cancer Control* 2000;7(2):111–119.
14. Kelly J, Payne R. Cancer pain syndromes. *Neuro Clin North Am* 1991; 9:937–953.
15. Roos DE, O'Brien PC, Smith JG, et al. A role for radiotherapy in neuropathic bone pain: preliminary response rates from a prospective trial (Trans-Tasmen Radiation Oncology Group, TROG 96.05). *Int J Radiat Oncol Biol Phys* 2000;46(4):975–981.
16. Raja SN. Role of the sympathetic nervous system in acute pain and inflammation. *Annals of Medicine*. 1995;27(2):241–246.
17. Bjurholm A, Kreicbergs A, Brodin E, et al. Substance P and CGRP: immunoreactive nerves in bone. *Peptides* 1988;9:165–171.
18. Cleeland CS, Janjan NA, Scott CB, et al. Cancer pain management by radiotherapists: a survey of Radiation Therapy Oncology Group physicians. *Int. J Radiat Oncol Biol Phys* 2000;47(1):203–208.
19. Cleary, FJ. Cancer pain management. *Cancer Control* 2000;7(2): 121–131.
20. Rutten EH, Crul BJ, van der Toorn PP, et al. Pain characteristics help to predict the analgesic efficacy of radiotherapy for the treatment of cancer pain. *Pain* 1997;69:131–135.
21. Advances in the Management of Cancer Pain. Reports from the 8th World Congress on Pain. *Oncology News* 1996;5(10):16.
22. Grossman SA, Staats PS. Current management of pain in patients with cancer. *Oncology* 1994;8(3):93–103.
23. Cleeland CS. Assessment of pain in cancer. *Adv Pain Res Ther* 1990; 16:47–55.
24. Fishman B, Pasternak S, Wallenstein S, et al. The memorial pain assessment card: a valid instrument for the evaluation of cancer pain. *Cancer* 1987;60:1151–1158.
25. Grossman SA, Sheidler VR, McGuire DB, et al. A comparison of the Hopkins pain rating instrument with standard visual analogue and verbal descriptor scales in patients with cancer pain. *J Pain Symp Manage* 1992;7:196–203.
26. Cleeland CS. Cancer related symptoms. *Sem Radiat Oncol* 2000; 10(3):175–190.
27. Advances in the Management of Cancer Pain. Reports from the 8th World Congress on Pain. *Oncology News* 1996;5(10):2–3.
28. Fidler M. Incidence of fracture through metastases in long bones. *Acta Orthop Scand* 1981;52:623–627
29. Body JJ. Metastatic bone disease: clinical and therapeutic aspects. *Bone* 1992;13:557–562.
30. Daffner RH, Lupetin AR, Dash N, et al. MRI in the detection of malignant infiltration of bone marrow. *AJR* 1986;146:353–358.
31. Jacobson H, Goran H. Radiological detection of bone and bone marrow metastases. *Med Oncol Tumor Pharmacother* 1992;8:25.
32. Hall, EJ. *Radiobiology for the radiologist*, 5th ed. Philadelphia, PA: JB Lippincott Co, 2000:5–111.
33. Bergonié J, Tribondeau L. Intrepretation de quelques resultats de la radiotherapie et essai de fixation d'une technique rationnelle. *Compt Rend Acad Sci* 1906;143:983.
34. Khan, FM. *The physics of radiation therapy*, 2nd ed. Baltimore, MD: Williams & Wilkins, 1994:45–68.
35. Bates T. A review of local radiotherapy in the treatment of bone metastases and cord compression. *Int J Radiat Oncol Biol Phys* 1992;23:217–221.
36. Macklis RM, Cornelli M, Lasher J. Brief course of palliative radiotherapy for metastatic bone pain: a pilot cost-minimization comparison with narcotic analgesics. *Am J Clin Oncol* 1998;21(6): 617–622.
37. Poulson HS, Nielson OS, Klee M, et al. Palliative irradiation of bone metastases. *Cancer Treat Rev* 1989;16:41–48.
38. Tong D, Gillick L, Hendrickson FR. Palliation of symptomatic osseous metastases: the final results of the study by the RTOG. *Cancer* 1982;50:893–899
39. Hill CS, Rogers AG, Audell LG, et al. Management of pain in special populations of cancer patients. *Oncology* 1998;12(4):573,576–569, 583–584.
40. Price P, Hoskin PJ, Easton D, et al. Prospective randomized trial of single and multifraction radiotherapy schedules in the treatment of painful bone metastases. *Radiother Oncol* 1986;6:247–255.
41. Blitzer PH. Reanalysis of the RTOG study of the palliation of symptomatic osseous metastasis. *Cancer* 1985;55:14468–1472.
42. Nielsen OS, Bentzen SM, Sandberg E, et al. Randomized trial of a single dose versus fractionated palliative radiotherapy of bone metastases. *Radiother Oncol* 1998;47:233–240.
43. Niewald M, Tkocz, H-J, Abel V, et al. Rapid course radiation therapy vs. more standard treatment: a randomized trial for bone metastases. *Int J Radiat Oncol Biol Phys* 1996;36:1085–1089.
44. Rassmusson B, Vejborg I, Jensen AB, et al. Irradiation of bone metastases in breast cancer patients: a randomized study with 1 year follow-up. *Radiother Oncol* 1995;34:179–184.
45. On behalf of the Bone Pain Trial Working Party. 8 Gy single fraction radiotherapy for the treatment of metastatic skeletal pain: randomized comparison with a multifraction schedule over 12 months of patient follow-up. *Radiother Oncol* 1999;52:111–121.
46. Anderson PR, Coia R. Fractionation and outcome with palliative radiation therapy. *Sem Radiat Oncol* 2000;10(3):191–199.
47. Ratanatharathorn V, Powers WE, Moss WT, Perez CA. Bone metastasis: review and critical analysis of random allocation trials of local field treatment. *Int J Radiat Oncol Biol Phys* 1999;44:1–18.

48. Bentzen SM, Hoskin P, Roos D, Nielsen OS. Fractionated radiotherapy for metastatic bone pain: evidence-based medicine or . . . ? Letters to the editor. *Int J Radiat Oncol Biol Phys* 2000;46(3):681–682.

49. Ratanatharathorn V, Powers WE, Moss WT, Perez CA. In response to Dr. Bentzen et al. Letters to the editor. *Int J Radiat Oncol Biol Phys* 2000;46(3):682–683.

50. Arcangeli G, Giovinazzo G, Saracino B, et al. Radiation therapy in the management of symptomatic bone metastases: the effect of total dose and histology on pain relief and response duration. *Int J Radiat Oncol Biol Phys* 1998;42(5):1119–1126.

51. Hartsell WF (PI). RTOG 97-14: Randomized trial of palliative radiation therapy for osseous metastases: a study of palliation of symptoms and quality of life. RTOG Headquarters, American College of Radiology, Philadelphia, PA. In press.

52. Rose C, Kagan R. The final report of the expert panel for the radiation oncology bone metastasis work group of the American College of Radiology. *Int J Radiat Oncol Biol Phys* 1998;40(5):1117–1124.

53. Smith TJ. Future strategies needed for palliative care. *Sem Radiat Oncol* 2000;10(3):254–261.

54. Kanner R. Pain treatment. In: Dutcher JP, Wiervik PH, eds. *Handbook of hematologic and oncologic emergencies*. New York: Plenum, 1987.

55. Nielsen OS, Munro M, Tannock IF. Bone metastases: pathophysiology and management policy. *J Clin Oncol* 1991;9:509–524.

56. Vikram B, Chu F. Radiation therapy for metastasis to the base of skull. *Radiology* 1979;130:465–468.

57. Wazer DE, Willett BL. Clinical consideration in palliative treatment of metastatic prostate carcinoma. *Int J Radiat Oncol Biol Phys* 1987;13:145–146.

58. Haberman TE, Lopez RA. Metastatic disease of bone and treatment of pathologic fractures. *Ortho Clin North Am* 1989;20:469–486.

59. Rose CM, Kagan RA. The final report of the expert panel for the radiation oncology bone metastases work group of the American College of Radiology. *Int J Radiat Oncol Biol Phys* 1998;40:1117–1124.

60. Cairacross JG, Posner JB. Neurologic complications of systemic cancer. In: Yarbro JW, Bornstein RS, eds. *Oncologic emergencies*. New York: Grune & Stratton, 1988:75–96.

61. Gilbert H, Apuzzo M, et al. Neoplastic epidural spinal cord compression. *JAMA* 1978;240:2771–2773.

62. Delaney TF, Olfield EH. Spinal cord compression. In: DeVita V, Helhnan S, Rosenberg S, eds. *Cancer principles and practice of oncology*, 4th ed. Philadelphia, PA: JB Lippincott, 1993:2118–2127.

63. Bruchman JE, Bloomer WE. Management of spinal cord compression. *Semin Oncol* 1978;5:135.

64. Findlay GFG. Adverse effects of the management of spinal cord compression. *J Neurol Neurosurg Psych* 1984;47:761–768.

65. Maranzano E, Latini P, Checcaglini F, et al. Radiation therapy in metastatic spinal cord compression: a prospective analysis of 105 consecutive patients. *Cancer* 1991;67:1311–1317.

66. Maranzano E, Latini P. Short-course radiotherapy (8 Gy × 2) in metastatic spinal cord compression: an effective and feasible treatment. *Int J Radiat Oncol Biol Phys* 1997;3 8(5):1037–1044.

67. Coia LR. The role of radiation therapy in the treatment of brain metastases. *Int J Radiat Oncol Biol Phys* 1992;23(1):229–238.

68. Coia LR, Hanks GE, Marts K, et al. Practice patterns of palliative care for the United States 1984–1985. *Int J Radiat Oncol Biol Phys* 1988;14:1261–1269.

69. DeAngelis L, Delattre J, Posner J. Radiation induced dementia in patients cured of brain metastases. *Neurology* 1989;39:789.

70. Kondziolka D, Patel A, Lunsford LD, et al. Stereotactic radiosurgery plus whole brain radiotherapy versus radiotherapy alone for patients with multiple brain metastases. *Int J Radiat Oncol Biol Phys* 1999;45(2):427–434.

71. Saitoh Y, Fujisawa T, Shiba M, et al. Prognostic factors in surgical treatment of solitary brain metastasis after resection of non-small-cell lung cancer. *Lung Cancer* 1999;24(2):99–106.

72. Smalley S, Schray M. Lans E, et al. adjuvant radiation therapy after surgical resection of solitary brain metastasis: association with pattern of failure and survival. *Int J Radiat Oncol Biol Phys* 1987;13:1611.

73. Pirzkall A, Debus J, Lohr F, et al. Radiosurgery alone or in combination with whole-brain radiotherapy for brain metastases. *J Clin Oncol* 1998;16(11):3563–3569.

74. Patchell RA, Tibbs PA, Regine WF, et al. Postoperative radiotherapy in the treatment of single metastases to the brain: a randomized trial. *JAMA* 1998;280(17):1485–1489.

75. Buschke F, Parker RG. Palliative radiation therapy of the patients with incurable cancer. In: Buschke F, Parker RG. *Radiation therapy in cancer management*. New York: Grune & Stratton, 1972:363–373.

76. Egelmeers A, Goor C, van Meerbeeck J, et al. Palliative effectiveness of radiation therapy in the treatment of superior vena cava syndrome. *Bull Cancer Radiother* 1996;83(3):153–157.

77. Saunders KB, Rudolf M, Banks RA, Riordan JF. Central airways obstruction in carcinoma of the bronchus treated by radiotherapy: a study of pulmonary function. *Br J Radiol* 1978;51(604):286–290.

78. Bleehen NM, Girling DJ, Machin D, et al. A Medical Reserach Council (MRC) randomized trial of palliative radiotherapy with two fractions or a single fraction in patients with in-operable non-small lung cancer (NSCLC) and poor performance status. *Br J Cancer* 1992;65:934–941.

79. Chetty KG, Moran EM, Sassoon CS, et al. Effect of radiation therapy on bronchial obstruction due to bronchogenic carcinoma. *Chest* 1989;95(3):582–584.

80. Mehta M, Shahabi S, Jarjour N, et al. Effect of endobronchial radiation therapy on malignant bronchial obstruction. *Chest* 1990;97(3):662–665.

81. Kraiphibul P, Srisupundit S, Kiatgumjaikajorn S, Pairachvet V. The experience in using whole pelvic irradiation in management of massive bleeding from carcinoma of the uterine cervix. *J Med Assoc Thai* 1993;76(Suppl 1):78–81.

82. Borgelt BB, Gelber IR, et al. Palliation of hepatic metastases. Results of RTOG pilot study. *Int J Radiat Oncol Biol Phys* 1978;7:587–591.

83. Sherman DM, et al. Palliation of hepatic metastases. *Cancer* 1978;41:2013–2017.

84. Scarantino CW, Caplan R, Rotman M, et al. A phase I/II study to evaluate the effect of fractionated hemibody irradiation in the treatment of osseous bone metastases-RTOG 88-22. *Int J Radiat Oncol Biol Phys* 1996;36:37–48.

85. Poulter CA, Cosmatos D, Rubin P, et al. A report of RTOG 8206: a phase III study of whether the addition of a single dose hemibody irradiation to standard fractionated local field irradiation is more effective than local irradiation alone in the treatment of symptomatic osseous metastases. *Int J Radiat Oncol Biol Phys* 1992;23:207–214.

86. Salazar OM, DaMotta NW, Bridgman SM, et al. Fractionated half-body irradiation for pain palliation in widely metastatic cancers: comparison with single dose. *Int J Radiat Oncol Biol Phys* 1996;36(1):49–60.

87. Morris DE. Clinical experience with retreatment for palliation. *Sem Radiat Oncol* 2000;10(3):210–221.

88. Eisbruch A, Dawson L. Re-irradiation of head and neck tumors. Benefits and toxicities. *Hematol Oncol Clin North Am* 1999;13(4):825–836.

89. McLean M, Chow E, O'Sullivan B, et al. Re-irradiation for locally recurrent nasopharyngeal carcinoma. *Radiother Oncol* 1998;48(2):209–11.

90. Cooper JS, Steinfeld AD, Lerch IA. Cerebral metastases: value of re-irradiation in selected patients. *Radiology* 1990;174(3 pt 1):883–885.

91. Eng, TY et al. High dose small field re-irradiation of brain tumors using a modified radiosurgery technique. *J Radiosurgery* 1998;1(4):273–279.

92. Jeremic B, Shibamoto Y, Igrutinovic I. Single 4 Gy re-irradiation for painful bone metastasis following single fraction radiotherapy. *Radiother Oncol* 1999;52(2):123–127.

93. Nieder C, Milas L, Ang KK. Tissue tolerance to reirradiation. *Sem Radiat Oncol* 2000;10(3):200–209.

94. International Commission on Radiation Units (ICRU). ICRU Report #38: Dose and volume specification for reporting intracavitary therapy in gynecology, ppl-16. Bethesda, MD, ICRU, 1985.

95. Saito M, Yokoyama A, Kurita Y, et al. Treatment of roentgenographically occults endobronchial carcinoma with external beam radiotherapy and intraluminal low dose rate brachytherapy. *Int J Radiat Oncol Biol Phys* 1996;34(5):1029–1035.

96. Kato H, Kagami Y, Tachimori Y, et al. Tumor bed implant brachytherapy for residual carcinoma after palliative esophagectomy. *J Surg Oncol* 1996;62(3):214–217.

97. Shasha D, Harrison LB. The role of brachytherapy for palliation. *Sem Radiat Oncol* 2000;10(3):222–239.

98. Huber RM, Fischer R, Hautmann H, et al. Palliative endo-bronchial brachytherapy for central lung tumors. A prospective, randomized comparison of two fractionation schedules. *Chest* 1995;107(2):463–467.

99. Sur RK, Donde B, Levin VC, Mannell A. Fractionated high dose rate intraluminal brachytherapy in palliation of advanced esopha-geal cancer. *Int J Radiat Oncol Biol Phys* 1998;40(2):447–453.

100. Jager J, Langendijk H, Pannebakker M, Rijken J, de Jong J. A single session of intraluminal brachytherapy in palliation of oesophageal cancer. *Radiother Oncol* 1995;37(3):237–240.

101. Montemaggi P, Morganti AG, Dobelbower RR Jr, et al. Role of intraluminal brachytherapy in extrahepatic bile duct and pancreatic cancers: is it just for palliation? *Radiology* 1996;199(3):861–6.

102. Brewster AE, Davidson SE, Makin WP, et al. Intraluminal brachy-therapy using the high dose rate microselectron in the palliation of carcinoma of the oesophagus. *Clin Oncol (R Coll Radiol)* 1995; 7(2):102–105.

103. Stitt JA. High dose rate brachytherapy in the treatment of cervical carcinoma. *Hematol Oncol Clin North Am* 1999;13(3):vii–viii, 585–593.

104. Bedwinek J, Petty A, Bruton C, et al. The use of high dose rate endobronchial brachtherapy to palliate symptomatic endobron-chial recurrence of previously irradiated carcinoma. *Int J Radiat Oncol Biol Phys* 1992;22:23–30.

105. Langendijk JA, Tjwa MK, de Jong JM, et al. Massive haemoptysis after radiotherapy in inoperable non-small cell lung carcinoma: is endobronchial brachytherapy really a risk factor? *Radiother Oncol* 1998;49(2):175–183.

106. Serafini AN. Current status of systemic intravenous radiopharma-ceuticals for the treatment of painful metastatic bone disease. *Int J Radiat Oncol Biol Phys* 1994;30(5):1187–1194.

107. McEwan AJB. Use of radionuclides for the palliation of bone metastases. *Sem Radiat Oncol* 2000;10(2):103–114.

108. Silberstein EB. Systemic radiopharmaceutical therapy of painful osteoblastic metastases. *Sem Radiat Oncol* 2000;10(3):240–249.

109. Robinson RG, Preston DF, Spicer JA, Baxter KG. Radionuclide therapy of intractable bone pain: emphasis on strontium-89. *Semin Nucl Med* 1992;22(1):28–32.

110. Silberstein, EB. The treatment of painful osseous metastases with phosphorous-32-labeled phosphates. *Sem Oncol* 1993;20(3)(Suppl 2):11–21.

111. Porter AT. Use of strontium-89 in metastatic cancer: US and UK experience. *Oncology* 1994;8 (11)(Suppl):25–29.

112. Bolger JJ, Dearnaley DP, et al. Strontium-89 (Metastron) versus external beam radiotherapy in patients with painful bone metas-tases secondary to prostatic cancer: preliminary report of a multi-center trial. *Sem Oncol* 1993;20(3)(Suppl 2):32–33.

113. Porter AT, McEwan, AJB. Strontium-89 as an adjuvant to external beam radiation improves pain relief and delays disease progression in advanced prostate cancer: results of a randomized controlled trial. *Sem Oncol* 199320(3)(Suppl 2):38–43.

114. Serafini AN, Houston SJ, Resche I, et al. Palliation of pain associ-ated with metastatic bone cancer using samarium-153 Lexidronam. a double-blind placebo-controlled clinical trial. *J Clin Oncol* 1998; 16(4):1574–1581.

115. Holmes RA. Radiopharmaceuticals in clinical trials. *Sem Oncol* 199320(3)(Suppl 2):22–26.

116. Knox SJ, Meredith RF. Clinical radioimmunotherapy. *Sem Radiat Oncol* 2000;10(2):73–93.

117. Buchsbaum DJ. Experimental radioimmunotherapy. *Sem Radiat Oncol* 2000;10(2):156–167.

118. Emami B, Lyman J, Brown A, et al. Tolerance of normal tissue to therapeutic irradiation. *Int J Radiat Oncol Biot Phys* 1991;21(1): 109–122.

119. Cox DJ, Stetz J, Pajak TF. Toxicity criteria of the Radiation Ther-apy Oncology Group (RTOG) and the European Organization for Research and Treatment of Cancer (EORTC). *Int J Radiat Oncol Biol Phys* 1995;31(5):1341–1346.

120. Ferrell, B. The cost of comfort: economics of pain management in oncology. *Oncology Economics* 2000;1(9):56–61.

CHAPTER **42**

Cancer Pain: Psychological Management

Janette L. Seville and Tim A. Ahles

Cancer pain impacts the quality of life of a significant proportion of patients with various types of cancer. Bonica (1) estimated that 20% to 50% of cancer patients experience pain at diagnosis and that approximately 50% of patients with advanced disease experience moderate to severe pain. Pain at or above a moderate level has been found to significantly impair patients' ability to enjoy life, including work, mood, sleep, general activity, walking, and relationships with others (2,3). Additionally, uncontrolled pain has been identified as a major factor contributing to suicidal ideation or the wish for a hastened death in cancer patients (4). Despite the significant negative impact of pain on the lives of cancer patients, evidence continues to suggest that cancer pain is not optimally managed in many cases. This stands in stark contrast to data suggesting that 80% to 90% of patients should receive good pain control through the application of the World Health Organization (WHO) guidelines (5,6).

Cancer pain has traditionally been managed through a unidimensional or medical model that generally assumes that pain is related to an identifiable pathophysiological process and that the amount of pain is proportional to the extent of tissue damage. The logical treatments associated with this model focus on pharmacological, surgical, and radiological approaches (7,8). Although medical treatment methods for cancer pain have significantly advanced, they have not entirely addressed the cancer pain problem because there continue to be limitations in effectiveness and problems with negative side effects/complications. These approaches also do not address the psychosocial impact of cancer pain.

Although medication management continues to be the mainstay of cancer pain treatment, a number of clinicians and researchers have recognized the importance of addressing psychological and behavioral factors related to coping with cancer pain as well. Recognition of the multifactorial nature of pain is not unique for cancer pain. In fact, multidimensional models of chronic nonmalignant pain have been accepted and described in the clinical and research literature for some time (9). Evidence supporting the use of this multidimensional treatment model for the treatment of cancer pain has been slower in coming. The evidence that is available suggests that the combination of medical, behavioral, and psychological pain management techniques represents the optimal approach for managing cancer pain. This chapter will review the multidimensional model of cancer pain management, psychological treatment strategies appropriate for cancer patients, and possible unique ways to deliver these interventions in a changing health-care system.

MULTIDIMENSIONAL PERSPECTIVE OF PAIN

Theories of pain perception have progressed from a unidimensional sensory model to a multidimensional model, in large measure due to the pioneering work of Melzack and Wall (10). The development of the gate control theory provided a conceptual framework for the development of multidimensional models of pain. Researchers examining noncancer-related pain have provided extensive data supporting the conceptual utility of the gate control theory in understanding how emotional and behavioral factors impact upon the perception and report of pain (9,11). From a multidimensional perspective, pain perception is conceptualized as an experience made up of several interacting components: (a) physiological, (b) sensory, (c) affective, (d) cognitive, and (e) behavioral. A comprehensive review of this model and its applicability to cancer pain research can be found in a previous publication (12). The components of the model are summarized below.

The physiological aspect of pain includes the pathophysiology and psychophysiology of the pain. All pain is not of the same quality, and the cause of the pain can greatly impact an individual's perception of the pain.

Bonica (1) has classified cancer pain into categories that include pain due to direct tumor involvement, pain syndromes associated with treatment (e.g., postmastectomy pain), and pain caused by cancer-induced pathophysiological changes (paraneoplastic syndromes). Whereas some of these pains may develop into chronic pain, others are relatively acute. Depending on the stage of disease and current treatment, a patient may have a combination of acute and chronic pains. Pain treatment, therefore, would vary depending on the source and potentially the chronicity of the pain.

Sensory aspects of pain include attributes such as the intensity, location, and quality of the pain. Pain intensity is the most commonly measured sensory parameter, and numerous self-report methods have been developed to try to assess this subjective aspect of pain (13). Pain intensity is usually the most salient aspect of pain for patients. However, because patients may have numerous sources and locations of pain they may find it difficult to accurately report the extent of pain. For example, Foley (14) found that cancer patients usually reported only their "worst" pain. A careful interview in conjunction with a pain diagram from the McGill Pain Questionnaire (15) can provide useful information about the extent and location of the pain.

Behavioral aspects of pain are the observable behaviors that communicate pain to other people. These typically include medication intake as well as behaviors such as guarding, bracing, groaning, and grimacing. Fordyce's (16) application of an operant conditioning model to pain behaviors posits that pain behaviors can be influenced by environmental factors such as attention, social support, or avoidance of unpleasant tasks (e.g., housework). Reliable and valid methods (e.g., Keefe & Block [17]) of assessing this aspect of patients has been developed and consists of videotaping and rating specific pain behaviors while the patient is doing set tasks such as lying down, sitting, standing, and walking. Whereas most research in this area has been done on observing patients with chronic nonmalignant pain, such as low back pain, similar observational methods have been developed for the study of cancer pain patients (18).

The affective and cognitive components of pain address the role that thoughts, attitude, mood, and attention play in the perception of pain. Several studies have supported the hypothesis that affective variables (i.e., patients becoming emotionally aroused) are influenced by cancer pain (see Ahles and Martin [19] for a broader review). For example, when people interpret pain as a disease threat they can become emotionally aroused. They may believe that an increase in pain intensity or a new pain location could be an indication of disease progression. However, pain is influenced by so many factors, physical overactivity being one factor, that pain is usually not the most reliable factor in determining disease progression.

There is evidence that these beliefs about the meaning of pain strongly influence how patients react emotionally. Ahles and colleagues (20) found that 61% of patients were concerned that changes in pain were indicative of a deteriorating condition. Those patients who believed that their pain was an indicator of disease progression had significantly higher scores on measures of anxiety and depression compared to patients who did not consider their pain as an indicator of a worsening condition. Spiegel and Bloom (21) reported that the belief that pain signals a worsening of their condition, and the related emotional distress, predicted the reporting of pain. However, the site of metastases in women with advanced breast cancer was not reliably associated with pain. Further, Daut and Cleeland (22) found that cancer patients who attributed their pain to causes other than cancer reported less interference in daily activities. Taken together, these studies indicate the importance of addressing cognitive and affective aspects of cancer pain in order to improve quality of life and cancer pain management.

Although many clinicians and researchers acknowledge the multidimensional nature of pain, often the patient has the unidimensional or medical model in mind, that is, the belief that pain intensity is equivalent to the amount of tissue damage or disease progression. Patients may not understand why they are being questioned about their mood, behaviors, feelings, and thoughts. A clear succinct explanation to patients can help them to better understand ways to control their pain, improve treatment adherence, and decrease their concerns that the health-care provider thinks that the pain may be "all in their head" or an "overreaction."

Stress-pain Cycle

The interactions of these pain components can be described to patients with verbal and visual representations of the gate control theory and the "stress-pain model." Most patients respond well to a clear explanation of the stress-pain cycle such as given here:

A number of factors can affect the pain you feel along with the extent of the injury (or tumor size). In fact, the way you feel emotionally can have a strong physical effect on your body and, in turn, on the degree of pain you feel. When a person is feeling stressed or worried, the body responds by increasing heart rate, blood pressure, releasing more chemicals like adrenaline, and by increasing muscle tension. This increased tension and physical response can lead to greater pain. Imagine having a severe low back pain and then trying to tighten up the back muscles even more. That would really increase the pain! The increased pain then becomes another source of stress to the body. As one can see from the following diagram, this becomes a vicious cycle of pain and stress that can seem endless.

We will work together to help you learn several ways to manage your pain better and to break up this vicious pain cycle. For example, relaxation strategies can help you reduce the strong physical responses that increase muscle tension and that release pain-enhancing chemicals in your body. By learning problem-solving strategies, improving communication skills, and learning ways to reduce worry and negative thinking, you can better manage stress. The pain itself can be better managed by learning ways to pace your physical activities so that you don't push yourself too hard physically or become too inactive.

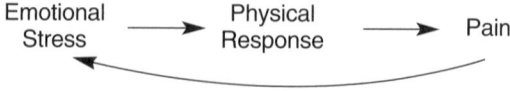

Patients with cancer pain may actively seek out treatment rather than worry that their pain is marginalized as being "in their head." Several researchers have demonstrated that cancer patients actively seek out strategies for managing their pain (23–26). However, the strategies utilized are often based on common sense or word of mouth from other patients rather than any empirically tested methods. Fortunately, there is gathering evidence as to the efficacy of some psychological interventions for cancer pain control.

REVIEW OF THE LITERATURE ON PSYCHOLOGICAL APPROACHES TO THE MANAGEMENT OF CANCER PAIN

Personal control has been shown to improve pain management (27). For example, Hill, Chapman, Kornell, Sullivan, Saeger, and Benedetti (28) demonstrated that bone marrow transplant patients with oral mucositis utilized less morphine when given control of narcotic administration through the use of patient-controlled analgesia (PCA) as compared to patients who received morphine by continuous infusion. Many psychological interventions, particularly cognitive behavioral, are designed to enhance personal control. Often cognitive-behavioral interventions are described to patients as pain "self-management" because the patient is taught specific techniques, strategies, and new habits that can reduce pain and prevent pain flareups.

One of the difficulties inherent in clinically providing psychological pain management for cancer patients, and for studying psychological approaches to the management of cancer pain, is that these techniques and habit changes typically require time to learn and become effective. There are several levels of psychological intervention available, however, to match patient needs and clinical resources. The range of interventions can be anywhere from simple educational pamphlets to multiple sessions of cognitive-behavioral coping skills training. In the next section we will review the various types of interventions and evidence supporting their efficacy for cancer pain management.

Educational Interventions

Several studies have examined the utility of educational interventions for nonmalignant pain (29–31). Most of these interventions have been developed from the theoretical perspective that providing accurate information allows for the development of accurate expectations, which, in turn, reduce distress and symptom focus (32). Educational interventions for cancer patients have primarily focused on knowledge about the disease, its progression, and various treatment options. Although there are educational materials available for cancer pain patients to view (e.g., Agency for Health Care Policy and Research [33]), few research studies have been published specifically demonstrating the efficacy of cancer pain education for patients. The studies that are available for review primarily focus on knowledge about pain medication. For example, Rimer and colleagues (34) assigned 230 mixed-diagnosis cancer patients to one of two groups: control or intervention. The intervention group received written information about pharmacological issues and 15 minutes of tailored individual counseling. One month later, members of the intervention group reported significantly better medication compliance and were more likely to believe they had some control over their pain than did the control group. In addition, intervention patients were less fearful of the possibility of addiction and tolerance to pain medications. There was no significant difference in pain reports between the two groups, however.

Ferrell and colleagues (35) did find an impact on pain ratings in their study where they stratified 40 cancer patients by age into either elderly (60–75 years) or oldest (older than 75 years) and then randomly assigned them to either the usual-care control group or intervention. The intervention consisted of three sessions that gave instruction regarding (a) general pain knowledge, (b) pharmacological management of pain, and (c) nondrug pain strategies such as relaxation/distraction, imagery, heat/cold, and massage. Caregivers for the intervention patients were encouraged to attend the sessions as well. The intervention resulted in increased knowledge about pain medications and increased pain medication use. Further, the patients receiving the intervention reported significantly decreased fear of addiction, pain intensity, perception of pain severity, and anxiety. Changes were also noted in caregiver behaviors such as the provision of adequate doses and consistent administration of pain medications.

Finally, De Wit and colleagues (36) selected 313 cancer patients in the Netherlands who either had district nursing or did not. These two groups of patients were then randomly assigned to one of two groups: care as usual or intervention. The content of the intervention was very similar to the Ferrell study (35) but was delivered in one session with two telephone followups. Longitudinal assessment indicated that patients who received the intervention had significantly greater pain knowledge. Some intervention patients also reported significantly less intense pain up to 8 weeks posttreatment, but this held true only for patients without a district nurse.

These three studies taken together suggest that cancer pain education alone appears to be especially helpful for patients to improve medication adherence and to reduce fear of addiction. This new knowledge can, in turn, lead to better overall pain management and less pain for some patients.

Hypnosis

One of the earliest descriptions of the use of hypnosis for pain relief in cancer was provided by a series of papers by Butler (37–40). Since that time, several additional case reports have appeared that suggest that hypnosis is effective for approximately 50% of the patients so treated (41–48). A close examination of the case reports suggests that a significant number of patients treated with hypnosis were experiencing psychological difficulties such as anxiety and depression. Therefore, hypnosis may reduce the self-report of pain by influencing the affective component of pain as well as by directly altering the sensory component of pain.

Support for this hypothesis was provided in the only control-group outcome study of hypnosis found in the literature. Spiegel and Bloom (49) studied a group of women with metastatic breast carcinoma. These women were randomly assigned to one of three groups: (a) psychological support group only, (b) psychological support group plus self-hypnotic training, and (c) a no-treatment control group. Their results demonstrated that the two treatments produced reduced reports of pain and suffering posttreatment as compared to the control group. Additionally, patients who received self-hypnosis training reported significantly less pain than patients who were treated with the support group alone. Finally, patients in the treatment groups reported an improvement in mood measured on the Profile of Mood States, and this improvement was inversely correlated with reports of pain.

These data support the hypothesis that hypnosis is effective in managing cancer-related pain and that reduction of pain is associated with elevations in mood. However, caution must be taken in interpreting this correlation because, as the authors point out, it is equally plausible to assume that decreased pain caused the elevation in mood as to assume that the elevation in mood caused the decrease in reported pain. Further caution must be taken in interpreting the results of the study because 41% of the patients reported no pain at baseline, and only six patients in the entire sample were taking prescription analgesics. Therefore, the patients in this sample appear to have been experiencing a relatively low level of pain. However, it is less clear, from these data, how effective these techniques would be for patients with moderate to severe pain. Interestingly, a close examination of the results reveals that patients receiving self-hypnosis training reported no increase in pain over time, whereas the control patients reported significantly more pain over time.

Relaxation and Biofeedback

Although relaxation and biofeedback techniques have been suggested for use with cancer patients, only two studies utilizing relaxation exercises and two studies utilizing biofeedback have examined the application of these techniques to the management of cancer-related pain. Fleming (50) reported that 36 of 58 patients with far-advanced cancer reported a reduction in several symptoms, including pain, after receiving relaxation training. However, no statistical analysis was reported that would allow an evaluation of the efficacy of the relaxation training in the control of pain specifically.

A methodologically stronger study (51) randomly assigned 60 hospitalized cancer patients experiencing pain to one of three groups. For 2 weeks each group received either routine care, progressive muscle relaxation and guided imagery training by audiotape, or progressive relaxation and guided imagery training by a live nurse instructor. Both intervention groups were found to have lower pain ratings and required less nonopioid pain medication than the control group.

Fotopoulos and colleagues (52) examined the utility of biofeedback techniques in the reduction of cancer-related pain. In their first study, these authors examined the influence of a combination of EMG and theta EEG biofeedback on the pain reports of seven cancer patients. All seven patients showed significant reductions in reported pain during biofeedback sessions; however, only two patients were able to obtain significant relief at home. In a similar study (53), these authors treated 12 patients with a combination of EMG and skin conductance level (SCL) biofeedback. Complete data were available on only five of the patients (two died, three became too ill to participate, and one moved from the area). Two of the five patients were able to reliably reduce their pain outside the biofeedback laboratory, and three of five reduced their use of analgesic medications.

The patients seen by Fleming had far-advanced cancer and were being cared for in a hospice. Additionally, the patients seen by Fotopoulos and colleagues had failed to respond to all other pain management modalities. Therefore, their pain was difficult to control, and many of them saw biofeedback as their last resort. Despite this, the results suggest that relaxation and biofeedback may hold promise for reducing the suffering of cancer-related pain. Control group outcome studies, particularly with patients who have not failed all other pain management attempts, are clearly necessary.

Multimodal Treatment Approaches

The studies described earlier have essentially utilized single modalities for the management of cancer pain; however, Ahles and colleagues (20) have argued that treatments need to be designed that target each of the multiple components of cancer pain. Table 42-1 demonstrates how treatment components can address all dimensions of pain.

Turk and Rennert (54) described a multicomponent, cognitive-social learning approach designed specifically for the management of cancer-related pain. The treatment package consists of four components: (a) pretreatment preparation, (b) conceptualization-translation, (c) coping skills training (e.g., relaxation and distraction techniques), and (d) rehearsal. Their goal was to design a treatment package that targeted the various components of the pain experience; however, they provided no data supporting the efficacy of their treatment package.

Dalton, Toomey, and Workman (55) randomized 16 mixed-diagnosis cancer patients with cancer-related pain to one of three groups. The three groups were: (a) relaxation alone, (b) relaxation plus distraction techniques and massage, (c) no-treatment control. Both treatment groups reported greater pain relief compared to the no-treatment group. Additionally, patients who reported high expectations of relief reported greater improvement in pain, suggesting the importance of cognitive factors in pain relief.

Although these results are interesting, there are two major problems: (a) The sample size was very small (16 patients divided among three groups), and (b) the intervention consisted of only one session, which could have limited the effectiveness of the intervention. Despite these limitations, the data support the hypothesis that cognitive-behavioral strategies may be effective in managing cancer

TABLE 42-1. *Components of the multidimensional model of pain with the treatment components*

Model component	Treatment methods
Physiological	• Guided imagery • Progressive muscle relaxation • Breathing strategies • Meditation
Sensory	• Activity pacing • Pain medication
Affective	• Challenging negative thoughts • Increasing pleasurable activities
Cognitive	• Education about cancer, medication, and pain • Distraction • Challenging negative thoughts
Behavioral	• Activity pacing • Exercise • Working with family members to ignore pain behaviors and reinforce well behaviors

pain and that individual differences (e.g., expectations of control) may be important mediating factors.

The importance of perceived control was also noted in a more recent study where 24 metastatic breast cancer patients were randomly assigned to one of three groups: (a) control; (b) relaxation and visualization; or (c) relaxation, visualization, and additional cognitive coping skills (56). The researcher found no differences in pain intensity ratings, distress level, or mood. The ratings of their perceived ability to decrease pain, however, were found to be significantly improved with a nurse's instruction on relaxation, distraction, visualization, and positive self statements. The limitations of this study are similar to the previous one in that sample size was small and the educational interventions extremely brief (75 minutes long for group 2 and 120 minutes long for group 3). Posttreatment measures were administered immediately after the intervention so patients had no time to utilize these skills in their daily lives for pain or mood management.

In a study (57) conducted at the Pain Relief Unit of Kidwai Memorial Institute of Oncology, Bangalore, India (52), patients were randomly assigned to two groups. The first group received "a combination of biofeedback-induced relaxation training and cognitive-behavioral techniques based on the principals of the operant and the stress inoculation methods," and the second group received medical management only. Sitaram (57) reported that at posttreatment the cognitive-behavioral group reported significantly reduced indices of pain (both visual analog scales and parameters from the McGill Pain Questionnaire), lower electrodermal activity, and improved mood compared to the medical management-only group.

To date, this study has been reported in abstract form only; therefore, many details are not available to completely evaluate the study (e.g., it is unclear which "cognitive-behavioral strategies" were used, and basic descriptions of the study population, including diagnosis and types of pain, are not available). Additionally, although the results appear very encouraging, patients were seen for 30 treatment sessions. Such an intensive treatment protocol is logistically impractical in most American cancer centers.

In more recent studies, Syrjala and colleagues (58,59) have published two reports comparing various combinations of psychological techniques for pain relief. The first study (58) compared 67 cancer patients with oral mucositis pain undergoing bone marrow transplant who were randomly assigned to either usual care, hypnosis, therapist support, or cognitive-behavioral skills other than guided imagery. They found that only hypnosis resulted in significant reduced pain reports, as compared to usual care, after transplant.

In a more recent publication, Syrjala and colleagues (59) tracked pain reports of 94 cancer patients receiving usual care as compared to three active interventions for patients with oral mucositis pain undergoing bone marrow transplant. One treatment group received therapist support, which consisted of active reassurance related to procedures and positive reframing of the patient's status. A second group received relaxation and imagery training. A third treatment group received the same training as the second plus additional cognitive-behavioral coping skills such as distraction, goal setting, and cognitive restructuring of negative thinking. It was concluded that relaxation and imagery training significantly reduced pain reports. The addition of other cognitive-behavioral coping strategies was not found to be additive to relaxation and imagery in terms of pain relief.

The studies investigating psychological treatment for cancer pain management do not show any one coping technique to be superior to all others in clinical populations. Given that the evidence in nonmalignant pain supports multidimensional approaches, such as cognitive-behavioral treatment, multidimensional approaches are currently considered state of the art for psychological cancer pain treatment. Several pamphlets, designed to inform patients and their families and/or health professionals about pain management, mention cognitive-behavioral strategies as being potentially effective (examples of pamphlets include *Pain Control in the Patient with Cancer*, American Cancer Society; *Cancer Pain Can Be Relieved: A Guide for Patients and Families*, Wisconsin Cancer Pain Initiative; *Coping with Pain at Home*, Du Pont Pharmaceuticals).

DESCRIPTION OF SELECTED PSYCHOLOGICAL TREATMENT COMPONENTS

Several publications (4,60–65) have described psychological interventions helpful for nonmalignant pain and, less frequently, cancer pain management. Selected psychological strategies will be reviewed here that appear most relevant for cancer pain management. A sample treatment protocol is included in Table 42-2 to demonstrate the sequence and typical breadth of techniques.

As can be seen in Table 42-2, pain education, stress management, and coping skills training are often combined for pain and distress reduction. The main focus of coping skills training is to help the patient acquire self-management skills that can be applied when needed to help prevent and reduce pain or psychological distress. The focus is not on resolving deeper emotional conflicts but more on developing skills to handle the day-to-day challenges of living with cancer and pain. This skill building can improve self-efficacy and lead to a greater sense of control over pain.

Relaxation and Imagery

The goal of relaxation strategies is to reduce overall emotional arousal and to reduce muscle tension. Relaxation has been found to decrease perceived pain intensity as well as increase tolerance to pain (66). Relaxation can be taught in many ways, including progressive muscle relaxation (67,68), diaphragmatic breathing, biofeedback

TABLE 42-2. *Sample treatment protocol*

Session 1
  Introduction of multidimensional model of cancer pain
  Introduction of self-management model of pain

Session 2
  Rationale for relaxation
  Breathing retraining
  Progressive muscle relaxation
  Guided imagery

Session 3
  Introduction to cognitive techniques
  Challenging unhelpful thoughts or decreasing
    catastrophizing
  Distraction

Session 4
  Physical activity regulation
  Importance of conditioning
  Inactivity versus overactivity
  How to pace activities optimally without overdoing it

Session 5
  The role of emotions in pain
  Enhancing mood with activity scheduling and problem
    solving
  Effective communication with family and health-care
    providers

Session 6
  Review and integration of techniques
  Preparing a pain flareup plan

assisted relaxation (69), and guided imagery (70,71). Probably the most frequently taught method of relaxation is a combination of diaphragmatic breathing and progressive muscle relaxation (PMR). PMR helps the patient reduce muscle tension by focusing attention on body sensations while systematically tensing and then relaxing a series of muscle groups.

Relaxation through imagery can be guided by the patient or by suggestion from someone else. The patient forms a mental image or picture associated with feelings of peacefulness and calm. Some patients, however, report that they are not able to form a mental picture or follow instructions such as "pretend you are lying on a warm tropical beach." It is important to have the patient include as many senses as possible into the image. For example, if patients are using a beach image, also suggest that they notice the smell of salt air, hear the waves come to the shore, feel the warm sand on their skin, etc.

Cognitive Restructuring

Cognitive restructuring is based on the model that emotional and physical responses to an event or symptom are based on the person's subjective interpretation of the event's meaning and the perceived ability to successfully handle to event (72). In the case of cancer, or cancer pain, the patient may very well be interpreting the cancer and pain as threats that cannot be effectively managed. Studies (58,59,73) that have already been reviewed in this chapter suggest that active cognitive coping skills can help cancer patients increase their perception of control and result in some reduction of pain and emotional distress. It should be emphasized that the goal of cognitive restructuring is not to convince patients that "everything is okay" but rather to help them focus on more helpful and active methods of reducing fear, pain, and suffering. An open discussion with patients can normalize the thoughts and feelings of fear and hopelessness while giving them skills to reduce the intensity of these negative feelings.

Creating new habits of thinking can reduce emotional distress and depression (74). Cognitive restructuring consists of teaching patients to challenge their own automatic negative thinking and coaching them to produce more helpful and accurate thoughts. Some clinicians incorrectly assume that this means simply giving patients positive affirmations, such as "I can handle this," to repeat to themselves. Rather, cognitive restructuring is a process that patients engage in to evaluate the accuracy of thoughts, possible alternative explanatory thoughts, and the helpfulness of their own thoughts in order to decide on the most adaptive attitude to adopt.

Introducing cognitive skills to patients in a way that is constructive is crucial in getting them to engage in the process. Following is an excerpt from one of our handouts that is used to provide the rationale to patients.

When pain does not go away quickly it is not unusual to worry about the pain or to worry more about other life problems. This worry, however, can negatively affect your physical recovery. Your thoughts about a situation determine how you feel emotionally and, in turn, affect how you physically react. Remember our pain cycle model from before:

Stress → Physical Response → More Pain.

Along with influencing the physical response and pain, your thoughts can also interfere with your behavior. For example, negative thoughts such as "nothing is going to help, so there's no point in even trying" can stop you from actively thinking through other ways to solve a problem. This type of negative thinking can also affect how motivated you are to do recommended exercise, take medication, or follow your doctor's advice. Although worry and negative "self-talk" about pain may feel as if it's beyond your control, there are ways to bring it under control.

This introduction is followed by specific instruction on how to identify and challenge negative thought patterns. Patients rate their degree of negative mood before and after their cognitive challenge to decide how effective the restructuring is for them.

Distraction

Another cognitive technique, known as *distraction,* encourages the patient to redirect attention away from pain or a perceived threatening situation (75). For example, playing video games, watching humorous videos, watching grandchildren play, and listening to music are sometimes useful distraction strategies. These strategies are most often used in acute procedural types of pain but are also helpful in reducing the suffering related to chronic pain.

Activity Pacing

Activity pacing, also known as *energy conservation,* is crucial for most cancer patients with pain. The increased fatigue that accompanies many treatments for cancer requires that patients do activities of daily living at a slower pace. In addition to the fatigue, if cancer patients are also experiencing pain, they must also figure out new ways to do tasks without significantly increasing their pain.

Many people find themselves becoming less active because it hurts to move, and they are fatigued, or they get frustrated with too little activity and push themselves even though it hurts. Both overactivity and inactivity can increase pain. The results of overactivity can be a sudden increase in pain and fatigue. On the other hand, if the patient is too inactive the muscles get deconditioned, and overall energy can drop. By pacing daily activities patients can gradually improve their ability to move around without causing pain flareups or setbacks. Therefore, they can actually be more functional by pacing activities because they won't spend as much time in extreme pain or with extreme fatigue, which can often stop them from doing daily activities.

Activity pacing is taught to patients by helping them break activities into smaller parts, encouraging frequent breaks, changing muscle groups, and planning these activities in such a way as to not overtax themselves at any one time. Many patients are told to "pace yourself" but do not know how to look at their daily habits in new ways. For example, doing a simple task such as washing the dishes may require washing only a few dishes at a time and then switching to relaxation practice or activities that use other muscle groups, such as making phone calls or paying bills.

Problem Solving

Problem solving is a structured method to identify pain-related or psychosocial problems and to systematically find ways to solve the problems that are contributing to emotional distress and pain. Problem solving consists of outlining the specific problem and then setting a specific goal designed to focus on some part of the problem. Goal setting is then followed by brainstorming possible solutions that could meet the specified goal. The pros and cons of each possible solution are then considered before deciding on a course of action. Although this strategy was traditionally researched in the context of depression management (76–78), it has also been applied to managing distress related to physical symptoms such as nonmalignant pain (79–82). Problem solving is not usually used in isolation for pain management but as a central component of a more comprehensive cognitive-behavioral treatment program; so it is difficult to determine its efficacy alone for general pain management.

The application of problem solving to cancer and cancer-related pain has been even more limited. Previous publications have proposed models for applying problem solving to family caregivers of cancer patients (83) and to cancer patients for managing general emotional distress (84). For example, Fawzy and colleagues (73) combined a modified problem-solving format, called "active coping," with communication skills training for patients with early stage melanoma. Patients who received the intervention had less emotional distress, had better survival rates at 6-year followup, and were using more active coping strategies than patients who received usual care. Pain was not measured in this study, however. As with the clinical research on nonmalignant pain, there are no specific studies related to the sole use of problem solving and cancer pain. Problem solving has been incorporated as one part of a larger package of cognitive-behavioral techniques for effective cancer pain management (e.g., Syrjala [58]).

CONTRAINDICATIONS FOR PROVIDING PSYCHOLOGICAL INTERVENTIONS FOR CANCER PAIN

Despite the general acceptance of the importance of psychological interventions for cancer pain management, there are some patients for whom these interventions are not appropriate. For example, psychological interventions are probably not appropriate if the patient is delirious, psychotic, rapidly deteriorating, vomiting, or experiencing severe uncontrolled pain (63). Appropriateness of timing for the intervention is usually determined through consultation of the treating physician with the behavioral specialist or psychologist trained to provide the psychological interventions.

There may be other challenges to providing appropriate psychological interventions for cancer pain, especially if there is no availability of appropriate specialists to provide assessment and treatment. If this is the case, medical staff may have to rely on educational materials only or alternative methods of service delivery. Patients may need alternative service delivery particularly if they are living in rural settings or if they are unable to travel to a central oncology center.

MODELS OF DELIVERY FOR PSYCHOLOGICAL PAIN TREATMENT

Traditional methods of delivering psychological pain management treatment include providing patients with educational materials, having them attend weekly pain groups facilitated by psychologists, or referring them for eight to ten individual counseling sessions with a psychologist or similarly trained behavioral specialist. These traditional methods have not been particularly effective for

some because of the lack of availability of professionals trained in cognitive-behavioral pain management techniques, particularly in rural settings. Additionally, physical status and multiple medical appointments of cancer patients frequently make attendance at individual or group pain management sessions logistically difficult. Finally, managed care has limited reimbursement for referrals to specialists in psychological pain management. These limitations have led to the investigation of new methods of delivery for psychological pain management that may be done within a practice and for less cost. In the past, most psychological treatments that have been practice-based have primarily been educational in nature. New models incorporate educational materials with brief specialized counseling to tailor the treatment plan for each patient. These models, however, are only proposed for investigation because they have not been clinically demonstrated in a cancer pain population.

Telephone-based and Minimal Contact Interventions

Although pain education may be an important part of pain management it has not proven to be sufficient to help all patients. One explanation of the limited effectiveness of pain education alone is that patients have difficulty applying it to their personal situation (85). One method to help tailor the strategies to individual patients so they can actually make lifestyle changes is to have a knowledgeable professional available to assist in identifying problem areas and to provide additional information when needed. These interventions need not be time intensive or even require an office visit. For example, some studies of headache treatment have demonstrated that minimal therapist contact interventions using phone appointments are as effective as office-based interventions (81,86) and can assist the patient in application of information and behavior change. Generally, these interventions include a structured intervention (e.g., books and/or tapes), two to three office visits spread over 2 to 3 months, and more frequent phone contact. The minimal therapist contact intervention with phone followups allows for more personal tailoring of the intervention.

In a recent preliminary study, Ahles and colleagues (82) randomly assigned patients with nonmalignant pain from primary-care settings to either care as usual or an intervention that included tailored educational materials and, for some patients, a nurse-educator intervention delivered over the phone. The nurse-educator intervention included training in basic pain management skills as described earlier and in a problem-solving approach designed to help patients cope with psychosocial problems. Chronic pain patients in the intervention group scored significantly better on the Pain, Physical, Emotional, and Social subscales of the SF-36 and on a measure of functional ability than did control patients. Examination of data from the process measure indicated that patients in the intervention group were slightly more knowledgeable about pain, felt more in control, were more satisfied with their treatment, and felt that the treatments provided were more effective than did the patients receiving usual care. Patients in the intervention group also evaluated their health-care team as better at providing a good explanation for the pain, listening to them about their pain, and providing help with stress and psychosocial problems. Based on this promising preliminary study showing that nonclinic-based interventions can be effective, a larger controlled trial is currently being conducted by Ahles and colleagues.

Group Medical Appointments, or Practice-based Intervention Groups

Group medical appointments (GMAs) are small group appointments that allow patients to interact with their physician/nurse team and receive education regarding their medical condition and self-management strategies in the context of a support group of patients who are coping with similar issues. GMAs offer a potentially effective and efficient approach to the management of chronic pain and cancer pain that has all the elements of an effective clinical encounter and can be integrated into primary-care settings or specialty care settings (87–89). The GMA approach appears to work particularly well for patients who have psychosocial problems and high need for emotional support (87)—a common situation in cancer patients. Researchers at Dartmouth are currently investigating the feasibility and efficacy of GMAs for pain management in primary care and hope to apply this approach to pain and symptom management in the oncology clinic.

SUMMARY AND CONCLUSIONS

Although pain medication will and should remain the mainstay of cancer pain treatment, there is growing evidence that psychological interventions can help provide pain relief and reduce suffering. Before psychological methods can gain widespread use and dissemination, however, their efficacy and effectiveness in practice must be established. Toward this end, this chapter has reviewed the current literature and highlighted the most promising strategies to date. In particular, comprehensive packages of coping skills implemented from a cognitive-behavioral model seem to be most helpful at present. Further research on matching treatments to patients and developing creative ways to deliver effective treatments is needed.

REFERENCES

1. Bonica JJ. Cancer pain. In: Bonica JJ, ed. *The management of pain.* 2nd ed. Philadelphia, PA: Lea & Febiger; 1990:400–460.
2. Cleeland CS. Assessment of pain in cancer: Measurement issues. In: Foley KM, Bonica JJ, Ventafridda V, eds, *Advances in pain research and therapy.* New York: Raven Press, 1990;16:47–56.
3. Wang XS, Cleeland CS, Mendoza TR., et al. The effects of pain severity on health-related quality of life: a study of Chinese cancer patients. *Cancer* 1999;86:1848–1855.
4. Breitbart W, Passik SD. Psychological and psychiatric interventions in pain control. In: Doyle D, Hanks GWC, MacDonald N, eds. *Oxford, textbook of palliative medicine.* Oxford: Oxford University Press, 1993:450–467.
5. Hill CS, Fields WS. *Advances in pain research and therapy (Vol.11): drug treatment of cancer pain in a drug-oriented society.* New York: Raven Press, 1989.
6. Jacox A, Carr DB, Payne R, et al. *Management of cancer pain. Clinical practice guideline number 9.* Rockville, MD: U.S. Department of Health and Human Services, Public Health Service, Agency for Health Care Policy and Research, AHCPR Pub. No. 94-0592, 1994.
7. Foley KM, Inturrisi, CE. Analgesic drug therapy in cancer pain: principles of practice. *Medical Clinics of North Americ,* 1987;71:207–232.
8. Portenoy RK. Practical aspects of pain control in the patient with cancer. *CA—Cancer Journal of Clinician,* 1988;38:327–352.
9. Turk DC, Meichenbaum D, Genest M. *Pain and behavioral medicine: a cognitive-behavioral perspective.* New York: Guilford Press, 1983.
10. Melzack R, Wall PD. Pain mechanisms: a theory. *Science* 1965;150:971–979.
11. Melzack R, Wall PD. *The challenge of pain.* New York: Basic Books, 1982.
12. Ahles T. Cancer pain: research from multidimensional and illness representation models. *Motivation and Emotion* 1993;17(3):225–243.
13. Tearnan B, Ward C. Assessment of the patient with cancer pain. *Hospice Journal,* 1992;8:49–72.
14. Foley K. Pain syndromes in patients with cancer. In: Bonica JJ, Ventafridda V, eds. *Advances in pain research and therapy.* New York: Raven Press, 1979;2:59–75.
15. Melzack R. The McGill Pain Questionnaire: major properties and scoring methods. *Pain* 1975;1:277–299.
16. Fordyce WE. *Behavioral methods of chronic pain and illness.* St. Louis, MO: Mosby, 1976.
17. Keefe FJ, Block AR. Development of an observation method for assessing pain behavior in chronic low back pain patients. *Behavior Therapy* 1982;13:363–375.
18. Ahles TA, Coombs DW, Jensen L, et al. Development of a behavioral observation technique for the assessment of pain behaviors in cancer patients. *Behavior Therapy* 1990;21:449–460.
19. Ahles TA, Martin JB. Cancer pain: a multidimensional perspective. *Hospice Journal,* 1992;8:25–48.
20. Ahles TA, Blanchard EB, Ruckdeschel JC. The multidimensional nature of cancer-related pain. *Pain* 1983;17:272–288.
21. Spiegel D, Bloom JR. Pain in metastatic breast cancer. *Cancer* 1983;52:341–345.
22. Daut RI, Cleeland CS. The prevalence and severity of pain in cancer. *Cancer* 1982;50:1913–1918.
23. Arathuzik D. Pain experience for metastatic breast cancer patients: unraveling the mystery. *Cancer Nursing* 1991;14:41–48.
24. Wilke D, Lovejoy N, Dodd M, Tesler M. Cancer pain control behaviors: description and correlation with pain intensity. *Oncology Nursing Forum* 1988;15:723–731.
25. Bressler LR, Hange PA, McGuire DB. Characterization of the pain experience in a sample of cancer outpatients. *Oncology Nursing Forum* 1986;13:51–55.
26. Donovan MI, Dillon P. Incidence and characteristics of pain in a sample of hospitalized cancer patients. *Cancer Nursin,* 1987;10:85–92.
27. Thompson SC. Will it hurt less if I can control it? A complex answer to a simple question. *Psychological Bulletin* 1981;90:89–101.
28. Hill HF, Chapman CR, Kornell JA, et al. Self-administered morphine in bone marrow transplant patients reduces drug requirement. *Pain* 1990;40:121–129.
29. Lindroth Y, Bauman A, Barnes C, et al. A controlled evaluation of arthritis education. *British Journal of Rheumatology* 1989;28(1):7–12.
30. Cherkin DC, Deyo RA, Street JH, et al. Pitfalls of patient education. Limited success of a program for back pain in primary care. *Spine* 1996;21(3):345–55.
31. Roland M, Dixon M. Randomized controlled trial of an educational booklet for patients presenting with back pain in general practice. *Journal of the Royal College of General Practitioners* 1989;39:244–246.

32. Leventhal H, Leventhal EA. Affect, cognition, and symptom perception. In: Chapman CR, Foley KM, eds. *Current and emerging issues in cancer pain: research and practice.* New York: Raven Press, 1993: 153–174.

33. Agency for Health Care Policy and Research. *Clinical practice guidelines on management of cancer pain: No. 9. Patient guide* (AHCPR Publication No. 94-0595). Rockville, MD: U.S. Department of Health and Human Services, 1994.

34. Rimer B, Levy MH, Keintz MK, et al. Enhancing cancer pain control regimens through patient education. *Patient Education Counseling* 1987;10:267–277.

35. Ferrell BR, Rhiner M, Ferrell BA Development and implementation of a pain education program. *Cancer* 1993;72(11):3426–3432.

36. de Wit R, van Dam F, Zanbelt L, et al. A pain education program for chronic cancer pain patients: follow-up results from a randomized controlled trial. *Pain* 1997;73:55–69.

37. Butler B. The use of hypnosis in the care of the cancer patient. *Cancer* 1954;1:1–14.

38. Butler B. The use of hypnosis in the care of the cancer patient (Part I). *British Journal of Medical Hypnotism* 1954;6:2:2–12.

39. Butler B. The use of hypnosis in the care of the cancer patient (Part II). *British Journal of Medical Hypnotism* 1955;6:3:2–12.

40. Butler B. The use of hypnosis in the care of the cancer patient (Part III). *British Journal of Medical Hypnotism* 1955;6:4:9–17.

41. Barber J. Hypnosis as a psychological technique in the management of cancer pain. *Cancer Nursing* 1978;11:361–363.

42. Barber J. Hypnosis. In: Bonica JJ, Chapman R, Rodyce E, Loeser J, eds, *The management of pain* (2nd ed.). Philadelphia, PA: Lea & Febiger, 1990:1733–1741.

43. Barber J, Gitelson J. Cancer pain: Psychological management using hypnosis. *Cancer* 1980;30:130–136.

44. Cangello V W. Hypnosis for the patient with cancer. *American Journal of Clinical Hypnosis,* 1962;4:215–226.

45. Hilgard ER, Hilgard JR. *Hypnosis in the relief of pain.* Los Altos, CA: William Kaufmann, 1975.

46. LaBaw W, Holton C, Tewell K, Eccles, D. The use of hypnosis by children with cancer. *American Journal of Hypnosis* 1975;17:233–238.

47. Sacerdote P. Additional contributions to the hypnotherapy of the advanced cancer patient. *American Journal of Clinical Hypnosis* 1965;1:308–319.

48. Sacerdote P. Theory and practice of pain control in malignancy and other protracted recurring painful illnesses. *International Journal of Clinical and Experimental Hypnosis,* 1970;18:160–180.

49. Spiegel D, Bloom JR. Group therapy and hypnosis reduce metastatic breast carcinoma pain. *Psychosomatic Medicine* 1983;45:333–339.

50. Fleming V. Relaxation therapy for far-advanced cancer. *The Practitioner* 1985;229:471–475.

51. Sloman R, Brown P, Aldana E, et al. The use of relaxation for the promotion of comfort and pain relief in persons with advanced cancer. *Contemporary Nurse* 1994;3:6–12.

52. Fotopoulos SS., Graham C, Cook MR. Psychophysiological control of cancer pain. In Bonica JJ, Ventafridda V, eds. *Advances in pain research and therapy,* Vol. 2. New York: Raven Press, 1979:231–244.

53. Fotopoulos SS, Cook MR, Graham C, et al. Cancer pain: evaluation of electromyographic and electrodermal feedback. *Progress in Clinical Biological Research* 1983;132D:33–53.

54. Turk DC, Rennert KS. Pain and the terminally ill cancer patient: a cognitive social learning perspective. In: Sobel H, ed. *Behavioral therapy in terminal care: a humanistic approach.* Cambridge, MA: Ballinger, 1981:95–124.

55. Dalton JA, Toomey T, Workman MR. Pain relief for cancer patients. *Cancer Nursing* 1988;11:322–328.

56. Arathuzik D. Effects of cognitive-behavioral strategies on pain in cancer patients. *Cancer Nursing* 1994;17(3):207–214.

57. Sitaram B. *Current status: assessment of psychological treatment of cancer pain.* Paper presented at the Satellite Meeting of the VI World Congress on Pain, Bombay, India, 1990.

58. Syrjala KL, Cummings C, Donaldson GW. Hypnosis or cognitive behavioral training for the reduction of pain and nausea during cancer treatment: a controlled clinical trial. *Pain* 1992;48:137–146.

59. Syrjala KL, Donaldson GW, Davis, et al. Relaxation and imagery and cognitive-behavioral training reduce pain during cancer treatment: a controlled clinical trial. *Pain* 1995;63:189–198.

60. Jacobsen PB, Hann DM. Cognitive behavioral interventions. In: Holland JC, ed. *Psycho-oncology.* New York: Oxford University Press, 1998:717–729.

61. Syrjala KL, Abrams J. Cancer pain. In: Gatchel RJ, Turk DC, eds. *Psychosocial factors in pain.* New York, NY: Guilford Press; 1999; 301–314.

62. Gatchel RJ, Turk DC, eds. *Psychological approaches to pain management: a practitioner's handbook.* New York: Guilford Press, 1996.

63. Loscalzo M, Jacobsen PB. Practical behavioral approaches to the effective management of pain and distress. *Journal of Psychosocial Oncology* 1990;8:139–169.

64. Turk DC, Feldman CS, eds. *Noninvasive approaches to pain management in the terminally ill.* New York: Hawthorn Press, 1992.

65. Thomas E, Weiss S. Nonpharmacological interventions with chronic cancer pain in adults. *Cancer Control* 2000;7(2):157–164.

66. Linton SJ, Melin L. Applied relaxation in the management of chronic pain, *Behavioral Psychotherapy* 1983;11(4):337–350.

67. Bernstein DA, Borkevec TD. *Progressive relaxation training: a manual for the helping professions.* Champaign, IL: Research Press, 1973.

68. Berstein DA, Carlson CR Progressive relaxation: abbreviated methods. In: Lehrer PM, Woolfolk RL, eds. *Principles and practice of stress management.* New York: Guilford, 1993: 53–88.

69. Basmajiian JV, ed. *Biofeedback: Principles and Practice for Clinicians,* 3rd ed. Baltimore: Williams & Wilkins, 1989.

70. Edwards DJA. Cognitive restructuring through guided imagery: lessons learned from Gestalt therapy. In: Freeman A, Simon KM, Beutler LE, eds. *Comprehensive handbook of cognitive therapy.* New York: Plenum, 1989;283–297.

71. Sheikh AA, ed. *Imagery: current theory, research and application.* New York: Wiley, 1983.

72. Lazarus RS, Folkman, S. *Stress, appraisal, and coping,* New York: Springer, 1984.

73. Fawzy FL, Fawzy NW, Hyun CS, et al. Malignant melanoma: effects of an early structured psychiatric intervention, coping, and affective state on recurrence and survival 6 years later. *Archives of General Psychiatry* 1993;50(9):681–689.

74. Beck AT, Rush AJ, Shaw BJ, Emery G. *Cognitive therapy of depression.* New York: Guilford, 1979.

75. McCaul, KD, Malott, JM. Distraction and coping with pain. *Psychological Bulletin,* 1984;95:516–533.

76. Barrett JB, Williams JW, Oxman TE, et al. The treatment effectiveness project: a comparison of paroxetine, problem-solving therapy, and placebo in the treatment of minor depression and dysthymia in primary care patients: background and research plan. *General Hospital Psychiatry* 1999;21:260–273.

77. Mynors-Wallis LM, Gath DH, Day A, Baker F. Randomised controlled trial of problem solving treatment, antidepressant medication, and combined treatment for major depression in primary care. *British Medical Journal* 2000;320(1):26–30.

78. Nezu AM. Efficacy of a social problem-solving therapy approach for unipolar depression. *Journal of Consulting and Clinical Psychology* 1986;57:4408–4413.

79. Von Korff M, Moore JE, Lorig K, et al. A randomized trial of a lay person-led self-management group intervention for back pain patients in primary care, *Spine* 1998;23:2608–2615.

80. Von Korff M, Saunders K. The course of back pain in primary care. *Spine* 1996;21:2833–2839.

81. Penzien DB, Ray SE, Holm JE, et al. *Home-based behavioral and cognitive-behavioral treatment of recurrent headache: preliminary findings.* Paper presented at the meeting of the Society of Behavioral Medicine, Boston, MA, 1988.

82. Ahles TA, Seville JL, Wasson J, et al. Panel-based pain management in primary care: a pilot study. *Journal of Pain and Symptom Management,* 2001;22(1);584–590.

83. Houts PS, Nezu AM, Nezu CM Bucher JA. The prepared family caregiver: a problem-solving approach to family caregiver education. *Patient Education and Counseling,* 1996;27(1):63–73.

84. Wood BC, Mynors-Wallis LM. Problem-solving therapy in palliative care. *Palliative Medicine* 1997;11(1):49–54.

85. Skelton AM, Murphy EA, Murphy RJL, O'Dowd, TC. Patient education for low back pain in general practice. *Patient Education and Counseling* 1995;25:329–334.

86. Blanchard EB, Andrasik F, Appelbaum Kaet al. The efficacy and cost-effectiveness of minimal therapist-contact, non-drug treatments of chronic migraine and tension headache. *Headache* 1985;25:214–220.

87. Noffsinger EB. Will drop-in medical appointments (DIGMAs) work in practice? *The Permanente Journal* 1999;3:58–67.

88. Scott J, Gade G, McKenzie M, Venhor I. Cooperative health care clinics: s group approach to individual care. *Geriatrics* 1998; 53:68–81.

89. Terry K. Should doctors see patients in group sessions? *Medical Economics* Jan 1997:70–95.

Pain and Medicolegal Issues

CHAPTER 43

Pain and the Social Security Disability System: The Validation of Pain

Will T. Dunn, Jr.

Several years ago I had a conversation with a high-ranking member of the Social Security Office of Hearings and Appeals, which is that part of the Social Security Administration that makes disability determinations. This individual observed that, more and more, psychiatrists and psychologists were being used to "quantify" pain. At the time, I was inclined to agree with that observation, but, in recent years, I've come to the conclusion that what is being accomplished is not a *quantification,* but rather a *validation* of pain. For purposes of this chapter, the Social Security Administration will be referred to as "the Agency." Readers, including some attorneys, will undoubtedly dispute some of the conclusions expressed herein. Suffice to say, the conclusions are my own, based upon successful representation of several thousand Social Security disability claimants before the Agency during the past approximately 30 years. In deference to detractors, I will concede that my practice has been restricted to hearing offices and, hence, administrative law judges within South Carolina and primarily within the Greenville, South Carolina, Office of Hearings and Appeals. Legal authorities cited are primarily from the Fourth Circuit Court of Appeals, which is the federal circuit within which I practice, but I have made an effort to cite Fourth Circuit decisions that, in my opinion, are representative of the law across the country, or at least what appears to be the national judicial trend.

MEDICAL SOURCES

The Agency, by regulation, will accept opinions only from certain "medical sources." These are defined in *20 CFR, §404.1513,* as physicians, osteopaths, and licensed psychologists (which, in South Carolina, would be licensed

clinical psychologists). The Agency will not, for example, consider itself bound by opinions from vocational experts, chiropractors, physical therapists, mental health counselors or therapists, or any of the growing army of personnel who perform "functional capacities assessments" at the request of physicians, insurance companies, etc. Opinions from all other than physicians, osteopaths, and psychologists are classified, in the regulations, as "information from other sources" and are considered useful only as they may "help" the Agency understand how impairments affect a claimant's "ability to work."

In proving disabling pain, statements from treating medical sources to the effect that a patient is disabled by pain may have an emotional impact on the adjudicator but, in reality, are entitled to little weight unless supported by objective clinical evidence or, in the case of the mental approach to proving pain, clinical opinions and/or results of psychological testing from examining or treating psychiatrists or psychologists.

Social Security Ruling *96-7P* is the Agency's published policy interpretation on assessment of pain in disability claims. Basically, *96-7P* specifies that factors to be considered in evaluating a claimant's credibility in reference to allegations of disabling pain include whether that individual has sought treatment, both for the physical and, in many cases, psychiatric aspects of the pain disorder and, more specifically, whether that individual is taking daily prescription pain medication. With regard to the daily consumption of prescription pain medication, what originated as a policy (*SSR 96-7P*) has been distilled into law, at least in the Fourth Circuit Court of Appeals, where the court has ruled that an administrative law judge is justified in disbelieving testimony of a claimant's pain on the basis that the claimant had not sought medical treatment from a physician for pain in more than a year and was taking only over-the-counter pain medications (*Mickles v. Shalala,* 29 F3rd 918, 4th Cir. 1994).

PAIN DEFINED

The Agency divides impairments into exertional and nonexertional. Pain, however, at least in the Agency's view, falls into neither category but instead is considered a "symptom" (*20 CFR §404.1529* and *SSR 96-7P*). The Fourth Circuit Court of Appeals apparently recognizes no such ambiguity and, in the 1989 case of *Walker v. Bowen* (876 F2d 1097, 4th Cir. 1989), declared that "Pain is a nonexertional limitation." In practice, the semantical distinction becomes irrelevant.

The approach to proving pain before the Agency can be bifurcated: On the one side, there is the *physical* approach, on the other, the nonphysical or *mental* approach.

On the physical side, pain can be proved—inferentially—by establishing that an individual suffers from a pain-generating physical disorder that meets the level of severity mandated by the *Social Security Regulatory Listing of Impairments,* that is, the so-called *Listings.* For example, §1.02 of the *Listings* provides criteria for proving the requisite level of severity in the case of an individual suffering from active rheumatoid or other inflammatory arthritis. Section 1.05 of the *Listings* deals with spinal disorders. Section 14.02 deals with proving disability based upon systemic lupus erythematosus, which usually, but not always, involves proving disability based upon pain. There are other examples within the *Listings* where pain may be proven inferentially on a physical, as opposed to a nonphysical, basis.

Proving the existence of pain on a nonphysical (nonexertional) basis is a different proposition and will almost always (at least in my practice) involve psychiatric evidence.

"PAIN DISORDER"

The diagnostic category of "Pain Disorder," along with inclusion criteria, is outlined in the *Diagnostic and Statistical Manual (DSM-IV)* of the American Psychiatric Association.

"Pain Disorder" appears as a subcategory in the *DSM-IV* under *Somatoform Disorders.* Somatoform disorder, or somatization, has been defined by the Fourth Circuit Court of Appeals as meaning, "In psychiatry . . . a conversion of mental experiences or states into bodily symptoms" (*Hooper v. Heckler* 752 F2d 83,87. 4th Cir. 1985).

Historically, a diagnosis of somatoform disorder carried with it the onerous implication that a patient was somehow exaggerating symptoms, with the result that, in certain cases, mental health examiners were reluctant to

make the diagnosis of somatization where there was evidence of a condition, such as rheumatoid arthritis, which could reasonably be expected to produce disabling pain. In other words, the diagnosis of somatoform disorder by the mental health provider was complicated by the prospect of suggesting that the patient was lying.

With the publication in 1994 of the *DSM-IV,* the American Psychiatric Association attempted to resolve this dilemma by, as noted, adding the subsection of "Pain Disorder" under "Somatoform Disorders" and specifically including §307.89: Pain disorder associated with both psychological factors and a general medical condition.

Section 307.89 deals with the claimant who has an objective basis (for example, residuals of spinal surgery) for pain, the degree of impairment imposed by the pain being in dispute, and who has developed a mood disorder, secondary to the chronic pain and resulting dysfunction.

Section 307.89 is not to be confused with §307.80 in the *DSM-IV:* Pain disorder associated with psychological factors, which, I submit, is the traditional somatoform disorder described in earlier editions of the *DSM.*

The advent of §307.89, I suggest, is a recognition of the somewhat simplistic view that depression (and, to a certain extent, anxiety) is caused by loss, and what greater loss, in the Social Security disability context, than the ability to work in the case of one who is motivated to work? Section 307.89 recognizes the reality of the pain-disabled patient and also recognizes the reality that pain is a purely personal, subjective experience, incapable of quantification or description.

Moreover, §307.89, although it attempts to assess psychological factors in pain cases, does not, I submit, require that the degree of depression and/or anxiety imposed by the pain be of a level mandated to prove disability based upon depression or anxiety alone. Rather, §307.89 attempts to define a condition where both pain and resulting psychological factors are considered.

Somatoform disorders fall within §12.07 of the *Social Security Listings of Impairments.*

Case in Point: Fibromyalgia

In the foreword to the 1994 edition of this book, Janet G. Travell, M.D., discussed what was, at that time, called myofascial syndrome, which she described as a:

> condition [that could] be demonstrated objectively by palpation of the muscles for trigger points and by recognition of their related referred pain patterns. The myofascial pain syndrome responds well to scientific local therapy if its multiple perpetuating factors are recognized and corrected. Stresses that are *both physical and emotional* usually must be dealt with if trigger-point therapy is to succeed.

Shortly after Dr. Travell wrote those words, the American College of Rheumatology recognized myofascial pain syndrome as fibromyalgia and thus initiated a consistent treatment approach to this renamed condition. Curiously, at approximately the same juncture, the *DSM-IV*, published in 1995, contained, for the first time, the condition of pain disorder.

The reason fibromyalgia warrants a subsection here is because it is representative of the problems encountered in proving the existence of disabling pain. The Social Security Administration, for example, does not recognize fibromyalgia (although individuals within the Agency may dispute this) and, I submit, cannot, under the present state of the law, ever recognize fibromyalgia or any similar condition. The reason why the Agency will not recognize fibromyalgia is because, although it is generically a pain condition, it is a pain condition that cannot be verified by traditional laboratory techniques, that is, serologic tests and/or x-rays, and the law is clear that the Agency will recognize only pain conditions that can be established by objective clinical proof.

If pressed psychiatrists and psychologists will opine that what the rheumatologists call fibromyalgia is what the mental health people have been treating as a type of somatoform disorder. The rheumatologists will argue intensely that fibromyalgia is, indeed, a physical, as opposed to a mental, disorder.

The example of fibromyalgia raises the question: What is pain? From a psychiatric standpoint, as noted herein, pain disorder is a mental condition. From the physical standpoint, fibromyalgia is a physical condition. I suggest that the mental health people, on the one hand, and the rheumatologists, on the other, are both correct and that pain is a biphasic phenomenon consisting of both physical and mental components. At the present time, however, and into the foreseeable future, the Social Security Administration recognizes fibromyalgia as the *DSM-IV* condition of pain disorder and is not likely to accept proof of fibromyalgia as a disabling condition unless there is psychiatric evidence of disabling pain.

PROVING PAIN

Proving pain from the physical side, as noted, involves establishing through a treating source (in the case of pain, usually an orthopedic or neurosurgeon, but it could be any licensed physician in any given instance) that the patient's pain meets the level of severity mandated by one of the Social Security regulations dealing with physical, as opposed to mental, impairments. Examples have previously been cited of rheumatoid and other types of inflammatory arthritis, disorders of the spine, and lupus.

Proving pain from a mental perspective is somewhat more complicated and is inevitably going to involve evaluations by psychiatrists and psychologists.

The regulations speak in terms of "clinical proof." In the case of purely physical approaches to pain, such proof will involve, for example, verification of spinal surgeries, MRIs, blood tests (in the cases of rheumatoid arthritis, lupus, etc.). On the other side, in patients with insufficient physical documentation, however, clinical proof will involve the "clinical observations of psychiatrists and psychologists" as well as results of certain types of psychological testing.

Psychological Testing

Psychological testing is becoming one of the most effective ways of proving disabling pain in disability cases. In this regard, the Minnesota Multiphasic Personality Inventory (MMPI) is presently the most useful tool in validating pain. The MMPI is likely the most widely utilized psychological test in the world. Although the MMPI does not purport to be able to prove or disprove the existence of pain, nor the degree of pain, nonetheless, in the hands of a capable examiner, it can verify that a patient is somatically concentrated or *convinced* he is disabled by pain. Additional aspects of the MMPI can verify that the patient is not malingering nor consciously exaggerating symptoms. In other words, the MMPI is very useful in *validating* the presence of disabling pain.

Moreover, the MMPI is one of the psychological tests specifically referred to as a source of objective clinical evidence in the preamble to the Social Security listings of mental disorders. Specifically, the regulations provide that the MMPI is one of the tests that "may be useful in establishing the existence of a mental disorder" or, in the pain case, the presence of a disabling somatoform pain disorder.

Somewhat less widely utilized and of more recent origin than the MMPI is the "Patient Pain Profile," or P-3. Unlike the MMPI, which covers the full spectrum of psychiatric disorders, the P-3, according to its developers, is designed to assess psychological functioning associated with pain, using samples of hundreds of patients in pain, as well as a national community sample.

The P-3 computerized interpretation compares a patient's score to both a national sample of normal community subjects and a national sample of patients in pain. It assesses the three clinical disorders most frequently encountered in patients with intractable pain, that is, depression, anxiety, and somatization.

The P-3 is presently used in thousands of hospitals, clinics, and private practices across the United States and Canada. Translation into several languages is under way. The test copyright is owned by National Computer Systems (NCS Assessments) of Minneapolis, Minnesota, which is the largest psychological test developer/supplier in the United States and also, incidentally, the marketer of the MMPI.

It is hoped that, in the future, more and more practitioners, both attorneys and physicians/psychologists, will utilize the P-3 as a supplement in pain cases to the MMPI and that results of the P-3 will come to be accepted by the Agency as a valid tool in evaluation of pain; which is not to say that pain cases that cannot be proved otherwise can be established by results of psychological testing. The present mind-set of the Agency is not such that one is going to be able to prove disability based upon pain on the results of a single psychological test or tests. Rather, the Agency looks for evidence that some treating source has identified psychological components in a particular claimant and that some effort has been made to treat these psychological components. A conundrum arises here, however, because, typically, somatoform patients do not respond well to attempts at treatment with psychotropic drugs or psychotherapy.

Somatoform pain disorder, as with other psychiatric conditions, is evaluated by the Agency utilizing a form called the Psychiatric Review Technique. This form was devised by the Agency several years ago as a means for the administrative law judges (read, Social Security judges) to evaluate mental disorders. However, the practice has evolved, in many areas of the country, of having mental health experts—treating and/or examining sources—complete the form. There are probably individual administrative law judges across the country who object to this practice, but it would seem reasonable that a psychiatrist or psychologist is better qualified to complete such forms than an administrative law judge.

SUMMARY AND CONCLUSION

Pain is, by its very nature, a purely personal experience. I submit it defies definition by lawyers, doctors, or bureaucrats. Pain is universally recognized as unpleasant, hence the presence of such words in our lexicon as *painful*. Nonetheless, I submit, the average Social Security claimant trying to describe his pain to even a sympathetic administrative law judge might as well be trying to describe the color red to a blind man. If an individual's pain has progressed to the point that that individual is no longer capable of being gainfully employed, that person is going to experience a substantial loss, which loss is going to manifest itself as depression/anxiety and which, as noted herein, is capable of producing a disability-qualifying condition, sometimes capable of proof at a physical level but, increasingly more often, at a psychiatric level.

CHAPTER **44**

Pain in Workers' Compensation and Personal Injury Law

Lynn Shook

Workers' compensation and personal injury laws are the American jurisprudence system's remedies for people who are injured on their jobs or because of the negligence or wrongdoing of others.

Although the purpose of both legal systems is to compensate the injured party by payment of medical bills, of lost wages, and for permanent bodily injuries, they are completely different in their legal requirements and fundamental purposes.

One of the most important role players in these types of legal claims and lawsuits are the physicians who treat the injured victims. Many kinds of diseases and injuries result from these accidents, and the medical treatment can be quite varied and extensive. It is not uncommon in some cases for patients to become chronically debilitated from the pain and require extensive pain syndrome management. Delays in medical treatment often occur when the injured victim's claims are legally denied by the defendants, compounding the medical outcome.

It is imperative that physicians understand these two completely different legal remedies and accept their important role, as well as understand how the medical evidence established by their treatment may affect their patients' legal rights.

Many physicians have complained that they did not go to medical school to get involved in the legal system. They want to practice medicine and be left alone by lawyers. Yet, any physician who treats patients who are injured on their jobs or as the result of someone else's negligence must accept that they will have to become legally involved because of the importance of the medical evidence in these cases.

To this end, I will describe these legal systems in a general nature so that the physician can understand their legal significance to the injured patient. This discussion will focus on workers' compensation laws and negligence actions that involve motor vehicle accidents (MVAs) and injuries sustained from falls in public places, referred to as "slip and falls."

WORKERS' COMPENSATION LAWS

On-the-job injuries are some of the most prevalent accidents in America. Each state's current workers' compensation systems are the result of social legislation that came about as a result of the rapid industrialization in the early twentieth century. This industrialization led to increasing numbers of serious on-the-job accidents. The first workers' compensation laws were enacted in the United States in 1911. Prior to this enactment of laws, an injured worker had to show that his or her employer was negligent or at fault in causing the injury.

This legal remedy was based on a well-established English common law principle that held that a master or employer was responsible for the injury or death of his servants or workers. This fault-based system was unduly onerous on injured workers, leading to delay or denial of medical care in many instances. Proving fault was difficult to do because it was timely and costly to hire an attorney to represent the injured worker in court and the wheels of justice have always turned slowly even in days of less litigious societies.

Most workers did not have the means to survive while they were unable to work, and they and their families suffered. The result was a social nightmare with the injured going without medical care and depending on what little governmental and charitable aid that was available.

By the close of the nineteenth century, it was apparent that a new legal system had to be developed for injured workers. Lawmakers wanted a system that was beneficent

672 VII / PAIN AND MEDICOLEGAL ISSUES

and remedial in character. The idea was to get away from the cumbersome procedures and technicalities of compensation based on the common law of England, which required fault. The workers' fault is not a defense. It is a system of "strict liability." In exchange, the employer's financial liability is capped, limiting their total payout, while lending predictability to the cost of doing business.

Social Objective of Workers' Compensation Laws

Historically, workers' compensation laws are based on these basic objectives:

1. To provide sure, prompt, and reasonable income and medical benefits to work-related accident victims, or income benefits to their families or dependents regardless of who was at fault;
2. To provide a single remedy and reduce court delays, costs, and judicial dockets arising out of personal injury litigation;
3. To relieve public and private charities of financial demands related to uncompensated occupational accidents;
4. To minimize payment of fees to lawyers and witnesses and long-drawn-out trials and court appeals;
5. To encourage employer interest in job safety and rehabilitation through an experience-rating mechanism;
6. To promote frank study of the causes of on-the-job accidents in an effort to reduce them and human suffering, rather than having employers tempted by the concealment of fault-caused accidents.

Although each state's compensation act varies, they typically have these features:

1. The basic operating principle is that the employee is automatically entitled to certain benefits whenever the employee suffers a "personal injury by accident arising out of and in the course of employment" or an occupational disease.
2. Negligence and fault are largely immaterial, both in the sense that the employee's contributory negligence does not lessen his or her rights and in the sense that the employer's complete freedom from fault does not lessen its liability.
3. Coverage is limited to persons having the status of employee, as distinguished from independent contractor.
4. Benefits to the employee include cash-wage benefits, usually around one half to two thirds of the employee's average weekly wage (AWW), and hospital, medical, and rehabilitation expenses; in death cases, benefits for dependents are provided; arbitrary maximum and minimum limits are ordinarily imposed.
5. The employee and dependents, in exchange for these modest but assured benefits, give up their common-law right to sue the employer for damages for any injury covered by the act.

6. The right to sue third persons whose negligence or fault caused the injury remains, however, with the proceeds usually being applied first to reimburse the employer for the compensation outlay, the balance (or most of it) going to the employee.
7. Administration is typically in the hands of the administrative commissions; and, as far as possible, rules of procedure, evidence, and conflict of laws are relaxed to facilitate the achievement of the beneficent purposes of the legislation.
8. The employer is required to secure its liability through private insurance, state-fund insurance in some states, or self-insurance; thus the burden of compensation liability does not remain with the employer but passes to the consumer, since compensation premiums, as part of the cost of production, will be reflected in the price of the product.

To receive benefits under the various state acts, the injured worker, or claimant as is usually the legal reference, must show that the injury was one "by accident" that "arose out of" the employment and "in the course of" the employment. And despite the social theory behind workers' compensation acts, the defendants in unusual and catastrophic injury cases often litigate these legal requirements.

"INJURY BY ACCIDENT"

Most typically this is not a difficult question for the worker who loses a finger or has a motor vehicle accident while in a company vehicle delivering a company's product. However, in more controversial injuries, such as ones associated with physical injuries accompanied by mental maladies or what is known as mental-mental claims where there is no physical injury, much litigation has ensued producing various legal requirements as well as defenses for the employer.

Traditionally, preexisting injuries that have been aggravated by a job injury are compensable. Therefore, claimants with prior knee surgeries may still recover damages for a subsequent leg injury involving the same knee. In most states, however, the defendants may receive a credit for prior disability awarded in a prior workers' compensation claim to that leg, especially if the injury occurred with the same employer.

If the prior knee injury did not involve an award for workers' compensation disability, then the defendant would usually be liable for the total impairment of the leg and the resulting disability. Most states have in place a fund from which to reimburse employers for awards of disability to workers with preexisting medical conditions. This fund is primarily generated from insurance companies and self-insured employers who are assessed fees based on set formulas. This fund is established by legislation and is typically administered by state or quasi-governmental entities. In South Carolina it is known as "The Second Injury Fund."

For the exacerbation of the prior medical condition to be compensable, the preexisting condition must combine with the job injury to make the disability of the individual greater and increase the costs of medical treatment greater than it would have been for the injury alone.

The idea is to encourage employers to hire workers with preexisting medical conditions. Most states include, under these provisions, certain listed diseases for which a legal presumption is that their existence constitutes a hindrance or obstacle to the injured worker in employment.

These diseases often include epilepsy, diabetes, cardiac disease, muscular dystrophy, cancer, pulmonary disease, ruptured intervertebral disc, deafness, ionizing radiation injury, and many other medical conditions individually set forth in the various state laws.

Traditionally, "injury" or "personal injury" used in some state laws is defined as an unlooked for, untoward event that is not expected or designed by the person who suffers the injury. An accident can involve many types of medical problems. It can be an occupational disease, from repetitive trauma, a heart attack, a stroke, a hernia, or a mental injury or any physical malady resulting from traditional accidents in the workplace.

The meaning of *undesigned* and *unforeseen* has been said to refer to the result produced and not its cause by a South Carolina Supreme Court case. "When a person lifts a heavy weight, they intend to do exactly what they do; nevertheless, if they strain a muscle, or rupture a blood vessel, the injury is due to an accident" (Green v. City of Bennettsville, 197 S.C. 313, 15 S.E.2d 334 [1941]).

Workers' compensation laws have evolved to keep pace with the workplace and developing accidental medical conditions. Heart attacks and strokes are considered accidental injuries in many states if the worker can show that they were subjected to either unusual or extraordinary physical exertion, violence, or strain in the employment or to unusual or extraordinary conditions of employment, and that there is medical causation showing that the unusual or extraordinary exertion, violence, or strain or unusual conditions resulted in the stroke or heart attack.

Examples of these conditions could include working in unusual and excessive heat, an unusual increase in work hours and or duties, or even a mild-mannered employee standing up for him- or herself with an offensive and demanding boss.

Many states have adopted the same standards for mental-mental injuries, or mental injuries unaccompanied by physical trauma, to be considered accidents. In most states, an occupational disease is defined as "a disease arising out of and in the course of employment that is due to hazards in excess of those ordinarily incident to employment and peculiar to the occupation in which the employee is engaged" (Section 42-11-10 SC Code of Laws Ann. [1976]).

Prime examples of such occupational diseases are black lung found in the coal mining industry and byssinosis found in the textile industry caused by the inhalation of cotton dust.

"ARISING OUT OF THE EMPLOYMENT"

Generally, "arising out of" refers to the cause or the origin of the accident. Nationwide, there are five tests for interpreting arising out of the employment:

1. The peculiar-risk doctrine that requires claimants to prove that the source of the accident was peculiar to their particular employment;
2. The increased-risk doctrine that requires claimants to prove that their employment was more likely to bring them into contact with the source of the accident;
3. The actual-risk doctrine that requires claimants to prove only that some aspect of their employment brought them into contact with the harm;
4. The positional-risk doctrine that requires claimants to prove that their injury would not have occurred but for some aspect of their employment that brought them into contact with the harm;
6. The proximate-cause test that requires claimants to prove that the harm was foreseeable as an incident of the employment and that the chain of causation was not broken by an intervening act, such as an act of God.

The increased-risk rule is the majority rule in the United States.

"IN THE COURSE OF THE EMPLOYMENT"

Generally, the "course of the employment" refers to the time, place, and circumstances of the accident. Generally, accidents that occur on the way to or on the way home from the workplace do not occur in the course of employment.

There are exceptions to this rule: when the means of transportation is provided by the employer or the time that is involved is paid for in the form of wages; where the employee is charged with a duty or task in connection with the employment; the way used is inherently dangerous and is the exclusive way of ingress and egress or is maintained by the employer.

The initial handling of claims is administrative in all but a few states. The intent was to reach a prompt decision regarding the worker's entitlement to benefits. State statutes vary, but most provide for fixed awards to the employees or their dependents in cases of employment-related accidents and diseases. Some of the acts go beyond the simple determination of the right to compensation and provide insurance systems, either under state supervision or otherwise. The various state acts vary as to the extent of coverage for accidents, as well as to the amount and duration of benefits. Typically independent contractors and farm and domestic labor are not covered.

If a workers' compensation claim is accepted or admitted, then workers in most states receives one half to sixty-six and two thirds of their average weekly salary as long as they are disabled or under care by a doctor who feels they cannot work. Workers will also receive payment of 100% of their medical bills that are related to the job injury. In most states, the employers are allowed to choose the physicians.

Originally, workers' compensation laws were designed to pay for medical treatment and to replace lost wages. As the system has evolved over the twentieth century, state legislatures began to pass what are known as "schedules" for the worth of various bodily extremities and internal organs. Implicit in these "schedules" is the presumptive "disability" entitling injured workers to compensation, regardless of the effect the injury had on their wages (Table 44-1).

Where the Workers' Compensation Act applies, it has been uniformly held that this remedy is exclusive and bars any common-law remedy against the employer that the employee may have had otherwise. As to the employer, the injured worker's remedy is limited to the compensation available under the act.

Each state's workers' compensation system varies, but the underlying concept is that the employer should assume the cost of occupational injuries. The resulting economic losses are considered costs of production, chargeable (to the consumer) as a price factor.

To get this highly controversial social legislation passed and accepted by the early industrial entrepreneurs, there had to be much negotiation and compromise. The result

was that workers' compensation benefits are financially capped in most states. This means that the injured worker, no matter how catastrophic the injury, can only receive a set number of weeks of compensation.

The compensation rate (CR) of the injured worker is typically one-half to two-thirds of their average weekly wage (AWW). This CR is the amount that the worker will draw on a weekly basis while unable to work. The cap means that no matter how much the worker made, this is all he or she may receive under the law.

In South Carolina, effective January 1, 2000, the maximum compensation rate for accidents that occurred in the year 2000, is $507.34. Regardless of the employee's income, the maximum they are eligible to receive weekly cannot exceed this weekly cap amount.

The impairment rating, a percentage assigned medically by a physician that signifies the loss of use of the injured extremity or body part, will usually form the basis for the amount of permanent disability awarded the injured worker. This disability award is typically paid in a lump sum of money to the injured worker. It is based on the amount of impairment given by the physician to the worker, and it is often based on the *American Medical Association's Guides to Permanent Impairment*, although in most jurisdictions this is not a legal requirement.

Disability awards are often higher than the assigned impairment rating or ratings because they are also based on the age, education, and work history of the injured

TABLE 44-1. *SC Code of Laws Ann. (1976) Title 42, Regulation 67–1101.*
Total or partial loss of use of a member, organ or part of the body

Organ, member, or body part	Total loss	Partial loss or loss of use	Organ, member, or body part	Total loss	Partial loss or loss of use
Breast	75	10–75	Fallopian tubes		10–100
Breasts	250	25–250	Heart		25–250
Coccyx	10	1–10	Intestine, small		10–400
Gall bladder	75	10–75	Larynx		25–400
Kidney	400	25–250	Liver		25–250
Lung	400	25–250	Mandible		10–100
Pancreas	500	10–250	Ovaries		10–100
Penis	350	25–250	Palate		25–250
Rib	10	1.5–10	Prostate		10–100
(Maximum award of 200 weeks for total loss of 4 ribs)			Rectum		10–250
Scrotum and testicles	350	30–300	Scapula		10–200
Spleen	25	2.5–25	Skin		5–300
Testicle	75	10–75	Spermatic cord		10–100
Testicles	250	25–250	Sternum		10–100
Tongue	500	50–500	Stomach		25–250
Tooth	2	0.5–2	Thyroid gland		10–100
Biliary tract		75–400	Ureter		10–100
Bladder		25–250	Urethra		10–100
Brain		25–250	Uterus		10–100
Bronchi or bronchus		25–400	Vagina		25–250
Esophagus		25–400	Vulva		25–250
Cervix		10–100	Nasal passage		10–75
Clavicle		10–100	Olfactory nerve		10–75
Colon		25–250	Sinus		5–30
Diaphragm		25–250	Zygomatic arch or facial nerve		
Duodenum		10–250	(in accordance with AMA "guides")		

individual. The extent of the injury and whether the worker can return to the same job can also be a factor.

The value of a workers' compensation claim is based on the body part or parts involved in the injury and the wages of the worker and the CR of the injured.

For example, a worker who injures his back in South Carolina where the back is worth up to 300 weeks (unless the worker is totally and permanently disabled and then it is worth 500 weeks) and is assigned a 10% impairment rating by the physician will have a rating worth $3,000.

In South Carolina, the leg is worth 195 weeks of compensation. So if a worker with a CR of $400 sustains an on-the-job injury to the leg and is assigned a 20% impairment rating by the physician, her impairment rating will be worth $15,600.

The caps on weekly compensation benefits can be financially detrimental to a worker with high wages. The cap means that no matter how much the injured worker made, he or she can only receive the maximum allowable in that state as weekly benefits.

In South Carolina, the maximum weekly compensation injured workers may receive if they are determined to be totally and permanently disabled is capped at 500 weeks times their CR. The same worker may, however, receive medical treatment for life that is causally related to the job injury. If killed on the job, the worker's legal dependants will share in the maximum compensation allowable of 500 weeks. A funeral benefit in the amount of $2,500 is also available in South Carolina to the deceased worker's dependants.

The issue of whether the medical treatment recommended is causally related to the on-the-job injury often becomes a source of litigation. Physicians should offer an opinion that the medical treatment is most probably related to the on-the-job injury in order for it to be paid for by the defendants. This opinion should be based, as much as possible, on objective findings and subjective complaints of the patient. Medical treatment is often delayed or denied, pending the outcome of this litigation. Generally, the injured worker or his or her attorney will hire a physician to provide an independent medical exam (IME) on this issue. Oftentimes when a doctor recommends a medical procedure that the insurance adjuster does not authorize for this reason, the result will be that the injured worker's medical treatment halts until the matter can be litigated.

Some states conduct their workers' compensation systems through the use of administrative hearings before hearing officers. These officers may or may not be attorneys. Other states have trials before judges alone, while some states require trials before juries. Regardless of the forum, injured workers have the burden of proof to show that their injury "arose out of and in the course of their employment." Additionally, they must show that the injury or resulting medical condition was caused by the accident.

For example, if a worker approaches another worker about the fact that he saw him talking to his girlfriend and a fight ensues resulting in injuries, then the injuries did not "arise" out of the work. The injuries may have resulted from something that happened "in the course of employment" because the fight took place at work. But to be compensable, the injury must both "arise out of" and "in the course of the employment."

So if the one worker approached the other worker in the plant and complained to her that she was not performing the work properly and a fight ensued resulting in injuries, then the injuries would have both "arose out of and in the course of employment."

Assume a worker develops a foot or lower-extremity pain while lifting at work. He reports the pain to his doctor the following day. Over the next few days, the worker's back begins to hurt. Two weeks later, he returns to the physician with the added complaint of back pain. An MRI is ordered and the results reveal a moderate herniated disc at L-5–S-1, with impingement on the nerve root. For the worker to receive treatment and related benefits for the injury, he must have the physician's opinion that the rupture was "most probably" caused by the lifting event at work.

When asked whether an injury was most probably caused by a specific event, many physicians are reluctant to commit to a firm opinion on such matters. Without this commitment, an injured worker's benefits may be denied. The physician should have no reservation in stating that, on the basis of information available to her, a specific event was the "most likely cause" of the medical condition being treated.

Workers' compensation laws are not designed to cover all workers and usually do not apply to very small businesses. There is a state minimum number of employees a business must have (in South Carolina the minimum number is four) before it must have workers' compensation insurance.

Federal employees are covered by the Federal Employees Compensation Act; seamen by the Jones Act; longshoremen and harbor workers by the Longshoremen's and Harbor Workers' Compensation Act.

ATTORNEYS' FEES

Most plaintiff and claimant attorneys take injury cases on a contingency fee arrangement, where the attorney gets usually 25% to 33% of the monies recovered, plus any costs that the attorney has paid associated with the claim or lawsuit.

In South Carolina, attorneys' fees for the injured worker are capped at one third the amount awarded. The worker's attorney must petition for approval of his or her fee and cannot receive the fee until the fee petition is approved. This amount usually does not include medical bills that are paid directly by the defendant. Other states cap attorney fees as low as 15%.

Medical charges are also capped under what is commonly referred to as "The Fee Schedule." The individual state's workers' compensation authorities outline the allowable charge for specific medical procedures and publish these schedules for medical providers.

Defense attorneys are generally paid by the insurer of the business and are typically paid at an hourly rate. The insurance company usually selects the attorney. A recent trend in the insurance industry is to submit these defense bills to companies who scrutinize these bills to determine whether they are fair and reasonable.

PERSONAL INJURY

A personal injury is considered a tort, which is defined as a private or civil wrong for which the court will provide a remedy in the form of an action for damages. There are many different torts that involve personal injuries: medical malpractice, toxic torts in environmental lawsuits, and injuries from defective products in product liability lawsuits.

The law of personal injury is based on negligence, strict liability, or acts of intentional misconduct. In negligence cases, the focus is whether the defendant failed to use ordinary care in the circumstances that caused the injury. In strict liability cases, manufacturers may be held legally responsible for injuries caused by defective products, if that product was unreasonably dangerous even when reasonable care was used in the manufacture or design of the product. Intentional misconduct cases include battery or harmful or offensive touching, false imprisonment or wrongful detention of a person and intentional infliction of emotional distress, or behavior that is outrageous to the degree that it results in severe emotional distress.

The basis of the legal remedy available in personal injury lawsuits is to right a wrong between the contestants. In most states, there is no legal monetary cap on the awards available to injured persons. In recent years, however, there has been much political pressure by various and sundry groups who have a financial stake in these awards to cap these awards. This has been referred to as "tort reform."

This discussion will be confined to personal injuries caused in motor vehicle accidents and accidents commonly referred to as "slip and falls" when the injury complained of results when the party falls or trips in a public place because of the negligence of the property owner.

The majority of personal injury cases involve motor vehicle accidents. In these cases the injured party must show not only that the injuries complained of are related to the accident, but also that the accident was caused by the negligence of another.

Personal injury insurance in tort liability is a familiar feature of modern law. In theory, the presence of insurance should not alter our conception of the rights and liabilities of the actual parties. Therefore, the mention of insurance coverage in trials of MVAs is strictly forbidden in most states.

Motor vehicle accident personal injury cases are usually a fight among the insurers of the vehicle in question. In some cases, the at-fault or negligent party will not have insurance coverage. In these accident cases, the injured party, if he or she has uninsured motor vehicle accident coverage, will deal with his or her own insurance company for compensation of damages.

It is important to recognize the importance of the insurance carrier in motor vehicle accidents. Unlike the statutory scheme of workers' compensation, negligence in motor vehicular accidents follows the common law, requiring the injured party to prove fault, medical causation, and damages to collect compensation from the at-fault driver. This means that even in the most obvious or egregious cases, the at-fault driver or his or her insurance company is under no legal obligation to pay the injured person until fault is proven. Consequently, until the claim is settled or adjudicated, the injured person will receive no payment to offset his or her actual out-of-pocket losses. This often has a profound impact on the injured with regard to the medical care received. It places an especially heavy and unfair burden on those without group health insurance or other financial resources to pay for necessary medical care pending resolution of the accident claim.

If an attorney is involved on behalf of the injured person, arrangements are often made with the health care provider to pay for medical treatment directly out of any settlement proceeds once a claim is concluded. This arrangement is mutually beneficial, assuring the provider that the medical bills will be paid (to the extent damages are recovered) while allowing the injured person to receive prompt, necessary, and adequate medical treatment.

The kinds of damages available under the American jurisprudence system vary and each contains technical requirements that the plaintiff or the injured party must show.

In motor vehicle accidents, the damages most often available to the injured cover medical costs, lost wages, property damage, pain and suffering, as well as whether the accident has left the injured victim disfigured or disabled. Other damages available in these cases include loss of family, loss of social and educational experiences, emotional damages, and property damage.

Pain and suffering is a subjective damage awarded by the jury based on the seriousness of the injury and accompanying pain of the individual party. Loss of consortium is a separate cause of action available to the spouse of the injured party. Damages for loss of consortium are awarded to reflect the loss of companionship of the injured party with his or her spouse as a result of the injury. Punitive damages that are awarded to punish the wrongdoer may also be available. A party who is unable to show negligence cannot usually recover punitive damages even though the party proves a personal injury or damage to property.

To get punitive damages in most states, one must show that the negligent party was also willful, wanton, or reckless. Willful or reckless conduct is usually defined as conduct exhibiting a consciousness and awareness from knowledge of existing conditions that injury would most likely result if certain acts are committed. In terms of "special damages," or ones associated with medical bills, the type of medical treatment will play a key role.

Medical treatment that is not directly provided by a physician is not valued as highly by the insurance company. This would include physical therapy, chiropractic treatment, and osteopathy. Given even less value by insurance companies are treatments such as massage and acupuncture.

The financial value of motor vehicle accidents is determined primarily by combining the total medical bills and lost wages, or actual damages, of the injured party. It is simple to add up the amount of lost wages and medical bills, but difficult to put a financial value on pain and suffering or on missed experiences or lost opportunities. The old adage that there is no amount of money that will compensate the injured party for his or her injuries is true, but nevertheless some figure must be derived.

Insurance companies generally use a formula for damages. First, the total medical expenses are calculated and these are called "specials." The adjuster next will look at the nature of the medical expenses: were they diagnostic; was treatment rendered by a specialist; was treatment by a physician versus a chiropractor; was treatment rendered immediately after the accident; was there emergency room treatment and was in-patient care necessary; if therapy wasn't done by physician referral or by licensed physical therapist versus chiropractor or massage therapist; were there objective injuries—broken bones, lacerations or scars, ruptured discs, etc.; what was the duration of treatment and was there consistency? All these factors and more are analyzed by the insurance adjuster in arriving at a fair valuation of the claim.

Besides the immediacy of treatment, the most important factor that the adjuster uses at determining the value of the medical expenses is the nature of the injury. Injuries that are objective in nature—lacerations, broken bones, etc.—are weighted much more heavily than soft tissue injuries. Consequently, myofascial pain resulting from whiplash that requires extensive therapy over a long period will have relatively less value than a broken arm from which the injured recovers fully in a matter of weeks.

Depending on the area of the country, the settlement value of these cases varies. The "settlement value," or the amount the insurance company will pay to avoid going to trial, is derived from factors that include past jury verdicts and the socioeconomic makeup of the community. Historically, jurors from areas primarily comprised of working-class, middle-income, and low-income people award the biggest jury verdicts.

Insurance companies and trial attorneys know this. However, insurance companies and trial attorneys also realize that one never knows what a jury will award, especially in emotionally tragic accidents. In reality, it is usually the lawyer's weakest accident cases (questionable liability, extensive treatment and expense outweighing medical findings, low or minimal impact cases) that will go to trial, because the parties most often settle the better cases.

In the real world, the amount of damages available to the injured plaintiff in MVAs is usually dictated by the amount of insurance on the at-fault vehicle, no matter what the amount of actual damages. Technically, in most states a jury award beyond the amount of insurance coverage can be recovered against the at-fault driver personally. Yet, many of these defendants are judgment-proof, with little, if any, financial assets. So it would be an exercise in futility for the trial attorney to attempt to collect more than the insurance coverage.

However, in many tractor-trailer accidents the liability coverage on the vehicle could be limitless or at least capped at several million dollars. The reason these vehicles are well insured to such limits is to protect these financially healthy companies and corporations. Tractor-trailer accidents are some of the most tragic MVAs and often involve several vehicles and multiple injured or dead plaintiffs.

SLIP AND FALL ACCIDENTS

In the negligence actions commonly called "slip and falls," the damages available are usually the same as those set forth above in MVAs. These accidents, also called business premises lawsuits, occur when someone falls and is injured in a public place. Damages in these cases are usually covered by commercial or property liability insurance policies.

Plaintiffs in these cases must prove that the storekeeper was negligent by showing a breach of duty of the owner to use reasonable care in order to win. To prove this, most courts require that the plaintiff show that the owner had either actual or constructive notice of a foreign object on the floor or of a hazardous condition that the defendant failed to remedy.

Slip and fall cases have flooded the courts over the past few decades. One reason is the demise of the local grocer and the development of giant self-service supermarkets. These large stores have given rise to more customers traversing the aisles and falling suffering injuries.

For example, a woman is shopping and as she turns to get a product off of the shelf she steps in ketchup, which has been dropped on the floor by another customer, and falls. She suffers a fractured hip and requires an ambulance to take her to the hospital. The above scenario is typical of these types of lawsuits.

Can the woman recover for her damages? She can if she can show that the store management was negligent or had knowledge of the ketchup and failed to clean it up. This is a difficult burden for the plaintiff. If the store's employees created the hazard, then recovery would be more likely.

Because of the increase in these types of lawsuits, many large food and retail chains have instituted procedures whereby employees conduct regularly scheduled "safety sweeps" of the premises to check for hazardous conditions. Some stores even document these checks in a notebook.

In reality, many slip and fall injuries that occur in public places are not the result of negligence, but because the individual tripped for no reason or had an idiopathic incident, one which is self-originated or from other causes. These legal burdens make these cases unattractive to personal injury lawyers who invest much time and money and receive no money in contingency contracts unless the plaintiffs prevail. Nevertheless, victims of these accidents can sustain serious and costly injuries and those without medical insurance suffer greatly.

In the past two decades, there has developed a belief among some legal theorists that the requirement of negligence should be eliminated in these cases and strict liability, or liability strictly because the injury occurred, should replace it. These theorists argue that cases where the roof falls in or the shelf falls over in a store and causes injuries are similar to defectively designed automobile cases where strict liability has been imposed. In some states, including Arizona, Washington, and Missouri, the judiciary seems to be willing to move in this direction when injuries occur in large self-service retail stores.

THE PHYSICIANS' ROLE IN DETERMINING DAMAGES IN WORKERS' COMPENSATION AND PERSONAL INJURY LAWSUITS

Many physicians do not realize the legal importance of their treatment relative to the injury case for the patient. It is the medical evidence on which the value of these cases will be determined. In workers' compensation claims, the acceptance of the case is often predicated on the first medical report. The focus is that the injured worker advise the physician how the accident occurred in the workplace. It is important that the physician get an accurate description from the patient as to how the injury occurred and document this in the medical narrative report. The medical welfare of the patient could depend on this, as well as the timeliness of payment of the physicians' medical charges.

The documentation of the extent of the injury by objective means such as x-ray, MRI, myelogram, and CT scans is also very important. The fact and notation that the patient will or may have recurring degenerative or future problems is important as well. Pain, immobility, weakness, discomfort, scarring, and permanent impairment should also be well documented by the physician.

DEFINITIONS USED IN WORKERS COMPENSATION AND PERSONAL INJURY CASES

1. Maximum medical improvement (MMI)—A legal-medical term that means that the injured worker has achieved a medical plateau so that further medical treatment will not help to return to the worker to the workplace.

2. Independent medical examination (IME)—A medical evaluation by a physician other than the one who has been treating the injured worker; it can be ordered by a judge or hearing officer, agreed to by the employer/insurance adjuster, or paid for by the injured worker or his or her attorney.

3. Company doctor—A physician who contracts with the employer to provide treatment for injured workers; oftentimes highly distrusted by the injured workers.

4. Third-party administrator (TPA)—Usually an insurance adjusting company that handles workers' compensation claims and personal injury claims for an employer who is self-insured or an insurance carrier.

5. Self-insured—Companies or groups of employers who elect to pay directly the compensation due an injured worker, rather than purchase insurance coverage; self-insurers are usually required to furnish satisfactory proof to the state of their financial ability to pay in conjunction with the requirement of an acceptable security, indemnity, or bond to secure the payment of liabilities as they occur.

6. Average weekly wage (AWW)—The average weekly wage, that an injured worker received prior to the job injury and is usually computed on the previous year's earnings.

7. Compensation rate (CR)—A figure that is $66\frac{2}{3}\%$ of the injured worker's average weekly wage; the weekly amount the injured worker receives; the figure on which the injured worker's disability lump-sum payment is based.

8. Negligence—The failure to use such care as a reasonably prudent and careful person would use under similar circumstances; it is the doing of some act that a person of ordinary prudence would not have done under similar circumstances or failure to do what a person of ordinary prudence would have done under similar circumstances (4).

9. Temporary total disability (TTD) benefits—Wages that injured workers draw on a weekly basis when they have been medically determined to be unable to return to work.

10. Temporary partial disability (TPD) benefits—Wages that injured workers receive on a weekly basis when they have been medically determined to be able to return to work, but at a lesser wage or for less hours per day than prior to the on-the-job injury; this wage makes up the difference in the wages earned prior to the injury and the wage that the injured worker is currently earning.

11. Permanent total disability (PTD) benefits—A monetary sum awarded or agreed upon based on the injured worker's compensation rate for loss of use or disability to the organ or body extremity injured on the job when

the worker is deemed medically capable of returning to the workforce although possibly to a less strenuous occupation.

12. Permanent total disability (PTD) benefits—A monetary sum awarded by a judicial body or agreed upon by the injured worker and the employer/insurance adjuster based on the worker's compensation rate when the worker has been deemed medically incapable of returning to the workplace in any job.

13. Malingerer—One who feigns sickness or any physical disablement or mental lapse or derangement, especially for the purpose of escaping the performance of a task, duty, or work; person who consciously feigns or simulates mental or physical illness for gain (2).

14. Deposition—A discovery device whereby testimony of a witness is taken under oath by a court reporter or someone commissioned to do so; a transcript or a word for word account is made of the testimony. Doctors usually participate in what is called a deposition *de bene esse,* which is one that takes the place of the physician at trial; the deposition could be read at trial, or in many workers, compensation matters submitted into the record as evidence.

15. Alternative dispute resolution (ADR)—The reference of a dispute to an impartial (third) person chosen by the parties to the dispute who agree in advance to abide by the arbitrator's award issued after a hearing at which both parties have an opportunity to be heard (2).

16. Mediation—Intervention; interposition; the act of a third person in intermediating between two contending parties with a view to persuading them to adjust or settle their dispute. The mediator is a neutral third party who does not give advice but acts to get the parties to resolve their issues.

17. Rehabilitation nurse—A nurse who is usually hired by the insurance carrier or often works for the insurance carrier directly or through a subsidiary owned by the insurance company and coordinates medical treatment for injured persons with the purpose of getting the injured persons to maximum medical improvement and/or returning to the workforce.

18. Private investigator (PI)—A person hired by the employer and/or insurance company to secretly follow and watch an injured person to determine (a) if the person is working at another job while drawing or claiming lost wages or (b) if the person is capable of doing physical activity that the person has denied being able to do. Often a PI will begin surveillance at a medical office, since the insurance adjuster will know in advance of the scheduled appointment.

19. Impairment—A number assigned by a physician for permanent loss of use of a body part of an injured person; the World Health Organization (WHO) defines impairment as "any loss or abnormality of psychological, physiological, or anatomical structure or function"; this is assessed by medical means and is a medical issue; often the American Medical Association (AMA) Guides to the Evaluation of Permanent Impairment (the Guides) is used by physicians to determine impairment; the Guides defines permanent impairment as one that has become static or stabilized during a period of time sufficient to allow optimal tissue repair, and one that is unlikely to change in spite of further medical or surgical therapy; in workers' compensation cases this number is most important for the injured worker because it is the basis for the award of disability; in personal injury cases this number signifies the long lasting effects of the injury.

20. Disability—A legal composite in workers' compensation claims that signifies the actual incapacity to perform the tasks encountered in one's employment and the wage loss that results; in determining disability, age, employment history, and education of the injured worker are taken into account.

21. Negligence—The omission to do something that a reasonable man, guided by those ordinary considerations that ordinarily regulate human affairs, would do, or the doing of something that a reasonable and prudent person would not do.

22. Actual damages or "out of pocket" damages—Real, substantial, and just damages or the amount awarded to an injured party for his or her actual and real loss or injury; synonymous with "compensatory damages" and with "general damages"; these damages would include medical bills casually related to the injury.

23. Punitive damages or exemplary damages—These damages are designed to punish or make an example of the negligent party; these are damages on an increased scale over and above what would compensate for the injury where the wrong done was committed willfully or with reckless disregard of another's rights.

24. Loss of consortium—The loss of conjugal fellowship of husband and wife, and the right of each to the company, society, cooperation, affection, and aid of the other in every conjugal relation. Damages for loss of consortium are commonly sought in wrongful death actions, or when spouse has been seriously injured through negligence of another.

25. Assumption of the risk—The doctrine of assumption of the risk means legally that a plaintiff may not recover for an injury to which he or she assents (i.e., that a person may not recover for an injury received when he or she voluntarily exposes her- or himself to a known and appreciated danger).

26. Comparative negligence—Under comparative negligence statutes or doctrines, negligence is measured in terms of percentage, and any damages allowed shall be diminished in proportion to the amount of negligence attributable to the person for whose injury, damage, or death recovery is sought.

27. Contributory negligence—The act or omission amounting to want of ordinary care on part of complaining

party, which, concurring with defendant's negligence, is proximate cause of injury. The defense of contributory negligence has been replaced by the doctrine of comparative negligence in many states.

28. Plaintiff—A person who brings an action; the party who complains or sues in a civil action and is so named on the record.

29. Defendant—The person defending or denying; the party against whom relief or recovery is sought in an action or suit or the accused in a criminal case.

30. Claimant—Analogous to plaintiff in workers' compensation claims; the injured worker who seeks medical, wage loss benefits, and or/ financial award for permanent disability related to an on-the-job injury and is so named on the record.

31. Uninsured motorist coverage—Protection afforded an insured by first-party insurance against bodily injury inflicted by an uninsured motorist, after the liability of the uninsured motorist for the injury has been established. Uninsured motorist coverage in automobile liability policies is designed to close the gaps inherent in motor vehicle financial responsibility and compulsory insurance legislation, and this insurance coverage is intended, within fixed limits, to provide financial recompense to innocent persons who receive injuries and dependents of those who are killed through the wrongful conduct of motorists who, because they are uninsured and not financially responsible, cannot be made to respond in damages.

32. Underinsured motorist coverage—Insurance coverage in an amount less than the value of the property insured or less than the risk exposure.

33. Automobile insurance—This term may embrace insurance against loss of or damage to a motor vehicle caused by fire, windstorm, theft, collision, or other insurable hazards, and also against legal liability for personal injuries or damage to property resulting from operation of the vehicle.

34. No-fault auto insurance—Type of automobile insurance in which claims for personal injury (and sometimes property damage) are made against the claimant's own insurance company (no matter who was at fault) rather than against the insurer of the party at fault. Under such state no-fault statutes only in cases of serious personal injuries and high medical costs may the injured bring an action against the other party or his or her insurer. No-fault statutes vary from state to state in terms of scope of coverage, threshold amounts, etc.

35. Proximate cause—A cause that is legally sufficient to result in legal liability; a cause that directly produces an event and without which the event would not have occurred.

36. Intervening event—An event that comes between the initial event in a sequence and the end result, thereby altering the natural course of events that might have connected a wrongful act to an injury.

37. Most probable cause—An effect or result that is more likely than not to have led to the conclusion in question in terms of legal proof (i.e., the lifting of the heavy box was the most probable cause of the herniated disc).

REFERENCES

1. Larson, A. *The law of workmen's compensation.* New York: Mathew Bender & Company, 1952–1992.
2. *Black's law dictionary*, 7th ed. St. Paul, MN: West Group, 1999.
3. *South Carolina Worker's Compensation Law annotated.* The State of South Carolina, Lawyers Cooperative Publishing, Rochester, New York, 1988–1997
4. *Black's law dictionary*, 5th ed. Henry Campbell Black, MA, West Publishing Company, St. Paul, Minnesota, 1979.

CHAPTER **45**

The Pain Physician's Role in Legal Proceedings

Gerald M. Finkel, Ralph C. McCullough, II and Erin M. Joyner

Pain is a medical concept. Pain and suffering is a legal concept. Although some legal commentators have attempted to create an ephemeral distinction between the concepts of pain and suffering, these attempts have been unsuccessful. Pain is the sensation of the body, whereas suffering is the consequence of pain to the individual. However, pain and suffering are so inextricably linked that it is often impossible to determine where one ends and the other begins. Therefore, courts treat pain and suffering as one concept with different components—past and present physical pain, future pain, and mental suffering.

The experience of pain has two consequences: the overt behavior of pain, and the subjective experience of pain (1). The job that faces physicians is determining the source of the pain and treating the pain. The job that faces the attorney is to help the patient, now the plaintiff, to be compensated for this pain. What is problematic for both professionals is the subjective nature of the pain. How does the physician separate the malingerer from the pain stricken? How does the attorney explain to the jury the subjective feeling of pain?

Physicians, like attorneys, oftentimes face the daunting task of assessing the legitimacy of their patient's, or client's, claims of pain. The physician's job in assessing the validity of these claims is primarily to diagnose and treat the underlying pathology. The physician, however, shares with the attorney, albeit secondarily, the task of assessing the legitimacy of these claims for the purpose of litigation. The attorney knows the law. The physician knows the medicine. Together, they can prove this pain. Thus, the physician not only occupies the unique position of healer, but also holds the financial future of the patient in his or her hands.

What makes this process somewhat easier is the growing recognition in the medical community of the concept of pain management. The multidisciplinary approach to

pain helps to alleviate in part the skepticism that used to accompany chronic pain. Although the alleviation of pain is still seen by some physicians as secondary to diagnosis and treatment of the underlying pathology, there are signs that the medical community may soon recognize the alleviation of pain as a primary duty. For example, the Joint Commission of Accreditation of Healthcare Organizations has proposed pain management standards. Standard PE (1.4) provides: "Pain is assessed in all patients" (2). Examples of implementation of this standard include the suggestions that physicians determine pain intensity through the use of a rating scale; "the onset, duration, variations and patterns," "alleviating and aggravating factors," and "effects of pain (impact on daily life, function, sleep, appetite, relationships with others, emotions, concentration, etc.)" (3). The very same factors that the physician must have in order to adequately treat the plaintiff's pain, the attorney must have to prove pain and suffering.

The purpose of this chapter is to bring to the practice of medicine the practical realities of the courtroom—how pain and suffering is proved, what is admissible, to what may the physician testify, and what can physicians include in medical records that may later help the patient prove his pain and suffering? To these ends, the chapter examines briefly several studies that attempt to analyze the jury decision-making process in pain and suffering cases. The chapter then discusses the basic legal principles of which physicians should be cognizant in order to help the patient in proving pain and suffering.

THE SUBJECTIVITY OF MONETARY VALUATION OF PAIN AND SUFFERING

Tort damages for pain and suffering is a controversial topic in the legal community. The disparity in awards for similar injuries has led many to the conclusion that these awards are excessive and arbitrary numbers (4). Thus, some conclude that pain and suffering awards should be done away with all together or, at the very least, capped (3). In the 1980s, this became the battle cry for many state legislatures, who passed legislation capping the available award for pain and suffering damages (3). Although such legislation spells bad news for plaintiffs, such proposals are based on well-founded criticisms of pain and suffering awards. Juries are given little, if any, guidance in how to reach their verdict. Methods, such as the per diem argument discussed later, can provide the jury some guidance, but the fact still remains that even such approaches cannot create a market price for pain and suffering (4).

The decision-making processes of juries are difficult to quantify, especially for the elusive concept of "pain and suffering." The same characteristics of pain that frustrate doctors and lawyers also frustrate jurors who are often given few guidelines in assessing the legitimacy of pain and in assigning a monetary value to it. Social scientists and legal commentators have attempted to quantify the mindset of the jury. What information, what details, influence juries' decisions? Although these questions are impossible to answer with absolute certainty, studies are helpful for attorney and lawyer alike in understanding how this complicated decision is made.

How Jury Instructions Are Formed

Kahneman and Spitzer examined how the framing of jury instructions can shape jury awards for pain and suffering (5). The study showed that although litigators typically use the "making whole" perspective in pain and suffering litigation, the more lucrative approach is the "selling price" perspective (5). The latter approach is disfavored by attorneys and courts alike, and may, in fact, be inappropriate in some jurisdictions (5). Thus, although this information may have little direct practical application in litigation, it does demonstrate the very important point that jurors' perceptions of pain and suffering are not static and can be influenced.

The "making whole" perspective asks the jury at what price can the plaintiff be made whole (5). The "selling price" asks the jury to determine at what price would the plaintiff sell her good health (5). Kahenman and Spitzer examined these approaches by asking groups to assign monetary values after being given various jury instructions. In both rounds, instructions based on the making whole perspective and the selling price perspective were given. In the second round, an additional instruction based on a hybrid approach was given. In both rounds, the "selling price" approach netted the largest award and the "making whole" perspective the smallest (5).

Injury Characteristics

The Wissler study (6) examined the way in which juries rated various injuries according to the following factors:

visibility, physical pain, duration of pain, mental suffering, duration of mental suffering, severity of injury, disability, disfigurement, and effect of the injury on everyday life (6). Test subjects were asked to rate several injuries, with varying degrees of information concerning the cause of the injury and plaintiff and defendant's respective fault levels, and to assign a monetary value to the injury. This study found that jurors' perceptions of injuries were sensitive to the characteristics of the injury as opposed to the cause and defendant's responsibility and that test subjects tended to be consistent in their ratings of the harm of each injury and the differences in degrees among the injuries (6). Thus, injury characteristics affected ratings on physical pain and mental suffering (6). The study also found that the monetary value assigned tended to be consistent with test subjects' severity ratings. The second part of the study, involving slight variation in the procedure and a larger test group, found results fairly consistent with the aforementioned results. This part of the study concluded that test subjects took into account the severity and duration of harm across the board in making a determination of the overall severity of the injury (6). The study concluded that, of all the factors considered, mental suffering and disability had the strongest impact on awards and pain had the weakest (6).

Inferences to be Drawn

These studies together suggest that pain and suffering awards are far from arbitrary and capricious and that the jury does not base the amount so much on which party they like better, but on their perception of the plaintiff's injury and how the issue of pain and suffering is framed. The Wissler study also suggests that people have a baseline of understanding in relation to human pain and suffering and that their awards reflect a commonsense, personal-experience approach to awarding these values. The practical application of this study is the demonstration that in order for the plaintiff to receive an award for an injury that is relatively benign in appearance but that causes great pain, the doctor and the lawyer must be prepared to show how this injury is disabling. As one legal source stated:

> Where it is not apparent to the jury that a particular injury . . . is painful, the physician . . . can give an illuminating medical and physiological explanation of why pain was experienced. By this means, doubts in the minds of the jury can be resolved" (7).

VALUATION WITHIN SOLE PROVINCE OF JURY

Valuation of pain and suffering is within the sole province of the jury. Much of the criticism of pain and suffering awards seems to stem in part from many legal commentators' fear of the jury and their seemingly omnipotent power. Many worry that jurors, when confronted by the savvy and sleek plaintiff's attorney, will disregard evidence and follow their hearts, ultimately awarding more than the pain and suffering is really worth. This fear is exacerbated by the fact that there is no real method to place a dollar amount on pain and suffering.

The principle that valuation is within the sole province of the jury has many implications in the actual trial. Most importantly, this means that the only power the court has over the award of damages is the power of correction when the award appears to be the result of abuse or passion (7).

DAMAGES AWARDS

Pain and suffering can be examined before, during, or after the actual pain experience. Implicit in the concept of pain and suffering is an awareness of the pain. Thus, to determine whether pain exists in the first place, plaintiff's level of consciousness must be determined (8).

Past and Present Pain

Damages for past and present pain can be established by plaintiff's own testimony and medical records (8). However, as will be discussed later in this chapter, such testimony often appears self-serving to the jury. Thus, additional testimony will be needed to buttress the plaintiff's claims regarding the pain and suffering.

Future Pain and Suffering

Future pain and suffering should be evaluated once the patient has stabilized so that the future pain and suffering can be determined with a reasonable certainty (8). Because damages must have a basis in evidence, courts have established legal thresholds. The majority rule—the reasonable certainty rule—is that future pain and suffering must be established by a reasonable certainty (9). The minority rule is that future pain and suffering awards are appropriate when this pain and suffering will, in reasonable probability, result from the injury. (9) Another minority approach has been adopted in Wisconsin (10). This standard requires that the future pain and suffering award be based on the "ordinary experience of mankind" in cases where the pain and suffering does not require "special learning, study and experience" (10).

Damages for future pain and suffering must usually be established by medical testimony. Unlike past and present pain and suffering, about which the plaintiff is competent to testify, future pain and suffering is generally a medical question. As stated by one court:

> Only a medical expert is qualified to express an opinion to a medical certainty . . . as to whether the pain will continue in the future, and, if so, for how long a period it will continue. In the absence of such expert testimony . . . the jury should be instructed that no damages may be allowed for future pain and suffering (11).

Two important components of future pain and suffering are the certainty that future pain will occur and the duration of the pain (11). Thus, where the pain is subjective, medical testimony is necessary (12). There are two exceptions made by many courts regarding the reasonable certainty of future pain component. First, expert medical testimony is not necessary when, based on the injury, it is common knowledge that future pain and suffering will result (13). Second, expert medical testimony is not necessary when the plaintiff establishes at trial the existence of pain and suffering (14).

Plaintiff, however, cannot testify regarding the duration of the pain and suffering or that his injuries are permanent (14). If the injury is permanent, mortality tables may be admitted to establish the duration of plaintiff's future pain and suffering (14).

Mental Suffering

Mental suffering is defined as the pain and suffering from the physical injury, "mental reaction" to the injury and "to the possible consequences of the injury" (15). Common examples of mental suffering include flight, nervousness, grief, anxiety, worry, mortification, humiliation, embarrassment, terror, and ordeal (15). There is no set rule or standard to be applied by juries when determining an award for mental suffering (15).

However, there are certain rules that can be gleaned regarding the availability of mental suffering damages. First, when the mental suffering accompanies a contemporaneous physical injury, the mental suffering is always compensable (14). Second, most jurisdictions allow recovery for mental suffering that can be traced back to the physical injury (14).

Mental suffering is probably the most difficult component of pain and suffering to prove. Obviously, the plaintiff, her family, and friends will testify as to this mental suffering. Additionally, in the absence of direct proof, the jury may infer the existence of mental suffering from the injury itself and compensate the plaintiff accordingly (14).

PERSONS WHO MAY RECOVER

Injured Persons

Only the injured person can recover pain and suffering damages in a personal injury suit (16). Although the injury and the resulting pain and suffering of the plaintiff obviously affect the plaintiff's family, the pain and suffering award is not a vehicle through which to compensate these people. Rather, causes of action such as loss of consortium are tailored toward such a goal. However, the pain and suffering award is meant to compensate the plaintiff for the pain that he has to endure through no fault of his own.

Injured Infants

Traditionally, courts denied infant plaintiffs the right to recover mental pain and suffering awards (16). However, courts today recognize that although a child may be unable to articulate her suffering as adults can, a child's pain is often clear and perhaps more poignant than the pain of an adult. Although a child may be too young to express this pain, it is often evidenced by crying and other outward manifestations of pain and discomfort. The pain is real even though the child cannot articulate it in the same way as an adult can, and the child is deserving of a monetary award for pain and suffering in the same way that an adult plaintiff is.

Thus, the absence of the infant plaintiff's testimony does not preclude recovery for pain and suffering. In *Capelouto v Kaiser Foundation Hospitals*, the Supreme Court of California held that the trial court erred in instructing the jury as follows: "You are not permitted to award Kim Capelouto damages for physical pain and mental suffering which, although possible, is under the law incapable of proof because of the age of the child" (17). The court drew a distinction between the capacity to experience pain with the ability to describe the pain or discover the cause of pain (17). Thus, an infant is not precluded from recovering pain and suffering damages simply because of an inability to articulate the pain to the doctor or the jury (18).

Survival Actions

Under the common law, the death of the defendant or the plaintiff in a tort case extinguished the case (19). In the case of the plaintiff's death, the courts made exceptions for tort actions involving personal property, but not for personal injury (19). Survival statutes abrogate the common-law rule that the cause of action is extinguished upon the death of the plaintiff or defendant (20). Thus, a personal injury cause of action that seeks damages for pain and suffering will survive the death of the plaintiff, unless the survival statute explicitly excludes pain and suffering damages. Currently, all 50 states and the District of Columbia have some form of survival statute (20). It is important to realize that these statutes do not create a new cause of action, but that the damages available to the decedent's family are derivative of the plaintiff's right to recover when living. It is also important to recognize that these statutes are not necessarily the same as statutes that provide a cause of action for wrongful death. However, survival statutes and wrongful death statutes have been merged by some legislatures (20).

Under survival statutes, the decedent's personal representative may recover the same damages the decedent would have in the personal injury lawsuit. However, the one caveat to this general rule is that some jurisdictions expressly preclude the recovery of pain and suffering damages (e.g., Arizona, California, Colorado, Washington). As an example, Arizona's survival statute provides as follows:

> Every cause of action, except a cause of action for damages for breach of promise to marry, seduction, libel, slander, separate maintenance, alimony, loss of consortium or invasion of the right of privacy, shall survive the death of the person entitled thereto or liable therefor, and may be asserted by or against the personal representative of such person, provided that upon the death of the person injured, damages for pain and suffering of such injured person shall not be allowed (21).

In the pain and suffering context, the compensable pain and suffering is the conscious pain and suffering from the moment of the accident to the death. The pain and suffering engendered on those left behind is not within the scope of the survival statute, but is left to the wrongful death statute. Thus, if death occurs instantly or the plaintiff never regains consciousness, there is no award of pain and suffering available (20).

Witnesses to Injuries of Another

Witnessing the personal injury of another is often traumatizing. Although no direct physical injury results, as it does to the victim, witnesses sometimes find that they too have been injured by the accident. These witnesses often have a cause of action as well (16).

However, this cause of action is somewhat new. Under the "impact" rule, which used to be the majority rule, recovery for mental suffering was not available absent direct physical injury to the plaintiff (14). Many courts have thrown this rule over for one of two rules, both allowing bystanders to recover for mental suffering (14). The first of these more liberal rules is the "zone of physical danger" rule (14). This rule is stated in Restatement (2d) of Torts §436(2):

> If the actor's conduct is negligent as creating an unreasonable risk of causing bodily harm to another otherwise than by subjecting him to fright, shock, or other similar and immediate emotional disturbance, the fact that such harm results solely from the internal operation of fright or other emotional disturbance does not protect the actor from liability.

The second of these more liberal rules in the "foreseeability test," which requires that the mental suffering be foreseeable at the time of the accident (14). The caveat to this provision is that in most jurisdictions, this mental suffering must result in a physical injury or physical manifestation of the mental suffering (14).

The "zone of physical danger" rule and the "foreseeability" test both deal with accidents resulting from negligence. When the injury sustained by the victim is the result of an intentional tort such as assault and battery, the witness may have a cause of action under Restatement (2d) of Torts §46, which provides:

(1) One who by extreme and outrageous conduct intentionally or recklessly causes severe emotional distress to another is subject to liability for such emotional distress, and if bodily harm to the other results from it, for such bodily harm.
(2) Where such conduct is directed at a third person, the actor is subject to liability if he intentionally or recklessly causes severe emotional distress
   (a) to a member of such person's immediate family who is present at the time, whether or not such distress results in bodily harm, or
   (b) to any other person who is present at the time, if such distress results in bodily harm.

This section is meant to apply to the most severe form of conduct. It is not meant to furnish a remedy to every person offended or otherwise angry over some trivial matter (22).

PROOF REQUIRED

Valuation

Valuation of pain and suffering, as previously discussed, presents the jury with the unique job of placing a value on the subjective feeling of another. Besides the requirement of reasonability, there appears to be no consensus as to how the jury is to reach its decisions. However, certain methods of valuation are common. Perhaps the most common is the per diem method.

The per diem approach has not been without controversy. Arguments in opposition to the per diem approach, which are echoed in many court opinions, include the following:

1. There is no evidentiary basis for converting pain and suffering into a monetary sum.
2. Suggesting monetary equivalents for pain and suffering is tantamount to giving testimony or expressing an opinion not disclosed by the evidence.
3. The per diem approach put the defendant at the disadvantage of having to rebut an argument that has no basis in evidence.
4. The per diem approach often misleads juries into awarding larger sums (23).

Arguments in favor of the per diem approach include the necessity to provide the jury with some reasonable considerations and the ability of defense counsel to suggest her own amount. Additionally, proponents argue that the per diem approach is merely a suggestion, not evidence, and is usually accompanied by a jury instruction to that effect (23).

Jurisdictions are divided into three categories regarding the per diem approach. Some jurisdictions do not allow the per diem approach as a matter of law (24). Some jurisdictions allow the use of this approach at all times (25). Finally, some jurisdictions have decided that the decision to allow the use of the per diem approach is within the sole discretion of the court. When this is the case, the per diem approach often must be accompanied by jury instructions that emphasize to the jury that the argument of plaintiff's counsel is not evidence (26), that the dollar amounts are merely suggestions (26), and that the jury need not adopt this approach (27). In addition to these jury instructions, the court may employ other protective features such as requiring plaintiff to notify the defense that the per diem argument is going to be used (28).

The following example of the per diem argument containing many of the aforementioned safeguards was upheld by the Supreme Court of Vermont:

During closing argument, plaintiff suggested that the jury think about the plaintiff's injury in terms of daily pain and suffering, and then determine what amount of damages would be appropriate compensation for each day of suffering. An average daily figure was suggested to the jury, which it could then multiply by the number of days plaintiff would live. . . . The jury was told to consider this figure only if it found the calculations useful in qualifying plaintiff's damages" (29).

Per Diem

The per diem approach involves the determination of two figures. First, the life expectancy of the plaintiff must be determined. Mortuary tables establish life expectancy based on statistical information of the population. Thus, the age of the plaintiff is subtracted from the life expectancy reflected in the mortuary table (16). Second, a value must be placed on some unit of time—a minute, hour, or day (30). These two numbers are multiplied to theoretically place a value on the plaintiff's pain and suffering.

Thus, the per diem approach works in this way:

Step 1:
Plaintiff's age (at the time of the accident):   X
Life expectancy (based on mortuary table):   L
$L - X = N$ (number of years plaintiff must endure pain and suffering)

Step 2:
The jury must assign a value to a pain-free unit of time (for the purposes of this example, the unit of time is one day):   D

Step 3:
Multiply the value by 365 in order to place a monetary value of one year.
$D(365) = Y$

Step 4:
$L * Y$ = Future pain and suffering award

Golden Rule

The Golden Rule approach is disfavored by practitioners (31) and inappropriate in most courts (19). Golden Rule approach, as the name suggests, asks the jury to base their pain and suffering award amount on an amount they would take to undergo the plaintiff's injuries (19). Essentially, this approach asks the jurors to place themselves in the plaintiff's place. Critics of this approach argue that this approach removes any objectivity from the already difficult task of assigning a value to pain, which has no market value, by encouraging jurors to base their award on personal bias (14). Use of this approach is reversible error (14).

Mortality Tables

Mortality tables, also called mortuary tables, are relevant when the plaintiff faces the prospect of lifetime pain and suffering. These tables "set up court-accepted standards of life expectancy based on statistical data establishing the norms of our population" (16). Although these tables are admissible to show life expectancy (14) (and indispensable when using the per diem argument), they are not conclusive (14). Life expectancy is a jury question, and the jury may disregard the tables or estimate the plaintiff's life expectancy based on their own criteria (14). It is also important to note that an accident may shorten the plaintiff's life expectancy and, while this is relevant for other damage components of the personal injury award, when awarding damages for future pain and suffering, the jury should consider the plaintiff s life expectancy in his injured condition (32).

Witnesses

Family Members and Co-workers

Pain and suffering, as previously discussed, is a subjective matter. The only direct proof that can be offered of this pain and suffering is the testimony of the plaintiff. However, because such testimony is sometimes seen as self-serving by juries that are skeptical of pain and suffering claims, additional testimony is often used to bolster the plaintiff's claims. Although the testimony of the physician is vital to giving the plaintiff's claims medical validity, the testimony of family members gives an inarguably less medical but sometimes more poignant look at the physical pain experienced by the plaintiff and how this effects his daily life. Family members and coworkers are able to offer a before-and-after comparison of the plaintiff that the physician and the medical records cannot (33).

Testimony given by the family members will likely include the plaintiff's initial reaction to his injury, what complaints he made directly following the injury, and the duration of his recuperation (34). The family member will also testify to plaintiff's activity level and hobbies before the injury in comparison to now (34). The family member will also testify as to the strain that plaintiff's injury has placed on other areas of his life and the family's welfare, including the financial situation of the family and the effect of plaintiff's pain on his relationships with family members (34). Coworkers can similarly testify as to how the injury has affected the plaintiff in the context of the workplace.

In some states, verbal expressions of pain (not made immediately preceding the accident so as to be a part of the res gestae) made to family, friends, and coworkers may be considered inadmissible hearsay (35). (However, the same verbal expressions may be admissible when made to a medical professional.) Many courts allow the introduction of such statements under various exceptions to the hearsay rule (36).

When the verbal expression involves objective manifestations of pain such as moaning or crying, consensus seems to exist that such testimony is admissible (36). When the verbal expression consists of a statement by the plaintiff, courts are less consistent in their approach (36). Some courts take the more liberal view that as long as the statement was made in such circumstances as to guarantee its reliability, it is admissible (36). Other states such as New York and Georgia take a more stringent approach, disallowing verbal statements made by the plaintiff to nonmedical professionals (36).

Additionally, some states allow such verbal expressions under the state of mind exception to the hearsay rule (33).

Physicians

The physician is perhaps the most important and credible witness the plaintiff can offer. The reason is obvious. Unlike the plaintiff and his family, who may have a motive to lie or exaggerate, the physician stands to receive no economic benefit from the ultimate verdict. Additionally, physicians, unlike other professions, are perceived by society as honest professionals bound by morality and their Hippocratic Oath to do good.

THE PHYSICIAN'S ROLE IN LITIGATION

The importance of the physician's testimony cannot be overstated. Given this importance, the physician should remain cognizant of certain legal principles in order to offer the best testimony possible.

Testimony as to Existence and Severity of Pain

The Physician's Belief

As noted above, the plaintiff's testimony concerning past and present pain is direct proof of the pain and suffering. However, physician testimony that, in the physician's opinion, the plaintiff's pain was real will help to bolster the plaintiff's claim. Physician testimony that the patient is feigning or malingering is admissible. The physician may also testify as to her opinion that the pain is real (37). Although it is an elementary principle, this principle warrants attention: The physician's belief in the patient is vital. As noted in *Lawyers' Manual Cyclopedia of Personal Injuries and Allied Specialities*:

> In the opinion of at least one medical expert, physicians are often the worst persons to testify at trial to the pain suffered by a plaintiff. After seeing thousands of patients complaining of pain over the course of years, many physicians view . . . pain in a relatively minor category (38).

Another's Expressions of Pain

As already discussed, the great difficulty in proving pain and suffering lies in the subjective nature of pain. As suggested by the Wissler study, jurors tend to better understand the pain and suffering associated with severe injury as opposed to less severe injury (33). Thus, although a physician cannot prove with certainty that a plaintiff's pain is genuine, that physician may testify as to the objective manifestations of pain by the plaintiff (39). These objective manifestations are particularly important when the patient appears relatively "physically sound" (33). Such objective findings include tears, perspiration, moaning, facial expressions such as grimacing, limitations in motion, and changes in vital signs (40). Thus, the physician and staff should include such objective behavior in the medical record of the patient.

Statements Made for the Purpose of Medical Diagnosis

The term *hearsay* is a technical, legal term that has become part of the American lexicon. Laypeople understand the word to mean that out-of-court statements are not admissible in court. This is, in fact, the correct understanding. However, the rule against the admission of hearsay is a rule that has been swallowed up by its exceptions. Rule of 803(4) of the Federal Rules of Evidence is just such an example. The rule provides:

> The following are not excluded by the hearsay rule, even though the declarant is available as a witness:
>   (4) Statements for Purposes of Medical Diagnosis or Treatment. Statement made for purposes of medical diagnosis or treatment and describing medical history, or past or present symptoms, pain, or sensations, or the inception or general character of the cause or external source thereof as reasonably pertinent to diagnosis and treatment.

This exception makes no distinction between examining and treating physicians. Thus, a physician examining the plaintiff for the purpose of testifying can testify as to statements made by the plaintiff concerning his condition. Thus, physicians should pay careful attention to the com-

plaints of the patients. It is important to note that this rule does not require the statement be made to a doctor. Thus, the physician should instruct her staff to be vigilant in listening to and recording these complaints (33).

Referral to Pain Management Treatment

A referral to pain management treatment strongly speaks to the physician's belief in the legitimacy of the plaintiff's pain. The case *City of Philadelphia v Shapiro* (41) is illustrative of this point. Plaintiff, Anthony Laurelli, was injured in an auto accident in 1954. Over the course of the next 9 years, plaintiff repeatedly received treatment for his pain. Defendant's argument on appeal was that the trial court erred in allowing the plaintiffs' doctors to testify as to plaintiffs' pain. The court noted that it is the jury's role to decide whether the doctor has been deceived. The court went on to state:

> Had Dr. Olsen in this case doubted the existence of the pain described by the plaintiff Laurelli, he certainly would not have drilled a hole in his head, lifted his brain, searched for a tiny nerve and snipped it with the scientific hope that by this cutting he would shut off the agony which was taking the patient in and out of hospitals, away from his work, away from his recreations, away from the pleasures of life he had enjoyed prior to the accident of 1954 (41).

Objective Tests

Although the doctor's testimony is key as to the doctor's belief in the sincerity of the patient's pain, the treating physician should conduct objective tests to reinforce her opinion (33). Also, it is important that physicians recognize that individuals have different levels of pain. Thus, unlike the use of pain as an indicator of an underlying ailment, pain also affects the quality of a patient's life and thus the degree of pain felt is relevant (42).

Patient's Threshold for Pain

As discussed above, a significant impediment to a truly effective claim for pain and suffering is the public perception that those suffering from pain and suffering are using the legal system to extort money from defendants. Although there are among the body of plaintiffs malingerers, such a perception ignores the medical reality that individuals have varying thresholds for pain (43). The defense will attempt to exploit this perception by offering medical evidence that the plaintiff is malingering (43). Therefore, the physician should be prepared to address the pain threshold issue (43) and should include in the medical record any pain threshold tests conducted.

Physiological factors, cultural factors, personality characteristics, and lifestyle factors contribute to the varying thresholds of individuals. Differences in the chemical makeup of individuals, as in the production of endorphins and serotonin, contribute (43). Also, one's culture, for example, whether one's culture teaches to maintain a stiff upper lip, contributes (43). Personality traits, such as how one handles stress, contribute (43). And, finally, lifestyle choices, such as one's level of physical fitness, contribute (43). Thus, a patient's complaints of pain cannot be dismissed because they seem out of proportion to the injury actually sustained.

No medical test can determine with certainty whether a patient is actually experiencing pain. However, some tests are available that may be helpful in drawing some type of conclusion in this regard (42). These tests include the superficial touch test, the superficial pain test, the temperature test, and the deep pressure test (42). Additionally, tests such as the Pain Index Predictor can be helpful (42).

Pain Indicators

Aside from determining the patient's pain threshold, the physician should undertake some objective tests to determine the existence of pain. Because pain is a subjective complaint, the jury may be unpersuaded by the plaintiff's testimony if no concrete medical evidence is presented to back up the plaintiff's claims. Thus, physicians should undertake objective tests, not only for her own purposes of diagnosis of pain and referral to pain management, but also to aid the patient's claim for pain and suffering.

Although such a step is obvious to the physician, what is not readily apparent is that objective tests undertaken may or may not be admissible, depending on the test's purported reliability and acceptance within the medical community. Thus, a new, experimental procedure may be an excellent diagnostic source and, yet, be inadmissible in court.

It is important for the physician to understand the criteria by which these procedures will be evaluated. Depending on the court, the objective test will have to pass muster with one of the following tests.

The first test is known as the Frye test, based on the 1923 case *Frye v United* States (44). There, the defendant, in a criminal case, sought to introduce a "deception test." The court held that these test results were inadmissible. The court stated:

> Just when the scientific principle or discovery crosses the line between experimental and demonstrable stages is difficult to define. Somewhere in the twilight zone the evidential force of the principle must be recognized, and while courts will go a long way in admitting expert testimony deduced from the well-recognized scientific principle or discovery, the thing from which the deduction is made is sufficiently established to have gained general acceptance in the particular field in which it belongs (44).

Under *Frye,* the test must be one that has crossed this line. Although this case offers little guidance in the way of factors to which one should look in order to determine whether the line has been crossed and the test has become an accepted procedure, a test commonly used by doctors will undoubtedly pass this test.

Many viewed the standards of *Frye* to be far too stringent. Thus, over 50 years after this decision, the Federal Rules of Evidence were adopted (45). Because it is not entirely clear whether the Federal Rules have superseded or merely liberalized *Frye* (45), the physician must be cognizant of both tests when deciding on which objective test to use. The Federal Rules of Evidence that are relevant here include rules 401, 403, and 702 (45). These rules provide as follows:

> Rule 401 Definition of Relevant Evidence
> Relevant evidence" means evidence having any tendency to make the existence of any fact that is of consequence to the determination of the action more probable or less probable than it would be without the evidence.

> Rule 403 Exclusion of Relevant Evidence on Grounds of Prejudice, Confusion, or Waste of Time
> Although relevant evidence may be excluded if its probative value is substantially outweighed by the danger of unfair prejudice, confusion of the issue, or misleading the jury, or by consideration of undue delay, waste of time, or needless presentation of cumulative evidence.

> Rule 702 Testimony by Experts
> If scientific, technical, or other specialized knowledge will assist the trier of fact to understand the evidence or to determine a fact in issue, a witness qualified as an expert by knowledge, skill, training, or education, may testify thereto in the form of opinion or otherwise, if (1) the testimony is based upon sufficient facts or data, (2) the testimony is the product of reliable principles and methods, and (3) the witness has applied the principles and methods reliably to the facts of the case.

Stated simply, evidence must be relevant, and even then it may be excluded in the face of time constraints or the possibility of prejudice.

The application of rules 401 and 403 requires a balancing by the court of relevance versus the possibility of unfair prejudice or delay. Some courts have articulated factors that may be considered when making this balance (46). The *Williams* court considered the potential rate of error (46), the existence and maintenance of standards (46), and "the care and concern with which a scientific technique has been employed, and whether it appears to lend itself to abuse" (46), and "the presence of 'fail-safe' characteristics" (46), as factors of reliability. Thus, the physician would be well-advised to consider these factors when deciding which objective tests to use.

Implicit in the requirement of relevance in Rule 401 and explicit in Rule 702 is the requirement of reliability. Thus, to meet this burden, the physician should take certain steps. The first most obvious is to choose a reliable and accepted test. (Although the Frye test has been superseded in some jurisdictions by the adoption of the Federal Rules of Evidence, acceptance in the medical community would obviously be a persuasive factor in determining the reliability of the procedure.) Secondly, the physician should be aware of any independent acts of the patient that could skew the results (45).

For example, the results of thermography, although generally considered reliable, may be altered by patients wishing to alter the test in their favor. Thus, the physician should include in his record the fact that the patient was given all relevant instructions before the test and that the patient indicated that she had complied with all these conditions (45).

Other Areas of Testimony

Thus far, we have discussed areas of testimony that are relevant for establishing the existence and severity of the plaintiff's pain. Other areas of testimony include the duration of treatment and future treatment that will be required (47). Future pain and suffering, as a general rule, must be established with medical testimony. Testimony regarding the duration of treatment, and the future treatment required, tend to help establish future pain and suffering damages with a reasonable certainty. Additionally, the physician should be prepared to explain to the jury the pain management approach.

Practical Suggestions

Essential to a successful personal injury case, especially those cases involving pain and suffering not readily apparent to the jury, is a thorough understanding, on the attorney's part, of the plaintiff's injury (33). Although attorneys who regularly work in the personal injury arena will likely have a good working knowledge of medical terms and procedures, this experience is no substitute for a medical degree. Thus, the physician should be prepared to help the attorney review and understand the medical records (33). Additionally, the physician should be prepared to offer the attorney referrals to medical literature (33).

CONCLUSION

In proving pain and suffering, the attorney faces the complicated task of making the jury understand what cannot be quantified or empirically shown. The attorney, in essence, must tell the story of the plaintiff's pain and suffering. Like all great storytellers, attorneys must not only give the facts, but also create the picture of pain. Attorneys use a number of devices in telling this story. First and most obviously, attorneys put the plaintiff on the stand to explain his pain and the effect that it has had on his life. The attorney also puts family, friends, and coworkers on the stand to testify as to what the plaintiff has said and how the pain has impacted his life and his relationships with others. However, the testimony of friends, family, and coworkers may be limited by the hearsay rule. Additionally, both the testimony of the plaintiff and his family and friends may be doubted by skeptical jurors. Thus, the physician's testimony is vital in bolstering the plaintiff's claims. Additionally, attorneys use demonstrative aids such as blown-up medical records and blown-up pictures of objective tests, such as the thermograph.

REFERENCES

1. Dennis C. Turk, Assessment of patients' reporting of pain: an integrated perspective, 353 The Lancet 1784, 1785 (May 22, 1999)
2. **Http://www.jcaho.org/standard/pm.html** (Visited Jan. 22, 2001).
3. Mark Geisfeld, *Placing a Price on Pain and Suffering: A Method for Helping Juries Determine Tort Damages for Nonmonetary Injuries,* 83 Calif. L. Rev. 773, 776 (1995). *See also* Oscar G. Chase, Helping Jurors Determine Pain and Suffering Awards, 23 Hofstra L. Rev. 763 (1995).
4. See DAN B. DOBBS, HANDBOOK ON THE LAW OF REMEDIES 545 (1973); Oscar G. Chase, *Helping Jurors Determine Pain and Suffering Awards,* 23 Hofstra L. Rev. 763, 769 (1995).
5. J. Kahneman & Matthew L. Spitzer, *Framing the jury: cognitive perspectives on pain and suffering awards,* 81 Va. L.Rev. 1341 (Aug. 1995).
6. Roselle L. Wisser, et al., Explaining "pain and suffering" awards: the role of injury characteristics and fault attributes, 21 Law and Hum. Beh. 181 (1997).
7. 31 Am Jur 2d Damages § 264.
8. *Conscious Pain and Suffering is not a Matter of Degree,* 74 Marq. L. Rev. 289, 302 (1991). 23
9. 22 Am Jur 2d Damages §245.
10. *Conscious Pain and Suffering is not a Matter of Degree,* 74 Marq. L. Rev. 289, 311 (1991).
11. See *Conscious Pain and Suffering is not a Matter of Degree,* 74 Marq. L. Rev. 289, 310 (19,91), quoting Diemel v. Weirich, 58 N.W.2d 651, 652–52 (1953).
12. 22 Am Jur. 2d Damages §915.
13. 22 Am Jur. 2d Damages §1006; 9 PERSONAL INJURY: ACTION, DEFENSES, DAMAGES §3.041[2][c] (Louis R. Frumer & Melvin I. Friedman, eds. 1998).
14. 9 PERSONAL INJURY: ACTION, DEFENSES, DAMAGES §3.04[2][c] (Louis R. Frumer & Melvin I. Friedman, eds. 1998).
15. 22 Am Jur.2d Damages §251.
16. RALPH C. MCCULLOUGH, CIVIL TRIAL MANUAL II 788 (1980).
17. 103 Cal.Rptr. 856, 858.
18. Cases allowing children to recover pain and suffering damages: Reale v. Wayne Tp., 332 A.2,d 236 (ICJ. Super. 1975); Hiraldo v. Khan, 699 N.Y.S.2d 456, 267 A.D.2d 205 (2 Dept. 1999); Williams v. Williams, 641 N.Y.S.2d 408, 226 A.D.2d 710 (2 Dept. 1996); Reid by Reid v. County of Nassau, 627 N. Y.S.2d 396, 215 A.D.2d 466 (2 Dept. 1995).
19. DAN B. DOBBS, HANDBOOK ON THE LAW OF REMEDIES 551 (1973)
20. 10 PERSONAL INJURY: ACTION, DEFENSES, DAMAGES § 1.02[2] (Louis R. Frumer At Melvin I. Friedman, eds. 1998).
21. Ariz. Rev. Stat. Ann. § 14–3110
22. RESTATEMENT (SECOND) OF TORTS §46, Cmt. d.
23. *See e.g.,* Giant Food v. Satterfield, 603 A.2d 877, 879 (Md.App. 1992).
24. *See e.g.,* Pool v. Bell, 209 Conn. 536, 551 A.2d 1254 (1989); Henne v. Balick, 51 Del. 369, 146 A.2d 394 (1958); Ferry v Checker Taxi Co., 165 Ill.App.3d 744,117 Ill.Dec. 382, 520 N.E.2d 733 (1987); Steel v Bemis, 121 N.H. 425, 431 A.2d 113 (1981); Cox v. Valley Fair Corp., 83 N.J. 381, 416 A.2d 809 (1980); Tate v. Colobello, 58 N.Y.S.2d 84, 459 N.Y.S.2d 422, 445 N.E.2d 1101 (1983); Ilosky v. Michelin Tire Corp., 172 W.Va. 435, 307 S.E.2d 603 (1983); Affect v. Milwaukee & S.T. Corp., 11 Wis. 2d 604, 106 NW.2d 274 (1960).
25. *See e.g.,* Beagle v. Vasold, 65 Cal.2d 166, 53 Cal. Rptr. 129, 417 P.2d 673 (1966); Paduach Area Public Library v. Terry, 655 S.W.2d 19 (Ky. App. 1983); Streeter v. Sears, Roebuck & Co., 533 So.2d 54 (La. App. 1988); Giant Food v. Satterfield, 603 A.2d 877 (Md. App. 1992); Cafferty v. Monson, 360 NW.2d 414 (Minn. App. 1985); Higgins v. Hermes, 89 N.M. 379, 552 P.2d 1227 (1976).
26. *See, e.g.,* Johnson v. Brown, 75 Nev. 437, 447, 345 P.2d 754 (Nev. 1959). See also 22 Am Jur 2d §265.
27. *See e.g.,* Debus v. Grand Union Stores of Vermont, 621 A.2d 1288,1290 (Vt. 1993).
28. 22 Am Jur 2d Damages §266.

29. Debus v. Grand Union Store of Vermont, 621 A.2d 1288,1290 (Vt. 1993).
30. Lawyers' Medical Cyclopedia of Personal Injuries and Allied Specialties §44A.44 (Richard M. Patterson, ed.)
31. J. Kahneman & Matthew L. Spitzer, Framing the Jury: Cognitive Perspectives of Pain and Suffering Awards, 81 Va. L. Rev. 1341, 1375 (Aug. 1995).
32. See 22 Am Jur 2d Damages §246; 9 PERSONAL INJURY: ACTION, DEFENSES, DAMAGES 3.04[7][b] (Louis R. Frumer & Melvin I. Friedman, eds. 1998).
33. Neil Sugarman & Charlotte Glinka, Explaining Pain: how you do it, who can help, Trial, 30 (Nov. 1994)
34. 8 Am Jur PoF3d 91 §§21–23.
35. See generally Admissibility in Civil Action, apart for res gestae, of Lay Testimony as to Another's Expressions of Pain, 90 ALR2d 1071 (1963); Neil Sugarman & Charlotte Glinka, Explaining Pain: how you do it, who can help, Trial, 30 (Nov. 1994).
36. See generally 90 ALR2d 1071 §2.
37. Expert and Opinion Evidence, 31A Am Jur 2d §§265–66.
38. Lawyers' Manual Cyclopedia of Personal Injuries and Allied Specialties 316 (Richard M. Patterson ed.)
39. 31A Am Jur.2d §264
40. 31A Am Jur.2d §266.
41. 416 Pa. 308, 206 A.2d 308 (Pa. 1965)
42. See generally Lawyers' Medical Cyclopedia of Personal Injuries and Allied Specialties §44A.41 (Richard M. Patterson, ed.).
43. 8 Am Jur PoF3d 91, §5
44. 293 F. 1013 (D.C. Ct. App. 1923)
45. Richard J. Byrne, Thermography: the double-edged sword which can either corroborate the existence of pain or weed out the malingerer, 38 Drake L. Rev. 355, 380 (Winter 1989).
46. See, e.g., United States v. Williams, 583 F.2d 1194 (2nd Cir. 1978), cited in Richard J. Byrne, Thermography: the double-edged sword which can either corroborate the existence of pain or weed out the malingerer, 38 Drake L. Rev. 355, 382–83 (Winter 1989).
47. 8 Am Jur PoF3d 91 §§24–31

CHAPTER **46**

Compliance for Pain Physicians

David M. Vaughn

Compliance for pain physicians is a difficult row to hoe. Cutting-edge technologies are evolving, yet there are often no CPT codes to bill for these technologies. When pain physicians finally do convince the American Medical Association (AMA) and the Health Care Financing Administration (HCFA) to include a new code in the CPT code for a pain procedure, often the local Medicare carriers will still deny the procedure as not medically necessary or as investigational. These denials, quite naturally, cause pain physicians an immense amount of consternation and frustration, often causing pain physicians to "creatively code" in order to obtain the reimbursement they believe is warranted. This is one of the reasons why pain physicians are investigated, audited, and prosecuted more prevalently than anesthesiologists.

Auditing thousands of pain records has revealed that the primary compliance issues with pain physicians involve coding, documentation, and kickback issues. Pain physician practices are rife with examples of unbundling, upcoding, billing for services not rendered, billing for services that are not medically necessary, not accurately documenting what was performed, not documenting according to the CPT descriptors for the CPT code billed, not using an accurate and complete Superbill, not accurately coding modifiers, and not taking kickback issues into account when dealing with hospital pain clinics.

These compliance deficiencies are commonly referred to as "fraud and abuse" by physicians and consultants; however, from a legal perspective, these violations transgress particular statutes for which a physician can be sued, prosecuted, or excluded from the Medicare program. Although there are a myriad of statutes and regulations that affect pain practitioners, the primary statutes affecting physicians are as follows:

1. *The Criminal False Claims Act*—This statute makes it a criminal offense to knowingly file a false claim with intent to defraud. An example of a criminal violation would be to purposefully code an epidurogram as a myelogram in order to obtain a higher payment. A violation is a felony, and the penalty is punishable by imprisonment.

2. *The Anti-Kickback Statute*—The anti-kickback statute makes it a criminal offense to receive or give anything of value in consideration for referring or receiving business that is paid in whole or in part by a federal health care program. An example might be referring patients to a hospital in exchange for receiving free space from the hospital to conduct office visits and consults.

3. *The Civil False Claims Act*—Sometimes the government decides to sue physicians for $10 000 per false claim (recently increased to $11 000 per false claim), rather than prosecute them criminally, based on false claims. For example, in *United States v Krizek,* the Justice Department sued a psychiatrist for $81 million for upcoding (billing a higher code than the service warranted). The $81 million was calculated on $10 000 per false claim times 8100 claims. The sad part about the case is that the 8100 false claims involved only one improper coding decision. The psychiatrist billed a 45-minute code for 15-minute visits. So, you can see how even one incorrect coding decision can lead to disastrous results. You should also be aware that judgments arising from the False Claims Act are not dischargeable in bankruptcy and that the government can seize from you any assets traceable to overpayments, including your house, your car, and your pension funds.

4. *The Stark Anti-Referral Statute*—The Stark statute is a civil statute that prohibits physicians from referring their patients for services or tests where the physician owns an interest in, or has a compensation arrangement with, the facility providing the service or test. An example might be an ownership in an ASC to which you refer pain patients for pain procedures. Before you enter into any financial arrangement with any health care entity, these arrangements must be examined to

determine whether the Stark statute is implicated, and if so, whether there is an applicable statutory exception.

EVALUATION AND MANAGEMENT ISSUES

Evaluation and management (E&M) services are those visits and consults provided in the inpatient and outpatient settings. Pain physicians are susceptible to noncompliance with regard to E&M services because almost all pain physicians provide office visits and consults, and most pain physicians still use the antiquated SOAP notes rather than the newer history, exam, and medical decision making used by the CPT code and HCFA. Upcoding has been so prevalent among all physicians, not just pain physicians, in regard to E&M coding that HCFA has announced several initiatives for auditing E&M codes. For example, in September 2000, the Office of Inspector General (OIG) advised that it was conducting focused audits on CPT codes 99214 and 99233, which are established patient visits in the outpatient and inpatient settings (1). E&M coding, in its present form, is primarily a function of documenting objective factors for the history and "bullet points" for the exam, as will be discussed in depth below.

HCFA E&M Documentation Guidelines

In determining how to code for E&M services, physicians should be aware of the latest HCFA E&M guidelines. HCFA has promulgated guidelines that instruct physicians as to what documentation is required for each level of E&M code. At the present time, HCFA has advised that physicians may use either the 1995 or the 1997 guidelines. The difference between the two sets of guidelines is that the 1995 guidelines do not contain any of the bullet items for the exam that the 1997 guidelines contain. In other words, the 1997 guidelines contain separate exam forms for a musculoskeletal exam, a neurological exam, and a multisystem exam. Each of these exam forms has specific items or "bullets" that must be performed to code a particular level of code. So, for example, a 99245 might require 25 bullet items for the exam, whereas a 99243 would only require 12 bullet items for the exam. As the 1997 guidelines are more objective, and more accurate to audit, I recommend the use of the 1997 guidelines.

New Test Pilot Guidelines

HCFA has advised that due to the outcry from the physician community, HCFA is going to test pilot a more "user friendly" set of guidelines. These guidelines are supposed to be put into a test practice in 2001. Based on this test, a new set of guidelines may be adopted in 2002.

Primary Components of E&M Service

At the current time, E&M codes consist of three primary components: history, exam, and medical decision mak-

ing. Each of these components has subcomponents. For example, the history has the following subcomponents: CC (chief complaint), HPI (history of present illness), ROS (review of systems), and PFSH (past, family, and social history). Each of these subcomponents has elements that must be met. For example, the HPI consists of eight factors, and each level of E&M coding requires a certain number of those factors to be documented in order to meet that level of coding. Similarly, the ROS consists of 14 systems, and each level of coding requires a certain number of those systems to be documented. Likewise, the PFSH consists of elements relating to the past history, the family history, and the social history of the patient. Each level of coding requires that some or all of these be addressed.

History of Present Illness (HPI)

According to both the 1995 and the 1997 E&M documentation guidelines, the elements of the HPI are the following (2):

Location
Quality
Severity
Duration
Timing
Context
Modifying factors
Associated signs/symptoms

Review of Systems (ROS)

The following systems, as stated in the E&M documentation guidelines, compromise a ROS (2):

Constitutional symptoms (e.g., fever, weight loss)
Eyes
Ears, nose, mouth, throat
Cardiovascular
Respiratory
Gastrointestinal
Genitourinary
Musculoskeletal
Integumentary (skin and/or breast)
Neurological
Psychiatric
Endocrine
Hematologic/lymphatic
Allergic/immunologic

Past, Family, Social History (PFSH)

The PFSH is comprised of (2):

Past history
Family history
Social history

All of the above sections—the HPI, the ROS, and the PFSH—are subcomponents of the history portion of an

E&M service. Once these are completed, the physician still needs to perform the other two components of the E&M service (i.e., the examination and medical decision making).

Three Types of Physical Exams

Insofar as the physical exam is concerned, pain physicians have the choice of three types of exam they can use to document the visit: (a) general multisystem exam, (b) musculoskeletal exam, or (c) neurologic exam. The multisystem exam, as its name suggests, is directed at performing a limited number of exam elements on a whole host of body parts, whereas the musculoskeletal and neurological exams focus on performing a concentrated exam on a limited number of systems. The documentation requirements of each of these exams differ depending on which of the three exams is performed and what level code is selected to be billed. Therefore, to properly document a particular level of E&M coding, you must first determine what type of exam you intend to perform, then determine the level you intend to perform, then review the relevant bullet points necessary for that exam, and then perform and document those bullet points.

Medical Decision Making

The third primary component of an E&M service, in addition to the history and the exam, is medical decision making. This is the plan component under the old SOAP note method of documentation. There are four levels of medical decision making according to the CPT code: straightforward, low, moderate, and high. The lower-level E&M services require only straightforward or low medical decision making, whereas the higher levels require moderate or high medical decision making (2).

Medical decision making is primarily comprised of four areas that should be documented: (a) the number of different diagnoses that bear on the physician's medical decision making; (b) the amount of data the physician must review in reaching his or her decision as to the patient's plan; (c) the severity, morbidity, and mortality of the patient; and (d) a documented plan.

Generally speaking, level 5 codes (or level 3 visits in the hospital setting) require a patient who is in an unstable condition with significant complications.

Difference in Documenting New Patients, Consults, and Established Patients

There is a significant difference in the documentation requirements for new patients and consults, on the one hand, and established patients on the other hand. For new patients, consults, and the admit visit into the hospital, the physician must document all three of the components of an E&M service—the history, exam, and medical decision making. However, for established patients in the office and for subsequent hospital care visits, the physician must only document two of the three components. The reason for this rule is HCFA expects the physician to perform a complete work-up for consults, new patients, and the initial admit visit to the hospital; however, for established patients and subsequent hospital care visits, the physician must only perform an interval service since the complete work-up has already been performed.

Accordingly, even if a physician does not perform an exam for an established patient or a subsequent hospital care visit, he or she could still meet the documentation requirements if a proper interval history and proper medical decision making were documented. Having said that, however, I recommend that all elements of the E&M service be documented on each occasion, even for established patients, in case the physician fails to document one of the E&M components, in which case the other two documented components will meet the documentation requirements.

Templates

Most E&M codes are overcoded by pain physicians because the physicians' forms do not contain all the "bullet points" required for the exam, or because the elements of the HPI, ROS, PFSH, and MDM (medical decision making) are absent. Quite frankly, it is no wonder that the exams do not measure up to HCFA's documentation requirements because there are so many factors and bullets to remember and perform. That is why we have created templates for our clients that track all of the bullet points that must be done for every level of visit and consult, inpatient or outpatient, that can be performed by pain physicians, regardless of whether they use the musculoskeletal exam, the neurological exam, or the multisystem exam. I recommend that all pain physicians use a template to capture all of the relevant factors required for the level of code they are billing.

Billing a Visit and a Procedure on the Same Date

One of the areas in which pain physicians get into trouble is billing for a visit and a procedure on the same date. Two rules apply here: First, if the patient is a new patient, most payors will pay for a procedure and a new patient visit on the same date because you must work up the patient in order to perform a procedure; otherwise, you face malpractice exposure. Therefore, a new patient visit and a procedure on the same date is generally considered appropriate.

However, the rule is just the opposite for established patient visits. The general rule for established patient visits is that you cannot bill for an established patient visit and a procedure on the same date. The only exception is where the visit is for a different purpose from the procedure.

For example, assume the dictation on a patient states, "the pain has been successfully treated with two prior epidural steroids and he requests another one." In this example, the reason the patient presents herself is specifically for an epidural steroid injection, and she is an established patient. Therefore, the only reason for the visit is for the procedure, and a separate visit should not be billed. Stated differently, there is a certain amount of visit already bundled into each procedure. You cannot perform a procedure without visiting with the patient. The only time you can unbundle the visit from the procedure and bill the visit separately from the procedure is when the visit is separate and distinct from the procedure either because the visit is new, or the symptoms on the established patient visit are different from the symptoms for the procedure.

An example of appropriate billing for a procedure on the same date as an established patient visit is where the patient presents for a LESI, but complains that she fell and hit her head on the floor since her last visit and has been having headaches and dizzy spells. In this example, the visit should be confined to the headaches and dizzy spells and not the LESI. In this instance there would be a different diagnosis code for the E&M code for the head injury as compared with the diagnosis code for the LESI. Also, the 25 modifier is required to be appended to the visit whenever it is billed in addition to the procedure. Local Medicare carriers sometimes do not want a 25 modifier on a new patient visit, but only on an established patient visit done on the same date as a procedure. Therefore, you must check your Local Medical Review Policies published by your local Medicare carrier in your state for its preference on this issue.

What Constitutes a New Visit

Another issue with regard to E&M coding is when a patient is a new patient and when he or she is an established patient. Billing a patient as a new patient, when the patient is actually an established patient is an upcode because reimbursement for a new patient visit is more than an established patient. Medicare has adopted the position that a patient who has not been to see you or anyone in your practice, within the same speciality, within the past 3 years is a new patient.

> A new patient is defined as a patient who has not received any professional services within the past three years from the billing physician or by another physician in the same group practice of the same speciality. Therefore, in a multi-speciality group practice, a patient referred to a different physician with a different specialty would be considered a new patient (3).

What Constitutes a Consult

One of the major compliance issues facing pain physicians in regard to E&M coding is whether to code a referral as a consult or a new patient visit. The reason this is a compliance issue is because coding a new patient as a consult is a 25 percent upcode due to higher reimbursement for consults. In 1999 HCFA relaxed the rules on billing consults to make it easier to code a consult. Before the new rules were adopted, a consult could not be billed if there was a transfer of part of the care to the consulting physician. Now that rule has changed so that a consult may be billed unless there is a complete transfer of care.

The Medicare Carriers Manual states:

> Payment [for a consult] may be made regardless of treatment initiation unless a transfer of care occurs. A transfer of care occurs when the referring physician transfers the responsibility for the patient's complete care to the receiving physician at the time of referral, and the receiving physician documents approval of care in advance. The receiving physician would report a new or established patient visit depending on the situation (a new patient is one who has not received any professional services from the physician or another physician of the same specialty who belongs to the same group practice, within the past three years) and setting (e.g., office or inpatient). A physician consultant may initiate diagnostic and/or therapeutic services at an initial or subsequent visit. Subsequent visits to manage a portion or all of the patient's condition should be reported as established patient office visits or subsequent hospital care, depending on the setting (4).

HIP, the Medicare carrier for Queens in New York, states, "When an anesthesiologist sees a patient referred from another physician for evaluation, a diagnosis and a recommendation for pain management procedures in an outpatient setting, it is appropriate for the anesthesiologist to bill a consult code (99241–99245). If the anesthesiologist renders any treatment, reimbursement will be made in addition to the consult (5)." However, the ASA warns that not all referrals are consults: "Many anesthesiologists have routinely billed all new patient encounters for pain management as consultations. This practice should be reviewed carefully (6)." I agree. Unless the referring physician is requesting an opinion of the consulting physician as to how to treat the patient, there is no consultation, only a new patient visit. Moreover, if the referring physician is simply turning the patient over to you, to handle all the patient's treatment, the referral is not a consult, but a new patient visit.

Inadequate Superbills

Superbills often are incomplete and do not contain every possible level of E&M coding. Some pain practices, for example, will only have 99204, 99205, 99244, and 99245 as the possible choices for new patient visits and consults, respectively. This deficiency resulted in a Midwest hospital being hit for $4.6 million in a settlement with the OIG. The OIG took the position that limiting the use of possible choices to only the highest level codes resulted in physicians being preordained to overcoding. Accordingly, all E&M codes for each level should be included as possible choices on the Superbill.

Macros

Another compliance problem with E&M coding is macros. Some pain practices have developed macros that have defaults that print data regarding a visit or consult that did not occur. For example, some software I have seen will select the average age, degrees of flexion, extension, and range of motion on exam, which if not changed will print out in the report. At one practice, certain parts of the exam were not performed on a routine basis, but the macros printed out the average results as if the patient had undergone the exam. In other words, results from unperformed tests were reported on a routine basis. Pain physicians must be careful in their attempts to reduce paperwork, not to create forms, macros, or software defaults that produce inaccurate.

Place of Service

The last problem we will discuss with regard to E&M coding is the place of service. For Medicare purposes, there are four primary places of service and reimbursement is different depending on the place of service. This is critical because a wrongly designated place of service can cause an upcode. The four primary places of service are: (a) office—place of service 11; (b) outpatient—place of service 22; (c) inpatient—place of service 21; and (d) ASC—place of service 24.

Medicare pays more for E&M services performed in the office setting because the physician has overhead there; conversely, Medicare pays less for services in the hospital setting because the physician has no overhead in that setting. On average, the office setting E&M codes pay one third more than the facility setting E&M codes.

Coding Issues for Pain Procedures

Let's explore some of the compliance and coding issues with regard to pain procedures.

Fluoroscopy

In CPT 2000, a fluoroscopy code, 76005, was added. There are several compliance issues surrounding this code. The first issue involves the relationship of the fluoroscopy code with the epidurography code, 72275, which was also added in 2000. The primary difference between the two codes is that the epidurogram code requires a formal interpretation and report, whereas the fluoroscopy code does not. One of the compliance issues that have confronted pain physicians is whether they can bill the fluoroscopy and the epidurogram together. The *CPT Assistant,* which is the AMA's coding newsletter, answered this question in January 2000, as follows:

> CPT code 76005 describes the fluoroscopic guidance to assist in accurately localizing specific spinal anatomy for placement

of a needle or catheter tip for spinal therapeutic or diagnostic injections. However, it is important to note that code 76005 does not represent a formal contrast study, such as myelography, epidurography or sacroiliac joint arthrography. If any of these formal contrast studies are performed, code 76005 is considered to be an inclusive component and should not be separately reported. For example, if epidurography is performed, you should report CPT code 72275. In this instance, it would be inappropriate to report 76005 in addition to code 72275, as the fluoroscopic guidance is considered an inclusive component of the epidurography code 72275 (7).

The second issue regarding fluoroscopy is determining which procedure codes can be coded with fluoroscopy, either 76005, or the previous existing code, 76000. According to CPT 2000, 76005 should be used with 27096 (SI joints), 62310–62319 (epidurals), 64470–64476 (facets), 64479–64484 (transforaminal epidurals), 62270–62273 (spinal puncture/blood patch), and 62280–62282 (neurolytic injection).

The third issue regarding fluoroscopy is the modifier -26, which must accompany it unless the pain physician owns his or her own C-arm. If the -26 modifier is appended to a radiological code, such as fluoroscopy, it signifies that the physician provided the professional component (reading the fluoro), but does not own the equipment. If the -26 modifier is not appended to the fluoroscopy code, the reimbursement is significantly higher because Medicare has built in more reimbursement to pay for the C-arm.

The fourth issue with regard to fluoroscopy is how many times can you bill in one day per patient. According to Texas Medicare, you are limited to billing fluoroscopy only once per day per patient unless the fluoroscopy is done both in the cervical and lumbar regions on the same date.

> If a true epidurogram is performed and medically necessary, Medicare would not expect to see this reported routinely more than one time, per patient, per session. In rare instances when both a lumbosacral epidurogram and cervical epidurogram are performed, two epidurograms might be reported on the same patient on the same day (8).

Bilateral Modifier

Another compliance issue that confronts physicians is the failure to properly capture the bilateral modifier on codes that accept bilateral procedures. The CPT code signifies by the terminology if the reimbursement is designed to apply to a procedure done unilaterally or bilaterally. If the code states "unilaterally or bilaterally" then only one code is billed and reimbursement is the same regardless of whether the procedure is performed unilaterally or bilaterally. Medicare has its own coding conventions regarding payment of bilateral procedures. This coding convention is known as the Correct Coding Initiative (CCI). The CCI is published each quarter and lists, among other things, which procedures can accept a -50 modifier, thus allowing bilateral procedures to be billed. Some of the bilateral pain procedures that can be billed include the facet and transforaminal epidural codes added in CPT 2000.

Unfortunately, even though these procedures can be performed and paid bilaterally, they are often not coded correctly due to flaws in the Superbill. Most of the pain Superbills I review have a checkoff line for the initial level and a separate checkoff line for additional levels. Since there are no lines to check off for bilateral procedures, the pain physicians check off the line designated as additional levels. Thus, in many pain practices a bilateral procedure is billed as an additional level, not a bilateral side. To correct this problem, the Superbill needs to add a checkoff line for bilateral procedures, not just additional levels.

Another issue is under what circumstances you can bill a bilateral injection. What if you can perform a bilateral injection without withdrawing the needle but just readjusting it while inserted? The *CPT Assistant*, a publication put out by the AMA CPT Advisory Committee, advises that you can bill for bilateral facet joint injections as long as you use the two-stick methodology, rather than the one-stick methodology (9).

The -51 Modifier

Another incorrect coding practice is the use of the -51 modifier with add-on codes. This incorrect coding practice has the effect of incorrectly reducing reimbursement. The coding conventions of the CPT code in the pain injections section incorporates the "add-on code" concept. The add-on code concept creates a separate code for the initial level of the injection and then an add-on code for second and subsequent levels. Any code identified as an add-on code should not append to it a -51 modifier.

The -51 modifier is a modifier used to tell the payor that you have performed a multiple procedure on the same date on the same patient. For example, if you injected five trigger points, the first trigger point would be billed with 20550 and the next four trigger points would be billed with 20550-51. The -51 modifier instructs the payor to reduce reimbursement by 50% for the second through fifth procedures.

However, a -51 modifier is not used with an add-on code because add-on codes already have a 50% reduction built into the code for the additional level injected. For example, the facet injections and the transforaminal injections contain an initial code for the initial level injected and a second code, referred to as an add-on code, for the second level injected. The Introductory Comments to the Surgery Guidelines (2) explain that add-on codes are identified with a "+" beside the code and "are exempt from the multiple procedure concept (modifier -51)." Modifier -51, found in Appendix A of CPT 2000, states that "this modifier should not be appended to designated add-on codes." As stated, the reason for this rule is that the add-on code is reimbursed based on a 50% reduction for an additional level. The -51 modifier also instructs the payor to reduce

50% If you append a -51 modifier to a code that is already reduced in reimbursement by 50%, you have instructed the payor to reduce payment to 25%, thereby unnecessarily depriving yourself of 25% of the proper reimbursement.

Facet Levels

What constitutes a facet level? Coding for facets is done per level. An additional code may be billed per each level injected. Does the vertebra or the interspace between each vertebra constitute a level? Some pain physicians believe that if they inject two nerves in an interspace, one of which emanates from L-3 and the other that emanates from L-4 that two facet codes can be billed, reasoning there are two nerves from two different levels, and the levels are the vertebrae from which the nerves emanate. Other clients of mine had indicated that each interspace was a level regardless of the number of nerves that are injected and the levels from which they emanate. To resolve this discrepancy, I wrote the *CPT Assistant* and asked how many levels should be coded if three separate nerves were injected at the L-3–4 interspace, but one emanated from L-3 and another emanated from L-4. I received the following response: "To specifically address your example, an injection given in the L-3–L-4 interspace constitutes one level, as this forms a single facet joint" (10).

Texas Medicare agrees, stating that, "Facet joints are supplied by nerves not only from the level of the joint but also from sensory nerves from the level above and the level below the particular joint. . . . As defined above, one procedure generally involves three levels of block" (11).

Accordingly, no matter how many nerves are injected at a particular interspace, only one facet code can be billed, regardless of whether the payor is Medicare or commercial insurance.

Procedure Place of Service

As discussed previously in the section on E&M coding, the place of service is important in regard to coding pain procedures. Medicare reimbursement is based on a reimbursement system known as Resource Based Relative Value Scale (RBRVS), a system developed by Harvard researchers. The RBRVS system incorporates three components into every pain procedure code: a work value, a practice expense value, and a malpractice expense value. The practice expense value differs greatly depending on whether the procedure is performed in the facility (hospital) or nonfacility (office) setting. Physicians have no practice expense when performing procedures in the hospital, since the hospital employs the staff, purchases the equipment, and supplies the drugs. Thus, the reimbursement for pain procedures is significantly lower in the facility setting than the nonfacility setting. Accordingly, it is crucial that billing staff correctly enter place of service 21 (inpatient) or place of service 22 (hospital outpatient), rather than place of service 11 (office) if a procedure is performed at the hospital. Otherwise, a significant upcode will occur.

For example, for the year 2000, the Medicare Fee Schedule is $91.53 for a lumbar epidural steroid injection (CPT 62319) performed in the hospital, but more than double that amount if performed in the office—$201.38 (unadjusted for geographic location). Similarly, for an SI joint injection, the Medicare Fee Schedule is $56.75 if performed in the facility, but $408.24 if performed in the office. The E&M codes we discussed earlier do not vary quite as much, but the difference is about one-third depending on the place of service. For example, a level four consult, CPT 99244, reflects a fee schedule of $127.78 in the facility setting and $161.83 in the nonfacility setting. The difference in Medicare reimbursement is one of the reasons that many practices are considering moving their pain practices out of the hospital pain clinic into their own private offices.

Pain physicians will want to review the HCFA 1500 forms to make sure that billing personnel are billing the correct place of service.

Physician Extenders

One of the primary bases on which physicians have been prosecuted and convicted is the improper use of physician extenders (i.e., nurse practitioners and physician assistants). Modifiers are no longer required to bill for these nonphysician practitioners; however, each must have their own Medicare UPIN. This rule became effective January 1, 1998, with the enactment of the Balanced Budget Act. "A summary of the changes [implemented by the Act] is as follows: (1) effective January 1, 1998, place of service restrictions were removed; (2) covered services are allowed at 85 percent of the Medicare Physician Fee Schedule amount; and (3) education, certification, and credentialing requirements are more specific" (12).

All claims for services rendered to Medicare beneficiaries must be filed by the employer on behalf of a physician assistant. Also, any physician assistant who renders services to beneficiaries for which claims will be made must have on file a Reassignment of Benefits Form 855R. A physician's assistant must be a W-2 employee (12).

One of the important points to note about compliance with regard to physician extenders is when to bill in the physician's name (for which Medicare pays 100% of the Physicians Fee Schedule), when to bill in the physician extender's name (for which Medicare pays 85% of the Physician's Fee Schedule), and most importantly, when not to bill in the physician's name (for which several physicians have been prosecuted). The two critical rules that a physician must follow in regard to billing for a PA or NP are that a physician may never bill in the physician's name for work done by a physician extender in the hospital setting and that a physician may not bill in the physician's name

for NP or PA work done in the office setting if the physician was not in the office suite when the NP or PA performed the work. Many physicians have been prosecuted for billing rounds done in the hospital, where the progress notes were written by the NP or PA and the bills were submitted in the name of the physician. That is illegal. The only time an NP or PA can bill in the name of the physician is if the service rendered is "incident to" the physician's service, and there is no "incident to" billing in the hospital setting. The rule is as follows: Medicare Part B allows coverage for services and supplies furnished "incident to" a nonphysician [or physician] practitioner's professional services. There have been no changes to these guidelines since their inception; however, they are often utilized incorrectly (e.g., in an inappropriate setting, such as a hospital) (13).

The safest billing methodology is to always bill in the name of the PA or NP at 85% of the Physicians Fee Schedule. This billing methodology significantly reduces the exposure for fraud and abuse because you never inadvertently upcode an NP's or PA's charge to the physician's rate. On the other hand, you may legally bill in the physician's name, at 100 percent of the Physicians Fee Schedule, even though the NP or PA performed the work, but only if the NP or PA services are "incident to" the physician's service and are performed in the office while the physician is present. I have been involved in several prosecutions where one of the allegations against the physician was that the service was performed by a nonphysician, but billed in the physician's name improperly. In these instances the prosecutor would subpoena the physician's calendar, determine all dates when he was on vacation or otherwise out of the office, and then ascertain if any bills were sent out of the office on that date in his name. If the prosecutor found any such bills, she concluded that these were fraudulent and indicted the physician. The physician would defend the case by claiming the services were performed by a physician extender, but the prosecution would counter that the physician was not in the office on the date the physician performed those services, or that the service was performed in the hospital where there is no "incident to" billing, so it was illegal to charge for those services in the name of the physician.

To understand this more fully, one must define "incident to" services. When may a physician bill at 100%, in the physician's name, for services rendered by an NP or PA? The Florida Medicare carrier recently discussed this rule at length, and restated the national rule on this issue as follows:

To be covered "incident to" the service of a physician or a nonphysician practitioner, a service or supply must meet all of the following conditions: (1) The service must be an integral, although incidental, part of the physician's or nonphysician practitioner's professional service; (2) of a type commonly furnished in a physician's office or clinic; (3) furnished under the physician's or nonphysician practitioner's direct supervision; and (4) furnished by an individual who qualifies as an employee of the physician or professional association/group.

Services performed by nonphysician practitioners incident to a physician's professional services include not only services ordinarily furnished by a physician's office staff, but also services ordinarily performed by the physician (e.g., minor surgery, reading X-rays, and other activities that involve evaluation or treatment of a patient's condition). However, the nonphysician practitioner must be licensed or certified to provide such services. . . . In addition, the physician must be in the office suite and immediately available to render assistance during the time the nonphysician practitioner is furnishing services which are incident to the physician's services.

A nonphysician practitioner such as a physician assistant or nurse practitioner may be licensed under state law to perform a specific medical procedure and may be able to perform the procedure without direct physician supervision and have the services covered by Medicare as a nonphysician practitioner's service. However, in order to have the same service covered as incident to a physician's service, it must be performed under the direct personal supervision of the physician as an incidental part of the physician's personal in-office service. . . . [This] does mean that there must have been a direct, personal, professional service by the physician to initiate the course of treatment of which the service being performed by the nonphysician practitioner is an incidental part, and there must be subsequent services by the physician of a frequency that reflects his/her active participation in and management of the course of treatment (13).

Local Medical Review Policies

One of the most critical compliance tools for pain practitioners is the Local Medical Review Policies (LMRP) that its Medicare carrier promulgates. Without these LMRPs, you cannot possibly code or document correctly. Each Medicare carrier publishes a newsletter, which is also duplicated on its Web site, that describes in detail the rules regarding particular pain procedures. For example, most states have policies regarding the following: epidurals, facets, trigger points, stims, pumps, IDET, electrical nerve blocks, fluoroscopy and epidurography, lysis of adhesions, and other nerve blocks.

Each of these LMRPs gives the criteria for:

1. Clinical indications that must exist in order to bill these procedures to Medicare;
2. Documentation requirements that must appear in the medical record on an audit in order to survive a repayment request;
3. Diagnosis codes that Medicare will authorize for this particular procedure;
4. How many times within a given time frame that the particular procedure may be performed;
5. Whether other procedures may be performed on the same date or not.

For example, regarding trigger points, some states such as New York have adopted a specific H&P form, requiring eight elements that must appear in the medical record in order to survive repayment on audit. For example, Empire Medicare Services in New York adopted an LMRP for trigger points in April 1999, which states as follow:

The diagnosis of trigger points requires a detailed history and thorough physical examination: (i) history of onset of the painful condition, and its presumed cause; (ii) distribution pattern of pain consistent with the referral pattern of trigger points; (iii) restriction of range of motion; (iv) muscular deconditioning in the affected area; (v) focal tenderness of a trigger point; (vi) palpable taut band of muscle in which trigger point is located; (vii) local taut response to snapping palpation; and (viii) reproduction of referred pain pattern upon stimulation of the trigger point.

This H&P was derived after these carriers determined that trigger points were being overutilized in those states. Accordingly, in these states, if the H&P is in the record but does not include the eight requirements stipulated by the LMRP, on an audit the provider will have to repay the trigger point reimbursement. Yet, other states do not contain such requirements. Unless you research your specific LMRPs for your state, you cannot possibly know whether you are meeting their documentation requirements.

As another example of differing LMRPs, again involving trigger points, Virginia has adopted an LMRP stating that there are eight body areas into which a trigger point can be injected. These areas generally correspond to the right and left upper and lower extremities, the head, and the three areas of the spine. Under the Virginia LMRP, multiple trigger points into the same body area constitutes one billable injection, regardless of the actual injections. You can bill up to five trigger points in a given encounter, but each must be in one of the eight different body areas (15). Georgia Medicare, on the other hand, only requires that trigger points be in different muscles to be reimbursable (16). Oklahoma has no requirement that different muscles or body areas be injected, but limits the diagnosis codes to 13 specific diagnoses (17). Arkansas Medicare requires the specific muscle to be identified (not a body area as in Virginia), limits the number of trigger points to three per session, three per patient per year, and eight diagnosis codes (18). The point is that each state's LMRP for the same procedure may vary widely. Relying on a general rule you heard at some national seminar can be misleading because it may be completely irrelevant to your state. Look up your LMRPs specific to your state for each of the pain procedures that you perform.

Lysis of Adhesions

For the year 2000 the CPT code added a new code, 62263, lysis of adhesions, primarily designed for the Racz catheter method of lysis. However, because pain practitioners were using epiduroscopy as a method to lyse adhesions, the *CPT Assistant* promulgated a coding article in August 2000 that severely limits the lysis code altogether and eliminates epiduroscopy as a method of billing for lysis of adhesions. Specifically, the *CPT Assistant* states, "there is no specific CPT code to describe 'epiduroscopy'" (19). *CPT Assistant* still recommends the use of 64999 "for placement of an endoscope in the epidural space for diagnostic or therapeutic epiduroscopy, since the reporting of 62263 should not be reported to describe a single procedure wherein diagnostic epiduroscopy and/or epiduroscopic mechanical lysis of adhesions is performed at a single session. . . ." However, if the use of the epiduroscope is "utilized as an adjunctive procedure specifically related to intent and use of 62263," then the epiduroscope does not preclude the use of 62263. According to *CPT Assistant,*

> Percutaneous lysis of epidural adhesions is a percutaneous epidural treatment involving targeted injection of various substances (e.g., hypertonic saline, steroid, anesthetic) via an epidural catheter. The catheter remains in place until treatment is completed. If required, the adhesions or scarring may also be lysed by mechanical means. Maneuvering of the catheter or an epiduroscope (inserted and removed in the same session) are examples of how "mechanical" adhesiolysis is accomplished. Therefore, the physician may opt to use an epiduroscope as an adjunctive mechanical-based technique performed in addition to the administration of neurolytic substance(s) via the initially- or previously-placed epidural catheter. . . . It would not be appropriate to additionally report 64999 for the insertion and use of the epiduroscope. Because the treatment goal involves a concerted effort to breakdown scar formation (adhesions) reduce edema, reduce inflammation, and block propagation of nociception (pain transmission) to the central nervous system, several separate treatments are frequently required. Code 62263 is reported once even though the treatment occurs over several days and may address several specific areas(s) of scarring and inflammation in the epidural space. . . . Code 62263 is intended to describe a procedure that involves placement of an epidural catheter that remains in place over a several-day period for the purpose of lysis of adhesions. Code 62263 may also include adjunctive use of a percutaneously-placed epiduroscope for intentional mechanical adhesiolysis. Code 62263 includes injection of contrast material for epidurography (use 72275 for formal interpretation) and subsequent fluoroscopic guidance and localization performed in association with the sequential lysis of adhesions treatment(s), thus precluding the additional reporting of code 76005 for either initial or subsequent adhesiolytic treatment. . . . The treatment involves catheter-based and adjunctive, mechanical-based (either by maneuvering the catheter or epiduroscope) adhesiolysis performed at multiple-day sessions (19).

Manufacturer's Suggested Codes

Be careful of equipment manufacturers who come bearing gifts. Some manufacturers have developed equipment designed to perform pain procedures. To sell this equipment, manufacturers will often suggest certain CPT codes for pain practitioners to use so that the physician can recoup their costs and ultimately make money using the equipment. Often, these codes are disputed by Medicare carriers and the AMA's coding sources. Often, the procedures are deemed investigational and will not be reimbursed by Medicare at all. Accordingly, prior to purchasing any equipment that suggested CPT codes, first determine from your specific Medicare carrier if the procedure will be reimbursed, and second, if the CPT codes rec-

ommended by the manufacturer will be reimbursed for that procedure.

For example, one of my clients reported to me that a particular manufacturer who had sold a piece of equipment designed to perform IDET had suggested that the IDET procedure be coded with various CPT codes, including 62292. I was concerned about this code, so I wrote the California Medicare Medical Director who warned, "Do not bill 62292 since Electrothermal Therapy uses heat not a chemical as required by 62292" (20). The *CPT Assistant*, which is the AMA's coding newsletter, has advised that there is no specific code for IDET, and that it should be billed with CPT 64999. The following question was asked of *CPT Assistant:* "My physician performs a procedure called intradiscal electrothermal coagulation, and I can't seem to find a specific code to report it. Can you please advise?" AMA comment: "From a CPT coding perspective, CPT does not contain a specific code for reporting intradiscal electrothermal coagulation (IDET). Therefore, the unlisted procedure code 64999, 'Unlisted procedure, nervous system,' should be reported. It is important to note that when an unlisted code is used, a copy of the operative report should be included when submitting to third-party payors" (21).

Other states have refused to pay for IDET, considering it investigational. For example, Arkansas Medicare has stated: "Intradiscal electrothermal therapy is considered investigational until more data on the mid- to long-term effectiveness is known, and randomized comparisons with more standard treatment has been completed. . . . There are no ICD-9 codes listed as applicable and thus, all such procedures will be denied" (22).

While other states and other carriers may pay for IDET, and none of my comments here should be taken to suggest otherwise, these are examples of the difficulties that pain providers face when purchasing new equipment for cutting-edge procedures. While I believe that eventually there will be a specific CPT code for IDET as more literature is developed on the efficacy of the procedure, submitted to Medicare, and a new code developed, at the present time 64999 is the appropriate coding route.

Another example of a manufacturer selling equipment with suggested CPT codes that have been rejected by some Medicare carriers involves an electrical nerve block, where the manufacturer has suggested that the electrical nerve block could be coded with the injection nerve block codes. Several carriers, such as New York Medicare, have rejected the manufacturer's suggested codes. New York Medicare has stated, "Noninvasive neuron blockade devices, electronic neuron blockade devices, bioelectric treatment systems or similar devices are not covered. CPT codes 64440–64450 (Introduction/injection of anesthetic agent [nerve block], diagnostic or therapeutic) specifically describe injection services. The use of these codes, or any other CPT codes, when the service is rendered by one of these devices is considered fraudulent"

(23). Texas Medicare has also indicated that billing an injection nerve block code for the use of electrical blockage of a nerve is considered improper and should not be billed: "It has come to our attention that providers may be billing CPT codes 64400–64450, introduction/injection of anesthetic agent (nerve block), diagnostic or therapeutic, when the actual service provided is an electrical nerve block. Currently, no CPT code exists for an electrical nerve block—a procedure where electricity is used as an anesthetic. Providers billing for this procedure should use a not otherwise classified code with a description to bill for this service" (24). The not otherwise classified code is 64999.

Some carriers may pay for IDET and electrical nerve blocks; some payors may allow the use of the codes suggested by the manufacturer; some payors may not consider these procedures investigational; however, the point is that a pain practitioner should not purchase equipment until she knows whether her Medicare carrier will require her to use 64999, a nonspecific code, and whether Medicare in her state might deny the procedure as investigational. Unless you learn these two facts, you not only will be making a less than fully informed purchasing decision, but also may miscode procedures that your Medicare carrier considers a false claim. Accordingly, write your Medicare carrier before purchasing new equipment to determine the reimbursement of the procedure and the appropriate CPT code. The problem with using 64999 is that it has no RBRVS fee schedule value, and the claim must be submitted in hard copy rather than electronically, with a copy of the procedure note, and the claim representative must individually determine how much, if anything, will be reimbursed for the procedure. Accordingly, using 64999 is considered extremely less effective in obtaining reimbursement than having a specific CPT code for the service.

Kickbacks and Paying Rent at the Pain Clinic

There are three areas in which the kickback statute may be implicated for pain physicians:

1. Conducting office visits and consults in the hospital pain clinic without paying rent;
2. Owning an ASC with other physicians or a hospital;
3. Waiving co-pays and deductibles.

Insofar as paying the hospital rent for the pain clinic is concerned, the reason that the kickback statute may be implicated in this scenario is that the pain physician is a referral source to the hospital. The pain physician refers patients to the hospital, for which the hospital is paid a facility fee by Medicare. Yet, the hospital does not charge the pain physician any rent for the office space used to conduct visits and consults. The hospital may not be charging patients for the office space that the pain physician uses for his consults and visits; therefore, the government could argue that the pain physician is receiving office space for free in exchange for referring patients to the hospital.

My opinion regarding this issue is twofold. First, as a general rule, and based on my experience with numerous clients on this issue, I do not believe that either the pain physicians or the hospitals have given much thought to the concept of free rent in exchange for pain patients. The kickback statute only makes it a crime where the intent of the parties is to receive free rent in exchange for referral of the pain patients to the hospital. I do not believe there is any intent in the situations that I have encountered; thus, I do not believe that the kickback statute has been violated. However, having said that, any health care lawyer worth her salt will tell you that intent is subjective, and the government can easily allege subjective intent and try to convince the jury of the parties' intent; therefore, it is not safe to idly sit by and do nothing when there is an available safe harbor to insulate a pain physician's exposure on this issue. The safe harbor is the rental safe harbor. The rental safe harbor requires a written contract, signed by the parties, for a term of one year or more, which pays rent to the hospital based on fair market value, and does not take into account the value or volume of referrals.

Some health care attorneys and consultants, the author being one, also believe that paying rent is not enough, and that because the pain physicians use the hospital personnel and equipment to schedule consults and visits, that the allocated fair market value of those services should also be included in the "rental" value.

There are some limitations and exceptions to this rent-paying scenario, however, in my opinion. First, there has been no OIG opinion on this exact issue; accordingly, those of us who hold this opinion are providing you with our personal opinion, without the benefit of a federal case or agency opinion to cite as authority. Second, if the hospital is charging the patient a fee for the use of the room in which the visit and consult is conducted, as some hospitals are now doing, I do not believe that the kickback statute is implicated, even if the pain physician does not pay rent. My opinion on this issue is predicated on the fact that since the hospital is charging a fee to the patient for the use of the premises, the hospital is already receiving "rent," and for the physician to pay rent as well would result in double payment to the hospital. Moreover, under this scenario, the pain physician is billing place of service 22 (outpatient hospital), not place of service 11 (office), which means that the pain physician is not receiving from Medicare the practice expense component of the visit or consult. Stated differently, visits and consults pay approximately one-third less in place of service 22, outpatient hospital, than they pay in place of service 11, office. The lower payment is based on Medicare's determination that the pain physician has no overhead. Accordingly, in my opinion, if the hospital is charging rent to the patient via a facility fee for the visit or consult, and if the pain physician is billing place of service 22, there is no kickback because the pain physician is not receiving anything free of value, as he is receiving a lower Medicare reimbursement for the visit or consult, and the hospital's "rent" is already being paid by the patient.

On the other hand, if the hospital is not charging a facility fee for the visit or consult to the patient, and the pain practice is not paying rent, then the hospital is not receiving any rent, and the pain practice is allowed to maintain an office practice of visits and consults without rent. While it is true that in this scenario, the pain physician is billing place of service 22, with a lower E&M reimbursement, that lower reimbursement does not address the fact that the landlord is not receiving any rent, and the landlord is making facility fees for procedures done in the pain clinic. Therefore, in my opinion, the safest and most compliant way to handle this scenario is to pay rent to the hospital for the limited space used for visits and consults, together with a rental value for personnel and equipment. The rental value should not include any space used to perform procedures, or any allocation of equipment and personnel related to pain procedures, as the hospital is already charging a facility fee to the patient for procedures.

At the same time the pain practice is paying rent to the hospital, the hospital should pay the pain physician a fee for being a medical director. In my opinion, the kickback statute is implicated if the hospital requests free services in the form of a medical directorship without paying the medical director. In most hospital pain clinics, the pain physician is essentially a hospital-based physician, and there is an OIG Fraud Alert, published in 1991, that cautions hospitals that the extraction of money, services, or equipment from hospital-based physicians may implicate the kickback statute (25). There is a safe harbor for personal services under which the medical directorship payment should be made, which requires that the medical directorship relationship be in writing, signed by the parties, that the amount of the medical directorship be based on an hourly rate, supported by time sheets turned in by the pain physician, with the contract having a term of at least one year, without any consideration of the value or volume of referrals between the two parties.

Thus, the pain clinic payments should be a two-sided coin. The pain practice should pay the hospital for any space, equipment, and personnel allocated to providing visits and consults, while the hospital should reciprocate and pay the pain practice a medical directorship fee for any administrative duties. While the reciprocal payments may, coincidentally, offset each other to some extent, each payment should stand on its own, and should not be geared to exactly set off the other. The rental payment to the hospital should be based on the fair market value of the rental space used, together with the time that the hospital personnel and equipment are used in dealing with the visits and consults of the pain practice. The medical directorship fee should be based on an hourly rate, and only paid for hours actually performed. The two payments

must be determined as an accounting exercise, independent of one another.

Kickbacks and Professional Courtesy

Another way in which the kickback statute is implicated is professional courtesy, or its cousin, "insurance only." In September 2000, the OIG released its compliance guidance to small physician practices (26). According to the OIG,

The term "professional courtesy" is used to describe a number of analytically different practices. The traditional definition is the practice by a physician of waiving all or a part of the fee for services provided to the physician's office staff, other physicians, and/or their families. In recent times, "professional courtesy" has also come to mean the waiver of coinsurance obligations or other out-of-pocket expenses for physicians or their families (i.e., "insurance only" billing), and similar payment arrangements by hospitals or other institutions for services provided to their medical staffs or employees. In general, whether a professional courtesy arrangement runs afoul of the fraud and abuse laws is determined by two factors: (i) how the recipients of the professional courtesy are selected; and (ii) how the professional courtesy is extended. If recipients are selected in a manner that directly or indirectly takes into account their ability to affect past or future referrals, the anti-kickback statute—which prohibits giving anything of value to generate Federal health care program business—may be implicated. If the professional courtesy is extended through a waiver of copayment obligations (i.e., "insurance only" billing), other statutes may be implicated, including the prohibition of inducements to beneficiaries, section 1128A(a)(5) of the Act (codified at 42 U.S.C. 1320a-7a(a)(5)). Claims submitted as a result of either practice may also implicate the civil False Claims Act (26).

These warnings by the OIG are the reason why health care lawyers advise their clients not to extend professional courtesy to anyone under any circumstances. This advice is given to protect the physician from getting confused regarding the limited circumstances in which professional courtesy is allowable, because the OIG, while acknowledging that there are circumstances in which professional courtesy is allowable, is so vague in its advice that healthcare lawyers are prone to take the easy way out and "Just say no." In regard to the circumstances in which professional courtesy is allowable, the OIG stated,

The following are general observations about professional courtesy arrangements for physician practices to consider: A physician's regular and consistent practice of extending professional courtesy by waiving the entire fee for services rendered to a group of persons (including employees, physicians, and/or their family members) may not implicate any of the OIG's fraud and abuse authorities so long as membership in the group receiving the courtesy is determined in a manner that does not take into account directly or indirectly any group member's ability to refer to, or otherwise generate Federal health care program business for, the physician. A physician's regular and consistent practice of extending professional courtesy by waiving otherwise applicable copayments for services rendered to a group of persons, would not implicate the anti-kickback statute so long as membership in the group is determined in a manner that does not take into account directly or indirectly any group member's ability to refer to, or otherwise generate Federal health care program business for, the physician. Any waiver of copayment practice does implicate section 1128A(a)(5) of the Act if the patient for whom the copayment is waived is a Federal health care program beneficiary who is not financially needy. The legality of particular professional courtesy arrangements will turn on the specific facts presented, and, with respect to the anti-kickback statute, on the specific intent of the parties (26).

I interpret the OIG's advice as allowing two types of professional courtesy: documented hardship, and free services (no payment to the physician) as long as the recipient is not an actual or potential referral source. I do not interpret the OIG as allowing insurance only to commercial insurers, and would caution against this practice, absent written consent from the insurer.

Kickbacks in Regard to Joint Ventures in ASCs

The kickback statute may also be implicated any time a pain physician owns an interest in an ASC. The OIG has issued an opinion letter regarding kickback issues where a pain physician owns an interest in the ASC, and more recently, new ASC safe harbors for ASCs have been adopted that detail with exact specificity the requirements that must be met in order for a pain physician to become an owner of the ASC (27). In a nutshell, these rules require that the pain physician generate one-third of her total medical practice income through procedures that are on the Medicare approved ASC procedure list, and that one third of all the pain physician's procedures are performed in the ASC in which she has an ownership interest. The nuances of these rules are too complex to discuss here other than to highlight the issues, so that you can contact counsel for an appropriate opinion should the need arise.

Refiling Denied Claims

The Health Care Financing Administration (HCFA) has set up a system of adopting national policies governing what medical conditions justify payment for particular procedures identified in the CPT code. Additionally, in the absence of national HCFA policy, many local Medicare carriers adopt local Medicare review policies governing what diagnoses will justify particular procedures. These policies address which clinical indications and diagnoses will justify payment for a particular CPT code. These policies also identify that diagnoses other than those stated in the policies will result in denial of payment.

Federal prosecutors have recently warned that claims that are denied due to lack of medical necessity (i.e., because the diagnosis code does not support the procedure code billed) are not generally to be recoded with a new diagnosis code and then resubmitted for payment. Specifically, these prosecutors have identified claims that have been denied and then resubmitted as a fraud and abuse target area. This prosecutorial warning has come about due to certain physicians, who in order to receive payment, are recoding and resubmitting denied claims with new diagnosis codes that were not present on examination, but which were placed on the resubmitted HCFA 1500 claim form solely to justify payment.

However, many times the recoding and refiling of a denied claim is appropriate because of human error that resulted in the first incorrect billing or because the data entry personnel left off a diagnosis that was documented in the record. Because refiling denied claims is a target area, I recommend that you institute and abide by the following procedures:

1. Do not add to the patient's chart any symptoms supporting diagnosis codes after the fact (i.e., after a claim has been denied due to an incorrect diagnosis code);
2. You may resubmit a denied claim with a new diagnosis code if patient conditions supporting the diagnosis were present in the chart but simply not recorded by the data entry personnel or not written down by the physician on the billing sheet given to the data entry personnel;
3. Either a hard copy or an electronic software note of all claims that are recoded and resubmitted after having been initially denied should be kept, containing an explanation by the data entry personnel as to the reason the claim was recoded (i.e., why the diagnosis code was not originally correct).

Recoding diagnosis codes should be a decision by the physician, not clerical staff.

Collection Procedures

The Medicare Carriers Manual states that during the collection process you are required to send a bill, a follow-up letter, a phone call that is documented listing the person to whom your staff talked, the date of the conversation, and what was stated. If those collection efforts have proved fruitless, and the patient is truly indigent, you should request that the patient send you documentation attesting to his or her indigence. Upon receipt of such information, you may legitimately write off the remaining debt.

Collection procedures should be handled the same for all patients; otherwise, you run the risk of being accused of purposeful discrimination against some patients in favor of others and improperly waiving copays and deductibles, thereby running afoul of the anti-kickback statute. If some patients are sent to collection when reaching a certain dollar threshold, then all patients, other than hardship patients, including Medicare patients, should be sent to collection at that threshold.

Documentation of Carrier Communications

Prosecutions of physicians are littered with the physician's excuse, "Medicare said I could bill that way." Unfortunately, the physician never has any documentation of his conversation with the Medicare person, nor any letter to or from Medicare supporting his defense. I cannot overstate how critical it is for pain practices to maintain copies of written communications with all of your carriers, which should be placed in a file designated as "Carrier Communications." Also, any phone conversations with payors regarding reimbursement issues need to be confirmed by letter sent via certified mail. I recommend that your letter contain a clause similar to the following: " This will confirm my conversation with you on today's date that you indicated that we should bill _____ by using CPT code _____. If I am incorrect in my understanding, please inform me in writing of such error; otherwise, our practice will rely on this information in our billing and documentation practices."

REFERENCES

1. HCFA Program Memo B-00-32.
2. *CPT 2000.*
3. Noridian, Medicare carrier for 11 western states, *Med B Issue* 178, September 1999.
4. HCFA Transmittal 1644, August 26, 1999; Medicare Carriers Manual, 14-3-15506, amended 1999.
5. HIP of New York Anesthesia Coding Guidelines, August 2000.
6. Anesthesia Answer Book Action Alert, June 1999, citing Robert Berenson, Director of HCFA's Center for Health Plans and Providers; Id., citing Conversation with ASA Practice Management Advisor, Karen Bierstein.
7. *CPT Assistant*, January 2000; CPT 2000, see comments immediately preceding 62263.
8. Medicare Part B Newsletter No. 145, August 30, 1996.
9. *CPT Assistant, Volume 6, Issue 4, April 1996.*
10. Letter from CPT Information Services to David Vaughn, August 21, 2000.
11. Texas Medicare Part B Newsletter No. 00-003, February 7, 2000.
12. HCFA Final Rule, Published in Federal Register, November 2, 1998.
13. The Florida *Medicare B Update!*, November/December 1999.
14. Reference deleted in text.
15. The *Medicare News Brief* (Part B), 99-3, April 1999.
16. *Georgia Medicare News*, November 1999, p. 21.
17. LMRP, No. 98-007, Oklahoma Medicare, Effective Date 3/15/98.
18. *Medicare Provider News,* Arkansas Blue Cross/Blue Shield, September 1998; *Medicare Provider News*, Arkansas Blue Cross/Blue Shield, December 1997.
19. *CPT Assistant*, August 2000.
20. Letter from California Medicare Director to Thomas B. Cocke, July 22, 1999.
21. *CPT Assistant*, January 2000.
23. The *Medicare News Brief*, 99-3, April 1999.
25. Fraud Alert, 59 FR 65372, December 19, 1994, OEI-09-89-00330.
26. Office of Inspector General Compliance Program Guidance for Individual and Small Group Physician Practices, September 2000.
27. OIG Advisory Opinion 98–12.

CHAPTER **47**

Evaluating and Rating of Physical Impairment

Kenneth Kemp and Martin Grabois

Perhaps one of the greatest challenges facing the clinician is to determine when maximum medical improvement has been obtained and then to provide an impairment rating. It not only is a time-consuming task, but also carries heavy responsibility (1). Yet we are often required to determine an impairment rating on which future benefits will be based and a report on which disability will be determined.

Although impairment ratings have been standardized using the American Medical Association's *Guides to the Evaluation of Permanent Impairment* (2), disability ratings have not enjoyed the same clarity. Much disagreement exists among physicians as to the specific evaluation and rating schedule to use when determining physical disability, and there are no clear guidelines or standardized measures that are uniformly accepted. Because of the adversarial nature of these determinations, some physicians attempt to evade the process altogether (1).

While this chapter will emphasize impairment ratings, it will also present generalized concept in regard to disability ratings.

DEFINITION

The disablement model of integrating impairment, disability, and handicap was noted by Gresham (3) (Fig. 47-1) Pathology is the alteration of anatomy and/or physiology (e.g., herniated disc) that exist at the tissue level. Impairment is an anatomic, physiologic, or psychological abnormality or loss at an organ or system level. These are objective and medically determinable through clinical and/or laboratory assessment as, for example, a contracture of a joint. Disability is a functional limitation or variance of what is considered normal, resulting from impairment, existing at the individual level (e.g., the inability to walk a significant distance because of a weak leg or lift 20 pounds because of a herniated nucleus pulposus). Disability, however, has another definition in the voca-

tional arena. It is the inability to engage in substantial, gainful, vocational activities by reason of any medical determinable physical or mental impairment. It is expected to last for a continuous period of not less than 2 to 12 months. This term is often used to provide justification for compensation for the inability to work. A handicap is something that an individual has to do and cannot do and exists at a societal level. The word came from the English beggar, standing cap in hand. Research and clinical experience has demonstrated that there is no clear relationship between pain and tissue damage and degree of functional disability.

IMPAIRMENT RATINGS INTRODUCTION

Prior to performing any impairment evaluation, one must consider which reference is to be used since several different rating systems have been developed and utilized (4–8). The *American Medical Association Guides to the Evaluation of Permanent Impairment* (2) was developed in an attempt to standardize the process of impairment rating. Originally, the text was a compilation of 13 separate articles in the *Journal of the American Medical Association* (JAMA) (9) and has been revised on several occasions. The fourth edition was printed in 1993 and is the most current; it will be used in this chapter. The fifth edition is scheduled for publication soon after this chapter was submitted. There have been a number of concerns raised about the AMA guides, including the lack of interrater reliability, the fact that true loss of function or "quality of life" is not judged, and the impairment rating does not reflect a full assessment of a worker's total loss after an injury (10). There may never be a perfect tool to assess impairment. Different states and agencies use different versions of the AMA guides and some states and jurisdictions do not use the guides at all (10). Therefore, it is important to understand where the AMA guides are deficient and use

The Disablement Model

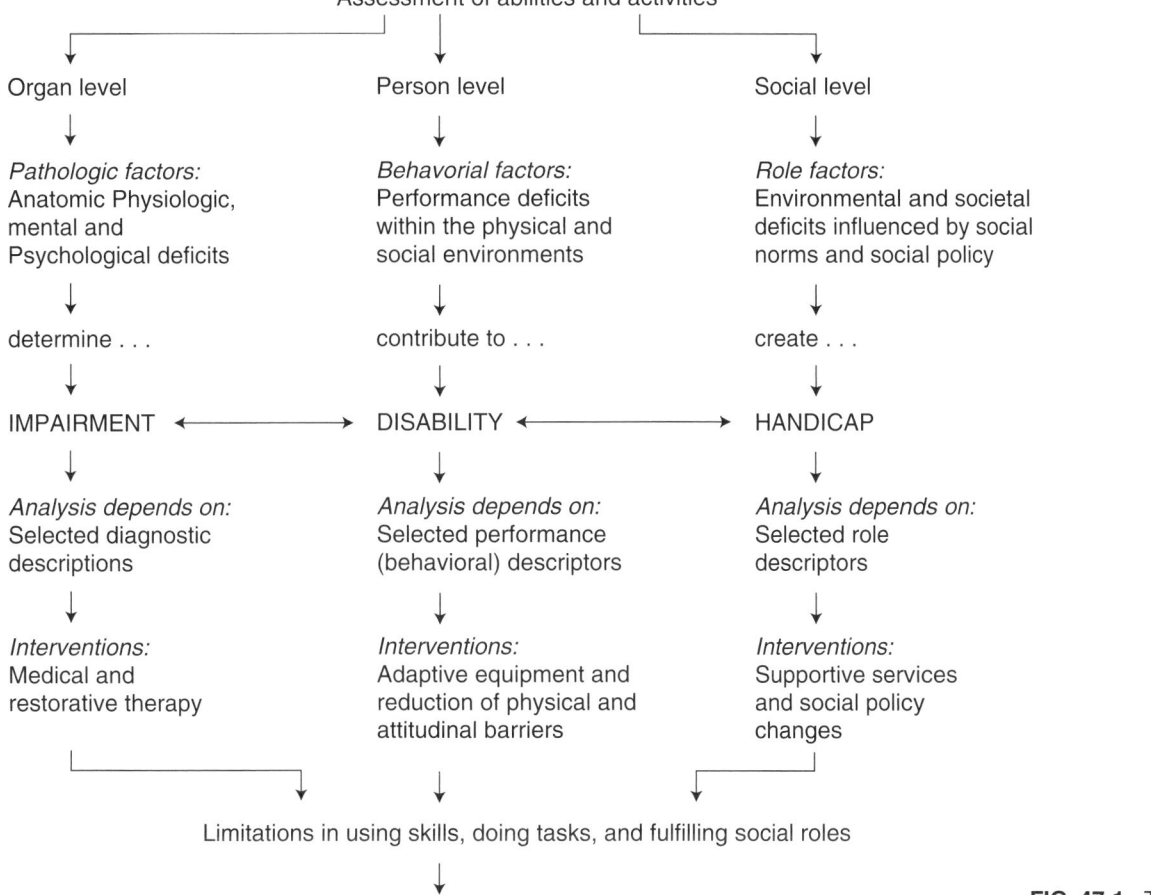

FIG. 47-1. The disablement model

reasonable medical probability and good medical judgment when assessing impairment. Thus, the AMA guides are a reference to assist you, but no guide will ever replace a physician's knowledge, judgment, and expertise. This is similar to the thought that a textbook of medicine will give a physician all the answers and the ability to diagnosis any problem.

Due to the detailed nature of impairment ratings, this chapter is only to assist you in the rating of pain. It is not meant to replace the AMA guides, and it is assumed that the reader will have access to the fourth edition as a reference.

IMPAIRMENT RATING HISTORY AND PHYSICAL EXAM

Since the impairment rating process can be time consuming, adequate time must be scheduled to complete the full assessment and its accompanying documentation. A successful evaluation begins with a complete review of all the examinee's medical records. This should include progress notes (hospital, office, emergency room), operative notes,

therapy notes, radiographic studies, and any other appropriate reports. It is important to establish and record the date of injury, the date an examinee sought treatment, and the dates the patient was unable to work. This information is important in many workers' compensation cases because funding guidelines are often based on injury dates or dates when benefits began to be paid. For example, in the Texas workers' compensation system, injured workers begin to receive temporary income benefits (TIBs) one week after they are unable to work. These benefits last for 104 weeks from the time TIBs begin or until maximum medical improvement (MMI) is reached, whichever comes first. At that time, an impairment rating must be done to determine what additional payments will be received and how long these payments will be received.

Before proceeding with the rating, it is important to explain to examinees the purpose of the evaluation. Examinees should understand that this is not a therapeutic relationship, and they have the ability or power to stop the exam at any point if they think they are being injured. However, in this situation examinees should be informed of the possible repercussions in regards to obtaining an impairment rating. The next step is to take a complete history of the examinees' case. Patients should be allowed to tell in their own words how they have been affected physically, functionally, socially, and psychologically. The history of the present illness should be a retelling of the events of the particular injury, including the mechanism of the injury, the treatment rendered, the current description of pain (character, location, exacerbating and alleviating factors, timing of pain with activities), and the current functional deficits left by the injury. Associated symptoms such as weakness, numbness, bowel difficulties, bladder difficulties, and sexual function should be noted. Other important information should include changes in weight, sleep, and vocational and recreational activities. The complete past medical history of surgeries and chronic illness is important to help establish contributing factors to the current impairment. A full social history, including return to work, financial stress, and family relationships, gives vital information about the possibility of secondary gain in the injured or ill person. Work and educational history, including past job performance and satisfaction and duration of employment are additional important ideas to note. These factors have been linked to prolonged recovery in certain types of injuries (11). By going through this lengthy history, the examiner can make judgments about examinees' ability to understand and cope with their injury or illness. This information can also provide information if examinees are amplifying the consequences of their illness.

Following the history, a complete physical exam is performed. By a thorough history and review of the medical records, the examiner should have a working diagnosis and concept of what will be found on the physical exam. It is important to do a complete exam, even outside of the specific injury areas. This assists the examiner in obtaining information on behavioral components related to the examinee's illness or injury (i.e., using Waddell's signs of nonorganic back pain) (10). However, particular attention is still paid to the injured areas in question including range of motion, motor or sensory nerve loss, atrophy, edema, crepitus, and limitation of use during the exam. Observation of the examinee's actions outside of the formal physical exam is extremely important. For example, a patient who cannot lift her hand over her head on an exam but was able to easily remove her shirt brings up questions on the patient's effort.

The next step is to assimilate all of the above information and answer some specific questions. Is this patient at maximum medical improvement (MMI)? This is important because now the examiner has to decide if the patient's past history and diagnosis is consistent with what is found during this evaluation. Are there any new diagnostic tests that could benefit this person or improve treatment that would affect functional outcome? If no new testing is needed and consistency is found, then have all appropriate treatments been rendered to this examinee? Will the examinee's impairment rating change significantly with new treatment? These questions are important because the impairment evaluation should only continue if the examinee is considered to be at maximum medical improvement. This means that the examinee's impairment is permanent, and all appropriate treatment has been rendered. Occasionally, a request is made for a temporary impairment rating. While this is acceptable, it must be specified in the report that further treatment or testing is necessary and that the number assigned to the Impairment Rating (IR) may change. This will happen in some states with statutory dates of MMI and impairment rating. For example, in Texas workers' compensation, a worker is at statutory MMI at 104 weeks from the date that TIBs began. An impairment rating must be done to continue the injured worker's benefits. If necessary, it must be clearly documented that the rating is not permanent and that future diagnostic testing and treatment are still necessary.

IMPAIRMENT RATING APPLYING THE AMA GUIDELINES

In regard to pain, the AMA guides do not specifically use pain as a diagnosis. Pain, in itself, is not an entity that can be rated in the fourth edition without an underlying impairment (2). Therefore, when doing the impairment evaluation, the examiner must, in reasonable medical probability, decide on a specific diagnosis. The AMA guides the state in several areas that "the impairment percents shown in the chapters considering the various organ systems make allowance for the pain that may accompany the impairing conditions" (2). An examiner must decide if the level of pain and disability displayed by the examinee is consistent with the diagnosis. If it is not consistent, one will need to consider whether the psychological components of pain and chronic pain syndrome have been addressed. If they have not been addressed, MMI has not been reached and further evaluation and treatment is necessary. When this treatment has been rendered and completed, then psychological impairment can be assessed and combined with the physical impairment. For comment on the psychological impairment of pain, see Chapter 53. If the examiner decides that the medical records, history, diagnostic tests, and physical exam, including pain, are all consistent with the established diagnosis, then it is time to apply the AMA guides for impairment ratings.

The AMA guides use the whole person concept of impairment. Each area of the body correlates to a certain unit of impairment of the whole person. All final impairment ratings must be in whole person units and all organ systems are addressed. The most common types of impairments to be evaluated are related to the neurological, muscular, or skeletal systems. The areas involved are the brain and spinal cord, upper extremities (dominant and nondominant), the lower extremities, cervical spine, thoracic spine, lumbar spine, pelvis, and sacrum. For example, in an injury to the thumb, first an impairment rating of the

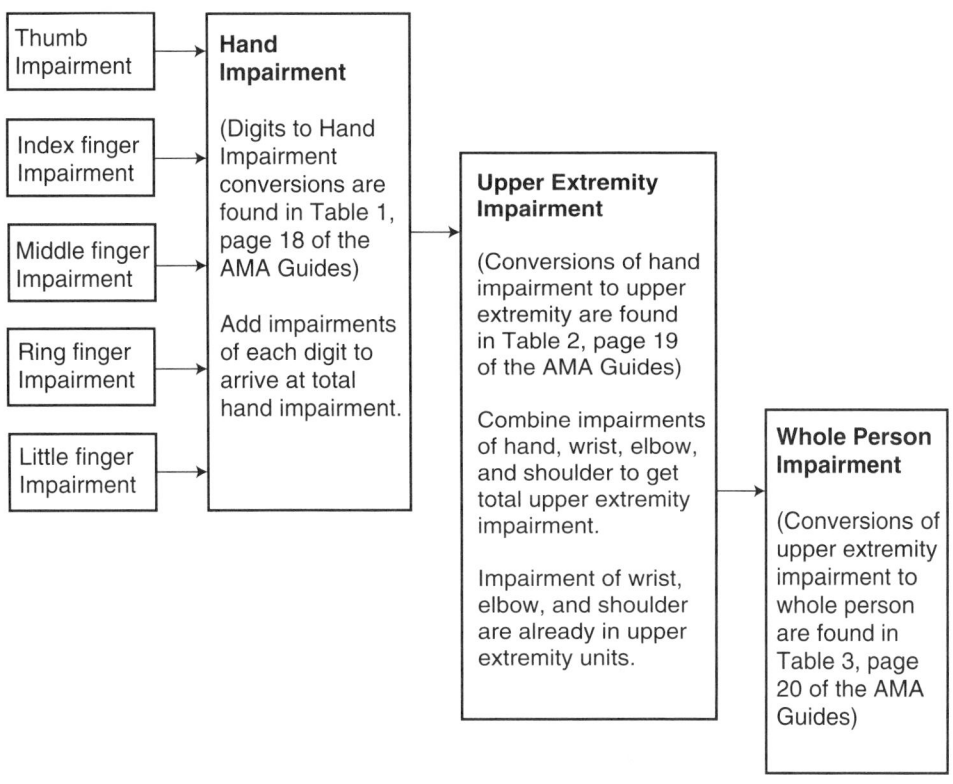

FIG. 47-2. Impairment of the hand

Thumb ROM Impairment

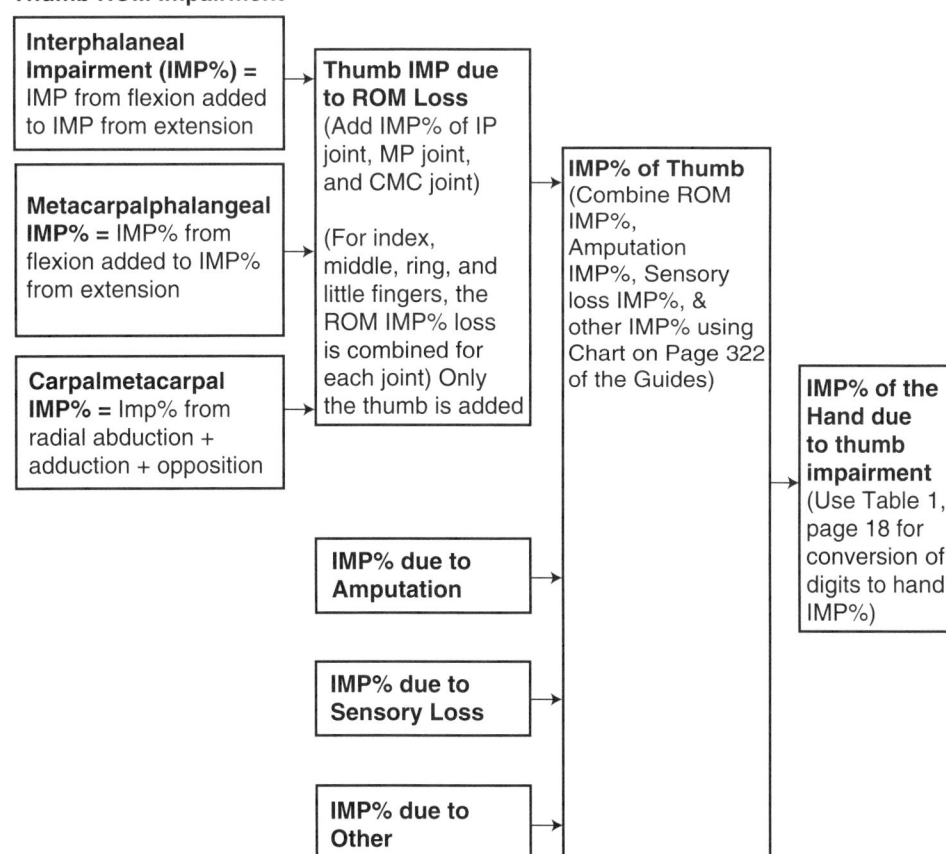

FIG. 47-3. Impairment of the thumb

---

thumb is assessed, then it must be converted to a percentage of hand impairment, then to upper extremity impairment, then finally to whole person impairment (Figs. 47-2 and 47-3). For nonmusculoskeletal impairments, the categories are respiratory, cardiac, hematopoietic, digestive, ENT (ear, nose, and throat), visual, endocrine, skin, mental illness, and urinary/reproductive systems. There are, however, several painful conditions that are not assigned impairment in the guides. These are, for example, fibromyalgia, dysmenorrhea, muscle contraction headache, and irritable bowel syndrome (12). The lack of objective diagnostic tests and the magnitude of subjective complaints make these clinical entities very difficult to quantify or establish.

IMPAIRMENT RATING APPLYING THE AMA GUIDELINES FOR UPPER AND LOWER EXTREMITIES

When beginning to assign impairment, it is important to have a working diagnosis that is documented in the past medical records and substantiated by the history and physical exam. In the fourth edition of the AMA guides, the musculoskeletal system impairments are evaluated by two different systems. Directly measurable or quantitative impairment such as range of motion (ROM) is the first system. The techniques delineated in the guides involve the use of active ROM measured by goniometers, since active ROM is thought to be a better measure of the examinee's true function. Some people (especially ones augmenting signs and symptoms) require a little assistance to give an accurate measure of ROM. While we use gentle assistance when measuring ROM, great care is taken to follow the examinee's request to stop testing if pain is experienced. Additionally, several series of measures are taken to assess reproducibility. The measurements taken are then compared to the normative data tables found in the guides (2). Measuring the uninjured side is sometimes also valuable. By comparing the uninvolved side, an examiner has a better idea of what the examinee's true ROM was prior to injury. We use the degrees lost method. First, measure the involved joint (IJ), then measure the comparison joint (CJ). The next stage is calculating the difference (CJ minus IJ) and then, using the AMA guides table for the specific joint in question, count back from the normal ROM value (i.e., 0% impairment). Finally, find the impairment percent that correlates with the difference (CJ minus IJ). For example, if an injured worker has right shoulder ROM in glenohumeral flexion of 130 degrees (IJ) and the worker's left shoulder flexion is 150 degrees (CJ), using Figure 38 on page 43 of the AMA guides, the worker has a 3% upper extremity ROM impairment in flexion. Using the degrees lost method: 150 degrees (CJ) – 130 degrees (IJ) = 20 degrees of ROM loss. Then, by beginning at 0% impairment and counting back 20 degrees, the injured worker has

a 1% upper extremity ROM impairment in flexion. It is felt using the worker's uninvolved side gives a more accurate assessment of ROM impairment (2).

The second component for evaluating impairment is qualitative impairment. These include diagnoses of specific disorders, motor and sensory loss, amputation, ankylosis, and disfigurement. Within this category, the AMA guides, at times, allow a practitioner to use the subjective complaints of pain and dysfunction to influence the impairment rating. These complaints need to be substantiated by objective findings (e.g., electromyographical studies, radiological studies, physical exam) and appropriate responses by the examinee given the specific injury or illness. Certain areas allowing subjective reports to affect impairment are in the areas of sensory nerve deficits or pain, peripheral vascular disease of the upper and lower extremity, trigeminal neuralgia, and hernia-related impairment as referenced in Table 47-1. For example, in Chapter 10, page 247, Table 7 (2) entitled "Classes of Hernia Related Impairment," a Class 2 impairment is defined as "palpable defect . . . and frequent or persistent protrusion . . . or frequent discomfort, precluding heavy lifting, but not hampering normal activity." The practitioner can estimate whole person impairment between 10% to 19%, depending on the subjective reports of pain or limited function. Again, this must be consistent with the examinee's diagnosis and physical exam. The practitioner must use reasonable medical probability when making these determinations.

With motor nerve loss estimates, objective, measurable, and reproducible deficits must follow known neuroanatomical pathways and be consistent with the examinee's established diagnosis and injury. In summary, all impairments of the extremities should take into account the specific disorder, the motor nerve loss, the sensory nerve loss, and the ROM loss. These impairments are com-

TABLE 47-1. *Tables in AMA guides allowing an examiner to judge functional effects of pain*

Table	Chapter	Page	Title
17	3	57	Upper Extemity Impairment due to Peripheral Vasuclar Disease
69	3	89	Lower Extemity Impairment due to Peripheral Vasuclar Disease
20	4	151	Deterring Impairment of Pain or Sensory Deficits Resulting from Peripheral Nerve Defects (Used for Root, Plexus, or Nerve Injury in the Upper or Lower Extremity)
9	4	145	Cranial Nerve V Impairment
14	4	148	Criteria for One Impaired Upper Extremity
7	10	247	Classes of Hernia Related Impairment

bined (see Combined Values Chart, page 322, AMA guides) and then converted from extremity impairment to whole person impairment (see Table 3, page 20, AMA guides for the upper extremity conversions). The lower extremity impairment conversions are integrated into the corresponding specific disorder, ROM, or nerve loss tables. In the fourth edition, several tables of diagnostic related estimates (DRE) for lower extremity hip or knee replacement, fractures, and skin grafting are available. Unlike spinal injury estimates (presented later in this chapter), in the lower extremity it is suggested to use both techniques to determine an impairment rating and take the higher of the two percentages rather than combining them both. In spinal trauma, only the DRE should be referenced. In previous editions of AMA guides, impairment percentages were reduced for the nondominant upper extremity; this is not the case in the fourth edition (except in Table 14, page 148, AMA guides). A thorough outline for rating of upper extremity impairment is found on page 66 of the AMA guides fourth edition (2).

Questions often arise in regard to the rounding of impairment values and when to add or combine values. First, in regard to rounding impairment percentages or degrees of ROM, it is generally accepted to round upper extremity ROM to the nearest 10 degrees. Rounding impairment percentages to the nearest 5% is not acceptable. Using the typical technique of: last digit < 4 = round down; 5–9 = round up is acceptable when there are decimal points in the impairment percentages. For example, final calculated impairment of 5.6% would round up to 6%. In regard to combining values, there are some simple rules to follow. An examiner can add values when dealing with motions of the same joint, digital impairments to establish hand impairment, spine motions of a particular region, the motions of the thumb, and giving credit for multiple surgeries and operative levels in spinal impairment. All other numbers should be combined. When combining values, always start with the two largest numbers and continue with the next largest number. For example, if an injured worker has an impairment of the right arm of 10%, impairment of the left arm of 30%, and impairment of the right leg of 40%, then the following calculation would apply.

Extremity Impairment		*Whole Person Impairment*
Right arm 10 %	=	6 %
Left arm 30 %	=	18 %
Right leg 40 %	=	16 %

Using the Combined Values Table (page 322, AMA guides), first combine 18 and 16 to equal 31. Next combine 31 and 6 to equal 35%. This injured worker would have an impairment of 35 percent.

(Conversions to whole person done using Table 3, page 20, AMA Guides and Chapter 3 tables regarding the lower extremity.)

IMPAIRMENT RATING APPLYING THE AMA GUIDELINES TO NERVE INJURY

When determining impairment due to motor or sensory loss, the examiner must make a judgment regarding the degree of loss. Tables 11 and 12 on pages 48 and 49 of the AMA guides (2) aid in this determination. These tables describe a range of percentages that can be given depending on the degree of motor or sensory loss. There are also multiple tables that give maximum values that can be attributed to certain damaged peripheral nerve, spinal nerve roots, or plexus lesions. For example, Table 13, page 51 of the AMA guides gives a maximum loss possible of 5% sensory and 30% motor due to damage of the C-5 nerve root. An examinee with 20% sensory loss and 20% motor loss of the C-5 root level as judged by the examiner, the impairment rating would be calculated as follows:

Root Level	*Maximum Possible Loss*		*Determined Loss*		*Percent Impairment*
C-5 sensory	5%	×	20%	=	1%
C-5 motor	30%	×	20%	=	6%

This combines to 7% upper extremity impairment. This converts to 4% whole person impairment.

IMPAIRMENT RATING: APPLYING THE AMA GUIDELINES TO SPINE DISORDERS

Earlier editions of the AMA guides use the ROM model for establishing impairment of injuries to the spine (13). This technique bases impairment on specific disorders, ROM, and nerve loss. However, the specific disorders table, when utilized, is based on diagnosis, x-ray changes, and whether or not surgery was performed. Extra percentage points are given for multilevel surgeries and multiple surgeries. Advanced degenerative changes on x-rays, possibly not related to the specific injury, are also considered in the rating system. The ROM technique used in these editions called for a dual surface inclinometer method. However, the validity of this method has been questioned (14). This is because spinal ROM testing can be influenced by examinee cooperation, soft tissue disorders not related to injury, congenital, or degenerative changes. The examinee's effort always needs to be scrutinized as compensation is based on percentage impairment. Symptom magnification and pain behavior can affect this evaluation. Thus, there are several validity criteria in the AMA guides to protect against this, but these are used in lumbar flexion and extension. In an attempt to remove these variables, the fourth edition emphasizes the use of a diagnostic-related estimate (DRE). The DRE method uses the diagnosis (based on objective testing) to establish impairment. In this model, an injured worker's response to treatment both good and bad is not considered in the impairment (2). For example, a worker diagnosed with lumbar radiculopathy without loss of motion segment integrity or evidence of cauda equina syndrome is given 10% impairment. This percentage is not altered if surgery is a component of the treatment. Additionally, the final outcome in regard to numbness, weakness, or pain is not evaluated in the fourth edition. The initial diagnosis determines the impairment percentage. The only time the ROM model is used is when the diagnosis is not covered in the DRE tables, which is rare. The DRE model removes the confounding factors of examinee cooperation, symptom magnification, and normal age related to changes.

The spine is divided into the cervicothoracic, thoracolumbar, and lumbosacral regions. The diagnosis-based ratings include the diagnoses of radiculopathy, loss of motion segment integrity, vertebral body compression, and fractures of the posterior elements. Severity of injury is graded into eight categories, depending on which disorder is present. The emphasis for severity is based on objective and reproducible findings of neurologic loss and abnormal changes in structural integrity (i.e., fractures, segmental stability) not in degenerative changes. The most important differentiators of impairment severity are EMG testing, urodynamic testing, and flexion extension x-rays for motion segment integrity. The less important are guarding, loss of reflexes, atrophy, loss of bowel or bladder control. Upper motor neuron signs can be combined with the diagnosis-related impairment in the cervicothoracic and thoracolumbar spine regions. The lumbosacral injuries, including cauda equina syndrome and paraplegia, are already integrated into Table 72 on page 100 of the fourth edition and therefore no combining of values is necessary (2).

THE IMPAIRMENT REPORT

When generating an impairment rating report, it is essential to be accurate and complete. Sections should contain medical history, analysis of an injury's impact on activities of daily living and work capacity, integration of medical judgment and impairment reference, physical examination, and calculation of the impairment percentage.

A complete narrative medical history should include all information obtained in the interview of the injured worker, review of medical records, treatment rendered, and current functional status of the worker. The physical exam should document all pertinent findings both positive and negative that support the working diagnosis and contribute to the examinee's impairment. Additionally, the examiner's thought process should be documented, including the important findings during the evaluation that give rise to the medical judgment and impairment rating given. A statement as to which reference is used in the rating and particular tables or figures from which information is derived should be specified. This allows other physicians, case managers, arbitrators, and lawyers to understand how

a decision or impairment was derived. It is important to submit all work sheets used in the evaluation for completeness. In the end, the report generated should be a synopsis of the case with logical progression from injury to diagnosis to treatment to functional outcome and finally impairment percentage.

The process of impairment rating can be irritating, confusing, and time consuming. Like many techniques and ideas in medicine, the best way to learn to do impairment ratings is to actually do them. Reading about how to do them is often tedious. Three case studies will be presented to assist with the practical application of the previous discussions. It is recommended that one do the ratings prior to reading the discussions because the best way to learn impairment ratings is to actually do them. The Guides Casebook is an excellent source for explaining the technique and thought processes that should be followed when completing impairment ratings.

IMPAIRMENT RATING— TRIGEMINAL NEURALGIA

Ms. N is a 48-year-old Caucasian female who has had a 1-year history of pain in the right side of her face. It is described as a brief shooting pain that begins in front of her ear and radiates to her chin. The episodes last for about 30 seconds. In the last year, a neurologist has followed her, and diagnostic testing, including an MRI (which showed no posterior fossa mass or lesions suggestive of multiple sclerosis), has been performed. She was diagnosed with trigeminal neuralgia and is taking carbamazepine. Currently, chewing and talking exacerbate her pain. The episodes of pain are intermittent, occur about three to four times a day, and are labeled a 5 on the scale of 10. She is still working as a secretary and supporting her three children, but is tired of constantly dealing with the pain. She is seeing a psychologist to help her cope with her current situation. The pain is better and she is able to sleep through the night. She has discussed other treatment options with her neurologist, and she is not interested in rhizotomy or injections.

On physical examination, her general neurological exam is normal to motor, sensory, and reflex testing, including sensation to the face and muscles of mastication. Ms. N was pleasant, cooperative, well groomed, and in no apparent distress. What is Ms. N's impairment rating?

In this case, there is truly no reason to establish a rating. If she was unable to work because of this diagnosis and severe pain, then it may be necessary to do impairment rating for disability purposes. The rating of trigeminal neuralgia is subjective and calls for sound medical judgment when establishing a percentage. Using Table 9, page 145 of the AMA fourth edition, this examiner placed this person in the first level, "mild impairment due to uncontrolled facial neuralgia pain" (2). Even in that category, the range for impairment is from 0% to 14% (whole person). Using the moderate degree of pain (Ms. N labeled it a 5 on a scale of 1 to 10), the continued level of function, and the patient's general appearance, this author would equate her condition to a 10% whole person impairment. Due to the subjective method of determining this impairment, there could be many debates over which category (mild, moderate, severe) to place Ms. N as well as what percentage to give within each category. Clinical judgment is paramount in developing Ms. N's impairment.

IMPAIRMENT RATING—CERVICAL RADICULOPATHY

Mr. C is a 38-year-old male who was injured on the job in April 1998. He was diagnosed with a right C-5 radiculopathy due to a herniated nucleus pulposus. Conservative treatment was initially tried, but he eventually underwent a microscopic discectomy in September 1998. Physical therapy was started 8 weeks after surgery; work hardening was completed in February 2000. He has returned to work as a welder. Currently, he has mild weakness of his right biceps, right-sided neck and shoulder pain (worse after a long day), and an occasional headache. Physical examination shows right C-5 weakness, subjective decrease in sensation over the lateral forearm, diminished right biceps reflex, and no evidence of upper motor neuron dysfunction. Otherwise, the examination is negative except for some right trapezius tenderness to palpation. What is Mr. C's impairment rating?

The fourth edition uses the DRE model of impairment. Mr. C has motor, sensory, and reflex testing evidence of right C-5 radiculopathy. However, the most important differentiator is EMG testing consistent with nerve root injury. By using Table 73, page 110 of the AMA guides, Mr. C is placed in category III for cervicothoracic impairment (radiculopathy). Additional information is necessary for an adequate impairment rating, including the lack of spinal instability, lack of long tract signs, and the lack of bowel or bladder involvement. If any of these are present, it would increase the impairment percentage. This worker's impairment is 15%. Another aspect of the DRE model is the fact that outcome of treatment is not included in the final impairment percentage. A worker left with no residual neurologic loss would have the same impairment as a worker who had to endure multiple surgeries. A dilemma may arise when an injured worker has a documented radiculopathy without evidence of long tract signs prior to surgery and develops them after surgery. If your examination documents upper motor neuron injury and there is no evidence in the medical records of this prior to surgery, can you combine this injury with the known radiculopathy? The answer would have to be no. Remember, page 100 of the fourth edtion of the AMA guides states that impairment percentage stays the same

following surgery regardless of the signs or symptoms that are a result of surgery (2). The outcome of the injury is irrelevant to impairment. It is the documented initial injury that matters.

IMPAIRMENT RATING—REFLEX SYMPATHETIC DYSTROPHY (RSD)

Ms. R is a 55-year-old right-handed female that suffered a laceration just below her elbow when falling through a plate glass window. She had an EMG documented incomplete injury to the right ulnar nerve. One week after surgery to repair the laceration and explore the nerve, Ms. R developed extreme pain and swelling in the fourth and fifth fingers of her left hand. A triple phase bone scan confirmed a diagnosis of RSD or complex regional pain syndrome Type II (CRPS2). Stellate ganglion blocks were attempted and multiple medications were attempted. The only medication that successfully dulled her constant burning pain was gabapentin. She is unable to tolerate light touch to her right hand. Ms. R does use her hand in basic-self care skills, but cannot grasp objects with her hand and has trouble sleeping at night and has been seen by a psychiatrist and is taking an SSRI. She is unable to work in any capacity as a florist, although she does take phone orders and assist with inventory counts on a part-time basis. Physical exam shows flexion contractures of the fourth and fifth digits. There is intrinsic hand atrophy and sensory changes and weakness are noted in the ulnar nerve distribution, although examination is difficult due to dysesthesias. Vasomotor and sudomotor changes are also noted. What is the impairment rating percentage assigned to Ms. R?

There are now two ways to assign impairment in a person with RSD. The first, and most cumbersome, and most widely used method is to combine ROM loss of all involved joints and peripheral nerve loss. The other method (Table 14, page 148 AMA guide) is to assign a rating based on criteria for "one impaired upper extremity." This method is best used when there is little documentation of actual nerve injury, but the physical findings and impact on the injured person's function are significant. We will go through both methods in this discussion.

First using Table 14, page 148 of AMA guides (2), "Criteria for One Impaired Upper Extremity" is a simple method to determine the impairment. By observing the use of a person's hand during the exam and specific questioning on their ability to do self-care activities, a rating can be obtained. Ms. R was able to use her hand, somewhat, in self-care tasks but was unable to grasp objects with her injured hand. Using this table, the whole person impairment could range from 25% to 39%. We awarded a 30% whole person rating based on the history and physical findings, including the examinee's ability to take off her shoes and jacket as well as manipulate several small objects with her hands.

TABLE 47-2. *Nerve loss impairment for RSD case study*

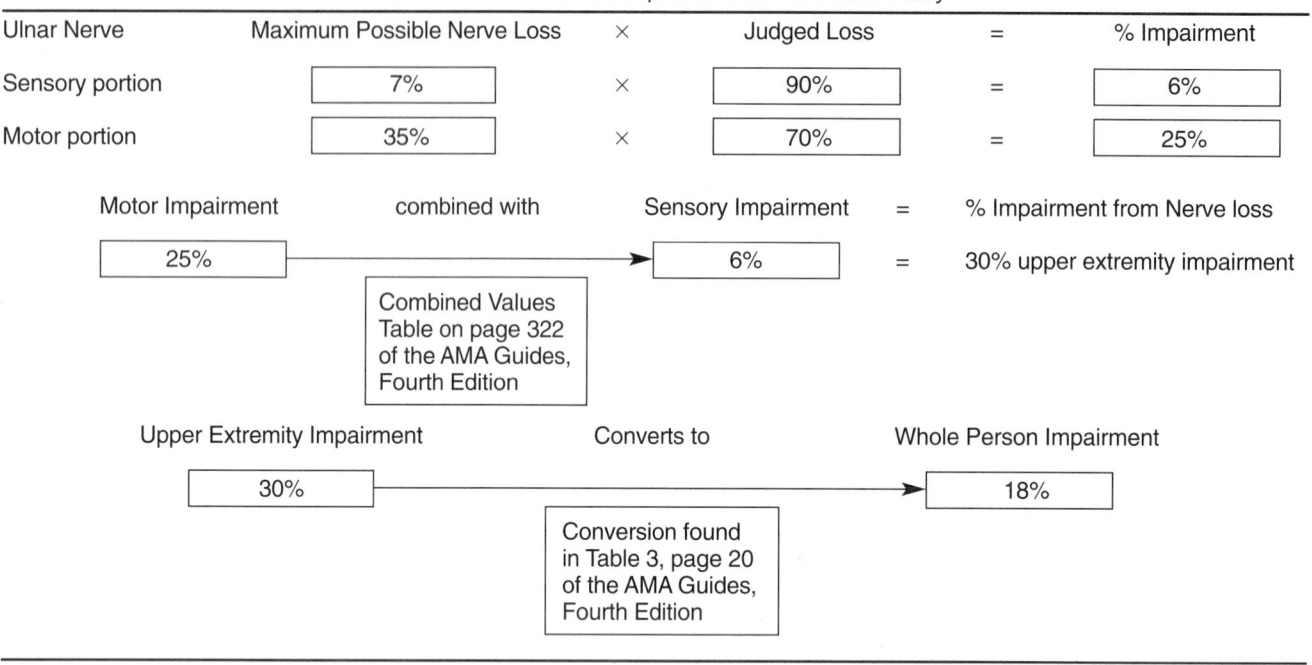

Ulnar Nerve	Maximum Possible Nerve Loss	×	Judged Loss	=	% Impairment
Sensory portion	7%	×	90%	=	6%
Motor portion	35%	×	70%	=	25%

Motor Impairment	combined with	Sensory Impairment	=	% Impairment from Nerve loss
25%		6%	=	30% upper extremity impairment

Combined Values Table on page 322 of the AMA Guides, Fourth Edition

Upper Extremity Impairment	Converts to	Whole Person Impairment
30%		18%

Conversion found in Table 3, page 20 of the AMA Guides, Fourth Edition

TABLE 47-3. *Impairment due to ROM loss for RSD case study*

Digits	Motion	ROM	ROM Impairment	Joint Impairment	Finger Impairment
Thumb	Normal	Normal	0%	Add IMP of ROM at each joint	Combine IMP of each joint within the digit (except the thumb—which is added)
Index	Normal	Normal	0%		
Middle	Normal	Normal	0%		
Ring	MP Flex	50 deg	22%	MP Joint 25%	Ring Finger 61%
	MP Ext	10 deg	3%		
	DIP Flex	40 deg	15%	DIP Joint 17%	Convert Finger to Hand IMP
	DIP Ext	−10 deg	2%		
	PIP Flex	50 deg	30%	PIP Joint 33%	Middle Finger 7%
	PIP Ext	−10 deg	3%		
Little	MP Flex	40 deg	27%	MP Joint 32%	Hand Impairment 14%
	MP Ext	0 deg	5%		
	DIP Flex	30 deg	21%	DIP Joint 23%	Little Finger 7%
	DIP Ext	−10 deg	2%		
	PIP Flex	40 deg	36%	PIP Joint 39%	Little Finger 68%
	PIP Ext	−10 deg	3%		

Add IMP of each finger

Convert Finger to Hand IMP (Table 1, page 18)

TABLE 47-4. *RSD case study*

Hand IMP	converts to	Upper Extremity IMP	converts to	Whole Person IMP
14%		13%		ROM loss 8%
	Use Table 2, page 19		Use Table 3, page 20	

Whole Person IMP for Nerve Loss	combines with	Whole Person IMP for ROM Loss
18%	Using the Combined Values Table on page 322	8%
	Ms. C's IMP 25%	

The next method would be to combine the motor and sensory loss of the extremity with ROM loss. Using Table 15, page 54 of the AMA guides indicates the maximum possible loss to the ulnar nerve is 7% sensory loss and 35% motor loss, whereas in Tables 11 and 12 on pages 48 and 49 Ms. R is judged to have a 90% loss of sensation and 70% motor loss. (Table 47-2).

Range of motion normative tables for the fingers and wrist are found on pages 32 through 34 of the AMA guides. One needs to determine impairment due to the range of motion loss for each motion at each joint of each digit involved (i.e., flexion and extension of the ring finger at the distal interphalangeal joint [DIP]) and then add the impairments together for each joint of a finger. If multiple joints of a finger are involved, the rater must combine the values of each joint to obtain the impairment percentage for that finger. When several fingers are involved, first determine the impairment of each digit, then convert to hand impairment. Once this is done, the examiner can add the hand impairments attributed to each digit for total hand impairment, then convert to upper extremity and finally to whole person impairment (Tables 47-2, 47-3, and 47-4).

The impairment percentage derived in this method is 25 percent. This is close to the judgment made using the first method. The examiner should use clinical judgment as to which method and number is the most appropriate. The Guides Casebook (12) states that the technique to be used depends on the injury. RSD is now defined as complex regional pain syndrome type I and II (CRPS 1 & 2). CRPS 2 has been known in the past as causalgia. If there is documented evidence of nerve injury as in Ms. R, then the most appropriate technique is assessing motor and sensory loss and ROM loss. If there is limited documentation of nerve injury (i.e., CRPS 1), then the assessment of the injury's impact on function is most appropriate.

DISABILITY RATING

Disability is defined by the World Health Organization as "any restriction or lack (resulting from an impairment) of ability to perform an activity in the manner or within the range considered normal for a human being" (15). In other words, disability is that function that the patient is "disabled" or unable to do in terms of his needs or desires. The AMA guidelines, unfortunately, can determine impairment rating but not disability. They have limited application for the disability evaluation. The AMA guides tend to place more importance on physical and laboratory findings instead of the client's history, functional assessment, and pain behaviors (16). Likewise, the definition of disability may vary from agency or organization making the determination.

To rectify these deficiencies and provide a more equitable rating system, there is a restructuring of the methodology whereby disability is evaluated and rated using the functional capacity evaluation.

The functional capacity evaluation (FCE) is a medical evaluative tool to assess the injured worker's physical capacity, functional limitations, and ability to return to a specific job. Harten (17) indicates that the reasons for doing an FCE are to identify when the patient's rehabilitative progress plateaus; to clarify when a difference exists between the patient's reported and observed function; when vocational planning calls for accounting of the patient's physical abilities; and to identify permanent restrictions when case closure is indicated by judgment or statues (18). The FCE may be useful to identify where there are inconsistencies in the patient's performance such as an increase or lack of increase in heart rate. If Waddell's signs are very prominent according to Harten (17), then there is a difference between what the patient reports and the function observed.

To determine whether someone can go back to work or is functionally disabled from doing that job, one must consider the essential functions of the job as well as accommodations. Both the patient and examiner are potentially subject to bias, thus having an impact on the validity of the evaluation when dealing with pain. As noted earlier, pain cannot be measured directly, as it is subjective. However, one needs to be objective in approaching disability in such patients. In determining what someone can do functionally, especially in relation to her job, one must go beyond merely considering the degree of impairment that can be medically and objectively determined. Walsh et al. (19) noted that functional evaluation measures the appropriateness of the patient's functional capacity for his level of impairment. Objective and quantitative measurements can also give a baseline with which to evaluate progress and a long-term outcome.

There are, however, scientific limitations to FCEs. These limitations include validity of an FCE to predict one's return to work (20) or the ability to predict a worker's success in actual job-related tasks (21). Remember that FCEs also may not correlate with a 6- to 8- or 12-hour working day. Additionally, the reliability of FCEs is also questionable (17).

There are many protocols for FCE testing but only three protocols are standardized according to Harten (17). However, these protocols have not been peer-reviewed according to Saunders (21). FCE includes an interview, similar to a medical history, a psychological battery, a musculoskeletal evaluation, functional testing, validation of sincerity of effort by various methods, and a summation report comparing the test to a specific job requirement (22–24). The musculoskeletal evaluation of a patient includes assessment of posture, flexibility, range of motion, endurance, dexterity, attitude, and consistency during the activity performance (24). The testing includes material-handling tasks, holding of static postures, and repetitive task performance (25). The FCE can also look at an isolated body part—for example, lumbar strength—while assessing several different functional units at the same time, such as lifting (23).

Velozo (26) and Wyman (27) noted that the work capacity evaluation and functional capacity evaluation must consider the work environment and the specific job criteria as defined by the employers and discuss the maximum amount of weight that needs to be lifted or carried. The employer should be able to provide this kind of information; if not, a health care worker may need to go to the job site to observe the job requirements.

It is important to note that the FCE is a tool that provides information about the injured worker's ability, as well as some insight as to what provokes symptomatology, and specific exertions at the time of testing. Functional capacity testing does not predict whether an individual can return to work. It will not evaluate motivation of an individual who is working in a rehabilitation program to return to work. It is, however, one useful tool that a physician can employ to evaluate what people can do and if they are making an effort to try to do it.

A worksheet can be used to aid the physician examiner and ensure that a consistent, systematic, and complete database is gathered during the IME. This evaluation, combined with the functional evaluation, leads to a functional assessment that can be helpful in determining disability. One needs to emphasize the lack of one-to-one correlation between clinical findings and disability. Through extensive reviews, a study by the Institute of Medicine demonstrated the poor relationship and the lack of correlation between objective identifiable pathology and impairments with an individual's function and disability (28).

Several authors have suggested measurement tools to assess pain and disability that should be considered in developing an ideal instrument. Many of these instruments provide valid and objective assessment of some of the psychological as well as social impairments and "disability." Information from such instruments is essential to reflect pain-related disability, in addition to the physical examination (29, 30).

However, to date, no instrument has been universally accepted as the "gold standard." Turk et al. (29) review the utilization of multiaxial pain assessment, which measures the impact of pain on an individual's functioning. This approach is a step toward providing an instrument that could be reliable, valid, and helpful in the classification of those individuals who report impairment and disability primarily due to pain.

Although physicians generally believe that they know when their patients are disabled, the fact remains that the term *disabled* does not have a universally accepted definition. Some clinicians use this term to denote an individual's inability to carry out a particular task, whereas others use it to indicate that the individual no longer has the capacity to perform prior work activity.

When communicating with disability adjudicators, it is important that the physician recognize that terms are used differently by the various programs and accept the need to clarify the terminology being used.

Status statements should be used to describe patients' overall functioning within their home and work environments. Each disability adjudicator must ultimately make a decision about the individual's total capacity to carry out physical and mental functions. Each disability decision is based on the assessment of a particular set of medical facts and any available descriptions of the applicant's physical and mental performance.

CONCLUSION

This chapter has provided a description of the challenges of determining impairment ratings and subsequent disability. The chapter describes the differences between the impairment rating, disability, and handicap and the role of the physician in determining impairment rating and disability.

A detailed discussion is presented on the impairment rating using the *AMA Guidelines to Evaluation of Permanent Impairments*. A comprehensive history and physical examination is described for determining impairment rating and disability, how the AMA guidelines are applied for impairment rating, and the impairment rating report. Three cases are utilized to explain and describe how impairment rating is determined for trigeminal neuralgia, a radiculopathy, and reflex sympathetic dystrophy.

Disability ratings are described and differentiated from impairment ratings. To adequately provide a disability determination, a functional capacity evaluation is desirable. The role of FCE in assessing the injured worker's physical capacity, functional limitations, and ability to return to a specific job is discussed.

There is a lack of consistency in the terminology used by different disability programs. Disability tools are needed to assess pain and resultant disability because there is no "gold standard" accepted to date. Turk describes a multiaxial pain assessment tool to improve the disability dilemma (29).

REFERENCES

1. Vernick SH, Sawyer J, Marin E, Rucker K. Evaluation and rating on physical disability. In: Rondinelli RD, Katz RT, eds. *Impairment rating and disability*. Philadelphia, PA: WB Saunders Co, 2000.
2. American Medical Association. *Guides to evaluation of permanent impairment*. 4th ed. Chicago, AMA 1993.
3. Gresham GE. Essential considerations of the disability evaluation. *J Musculoskel Med* 1986;3(5):43–50.
4. American Academy of Orthopedic Surgeons. *Manual for orthopedic surgeons in evaluating permanent physical impairment*. Chicago: American Academy of Orthopedic Surgeons, 1975.
5. Smith WC. *Principles of disability evaluation*. Philadelphia, PA: JB Lippincott, 1959.
6. Rice CO. *Calculation of industrial disability of the extremities and back*, 2nd ed. Springfield, IL: Charles C. Thompson, 1968.
7. McBride ED. *Disability evaluation: principles of treatment of compensable injuries*, 6th ed. Philadelphia, PA: JB Lippincott, 1963.
8. Kessler HH. *Disability determination and evaluation*. Philadelphia, PA: Lea & Fibiger, 1970.
9. Grabois M, Garrison SJ, Hart K, et al. *Physical medicine and rehabilitation: the complete approach*. Malden, MA: Blackwell Science, 2000.
10. Waddell G, McCulloch J, Jemmel E, et al. Nonorganic signs in low back pain. *Spine* 1980;5:117–125.
11. Bigos SH, Bathe M, Spengler DM, et al. A prospective study of work perceptions and psychosocial factors affecting the report of back injury. *Spine* 1991;16:1–6.
12. American Medical Association. *The guides casebook*. AMA, Chicago, 1999.
13. American Medical Association. *Guides to the evaluation of permanent impairment*, 3rd ed, 2nd print. AMA, Chicago 1003.
14. Rondenelli R, Murphy J, Esler A, et al. Estimation of normal lumbar flexion with surface inclinometry: a comparison of three methods. *Am J Phy Med Rehab* 1992;71:219–224.
15. World Health Organization. *International classification of impairments, disabilities, and handicaps*. Geneva: WHO, 1980.
16. Rucker K, Metzler H, Wehman P, et al. Pain literature and social security policy. *J Back Musculoskel Rehab* 1991;1:62–73.
17. Harten JA. Functional capacity evaluation. Occupational medicine: *State of the Art Reviews* 1998;13(1):209–212.
18. Bloodworth D, Calvillo O, Smith K, Grabois M. Chronic pain syndromes: evaluation and treatment. In: RL Braddom, ed. *Physical medicine and rehabilitation*, 2nd ed. Philadelphia, PA: WB Saunders, 2000.
19. Walsh NE, Dumitru D. Ramamurthy S, Schoenfeld LS. Treatment of patient with chronic pain. In: DeLisa JA, ed. *Rehabilitation medicine: principles and practice*, 2nd ed. JB Lippincott Company, Philadelphia, PA: 1993.
20. King PM, Tuckwell N, Barrett TE. A critical review of functional capacity evaluations. *Phys Ther* 1998;78(8):852–866.
21. Saunders RL, Beissner KL, McManis BG. Estimates of weight that subjects can lift frequently in functional capacity evaluations. *Phys Ther* 1997;77(12):1717–1728.
22. Hazard RG, Bendix A, Fenwick JW. Disability exaggeration as a predictor of functional restoration outcomes for patients with chronic low back pain. *Spine* 1991;16(9):1062–1067.
23. Strang JP. Chronic disability syndrome: In: Aronoff GM, ed. *Evaluation and treatment of chronic pain*. Baltimore, MD: Urban & Schwarzenberg, 1985.
24. Turk DC, Okifuji A. Perception of traumatic onset, compensation status, and physical findings: impact on pain severity, emotional distress, and disability in chronic pain patients. *J Behav Med* 1996;19(5): 435–453.
25. Portenoy RF, Kanner RM. Definition and assessment of pain. In: Portenoy RK, Kanner RM, eds. *Pain mechanism theory and practice*. Philadelphia, PA: FA Davis CO, 1996.
26. Wall Street Journal, Friday June 2, 2000 page B1.
27. Wyman DO. Evaluating patients for return to work. *AFP* 1999; 59(4):844–848.
28. Osterweis M, Leinman A, Mechanic D. *Pain and disability—clinical behavioral and public policy perspective*. Committee on Pain, Disability and Chronic Illness Behavior. National Academy Press, Washington, DC.
29. Turk DC, Rudy TE, Strieg RL. The disability determination dilemma: toward a multiaxial solution. *Pain* 1989;34:217–229.
30. Vasudevan SV, Monsein M. Evaluation of functional and disability in the patient with chronic pain. In: PP Raj, ed. *Practical management of pain*, 2nd ed. St. Louis, MO: Mosby-Year Book, Inc. 1992.

CHAPTER **48**

Evaluation and Rating of Psychological Impairment and Disability

C. David Tollison and Donald W. Hinnant

Clinical psychologists and psychiatrists, particularly those specializing in pain management, are being asked with increasing frequency to assume responsibility for assessing the patient in pain for psychological impairment. This requirement of psychological pain management is primarily limited to patients covered under workers' compensation and those patients applying for Social Security disability. However, the assessment of psychological impairment may also be required in the evaluation and treatment of patients suffering personal injury, such as motor vehicle accidents and "slip and fall" or other injury with potential liability. In addition, a growing number of long-term disability insurance companies are requesting the formal assessment of psychological impairment in patients applying for insurance benefits. Given that the assessment of psychological impairment is, historically, no more a subject of instruction in mental health training than is assessment of physical impairment a curriculum topic in medical training, it is hardly surprising that most clinical psychologists and psychiatrists often find the responsibility of assessing psychological impairment a topic of some complexity and confusion.

In this chapter we shall briefly review the basics of psychological impairment within the existing medical-legal system, focusing on the applied mechanics of performing an impairment evaluation, and utilizing the American Medical Association *Guides to the Evaluation of Permanent Impairment* (1), the American Psychiatric Association *Diagnostic and Statistical Manual of Mental Disorders* (4th ed.) (2), and Social Security Administration *Disability Evaluation Under Social Security* (3) as directional guides.

DISABILITY VERSUS IMPAIRMENT

Disability is, in general terms, a system of either social legislation or private insurance designed to protect individuals from suffering undue financial hardship when they are unable to work. Consequently, disability may result from physical, psychological, or a combination of physical and psychological disorders.

More specifically, disability is not a system, but a number of systems that include commercially available disability and wage protection insurance, personal injury liability, Social Security disability benefits (title II) and supplemental security income (title XVI), and workers' compensation. Workers' compensation laws differ in each of the 50 states, the District of Columbia, and various U.S. territories. In addition, federal laws provide disability coverage for federal employees, and many maritime workers are covered under the federal Longshore and Harbor Workers' Compensation Act.

Despite the multiplicity of laws, jurisdictions, and workers' compensation versus tort-based versus social legislative systems, the determination of impairment/disability is sufficiently similar that we can, for purposes of this chapter, discuss the clinical and administrative determination of psychological impairment/disability as if it were a single general system. Variances to this approach will be noted when applicable. The interested reader is urged to consult the appropriate chapters in this text for additional and detailed information on workers' compensation and Social Security disability.

A basic premise underlying the determination of psychological functioning is the distinction between "impairment" and "disability." The definition of disability is based on an individual's ability (or inability) to engage in "substantial gainful activity" or to work (4). Thus, the adjudication of disability claims is fundamentally a vocational/administrative issue rather than a medical one (4). This position has been supported as far back as 1958 when the American Medical Association Committee on the Rating of Mental and Physical Impairment wrote in their *Guides to the Evaluation of Permanent Impairment, the Extremities and Back* that the determination of impairment is purely a medical decision and that whether a given impairment represented a disability was an administrative responsibility and function, rather than a medical one (5). Consequently, a physician or clinical psychologist is charged with a responsibility of determining and documenting *impairments*, a term considered to be of medical parlance. *Disability*, on the other hand, is generally considered a legal term and the determination of a ruling board, agency, court, or other authority. Therefore, an evaluating clinical psychologist or psychiatrist is responsible for determining the presence or absence of psychological impairment that is subsequently considered in the nonmedical determination of whether an impairment constitutes a disability. The Social Security Administration, in fact, unequivocally states that "the physician is neither asked for nor expected to make a decision as to whether a patient is disabled" (3).

PSYCHOLOGICAL IMPAIRMENT IN THE MEDICAL-LEGAL SYSTEM

There are numerous disability jurisdictions in the United States that oversee disability determination and monitor their own policies and procedures. Each jurisdiction has its own criteria for disability, as determined by administrative philosophy and policy, and there is considerable variation across jurisdictions. Likewise, the covered conditions, length and amount of payments, and review procedures also vary, as does the degree to which nonmedical factors (e.g., age, education, and social environment) are considered. For example, in certain situations, an individual may qualify for more than one form of disability compensation.

Despite the array of disability systems and the variability in criteria and structure, there appear to be two common factors across systems. The first is that physicians and clinical psychologists do not determine disability, although their findings are considered relevant. Health professionals may render a medical opinion in individual cases about the degree of impairment, treatment, and prognosis but, as previously mentioned, disability (work incapacity) remains an administrative or judicial determination following input from various sources (6). A second common threat across disability systems is the general recognition of two types of disability: physical and psychological.

Because the determination of psychological disability is based in part on the responsibility of psychiatrists and clinical psychologists to provide specific information on impairment, we should have a basic familiarity with the procedures, regulations, and philosophy of the particular agency and the criteria for disability determination currently in use. However, because an analysis of every current disability system is far beyond the limitations of this chapter, we shall restrict our discussion to a brief overview of three primary systems: (1) workers' compensation, (2) Social Security, and (3) personal injury.

Workers' Compensation

In general, workers' compensation is a system of state and federal legislations designed to protect workers from suffering undue financial hardship when they are unable to work as the result of a work-related injury. Although workers' compensation is intended to protect injured workers from financial hardship, the system is not designed to totally replace lost income. Thus, under the most typical benefit scheme, a totally disabled worker will receive only two-thirds of his average weekly wage, subject to a state maximum benefit. In the majority of workers' compensation cases, the system functions almost automatically: upon receipt of notice that an employee has been injured, the employer arranges with the workers' compensation insurance company to initiate payment of the employee's medical bills and begins making weekly payments of benefits to which the employee is entitled until he is able to return to work. Nevertheless, there remain many cases in which there is disagreement between the parties as to whether the employee has sustained a compensable injury, and, if so, what benefits he is entitled to receive. In the experience of the authors, the frequency of disagreement among the employer, workers' compensation insurance company, injured employee, and legal representative of the injured employee is particularly high in cases involving a psychological component (e.g., posttraumatic stress disorder, depression in reaction to pain intensity, duration, and lifestyle alteration).

In most states, determination on contested proceedings is conducted before a hearing officer (often termed a referee, administrative law judge, or commissioner). Because the procedure is an administrative-type hearing rather than a court trial, the rules of evidence may be less strictly applied than would be in court action. Psychiatrists and clinical psychologists should remember that hearing officers rarely have any medical or psychological training. Therefore the psychiatrist or clinical psychologist called on to render expert opinion in a workers' compensation case must remember to be clear in explaining her diagnosis, impairment findings, and prognosis. The psychiatrist/clinical psychologist should be prepared to explain an official diagnosis in nontechnical terms, avoid unnecessary medical terminology, and spell out in detail the causal relationship between the events of the work-related injury and the employee's current impairment. With regard to a rating of the degree of psychological impairment sustained by a claimant, the psychiatrist/clinical psychologist should be aware that insurance companies and hearing officers expect to have ratings based on standard AMA guidelines (Table 48-1).

TABLE 48-1. *Classes of impairment due to mental and behavioral disorders*

Area or aspect of functioning	Class 1— No impairment	Class 2— Mild impairment	Class 3— Moderate impairment	Class 4— Marked impairment	Class 5— Extreme impairment
Activties of daily living Social functioning Concentration Adaptation	No impairment noted	Impairment levels are compatible with most useful functioning	Impairment levels are compatible with some, but not all, useful functioning	Impairment levels significantly impede useful functioning	Impairment levels preclude useful functioning

(From *Guides to the Evaluation of Permanent Impairment*, 5th ed. American Medical Association. November 2000, with permission.)

Workers' compensation benefits are paid during the period in which the injured employee is disabled from returning to work and, in some instances, for presumed future disability. Assuming a period of temporary total disability, it will be determined at some point that the injured worker has attained the maximum medical improvement (MMI) that can be expected. This does not necessarily mean that the injured worker is fully recovered or symptom-free, only that improvement has reached a level of plateau and no additional treatment is likely to significantly improve the patient's condition in the foreseeable future. In cases involving psychological symptoms, MMI is determined by the clinical psychologist/psychiatrist. Often there is significant pressure brought on the mental health professional by the insurance company, wishing to close the case and avoid payment of additional treatment charges, and the patient or patient's legal representative, wishing to benefit from treatment intended to improve the patient's condition.

Once MMI has been reached, a determination must be made, with assistance of psychiatric/psychological opinion, as to whether the injured worker has sustained any permanent impairment and, if so, the extent of that impairment. If it is determined that the worker will be unable to return to work in the foreseeable future, he may be classified as permanently and totally disabled and will be awarded benefits accordingly. If the worker is able to return to work, but has some residual psychological disability attributable to the injury, he is likely to receive an award based on the state's "schedule" of injuries.

At this point the reader will likely have noted three points in the above process at which psychiatric/psychological opinion is not only necessary, but almost always indispensable: (a) determining a causal relationship between the worker's injury and psychological symptoms, (b) determining when the injured worker has reached MMI, and (c) "rating" the degree of permanent impairment, which includes diagnosing whether residual symptoms will cause permanent partial or permanent total psychological impairment (Table 48-1). Psychological impairment may occur with no physical injury or impairment, or may occur in addition to physical impairment.

Social Security

Disability has been defined for the purposes of Social Security claims adjudication under the Social Security Act as an "inability to engage in any substantial gainful activity by reason of a medically determinable physical or mental impairment which can be expected to result in death or can be expected to last for a continuous period of not less than 12 months" (3). The adjudication of claims for disability benefits under Title II (Social Security Disability Benefits) and Title XVI (Supplemental Security Disability and Income) of the Social Security Act is based on the use of established medical criteria as described in the Listing of Impairments. As in other systems of disability determination, however, clear differences exist between what constitutes an "impairment" and what constitutes a "disability" within the context of the Social Security regulations, and it is on the interpretation of these differences that the Social Security Administration has placed considerable focus in the last several years.

The use of objectively demonstrable signs, symptoms, and medical findings at a disability adjudication has served the intent of the law relatively well in problems related to acute medical conditions, but the law does not provide an objective mechanism for evaluating the patient in pain. Because the pain experience is a perception and because perceptions are not directly and objectively quantifiable, pain was considered in the evaluation of disability only as a secondary factor associated with a medically determinable impairment. The Social Security Administration has had increasing numbers of court cases challenging this policy regarding the evaluation of pain because chronic pain sufferers often present with allegations of pain that are not consistent with medically determinable impairment.

For patients in pain who also develop psychological symptoms and disorders, the diagnostic category of somatoform pain disorder, included in the fourth edition of the *Diagnostic and Statistical Manual (DSM-IV)* of the American Psychiatric Association (2), has provided an avenue of adjudication under the umbrella of mental disorders. Psychological impairment/disability is recognized by a variety of disability agencies and sources, but probably none more readily or with greater complexity than in Social Security disability. The evaluation of Social Security disability on the basis of mental disorders requires the documentation of a medically determinable impairment as well as consideration of the degree of limitation such impairment may impose on the individual's ability to work, and whether these limitations have lasted or are expected to last for a continuous period of at least 12 months. The listings for mental disorders under Social Security disability are arranged in eight diagnostic categories: (a) Organic Mental Disorders, (b) Schizophrenia, Paranoid, and Other Psychotic Disorders, (c) Affective Disorder, (d) Mental Retardation and Autism, (e) Anxiety-Related Disorders, (f) Somatoform Disorders, (g) Personality Disorders, and (h) Substance Addiction Disorders. Each diagnostic category, except Mental Retardation and Autism and Substance Addiction Disorders, consists of a set of clinical findings (paragraph A criteria), one or more of which must be met, and which, if met, leads to an assessment of functional restrictions (paragraph B criteria), or which two or three must also be met. There are additional considerations (paragraph C criteria) in the categories of Schizophrenia, Paranoid, and Other Psychotic Disorders and Anxiety-Related Disorders.

The purpose of including criteria in paragraph A of the listings for mental disorders is to medically substantiate the presence of a mental disorder. The purpose of including criteria in paragraphs B and C is to describe those functional limitations associated with mental disorders that are incompatible with the ability to work. The restrictions listed in paragraphs B and C must be the result of the mental disorder that is manifested by the clinical findings outlined in paragraph A. The criteria included in paragraphs B and C of the listings for mental disorders have been chosen by the Social Security Administration because they represent functional areas deemed essential for work. An individual who is significantly limited in these areas as a result of an impairment identified in paragraph A is presumed to be unable to work.

The existence of a medically determinable impairment of the required duration must be established by medical evidence consisting of clinical signs, symptoms, and/or laboratory or psychological test findings. These findings may be intermittent or persistent, depending on the nature of the disorder. Clinical signs are medically demonstrable phenomena that reflect specific abnormalities of behavior, affect, thought, memory, orientation, or contact with reality. Social Security typically expects such an assessment to be performed by a psychiatrist or clinical psychologist. A growing trend is the increasing requirement of objective psychological testing, such as the Minnesota Multiphasic Personality Inventory (MMPI) or, in cases of claimants with complaints of pain, the Pain Patient Profile (P-3).

In the following section we will outline four of the eight categories of mental disorders and impairments considered to constitute evidence for psychological disability by the Social Security Administration. The categories of Affective Disorders, Anxiety-Related Disorders, Somatoform Disorders, and Personality Disorders are the four categories most frequently encountered by professionals determining psychological impairment as a result of or in association with pain.

Four Social Security Administration Categories of Mental Disorders

Affective Disorders

Affective disorders are characterized by a disturbance of mood, accompanied by a full or partial manic or depressive syndrome. Mood refers to a prolonged emotion that colors the whole psychic lift; it generally involves either depression or elation.

The required level of severity for these disorders is met when the requirements in both A and B are satisfied.

A. Medically documented persistence, either continuous or intermittent, of one of the following:
  1. Depressive syndrome characterized by at least *four* of the following:
      a. Anhedonia or pervasive loss of interest in almost all activities; or
      b. Appetite disturbance with change in weight; or
      c. Sleep disturbance; or
      d. Psychomotor agitation or retardation; or
      e. Decreased energy; or
      f. Feelings of guilt or worthlessness; or
      g. Difficulty concentrating or thinking; or
      h. Thoughts of suicide; or
      i. Hallucinations, delusions, or paranoid thinking; or
  2. Manic syndrome characterized by at least *three* of the following:
      a. Hyperactivity; or
      b. Pressure of speech; or
      c. Flight of ideas; or
      d. Inflated self-esteem; or
      e. Decreased need for sleep; or
      f. Ease of distractability; or
      g. Involvement in activities that have a high probability of painful consequences that are not recognized; or
      h. Hallucinations, delusions, or paranoid thinking; or
  3. Bipolar syndrome with history of episodic periods manifested by the full symptomatic picture of both mania and depressive syndromes (and currently characterized by either or both syndromes)
  AND

B. Resulting in at least *two* of the following:
1. Marked restriction in activities of daily living; or
2. Marked difficulties in maintaining social functioning; or
3. Deficiencies of concentration, persistence, or pace resulting in frequent failure to complete tasks within a timely manner (in work settings or elsewhere); or
4. Repeated episodes of deterioration or decompensation in work or work-like settings that cause the individual to withdraw from that situation or to experience exacerbation of signs and symptoms (which may include deterioration or adaptive behaviors).

Anxiety-Related Disorders

In these disorders, anxiety is either the predominant disturbance or it is experienced if the individual attempts to master symptoms; for example, confronting the dreaded object or situation in a phobic disorder or resisting the obsessions or compulsions in obsessive-compulsive disorders.

The required level of severity for these disorders is met when the requirements in both A and B are satisfied, or when the requirements in both A and C are satisfied.

A. Medically documented findings of at least *one* of the following:
1. Generalized persistent anxiety accompanied by three out of four of the following signs or symptoms:
   a. Motor tension; or
   b. Autonomic hyperactivity; or
   c. Apprehensive expectation; or
   d. Vigilance and scanning; or
2. A persistent irrational fear of a specific object, activity, or situation that results in a compelling desire to avoid the dreaded object, activity, or situation; or
3. Recurrent severe panic attacks manifested by a sudden unpredictable onset of intense apprehension, fear, terror, and sense of impending doom occuring on the average of at least once a week; or
4. Recurrent obsessions or compulsions that are a source of marked distress; or
5. Recurrent and intrusive recollections of a traumatic experience, which are a source of marked distress; and
B. Resulting in at least *two* of the following:
1. Marked restriction of activities of daily living; or
2. Marked difficulties in maintaining social functioning; or
3. Deficiencies of concentration, persistence, or pace resulting in frequent failure to complete tasks in a timely manner (in work settings or elsewhere); or
4. Repeated episodes of deterioration or decompensation in work or work-like settings that cause the individual to withdraw from that situation or to expe-

rience exacerbation of signs and symptoms (which may include deterioration of adaptive behaviors); or
C. Resulting in the complete inability to function independently outside the area of one's home.

Somatoform Disorders

Physical symptoms for which there are no demonstrable organic findings or known physiologic mechanisms are considered somatoform disorders.

The required level of severity for these disorders is met when the requirements in both A and B are met.

A.
1. A history of multiple physical symptoms of several years duration beginning before age 30, and that have caused the individual to take medicine frequently, see a physician often, and alter life patterns significantly; or
2. Persistent nonorganic disturbance of one of the following:
   a. Vision; or
   b. Speech; or
   c. Hearing; or
   d. Use of a limb; or
   e. Movement and its control (e.g., coordination disturbance, psychogenic seizures, akinesia, dyskinesia); or
   f. Unrealistic interpretation of physical signs and sensations associated with the preoccupation or belief that one has a serious disease or injury; and
B. Resulting in *three* of the following:
1. Marked restriction of activities of daily living; or
2. Marked difficulties in maintaining social functioning; or
3. Deficiencies in concentration, persistence, or pace resulting in frequent failure to complete tasks in a timely manner (in work settings or elsewhere); or
4. Repeated episodes of deterioration or decompensation in work or work-like settings that cause the individual to withdraw from that situation or to experience exacerbation of signs and symptoms (which may include deterioration of adaptive behaviors).

Personality Disorders

A personality disorder exists when personality traits are inflexible and maladaptive and cause either significant impairment in social or occupational functioning or subjective distress. Characteristic features are typical of the individual's long-term functioning and are not limited to discrete episodes of illness.

The required level of severity for these disorders is met when the requirements in both A and B are satisfied.

A. Deeply ingrained, maladaptive patterns of behavior associated with *one* of the following:
1. Seclusiveness or autistic thinking; or
2. Pathologically inappropriate suspiciousness or hostility; or
3. Oddities of thought, perception, speech, and behavior; or
4. Persistent disturbance of mood or affect; or
5. Pathologic dependence, passivity, or aggressivity; or
6. Intense and unstable interpersonal relationships and impulsive and damaging behavior;
    AND
B. Resulting in *three* of the following:
1. Marked restriction of activities of daily living; or
2. Marked difficulties in maintaining social functioning; or
3. Deficiencies of concentration, persistence, or pace resulting in frequent failure to complete tasks in a timely manner (in work settings or elsewhere); or
4. Repeated episodes of deterioration or decompensation in work or work-like settings that cause the individual to withdraw from that situation or to experience exacerbation of signs and symptoms (which may include deterioration of adaptive behaviors).

Personal Injury

Anglo-Saxon law dictates, in legal parlance, a tort system for adjudication of personal injuries. Tort systems are designed to provide compensation (in the form of damages awards) from wrongdoers to those injured because of the wrongdoer's fault or negligence. Personal injury litigation allows the victim to sue for direct punitive damages as the result of wrongdoing, as well as for residual pain and suffering.

Differences between tort systems and workers' compensation may be illustrated in an example of an individual who slips in a puddle of water and injures herself while walking through a building. In a tort system, whether the injured person could recover from someone else for her injuries would depend on how the water got on the floor, whether the owner of the building knew or should have known that the water was there, whether the injured individual or other individuals should have been walking in the wet area, and whether the injured individual should have been able to see the water and avoid stepping in it. If all of these issues were resolved in the injured person's favor, she could recover her medical expenses in treating the injury, her past and future lost wages attributable to the injury, and her pain and suffering. In addition, her husband could recover for loss of consortium, that is, the diminution in value of her services to him as a result of the injury. The injured individual might also recover punitive damages if the judge or jury found that the defendant's conduct was especially blameworthy; for instance, if the puddle had been on the floor for a prolonged period and in

an area heavily frequented by the public and the building owner had refused to clean it up.

In contrast, if an individual had slipped in a puddle while he was working, questions of whose fault the accident was and who knew or did not know about the puddle would be generally irrelevant. The only issues would be whether his injuries were sufficiently work related and whether those injuries kept him from working. His recovery, however, would be limited to payment of his medical bills, payment of compensation benefits for the weeks he was unable to work and, in most states, a schedule award for his presumptive loss of wages if, after reaching maximum medical improvement, it was determined that he had a residual permanent loss of function (physical and/or psychological) attributable to his injuries.

In a general sense, personal injury litigation cases often rely heavily on "pain and suffering" and other reactive psychological ramifications that may result from physical injuries received. Typically, such legal cases require that the psychiatrist/clinical psychologist testify as to the diagnosis, prognosis, and psychological impairment (temporary or permanent) resulting from the injury, and attribute any reactive psychological dysfunction in a causal manner to an accident or injuries received. For example, a claimant is a passenger in an automobile driven by a friend. Because of the wrongdoing and fault of the driver of another vehicle that strikes the car of the claimant, the claimant's friend is killed. The claimant may then bring personal injury suit against the driver of the other car for psychological injuries received as a result of being pinned in the car and forced to watch the slow and gruesome death of his friend.

NOSOLOGY: DIAGNOSTIC AND STATISTICAL MANUAL OF MENTAL DISORDERS

The determination of psychological impairment is predicated on the recognition of psychological impairment/disability either in combination with physical impairment/disability or as a distinct entity that does not require the determination of an organic or physical component. In the determination of psychological impairment following painful accidents or injuries, the busy clinician will likely encounter both.

To accurately communicate the determination of psychological impairment, a nosology that provides a common language is required. In determination of psychological functioning, this nosology is the *Diagnostic and Statistical Manual of Mental Disorders* (*DSM*).

The *DSM* has undergone four revisions since originally published in 1952. The last revision (*DSM-IV*) was published in 1994 (2). Although developed for use with psychiatric and not pain patients, selected nomenclature in the *DSM-IV* is applicable to patients and psychological aspects of symptoms. Diagnostic criteria from the *DSM-IV* are reprinted with permission of the American Psychiatric Association, whose cooperation and commitment to continuing education is appreciated.

SOMATOFORM DISORDERS

The essential feature of this group of disorders is the presence of physical symptoms that suggest a somatic (general medical condition) condition. However, the symptoms are not fully explained by a known general medical condition, the effects of substance, or other mental disorder. Patients may be diagnosed with a somatoform disorder who present with physical symptoms with no organic findings from laboratory, radiologic, or other objective assessment. Alternatively, patients may be diagnosed with a somatoform disorder who present with an objective basis for nociceptive pain, but the patient's overall symptomatology is not fully explained by objective data. In both cases, psychological factors are presumed to be influential and symptoms are not judged to be under voluntary control (e.g., malingering).

Somatization Disorder

Historically referred to as hysteria or Briquet's syndrome, somatization disorder is a polysymptomatic disorder that begins before age 30, extends over a period of years, and is characterized by a combination of pain, gastrointestinal, sexual, and pseudoneurological symptoms. Somatic complaints are considered significant if they result in medical treatment or cause substantive impairment in social, occupational, or other important areas of functioning. The multiple complaints cannot be fully explained by any known general medical condition or effects of substance or, if the complaints occur in association with a general medical condition, the complaints and symptoms are excessive to what would be expected given the objective medical evidence.

Clinically, patients with a diagnosis of somatization disorder frequently present as the "worried well." An objective basis to explain the multiple visits to health professionals and impairment in function is either lacking or insufficient to fully account for the patient's pattern of illness or pain behavior. These individuals often present with a lifetime pattern of "doctor shopping" and frequently subject themselves to multiple (and painful) diagnostic procedures, somatic treatments, and surgeries. Occasionally these patients are under the care of several medical professionals simultaneously and typically describe symptoms in a vague and dramatic fashion. While psychological factors are judged to play a significant role in this diagnosis, the patient is not considered to be consciously magnifying symptoms or malingering. In addition to a standard psychological diagnostic assessment, the clinical psychologist or psychiatrist should, obviously, have available for review the medical records of the patient and should develop a detailed medical history (Table 48-2).

TABLE 48-2. *Diagnostic criteria for somatization disorder*

A. A history of many physical complaints beginning before age 30 that occur over a period of several years and result in treatment being sought or significant impairment in social, occupational, or other important areas of functioning.
B. Each of the following criteria must have been met, with individual symptoms occurring at any time during the course of the disturbance:
  (1) *four pain symptoms*: a history of pain related to at least four different sites or functions (e.g., head, abdomen, back, joints, extremities, chest, rectum, during menstruation, during sexual intercourse, or during urination)
  (2) *two gastrointestinal symptoms*: a history of at least two gastrointestinal symptoms other than pain (nausea, bloating, vomiting other than in pregnancy, diarrhea, or intolerance of several different foods)
  (3) *one sexual symptom*: a history of at least one sexual or reproductive symptom other than pain (sexual indifference, erectile or ejaculatory dysfunction, irregular menses, excessive menstrual bleeding, vomiting throughout pregnancy)
  (4) *one pseudoneurological symptom*: a history of at least one symptom or deficit suggesting a neurological condition not limited to pain (conversion symptoms such as impaired coordination or balance, paralysis or localized weakness, difficulty swallowing or lump in throat, aphonia, urinary retention, hallucinations, loss of touch or pain sensation, double vision, blindness, deafness, seizures, dissociative symptoms such as amnesia, or loss of consciouness other than fainting)
C. Either (1) or (2)
  (1) after appropriate investigation, each of the symptoms in Criteria B cannot be fully explained by a known general medical condition or the direct effects of a substance (e.g., a drug of abuse, a medication)
  (1) when there is a related general medical condition, the physical complaints or resulting social or occupational impairment are in excess of what would be expected from the history, physical examination, or laboratory findings.
D. The symptoms are not intentionally produced or feigned (as in Factitious Disorder or Malingering).

Undifferentiated Somatoform Disorder

The essential feature of this diagnostic category is one or more physical complaints that persists for 6 months or longer. There may be a single circumscribed symptom or, more commonly, multiple physical complaints, such as fatigue, loss of appetite, and nonspecific complaints of pain. Like somatization disorder, symptoms cannot be fully explained by known medical conditions or physical complaints are in excess of what would be expected from the history, physical examination, or laboraratory findings. Unlike somatization disorder that requires multiple physical complaints and onset before age 30, undifferentiated somatoform disorder may involve only one physical complaint and onset may be at any age. This diagnosis should be considered only for those persistent somatoform presentations that do not meet the full criteria for somatization

TABLE 48-3. *Diagnostic criteria for undifferentiated somatoform disorder*

A. One of more physical complaints (e.g., fatigue, loss of appetite, gastrointestinal or uninary complaints)
B. Either (1) or (2)
  (1) after appropriate investigation, the symptoms cannot be fully explained by a known medical condition or the direct effects of a substance (e.g., a drug of abuse, a medication)
  (2) when there is a related general medical condition, the physical complaints or resulting social or occupational impairment is in excess of what would be expected from the history, physical examination, or laboratory findings
C. The symptoms cause clinically significant distress or impairment in social, occupational, or other important areas of functioning.
D. The duration of the disturbance is at least 6 months.
E. The disturbance is not better accounted for by another mental disorder (e.g., another Somatoform Disorder, Sexual Dysfunction, Mood Disorder, Anxiety Disorder, Sleep Disorder, or Psychotic Disorder).
F. The symptom is not intentionally produced or feigned (as in Factitious Disorder or Malingering).

TABLE 48-4. *Diagnostic criteria for conversion disorder*

A. One or more symptoms or deficits affecting voluntary motor or sensory function suggest a neurological or other general medical condition.
B. Psychological factors are judged to be associated with the symptom or deficit because the initiation or exacerbation of the symptom or deficit is preceded by conflicts or other stressors.
C. The symptom or deficit is not intentionally produced or feigned (as in Factitious Disorder or Malingering).
D. The symptom or deficit cannot, after appropriate investigation, be fully explained by a general medical condition, or by the direct effects of a substance, or as a culturally sanctioned behavior or experience.
E. The symptom or deficit causes clinically significant distress or impairment in social, occupational, or other important areas of functioning or warrants medical evaluation.
F. The symptom or deficit is not limited to pain or sexual dysfunction, does not occur exclusively during the Somatization Disorder, and is not better accounted for by another medical disorder.

disorder or another somatoform disorder (e.g., pain disorder) (Table 48-3).

Conversion Disorder

The essential feature of this diagnosis is the presence of symptoms or deficits affecting voluntary motor or sensory function that suggest a neurological or other general medical condition, but that, instead, is apparently an expression of a psychological conflict or need. The symptoms are not intentionally produced or feigned and the disorder is not diagnosed if symptoms are limited to subjective pain (see "Somatoform Disorder"). However, conversion disorder may be considered a diagnosis, in association with pain, to explain a concrete "physical" disorder generated by a psychological etiology.

Symptoms of conversion disorder usually develop in a setting of extreme psychological stress and appear suddenly. Prolonged loss of function of a body part (e.g., arm) may produce serious complications, such as contractures or disuse atrophy. The differential diagnosis of conversion disorder is sometimes difficult given that knowledge of anatomical and physiological mechanisms is incomplete and methods of objective assessment have limitations (Table 48-4).

Hypochondriasis

The essential feature of this disorder is preoccupation with a fear of having, or the belief that one has, a serious disease, based on the person's interpretation of physical signs or sensations as evidence of the physical disease. A thorough medical evaluation does not identify a general med-

ical condition that fully accounts for the person's concerns about disease or for the physical signs or symptoms (although a coexisting general medical condition may be present). The unwarranted fear or belief of having a disease persists despite medical reassurance, but is not of delusional intensity, in that the person can acknowledge the possibility that she may be exaggerating the extent of the feared disease or that there may be no disease at all.

The preoccupation may be with bodily functions, such as heartbeat, sweating, or peristalsis, or with major physical abnormalities. In patients who have suffered trauma with residual pain and functional limitations, the presence of discomfort and physical signs, particularly radicular sensations, may be interpreted as the result of having cancer or other dreaded disease. The medical history is often presented in great detail and at length. "Doctor shopping" and deterioration in doctor–patient relationships, with frustration and anger on both sides, are common. Patients with this disorder often believe that they are not getting proper care and that physicians have simply not found the true "cause" of their symptoms. As a rule, these patients are highly resistant to a psychological explanation of their situation.

The most important differential diagnostic consideration in hypochondriasis is the presence of true organic disease, such as early neurologic disorders, endocrine disorders, or neurologic disorders resulting from trauma. The presence of true organic disease does not, however, rule out the possibility of coexising hypochondriasis. In somatization disorder there tends to be preoccupation with symptoms rather than fear of having a specific disease. When the criteria for both somatization and hypochondriasis are met, both diagnoses should be given (Table 48-5).

TABLE 48-5. *Diagnostic criteria for hypochondriasis*

A. Preoccupation with fears of having, or the idea that one has, a serious disease based on the person's misinterpretation of bodily symptoms.
B. The preoccupation persists despite appropriate medical evaluation and reassurance.
C. The belief in Criteria A is not of delusional intensity (as in Delusional Disorder, Somatic Type) and is not restricted to a circumscribed concern about appearance (as in Body Dysorphic Disorder).
D. The preoccupation causes clinically significant distress or impairment in social, occupational, or other important areas of functioning.
E. The duration of the disturbance is at least 6 months.
F. The preoccupation is not better accounted for by Generalized Anxiety Disorder, Obsessive-Compulsive Disorder, Panic Disorder, a Major Depressive Episode, (Separation Anxiety, or another Somatoform Disorder).

TABLE 48-6. *Diagnostic criteria for somatoform pain disorder*

A. Pain in one or more anatomical sites is the predominant focus of the clinical presentation and is of sufficient severity to warrant clinical attention.
B. The pain causes clinically significant distress or impairment in social, occupational, or other important areas of functioning.
C. Psychological factors are judged to have an important role in the onset, severity, exacerbation, or maintenance of the pain.
D. The symptom or deficit is not intentionally produced or feigned (as in Factitious Disorder or Malingering).
E. The pain is not better accounted for by a Mood, Anxiety, or Psychotic Disorder and does not meet criteria for Dsypareunia.

Somatoform Pain Disorder

Somatoform pain disorder is one of the most frequent diagnoses presenting to clinical psychologists and psychiatrists who specialize in pain management. The essential feature of this disorder is pain that is a predominant focus of the clinical presentation and is of sufficient severity to warrant clinical attention. The pain must be of sufficient severity to result in distress or impairment in social, occupational, or other important areas of functioning. While psychological factors are judged to play a significant role in pain onset, severity, exacerbation, or maintenance, the pain and symptoms are not intentionally produced or feigned (as in factitious disorder or malingering). Examples of impairment resulting from the pain include inability to work or attend school, frequent use of the health care system, the pain becoming a major focus of the individual's life, substantial use of medications, and relational problems such as marital discord and disruption of the family's normal lifestyle (Table 48-6).

Somatoform pain disorder is divided into three subtypes, depending on which of the three best characterize the factors involved in the etiology and maintenance of the pain. *Pain Disorder Associated with Psychological Factors (DSM-IV 307.80)* is used when psychological factors are judged to have a major role in the onset, severity, exacerbation, or maintenance of the pain. In this subtype, general medical conditions play either no role or a minimal role in the onset or maintenance of the pain. *Pain Disorder Associated with Both Psychological Factors and a General Medical Condition (DSM-IV 307.89)* is used when both psychological factors and a general medical condition are judged to have important roles in the onset, severity, exacerbation, or maintenance of the pain. *Pain Disorder Associated with a General Medical Condition* is *not* considered a mental disorder and is used when psychological factors are judged to play either no role or a minimal role in the onset or maintenance of the pain.

Malingering

The essential feature of this diagnostic category is the intentional production of false or grossly exaggerated physical or psychological symptoms, motivated by external incentives such as obtaining financial compensation, evading criminal prosecution, or obtaining drugs. Malingering is considered a subset of the major diagnostic category *Additional Conditions that may be a Focus of Clinical Attention* in the *DSM-IV*. According to the *DSM-IV*, malingering should be strongly suspected if any combinations of the following is noted:

1. Medicolegal context of presentation (e.g., the patient is referred by an attorney to the clinician for examination.
2. Marked discrepancy between the person's claimed stress or disability and the objective findings.
3. Lack of cooperation during the diagnostic evaluation and in complying with the prescribed treatment regimen.
4. The presence of antisocial personality disorder.

In the experiences of the authors (with a combined experience in pain management of over 40 years), the malingering patient is uncommonly encountered. When infrequently encountered, the malingering patient usually presents with lack of intellectual sophistication and a symptom presentation that is unchallenging and uncomplicated for an experienced clinician. It is should be remembered that a diagnosis of malingering is based on *conscious* and *intentional* production or exaggeration of symptoms as motivated by external incentives. Malingering differs from factitious disorder in that the motivation for the symptom production in malingering is an external incentive, whereas in factitious disorder external incentives are absent. Evidence of an intrapsychic need to maintain the sick role suggests factitious disorder. Malingering is differentiated from conversion disorder and other somatoform disorders by the intentional production of symptoms and by the obvious, external incentives associated with it.

AMA GUIDELINES TO THE EVALUATION OF PERMANENT IMPAIRMENT

In late 2000, the American Medical Association published the fifth edition of the *Guides to the Evaluation of Permanent Impairment*. Few changes have been made in the newest edition chapter on mental and behavioral disorders, in comparison with the fourth edition. In the fifth edition, the section on Social Security disability assessment that appeared in the fourth edition has been removed. Additions to the fifth edition include more case examples exemplifying the relationship among diagnosis, typical symptoms and signs of a disorder, and the impact on the ability to perform activities of daily living. In addition, a template of factors to be included in a psychiatric assessment has been added.

The fifth edition of the *Guides*, like the fourth edition, avoids the use of numerical impairment ratings. Rather, impairment in mental and behavioral functioning is assessed using a continuum of severity from Class 1 (no impairment) to Class 5 (extreme impairment). Areas or aspects of functioning include (a) activities of daily living, (b) social functioning, (c) concentration, persistence, or pace, and (d) adaptation to stressful conditions (Table 48-1).

Unfortunately, the fifth edition of the AMA *Guides* does not solve the obvious problem of interrater reliability in assigning impairments. Furthermore, and from a practical perspective, the lack of numerical percentages of impairment in mental and behavioral disorders creates confusion among attorneys, judges, agencies, and others accustomed to dealing with numeric values assigned to all anatomic segments of the human body.

CONCLUSIONS

Psychological impairment and resulting disability, which often occur in association with pain, will probably continue to be a controversial topic among health professionals for years to come. Historically, our litigious society has intentionally or unintentionally complicated the combination of physical and psychological consequences following injury. It is becoming common practice, however, for health professionals who evaluate and treat accident victims to secure a multidisciplinary evaluation of the patient. Such an approach best addresses the patient's total sphere of functioning.

REFERENCES

1. American Medical Association, *Guides to the evaluation of permanent impairment*, 5th ed. Chicago, IL: American Medical Association, 2000.
2. American Psychiatric Association. *Diagnostic and statistical manual of mental disorders*, 4th ed. Washington, DC: American Psychiatric Association, 1994.
3. United States Department of Health and Human Services, Social Security Administration. *Disability Evaluation Under Social Security, SSA.* Pub. No. 64–039. Washington DC: U.S. Government Printing Office, May 1992.
4. Nadolsky JM. Social Security: In need of rehabilitation. *J Rehabil* 1984;50:6–8.
5. AMA Council on Rating Mental and Physical Impairment. Guides to the evaluation of permanent impairment—the extremities and back. *JAMA* 1990;169.
6. Crook PL. Worker's compensation. In Tollison CD: *Handbook of pain: chronic pain management*. Baltimore, MD: Williams & Wilkins, 1989.

SECTION VIII

Selected Topics

CHAPTER **49**

Pain Management in Primary-Care Medical Practice

Tom Parrott

Pain of all types is one of the most frequently encountered problems in primary-care medical practice. Nine of ten Americans aged 18 or older report suffering pain at least once a month, and 42% of adults reported experiencing pain every day (1). Chronic pain (defined as pain lasting or recurring over 6 months or longer) affects 22% of primary-care patients worldwide (2). An estimated 75 million U.S. citizens experience chronic pain (3). It is estimated that 9% of the U.S. adult population suffers from moderate to severe noncancer pain (4).

In a World Health Organization (WHO) study the most frequent sites of pain for patients presenting to primary-care practices were, in descending order, back pain, headache, joint pain, pain in the extremities, chest pain, abdominal pain, and pain elsewhere; 68% had pain at two sites. Patients with persistent pain were more likely to have an anxiety or depressive disorder, to have an unfavorable perception of their health, and to have moderate to severe work role interference (2). Patients with chronic pain are five times more likely than patients without chronic pain to utilize health-care services (5).

Treatment options for acute and chronic pain in the primary-care setting include all of the therapeutic modalities available to ambulatory patients. The type of therapy that primary-care physicians are called upon most frequently to provide is pharmacologic therapy with oral medications that fall into four categories: acetaminophen, nonsteroidal antiinflammatory drugs (NSAIDs), adjuvant pain medication, and opioid analgesics.

In considering different treatment modalities, acute and chronic pain has often been divided into pain deriving from cancer and pain deriving from noncancer (often termed *nonmalignant*) sources. Although pain from any etiology presents unique challenges in diagnosis and treatment, the vast majority of chronic pain patients suffer

from noncancer pain. It is important to maintain an objective approach to the diagnosis and treatment of acute and chronic pain regardless of its etiology. In the last half of the twentieth century physicians have felt free to use the first three categories of pain medicines much the same as they would prescribe for any other medical condition. On the other hand, physicians have been reluctant to use opioids because of cultural views that this class of medicines is addicting and sedating and that government regulators would penalize the doctors prescribing them. During the past 15 years, the World Health Organization and the U.S. Department of Health and Human Services have urged physicians to use opioids in effective doses against cancer pain. Experience gained in the treatment of cancer pain has allowed many of the same concepts to be applied to noncancer pain as well (6,7).

Despite advances in knowledge during the past century, as recently as the past decade large groups of patients with pain problems have been inadequately treated. Cleland et al. found that 40% of outpatients with metastatic cancer pain did not receive effective pain relief (8). Benabei et al. reported that 40% of nursing home patients with cancer had daily pain but that 25% received no analgesics. Patients in minority groups and women were most likely to receive inadequate analgesia (9). Breibart et al. found that 85% of HIV-infected adults sampled did not receive adequate analgesia for their level of pain (10). The American Pain Society released a study of 805 people who suffered from noncancer pain; 56% of all individuals with chronic moderate to severe pain had been suffering for more than 5 years. The majority of individuals were being seen by primary-care physicians for treatment of their pain, including 49% of persons with the most severe pain. Most of those with the most severe pain described their pain as out of control; 47% had changed doctors at least once since their pain began. The reasons given were the following: continued suffering (42%), doctor's lack of knowledge (31%), doctor's not taking their pain seriously enough (29%), and doctor's unwillingness to treat it aggressively (27%) (4).

This chapter will review several aspects of pain diagnosis and treatment that are frequently encountered in the outpatient setting. This will include a classification of pain, methods to measure pain severity, and social and psychological influences on pain perception in the outpatient setting. Alternative medical treatments and nonpharmacologic treatments for pain will be listed but are discussed in detail in the previous chapters of this text. Allopathically trained physicians and practitioners are primarily called on to provide pharmacologic treatments for their primary-care patients, therefore a discussion of the pharmacologic treatment of acute and chronic pain will form the focus of this chapter. The treatment of pain is very often only one of several important problems that patients bring to their primary-care providers. Effective pain treatment will require coordination of care for all of the patient's problems in an integrated manner.

CLASSIFICATION OF PAIN

Pain encountered in the outpatient setting can usually be classified into four general categories. These account for the overwhelming majority of pain syndromes we see. This is useful in understanding the etiology and prognosis and in selecting the best treatment (11).

- Somatic pain: caused by activation of nociceptors in cutaneous and deep musculoskeletal tissue. The patient can usually point to the pain. This is the most common type of pain encountered in the primary-care setting and is the type of pain associated with skin, muscle, and bone injuries from trauma and surgery. If it is from a noncancer etiology this pain has the highest potential for healing and therefore to be self-limiting.
- Neuropathic pain: caused by injury to peripheral nerves, the spinal cord, or the brain. Very often it is extremely severe: "Sharp," "burning," "electrical shock," "viselike," "can't really describe it" are adjectives often used by patients. May occur spontaneously for years after original damage has occurred. "Excessively sensitive" (hyperesthesia), "unpleasantly sensitive," "painful" (dysesthesia), and "numbness" are common terms used to describe the area affected. Because of limited healing potential of nerve tissue, it is most difficult to treat and most likely to become chronic.
- Complex regional pain syndrome (formerly called reflex sympathetic dystrophy): often involves an extremity. Involves pain and abnormal autonomic/vascular dysfunction. Can occur without obvious nerve injury. Often has neuropathic pain features.

- Visceral pain: pain from thoracic, abdominal, and pelvic viscera. It may be referred. Often associated with nausea, diaphoresis. Difficult for the patient to localize.

MEASUREMENT OF PAIN

Perhaps one of the most difficult aspects of treating pain is the fact that it is one of the most subjective of all medical conditions. The stakes are higher for patients who seek pain relief because of the immediate suffering that they are experiencing. In the case of chronic pain, this is in contrast to chronic conditions such as diabetes and hypertension, where many of the benefits of treatment would be realized years in the future. Pain produces a multitude of emotional and behavioral responses that confound the clinician's ability for precise measurement.

The best technical modalities for the measurement of pain are positron emission tomography and ultrafast magnetic resonance imaging. These modalities measure the response of the brain during a variety of conditions, including the presence of pain. Neither technology is readily available or affordable to primary-care patients.

What is available in the primary-care setting is a wide variety of questionnaires and instruments to measure the intensity of pain (12). By far the simplest and most useful measurement of the intensity of pain is the scale of 1 (minimal pain that comes and goes) to 10 (worst pain imaginable, present all of the time). Most patients in the primary-care setting can understand this concept. It is extremely useful in monitoring response to treatment in the same patient over a period of time. Because pain ratings are highly individual and influenced by a wide variety of factors, it is difficult to compare one patient's rating of 7 out of 10 to another patient's 4 out of 10 for the same diagnosis. The American Pain Society has identified a number of principles that aid in effective pain management. Among the most important of these principles is to trust the patient's report of pain. The best operating definition is: Pain is what the patient says it is regardless of actual or potential tissue damage (13).

This 1 to 10 rating scale also works well for acute pain from injury and for the postoperative setting (14). Treatment of acute pain (e.g., ankle sprain, postop abdominal surgery, tooth extraction, etc.) is often based on the clinician's experience (i.e., likely to produce mild, moderate, or severe pain) in addition to the patient's specific number rating regarding the intensity and duration of pain. Basing pain treatment on physician expectations works well most of the time when the pain is self-limited. It becomes more important to use a score to measure relative improvements or deteriorations when following patients with chronic pain.

Riley et al. have identified a four-stage model of pain processing (15). Stage 1 is the perceived intensity of the pain sensation, which is scored on a scale of 1 to 10, as discussed earlier. Stage 2 is termed *immediate unpleasantness* and reflects the individual's immediate affective response, involving limited cognitive processing. This dimension of pain is hard for many patients to clearly verbalize. Stage 3 of pain processing involves longer-term reflective or cognitive processes that relate to the meanings or implications that pain holds for one's life. This would involve emotions such as depression, frustration, anxiety, fear, and anger. Stage 4 is the overt behavioral expression of pain: moaning or crying during the exam or at home, lying down during the day, and interference in work or home responsibilities. Patients may try to express some or all of these aspects of their pain during a visit to the primary-care doctor. A spouse, family member, or friend can be invaluable in helping to quantify various aspects of the pain response.

Riley and his group found that different age groups showed variable responses over these four stages. Their study looked at younger (18–44 years old), middle-aged (45–64 years old), and older (65–85 years old) adults. The older adult group reported less emotional response to pain and less pain behavior than the younger or middle-aged groups. Members of the middle-aged group showed the highest association between their emotional responses to pain and their pain behaviors, and the older group showed the least association. All groups described intensity of pain (on the scale of 1 to 10) in a similar fashion. The primary-care physician is often presented with a complex description of global suffering from pain involving aspects of these four stages. Being able to identify components that come from the pain itself (rating of pain) and the normal emotional and psychological aspects of the pain response is very valuable in order to tailor effective treatment. Patients are heavily influenced by the preceding factors in their ability to clearly communicate their history.

To make matters more challenging, the clinician's responses to the patient are often influenced by the patient's personality. A minority of patients in the primary-care setting have personality disorders that can make their pain much more difficult to evaluate. These are grouped as Cluster B Personality Disorders in the *Diagnostic and Statistical Manual IV* published by the American Psychiatric Association (16):

• Antisocial personality disorder: pervasive pattern of disregard for and violation of the rights of others. A pattern of lying may cause exaggeration of level of pain in order to obtain opioids or antianxiety medications, which are later sold.
• Borderline personality disorder: a pervasive pattern of instability of interpersonal relationships, self-image, and affects. Relationships with care providers alternate between extremes of idealization and devaluation (provider may be highly praised or condemned for the patient's pain treatment). Impulsivity manifested by self-damaging behavior such as drug abuse, reckless driving, injuries due to accidents, self-mutilation, and reckless spending.

• Histrionic personality disorder: pattern of excessive emotionality and attention seeking. These patients wish to be the center of attention, and pain can create a pretext for this. Their style of speech is excessively dramatic, clouding objective assessment of pain and its treatment.
• Dependent personality disorder: has an excessive need to be taken care of that leads to submissive and clinging behavior. All patients will depend on their medical care providers for assessment and effective treatment of pain. Dependent personalities, however, are less capable of assuming the level of responsibility for decision making and self-reliance necessary for optimal treatment of pain.

TREATMENT OF PAIN

In our society treatment for pain available to primary-care patients can be grouped into five broad categories:

1. Alternative medical treatments: generally those treatments provided by practitioners trained outside of traditional (allopathic) medical schools (Table 49-1)
2. Scientifically based nonpharmacologic pain treatments: provided by those trained in traditional (allopathic) medical schools using such modalities as relaxation

TABLE 49-1. *Nonmedical pain treatments used by primary-care patients*

Alternative medical treatments (17)
1. Acupuncture
2. Applied kinesiology
3. Aromatherapy
4. Bodywork: The Alexander method
          The Feldenkrais method
          Rolfing
          Reflexology
5. Chiropractic
6. Craniosacral therapy
7. Detoxification therapy
8. Herbal medicine
9. Homeopathy
10. Magnet therapy
11. Naturopathic medicine
12. Reconstructive therapy

Scientifically based nonpharmacologic pain treatments (18)
1. Relaxation techniques
2. Hypnosis
3. Cognitive-behavioral therapy
4. Biofeedback

Osteopathic manipulation

Physical therapy
1. Heat
2. Ice
3. Massage
4. Phonophoresis
5. Strengthening
6. Stretching
7. TENS units

techniques, hypnosis, cognitive-behavioral therapy, and biofeedback (Table 49-1)

3. Physical therapy, osteopathic manipulation, exercise, and topical therapy (Table 49-1)
4. Pharmacologic therapy: oral and parenteral
5. Therapeutic injection therapy and surgical therapy: removing diseased or displaced (e.g., intervertebral discs) tissue, peripheral, and central nervous system destructive procedures

In primary care it is important for us to help our patients take advantage of those modalities that are available to them in a manner that is affordable and appropriate to their needs. This section will only briefly mention all except pharmacologic treatments. Many primary-care patients can benefit by integrating nonpharmacologic treatments into an overall treatment plan. A detailed discussion of these modalities occurs elsewhere in this text.

The guiding philosophy in the treatment of acute pain is similar to the guiding philosophy in the treatment of any acute medical condition: Remove or allow healing of the cause of the pain by the most effective means possible while alleviating suffering by the most effective means possible.

The guiding philosophy in the treatment of chronic pain is similar to the guiding philosophy in the treatment of other chronic medical conditions: Try to control the source of tissue damage, optimize overall health, extend life expectancy, and relieve suffering to whatever extent possible without producing unacceptable side effects from treatment. Many sources of chronic pain can be expected to last months, years, or even a lifetime. It is very helpful, therefore, if the clinician adopts an approach similar to the management of other chronic illnesses. This is a stepwise approach beginning with nonpharmacologic treatment and/or alternative therapies, progressing to over-the-counter analgesics, nonsteroidal antiinflammatory drugs (NSAIDs), adjuvants (tricyclics, anticonvulsants), then to opioids, nerve blocks, and, as a last resort, invasive methods such as CNS ablation or nerve stimulators. Keeping these different levels of therapy in mind, and informing the patient of their availability, makes a big difference in how discouraged both patient and physician can become if the pain is uncontrolled or if the condition worsens over time.

Alternative medical treatments (Table 49-1) are provided by a variety of practitioners trained in methods not normally taught in allopathic medical schools. The American Pain Society found that the majority of chronic pain sufferers, especially those with severe pain, had already turned to nonpharmacologic and/or alternative therapies by the time they visited a primary-care physician (4). If patients find the treatment(s) effective and affordable, they should be incorporated into the overall care plan.

Scientifically based nonpharmacologic pain treatments (Table 49-1) were rated by an expert panel of physicians looking for scientific evidence in support of their effectiveness (18). It is notable that they have not shown effectiveness similar to pharmacotherapy in more severe noncancer pain states such as myofascial back pain and neuropathic pain.

There are several practical drawbacks to the use of scientifically based nonpharmacologic pain treatments for the average primary-care patient. Most importantly, therapists with time and training to provide the therapy are not available in many (probably most) communities. Many medical insurance companies do not pay for this form of therapy. It is quite time consuming, depending on the condition being treated, and unless the patient is unemployed, it is difficult to schedule. Finally, many patients are from a culture that is biased against using psychological approaches to physical problems.

Physical therapies (Table 49-1), when provided by a licensed physical therapist, require authorization by an allopathically trained physician. They can play an important role in the treatment of acute pain following injury and surgery. The expense and physical difficulties of going to the hospital or physical therapist's office make them much less practical for patients with chronic pain. The availability of physical therapy in the home is extremely valuable. In some cases, physical therapists are associated with visiting nurse organizations and can provide service in the home. In many cases patients can use a variety of physical therapy modalities at home on a daily basis once trained to do so.

There is ongoing research in the role of exercise in the treatment of pain. It is known that exercise releases hormones, including epinephrine, norepinephrine, cortisol, and glucagon. It is associated with the release of blood glucose from glycogen stores. It may be associated with the release of endorphins at both central and peripheral sites. Competition has been shown to alter the perception of noxious stimuli (19). It is known that contact and endurance athletes have better pain tolerance to certain types of pain than do recreational athletes or nonathletes (20). In many cases of acute pain coming from an injury, rest of the injured structure is paramount to recovery. However, if exercise using noninjured muscle groups can continue, blood flow is promoted to the injured structures, thereby reducing healing times. If regular exercise can be incorporated into the care plan of primary-care patients with chronic pain, it provides a variety of health benefits, including improved pain tolerance, improved cardiorespiratory fitness, improved sleep pattern, improved appetite, and overall enhancement of self-esteem.

PHARMACOLOGIC TREATMENT FOR ACUTE AND CHRONIC PAIN

Acute Pain

According to current classifications, acute pain is resolved in less than 6 months. This follows tissue injury and generally disappears when the body heals. Somatic pain from tissues with a high potential for healing (skin, muscle, bone, etc.) and certain visceral pain (peptic ulcer disease) account for the majority of acute pain syndromes. Acute pain is often, but not always, associated with objective signs of autonomic nervous system activity such as tachycardia, hypertension, diaphoresis, mydriasis, and pallor. In cases in which the cause of acute pain is uncertain, establishing a diagnosis is important, but symptomatic treatment of the pain is a priority while the investigation is proceeding. It is rarely justified to defer analgesia until a diagnosis is made (21).

Chronic Pain

Chronic (also called *persistent*) pain is defined by the World Health Organization (WHO) as pain that has recurred or lasted longer than 6 months (2). This form of pain can derive from cancer, but in the vast majority of cases it derives from noncancer sources. Tissue damage to structures with more limited healing capacity (peripheral and central nervous system, joints, etc.) is more likely to produce chronic pain. Chronic cancer pain, in contrast to acute pain, rarely is accompanied by signs of central nervous system arousal. The lack of objective signs may prompt the inexperienced clinician to say that the patient does not look like he or she is in pain (21). In both acute and chronic pain an objective assessment with the patient's self-report is the most reliable in quantifying the severity of pain.

The World Health Organization Analgesic Ladder

In 1986 the WHO published a three-step analgesic ladder intended to provide guidelines for clinicians to provide effective pain relief for cancer patients (Fig. 49-1) (22). These guidelines were intended to encourage more effective pain control using inexpensive and readily available medications. Reluctance to use opioids had resulted in suffering by numerous patients worldwide. As mentioned, it is

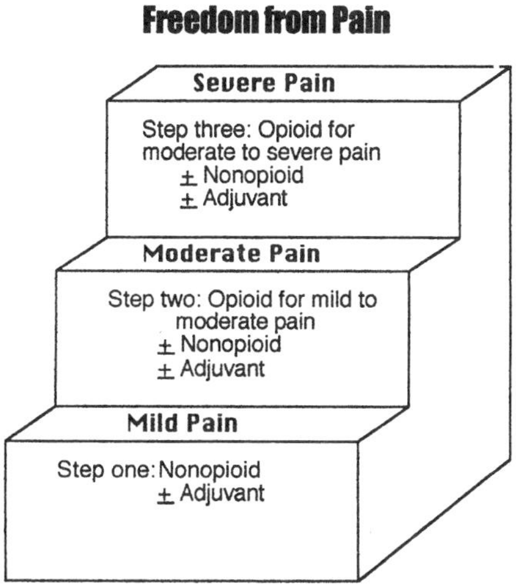

FIG. 49-1. "Three-step analgesic ladder."

inappropriate to restrict effective treatment of pain to only those patients who have a socially acceptable source of pain such as cancer (i.e., cancer pain patients are "good patients," whereas noncancer pain patients are complainers, drug seekers—"bad patients"). Several authors have advocated use of the pain treatment approach expressed in the WHO ladder regardless of the source of pain (6,7,23,24).

The WHO ladder discusses three categories of medicines that can be used for pain treatment: nonopioids, adjuvants, and opioids. The pharmacology of these groups of medicines with a detailed discussion of side effects, withdrawal protocols, etc. is discussed elsewhere in this text. Commonly used representatives of these groups of medicines will be discussed in this chapter related to their use in primary care.

NONOPIOIDS

This large category of pain relievers includes nonsteroidal antiinflammatory drugs (NSAIDs) and acetaminophen. Nonopioids are the most commonly employed agents both in nonprescription and prescription form for both acute and chronic pain. Aspirin, acetaminophen, ibuprofen, naproxen, and other NSAIDs are active ingredients in many nonprescription pain relievers. An American Pain Society survey found that 63% of chronic pain sufferers were currently using nonprescription pain relievers, and 29% were taking prescription NSAIDs (4). Nonopioids are currently in the standing orders of hospitals and nursing homes as the starting analgesics for institutionalized patients with mild to moderate pain. Pharmacologic management of mild to moderate pain following injury and postoperative pain should begin with an NSAID (25).

Acetaminophen

Acetaminophen is as effective as aspirin, similar in potency, and, in single analgesic doses, has the same time-effect curve but does not have the adverse effects characteristic of aspirin. It is the most widely used analgesic by primary-care patients, most commonly as an ingredient in over-the-counter medications.

Large overdosage with acetaminophen can cause serious or fatal hepatic injury. Some patients, such as patients who are alcoholics, patients who are fasting, and patients who are taking cytochrome P-450 enzyme-inducing drugs concurrently, may develop hepatic injury after moderate overdosage or even high therapeutic doses (26). Most patients can take up to 4 grams a day without adverse effects. This is an important consideration with pain relievers that contain a combination of acetaminophen and another active ingredient (e.g., Percocet, Lorcet, Fioricet). A total of 13 regular acetaminophen tablets or Percocet tablets would provide 4225 mg of acetaminophen per 24 hours, increasing the risk of toxicity.

Acetaminophen, aspirin, or NSAIDs can be given concurrently with opioids for an additive effect. Even when insufficient alone to control pain without exceeding potentially toxic doses, these agents often permit using lower doses of opioids (26).

Nonsteroidal Antiinflammatory Drugs

This group of medications is discussed in detail in an earlier chapter of this text. It comprises the mainstay of nonopioid prescription pain medications available to primary-care patients. All members of this group are available in oral preparations and are therefore suitable for use in ambulatory patients for both acute and chronic pain treatment. After efficacy of an NSAID has been established, selection is determined by side-effect profile, potential for drug interactions, dosing frequency, and cost. Primary-care providers can become familiar with a few effective and affordable NSAIDs that are useful in a variety of situations. This discussion of nonopioid medication will concentrate on considerations that are most commonly encountered in the primary-care setting.

NSAIDs have antipyretic and analgesic properties as well as antiinflammatory effects (27). The antiinflammatory effect is due mainly to inhibition of the two isoforms of cyclooxygenase (COX-1, COX-2), which promote the formation of inflammation and pain-producing prostaglandins. These enzymes also inhibit the formation of protective prostaglandins in the gastrointestinal tract, kidney, and other organs.

Their therapeutic effects and side-effect profiles are based on which enzymes are inhibited. COX-1 is expressed in most tissues and is thought to protect the gastric mucosa. COX-2 is expressed in the kidney, brain, uterus, ovary, cartilage, bone, and at various sites of inflammation. Older NSAIDs, in varying degrees, block both COX isoforms. Celecoxib (Celebrex) and rofecoxib (Vioxx) in therapeutic doses selectively inhibit COX-2 but not COX-1 (28).

The issues that come up most frequently for primary-care patients using nonopioid pain medications are cost and gastrointestinal side effects. Additional issues of concern to primary-care providers are inhibition of platelet function, serious gastrointestinal bleeding, renal failure, central nervous system side effects (depression, disorientation, headache), hepatic injury, and interference with the use of other medications (decreased effectiveness of antihypertensives and warfarin) (see Chapter 18).

Salicylates are commonly available in acetylated (aspirin) and nonacetylated (choline magnesium trisalicylate—[Trilisate] and salsalate—[Disalcid]) forms. Aspirin has been shown to be effective in most types of pain, including cancer pain. Many primary-care patients have already been taking OTC products containing aspirin but don't think that it is important to mention it to their provider. The most common mode of aspirin use among primary-care patients is the use of a low daily dose to prevent

myocardial infarction. Considering the cost effectiveness of aspirin, provided that no side effects are being encountered, the history of existing aspirin use could encourage the clinician to suggest a therapeutic dose of aspirin for acute or chronic pain treatment. Nonacetylated salicylates may be used as alternatives to other NSAIDs because they are associated with a low rate of gastrointestinal upset (27).

All NSAIDs, with the exception of nonacetylated salicylates, selective COX-2 inhibitors, and possibly meloxicam (Mobic) and nabumetone (Relafen), can interfere with platelet function and prolong bleeding time (28). A single therapeutic dose of aspirin irreversibly inhibits platelet function for the 8- to 10-day lifetime of the platelet, inhibiting hemostasis and prolonging bleeding time. Other NSAIDs such as ibuprofen and piroxicam reversibly interfere with platelet function. The duration of this interference is related to their half-life, which is 24 hours for ibuprofen but 2 weeks for piroxicam (27). This is extremely important for patients with serious NSAID-associated gastrointestinal hemorrhage and for those scheduling elective surgery.

The use of older (COX-1 and 2 inhibitors) NSAIDs is associated with gastrointestinal side effects in 15% to 25% of patients (27). These can generally be treated empirically with an H2-receptor antagonist or a proton pump inhibitor. If a gastroduodenal ulcer develops, the most prudent approach is to discontinue the NSAID and substitute therapy with acetaminophen or a nonacetylated salicylate. After the ulcer has healed, if it has been determined that NSAID therapy must be continued, the most effective prophylaxis against recurrent ulcers is the concomitant administration of misoprostol (at least 200 micrograms given three times a day), a proton pump inhibitor, or the use of an NSAID that selectively inhibits cyclooxygenase-2 (29). Elderly patients are at greatest risk of serious gastrointestinal bleeding.

Commonly used NSAIDs for primary-care patients, when used at full antiinflammatory doses, reduce urinary prostaglandin excretion by at least 50% with a maximal reduction of 60% to 80%. This does not produce a significant change in renal function in otherwise healthy patients. However, in those patients over the age of 60, those using diuretics, and those with intravascular volume depletion, hypertension, diabetes mellitus, or atherosclerosis, glomerular blood flow is decreased, and renal failure may occur (27). This form of renal failure is largely reversible. The effects of habitual use of analgesics alone or in combination on the progression to more chronic forms of renal disease are unclear. Prolonged regular use of NSAIDs should be discouraged in all patients, and if such use is necessary, renal function should be monitored (30).

After a patient shows an allergy to a nonsteroidal agent, further use of that drug or other NSAIDs is contraindicated (27). A single dose of aspirin can precipitate asthma in sensitive patients (26). There is a high degree of cross sensitivity between aspirin and other NSAIDs in patients

TABLE 49-2. *Commonly used NSAIDs in primary care (28)*

	Dose range for arthritis	Cost for 30 days*
Inexpensive generics		
Ibuprofen	1200 to 3200 mg/day in 3 or 4 doses	$ 2.30
Sodium salicylate	3.6 to 5.4 gm/day	8.80
Naproxen sodium	275 or 550 mg b.i.d.	10.94
Indomethacin	25 to 50 mg t.i.d.-qid	17.10
Enteric-coated aspirin	975 mg qid	18.00
Naproxen	250 to 500 mg b.i.d.-t.i.d.	21.00
Salsalate	3 to 4 gm/day in 2 to 3 doses	25.20
Piroxicam	20 mg once/day	31.80
Diclofenac	150 to 200 mg/day in 2 to 3 doses	46.20
More expensive brands		
Oxaprozin (*Daypro*)	600 to 800 mg/day	43.80
Meloxicam (*Mobic*)	7.5 to 15 mg/day	59.70
Nabumetone (*Relafen*)	1000 to 2000 mg/day	71.40
Rofecoxib (*Vioxx*)	25 to 50 mg once/day	72.00
Celecoxib (*Celebrex*)	100 to 200 mg b.i.d.	84.00
Diclofenac (*Arthrotec*) + Misoprostol	50 mg diclofenac + 200 mcg misoprostol t.i.d.-qid	126.90

*Average cost to the patient for 30 days' treatment with the lowest recommended dosage, based on data from retail pharmacies nationwide provided by Scott-Levin's *Source™ Prescription Audit (SPA)*, June 1999 to May 2000.

who have symptoms of rhinitis or asthma. For patients who develop urticaria upon exposure to aspirin, an immunologic mechanism is probably involved, and all salicylates should be avoided. In the production of urticaria there is no cross reactivity with the structurally dissimilar NSAIDs, but it is prudent to avoid their use until more definite data are available (27).

Table 49-2 lists some of the NSAIDs that are commonly used in primary care. They are grouped with less expensive generics first, progressing down the list to more expensive drugs available only as brand names. The brand name prices are not listed for the drugs readily available as generics.

It is uncommon for patients to be able to distinguish differences in effectiveness or side effects between generic and brand name NSAIDs, but it does occur. Generally the least expensive medication that is effective without unacceptable side effects is going to be the best received by the patient. No NSAID is consistently more effective than any other for all patients, but some patients who do not respond to one drug may respond and tolerate another (28). If one drug does not prove effective after 1 to 3 weeks at the maximally tolerated dose, another drug should be substituted. A favorable response from the same NSAID class is not precluded (27).

Despite their considerable potential for side effects and toxicity, acetaminophen and the NSAIDs are the mainstay of nonopioid therapy for acute and chronic pain.

Although NSAIDs would ideally be taken only on an as-needed basis for all forms of pain, the vast majority of primary-care patients have been able to use them safely for both acute and chronic pain.

ADJUVANT MEDICATIONS FOR PAIN

Adjuvant medications for pain are part of the WHO three-step analgesic ladder. Those that are available in oral form are suitable for ambulatory patients and can play a strong role in primary-care pain management. They are mentioned elsewhere in this text (Chapters 16–18) but will be mentioned here briefly as they apply to problems frequently encountered in primary care. This group of medications has been developed to treat different (although in many cases closely associated) clinical problems. They fall into five general categories: antidepressants, anticonvulsants, caffeine, antihistamines, and corticosteroids.

The subset of antidepressant medications that has had the strongest scientific support as adjuncts for pain are the tricyclic antidepressants. Amitriptyline (Elavil), desipramine (Norpramin), doxepin (Sinequan), and nortriptyline (Pamelor) have been studied for their role in treating neuropathic pain. Low doses of tricyclic antidepressants have been demonstrated to be beneficial in postherpetic neuralgia and poststroke pain syndromes (31). Selective serotonin reuptake inhibitors such as fluoxetine (Prozac) have been shown to be effective in reducing pain and improving global wellness scores in patients with fibromyalgia, especially when used in combination with amitriptyline (32). Antidepressants with more favorable side-effect profiles (e.g., nortriptyline, desipramine, and trazodone) are preferred over amitriptyline.

Because enhancement of sleep is always desirable, increase in dosage to improve sleep pattern will often be necessary in chronic pain states. Although tricyclic antidepressants were initially recommended to be used in low doses to treat chronic pain, current guidelines call for chronic pain patients to receive doses normally used for depression with disordered sleep (50 to 100 mg of amitriptyline, 50 to 200 mg of desipramine, 50 to 300 mg of trazodone at bedtime) (33). An added bonus of this class of medicines is reduction in depression, which is a frequent concomitant of chronic pain (2).

The anticonvulsants carbamazepine (Tegretol), clonazepam (Klonopin), phenytoin (Dilantin), and gabapentin (Neurontin) can relieve neuropathic pain from diabetic neuropathy, trigeminal neuralgia, postherpetic neuralgia, glossopharyngeal neuralgia, and neuralgias arising from nerve trauma or from cancer (26).

Caffeine in doses of 65 to 200 mg has been shown in controlled trials to enhance the analgesic effect of acetaminophen, aspirin, or ibuprofen. This has been shown to be helpful in the treatment of headache, postoperative, and postpartum pain (26). This is an important ingredient in a recent group of over-the-counter medications marketed to treat migraine headache (Bufferin, Excedrin migraine).

Hydroxyzine (Vistaril and others) in doses of 50 to 100 mg IM may add to the analgesic effect of opioids in postoperative and cancer pain while reducing the incidence of nausea and vomiting (26).

Through their antiinflammatory effect corticosteroids can produce analgesia in some patients with inflammatory diseases (26). In pain due to soft tissue infiltration, acute nerve compression, visceral distension, and increased intracranial pressure due to cancer, corticosteroids can be used (33).

Capsaicin (Zostrix), a pungent and irritating compound found in red peppers, has been used topically for centuries to relieve pain (34). Capsaicin has been used to help manage pain in many conditions, including diabetic neuropathy, postherpetic neuralgia, rheumatic diseases, postmastectomy pain, and cluster headaches. Clinical trials performed in patients with diabetic neuropathy demonstrated a 50% improvement in pain status with the use of capsaicin for 22 weeks (35).

OPIOID ANALGESICS

Opioid analgesics are recommended by the WHO for the treatment of moderate to severe cancer pain. Applying the same general principles of treatment to pain deriving from any source gives the clinician the opportunity to use what is by far the most effective class of medications available for moderate to severe pain. Along with this opportunity, however, goes a unique set of problems and challenges. This derives from the fact that in addition to unique pharmaceutical problems such as tolerance and physical dependency with potential withdrawal symptoms, the use of opioids is associated with social problems, including addiction, drug abuse, and diversion. Throughout the world these social problems have resulted in government regulations that restrict the amounts and the manner in which opioids are prescribed in an effort to limit their overall consumption in society. As mentioned, this has often resulted in a large number of patients receiving less than optimal pain relief.

Using opioids for acute pain based on the WHO ladder is straightforward. Agents for mild to moderate pain (Table 49-3) are usually prescribed in a dose adequate to provide pain relief over a few days to a few weeks at most. Most clinicians prescribe what their experience has told them is an effective dose of short-acting opioid for an appropriate duration to allow healing of acute pain.

The effects of chronic pain on the patient's health and function are much greater, and the social and regulatory difficulties the clinician faces in using opioids for chronic pain are significantly greater than in using them for acute pain treatment.

In a survey conducted for the American Pain Society, chronic noncancer pain sufferers were asked to rate the

TABLE 49-3. *Common oral opioids mild to moderate pain (ranked in descending order of effectiveness and dependency potential)*

Drug	DEA schedule	Starting dose/ 24 hours* (opioid naive patients)
Hydrocodone (*Vicodan, Lortab*)	III (Phone prescription can refill up to 6 months)	10 to 60 mg
Codeine 30 mg	"	120 to 240 mg
Propoxyphene (*Darvon*)	IV "	260 to 780 mg
Propoxyphene Napsylate (*Darvocet*)	"	400 to 600 mg
Tramadol (*Ultram*)	Unscheduled	200 to 400 mg
Opiate agonist/antagonist Pentazocine (*Talwin*) III		200 to 300 mg

Management of cancer pain in adults: Quick reference guide for clinicians no. 9. Rockville, MD: Department of Health and Human Services, Public Health Service Agency for Health Care Policy and Research, 1994; AHCPR publication no. 94-0593.

effectiveness of the medications they were taking for pain control. On a scale of 0 to 10 with 10 representing complete relief, users of three groups of medication assigned them these scores: opioids 7.6; prescription NSAIDs 6.2; and nonprescription medications 5.2. The gap between these ratings widened among persons with very severe pain: opioids 7.4; prescription NSAIDs 5.3; and nonprescription medications 4.4. Regardless of pain severity, 63% of chronic pain sufferers used nonprescription medications; 29% used prescription NSAIDs; and 16% used opioids. Among those with very severe pain, the use of opioids (26%) almost equaled that of prescription NSAIDs (31%) despite the higher potency of opioid medications. Approximately one half (49%) of respondents who had taken opioids reported concerns about addiction—fears that experts believe are often exaggerated or misplaced (4).

The pharmacology of opioids is discussed in detail in Chapter 15. There are several pharmacologic principles that are extremely important in the primary-care setting, and these will be discussed here.

Some clinicians believe that opioids exert their effects only on the brain and that their pain-relieving properties are directly proportional to their sedative effects. In our society this is a less culturally acceptable practice than the practice of using a medicine that works directly on the problem (i.e., reduces inflammation directly at the source in a manner similar to NSAIDs). Recent research, however, is forcing us to expand our understanding of how opioids work. We now realize that they have both peripheral and central effects (36).

The actions of systemically delivered opioid analgesics have been extensively studied. Their effects are based on stimulation of mu, kappa, and delta opioid receptors and receptor selective opioid peptides that are concentrated in several sites, including the brain and spinal cord. Injection of opioids at the level of the spinal cord does not require high systemic levels that affect the brain. This peripheral action of opioids allows them to be used for the relief of labor pain, postoperative pain, and cancer pain (37).

Milder opioids (Table 49-3) such as codeine, propoxyphene, and pentazocine, when taken alone in usual doses are no more effective than aspirin or acetaminophen (26). Tramadol (Ultram) is a centrally acting analgesic that binds to mu opioid receptors. The analgesic efficacy of tramadol is considered equivalent to Tylenol with Codeine #3 (30 mg of codeine + 650 mg of acetaminophen) (33). In elderly patients and those intolerant of NSAIDs a mild opioid for step 1 pain is often ideal. These agents are often combined with aspirin or acetaminophen to treat moderate pain. Morphine, hydromorphone, methadone, levorphanol, fentanyl, and large doses of oxycodone are used for more severe pain (26) (Table 49-4).

Tolerance is a unique problem that occurs with opioid analgesics. The patient first notices a shorter duration of analgesia and then an increase in pain. In my experience this problem has affected a relatively small number of patients who are experiencing the most severe pain. Tolerance can be delayed by giving nonopioid analgesics and adjuvant therapy (e.g., tricyclic antidepressants) concurrently (33). Tolerance to most adverse effects of opioid analgesics, including respiratory and central nervous system depression, develops at least as rapidly as the analgesic effect. Cross tolerance exists among all full agonists, but it is not complete, and starting with one half the dose when

switching to another opioid agonist is advised. Switching to a partial agonist or a mixed agonist-antagonist can precipitate withdrawal in a patient whose pain has been treated with one of the morphine- or codeine-related or synthetic agonists (26).

Both short- and long-acting versions of oxycodone and morphine are now available in oral forms. As a general principle, acute pain is treated with short-acting opioids over days to weeks. Chronic pain is better treated with long-acting preparations and is better managed if doses can be scheduled. Many chronic pain patients do well with scheduled doses of long-acting agents, using short-acting agents for breakthrough pain. It is often not possible to control pain as well using only long-acting agents as with a combination of long- and short-acting opioids. The goal in therapy is to develop a regimen that makes patients feel that they are in maximum control of their pain.

When opioids are used, the easiest way to monitor the dose is to look at the mg per 24 hours. It is recommended that the dose per 24 hours be adjusted every 2 to 3 days until effective pain control is achieved. If the patient is using mostly short-acting medication (e.g., oxycodone), as much of the 24-hour dose as possible can be switched over to the long-acting form. In some cases a combination of different opioid preparations works best for the patient, e.g., daytime oxycodone (less sedating) and bedtime methadone (more sedating). Recommended starting doses for opioid naive patients with different levels of pain are listed in Tables 49-3 and 49-4. Recommended doses should be given in formulations (short vs. long acting) when they will be most useful for pain relief and allow patients to optimize normal function. It is important to emphasize to patients with chronic pain that the pain medication will most often not take their pain away completely but that it will allow them to improve their functional level (7). Normally the mildest agents are prescribed first for mild to moderate pain, reserving the strongest agents for the most intractable pain.

There is a certain amount of variation in the tolerability (side effects such as sedation, mental clouding, constipation) of a given opioid among different patients. My experience has been that oxycodone is the opioid that is most effective and best tolerated by the largest group of patients. Oxycodone is a Schedule II narcotic (normally used for moderate to severe pain with starting doses between 60 and 80 mg/24 hours), but it is also useful in the treatment of mild to moderate pain in doses of 20 to 60 mg/24 hours. Methadone and long-acting morphine (MS Contin) tend to be the most sedating, which makes them ideal to use at bedtime.

Prescribing for chronic pain varies somewhat between cancer pain, which is often progressively more severe, and noncancer pain, which often starts out in the moderate to severe range and remains there. With cancer pain, progression of the cancer with increased pain intensity is the most common reason to have to use a stronger opioid or to

TABLE 49-4. *Common oral opioids for moderate to severe pain (ranked in descending order of effectiveness and dependency potential)*

Drug	DEA schedule	Starting dose/ 24 Hours* (opioid naive patients)
Morphine (*MS IR, MS Contin*)	II (Need written prescription 1-month supply limit)	180 to 240 mg
Fentanyl (*Duragesic*)	"	50 to 75 mcg/hour
Meperidine (*Demerol*)	"	Not recommended**
Hydromorphone (*Dilaudid*)	"	45 to 60 mg
Methadone	"	60 to 80 mg
Oxycodone (*Percocet, OxyContin*)	"	60 to 80 mg
Codeine 60 mg	"	360 to 480 mg

*Management of cancer pain in adults. DHHS, 1994.
**Oral meperidine not recommended for chronic use because of possible accumulation of normeperidine, a toxic metabolite.

increase the opioid dose. With noncancer pain, tolerance is the most common reason to have to go to stronger opioids or to increase the dose above the starting dose. Experts have pointed out that there is no optimal or maximal dose of a step 3 opioid analgesic drug. The appropriate dose is one that relieves a patient's pain throughout its dosing interval without causing unmanageable side effects (33). Many pain patients have other illnesses, and interaction of opioid analgesics with other medications will need to be considered.

Constipation, sedation, dizziness, nausea, and vomiting are the most common adverse effects of opioid analgesics. Sedation can be ameliorated by decreasing the dose and increasing the frequency of administration, i.e., switching to shorter-acting preparations of the same opioid (26). Constipation is the most frequent side effect with chronic use, particularly in the elderly and in those who are extremely inactive. Constipation should be anticipated and managed prospectively if possible. Some patients may already have a favorite stool softener, laxative, or dietary regimen high in fiber that they can augment. A suggested program might include docusate 1 to 4 tablets b.i.d. with a bisacodyl 10 mg (Dulco-lax) suppository or magnesium citrate 8 oz every other day PRN. More detailed suggestions regarding its management are published elsewhere (23).

All patients who take opioid analgesics will develop some degree of physical dependence and will develop withdrawal symptoms if the drug is withdrawn suddenly. Patients who take opioid analgesics for acute pain or cancer pain rarely experience euphoria and even more rarely develop psychic dependence or addiction to the mood-altering effects of the narcotics (26). A 1996 review of case studies in which opioid analgesics were used to treat chronic noncancer back pain found that abuse behaviors occurred in less than 5% of 566 patients during periods ranging from 6 months to 16 years (38). The degree of physical dependence is directly proportional to the strength and effectiveness of the opioid analgesic being used. Symptoms of opioid withdrawal include intense desire for drugs, muscle cramps, arthralgia, anxiety, nausea, vomiting, and malaise. Signs of withdrawal include drug-seeking behavior, mydriasis, piloerection, diaphoresis, rhinorrhea, lacrimation, diarrhea, insomnia, and mild elevation of blood pressure and pulse rate (39). These symptoms and signs would typically be observed during withdrawal from the use of intravenous heroin. The medical examiner's office in the author's state has never recorded a case where a person died of opioid withdrawal syndrome, even heroin withdrawal (40). With long-term use of oral opioids, it is common for patients to run out of medication from time to time. Even in patients taking higher doses of medications, the withdrawal symptoms (most commonly anxiety, insomnia, and muscle cramps) are described as less of a problem than the return of pain.

Opioid detoxification protocols using clonidine or methadone are available (39). If opioid analgesic withdrawal is the primary diagnosis, federal regulations allow the use of methadone for opioid detoxification only at facilities specifically designated for this purpose. Methadone may be used for withdrawal, however, if the primary diagnosis is a medical condition and the secondary condition is opioid withdrawal.

The U.S. Drug Enforcement Administration has established schedules for opioid medications. The lower the schedule number, the more powerful the opioid analgesic. Tramadol (Ultram) is unscheduled. Schedule IV medications include propoxyphene (Darvon), and pentazocine (Talwin). Schedule III medications include hydrocodone (Lortab, Vicodan, others) and codeine 30 mg. Schedule IV and III medications are considered less addicting, and prescriptions can be called in to the pharmacy. Schedule II medications are considered more addicting, need a written prescription (with a DEA number) and are limited by state regulations to a total number of pills per prescription. Codeine 60 mg, oxycodone (Percocet, Tylox, OxyContin, others), methadone, hydromorphone (Dilaudid), meperidine (Demerol), fentanyl (Duragesic), and morphine (MSIR, MS Contin) are all Schedule II narcotics.

The selection of an opioid analgesic should be guided by factors such as (a) the type, location, and cause of pain (e.g., headache, inflammation, posttraumatic, abdominal-pelvic, neuropathic, etc.); (b) how long during the night or day the pain is active and which of the patient's activities are influenced by pain; (c) associated medical and psychological conditions; (d) how effective it is in relieving pain and what side effects it produces; and (e) the complex emotional and social context in which the patient, the patient's family, and the medical care providers view this type of medication.

There is perhaps no other patient care situation in which honest communication and the informed consent of the patient are more crucial than with the use of opioids. The patient is the best judge of the effectiveness of treatment in reducing pain, and the clinician must trust the patient's assessment. The practice of patient-centered medicine in which the patient shares heavily in the decision making is the ideal we as clinicians should strive for (41,42).

OPIOID ANALGESIC ABUSE AND ADDICTION

Drug abuse is defined in several ways. The National Institute of Drug Abuse considers drug abuse to occur when psychoactive medication (prescribed or nonprescribed) is used for nonmedical reasons, i.e., to become high (stimulated, intoxicated, or euphoric) (43). The Drug Abuse Warning Network (DAWN—sponsored by the Substance Abuse and Mental Health Services Administration in the U.S. Department of Health and Human Services) provides estimates of the health consequences of the nonmedical use of individual drugs. This agency also includes drug dependence and use of the drug in a suicide attempt or gesture as criteria for drug abuse (44). According to the

1998 National Household Survey on Drug Abuse, opioid analgesics were used for nonmedical purposes at least once during the previous year by 1.9% of the respondents (45). The number of respondents who reported that they had experienced problems related to nonmedical analgesic use, such as feelings of depression, isolation, and irritability, or whose drug use had caused problems with their health, work, or school activities was too infrequent to yield reliable estimates (43). To put the abuse of opioid analgesics into perspective with the abuse rates of other substances monitored by the National Household Survey, the percentage of respondents reporting binge or heavy alcohol use (defined as drinking five or more drinks on the same occasion) during the previous year was 64%. The percentage reporting marijuana and hashish use was 8.6%, the percentage reporting the use of cocaine was 1.7%, and the percentage reporting the use of hallucinogens (PCP, LSD) was 1.6% (45).

From 1990 to 1996 there were increases in the medical use of opioid analgesics. During this same period the percentage of drug abuse mentions (visits to U.S. emergency rooms as a result of nonmedical use) relative to mentions of all drugs monitored fell from 5.1% to 3.8%. In 1996 the percentage of visits to emergency rooms due to the use of other drugs (amphetamines, antidepressants, antipsychotics, benzodiazepines) was 36.1%, the visits due to illicit drugs (cocaine, heroin, LSD, marijuana, amphetamines, methaqualone, PCP) was 33.2%, the visits due to alcohol in combination with other drugs was 18.3%, and the visits due to nonopioid analgesics (butalbital, NSAIDs, acetaminophen) was 8.6% (44). It appears that although medical use of opioids has increased during the past decade, the abuse of opioids has actually declined.

Monitoring patient drug use can be difficult. Patient behavior patterns in a given population are influenced by such factors as population mobility, incidence of drug abuse and criminal activity in the community, and access to and the quality of ongoing relationships to medical providers. I practice in a suburban to rural environment in northern New England. The size of the population in our service area, roughly 35,000, facilitates close communication with pharmacists and police agencies in the community. It is extremely important for patients to fill opioid prescriptions at only one pharmacy (must be within a 2-hour radius) for this reason.

Characteristic patient behaviors that suggest the possibility of opioid intoxication or diversion would be the following: (a) obtaining opioid prescriptions from more than one provider or pharmacy; (b) appearing intoxicated when arriving for office visits, at home, at work, or in the community; (c) being arrested for driving under the influence of drugs or alcohol; (d) repeatedly losing (or having stolen) their opioid prescription and then requesting refills from the physician on call or from doctors in emergency rooms or urgent care facilities; (e) engaging in any illegal activities such as selling the drugs, distributing them for recreational

purposes, altering or forging prescriptions, etc. As is the case with alcoholism, a family member or close friend, if the patient lives alone, is an invaluable source of information about adverse effects of opioids.

Recent guidelines for the use of controlled substances for the treatment of pain have been published by the Federation of State Medical Boards of the United States (46). These are appropriate for patients receiving opioids for chronic pain and represent sound principles of medical practice and record keeping for patients with any illness. Physicians are expected to perform and document the following:

1. The physician should obtain a complete history and physical examination. The record should include details about the intensity of pain, current and past pain treatments, the effect of pain on physical and psychological functioning, and history of substance abuse.
2. The patient's treatment plan should be documented, including ways to measure response to treatment. Treatment with modalities other than opioid analgesics and treatment of other medical and psychological conditions should be mentioned.
3. The physician should document a discussion with patients of the risks and benefits of their pain treatment using controlled substances (obtain an informed consent). Expectations for appropriate blood and/or urine tests should be documented. A contract or written agreement describing dosage of opioids, frequency of visits, and number of prescription refills is recommended.
4. The physician should see the patient at appropriate intervals.
5. Consultations with other specialists (e.g., pain treatment specialists, mental health experts, neurosurgeons) should occur as appropriate.
6. There should be an accurate record of medications prescribed (date, type, dose, and quantity) and followup visits planned.
7. The physician must be licensed in the state and be in compliance with federal and state regulations.

The Federation of State Medical Boards guidelines also clarify three important concepts regarding opioid use:

1. Addiction is a neurobehavioral syndrome with genetic and environmental influences that results in psychological dependence and the use of substances for their psychic effects and is characterized by compulsive use despite harm. Physical dependence and tolerance are normal physiological consequences of extended opioid therapy for pain and should not be considered addiction.
2. Pseudoaddiction is a pattern of drug-seeking behavior of pain patients who are receiving inadequate pain management that can be mistaken for addiction.
3. Physical dependence on a controlled substance is a physiologic state of neuroadaptation that is characterized by the emergence of a withdrawal syndrome if drug use is stopped or decreased abruptly, or if an

antagonist is administered. Physical dependence is an expected result of opioid use. Physical dependence, by itself, does not equate with addiction (46).

AN OFFICE PROGRAM TO USE OPIOID ANALGESICS FOR CHRONIC PAIN

Chronic pain is similar to other chronic illness in many ways, and the goals for treating it are similar. Ideally, medications prescribed should be the lowest dose of the most effective, least expensive agent associated with the fewest undesirable side effects.

Patients suffering from moderate to severe pain are the most symptomatic encountered in the primary-care set-ting. As a result they require more time than patients who are less symptomatic. If opioid analgesics are prescribed, it becomes more time consuming because of the need to document complicated history and physical findings, to provide patient education and support, and to include the patient in what can be a difficult decision-making process. Needless to say, this can be very disruptive to the physician and office staff in a busy primary-care office.

To better meet the needs of the patients and to make rules of conduct and treatment expectations clear to my patients, office staff, and physician partners on call, I developed a simple program on four pages of the patient record (Figs. 49-2–49-5). This provides a time-efficient way to implement the Federation of State Medical Boards guide-

---

Contract for Long-Term Use of Opiold (Narcotic) Analgesics

You have agreed to use opioid analgesic therapy for the relief of pain. The reason(s) you have pain is (are): _____

_____

The goals for using this medication are (1) to relieve suffering, (2) to improve sleep and functioning during the day, and (3) to work along with other treatments to allow your body to heal as much as possible. This class of medicines can produce the following adverse effects: drowsiness, nausea, confusion, constipation, tolerance (requires more and more of the medicine to provide the same amount of pain relief), physical dependence (a withdrawal syndrome might occur when you stop using it), increased sensitivity to all pain, and addiction (loss of control over the amount of medicines used, constantly seeking more medicine, and adverse effects on important portions of your life).

Prescribing this class of medications is regulated by state and federal law. It is very important that you agree to the following guidelines:

I will obtain medication from only one physician: _____

If my regular physician is not available, I will contact the physician from White River Family Practice who is on call and explain the circumstances. I might be asked to come to the office for evaluation. Normally only enough medication to last until my next appointment with my regular physician will be prescribed. If my pain can be controlled with rest and other measures for a few days, that is far better than asking for an "emergency supply." I will not visit the emergency department or any doctors outside this office for opioid medicaton.

I will purchase my prescriptions from only one pharmacy: _____

I agree that this pharmacy will have a copy of this contract so that the pharmacist is clear on what to expect. If I use other physicians or pharmacies to obtain opioid analgesic medication, it could result in discontinuation of all treatment from any of the doctors at White River Family Practice. I also agree that the doctor may tell other area pharmacies about my contract.

The opioid analgesic medication(s) and doses will be: _____

_____

_____

_____

The frequency of visits to the office will be: _____

Don't change the frequency or dose of your medication unless you check with your regular physician. If your opioid medication is stolen, it must be reported to the police. Repeatedly lost or stolen medication or frequently missed appointments could result in discontinuation of treatment.

Signature of patient _____ Date: _____

Signature of physician _____ Date: _____

FIG. 49-2. Contract for long-term use of opioid (narcotic) analgesics

---

Instructions for Patients Receiving Opioid (Narcotic) Medication

The amount and type of pain medication must be agreed upon and a contract signed during your office visit with your doctor. The number of pills will be calculated to last until your next visit. If you run out or lose your medication you may experience withdrawal symptoms (muscle cramps, nausea, diarrhea, nervousness). These symptoms are not dangerous (no one has ever died from them), but they are uncomfortable. If your pain returns you may contact your doctor or the doctor on call for help. No opioid medications will be called in. Advil, aspirin, Tylenol, or a nonopioid prescription to be called in can be used until you can visit your regular doctor. If your opioid medicine has been stolen you must report this to the police and bring a police report with you at your next office visit. Repeatedly lost or stolen prescriptions will result in no further opioid prescriptions, and/or dismissal from the practice.

If you arrive at the office having taken too much pain medication, psychiatric medicine, or drunk too much alcohol, and you appear intoxicated (sluggish and sleepy) your medication dosage will be reduced. If you have driven to the office yourself and are intoxicated, a ride will be arranged for you to go home—cab, relative, or friend. The police will be called if you refuse and you look like you will be a danger while driving.

You will be dismissed and not able to get any care from our practice if any of the following occur:

a.) Verifiable report(s) that you have sold or given your medication to another person.

b.) You lie or are rude to our office staff or to the doctors.

c.) You are disruptive while in the office or make our other patients uncomfortable.

d.) You obtain opioid prescriptions from other doctors.

e.) You refuse to have your blood tested for levels of your medicines or the bad effects that they may cause.

FIG. 49-3. Instructions for patients receiving opioid (narcotic) analgesics

lines. It simplifies taking a focused history, performing a focused physical examination, formulating a treatment plan based on decisions with which the patient is informed and compliant, and documenting complex medication schedules. The clinician may elect to use this program only for those patients taking higher doses of opioids, those with complicated pain and other medical problems, and/or those with a history of drug dependency. The history sheet (Fig. 49-4) summarizes the most important elements of the patient's history, physical findings, initial laboratory and radiographic findings, and adjuvant and nonmedical treatments for pain. The contract for long-term use of opioid medication (Fig. 49-2) serves as an informed consent and as an educational tool for the patient. The instructions for patients receiving opioid (narcotic) medication (Fig. 49-3) are printed on the back of the contract. Two copies of this sheet are made as the patient checks out: one to give to the pharmacist, one for the patient to keep.

The flow sheet (Fig. 49-5) is perhaps the most time-conserving portion of the program from the clinician's point of view. It records date of visit, total opioid dose per 24 hours, exact amounts prescribed, date of next visit,

pharmacy, peak pain scores with response to medication, hours of sleep per 24 hours, hours of work or useful activity during the day, minutes spent each day in exercise (used as an adjunct for pain control), patient's view of quality of life, contact with family or friends, reliability of keeping appointments, any adverse effects (intoxication, illegal acts, side effects), laboratory findings (opioid levels to ensure that opioids are being taken as expected, not sold; hepatic and renal functions if acetaminophen and/or NSAIDs are also in use), and comments. Not every issue is discussed at each visit, but it provides a very quick way to assess overall success of treatment, frequency of problems, and how closely the patient has followed the treatment plan.

PRIMARY-CARE PRACTICE EXPERIENCE IN TREATING CHRONIC PAIN

Over 24 years of family practice I have developed a patient population of approximately 3500 patients who consider me their primary-care provider among our group of five physicians. Roughly 3000 of these patients are over the age of 18. Over a 6-month period I audited the practice to

---

Chronic Pain History and Exam Sheet

Name: _____   Date of birth: _____

Diagnosis(es): _____

Date of pain onset: _____   Today's date: _____

Pertinent history and physical findings: _____

_____

Lab and X-ray results: _____

_____

Consultations & dates: _____

_____

Current habits or conditions affecting healing (smoking, alcohol, diet, etc.): _____

_____

History of substance abuse: _____

History of opioid analgesic use: _____

Date opioid analgesics were started: _____   Opioid contract date: _____

Nonopioid and adjunct pain medication: _____

Nonmedical treatments (physical therapy, behavioral/relaxation, etc.): _____

Other important medical problems and medications: _____

_____

Social support (family, friends): _____

Education: _____   Occupation: _____

Religious and community activities: _____

Leisure pursuits and interests: _____

Comments: _____

_____

_____

_____

FIG. 49-4. Chronic pain history and exam sheet

identify those patients who were using medications daily for control of chronic pain and whose medical records indicated a chronic pain diagnosis on the problem list. There were three patients being treated at that time for cancer pain. In addition there are perhaps a hundred or more who use medications (both prescription and nonprescription) intermittently on an as-needed basis as they suffer from recurrent pain. This latter group of irregular analgesic users comprises the largest group of pain sufferers in the practice but was not analyzed for the audit.

An analysis of the noncancer patients using nonopioid and opioid medications on a daily basis is presented in Tables 49-5–49-8; 129 patients (4.3% of adult patients in the practice) were using nonopioids, and 52 (1.7%) were using opioids on a daily basis. All groups had a high per-

centage of other significant medical problems. The patients using nonopioid medications and the WHO step 1 patients using opioids for mild chronic pain were quite similar in terms of age (average age of 60 and 59) and pain diagnoses. Degenerative sources of pain led the list for both groups. Of the 14 patients in the step 1 group using opioids, seven were either allergic to NSAIDs or had experienced significant gastrointestinal bleeding on NSAIDs. The other seven had simply found opioids more affordable and effective. The information that older patients tolerate chronic pain with less emotional response may explain why older pain patients can receive adequate analgesia with less potent agents.

The high frequency of unresolved lumbosacral nerve root irritation as the leading pain diagnosis in the step 2

Opioid Analgesic Flow Sheet

Patient name: _____   Diagnosis: _____

Visit dates				
Opioid dose per 24 hrs.				
Amount prescribed this visit with dates of Rx				
Date of next visit				
Pharmacy				
Pain intensity peak lowest				
Hours sleep per 24 hrs				
Minutes per day exercise extra rest				
Hours per day of work/useful activity				
Quality of life				
Contact with family/friends				
Reliably keeps appointments				
Adverse events sedation/illegal acts				
Laboratory				
Comments				

FIG. 49-5. Opioid analgesic flow sheet

and 3 groups confirms data recently published about the often poor prognosis of this injury in the primary-care population (47).

Patients receiving opioids are among the sickest of my practice population. In a previous report it was noted that patients in the 20-to-60 age group averaged three to four times as many office visits per year as age-matched controls. The chronic pain patients in the over-60 age group averaged the same number of visits per year as patients their age with other chronic illnesses (6).

Because state laws restrict the amount of Schedule II opioids that can be prescribed at one time and prohibit refills, chronic pain patients have needed predated written prescriptions. For example, following U.S. Department of Health and Human Services guidelines to treat moderate to severe pain, 60 to 80 mg per 24 hours of oxycodone

TABLE 49-5. *Chronic pain patients using daily nonopioid medication*

	Prescription NSAIDs	OTC meds	Total
Total patients	107	22	129
Average age	60	68	61
Percent with other significant medical or psychiatric problems	83 (78%)	11 (77%)	100 (76%)
Diagnoses: (some patients with two sources of pain)			
Degenerative arthritis	76	16	92
Myofascial pain (fibromyalgia)	11	3	14
Nerve root irritation	8	1	9
Rheumatoid arthritis	6		6
Diabetic neuropathy	4	1	5
Headaches	2		2
Osteoporosis	2		2
Complex regional pain syndrome	1		1
Cervical spondylosis	1		1

TABLE 49-7. *Chronic pain patients using daily opioids—step 2: moderate pain*

Total patients	28
Average age	49 years
Number with other significant medical problems	22 (78%)
Duration of therapy: range 1 to 24 years	(average 5 years)
Diagnoses	
Nerve root irritation (lumbosacral [11], cervical radicular [3] syndrome)	14
Degenerative arthritis	10
Myofascial pain	1
Diabetic neuropathy	1
Ankylosing spondylitis	1
Postconcussion syndrome	1
Opioids used and doses (two patients on two opioids)	
Oxycodone 20 to 60 mg/24 hours	16
Propoxyphene 520 to 650 mg/24 hours	5
Hydrocodone 15 to 60 mg/24 hours	4
Codeine 120 to 240 mg/24 hours	3
Morphine 30 mg/24 hours	1
Tramadol (Ultram) 300 mg/24 hours	1

might be required for adequate pain control. Many of my patients fill prescriptions in New Hampshire, where patients are limited to 100 tablets (or a month's supply, whichever is smaller) of 5-mg oxycodone per prescription. Taking 12 to 16 5-mg tablets per day would exhaust a prescription in 6 to 8 days, necessitating very frequent visits to the doctor's office for written prescriptions. To deliver the same dose in the form of long-acting oxycodone (e.g., OxyContin 40 mg b.i.d.), a written prescription for 60 tablets could last for 30 days. Long-acting opioids are not yet available in generic form and are extremely expensive to use over several months, so some patients will still need

short-acting forms in larger numbers to reach adequate dosage levels.

Ideally, the visits to the clinician for written prescriptions could be scheduled in a time frame similar to those needed to manage other chronic illnesses (e.g., every 3 months recommended for diabetic patients). For the patients with WHO step 3 chronic pain taking very high doses of oral opioids, visits once a month have proven to be the maximal interval that is practical. For patients with

TABLE 49-6. *Chronic pain patients using daily opioids—step 1: mild pain*

Total patients (7 NSAID intolerant)	14
Average age	59 years
Number with other significant medical problems	12 (86%)
Duration of therapy: range 1 to 12 years	(average 5 years)
Diagnoses	
Degenerative arthritis	8
Myofascial pain	4
Visceral pain	1
Headaches	1
Opioids used and doses	
Oxycodone 10 to 20 mg/24 hours	6
Propoxyphene 260 to 650 mg/24hrs	5
Hydrocodone 15 to 20 mg/24hrs	2
Codeine 60 mg/24hrs	1

TABLE 49-8. *Chronic pain patients using daily opioids—Step 3: severe pain*

Total number of patients	10
Average age	48 years
Number with other significant medical problems	8 (80%)
Duration of therapy: range 2 to 18 years	(average 7 years)
Diagnoses (some patients with two sources)	
Lumbosacral nerve root irritation	4
Peripheral nerve injury	2
Myositis/myofascial pain	2
Comminuted femur fracture/ intramedullary rod	1
Surgical injury to celiac plexus	1
Osteoporosis with pathologic fractures	1
Opioids used and doses (three patients use two opioids)	
Oxycodone 100 to 800 mg/24 hours	7
Morphine 60 to 480 mg/24 hours	2
Hydrocodone 100 mg/24 hours	1
Hydromorphope (Dilaudid) 24 mg/24 hours	1
Methadone 4 mg q.h.s.	1

step 2 pain requiring a lower number of pills, visits every 2 to 3 months have worked out well.

This plan will need to be reviewed with the pharmacist and is one of several aspects of prescribing opioids for chronic pain that the clinician and pharmacist should discuss. In most cases the pharmacists have been willing to keep predated prescriptions on file for the patient. In a few cases the patients have preferred to hold the prescriptions at home and present them at the appropriate time. Both plans have worked well as long as the expectations are clear to all parties concerned. It is important to note that in many areas, predated prescriptions are not legal. Check with local authorities for clarification.

It has been helpful to monitor blood levels of opioid medications in patients using high doses for step 2 and step 3 pain. Blood levels are more expensive than qualitative urine screens but provide better information on the effects of the medication at the time of the patient's visit. Blood levels have often reflected lower than expected values if tolerance is present. Effectiveness and/or toxicity from opioids have been better correlated with clinical findings than with blood levels. Drawing blood tests for opioids has given important information that opioids are being taken by the patient and not diverted, and tests for renal and hepatic toxicity could be run at the same time if the patient was using acetaminophen or NSAIDs.

Qualitative urine tests for "drugs of abuse" test for the presence of opioids (as expected) and screen for illegal substances. If illegal substances are present it identifies patients in contact with those who deal in illegal drugs.

My experience in treating chronic noncancer pain with opioid medications has been generally very favorable. Even patients receiving moderate to high doses of opioids for step 2 and 3 chronic pain have been able to use opioids safely over periods as long as 24 years. All patients have achieved significant pain relief, and most have been able to function at a level necessary to continue with employment, family responsibilities, and community activities. All patients in this treatment group have expressed gratitude for being listened to and allowed to participate in decisions about which treatments work best for them. In no cases has treatment of pain with opioid analgesics by itself led to psychoactive substance abuse disorders involving prescribed or illegal drugs.

Although experience treating my primary-care patients has been generally positive, several of the patients receiving treatment for chronic pain have been engaged in self-destructive behaviors much of their adult life. As these behaviors began to involve opioids that I was prescribing, it became in everyone's best interest that they be dismissed from the practice. Table 49-9 identifies several salient characteristics of patients who have been dismissed. It is noted that they all manifested objective evidence of pain. These patients were between the ages of 28 and 40. The American Pain Society identifies this group of individuals (those with psychosocial disarray manifested by a history of

TABLE 49-9. *Factors leading to patient dismissal (several patients with multiple factors)*

Number dismissed in past 10 years	9
Number with objective evidence of injury/pain	9
1. Psychosocial disarray: unmarried, variable employment, transient, history of psychiatric hospitalization, history of jail time, psychiatric diagnosis, personality disorders (sociopathic), poor	8
2. Appeared intoxicated in office or to family	5
3. Illegal, dishonest activities: distributing/selling opiates, altering/forging prescriptions	4
4. Lying or being disruptive to office staff	3
5. Repeatedly losing medication (stolen), using medications faster than agreed upon	3
6. Prescriptions from multiple doctors/pharmacies	2
7. Stops for driving under the influence	1

poverty, substance abuse/addiction, personality disorders, certain mental illnesses, and those who are disenfranchised from medical care) as the group of pain sufferers most difficult to effectively treat in our present medical system. In my practice some of these patients who were dismissed knew each other as members of a small criminal subculture that exists in the communities of our service area. In the five cases where intoxication was noted, the patients were currently using potentially sedating medication along with opioids (benzodiazepines 3, butalbital 1, carisoprodol 1). Two of the four cases dismissed for illegal activities were reported by police, two were reported by another patient. In the majority of cases dismissed, multiple factors were involved in the decision to no longer provide care for the patient.

Patients are expected to receive all of their primary care through my office after they are enrolled as regular patients. This requirement has usually made management of pain one component of the management of several chronic medical problems. It is made clear to patients that (Schedules IV and III) opioid medications cannot be prescribed by telephone outside the service area (a radius of roughly 100 miles) and that in no case can the prescriptions be filled in states where I am not licensed. These restrictions have limited the tendency for patients to migrate to my practice specifically for the purpose of obtaining opioid prescriptions.

In many cases opioids have been used with success following surgery. Some patients are unable to resolve pain following surgery, and it becomes difficult for the surgeon to continue monitoring and prescribing analgesics beyond a certain point in time (usually 6 to 12 weeks). Good communication between surgical and primary-care specialists regarding short- and long-term pain management is important, particularly if the patient will require treatment for chronic pain. Further work to improve this communication process is needed in many medical communities.

None of my patients has died as a result of using opioids, and there have been no deaths recorded in Vermont as a result of opioid withdrawal (40). However, prescription narcotics were second only to toxic effects of alcohol (not alcohol-related traffic deaths) on the list of drug-related deaths evaluated by the state medical examiner's office. Most of the prescription narcotic-related deaths were intentional, and the narcotic most often involved was propoxyphene (48).

The goal of using opioid medications and all other components of a pain management program (nonopioids, adjuvants, and nonmedical treatments) has been to reduce suffering and to improve patient function and quality of life while natural healing to whatever extent possible takes place. When opioids were used, the goal has not been to stop the addicting medicines as soon as possible.

Pain has a tremendous adverse impact on patients' ability to order their lives. Because the patients' informed participation has been essential in developing a safe and effective treatment program, much education, discussion, and negotiation has been required. To arrive at an effective program of pain control most often has taken several months. The patients' clinical condition has sometimes changed, necessitating further modification in their pain control program. If a patient has had an effective pain management program using opioids before coming to my office, it has been best to maintain that program until rational changes can be agreed upon between clinician and patient.

There is a specialty pain treatment facility at the tertiary care hospital in our community that is staffed by three anesthesiologists (two of whom spend time in other activities) and two fellows. Appointments are scheduled for one or two physicians to see patients 5 days a week, with an average wait for a new patient of one month. Invasive treatments presently available at this center include nerve blocks and injection of intrathecal medications, including opioids, anesthetics, and antiinflammatory agents.

Referrals to this pain center come most frequently from neurosurgeons, followed by orthopedists, then primary-care physicians. The program director's preference is to provide invasive treatments as appropriate but to provide consultation so that the day-to-day management of the patient remains with the primary-care doctor. This approach requires the primary-care doctor to be the one to prescribe all oral medications, but in certain cases the pain treatment program physicians are willing to assume the responsibility for opioid prescriptions. To clarify this responsibility, the program director insists on effective communication at both ends of the referral and consultation process. A directory of pain treatment facilities is available through the American Pain Society, 4700 W. Lakeview Ave., Glenview, IL 60025-1485.

Pain management in primary-care medical practice brings with it many challenges and rewards. Pain of all types is one of the most frequent reasons for visits to primary-care clinicians. Using a stepwise approach, starting with nonmedical therapies, adding pharmacologic treatments that are affordable and readily available, and then in some cases referral to include therapeutic injections and invasive therapy, allows the physician to design a comprehensive pain management program that will meet the needs of almost all patients. Primary-care physicians are often fortunate to enjoy strong therapeutic relationships with their patients over a long period of time. Accordingly, primary-care providers, perhaps more than any other specialty, are in a uniquely qualified position to provide the best care to patients suffering from both acute and chronic pain.

REFERENCES

1. Gallup Inc. Pain in America: highlights from a Gallup survey. June 9, 1999. Also available at Arthritis Foundation website: www.arthritis.org/Answers/sop factsheet.asp.
2. Gureje O, Von Korff M, Simon G, Gater R. Persistent pain and well being—a World Health Organization study in primary care. *JAMA* 1998;280:147–151.
3. Schnitzer T. Non-NSAID pharmacologic treatment options for the management of chronic pain. *Am J Med* 1998;105:45S–52S.
4. American Pain Society. Chronic pain in America: roadblocks to relief-survey highlights. Feb.19 1999. Chronic Pain in America—Roadblocks to Relief a survey conducted by Roper-Starch Worldwide for the American Academy of Pain Medicine/American Pain Society and Janssen Pharmaceutica, 1999. Available at American Pain Society website: www.ampainsoc.org/whatsnew/conclude road.htm
5. Becker N, Bondegaard-Thomsen A, Olsen A, et al. Pain epidemiology and health related quality of life in chronic non-malignant pain patients referred to a Danish multi-disciplinary pain center. *Pain* 1997;73:393–400.
6. Parrott T. Using Opioid analgesics to manage chronic noncancer pain in primary care. *J Am Board Fam Pract* 1999;12:293—306.
7. Marcus D. Treatment of nonmalignant chronic pain. *Am Fam Physician* 2000;61:1331–1138.
8. Cleland C, Gonin R, Hatfield A, et al. Pain and its treatment in outpatients with metastatic cancer. *N Eng J Med* 1994;330:592–596.
9. Benabei R, Gambassi G, Lapane K, et al. For the SAGE study group. Management of pain in elderly patients with cancer. *JAMA* 1998; 279:1877–1882.
10. Breibart W, Rosenfeld B, Passik S, et al. The undertreatment of pain in ambulatory AIDS patients. *Pain* 1996;65:243–49.
11. Payne R, Allen R. *Pain. Scientific American Medicine.* 2001;11:XIV,1–2.
12. Cancer Pain Guideline Panel, Rockville Maryland. Management of cancer pain: adults. *Am Fam Physician* 1994;49:1853–1868.
13. Whitecar P, Jonas P, Clasen M. Managing pain in the dying patient. *Am Fam Physician* 2000;61:755–764.
14. Carpenter R. Optimizing postoperative pain management. *Am Fam Physician* 1997;56:835–844.
15. Riley J, Wade J, Robinson M, Price D. The stages of pain processing across the adult lifespan. *The Journal of Pain* 2000;1:162–170.
16. American Psychiatric Association. Diagnostic Criteria from DSM-IV. Washington, DC, 1994:279–284.
17. Saberski L. Alternative medicine and pain management. *The Pain Clinic* Aug 1999:10–18.
18. NIH Technology Assessment Panel. Integration of behavioral and relaxation approaches into the treatment of chronic pain and insomnia. *JAMA* 1996;276:313–318.
19. Sternberg W, Bailin D, Grant M, Gracely R. Competition alters the perception of noxious stimuli in male and female athletes. *Pain* 1998;76:231–238.
20. Janal M, Glusman M, Kuhl J, Clark W. Are runners stoical? An examination of pain sensitivity in habitual runners and normally active controls. *Pain* 1994;58:109–116.
21. American Pain Society. Principles of Analgesic Use in the Treatment of Acute Pain and Cancer Pain. Glenview, IL, 1999.
22. World Health Organization. *Cancer pain relief,* 2nd ed. With a guide to opioid availability. Geneva, Switzerland: WHO, 1996:12–15.
23. Montauk S, Martin J. Treating chronic pain. *Am Fam Physician* 1997;55:1151–1160.
24. Morgan GJ. Review of available therapy for management of chronic nonmalignant pain. Challenges facing clinicians in managing chronic pain *A Postgraduate Medicine Special Report* 1998.

25. Agency for Health Care Policy and Research. Acute pain management in adults: operative procedures. *Am Fam Physician* 1992;46: 128–138.

26. The Medical Letter. *Drugs for Pain* 1998;40:79–84.

27. Miller L, Pritchard J. Selecting nonsteroidal anti-inflammatory drugs pharmacologic and clinical considerations. *J Am Board Fam Pract* 1989;2:257–270.

28. The Medical Letter. *Drugs for rheumatoid arthritis.* 2000;42:57–59.

29. Wolfe M, Lichtenstein D, Singh G. Gastrointesinal toxicity of nonsteroidal antiinflammatory drugs. *N Engl J Med* 1998;338:1888–1898.

30. DeBroe M, Elseviers M. Analgesic nephropathy. *N Engl J Med* 1998;338:446–452.

31. McQuay H, Carroll D, Glyn C. Low dose amitryptiline in the treatment of chronic pain. *Anaesthesia* 1992;47: 646–652.

32. Goldenberg D, Mayskiy M, Mossey C, et al. A randomized double blind crossover trial of fluoxetine and amitryptyline in the treatment of fibromyalgia. *Arth Rheum* 1996;39:1852–1859.

33. Levy M. Pharmacologic treatment of cancer pain. *N Engl J Med* 1996;335:1124–1132.

34. Fusco B, Giovasco M. Pepper and pain: the promise of capsaicin. *Drugs* 1993;56:909–914.

35. Tandan R, Lewis G, Krusinsky P, et al. Topical capsaicin in painful diabetic neuropathy: controlled study with long term follow up. *Diabetes Care* 1992;15:8–14.

36. Stein C, Comisel K, Haimerl E, et. al. Analgesic effect of intraarticular morphine after arthroscopic knee surgery. *N Engl J Med* 1991; 325:1123–1126.

37. Basbaum A, Levine J. Opiate analgesia—how central is the peripheral target? *N Eng J Med* 1991;325:1168–1169.

38. Brown R, Patterson J, Rounds L, Papasouliotis O. Substance abuse among patients with chronic back pain. *J Fam Pract* 1996;43: 152–160.

39. Miller N, Gold M. Management of withdrawal syndromes and relapse prevention in drug and alcohol dependence. *Am Fam Physician* 1998; 58:139–146.

40. Morrow P. Personal communication 10/4/99.

41. Laine C, Davidoff F. Patient centered medicine—a professional evolution. *JAMA* 1996;275:152–156.

42. Woolf S. Shared decision making: the case for letting patients decide which choice is best. *J Fam Pract* 1997;45:205–208.

43. Cooper J, Czechowicz D, Peterson R, Molinari S. Prescription drug diversion control and medical practice. *JAMA* 1992;268: 1306–1310.

44. Joranson D, Ryan K, Gilson A, Dahl J. Trends in medical use and abuse of opioid analgesics. *JAMA* 2000;283:1710–1714.

45. Substance Abuse and Mental Health Services Administration Population Estimates in: National Household Survey on Drug Abuse, 1998, Number H-10. Rockvill, MD: Public Health Service, US Dept Health and Human Services, Office of Applied Studies, 1999. SMA publication 99-3328.

46. Model guidelines for the use of controlled substances for the treatment of pain recommendations by the Federation of State Medical Boards of the United States, Inc. 1998. www.fsmb.org/pain.

47. Croft P, Macfarlane G, Papageorgiou A, et al. Outcome of low back pain in general practice: a prospective study. *BMJ* 1998;316:1356–1359.

48. Office of the Chief Medical Examiner. Drug related deaths in Vermont 1992 to 1996. *Medical Examiner Issues* 1997;8:2–7.

CHAPTER **50**

Pain in Infants and Children

Gary A. Walco, Steven L. Halpern and Paola M. Conte

Over the past two decades, there has been increasing recognition of the need to adequately assess and treat pain in children. The focus of this chapter will be developmental aspects of pain in the young, pain assessment strategies commonly used in infants and children, and aspects of pharmacological and nonpharmacological management strategies that pertain to infants and children.

PHYSIOLOGICAL DEVELOPMENT OF PAIN NETWORKS

For many years it was believed that infants lack the neurological mechanisms to experience pain. Recent evidence indicates, however, that nociceptive pathways, although still developing, are in place and functional in premature neonates even as young as 26 weeks, gestation (1). The peripheral and central nervous system structures involved in nociception develop during the second and third trimesters of gestation (2). Focus on the development of pain pathways *per se* is a relatively new endeavor; much has been inferred based on what is known about adult pain systems and the development of critical neuroanatomical substrates in the fetus (2). In addition, animal models, specifically rat pups, have provided a great deal of the data on the specific biological aspects of pain development (3). Although the timetable is compressed, the same developmental progression takes place in both species, and thus reasonable comparisons may be made.

Fitzgerald has conducted a series of studies with rats that maps out the essential elements of the developmental neurophysiologic processes related to pain. Peripheral nociceptors, those with both Aδ and C fibers, develop soon after cutaneous axons reach the skin (a process occurring between 7 and 20 weeks, gestation in humans), and at birth their function parallels mature nociceptors (4). Large-diameter dorsal root fibers grow into the spinal cord first, followed by small-diameter C fibers, which occurs just before birth (corresponding to about 24 weeks,

gestation in humans). There is a discrepancy in developmental patterns between Aδ and C fibers, however (5). As Aδ fibers grow into the spinal cord, they rapidly produce synaptically evoked activity in dorsal horn cells. C fibers do not produce such activity until the end of the first postnatal week (which roughly translates to several weeks in the human neonate). Thus, relatively low-level tactile stimulation may lead to reflexive "pain" responses in young human neonates. In addition, the more typical adult pattern of rapid Aδ firing followed by C fiber stimulation in response to tissue damage would not be so clear-cut at this stage.

A critical question focuses on the long-term impact of pain experiences early in life. In their discussion of neural development, Anand and Carr (2) state, "importance of this phase of development in the maturation of the pain system is underscored by the high index of 'brain plasticity' present during this period. Clearly the cellular, synaptic, and molecular mechanisms determining brain plasticity are highest during infancy and early childhood. Painful and other experiences during this period therefore may determine the final architecture of the adult pain system, with subtle and presently undefined characteristics responsible for the clinically evident individual variation" (p. 800).

Fitzgerald and colleagues, through studies both with rats and human neonates, have shed light on this issue. With rats, it was shown that tissue damage in the early postnatal period causes a profound and lasting sprouting response of local sensory nerve terminals (6). This in turn results in hyperinnervation, which remains evident in adult rats well after the wound has healed. Analysis indicated that both Aδ and C fibers are involved in this process, which may account for the extensiveness of the observed hyperinnervation. The implication is that in the neonatal period, peripheral nerve networks are going through a process of increasing differentiation. When repeatedly insulted with painful stimuli, that process is altered such that lower levels of stimulation potentiate relatively significant nociceptive responses. Indeed, human neonates

748

undergoing repeated heel lancing demonstrated a similar hyperalgesic response (7).

Other clinical research findings support these concerns. Taddio et al. (8) focused on reactions to routine vaccination at 4 and 6 months of age among three groups of boys: those who were uncircumcised, those who were circumcised within 5 days of birth using EMLA cream (a topical anesthetic) for pain management, and those who were circumcised with a placebo topical cream. When these children came in for their routine vaccinations, they were videotaped so that a number of pain behaviors could be evaluated, including facial action (brow bulge, nasolabial furrow, eyes squeezed shut) and cry duration, and a visual analog scale score for pain was assigned. Analysis showed greater pain responses across the board in boys who were circumcised without local anesthesia in contrast to those who were uncircumcised. In addition, visual analog scores were significantly different between boys circumcised with EMLA versus those with the placebo. Relevant variables, such as temperament, age, weight, time since last feeding, time of last sleep before vaccination, and ingestion of paracetamol, did not correlate with pain indices. Thus, early untreated pain experiences appear to sensitize the child to subsequent painful experiences.

Similar possibilities were raised in a study by Walco and colleagues (9), who assessed pain threshold values in four groups of children: those with juvenile rheumatoid arthritis (JRA, a chronic illness in which chronic pain is a common feature), those with sickle cell disease (SCD, a chronic illness in which recurrent episodes of acute pain are a common feature), those with asthma (a chronic illness in which pain is typically not a feature), and healthy controls. Pain threshold was measured in two modalities: direct mechanical pressure stimulation of a digit and circumferential pressure of the upper arm. Results showed that children who experience clinical pain on a regular basis (those with JRA and SCD) had lower pain thresholds than their healthy peers.

Certainly a great deal more research on the development of pain pathways needs to be conducted in order to understand these findings. We currently know very little about the development of central components to pain systems, especially in the areas of the thalamus, cortex, and cingulate gyrus of the limbic system. In addition, however, cognitive and affective factors, both of which have their own developmental pathways, play a major role in the pain experience and should be considered.

COGNITIVE AND EMOTIONAL DEVELOPMENT

Similar to the development of pain networks on a physiological level, both cognition and emotion develop with increasing differentiation and integration. A thorough review of potential cognitive and socioemotional influences on pain is well beyond the scope of this chapter. Thus, we will highlight areas where there has been a spe-

cific focus on developmental aspects of pain as related to concept development and to temperament.

It is well known that as children's cognitive abilities increase, their concepts of illness become increasingly differentiated and integrated. Bibace and Walsh (10) showed that there is a strong relationship between Piagetian cognitive stage and concept of illness. Thompson and Varni (11) elaborated on this model and discussed the relationship between emerging concepts of illness and related concepts of pain. Although implications for assessment were described, no data were offered demonstrating the precise nature of this relationship.

Ross and Ross (12) conducted semistructured interviews with almost 1000 children between the ages of 5 and 12 years in school, hospital, or clinic settings. Interestingly, they found no age trends in children's pain concepts. Definitions of pain were "unidimensional" as pain was defined in the context of general discomfort or specific pain events. Children failed to comprehend the warning or diagnostic value of pain, and secondary gains or other values of pain were rarely recognized. Specific pain experiences were attributed to immediate causes (e.g., accidents, illness, surgery). Noticeably absent was the notion of pain related to imminent justice; if pain was seen as a punishment, it was in relation to immediate and proximal, not remote, events. Pain descriptors were used meaningfully, and children could recollect various contextual aspects of previous pain experiences.

In contrast, Gaffney and Dunne (13) showed that children's understanding of pain follows a Piagetian developmental model. They used a sentence completion item of "Pain is . . ." in the context of a broader assessment of children between the ages of 5 and 14 years. Three composite categories were derived to responses, reflecting concrete definitions, semiabstract definitions, and abstract definitions. Data showed statistically and clinically significant differences as there was increasing abstraction and generalization with age. The authors noted that the three coding categories for definitions of pain correspond to the Piagetian stages of preoperational, concrete operational, and formal operational thought, respectively, and the age distributions observed were consistent with expectations. Thus, children's concepts of pain begin in toddlerhood and are quite illogical and egocentric in nature. With development, concepts become increasingly realistic, integrated, and abstract.

In a second study (14), causality of pain was the focus. Twelve categories were derived, including illness, malfunction, transgressions involving eating, transgressions involving other activities, transgressions in general, psychological factors, need states, physiological explanations, and contamination or contagion. Developmental patterns were observed in that the frequency of objective, physical explanations of pain (trauma, malfunction) increased significantly with age, as did abstract, psychological explanations. Physiological explanations were noticeably scarce.

The issue of transgression was apparent as children often attributed pain to carelessness or misdeed. Of note, however, is that the authors viewed these explanations as arising much more from intrinsic processes of cognitive development than from environmental influences, such as statements from parents.

We know of no research that specifically examined the relationship between children's understanding of pain and actual clinical pain experiences. However, data from one study appears to support the notion that increasing levels of cognition and awareness, as well as concurrent emotional development, have a significant impact on pain experience. Ilowite, Walco, and Pochaczevsky (15) used liquid crystal thermography to measure the heat of joints affected by juvenile rheumatoid arthritis in children between the ages of 4 and 16 years. By comparing affected joints with contralateral unaffected joints (or adjacent nonarticular tissue in cases of bilateral disease) specific values representing changes in temperature due to disease (ΔT) could be established. These ΔT values were then correlated with visual analog scales for pain intensity provided by the patient, parent, and physician. For the latter two, significant correlations were observed. Although this correlation was also highly significant in younger patients (less than about 8 years of age), it was much lower in older patients. The authors concluded that in older patients, many more variables, including cognitive and emotional processes, come into play and impact on subjective pain experiences.

A significant literature exists on the relationship between psychological functioning, personality variables, and aspects of the pain experience in adults (16). In contrast, very little has been published on these elements in children. Increasingly, however, it is becoming recognized that many of the same functional elements that comprise temperamental styles in general may apply to pain as well. Consistent, inherent predispositions underlie and modulate the expression of activity, reactivity, emotionality, and sociability (17). Clearly these factors are critical in understanding individual differences in pain response. Recently, attention has been turned to the manner in which temperamental variables affect reactivity and self-regulation, including as related to self-focus as a coping style for pain (18). This literature is in its infancy, and laboratory and clinical studies are needed to further delineate specific relationships among temperament, pain responsiveness, and pain coping. Finally, it is clear that affect plays a significant role in the pain experience. Studies comparing the increasing differentiation and integration of affect with elements of the pain experience, including differentiation of those responses, will be extremely helpful.

ASSESSMENT OF PAIN IN CHILDREN

The accurate and comprehensive assessment of the child's pain experience and contextual factors is a necessary first step in pain management. The three major modalities available to the clinician and researcher are self-reports of the child (and sometimes others), behavioral observations, and monitoring of physiological parameters (19). The specific modalities invoked depend upon the child's developmental level, especially among those who are preverbal, and the nature of the pain that is to be assessed, e.g., acute, procedural, neoplastic, recurrent, or chronic. In addition, these factors will dictate the degree to which contextual factors will be highlighted. For example, in evaluating a chronic pain syndrome, it is important to evaluate family and social factors that may be influencing the frequency, intensity, and duration of pain difficulties.

Although the focus of subsequent discussion here will be on the assessment of pain as a symptom *per se,* it is important to stress the significance of an array of contextual factors, including nature of the medical condition, developmental level, previous pain experiences, comprehension of medical condition and treatments, temperament, ethnocultural background, affective states, and coping styles. In addition, data on pain responsiveness (pain threshold, typical pain reactions) are also extremely helpful (9,20). It is imperative to acknowledge that whether the focus is pain symptoms or contextual factors, one must consider the reliability, validity, and clinical sensitivity of the measures used, as well as the feasibility of use in the clinical setting (19,21).

Assessment of Pain by Self-report

Because pain is a subjective experience, self-report methods are considered to be optimal for pain assessment in children mature enough to do so (22). Children have words for pain by approximately 18 months of age and are cognitively proficient at reporting the degree of pain (i.e., little, a lot) by age 3 or 4 years (23). Children can accurately report on the location, sensory quality (e.g., aching, burning, tearing, gnawing, stinging, throbbing, sharp or dull), intensity, affective elements, and tolerability of pain if probed in a developmentally sensitive manner.

Pain quality can be assessed using adjective checklists. Word lists facilitate verbalization of the sensory component of pain (e.g., squeezing, burning, pins and needles), tolerability of pain (e.g., unbearable, horrendous), and affective qualities of pain (e.g., scary, sad). Scales such as the Children's Anxiety and Pain Scale (24), which use pictures to assess anxiety and pain in the same context, or the Children's Somatization Inventory (25), may enable the child to communicate a broad range of physical symptoms.

A measure that is useful in assessing pain intensity with young children (4 to 8 years) is the Poker Chip Tool (26), in which children rate pain concretely as "pieces of hurt" (the more pieces, the greater the intensity). On the Oucher Scale, respondents rate their own pain intensity by anchoring it to photographs of the faces of children depicting increasing levels of pain (27). The location and relative intensity of pain might be ascertained with body outlines on which patients can mark areas of discomfort and rate them for relative intensity; colors might facilitate relative rankings (28).

Children over 4 years can rate pain intensity reliably using a "pain thermometer" (29) or a visual analog scale (VAS), which is a line with verbal, facial, or numerical anchors at the extremes. These instruments may be pencil and paper based or of a slide rule type, and children are asked to indicate their level of pain on those continua (19). The utility of these scales lies in the fact that they have been shown to be rational in nature; that is, there is an absolute zero point, and the distances along the scale may be treated arithmetically. This is very important when it comes to documenting the efficacy of interventions. Only in instances when the child is too impaired or too young should parents or significant others provide these ratings. In addition to intensity, recent data indicate that the affective component of pain is crucial because it cannot be separated from nociceptive responses, and it correlates highly with tolerability (30). The Faces Scale provides a series of facial expressions depicting gradations of pain, and children choose the one that approximates their own pain experience (31). Although useful and reliable, these scales are limited because the specific affective components (e.g., sadness, anxiety, distress) involved are unclear.

Standardized assessment of chronic pain continues to pose a challenge. The Varni-Thompson Pediatric Pain Questionnaire (32) was first used to assess chronic pain in children with juvenile rheumatoid arthritis but has been utilized with a broad range of chronic pain syndromes (33,34). Pain symptom diaries are also useful in the assessment of chronic pain (35). Critical in these endeavors is capturing elements of the broader pain experience and not simply elements of the symptom itself.

In some circumstances, psychological testing among children and adolescents with chronic pain may be beneficial in providing information about problem-solving skills, other psychological symptoms, and problems that may not be revealed during an interview about additional areas of stress being experienced by the child. Intelligence testing reveals cognitive deficits and relative strengths and weakness, and academic testing assesses whether the child is functioning at grade level and whether school is a potentially important source of stress (36).

Observational Pain Assessment

Specific behaviors associated with pain (e.g., vocalizations, facial expressions, body movements) provide an additional window through which pain and distress may be evaluated. The reliability and validity of behavioral observations are highest when the pain being measured is short in duration and acute in nature, such as pain associated with procedures (37). It is critical to note that these indices should be used as an adjunct to self-report, not necessarily in its place, because multidimensional assessments are deemed more accurate than are single parameters (38).

Research suggests discordance between self-report and observed pain behaviors, indicating that measurement of both dimensions may yield a more comprehensive evaluation of the pain experience (39). This is likely due to the fact that there is not necessarily a direct relationship between one's internal subjective experience and behavioral manifestations (40).

A developmental dimension has been appreciated with a general trend toward increasing differentiation and specificity of pain responses. Infants' responses to acute pain may include general body movements, specific facial expressions (furrowed brow, nasal flaring, quivering lips), and crying patterns (41). In infants, facial expression has been found to be a reliable and consistent indicator of pain across populations and types of nociceptive stimulation and thus has become a major focus of assessment (42).

An array of behavioral coding scales has been developed for infants. The Neonatal Facial Coding System is a valid and reliable coding system for measuring facial actions associated with acute pain in infancy (43). Behavioral assessment tools developed for older infants (4 to 6 months) include the Modified Behavioral Pain Scale (44) and the Neonatal Assessment of Pain Inventory (45) for use in children aged 1 to 36 months.

Toddlers' and young children's responses to acute pain include specific body reactions that are more precisely localized and are accompanied by verbalizations. The FLACC (facial expression, leg movement, activity, cry, and consolability) is gaining in popularity as a reliable and valid means to assess pain behavior (initially postoperative pain) in children between the ages of 2 months and 7 years (46).

Children's distress responses to invasive medical procedures have been a focus of studies on pain behavior. Behaviors prior to, during, and after noxious stimulation are noted in order to define distinct patterns that represent responses to pain. In these scales, specific pain behaviors are operationally defined and are then tallied as they occur during set intervals or phases of a procedure (37). The Procedural Behavior Rating Scale revised (PBRS-r) (47) and the Observational Scale of Behavioral Distress (OSBD) (48) are the most utilized observational distress scales for pediatric oncology patients during lumbar punctures and bone marrow aspirations. For the PBRS-r, the observer records the occurrence of 11 behaviors during three time periods within the medical procedure, whereas the OSBD continually samples the same 11 behaviors throughout the procedure. The behaviors include crying, screaming, physical restraint, verbal resistance, requests for emotional support, muscular rigidity, verbal fear, verbal pain, flailing, nervous behavior, and information seeking.

Physiological Indices of Pain

Children's pain and distress can be evaluated with objective physiological measures. Traditionally, the focus has been on sympathetic nervous system indicators of arousal, including heart rate, respiratory rate, blood pressure, and palmar sweating. More recently, it has been recognized that these factors are nonspecific for pain or stress, and increasing attention has been paid to parasympathetic responses, such as heart rate variability and vagal tone, and hypothalamic-pituitary-adrenocorticosteroid (HPA) responses, such as circulating cortisol levels (49,50).

Threats to an animal elicit a "fight or flight" reaction. Thus, the organism responds to acute stress by being prepared to react with vigor. This accounts for increases in heart rate, respiration rate, blood pressure, and sweating, with concomitant decreased blood flow to the gut. Children undergoing invasive procedures demonstrate such stress responses. In addition, however, the parasympathetic nervous system works to regain a state of homeostasis. Thus, during acute threats it is relatively inactive compared to its counterpart. As the stress or pain continues, the parasympathetic nervous system may attempt to become more active. It is through indicators of exaggerated variability, such as in heart rate and vagal tone, that one can measure the impact of stress on this system (50).

Additionally, the body prepares itself to react to stress with hormonal and metabolic changes. Central here is the activity of the HPA system, which makes glucose more available for consumption in service of "fueling" the response. Cortisol plays a central role in this process and may be found in the blood, urine, and saliva. Thus, by measuring cortisol approximately prior to and then 20 to 30 minutes after the onset of acute stress, one has a reliable index of the HPA system response (49). The relationship among sympathetic, parasympathetic, and HPA system responses in children undergoing lumbar punctures and bone marrow aspirations is complicated, apparently mediated by an array of factors (40).

It is important to note that some investigators have begun to integrate various components of pain assessment into a single instrument. For example, the Neonatal Infant Pain Scale includes five behavioral and one physiological parameter of pain (51). The Premature Infant Pain Profile has behavioral, physiological, and contextual factors to assess pain in both clinical and research contexts (52).

The concept of multidimensional assessment is ideal to account for multiple aspects of the pain experience. It is recognized, however, that physiological parameters such as vagal tone and cortisol release are not practical in most clinical settings. Ultimately, it is important to understand the relationship among self-report, behavioral indicators, and physiological responses to pain so that we can match individual patients to specific pain treatment protocols that involve pharmacological and psychological strategies.

PHARMACOLOGICAL INTERVENTIONS

The principles of the treatment of pain in the pediatric population parallel those of the adult population—drug and nondrug therapies should be employed judiciously with the intent to eliminate discomfort. Although it has been demonstrated that beyond the neonatal period, the pharmacology of most analgesics is similar between children and adults (53–58), many of these drugs are not approved for younger children due to their lack of inclusion in clinical trials. Thus, practitioners must rely on clinical guidelines for direction, incorporating knowledge of dosages, half-life, and frequency of administration, routes of administration, side effects, and potential interactions with other medications.

As with adults, in formulating a treatment pain utilizing analgesic therapy in children a model often invoked is the World Health Organization (WHO) three-step analgesic ladder: step 1, mild pain, nonopioid analgesics +/– adjuvant; step 2, moderate pain, opioid for mild to moderate pain +/– nonopioid +/– adjuvant; step 3, severe pain, opioid +/– nonopioid +/– adjuvant (59). Note that nonopioid drugs can be used concurrently to potentiate the beneficial effects of the opioids. Also, a fourth step, invasive therapy, has been advocated, especially in the context of severe pain in children with terminal illnesses. The goal is freedom from pain.

Nonopioid Analgesics

Nonopioid drugs include paraamino phenol derivatives such as acetaminophen, salicylates such as aspirin and choline magnesium trisalicylate, and the nonsteroidal antiinflammatory drugs (NSAIDs) such as ibuprofen, naproxen, ketorolac, indomethacin, diclofenac, and piroxicam. At present acetaminophen is the most commonly prescribed analgesic for mild to moderate pain because of the lack of serious side effects on renal, gastrointestinal, and platelet function. It has been demonstrated to have additive effects when used in conjunction with opioids. The usual dose is 10 to 15 mg/kg every 4 hours with a maximal dose of 60 mg/kg per day (60). It also has the advantage of being available as a rectal suppository.

Salicylates, primarily aspirin, had been widely used until the past 20 years as an analgesic and antipyretic, but their use has been markedly curtailed because of association with Reye's syndrome (a rare but possibly fatal illness involving the liver and central nervous system) (61). Aspirin is also associated with platelet dysfunction and bleeding, which make it an inappropriate choice for children with malignancy. However, it is still used in children with rheumatic disease because of its antiinflammatory properties. The dose is 10 to 15 mg/kg per dose given every 4 hours. Ibuprofen is another NSAID used in children, and some studies have suggested it is a more effective analgesic than acetaminophen (62,63). It has also been shown that when used with narcotics, ibuprofen can significantly decrease the total amount of opioids needed for effective postoperative pain control (64,65). The dose of ibuprofen is 5 to 10 mg/kg with a maximal dose of 40 mg/kg per day (60).

Ketorolac is the only NSAID available for intravenous use. Studies have demonstrated its safety and its use as an adjuvant therapy with narcotics in children experiencing vasoocclusive pain from sickle cell disease (66) and postoperative pain (67). The dose is 0.5 mg/kg given every 6 to 12 hours, with a maximal dose of 60 mg. The main limitation is that ketorolac cannot be used for more than 5 days nor in patients with renal dysfunction. Finally, there are initial studies on the use of cyclooxygenase-2 (COX-2) inhibitors such as celecoxib, primarily in children with rheumatologic diseases, to demonstrate indication for its use.

Opioid Analgesics

Narcotics are the mainstay for treatment of moderate to severe pain. These drugs are reliable with predictable efficacy, onset of action, half-life, and side effects. Two major barriers have previously minimized the use of these medications with young children—respiratory depression and risk of addiction—but data have shown that both are extremely rare and that children are at no greater risk for these complications than are adults (68). With proper dosing and monitoring, risks of respiratory difficulties are minimal.

The weaker opioids are usually administered orally and are most often given in combination with acetaminophen or NSAIDs. They include codeine (1 mg/kg every 4 hours), oxycodone (0.1 mg/kg every 4 hours), and hydrocodone (0.1 mg/kg every 4 hours) (69). Among stronger opioids, morphine has the widest usage in the pediatric population, with a predictable onset of action and duration. Other commonly used drugs in this class are methadone, hydromorphone, and fentanyl. Meperidine is not recommended for use in children because of the excessive buildup of one its metabolites, normeperidine, which can cause central nervous system irritability and seizures.

As a general rule, opioids should be administered on an around-the-clock regimen or as a continuous infusion when given intravenously to avoid peaks and valleys in the levels of the drug. The starting dose of morphine is 0.1 mg/kg given every 3 to 4 hours, methadone 0.1 mg/kg given every 6 to 24 hours, hydromorphone 0.01 to 0.02 mg/kg given every 3 to 4 hours, and fentanyl 0.001 mg/kg given every 1 hour. There are no maximal dosages for narcotics. As with adults, tolerance is a common phenomenon seen with the steady use of narcotics, and there have been reports of even small children requiring over 500 mg/kg per hour of morphine to control severe cancer pain (70). As is the case with adults, one should be aware of the side effects commonly seen, which include constipation, nausea, sedation, confusion, pruritus, and urinary retention.

Patient-controlled analgesia (PCA) has been used successfully in children as young as 6 or 7 years (71). It has been used extensively for analgesia in the postoperative setting (71) and for children with burns (72), sickle cell anemia (73), and cancer (74). In younger patients, some have suggested parent-assisted or nurse-controlled analge-

sia, but this is still somewhat controversial (75). The narcotics that are commonly used for PCA include morphine, fentanyl, and hydromorphone. A typical regimen may include a loading dose of 0.1 mg/kg of morphine, followed by a basal infusion rate of 0.015 to 0.02 mg/kg (74). The child is then able to administer small frequent boluses of approximately 0.02 mg/kg, delivered every 5 to 10 minutes (lockout interval) with a maximum of approximately 0.15 mg/kg per hour. If the child is utilizing the maximum allowable amount of medication, consideration should be made to either increase the basal rate or the amount of bolus dosing. Careful monitoring of respiratory status using a pulse oximeter to maintain an oxygen saturation > 92%, as well as ensuring adequate blood pressure and heart rate, is essential.

Adjuvant Medications

Other medications that are used in conjunction with the analgesics include tricyclic antidepressants (e.g., imipramine, amitriptyline, nortriptyline), anticonvulsants (e.g., carbamazepine, gabapentin), antihistamines (e.g., diphenhydramine and hydroxyzine), and psychostimulants (e.g., dextroamphetamine, methylphenidate). As with adults, with children tricyclic antidepressants can have a role in treating chronic pain, such as in fibromyalgia syndrome (76) and neuropathic pain. The latter is also treated with anticonvulsants, antiarrhythmics (mexiletine), and capsaicin cream (77).

PROCEDURAL PAIN

Managing the acute distress associated with invasive procedures is an area in pediatric pain management that has shown considerable strides in the last 10 years (78). A model for addressing these issues is the child with cancer who frequently undergoes diagnostic procedures such as venipuncture, bone marrow aspiration and biopsy, and lumbar puncture. In 1990, the Report of the Subcommittee on the Management of Pain Associated with Procedures in Children with Cancer (79) stated that the vast majority of pediatric oncology centers had no formal protocols for procedural distress, despite the fact that anxiety associated with such procedures could have significant impact on coping with subsequent medical interventions. In that report, various psychological strategies were described (see following), and guidelines were suggested for the use of sedation along with analgesics for the apprehensive child undergoing these procedures. Over the last 10 years it has become the standard of practice in most pediatric oncology centers to offer some form of sedation to these children. These principles are now being applied to procedural pain outside the realm of cancer and include the pediatric emergency room for suturing of lacerations and setting of fractures and the hospital inpatient area for burn and wound care, joint aspirations, and chest tube placement (78).

The level of sedation that is employed can vary from conscious sedation, defined as a "medically controlled state of depressed consciousness that allows protective reflexes to be maintained, retains the patient's ability to maintain a patent airway and permits appropriate response by the patient to physical stimulation or verbal command," to deep sedation, defined as a "medically controlled state of depressed consciousness or unconsciousness from which the patient is not easily aroused" (80). Deep sedation may be accompanied by a loss of protective reflexes and includes the inability to maintain a patent airway independently and respond purposefully to physical stimulation or verbal stimuli.

The personnel responsible for administration of these drugs should be familiar with the pharmacology of the medications. They should also be proficient in airway management and cardiopulmonary resuscitation. The child should be closely monitored with continuous pulse oximetry, as well as frequent determinations of blood pressure, heart rate, and respiratory rate (80).

A decade ago, conscious sedation strategies were rather crude. Common practices included the combination DPT (demerol, phenergan, and thorazine) or chloral hydrate, both of which are now discouraged because of the unpredictability of onset of action, high incidence of side effects, and lack of analgesic properties (81). More commonly today, conscious sedation is achieved with a combination of drugs that includes an anxiolytic, typically midazolam at an initial dose of 0.025 to 0.1 mg/kg with a maximum dose of 0.4 to 0.6 mg/kg, in tandem with an opioid, such as fentanyl at a dose of 1 µg/kg (78). Other sedative/hypnotic agents that are utilized include pentobarbital and thiopental. For the more cooperative child who nevertheless requires some level of sedation and pain control beyond that provided by a local anesthetic, a safe and effective alternative to conscious sedation is the administration of transmucosal fentanyl citrate (Fentanyl Oralet) (82). A dose of 0.005 to 0.015 mg/kg given 15 to 20 minutes in the buccal pouch provides adequate relief for many older children.

An increasingly popular method of providing deep sedation in children undergoing these procedures is the use of general anesthetic agents. Until recently, these agents could be given only in the setting of an operating room or recovery room. It is now common practice in many institutions for an anesthesiologist or pediatric intensivist to administer these drugs in an outpatient area or emergency room.

Ketamine is a general anesthetic with an extensive track record, especially in the emergency room, for procedures such as setting fractures or laceration repairs (83,84). Its main advantage is that it provides significant analgesia and can be given by the intramuscular, intravenous, or oral route. The disadvantages of ketamine are that it increases production of secretions, can cause laryngospasm, and can elevate blood pressure and increase intracranial pressure. It is therefore contraindicated in children with upper airway disease or head trauma. Ketamine is also known to cause unpleasant dreams and hallucinations, although this side effect is less commonly seen in children than adults (83). Ketamine is usually administered in combination with atropine as an antisialagogue and midazolam to decrease the spasmodic movements associated with ketamine as well as the concomitant hallucinations. Ketamine can be given intramuscularly at a dose of 2 to 3 mg/kg or intravenously at 0.5 mg/kg, which are sedating doses, or 1 to 5 mg/kg to induce general anesthesia.

Propofol is the preferred drug at many pediatric oncology centers across the country (81). Propofol is an anesthetic and must be given intravenously, preferably as a continuous infusion. It has a rapid onset of action, a short half-life, is easy to titrate, and has antiemetic effects. The initial dose is 2 to 5 mg/kg, given over 15 seconds with an intravenous infusion of 0.05 to 0.3 mg/kg per minute. Because propofol has no analgesic properties, a short-acting opioid such as fentanyl is often given in conjunction. After cessation of administration, the child is usually fully awake within 15 minutes.

The major advantage of propofol is that it is a safe, highly effective way of achieving sedation. It is associated with respiratory depression and apnea, which usually resolves quickly because of its short half-life. However, it must be given by someone with experience with airway management and tracheal intubation. There are reports confirming its safety and efficacy in the outpatient setting, administered by either an anesthesiologist or pediatric intensivist (85,86). It is suspended in an egg-based medium so that it is contraindicated in patients allergic to eggs. It is also irritating, so it should be given with a local anesthetic such as lidocaine when given via a peripheral vein.

In some situations an inhalation agent such as nitrous oxide can be used for sedation for painful procedures such as wound debridement or laceration suturing in the emergency room (87,88). The advantage of this approach is that it can be given without starting an intravenous line, it has a rapid onset of action and short half-life, and it has both anxiolytic and analgesic properties. Disadvantages include the necessity of having special equipment and a high incidence of vomiting.

An effective way of providing local anesthesia, prior to lumbar puncture or bone marrow aspiration in children not requiring sedation, or prior to venipuncture or intramuscular or subcutaneous injections, is the topical anesthetic EMLA cream. EMLA is a eutectic mixture of lidocaine and prilocaine in a water-based cream (89,90). When applied topically under an occlusive dressing, effective local anesthesia is achieved within 60 to 90 minutes. The major disadvantage therefore is the extended time needed for application prior to the procedure. It is also contraindicated in patients who are receiving other medications that can induce methemoglobinemia.

When more rapid local anesthesia is required, an alternative to EMLA cream is Numby Stuff (91). This is a system for delivering topical lidocaine using iontophoresis, a technique for achieving transdermal delivery of a local anesthetic via a low-intensity electrical current. Two electrodes are placed, one on the procedure site where 1 cm of lidocaine has been placed, and the other on a major muscle, at least 15 cm from the procedure site. Its advantage over EMLA cream is its rapidity of efficacy (less than 15 minutes). It may not be suitable for some children because of the mild discomfort caused by the tingling feeling of the small electrical current. Studies have demonstrated that these techniques are an effective way of reducing or eliminating the pain and anxiety associated with needle sticks.

Procedural Pain in Neonates

Neonatal pain is an area of particular interest as it continues to be severely undertreated. Because of these concerns the American Academy of Pediatrics in association with the Canadian Paediatric Society released a policy statement in February 2000 (92). The main concepts of that statement are: (a) Neuroanatomical components and neuroendocrine systems are sufficiently developed to allow transmission of painful stimuli in the neonate, (b) exposure to prolonged or severe pain may increase neonatal morbidity, (c) infants who have experienced pain during the neonatal period respond differently to subsequent painful events, (d) severity of pain and effects of analgesia can be assessed in the neonate, (e) neonates are not easily comforted when analgesia is needed, and (f) a lack of behavioral responses (including crying and movement) does not necessarily indicate a lack of pain.

This policy statement strongly advocates the avoidance of painful or noxious stimuli, when possible, and *adequate* pain management through the aggressive use of analgesics and anesthesia when indicated. The painful procedures that neonates undergo include venipunctures, arterial punctures, placement of arterial venous lines, insertion of chest tubes, bladder catheterization, suprapubic bladder punctures, lumbar puncture, circumcision, heel sticks, and intubation. Until recently most of these procedures were performed with little or no analgesia or sedation.

For some procedures such as arterial sticks or chest tube insertion, local anesthesia, including superficial infiltration of lidocaine or bupivacaine or application of EMLA cream, is sufficient. Although EMLA cream was initially contraindicated in the newborn because of concerns of development of methemoglobinemia, recent studies have proven its safety when used as a single dose of less than 2 grams (93). However, EMLA cream should be avoided when the neonate is receiving systemic drugs, such as acetaminophen, which are known to cause methemoglobinemia.

Narcotics have been used a great deal in the neonatal intensive care unit (94). One must be aware of the differences in the pharmacokinetics, i.e., metabolism and clearance, of these drugs among the premature newborn,

full-term newborn, and older infant. The opioids that have been prescribed most often are morphine and fentanyl. The half-life of morphine in the newborn is seven times that of the older infant, leading to levels two to three times higher. In addition, the half-life is even more prolonged in the premature infant. Therefore, the initial starting dose is about half that used in older children (0.05 mg/kg). When given as a continuous infusion in the term infant a dose of 0.01 to 0.02 mg/kg per hour usually provides sufficient analgesia, whereas in the preterm newborn the dose is 0.005 to 0.010 mg/kg per hour.

Fentanyl is an alternative to morphine and is particularly useful for infants with pulmonary hypertension or infants undergoing extracorporeal membrane oxygenation (ECMO) because it decreases pulmonary vascular resistance in the neonate (95). The starting dose is similar in term and preterm infants (0.001 mg/kg per hour). However, because of the development of tolerance it is not unusual to see a requirement for rapidly increased doses after a few days. Also one should be aware of the development of physical dependence and possible withdrawal symptoms with prolonged use. Accordingly, the medication should be slowly weaned when being used for more than a few days. Other narcotics that have been used in newborns, especially those undergoing surgery, are sufentanil and alfentanil because of their high potency, very rapid onset of action, and short half-life, which usually leads to rapid recovery from side effects (96).

Respiratory depression is the major side effect of opiates among newborns. Therefore, careful monitoring of respiratory status and oxygen saturation is mandatory. Ideally the infant should be in a setting where there is capability for intubation should apnea develop.

For milder pain, studies have shown that acetaminophen can be safely administered to neonates (94). Unfortunately, there is some question of its efficacy as an analgesic when used alone, and, as in older children, it may potentiate the effects of narcotics. The dose is 10 to 15 mg/kg when given orally and 20 to 25 mg/kg when given rectally. Other NSAIDs and aspirin are not recommended for the newborn. As adjuvants to analgesics, sedatives are often given in the neonatal unit (94). Benzodiazepines are most commonly prescribed. The drugs of choice are midazolam and lorazepam because of their short half-life.

Circumcision

Perhaps the best example of how attitudes have changed toward pain relief in children is the use of analgesia for circumcision. Until recently the prevailing feeling was that the pain with this procedure was insufficient to justify treatment. However, it has been clearly demonstrated that untreated pain during and following circumcision can lead to physiologic changes consistent with stress (elevated cortisol level, increased blood pressure and heart rate) and perhaps an exaggerated response to pain later in life (8).

EMLA cream has been found to be beneficial in ameliorating these responses in the newborn (93). One to two grams is applied with an occlusive dressing to the distal half of the penis for 60 to 90 minutes prior to the procedure.

A more effective way of achieving analgesia is the dorsal penile nerve block (97,98). When administered by someone skilled in this technique it has been shown to be both safe and effective. A 27-gauge needle is placed at the base of the penis, just cephalad to the pubic bone. After the needle penetrates Buck's fascia a local anesthetic such as lidocaine or bupivacaine is injected at the 10 o'clock and 2 o'clock position relative to the base of the penis. Epinephrine should never be given because of its vasoconstrictive effect.

A third alternative is the placement of a subcutaneous ring of a local anesthetic (without epinephrine) around the midshaft of the penis (99). Along with the local anesthetic, sucrose on a pacifier along with oral acetaminophen have been found to decrease the pain (100).

PSYCHOLOGICAL INTERVENTIONS

Over the last two decades, numerous studies have demonstrated the efficacy of cognitive-behavioral therapy (CBT) interventions for decreasing anxiety and distress related to procedural pain in children (101–107). Although CBT may be comprised of various specific strategies, in all cases the aim is to provide children with a specific set of responses that may be used to master the distressing situation, ideally in a manner consistent with their basic coping strategies.

Simple educational preparation is widely used to help children cope with anticipatory anxiety. The patient is provided with information, both procedure related (what will be done) and sensory (what it will feel like) throughout the phases (pre-, during, post-) of the procedure. Procedure-related information describes the steps of the procedure in some detail, whereas sensory-related information focuses on the child's subjective experiences. An example of sensory information for children being prepared for a lumbar puncture might include telling the children that they will feel a "pinch" as the needle goes in. The nature and amount of information given depend on the child's developmental stage, level of anxiety, and available coping strategies (108). With regard to the latter, children who are principally "attenders" focus on the stressor and generally seek out information in order to master the challenge. Conversely, "distracters" orient away from the procedure and cope more effectively when attention is diverted.

Anticipatory distress or acute fears of medical procedures can be treated with systematic desensitization. With this technique, children are gradually exposed to stimuli associated with the procedures in a hierarchical fashion from least to most threatening. The key is to provide an alternative response to the threatening stimuli such that what used to result in acute anxiety responses is replaced with calm or relaxation. The ultimate goal is to generalize these gains to the actual treatment setting, thereby promoting mastery and coping (30).

Positive incentive techniques involve presenting children with a small token reward (e.g., stickers, prizes) for their attempts at mastery during the painful procedure. Patients are encouraged to lie still, which significantly reduces the likelihood of complications in conducting the medical procedure, and to do breathing exercises aimed at preventing acute behavioral distress such as kicking and screaming. The purpose of the reward is to provide an incentive for engaging in positive coping behaviors and to enable the child to reframe, at least in part, the meaning of the pain as a challenge. Ultimately, all children receive positive reinforcement for their efforts, thereby using tokens as an incentive rather than a reward *per se* (101, 103,106). It is preferable to encourage children verbally during the procedure and to present concrete rewards following the procedure, pointing out the cooperative behavior or coping efforts.

Distraction refers to activities intended to divert a patient's attention away from distressing stimuli. In some cases, patients are asked to form a mental image of a strong capable character, such as a superhero, and to incorporate that character into the painful procedure in some adaptive manner (101,103,106). In other cases, distraction refers to specific activities in which a child can engage, such as coloring, watching a video, or putting a puzzle together (104).

Hypnosis is a frequently used distraction technique that involves helping the child to become as intensely involved in a fantasy experience as possible. Hypnosis involves a more elaborate process as patients are taught an initial induction technique, such as eye fixation or hand levitation, then a deepening strategy, such as progressive muscle relaxation. Finally, patients "visualize" or "experience" being in a special place and are encouraged to imagine a story around that place (109). In some instances, hypnoanalgesia or hypnoanesthesia may be introduced as a means of altering the subjective sensory experience (110). After a promising combination of strategies is found, patients are encouraged to practice on their own (self-hypnosis) (109) in an effort to facilitate generalization to the actual distressing situation (107,111). Additionally, these strategies may be implemented at home, in school, or in peer settings and might be used to facilitate pain relief, reduction of anxiety, or transitions to sleep, which may occur with chronic or recurrent pain (36).

Teaching a child to implement simple relaxation strategies, such as deep breathing or progressive muscle relaxation, is especially useful for reducing anxiety. The specific elements of the deep breathing technique used depend on the child's age. For example, older children may be given simple verbal suggestions to take a deep breath and to let it out slowly (103). Younger children require more concrete images and thus may use a party blower to facilitate the same breathing patterns during painful procedures (102,104). Relaxation can also be achieved through the use of imagery as children are guided through a scene where they are floating on a fluffy cloud (30), or they may be asked to be like a rag doll.

Modeling and rehearsal are key components for teaching and reinforcing coping prior to and during a procedure. Patients are shown a video of a similarly aged child who models positive coping behaviors (breathing exercises and imagery) and positive coping self-statements ("I know I can do it"). Typically, a child's voice narrates the steps of the procedures along with thoughts and feelings at critical points (103).

In behavioral rehearsals, children are encouraged to practice positive coping behaviors with "pretend" medical staff. Typically, one therapist will play the role of the doctor, while another plays the role of the patient's coach. Similarly, sometimes children are asked to "pretend doctor" (younger children) or to conduct a demonstration of the painful procedure using a doll (older children). While the child administers the procedure, the doll is coached to lie still and engage in deep breathing and imagery exercises (103).

Biofeedback could be used as an adjunct to self-regulatory strategies as a means of providing immediate information to children concerning the relative success of their efforts. Biofeedback has been used successfully for a variety of pain states, including headaches and generalized muscle tension. Children quickly learn the significance of the auditory and/or visual feedback and can be taught to use the modality independently at home.

The clinical usefulness of psychological strategies for various pain syndromes related to chronic illness has been documented. Specifically, these strategies have been successful in treating children with sickle cell disease (112), headaches (113), and musculoskeletal pain syndromes (34,114,115).

Finally, recent data indicate that a variety of staff (physicians, nurses, social workers, child life specialists) may be taught these techniques in a systematic way and then use them successfully in clinical settings (116). Thus, the need for individuals with advanced training in this area is reduced when children present with relatively straightforward concerns.

In summary, cognitive-behavioral interventions have a number of advantages. They facilitate a sense of mastery over a stressful situation that may be generalized to future coping. Parents may be given specific roles to assist their children with the behavioral techniques, which may be gratifying to both parents and children. Unlike pharmacological interventions, there are virtually no untoward side effects. These strategies are by no means a panacea, however, because some children may lack the motivation, cognitive ability, or emotional temperament to utilize them. Clearly, one does not need to choose pharmacological *versus* psychological strategies; rather, combinations tailored to the needs of individual patients are most reasonable.

In order to manage pain adequately in children, a multimodal approach to its assessment and management, which includes pharmacological, psychological, and physical components, has been recommended by the American Pain Society and the American Academy of Pediatrics (117,118). The specific interventions implemented should be tailored to the needs and interests of individual patients. Standardized protocols that merely reflect hospital policy or physician preference, without strong empirical support, have no place in current pediatric practice.

REFERENCES

1. Andrews K, Fitzgerald M. The cutaneous withdrawal reflex in human neonates: sensitization, receptive fields, and the effects of contralateral stimulation. *Pain* 1994;56:95–101.
2. Anand KJS, Carr DB. The neuroanatomy, neurophysiology and neurochemistry of pain, stress, and analgesia in newborns, infants, and children. *Pediatric Clinics of North America* 1989;36:795–822.
3. Fitzgerald M, Anand KJS. Developmental neuroanatomy and neurophysiology of pain. In: Schechter NL, Berde CB, Yaster M eds. *Pain in infants, children, and adolescents.* Baltimore, MD: Williams and Wilkins, 1993:11–31.
4. Fitzgerald M. Cutaneous primary afferent properties in the hindlimb of the neonatal rat. *Journal of Physiology,* 1987;383:79–92.
5. Fitzgerald M. The development of activity evoked by fine diameter cutaneous fibres in the spinal cord of the newborn rat. *Neuroscience Letter* 1988;86:161–166.
6. Reynolds M, Fitzgerald M. Long term sensory hyperinnervation following neonatal skin wounds. *Journal of Comparative Neurology* 1995;358:487–498.
7. Fitzgerald M, Millard C, McIntosh N. Cutaneous hypersensitivity following peripheral tissue damage in newborn infants and its reversal with topical anaesthesia. *Pain* 1989;39:31–36.
8. Taddio A, Katz, J, Ilersich AL, Koren G. Effect of neonatal circumcision on pain response during subsequent routine vaccination. *Lancet* 1997;349:599–603.
9. Walco GA, Dampier CD, Hartstein G, et al. The relationship between recurrent clinical pain and pain threshold in children. In: Tyler DC, Krane, EJ eds. *Advances in pain research and therapy. Pediatric pain.* New York: Raven, 1990;15:333–340.
10. Bibace R, Walsh ME. Development of children's concepts of illness. *Pediatrics* 1980;66:912–917.
11. Thompson KL, Varni JW. A developmental cognitive-biobehavioral approach to pediatric pain assessment. *Pain* 1986;25:282–296.
12. Ross DM, Ross SA. Childhood pain: the school-aged child's viewpoint. *Pain* 1984;20:179–191.
13. Gaffney A, Dunne EA. Developmental aspects of children's definitions of pain. *Pain* 1986;26:105–117.
14. Gaffney A, Dunne EA. Children's understanding of the causality of pain. *Pain* 1987;29:91–104.
15. Ilowite NT, Walco GA, Pochaczevsky R. Pain assessment in juvenile rheumatoid arthritis: relation between pain intensity and degree of joint inflammation. *Annals of the Rheumatic Diseases* 1992;51: 343–346.
16. Bradley LA, Haile M., Jaworski TM. Assessment of psychological status using interviews and self-report instruments. In: Turk DC and Melzack R, eds. *Handbook of pain assessment.* New York: Guilford, 1992: 193–213.
17. Goldsmith H, Buss A, Plomin R, et al. Roundtable: what is temperament? Four approaches. *Child Development* 1987;58:505–529.
18. Zeltzer L, Bursch B, Walco, G. Pain responsiveness and chronic pain: a psychobiological perspective. *Journal of Developmental and Behavioral Pediatrics* 1997;18:413–422.
19. McGrath PA, Brigham MC. The assessment of pain in children and adolescents. In: Turk DC, Melzack R, eds. *Handbook of pain assessment.* New York: Guilford Press, 1992:295–314.
20. Adesman AR, Gootman CS, Walco GA. *Comparison of parent and child measures of children's characteristic pain response.* Paper presented at the 9th Annual Scientific Meeting of the American Pain Society, St. Louis, MO, 1990.
21. Franck LS, Greenberg CS, Stevens B. Pain assessment in infants and children. *Pediatric Clinics of North America* 2000;47:487–512.

22. Acute Pain Management Guideline Panel. Acute Pain Management: Operative or Medical Procedures and Trauma. Clinical Practice Guideline. AHCPR Pub. No. 92-0032. Rockville, MD: Agency for Health Care Policy and Research. Public Health Service, U.S. Department of Health and Human Services, 1992.

23. Harbeck C, Peterson, L. Elephants dancing in my head: a developmental approach to children's concept of specific pains. *Child Development* 1992;63:138–149.

24. Kuttner L, LePage, T. Faces scales for the assessment of pediatric pain: a critical review. *Canadian Journal of Behavioral Science* 1989;21:198.

25. Garber J, Walker LS, Zeman J. Somatization symptoms in a community sample of children and adolescents: further validation of the Children's Somatization Inventory. *Psychological Assessment,* 1991;3:588–595.

26. Hester NO, Foster R, Kristensen K. Measurement of pain in children: generalizability and validity of the pain ladder and the poker-chip tool. In: Tyler DC, Krane EJ, eds. *Advances in pain research and therapy. Pediatric pain.* New York: Raven Press, 1990:79–84.

27. Brieri D, Reeve RA, Champion GD, et al. The face pain scale for the self assessment of the severity of pain experienced by children: development, initial validation, and preliminary investigation for the ratio scale properties. *Pain* 1990;41:139–150.

28. Eland JM, Anderson, IF. The experience of pain in children. In Jacox AK, ed. *Pain: a source book for nurses and other health professionals.* Boston: Little Brown, 1977:453–476.

29. Szyfelbein, SK, Osgood, PE, Carr, DB. The assessment of pain and plasma B-endorphin immunoactivity in burned children. *Pain* 1985;22:173–182.

30. Anderson CTM, Zeltzer LK, Fanurik D. Procedural pain. In: Schechter NL, Berde CB, Yaster M, eds. *Pain in infants, children and adolescents.* Baltimore, MD: Williams & Wilkins, 1993:435–458.

31. McGrath PA. *Pain in children: nature, assessment and treatment.* New York: Guilford Press, 1990:466.

32. Varni JW, Thompson KL, Hanson. The Varni/Thompson Pediatric Pain Questionnaire:I. Chronic musculoskeletal pain in juvenile rheumatoid arthritis. *Pain,* 1987;28:27–38.

33. Walco GA, Dampier CD. Pain in children and adolescents with sickle cell disease: a descriptive study. *Journal of Pediatric Psychology* 1990; 15:643–658.

34. Walco GA, Varni JW, Ilowite NT. Cognitive-behavioral pain management in children with juvenile rheumatoid arthritis. *Pediatrics* 1992;89:1075–1079.

35. Shapiro BS, Dinges DF, Orne EC, et al. Home management of sickle cell related pain in children and adolescents: natural history and impact on school attendance. *Pain* 1995;61:139.

36. Bursch B, Walco GA, Zeltzer L. Clinical assessment and management of chronic pain and pain-associated disability syndrome. *Journal of Developmental and Behavioral Pediatrics* 1998;19:45–53.

37. Mathews JR, McGrath PJ, Pigeon H. Assessment and measurement of pain in children. In: Schechter NL, Berde CB, Yaster M, eds. *Pain in infants, children and adolescents.* Baltimore, MD: Williams & Wilkins, 1993:97–111.

38. Stevens B. Composite measures of pain. *Progress in pain research and measurement* 1998;10:161–178.

39. Beyer JE, McGrath PJ, Berde CB. Discordance between self-report and behavioral pain measures in children aged 3–7 years after surgery. *J Pain Symptom Manage* 1990;5:350–356.

40. Walco GA, Conte PM, Labay LE, et al. *Procedural distress in pediatric oncology.* Paper presented at the 5th International Symposium on Pediatric Pain, London, Great Britain, 2000.

41. Grunau RVE, Craig KD. Pain expression in neonates: facial action and cry. *Pain* 1987;28:395–410.

42. Craig KD. The facial display of pain in infants and children. *Pain Research and Management,*1998;10:103–121.

43. Grunau RVE, Johnston, CC, Craig, KD. Neonatal facial and cry responses to invasive and non-invasive procedures. *Pain* 1990;42: 295–305.

44. Taddio A, Nulman,I. Koren BS. A revised measure of acute pain in infants. *J Pain Symptom Manage* 1995;10:456–463.

45. Schade JG, Joyce BA, Gerkensmeyer,J. Comparison of three preverbal scales for postoperative pain assessment in a diverse pediatric sample. *J Pain Symptom Manage* 1996;12:348–359.

46. Merkel SI, Voepel-Lewis T, Shayevitz JR, Malviya S. The FLACC: A behavioral scale for scoring postoperative pain in young children. *Pediatric Nursing* 1997;23:293–297.

47. Katz ER, Kellerman J, Siegel SE. Behavioral distress in children with cancer undergoing medical procedures: developmental considerations. *Journal of Consulting and Clinical Psychology*, 1980;48:356–365.

48. Jay SM, Ozolins M, Elliott C, Caldwell, S. Assessment of children's distress during painful medical procedures. *Journal of Health Psychology*1983;2:133–147.

49. Gunnar MR. Reactivity of the hypothalamic-pituitary-adrenocortical system to stressors in normal infants and children. *Pediatrics* 1992;90:491–497.

50. Porges SW. Vagal tone: A physiologic marker of stress vulnerability. *Pediatrics* 199290:498–504.

51. Lawrence J, Alcock D, McGrath P, et al. The development of a tool to assess neonatal pain. *Neonatal Network*1993;12:59–66.

52. Stevens B, Johnston CC, Petryshen P, Taddio A. Premature infant pain profile: developmental and initial validation. *Clin J Pain* 199612:13–22.

53. Olkkola KT, Hamunen K, Maunuksela EL. Clinical pharmacokinetics and pharmacodynamics of opioid analgesics in infants and children. *Clinical Pharmacokinetics* 1995;28:385–404.

54. Olkkola KT, Maunuksela EL. The pharmacokinetics of postoperative intravenous ketorolac tromethamine in children. *British Journal of Clinical Pharmacology* 1991;31:182–184.

55. Korpela R, Olkkola KT. Pharmacokinetics of intravenous diclofenac sodium in children. *European Journal of Clinical Pharmacology* 1990;38:293–295.

56. Miller RP, Roberts RJ, Fischer LJ. Acetaminophen elimination kinetics in neonates, children, and adults. *Clinical Pharmacology and Therapeutics* 1976;19:284–294.

57. Peterson RG, Rumack BH. Pharmacokinetics of acetaminophen in children. *Pediatrics* 1978;62:877–879.

58. Kauffman RE, Nelson MV. Effect of age on ibuprofen pharmacokinetics and antipyretic response. *Journal of Pediatrics* 1992;121:969–973.

59. Cancer Pain Relief and Palliative Care in Children. Geneva: WHO, 25, 1998.

60. Maunuksela, EL. Nonsteroidal anti-inflammatory drugs in pediatric pain management. In Schechter NL, Berde CB, and Yaster M, eds. *Pain in infants, children, and adolescents.* Baltimore, MD: Williams and Wilkins, 1993:135–143.

61. Hurwitz ES, Barrett MJ, Bregman D, et al. Public Health Service study on Reye's syndrome and medications. Report of the pilot phase. *New Engl J Med* 1985;313:849–857.

62. McGraw T, Raborn W, Grace M. Analgesics in pediatric dental surgery: relative efficacy of aluminum ibuprofen suspension and acetaminophen elixir. *ASDC Dentistry for Children* 1987;54:106–109.

63. Rumack BH. Aspirin versus acetaminophen: a comparative view. *Pediatrics* 1978;65:943–946.

64. Pang W, Mok MS, Ku MC, et al. Patient-controlled analgesia with morphine plus lysine acetyl salicylate. 1999;89:995–998.

65. Plummer JL, Owen H, Ilsley AH, et al. Sustained-release ibuprofen as an adjunct to morphine patient-controlled analgesia. 1996;83: 92–96.

66. Perlin E, Finke H, Castro O, et al. Enhancement of pain control with ketorolac tromethamine in patients with sickle cell vaso-occlusive crisis. *American Journal of Hematology* 1994;46:43–47.

67. Vetter TR, Heiner EJ. Intravenous ketorolac as an adjuvant to pediatric patient-controlled analgesia with morphine. *J Clin Anesth* 1994;6:110–113.

68. Walco GA, Cassidy RC, Schechter NL. Pain, hurt, and harm: the ethical issue of pediatric pain control. *New Engl J Med* 1994;331: 541–544.

69. Golianu B, Krane EJ, Galloway KS, et al. Pediatric acute pain management. *Pediatric Clinics of North America* 2000;47:559–585.

70. Collins JJ, Grier H, Kinney HC. Control of severe pain in children with terminal malignancy. *Journal of Pediatrics* 1995;126:653–657.

71. Berde CB, Lehn BM, Yee JD, et al. Patient controlled analgesia in children and adolescents: a randomized, prospective comparison with intramuscular administration of morphine for postoperative analgesia. *J Pediatrics* 1991;118:460–466.

72. Gaukroger PB, Chapman MJ, Davey RB. Pain control in paediatric burns—the use of patient-controlled analgesia. *Burns* 1991;17: 396–399.

73. Trentadue NO, Kachoyeanos MK, Lea G. A comparison of two regimens of patient-controlled analgesia for children with sickle cell disease. *Journal of Pediatric Nursing* 1998;13:15–19.

74. Guakroger, PB. Patient-controlled analgesia in children. In: Schechter NL, Berde CB, and Yaster M, eds. *Pain in infants, children, and adolescents.* Baltimore, MD: Williams and Wilkins, 1993: 203–211.

75. Monitto CL, Greenberg RS, Kost-Byerly S. The safety and efficacy of parent-/nurse-controlled analgesia in patients less than six years of age. 2000;91:573–579.

76. Yunus MB, Masi AT. Juvenile primary fibromyositis syndrome. A clinical study of thirty-three patients and matched normal controls. *Arth Rheum* 1985;28:138.

77. Olsson, GL. Neuropathic pain in children. In: McGrath PJ, Finley, GA, eds. Chronic and recurrent pain in children and adolescents. *Progress in pain research and management.* Seattle, WA: IASP Press, 1999;13:75–98.

78. Krauss B, Green S. Sedation and analgesia for procedures in children. *New England Journal of Medicine* 2000;342:938–945.

79. Zeltzer LK, Altman A, Cohen D. American Academy of Pediatrics report of the subcommittee on the management of pain associated with procedures in children with cancer. *Pediatrics* 1990;86:826–831.

80. Committee on Drugs. Guidelines for monitoring and management of pediatric patients during and after sedation for diagnostic and therapeutic procedures. *Pediatrics* 1992;89:110–115.

81. Conte PM, Walco GA, Sterling CM, et al. Procedural pain management in pediatric oncology: a review of the literature. *Cancer Investigation* 1999;17:448–459.

82. Schechter NL, Weisman SJ, Rosenbaum M. et al. The use of oral transmucosal fentanyl citrate for painful procedures in children. *Pediatrics* 1995;95:335–339.

83. Green SM, Rothrock SG, Harris T, et al. Intravenous ketamine for pediatric sedation in the emergency department: safety profile with 156 cases. *Academic Emergency Medicine* 1998;5:971–976.

84. Kennedy RM, Porter FL, Miller JP. Comparison of fentanyl/midazolam with ketamine/midazolam for pediatric orthopedic emergencies. *Pediatrics* 1998;102:956–963.

85. Havel CJ Jr, Strait RT, Hennes H, et al. A clinical trial of propofol vs midazolam for procedural sedation in a pediatric emergency department. *Academic Emergency Medicine* 1999;6:989–997.

86. Hertzog JH, Dalton HJ, Anderson BD, et al. Prospective evaluation of propofol anesthesia in the pediatric intensive care unit for elective oncology procedures in ambulatory and hospitalized children. *Pediatrics* 2000;106:736–741.

87. Griffin GC, Campbell VD, Jones R. Nitrous oxide-oxygen sedation for minor surgery, experience in a pediatric setting. *JAMA* 1981; 245:2411–2413.

88. Gamis AS, Knapp JF, Glenski JA. Nitrous oxide analgesia in a pediatric emergency department. *Annals of Emergency Medicine* 1989;18: 177–181.

89. Halperin SA, McGrath P, Smith B, et al. Lidocaine-prilocaine patch decreases the pain associated with the subcutaneous administration of measles-mumps-rubella vaccine but does not adversely affect the antibody response. *Pediatrics* 2000;6:789–794.

90. Juarez Gimenez JC, Oliveras M, Hidalgo E, et al. Anesthetic efficacy of eutectic prilocaine-lidocaine cream in pediatric oncology patients undergoing lumbar puncture. *Annals Of Pharmacotherapy* 1996;30: 1235–7.

91. Squire SJ, Kirchhoff KT, Hissong K. Comparing two methods of topical anesthesia used before intravenous cannulation in pediatric patients. *Journal of Pediatric Health Care* 2000;14:68–72.

92. Policy Statement American Academy of Pediatrics. Prevention and management of pain and stress in the neonate. *Pediatrics* 2000;105: 454–461.

93. Taddio A, Stevens B, Craig K, et al. Efficacy and safety of lidocaine-prilocaine cream for pain during circumcision. *New England Journal of Medicine* 1997;336:1197–1200.

94. Franck LS, Gregory GA. Clinical evaluation and treatment of infant pain in the neonatal intensive care unit. In: Schechter NL, Berde, CB and Yaster M, ed. *Pain in infants, children, and adolescents.* Baltimore, Williams and Wilkins. 1993:519–535.

95. Saarenmaa E, Huttunen P, Leppaluoto J, et al. Advantages of fentanyl over morphine in analgesia for ventilated newborn infants after birth: a randomized trial. *Journal of Pediatrics* 1999;134:144–150.

96. Anand KJ, Hickey PR. Halothane-morphine compared with high-dose sufentanil for anesthesia and postoperative analgesia in neonatal cardiac surgery. *New England Journal of Medicine* 1992;326:1–9.

97. Kirya C, Werthmann MW. Neonatal circumcision and penile dorsal nerve block—a painless procedure. *Journal of Pediatrics* 1978; 92:998–1000.

98. Mintz MR, Grillo R. Dorsal penile nerve block for circumcision. *Clinical Pediatrics* 1989;28:590–591.

99. Masciello, AL. Anesthesia for neonatal circumcision: local anesthesia is better than dorsal penile nerve block. *Ostetrics and Gynecology* 1990;75:834–838,.

100. Blass EM, Hoffmeyer LB. Sucrose as an analgesic for newborn infants. *Pediatrics* 1991;87:215–218.

101. Jay S, Elliot C, Ozolins M, et al. Behavioral management of children's distress during painful medical procedures. *Behavioral Research and Therapy* 1985;23:513–520.

102. Manne S, Redd W, Jacobsen P, et al. Behavioral intervention to reduce child and parent distress during venipuncture. *Journal of Consulting and Clinical Psychology* 1990;58:565–572.

103. Jay S, Elliot C, Woody P, Siegel S. An investigation of cognitive-behavioral therapy combined with oral valium for children undergoing painful medical procedures. *Health Psychology* 1991;10: 317–322.

104. Blount R, Powers S, Cotter M, et al. Training pediatric oncology patients to cope and their parents to coach them during BMA/LP procedures. *Behavior Modification* 1994;18:6–31.

105. Powers S, Blount R, Bachanas P, et al. Helping preschool leukemia patients and parents cope during injections. *Journal of Pediatric Psychology* 1993;18:681–695.

106. Jay S, Elliot C, Katz E, Siegel S. Cognitive-behavioral and pharmacologic interventions for children's distress during painful medical procedures in children. *Journal of Consulting and Clinical Psychology* 1987;55:860–865.

107. Smith J, Barabasz A, Barabasz M. Comparison of hypnosis and distraction in severely ill children undergoing painful medical procedures. *Journal of Counseling Psychology* 1996;43:187–195.

108. Siegal LJ. Preparation of children for hospitalization: a selected review of research literature. *Journal of Pediatric Psychology* 1976; 1:26–30.

109. Kellerman J, Zeltzer L, Ellenberg L, Dash J. Hypnosis for the reduction of the acute pain and anxiety associated with medical procedures. *Journal of Adolescent Health Care* 1983;4:85–90.

110. Olness K, Kohen DP. *Hypnosis and hypnotherapy with children,* 3rd ed. New York, Guilford, 1996.

111. Zeltzer L, LeBaron S. Hypnosis and nonhypnotic techniques for reduction of pain and anxiety during painful procedures in children and adolescents with cancer. *Journal of Pediatrics* 1982;101: 1032–1035.

112. Zeltzer LK, Dash J, Holland JP. Hypnotically induced pain control in sickle cell anemia. *Pediatrics* 1979;4:533–536.

113. Cozzi L, Tryon WW, Sedlacek K. The effectiveness of biofeedback-assisted relaxation in modifying sickle cell crisis. *Biofeedback and Self Regulation* 1987;12:51–61.

114. Varni JW. Self-regulation techniques in the management of chronic arthritic pain in hemophilia. *Behavior Therapy* 1981;12:185–194.

115. Walco GA, Ilowite NT. Cognitive-behavioral intervention for juvenile primary fibromyalgia syndrome. *Journal of Rheumatology* 1992; 19:1617–1619.

116. Solomon R, Walco GA, Robinson MR. Pediatric pain management: program description and preliminary evaluation results of a professional course. *Journal of Developmental and Behavioral Pediatrics* 1997;19:193–195.

117. American Academy of Pediatrics, American Pain Society. Policy Statement: The assessment and management of acute pain in infants, children, and adolescents. *Pediatrics* 2001;108:793–797.

118. American Pain Society Task Force on Pain in Children. Policy Statement on Pediatric Chronic Pain. *APS Bulletin,* 2001;11:10–12.

CHAPTER 51

Office and Hospital Pain Consultations

Victor C. Lee

The pain management specialist assists in the treatment of pain problems by providing consultation to physicians and other health-care providers who are involved with medical and surgical care of patients. Pain problems arise in the context of routine medical and surgical care. Pain symptoms must be considered in order to formulate a diagnosis and a plan of treatment. The traditional model of medical practice is based on correctly diagnosing the underlying pathophysiology responsible for the patient's pain symptoms and then treating the pathophysiologic condition in order to relieve the pain. Fortunately, in most cases this medical model achieves its goals: Pathophysiology is identified, and with appropriate treatment there is indeed resolution of pain. When the traditional medical model of diagnosis and treatment fails to alleviate the patient's pain, however, the pain management specialist is called upon. How the pain management specialist goes about providing such consultation is the subject of this chapter.

The pain management specialist offers special expertise in the management of pain problems and the issues surrounding pain problems. Consultation with the pain specialist is required when merely identifying pathophysiology and instituting standard treatments fail to adequately deal with the pain experience and its impact upon the patient. There are several well-appreciated scenarios in which this situation arises:

1. Pathophysiology is identified but is not reversible by standard treatments (e.g., pain of advanced malignancy, diabetic neuropathy, end-stage peripheral vascular disease, sickle cell crises, AIDS, severe rheumatoid arthritis or other connective tissue disorders, etc.). In such situations, chronic persistent pain accompanies chronic progressive illness and remains a significant problem in spite of appropriate medical care.
2. Pain is experienced acutely during institution of standard medical or surgical care (e.g., postsurgical pain).

Although analgesics are prescribed, this pain may respond poorly to routine methods of analgesic administration. In the case of postsurgical care, inadequately treated pain can increase perioperative morbidity when complications such as respiratory impairment or hypertension result from pain.
3. Pain persists in spite of medical or surgical intervention (e.g., postlaminectomy back pain, postsurgical sympathetic dystrophies, and postamputation phantom pain). When surgical interventions have failed to relieve the pain or have worsened the pain, the surgeon will often consult with a pain specialist.
4. The etiology of pain and precise medical diagnosis remain elusive, with standard medical and surgical approaches unable to offer any respite from chronic pain. Examples of this would include patients with back pain, headache pain, or abdominopelvic pain of obscure etiology. Patients with the poorly understood generalized musculoskeletal pain syndrome called *fibromyalgia* would be included in this group. Such patients may have been subjected to numerous diagnostic tests and have been told that nothing is wrong with them. Such patients may be on chronic analgesic medications, with dependency issues. Such patients may also be manifesting maladaptive chronic pain behaviors, depression, and other psychological consequences of unrelieved pain.

The pain consultant plays an important role in assisting with the acute and chronic management of a pain experience that is otherwise inadequately controlled. The pain consultant offers expertise in the following areas: identifying physiological and nonphysiological factors important in sustaining severe pain, instituting specialized interventions to supplement ongoing medical or surgical care, and identifying a plan for managing chronic issues. These are the essential elements of a pain management consultation.

MOST COMMON REASONS FOR INITIATING A PAIN CONSULTATION

Office Consultations

Pain Problems Typically Requiring Consultation

The pain specialist who is consulted in the outpatient setting is dealing in most cases with established chronic pain problems. The pain diagnoses in Table 51-1 comprise a typical mix of musculoskeletal and soft tissue pain, headaches, neuropathic pain, pain of malignancy, and other pain syndromes that are referred for consultation in a multidisciplinary pain management setting. Such patients are referred by a primary treating physician, whether that physician is in general medical practice or is a specialist. The consultation is initiated when the referring physician feels that a pain specialist has something to contribute to the care of the patient that the referring physician is not able to provide. This is not to supplant the role of the primary physician in diagnosing and treating pain. To the contrary, the primary treating physician is indispensable in assuring that a comprehensive and appropriate evaluation of the patient's pain disorder is initiated and that appropriate medical care has been given and consults the pain specialist only when such routine medical care fails to alleviate the pain. This is another way of saying that the pain specialist should not be the first care provider to work with the patient's pain problem and that all such patients should be screened for treatable medical problems prior to being seen by a pain specialist.

How and When a Pain Consultation Is Initiated

As "gate keeper" of medical resources, the primary treating physician determines at what point a patient's pain problem exceeds the conventional domain of medical diagnosis and treatment. The pain specialist should not be consulted prematurely, before appropriate diagnostic studies and routine medical care have been instituted. On the other hand, it is not really desirable to delay a pain consultation. For example, the pain experience may sometimes become unmanageable for the patient during the course of a routine medical workup. This may become manifest as rapid escalation of analgesic medication use or extremely exaggerated pain behaviors during the course of a medical workup, even before all of the tests are completed and a final diagnosis made. It is probably best to consult with a pain specialist earlier than later in these situations. A patient hospitalized for evaluation of a severe pain disorder, for example, may be well served by a consultation with an acute pain service, even though the medical workup is not yet completed. Certain pain behaviors may become entrenched in a patient's behavioral repertoire if allowed to go unaddressed for prolonged periods: Successful intervention in the pain problem may become more difficult to achieve as certain behavioral and emotional consequences of untreated pain impact upon the patient's psyche.

It may also be prudent to consult with pain specialists prior to instituting treatments with irreversible consequences, such as back surgery or neuroablative surgery. The demise of the "low back loser" (1) is a case in point: A patient with back pain undergoes, for better or for worse, lumbar spine surgery that fails to achieve beneficial results and results in worsened pain. The hapless surgeon, not knowing what else to do for the miserable patient, proposes further back surgery, which commences only a downward spiral of worsening pain and dysfunction. Perhaps a pain management consultation, with psychological screening when indicated (2), may help steer some of these patients away from such a demise, especially when more conservative options appear to be indicated as an alternative to such surgery.

Diagnostic and Therapeutic Nerve Blocks

This discussion acknowledges that nerve blocks are frequently requested during the course of a pain consultation and have come to play a role in pain management—either in the diagnosis or the treatment of pain. Often the referring physician desires a nerve block be administered in order to either eradicate the patient's pain or to determine whether the patient's pain is "real." Unfortunately, neither represents a completely realistic role for nerve blocks in the management of pain.

Whether or not a patient's pain may be blocked (i.e., is "blockable") by a regional anesthetic technique has come to mean different things to different care providers. The issue of "blockability" of a particular pain syndrome is a complex one. It is incumbent upon the pain specialist to define to the referring physician the proper role of nerve blocks in the care of the patient. The pain specialist needs to specify whether a nerve block is indicated, whether it is expected to be of long-lasting therapeutic benefit, and whether it would provide any useful diagnostic or prognostic

TABLE 51-1. *Common diagnoses encountered at the Augusta pain management center*

Diagnosis	ICD9 Code
Extremity pain	729.5
Lumbosacral radiculopathy	724.4
Low back pain	724.2
Herniated lumbar disc	722.10
Postlaminectomy syndrome	722.83
Lumbosacral spinal stenosis	724.02
Lumbar strain/sprain	847.2
Lumbar spondyloarthropathy	721.3
Myofascial pain, fibromyalgia	729.1
Cervicalgia	723.1
Headache	784.0
Sacroiliac strain	724.6

information. A particular pain syndrome may have multiple contributing elements, and a specific nerve block may have little or no ability to alleviate all of the elements. The pain consultant should be able to fully convey the reasons for a "failed" nerve block. For example, a sympathetic nerve block may block either the burning pain or the allodynia, but not necessarily both of these elements of reflex sympathetic dystrophy (3) and may not block the accompanying myofascial pain or the joint pain. On the other hand, nerve blocks may "succeed" for unintended reasons. For example, a nerve block may prompt patient reporting of relieved pain for a variety of reasons that may or may not be specific to the underlying mechanisms of the original pain problem, not the least of which is placebo effect. Extreme care must be taken if a positive response to a nerve block is taken to be a positive prognosticator of the outcome of proposed surgery. The nonspecific effects of a local anesthetic nerve block, although seemingly promising, may fail to be duplicated by a followup surgical procedure, much to the disappointment of both patient and surgeon. The intentions of performing diagnostic nerve blocks should be made very clear, and the interpretation of the results of such blocks should be done very carefully. Otherwise, nerve block results not interpreted very thoughtfully serve to create only greater confusion in the care of patients who prove to be far more complex than the paradigm of diagnostic nerve blocking usually allows.

In addition, a more global view of a particular pain problem may reveal that psychosocial and physical rehabilitation issues may predominate for a particular patient and that a focus on nerve blocks as a "curative" intervention may be improperly placed. Nerve blocks should probably be considered adjunctive rather than the primary mode of therapy (which would inappropriately link the success of pain management to the success of the block itself). With reflex sympathetic dystrophy, for example, appropriately administered physical therapy is often the key therapeutic intervention, with nerve blocks being given largely to control symptoms and to assist with the physical therapy (4). Finally, if any progress is to be made with patients suffering from chronic pain, it is important not to invalidate a patient's claim of pain; hence, nerve blocks should never be used as a "litmus test" to discriminate "real" pain from psychogenic or surreptitious pain.

Medication Issues

Patients are often referred for pain management consultation when treatment of chronic pain with opioid analgesics has become an issue. It is certainly a highly desirable goal to have a patient's chronic pain managed without the use of dependency-producing medications. The pain consultant must therefore be able to suggest or provide the means for decreasing the dependence on such medications and, indeed, the means for decreasing the patient's dependence on costly medical resources in general. On the other hand, it is an equally important role of the pain specialist to determine when the use of chronic opioid medication is, in fact, an appropriate option.

The use of opioid medication to treat chronic pain problems of nonmalignant origin is problematic for a number of reasons, not the least of which is controversy within the medical community itself (5). The lack of efficacy of opioid medications in certain types of chronic pain problems (6), the development of opioid tolerance, illicit drug diversion, dose escalation, and drug dependence all become issues when opioid medications are used chronically. On the other hand, the physician's fear of being audited for opioid prescribing practices that can lead to suspension of license or other penalties often leads to arbitrary limitations and the underprescribing of opioids. Sadly, there are physicians who underprescribe opioid medication even when such medications are highly appropriate (e.g., the treatment of cancer pain). Many patients referred to a pain specialist with chronic nonmalignant pain have already been receiving opioid analgesics for years with unsatisfactory consequences. This is not to reject the notion that certain carefully selected patients with chronic nonmalignant pain may benefit from chronic opioid medication. However, certain patients seem to develop only worsening pain and pain-related issues when they come to depend on opioids chronically for management of pain. Whether or not a given patient should be prescribed chronic opioid medication is not a simple question to answer, and the pain specialist must be willing to take the time and effort to lead the patient as well as the referring physician through the maze of complex issues.

Psychological Issues

When the primary care physician or specialist colleague is confounded by a patient with seemingly enigmatic pain, the question often arises: Is the patient's pain "real," or is it "psychological" in origin? Often the object of a pain management consultation is to shed light on this very question. Although most patients present a spectrum of degrees of somatic or nociceptive contributing factors as well as psychoemotive contributing factors, the notion of a dichotomy between "real" and "imagined" serves no useful purpose in pain management. In fact, such a diagnostic dichotomy only inflames the relationship between the physician and patient. The physician would logically conclude that the patient with "psychological pain" is making the whole thing up and is not to be trusted. On the other hand, the patient or the patient's family spreads the word that the physician either doesn't have enough medical knowledge to correctly diagnose the problem or simply doesn't care. In the end, nobody benefits.

The most useful approach, with regard to management of psychological issues in the pain patient, is to identify which factors may play a role in creating or sustaining chronic pain expressions and behaviors rather than to distinguish between psychogenic pain and "genuine" somatic pain. Consultation with a pain psychologist will often lead to counseling or training in such techniques as biofeedback and self-relaxation. When a pain psychologist works hand-in-hand with the patient's pain management physician as well as the patient's primary physician, a strong therapeutic relationship develops along the lines of a team, or interdisciplinary, approach. Such an interdisciplinary approach is likely to have more of an impact upon the patient's pain problems than will seeing disconnected multiple providers who communicate minimally with each other.

Back to Work and Disability Issues

Another frequently encountered question posed to the practitioner involved in the management of a chronic pain problem is, "When will the patient be able to return to work?" It is a complex issue that embodies many questions:

1. To what extent is the patient's physical functioning limited by pathophysiology? By pain? By both?
2. Is improvement expected with treatment or rehabilitation? When is maximal improvement (MMI) expected?
3. Will there be some residual functional impairment that would prevent the patient from resuming his or her original work duties?
4. If unable to resume original duties, what sort of work can the patient be expected to perform?
5. When will a treatment course be completed (i.e., when is MMI achieved), and what maintenance therapy may be needed after this?
6. If there is to be a permanent disability, what is the extent of this disability?

These questions are familiar enough to any health practitioner who has worked with the work-injured patient, regardless of whether there is an ongoing pain problem. And yet they are often the most difficult questions to answer, particularly when there is a significant limitation imposed by pain alone, in absence of "hard" pathophysiology. For example, an orthopedist may be able to quantify the limitations imposed by specific musculoskeletal or neuromuscular lesions. It is relatively straightforward to assign impairment based on, say, a C-5 spinal cord transection. On the other hand, chronic pain itself may impose functional limitations even when it is not possible to demonstrate a specific lesion or pathophysiology leading to a quantifiable impairment. In such a situation it becomes necessary to obtain an opinion from a pain specialist regarding the limitations imposed by pain itself upon the patient. Although this is an area of medical determination fraught with ambiguity and inadequacy (7), increas-

ing demands are being placed upon the pain specialist to render an opinion regarding the impact of pain upon the patient's ability to work. A pain consultant can expect to be confronted by such questions during the course of a clinical pain practice and must be able to formulate some kind of satisfactory response to such questions.

Hospital Consultations

The patient may be suffering from pain that is directly related to his being hospitalized or that is coincidental with the hospitalization. The emergence of hospital-based acute pain management services is increasing the availability of pain specialists to assist with pain problems encountered in the hospital setting and to respond to such problems in a timely fashion.

Postsurgical Pain Management

The management of acute pain problems in the hospital setting is best exemplified by the recent emphasis on the treatment of acute postoperative pain, motivating the 1992 release of the guidelines for acute pain management by the Agency for Health Care Policy and Research, Public Health Service, U.S. Department of Health and Human Services (8). The pain experienced following surgery often exceeds treatment by conventional analgesic regimens and poses special problems in certain situations (i.e., systemic opioids administered to ventilator-dependent patients may delay or prevent weaning from mechanical ventilation). Consultation with a pain management specialist (such as an anesthesiologist) possessing expertise in managing pharmacological techniques such as continuous opioid infusions, patient-controlled analgesic regimens, perispinal opioid analgesia, and continuous local anesthetic infusions may be extremely beneficial for the surgical patient. Nonpharmacological techniques such as transcutaneous electrical nerve stimulation (TENS) may be helpful. Increasing use is being made of alternative and complementary medicine in the management of postsurgical pain. Such techniques might include audio recordings of music, guided imagery for distraction or relaxation, hypnotherapy, massage therapy, and acupuncture. The pain specialist should be aware of such resources that may be available locally and know which of these resources, if any, may be appropriate for a given patient.

Other Hospital-based Pain Problems

Besides postsurgical pain, a variety of other scenarios may prompt a hospital consultation for pain management services. Such scenarios may include the following: acute escalation of cancer pain, management of burn pain, trauma pain, pain of sickle cell crisis, pain of acute pancreatitis, intractable headache pain, and pain crises experienced during the workup of acute musculoskeletal, abdominopelvic, or neurovascular pain. A hospitalized patient may require management of a coexisting chronic pain problem (e.g., low back pain) during the course of hospitalization for an unrelated ailment. Occasionally, a patient who chronically receives opioid medication may require special medical management during the course of a hospitalization, necessitating specific advice regarding concurrent analgesic pharmacotherapy.

RESPONDING APPROPRIATELY TO A PAIN CONSULTATION

Providing Answers to the Questions

Responding appropriately to a pain consultation demands an appreciation of what questions are being asked by the referring physician. It is important to appreciate the original course of diagnostic workup and treatment of the patient, and a mechanism for receiving this information from the referring physician is imperative. Professional acknowledgment of the referring physician's interventions is essential in a continuum of care. Although the consulted pain specialist may formulate an alternative hypothesis for the nature of the patient's pain complaints, the original questions raised by the referring physician should be addressed in a satisfactory manner. For example, a patient referred for conservative management of lumbar radiculopathy and epidural steroid injections may be found by the consulted pain specialist to be manifesting a myofascial pain syndrome, which is not likely to respond to such epidural injections. Perhaps a patient has been referred for evaluation of a suspected reflex sympathetic dystrophy and treatment by sympathetic nerve blocks; but the pain specialist instead determines that the patient's pain, although it may bear neuropathic features, is not a sympathetically maintained pain syndrome and therefore not likely to respond to sympathetic nerve blocks. Reasons for reformulating the working pain hypothesis must be detailed in a thorough and professional manner, including a courteous and thoughtful explanation of why the pain consultant has chosen not to implement the treatment requested by the referring physician. Such an explanation should educate the referring physician to the perspective of the pain specialist but at the same time not be so patronizing as to discourage further referrals. Alternative approaches for managing the pain problem should be outlined in detail.

Communicating with the Patient

Perhaps the most crucial element to successful intervention in a pain problem is communication with the patient. Often the greatest strides in pain intervention are made when the nature of the pain problem itself is explained to the patient. In a highly technical and impersonal age of medical practice, the patient is most often left in the dark

after a battery of tests turns out negative and the patient is never presented with the negative results or what it means to have negative test results. The patient is left to brood upon what is "wrong" with his or her body, why the pain persists, why no more tests have been ordered, why multiple specialists have failed to provide answers, and why a "pain specialist" is being consulted. The primary referring physician may not have taken the time to discuss these issues with the patient. Patients are often never called when test results are negative and have no way of knowing if the test really showed anything, whether the test was adequate, or if the doctor simply forgot about the patients.

First of all, the intentions of the referring physician should be explained to the patient, if this has not already been done. The patient may already have perceptions, rightly or wrongly, verified or unverified, about what is causing his or her pain. Before a successful plan of intervention can be instituted, the patient must be convinced that a thorough and systematic evaluation of treatable pathophysiology has been conducted. Patients are unlikely to become invested in a program of pain management if they feel that something about their body is still "wrong." Dissatisfied patients often feel that a pathologic process has been overlooked and that all this business about pain management and "dealing with pain" is simply a diversion from getting the real problem "fixed." Patients are not likely to trust a pain consultant who is not in touch with all aspects of the original diagnostic workup (e.g., "Did you also get to see my x-rays, Doctor?"). The following elements constitute an essential beginning in initiating a relationship between a pain specialist and a patient: effective communication with the patient concerning the development and rationale of the medical workup, the nature of the pain problem, whether acute or chronic, the reasons for initiating a consultation with a pain specialist, and the role of the pain specialist in the ongoing medical care.

The nature of chronic pain is often the most difficult concept for a patient to grasp. The patient may become distrustful of a medical system that simply doesn't know how to fix the problem. When a pain specialist is consulted, sometimes the patient may feel "written off," or worse, think that the care providers believe the pain to be imaginary. On the other hand, the patient may view the pain consultant as the ultimate rescuer who will eliminate the pain that has caused immeasurable suffering for many years. Not only must the patient be educated in the nature of chronic pain, but also a realistic picture of the goals of pain management must be painted. Acceptance by the patient of the diagnosis of "chronic pain" is the first, and often most difficult, step. After acceptance by the patient is achieved, a set of realistic goals should be spelled out in great detail for the patient, e.g., decreasing medications, increasing activity, increasing tolerance for pain, normalizing sleep patterns, etc. Table 51-2 summarizes therapeutic goals embraced by the Augusta Pain Management Center in Fishersville, Virginia. The pain specialist should never

TABLE 51-2. *Primary objectives of the Augusta pain management center*

1. Formulate a diagnostic and treatment framework in which patients may interface with appropriate medical, surgical, allied health care, and complementary treatment resources appropriate to the management of their pain problem.
2. Reduce pain intensity as practicable by means deemed appropriate by the care standards established within the pain management specialty.
3. Return patients to the highest level of functional status possible, given the limitations of their particular pathophysiology and the limitations of medical treatment.
4. Promote patients' ability to deal with and manage their pain independently, reducing dependence on often costly medical resources to the extent that is possible (e.g., reduction of dependence on excessive drug therapy or repeated visits to physician's offices or emergency departments).

promise total elimination of pain because it is impossible to guarantee such a result to the patient and likely to leave the patient very disappointed when such a goal is not achieved.

Reasons for Unsatisfactory Pain Consultations

The pain consultant does not practice in a vacuum; rather, the pain consultant works within a network of primary and specialty physicians who are reliant upon each other for effective management of particularly difficult cases. The multidisciplinary, or interdisciplinary, model of pain management is built upon the premise that no single specialist possesses all of the tools that may be necessary for the effective management of difficult cases of chronic pain. The consultant in pain medicine must necessarily rely upon primary physicians for referrals and must also have the appropriate resources for invoking treatments that may be outside of his or her own particular discipline (e.g., physiatrist, neurologist, psychologist, anesthesiologist, neurosurgeon, etc.). Such a consultant must know how to network effectively within a referral base as well as with allied and complementary disciplines in pain management in order to serve the patient well.

Unsatisfactory pain consultations often occur as a result of inadequate communication. The referring physician may feel that inadequate answers have been provided to the pain issues at hand or that inadequate followup in the form of ongoing pain management has been provided. For example, the pain specialist may have performed a nerve block that provided no relief or only temporary relief; the referring physician still expects the pain specialist to try to shed light on the reasons for persistent pain and to assist in providing care for the patient. Pain specialists who simply do procedures, whether or not the results are successful, and then provide no followup care are likely to be judged as unsatisfactory pain management consultants. Inadequate communication between the pain special-

ist and the patient is also problematic. The patient may feel that his or her questions about what is causing the pain have not been adequately addressed or that too many ongoing care issues have been left up in the air and that nobody is really taking care of the patient. For example, the pain specialist may have indicated during the course of consultation that it is appropriate for the patient to receive chronic opioid therapy. The patient becomes very confused and frustrated when he or she returns to the referring physician, who then tells the patient to get these prescriptions from the pain specialist, but then the pain specialist tells the patient that the referring physician is responsible for these prescriptions.

Ineffective networking also accounts for many pain consultations that are perceived as unsatisfactory. Effective networking requires effective professional conduct at both ends of a consultative relationship, involving both referring physician and consulted pain specialist. The referring physician has the responsibility of assuring that a complete picture of the patient is conveyed to the pain specialist, including full medical records and summaries, and the reasons for seeking a pain management consultation. The referring physician must make it clear what questions are to be answered by the pain specialist and what services are sought. The pain specialist must also assure that specific questions raised by the referring physician are answered in a satisfactory manner, as discussed in the previous sections. The referring physician's original working hypothesis for the patient's pain problem must be acknowledged in a professional way, even though this hypothesis may change during the course of a pain management consultation. The pain specialist is also obliged to facilitate networking with other allied pain management disciplines that will support the management of a particular patient's case (for example, referral to a physical therapist for a functional capacity evaluation in a work-injury case). The inability of the pain specialist to facilitate such a connection in a prompt and professional manner is likely to be viewed as ineffective networking.

It must also be worked out in advance which followup issues will be handled by the consulted pain specialist and which followup issues will be directed back to the referring physician. Such followup issues would include who is responsible for medication prescriptions, subsequent diagnostic studies, additional specialty referrals, and disability reports. If the pain specialist is unprepared to deal with all of these issues, the referring physician needs to be so informed. Inattention to such issues results in inadequate followup, which is frustrating for both referring physician and patient.

Without effective networking and communication regarding these matters, the patient is likely to "fall through the cracks," to be "left hanging," or to be "lost to followup." The pain consultant may begin to see fewer consultations directed to his or her practice. Inadequate communication, inadequate networking, and inadequate followup will likely result in unsatisfactory pain management consultations.

PROVIDING SERVICE: *CPT* CODES AND WHAT THEY REPRESENT

In order to establish uniform guidelines for providing and billing for medical and surgical services, the American Medical Association has established the *Current Procedural Terminology* (*CPT*) handbook, which is by now familiar to most physicians. Medical reimbursement has become a quite complex science of its own, and changes in reimbursement practices occur practically on a monthly basis. The following section contains suggestions for how pain consultation services may be provided within the structure defined by the AMA's *CPT 2000* codes (9).

The following section deals with services provided by a pain consultant. Whenever consultations and procedures are performed, they must be rendered in conjunction with a medical diagnosis. Most medical reimbursement of services is based upon standardized diagnostic terminology as provided by the ICD9 listings (10); Tables 51-3 and 51-4 illustrate typical primary and secondary diagnoses utilized by pain consultants.

The crucial elements in office and hospital consultations are "history," "physical exam," and "medical decision making," which are graded as to level of complexity by descriptors provided in the *CPT* handbook (Table 51-5). In order for a consultation to merit reimbursement, it must contain all three of these elements and provide adequate documentation. In the subsequent discussion, suggestions are provided for how to structure a pain consultation along these guidelines. These are suggestions only and not intended to be all-inclusive or exclusive of any tools that may be utilized by the great spectrum of clinician specialists who are pain consultants.

History: History taking by a pain consultant should discuss elements of the pain complaint itself, i.e., precipitating events, exacerbating factors, pain intensity (often quantified by numeric scale), sensory qualities of the pain (e.g., dull, sharp, burning, shooting), and spatiotemporal aspects of the pain complaint (including day-to-day variations). The patient should be asked about his medical

TABLE 51-3. *Pain diagnoses by location (typically used as primary diagnoses)*

Diagnosis	ICD9 code
Head or face	784.0
Abdomen	789.0
Any extremity	729.5
Back (lumbar)	724.2
Chest (central)	786.50
Neck	723.1
Shoulder	719.41
Muscle	729.1

TABLE 51-4. *Pain diagnoses by presumed etiology (typically used as secondary diagnoses)*

	ICD9 code
Low back pain	
Lumbar strain/sprain	847.2
Sacroiliac strain/sprain	846.1
Arachnoiditis	349.2
Postlaminectomy syndrome	722.83
Lumbar stenosis	724.02
Lumbar disc herniation	722.10
Lumbosacral radiculopathy	724.4
Lumbar spondyloarthropathy	721.3
Cervical pain	
Cervical strain/sprain	847.0
Cervical radiculopathy	723.4
Postural neck pain	723.9
Herniated cervical disc	722.0
Postlaminectomy syndrome	722.81
Neuropathic pain diagnoses	
Carpal tunnel syndrome	354.0
Causalgia, upper extremity	354.4
Reflex sympathetic dystrophy, upper extremity	337.21
Phantom limb syndrome	353.6
Intercostal neuralgia	353.8
Myofascial pain diagnoses	
Myofascial pain or fibromyalgia	729.1
Muscle wasting, atrophy, disuse	728.2
Muscle spasm	728.85

workup, what has or has not alleviated the pain, the impact of the pain upon work and pleasure activities, social and family relations, and, perhaps most important of all, the perception the patient has concerning his pain problem. Based on how many of these elements are evaluated, the level of history taking is rated as "problem focused," "expanded problem focused," "detailed," or "comprehensive" (Table 51-5). Most initial office consultations should be conducted at the "detailed" and "comprehensive" levels, and most initial hospital consultations should be conducted at the "expanded problem focused" and "detailed" levels. As mentioned, documentation must be provided.

Examination: Most examinations conducted by pain specialists focus initially on painful body regions; evaluation of tenderness and limitations in range of motion and motor effort by pain; and alterations in the integument, including edema, temperature, and trophic changes. Evaluation of trigger points is also included in such an examination ("problem focused"). The examination is expanded ("expanded problem focused") when a neurologic exam is performed to evaluate sensory, motor, and reflex functions. Pain syndromes producing perceived sensory alterations should prompt a "detailed" sensory examination: Qualities of sensation such as allodynia, mechanical and thermal hyperalgesia, and hyperpathia should be reported in

TABLE 51-5. *Office and hospital consultations and their corresponding CPT codes*

CPT code	History and physical exam	Medical decision-making complexity	Suggested times
New or established office consultations			
99241	problem focused	straightforward	15 minutes
99242	expanded	straightforward	30 minutes
99243	detailed	low complexity	40 minutes
99244	comprehensive	moderate complexity	60 minutes
99245	comprehensive	high complexity	80 minutes
Initial hospital consultations			
99251	problem focused	straightforward	20 minutes
99252	expanded	straightforward	40 minutes
99253	detailed	low complexity	55 minutes
99254	comprehensive	moderate complexity	80 minutes
99255	comprehensive	high complexity	110 minutes

Refer to the AMA's *Current Procedural Terminology* for definitions of the above descriptors. All consultations should provide documentation of history taking, physical examination, and medical decision making. The suggested times are for comparison purposes only and should not be used as a basis for establishing a level of consultation.

addition to the basic sensory modalities of pinprick, thermal, vibratory, etc. The terminology used to describe pain-associated sensory alterations is defined in the International Association for the Study of Pain's published listing of pain terminology (11). Any report of headache, dizziness, altered special senses, or altered mentation should prompt an evaluation of the cranial nerves. A "comprehensive" examination may possibly involve detailed kinetic and functional examinations in addition to the preceding.

Medical decision making: The clinician should probably take care to provide a level of decision making that is commensurate with the amount of work put into her history and physical examination. The AMA descriptors of complexity of medical decision making are "straightforward," "low complexity," "moderate complexity," and "high complexity." A recommendation of "continue present therapy and send patient back to me for followup in a month" is not likely to rate a very high level of medical decision making, regardless of how many trigger points were examined or how many sensory modalities were tested.

The pain consultant's suggestions should, of course, incorporate a rationale and a plan of action based on a working pain hypothesis that would be presented in his or her "impressions" or "assessment" statement. This assessment should acknowledge that the referring physician has indeed performed a complete medical evaluation and provided correct medical care. Otherwise, if the pain consultant suspects that further workup is needed, this should be made clear in his or her recommendations for further evaluations and diagnostic workup. As stated before, pain consultants do occasionally find previously undetected pathology such as malignancy, thus reverting the case back to a

traditional medical model at least until the pathology can be adequately worked up and correct treatment initiated.

The consultant's recommendations should address the patient's pharmacotherapy: continuing or discontinuing medications, instituting a different medical regimen, etc. If pharmacological adjuncts (e.g., antidepressants, anticonvulsants, skeletal muscle relaxants) are recommended, guidelines concerning medication selection, dosing, and projected duration of therapy should be provided. If the pain consultant disagrees with the use of opioid or sedative-tranquilizer medications, this should be indicated and the reasons provided. If a drug withdrawal program is advised, the consultant should provide detailed guidelines concerning how this should be done and how pain escalation should be dealt with if this occurs during detoxification. If the pain consultant agrees that some level of drug maintenance is indicated or that alternative pharmacotherapy should be tried, then guidelines for this should also be provided.

The need for specialized interventions such as nerve blocks, stimulation techniques, physical therapy training and modalities, diet counseling, psychological counseling, and self-regulation techniques should be addressed if these are indicated (examples of *CPT* codes for some of these interventions appear in Table 51-6). The means for implementing such interventions (i.e., what other referrals are needed) should be described as well, if the consultant is not in a position to provide all of the services proposed. Pain specialists are occasionally consulted regarding advisability of performing surgery, and a discussion and recommendations should be provided if this is the case. Finally, the consultant should provide some guidelines concerning followup care and what kind of response and long-term prognosis is projected, recognizing that this is fraught with some uncertainty and usually subject to change. Such guidelines should address such issues as ability to return to

TABLE 51-6. *Examples of pain management procedural CPT codes*

	CPT code
Injection procedures	
Trigger point injections	20550
Epidural block	62311
Other peripheral nerve block	64450
Physical therapy procedures	
Physical performance test	97750
Therapeutic exercise	97110
Functional activities	97530
TENS application	97014
Psychological services	
Psychological evaluation	90801
Psychotherapy 20–30 minutes	90804
Psychotherapy 45–50 minutes	90806
Psychotherapy 75–80 minutes	90808
Biofeedback training	90901

work, need for psychological or marital counseling, need for vocational rehabilitation, and the possibility of persistent functional impairment due to pain. Provision of most of the preceding elements in a pain consultation is likely to merit a level of "high complexity" of medical decision making, and anything less should be scaled down accordingly.

SUMMARY

Pain consultation services are playing an increasingly important role in modern medical practice. Pain specialists provide special expertise in the management of patients for whom routine medical diagnosis and treatment (the traditional medical model) have failed to adequately deal with the experience of pain and the consequences of that pain. It is still incumbent upon the referring physician to provide a thorough medical evaluation and appropriate medical care prior to consulting with a pain specialist. However, if the pain experience becomes unmanageable during the course of a medical workup it is probably better to consult with a pain specialist sooner than later.

Pain consultations are initiated when the patient's pain defies usual medical diagnostic and treatment approaches. Such pain problems can include acute as well as chronic pain problems, and the pain specialist is often requested to provide specialized pain interventions that may help decrease the patient's pain, reduce the need for opioid pain medications, and help restore the patient to a functioning existence. Whereas most office pain consultations deal with chronic and subacute pain problems, hospital pain consultations deal in acute pain issues such as traumatic or postsurgical pain and intercurrent chronic pain problems or medication issues that may be coincidental to the primary reasons for hospitalization.

The pain specialist should be able to review and acknowledge the patient's ongoing medical workup and treatment and respond to specific questions raised by the referring physician. The consultation should be circumspect in its scope and specific with regard to the actual recommendations made. If interventions outside of the pain specialist's actual discipline or practice base are recommended, the consultant should provide specific instructions regarding the implementation of such interventions.

Adequate communication should effectively link the pain consultant with the patient, referring physician, and associated specialists in the allied and complementary disciplines. The most common causes for unsatisfactory pain consultations are inadequate communication, inadequate networking, and inadequate followup.

Pain consultation services can be structured within the AMA's *CPT* guidelines. Consultations must provide three elements: history, physical examination, and medical decision making. Descriptors for levels of detail or complexity of each of these elements are also found in the AMA guidelines. Reimbursement for different levels of consultation services will require adequate documentation of care in most cases.

REFERENCES

1. Sternbach RA, Wolf SR, Murphy RW, Akeson WH. Traits of pain patients: the low-back "loser." *Psychosomatics* 1973;14:226–229.
2. Pondaag W, Oostdam EMM. Predicting the outcome of lumbar disc surgery by means of preoperative psychological testing. In: Bonica JJ, Liebeskind JC, Albe-Fessard DG, eds. *Advances in pain research and therapy*. New York: Raven Press, 1979;3:713–717.
3. Lee VC. When sympathectomy fails to relieve causalgic burning pain. *Anesth Analg* 1990;71:313–314.
4. Bonica JJ. Causalgia and other reflex sympathetic dystrophies. In: Bonica JJ, ed.: *The management of pain*, 2nd ed. Philadelphia: Lea & Febiger, 1990;1:220–243.
5. Portenoy RK. Chronic opioid therapy in nonmalignant pain. *J Pain Symptom Manage* 1990;5(1S):S46–S62.
6. Arner S, Meyerson BA. Lack of analgesic effect of opioids on neuropathic and idiopathic forms of pain. *Pain* 1988;33:11–23.
7. Osterweis M, Kleinman A, Mechanic D, eds. *Pain and disability: clinical, behavioral, and public policy perspectives*. Washington, DC: National Academy Press, 1987:211–231.
8. Acute Pain Management Guideline Panel. *Acute pain management: operative or medical procedures and trauma*, AHCPR Publication No. 92-0032. Rockville, MD, Agency for Health Care Policy and Research, Public Health Service, U.S. Dept. Health and Human Services, 1992.
9. Gordy TR, AMA CPT Editorial Panel. *CPT 2000, physician's current procedural terminology, standard edition*. Chicago: American Medical Association, 1999.
10. Baierschmidt C, Ericson B, Miller A, et al. *ICD-9-CM, International classification of diseases, 9th revision, clinical modification*, 5th ed., Salt Lake City, UT: Medicode Inc., 1998.
11. Merskey H, Bogduk N. Pain Task Force on Taxonomy of the International Association for the Study of Pain. *Classification of chronic pain, descriptions of chronic pain syndromes and definitions of pain terms*, 2nd ed., Seattle: IASP Press, 1994.

CHAPTER **52**

Outpatient Rehabilitation Programs for Patients with Chronic Pain

Stanley L. Chapman

Pain has been defined by the International Association for the Study of Pain (1) as "an unpleasant sensory and emotional experience, primarily associated with tissue damage, defined in terms of such damage or both . . ." This definition is important in defining pain as an experience and therefore subjective and intimate to the sufferer. It also calls attention to the involvement of both the senses and the emotions. The role of emotions and attitudes becomes especially important in chronic pain, which often requires different treatments from acute pain. The word *chronic* comes from the Greek *kronos* meaning "time," and the term is usually reserved for pain that outlasts the healing period of 3–6 months following an accident, injury, or disease. "Acute" pain, on the other hand, is of recent onset. With acute pain, the role of the health professional consists largely of evaluating and treating the cause(s) of the painful condition while keeping the patient as comfortable as possible until the condition reverses through treatment or the passage of time. Most commonly, patients resume normal function without psychosocial or interdisciplinary treatment.

Medical evidence to account for the presence of pain and associated dysfunction is more often weak or ambiguous in chronic than in acute pain (2). Flor and Turk's (3) review found that even in cases in which medical conditions assumed to be the cause of pain can be identified, they often bear little relationship to the level of pain and dysfunction reported. The medical conditions reviewed included inflammatory processes, degenerative processes (such as disc herniation and osteoarthritis), structural problems (such as postural abnormalities and spinal deformities), the extent of traumatic injury, and muscular and ligamentous dysfunction.

COST OF PAIN

Pain is very costly. Frymoyer and Durett (4) estimated in 1997 that back pain in the United States cost $33.6 billion for medical payments, $11–$43 billion for disability compensation, $4.6 billion for lost productivity, and $5 billion in legal services. The bulk of these costs came from a relatively small percentage of individuals. A small number of patients create a very disproportionate amount of this cost. A massive study across many years that evaluated costs of pain in Quebec revealed that 7.4% of injured workers accounted for 75.6% of medical and compensation costs (5), and a similar cost analysis from the Boeing plant revealed that 10% of injured workers accounted for 79% of such costs (6). Of course, any financial accounting of the costs of pain cannot include the emotional costs involved to the sufferer and his or her family.

EVOLUTION OF COMPREHENSIVE REHABILITATION PROGRAMS

Awareness of such costs of pain has given impetus to the development of treatments for chronic pain; however, chronic pain was hardly even recognized as an entity until 1953, when John Bonica (7) published a landmark text, *The Management of Pain.* This book identified chronic pain as an entity distinct from acute pain, with its own set of characteristics and treatment needs. Melzack and Wall (8) published in 1965 the influential "gate theory of pain," which holds that pain not only is influenced by physiological events occurring in the body, but also is intimately linked to the functioning of the central nervous system, which can open or close the "gate" that influences its experience and perception. Their work showed pain to be a complex interaction of physical, emotional, and behavioral events.

In 1976, Wilbert Fordyce (9) published *Behavioral Methods for Chronic Pain and Illness,* which posited that many of the behaviors found in patients with chronic pain (such as verbally and nonverbally expressing pain, remaining inactive and unemployed, and taking medications) are conditioned not only by the presence of pain and/or medical problems, but also by responses to these behaviors in the patients' environment. He and other behavioral psychologists demonstrated that these behaviors could be changed with treatment designed to alter such responses in the absence of any medical treatment to alter the underlying painful condition (9).

These data and writings played a major role in the establishment of comprehensive interdisciplinary rehabilitation programs for patients with chronic pain. Because many patients' pain and associated dysfunction are related to so many factors, it became clear that a health professional with training only in one discipline was inadequate to treat them. Furthermore, if pain could not be related clearly to medical findings, alteration of one's medical condition could hardly be expected by itself to alleviate pain. Multidisciplinary pain centers (MPCs) thus were established to address many of the factors found to influence pain and dysfunction. These centers, which became prevalent in the 1970s, were based largely on the work of Fordyce and other behavioral psychologists. They employed strict behavioral principles designed to replace pain-related behaviors with alternative health behaviors. Patients thus were guided not to talk about their pain and had to meet gradually more rigorous quotas for increasing physical activities, working toward vocational goals, and tapering use of habit-forming medications to zero. Families and other members of the patient's support system were trained to reinforce more normalized and healthy function rather than to reward pain and inactivity with sympathy or attention. The nature and length of treatment often were highly structured, if not predetermined. Most patients were seen as inpatients, and programs averaged 3–6 weeks in length.

The nature and duration of such programs gradually changed over time. Explosions in the cost of health care gave rise to efforts to cut costs, and data failed to show that inpatient treatment was required over less costly outpatient approaches to produce favorable outcomes (10,11). Moreover, the strict behavioral approach employed in the 1970s gradually was modified in several ways. Treatment began to focus on cognitions (beliefs, attitudes, and self-statements) as researchers found that patients benefited from learning and applying adaptive cognitions in controlling pain and related problems (12,13).

In addition, the concept that treatment of pain itself should not be a major focus within rehabilitation was altered. Treatments that alleviated pain directly, such as medications and stimulation methods, became increasingly integrated with therapies designed to teach the individual skills leading to better self-control of pain and function. The prescription of opioid medication, which earlier had been viewed as antithetical to rehabilitation, gradually became viewed as a possible tool to enhance function.

The proper role of such medication for patients with chronic pain remains a hot topic of controversy today. Some experts have cited data and argued that such medication can effectively relieve pain for many subjects, with minimal risk of tolerance or addiction and a very low frequency of patient abuse (14,15). Others have cited limitations and dangers of opioid use, such as low levels of benefit, increased depression, impaired neuropsychological function, and a medication-centered lifestyle (16,17).

CURRENT STATUS OF MPC PROGRAMS

After a period of very rapid growth from the 1970s through the mid-1990s, comprehensive rehabilitation programs are no longer growing in number and may even be in decline. From early 1999 to 2000, the number of inpatient or intensive (defined as requiring 25 hours of treatment per week or more) outpatient chronic pain management programs accredited by the Commission on Accreditation of Rehabilitation Facilities (CARF) actually decreased from 122 to 113. Concurrent with this decrease has been the increasing use of procedural interventions and medication, which receive a great deal of support from medical technology and pharmaceutical companies.

Much of this apparent decline appears related to the rules and policies related to managed care insurance. This insurance places an emphasis on treatment from primary-care physicians and uses specialists primarily as consultants rather than as providers. Many primary-care providers, who are gatekeepers for treatment, have limited awareness of rehabilitation approaches. An additional hurdle for financing MPC treatment is the fact that insurance companies frequently have separate divisions for approval of physical and mental-health components, which require a facility to make application for both. Furthermore, one or more professionals staffing an MPC may not be on the approved list of providers, and companies generally are not organized to approve a package of treatments. A cohesive structured program cannot be designed if some patients are given approval for 6 group visits or 6 physical therapy sessions when the program structure calls for 15, and others are approved only for individual and not group psychological therapy. In many cases, authorization is given for a very limited number of sessions, with an "offer" that more visits can be applied for after lengthy documentation of patient progress and continuing need. This offer effectively negates a rehabilitation program that requires advanced planning and continuity. Moreover, virtually no plans cover housing for patients who live too far from a center for driving.

Owing partly to these problems, many MPCs had treated primarily patients with worker's compensation insurance, but even that insurance plan has become more hostile to financing MPC programs. The situation varies among states, each of which has its own policies regarding worker's compensation; however, the trend is for less liberal payments to care providers, with some states reducing payments to be equivalent to Medicare. Another trend is toward limitation of the term of liability for insurers, creating reduced incentive for them to value the long-term benefits and cost savings that characterize rehabilitation. The availability of Social Security disability income for patients also provides an incentive for them to settle quickly with the worker's compensation insurer, offering still another reason for the latter to focus on short-term rather than long-term results.

EVALUATION OF PATIENTS FOR INCLUSION IN MPC PROGRAMS

There are literally millions of patients who have chronic pain but are not candidates for comprehensive chronic pain rehabilitation. Most chronic pain sufferers are able to cope with their medical conditions through fairly simple means, such as taking antiinflammatory medication or a pain reliever when the condition flares up. MPCs are specifically designed to treat those who have what CARF characterizes as "chronic pain syndrome," identifiable by the following four criteria: enduring pain, pain different from premorbid status, lack of response to previous appropriate medical and/or surgical treatment, and interference with physical, psychological, social, and/or vocational functioning (18). Generally speaking, MPCs treat patients for whom the duration of pain has outlasted the normal healing period following an injury. Morse (19) coined the term "Disease of the *D*s" to describe the problems of patients who are likely to require MPC treatment. The "*D*s" described by Morse include display of pain, reliance on doctors and drugs, physical disuse, depression, disability, and dependency. To this list could be added physical deconditioning, disharmony in relationships, demoralization, and many dollars of previous health-care costs. Generally, the more *D*s that are present, the more likely it is that the patient needs MPC treatment.

Psychometric Testing

Psychometric testing has the advantage of providing standardized information about a patient that allows comparison of that patient's responses to those of the normative sample of the test battery. Though test results can be biased by the way in which directions are given or how the patient perceives the test-taking situation, they are less likely to depend on the personality or presentation of another person than are results gathered from an interview. In addition, some patients may be more willing to

disclose information on a written form than to discuss it with a professional.

Multidimensional Pain Inventory

A variety of psychometric instruments are available to evaluate the candidacy of a patient for MPC programs. One of the best designed is the Multidimensional Pain Inventory (MPI), devised by Kerns, Turk, and Rudy (20). This test includes 61 items, each scored on a 0 to 6 scale, requiring about 15 to 20 minutes for the average patient to complete. Unlike many other instruments commonly employed, it has the advantage of having been normed on and specifically devised for patients with chronic pain and of evaluating those factors most relevant in determining the nature and comprehensiveness of treatment needed. Scores are presented in several sections. The "psychosocial" section includes scales measuring pain severity, interference of pain in activities, perceived overall control of life, emotional distress, and level of interpersonal support given by the spouse or significant other related to pain. The "behavioral" section provides data regarding the frequency of three types of responses by the spouse/significant other to pain: "punishing" (i.e., angry or irritated), "solicitous" (asking how he/she can be helpful) or "distracting" responses. This section also includes scales measuring the extent of the patient's participation in household chores, outdoor tasks, activities away from home, and social activities, as well as the overall level of activity.

From their overall pattern of scores, patients can be divided into one of several categories that have been found to be predictive of treatment response (21). Those categorized as "adaptive copers" have a high likelihood of responding well to appropriate simple interventions for pain and are not likely to need MPC treatment. On the other hand, "dysfunctional" patients merit psychological interviewing and often are candidates for MPCs because they often do not respond well to simple medical intervention for pain without any behavioral treatment. A third category, "interpersonally distressed," includes patients who have felt or experienced a loss or lack of social and emotional support from their spouse or significant other in the context of pain and related problems. Involving the spouse/significant other often is critical for successful outcome for these patients.

Beck Depression Inventory

Because depression often is treatable and predicts failure with medical treatment (22), another useful screening tool for the need for more comprehensive treatment is the short form of the Beck Depression Inventory, which includes only 13 questions and is very highly correlated with the longer version of the inventory (23). Each question relates to a particular aspect of depression and includes four statements representative of given levels of depression, from which the patient selects the most applicable. The inventory includes items relating to negative affect (such as sadness and dissatisfaction with life), negative cognition (such as guilt, a perception of being a failure, and pessimism), and somatic factors (such as low energy, poor appetite, and difficulty getting started). In addition, one item addresses suicidal ideation and potential. A score indicating significant depression (10 or higher on the short form) and/or the presence of suicidal ideation suggests the need for further psychological evaluation.

Other Tests

Many other tests can serve as useful screening or assessment tools for patients with chronic pain. These tests can be divided into tests specifically devised for patients with pain and medical conditions and tests that assess more general psychological status. Among the former is a database devised by the International Association for the Study of Pain (IASP), which provides a good overview encompassing the location and perception of pain, its onset, the history of treatment, medication, nicotine and alcohol use, sleep patterns, demographic data, and family, social, vocational, and legal/disability issues. Another test, the Coping Strategies Questionnaire (CSQ) (24), includes 50 items and evaluates the types of cognitive and behavioral strategies that a patient may utilize in coping with chronic pain. Those patients using any of a variety of maladaptive strategies may require cognitive intervention to achieve optimal outcome. A related questionnaire is the Survey of Pain Attitudes (25), which includes 57 questions that assess beliefs related to perceived control of pain, one's disability from pain, the possibility of a medical cure, the desired responses from family members, the appropriateness of medications to manage pain, the effects of emotions on pain, and the belief that pain indicates damage and that activities can cause harm. The Psycho-Social Pain Inventory (26) is an interview guide that consists of 25 scored items pertaining to pain history and treatment and the effects of pain on job, home, and family support. The authors suggest that the inventory can predict poor response to medical interventions for pain.

The McGill Pain Questionnaire (27) includes 20 lists of words, from each of which the patient may choose one that describes his or her pain. Words within lists represent different levels of severity, and each list reflects sensory, affective, or evaluative components of pain. A simple visual analog scale (28), on which the patient makes a mark along a line with end points with labels such as "no pain" and "pain as bad as it could be," can yield a very simple and reliable measure of the current, worst, usual, and least pain experienced. It also can be easily repeated to evaluate patterns of pain during the day or following treatments.

Among tests devised for general medical populations are two tests useful to evaluate the impact of health prob-

lems on quality of life. The 136-item Sickness Impact Profile (29) assesses the impact of health problems on multiple areas of functioning within categories of physical, psychosocial, and "other" (i.e., sleep, management of the home, work, recreational activities, and eating). The 36-item Medical Outcomes Study Short Form-36 Questionnaire, often referred to as SF-36 (30), includes scales measuring such dimensions as overall physical functioning; how it is impacted by health; the intensity, frequency, and duration of pain; self-evaluation of overall health; vitality; the effect of health on social functioning; the interference of emotional health on daily activities; and composite mental health.

A frequently used test for psychological assessment of patients with and without pain, the Minnesota Multiphasic Personality Inventory-2, identifies psychological problems along many dimensions, with clinical scales measuring hypochondriasis, depression, conversion hysteria, psychopathic deviance, masculinity-femininity, paranoia, psychasthenia (i.e., anxiety), schizophrenia, mania, and introversion-extroversion. The test is very lengthy, with 370 questions providing the minimum database for scoring these scales. Advantages of the MMPI-2 include its comprehensiveness, the use of scales to measure the validity of the profile derived, and a research database from the original and revised MMPI versions that includes literally tens of thousands of studies, with hundreds conducted with patients with chronic pain. Besides its length, disadvantages include its intrusiveness for many patients and the fact that the test was not normed on individuals with pain and can yield distortions in interpretation.

The Symptom Checklist 90-Revised (31) includes 90 symptoms of physical and emotional distress rated according to how much each bothers the patient, from 0 (never) to 4 (always). It generates measures of somatic preoccupation, obsessiveness, interpersonal sensitivity, depression, anxiety, hostility, paranoid ideation, phobia, and psychoticism, as well as several scales of overall responding style.

By no means is this summary of test batteries and questionnaires exhaustive. The health professional who is evaluating the patient with chronic pain must choose test(s) based on the purpose of the evaluation. A test such as the Beck Depression Inventory is easy to administer to provide a quick screen for depression, but the evaluator interested in evaluating the possibility of a personality disorder would likely rely instead on the MMPI-2. Similarly, the need for cognitive therapy might best be assessed by the CSQ, whereas a general pain-related history might best be provided by the IASP database. For consideration of the applicability of a comprehensive rehabilitation approach, the MPI would be particularly helpful, whereas evaluation of how pain varies throughout the day or following treatment might be addressed most directly using a visual analog pain scale.

Psychosocial Interview

Whereas psychometric testing provides standardized and quantifiable information about a patient, an interview has the advantage of allowing in-depth exploration of significant areas of patient functioning and providing a live sample of a patient's affect, cognition, and ability to relate to an interviewer. An adequate understanding of a patient's history and functioning often necessitates interviewing not only the patient, but also significant members of his/her support system, particularly the spouse or significant other. Sources of relevant information may also include past and present treating professionals, the case manager (if one exists), and the attorney.

It is often particularly revealing to interview family members separately from the patient so that they may feel most free to reveal relevant information. Important information to gather from family members includes their observations of the patient's verbal complaints, activity level, substance use, compliance with treatment, attitudes expressed toward pain and its treatment, and social, medical, and family history. The degree of concordance between the patient's and the family's perceptions can be an important factor in assessing the credibility of the patient's self-reports, on which many treatment decisions may depend.

In addition, significant others' responses often affect the patient's behaviors significantly. Sympathy and support may be appropriate compassionate responses, but when provided contingent on pain behavior, they can increase the frequency of such behavior. On the other hand, withdrawal from the patient can heighten his/her isolation or depression. Such withdrawal or anger may occur because family members do not perceive the pain as "real" or have become frustrated by losses of patient function or family income. Some family members reinforce adaptive responses, such as focusing away from pain or maximizing function and activity within limitations, whereas others may reinforce or model anger, helplessness, or negative cognitions. Their advice and opinions regarding the nature and reality of pain and what treatments or strategies should be used to treat it also can be very influential. Examples of areas of important inquiry include the family's views regarding whether treatment should be directed toward the "cause" of the pain versus managing it more effectively, whether the patient should work to increase activity or return to work, and what medication use is best.

Basic information to be gathered from the interview with the patient includes the pain and its history, activities and work, sleep, and psychosocial functioning. In evaluating information from an interview, it is important to be very thorough and careful in drawing conclusions, particularly in view of the poor understanding of factors that create or contribute to pain.

Pain Complaints

The origin of pain complaints can provide important information about factors involved in its occurrence, particularly if pain began during a particularly stressful time in the patient's life. Pain complaints that are vague, diverse and diffuse, poorly described, or presented with highly dramatized language suggest an increased likelihood of the importance of environmental, emotional, or behavioral factors; however, some conditions, such as certain forms of arthritis, are characterized by diffuse pains and vague patterns of occurrence, so conclusions must be drawn with care and based on multiple sources of information. Keefe and his colleagues (32,33) have devised a system for quantifying the occurrence of overt pain behaviors, such as bracing, guarding, rubbing painful areas, and sighing. It is important to evaluate patterns of occurrence of these nonverbal pain behaviors as well as verbal expressions of pain with regard to their relationship to medical findings and to such variables as stress levels, sleep problems, environmental reinforcers, medication use, weather, time of day, etc. Such analysis can help to determine what medical, physical, and psychosocial treatments may be effective in altering them.

Activity Levels and Patterns

Inactivity represents one of the most insidious aspects of chronic pain. Some effects of inactivity include muscular weakness, reduced cardiac function and circulation, urologic and gastrointestinal problems, obesity, increased risk of depression, cognitive dullness, and reduced ability to sleep (34,35). Endorphins associated with aerobic activity may help control pain (36). Chronic pain patients often report increased pain with activity, which can occur because of an inappropriate choice of activity for the medical problem, poor body mechanics, poor pacing, and/or a pattern of inconsistent activity with alternate inactivity and overdoing. In many cases, patients may stay inactive because they are mistakenly afraid that activity may cause additional permanent medical damage.

It is thus important to evaluate patients' behaviors, experiences and beliefs regarding physical and recreational activities, and how they have changed since the onset of pain. The cessation of recreational activity and participation in hobbies may be important in depression and reduced quality of life. Patient diaries of daily activities are useful supplements to interview data.

Work

Inasmuch as most working adults spend one third to one half of their waking hours at work, loss of work associated with pain makes a critical difference, both economically and psychologically. Self-esteem can be highly related to feelings of productivity associated with work, and many individuals derive many social relationships from the work setting. A study of over 27 000 workers at the Boeing plant revealed poor supervisor rating of work performance to be a significant precursor of work-related injury and failure to return to work (37). A comprehensive interview needs to address the role of work-related issues in patients' lives, including work history and performance, relationships with supervisors and employers, and job satisfaction. Evaluation of patients' attempts to return to work and perceived job abilities is critical. Psychologically functional individuals are likely to have evaluated their work skills and limitations carefully and to have developed a plan to return to some kind of employment if their physical condition allows it. Patients who have not done so may be depressed, have low confidence in their abilities to be successful, fear of failure or reinjury with return to work, or may have significant secondary gain issues.

Factors related to disability and compensation issues need to be evaluated carefully. Some disability systems have inherent disincentives for return to work, including payments competitive with that available through work, delays in litigating claims, absence of provisions for gradual return to work or partial disability for return to a different job, and immediate loss of disability with reemployment. Sometimes coached by attorneys, some patients may wish to increase a financial settlement through maximizing the negative effects of an accident or injury. Failure to return to work may also relate to the lack of available work within a patient's physical limitations. Also, the employer may be unwilling or hesitant to make provisions to accommodate the patient in the workplace, such as different job hours or responsibilities, a modified pace of work, or physical changes to improve the ergonomics of the work setting.

Decisions that patients make regarding disability issues doubtless depend on a great variety of factors. Research regarding the role of disability and financial issues in affecting rehabilitation suggests the importance of the professional's avoiding facile conclusions (38,39). By no means is it true either that all patients receiving disability contingent on dysfunction will not make efforts to increase their function or that financial considerations have no effect on patient behavior.

Sleep

Lack of sleep frequently accompanies chronic pain and, in turn, affects patients' quality of life and their ability to cope with it. Irritability, impaired memory, and fatigue often accompany poor sleep. Some medical conditions, such as fibromyalgia or restless legs syndrome, have specific relationships with sleep disturbances. Information about patients' sleep patterns also may help to identify psychosocial factors that may need to be addressed during treatment. Some patients sleep extensively during the day, which may represent an avoidance behavior as well as preclude effective sleep at night. Difficulty getting to sleep can be associated with many factors, including anxiety and stress, caffeine use, or inactivity. Although a frequent hallmark of depression, early morning awakening also may reflect dependence on medication and/or increase in pain during the night, often related to posture and lack of movement.

Social Relationships and History

Patients' relationships often suffer with pain as patients become more irritable and withdrawn. Some wish to avoid being a burden on others or feel shameful about their difficulties. Others avoid social activities out of fear that their condition may necessitate having to cancel the activities or leave early or because they do not want to arrange special provisions to control the pain. Needed friendships can suffer as a result. An added problem for many patients with pain is reduced sexual function, which can result from increased pain upon sexual activity and/or be associated with depression, interpersonal stress, or medication use.

A comprehensive interview should address a patient's social support system and relationships, both historically and presently. The interview itself can be looked upon as a sample of social behavior, allowing evaluation of eye contact, listening and communication skills, appropriateness of responses, affect, use of humor, etc.

Emotional and Cognitive Status

Physical responses are closely interconnected with emotions and cognitions. A growing body of evidence suggests that histories of emotional disturbance and of sexual or physical abuse can predispose some individuals to pain (40,41). An individual's effectiveness in dealing with major health problems productively clearly is related to his/her emotional and cognitive status. A comprehensive interview thus addresses the patient's emotional history and function and how they relate to the patient's current management of pain and related problems. Symptoms of anxiety, depression, and anger frequently accompany pain and loss and need to be addressed in treatment for optimal outcome.

Similarly, a patient's beliefs and attitudes regarding the causes and contributants of pain and related problems and how they can or should be treated are often critical determinants of effort and return to function. Beliefs regarding "self-efficacy," or the ability to control health and function through one's own behavior, may be particularly critical in determining participation and success in rehabilitation (13,42). Patients with distorted beliefs, low self-esteem, undue pessimism, and/or a tendency to "catastrophize" (i.e., see the future as getting worse and worse) are likely to require intervention that alters these cognitions (43).

Cognitive changes, such as distractibility, poor memory, and concentration, often accompany pain as well. They can be affected positively or negatively by medications. Poor memory, attention, and concentration often are associated with a great deal of emotional distress and obviously can be very important factors in determining quality of life and work potential. Although standardized tests can be employed to assess them, the interviewer also can assess them through observation of responses to interview questions. It is often useful to conduct some brief screening of such functions.

Psychophysiological Evaluation

Measures of biofeedback can be helpful to measure physiological correlates of pain and of anxiety and to help determine whether biofeedback therapy is appropriate to help with function and pain control. Such evaluation should be conducted under a variety of situations, including while the patient is in a natural state with no instructions, while the patient is attempting to relax, while the patient is engaging in a typical activity (such as while a secretary is typing), and while under stress. The latter can include having the patient imagine a relevant stressful situation or having him or her placed in such a situation, such as having to do difficult mental arithmetic. Because measures often vary across time periods and situations (44), taking repeated measures across different situations is necessary.

Because of the assumed relevance of muscle tension to the presence of pain, electromyographic (EMG) biofeedback is commonly employed. This involves placing electrodes on the skin surface to measure the tightness of a muscle below. Tightness can relate to medical conditions, the patient's bracing or guarding against pain, posture, and/or anxiety. Levels of tension are most accurately measured in muscles near the skin surface. A comprehensive evaluation would include muscle activity measured while the patient is engaged in typical movement (dynamic EMG) and while the patient is stationary in a variety of typical postures (static EMG). Readings can be compared against normative values to evaluate the degree of abnormal tightness found.

Thermal biofeedback involves measurement of skin temperature through a sensor placed on the surface of the skin, usually on a finger or hand, occasionally a foot. Temperature is reflective of blood flow, and a cold temperature can be associated with increased pain. Indeed, some chronic pain problems, such as Raynaud's disease or complex regional pain syndrome, are linked with reduced blood flow and cold extremities. In addition, increased anxiety is often associated with reduced peripheral blood flow. Temperature can also be influenced greatly by extraneous factors, including the temperature of the room, recent exercise, and caffeine; an adaptation period of at least 10 minutes is needed for evaluation.

Other physiological measures correlate with anxiety and may be evaluated, including electrodermal responses, heart rate, and blood pressure. Photoplethysmographic measurements have been used to measure dilation of blood vessels important in migraine headache and erectile dysfunction, whereas electroencephalographic (EEG) biofeedback can provide information about quality of sleep, states of consciousness, and ability to relax.

Research findings suggest a complex and often uncertain and variable relationship between many of these physiological measures and the presence of pain, both in evaluating across times within a given individual and in evaluating between different individuals (45–47). Thus, a great deal of caution must be exercised in generating conclusions about the causes or contributants to pain solely from such physiological measures. It may be that the office setting does not allow measurement of such parameters as they generally vary in a typical day. Measurement of such parameters in the patient's home environment and in individualized situations that give rise to pain (perhaps during a stressful event or during movement) may increase the magnitude of the relationship found between biofeedback parameters and pain levels.

TREATMENT

Goals of MPC Programs

The goals of pain programs frequently differ among different interested parties. For the patient, decreased pain often is given as the principal goal, and one frequently hears statements such as, "I would like to get rid of this problem once and for all so that I can go on with my life." The referring source may be most interested in removing a difficult patient from his/her care, the insurance company in reducing costs, and the patient's attorney in documenting difficulties so that a favorable settlement can be achieved. The patient's family often wishes for restoration of the patient's function and improvement in his/her emotional status so that he/she again can participate fully in family life.

It is very important that the goals of treatment be defined at the outset and be appropriate to the treatment offered. A contract that outlines the goals and the responsibilities of the treatment team and the patient, signed by both, often can formalize and clarify this process. The goals that most MPCs address include the following: (a) maximize physical function and activity level within medical limitations; (b) minimize medication use so that only those medications necessary for enhancing patient functioning are utilized; (c) reduce reliance on the health-care system through increased independent management of pain and related problems; (d) improve emotional function to reduce depression, anger, and other harmful emotional states associated with pain; (e) find suitable employment, if possible; (f) help in the fair settlement of disability issues, if applicable, and (g) reduce subjective pain intensity.

Treatment must be individualized to meet the goals of each patient. It is likely that an intensive treatment is necessary for patients found to be "dysfunctional" on the MPI or found to have many of the *D*s listed earlier. Other patients may benefit from a less intensive and targeted treatment approach. For example, those who do not have significant depression or emotional disturbance but are very physically deconditioned or inactive may benefit from physical therapy, education in the role of activities in pain management, and, perhaps, brief instruction in relaxation therapy. An intensive psychological therapy program for them may waste money and time and decrease the credibility of the rest of treatment. In general, comprehensive rehabilitation programs are not appropriate for patients who have acute pain and are still healing, those who are clearly surgical candidates, those who cannot learn or apply basic information, or those who are not willing to work on behavioral, emotional, and attitudinal changes to enhance their coping with pain and related problems.

Programmatic Requirements for Successful Outcome

Comprehensive rehabilitation programs should be goal oriented, coordinated, interdisciplinary, and inclusive. Goals and decisions are formulated together by the patient and treatment team, who stay in close communication throughout treatment. Professionals meet regularly at specified intervals (usually weekly) in a team conference to discuss and coordinate treatment. All relevant individuals involved in the patient's care generally need to be involved in the treatment process, including the patient's family, physician(s) or other treating professional(s), attorney, and prospective or current employer. The insurance adjuster or rehabilitation provider (if one exists) often needs to stay informed about treatment needs and requirements. The patient remains accountable for working toward clear and realistic goals. Diaries of activity levels, completion of assignments, and use of recommended methods such as physical therapy and relaxation can help assess and foster sustained patient effort.

Treatment is often most effective when provided concurrently rather than sequentially because different modalities of treatment can often provide synergies absent in a consultative or piecemeal approach. Examples of such synergies include teaching alternative methods of pain control (such as relaxation methods or proper use of pacing or heat or ice) while reducing medication or providing group support and encouragement and some pain-relieving procedures while the patient works at reestablishing difficult activities. Because the pain is chronic, treatment must be directed toward long-term management of pain and related problems and development of enduring skills. Interventions for pain relief are applied depending on whether they contribute toward the development of enhanced long-term function.

Followup must be planned carefully. Treatment should often be tapered to allow evaluation and reinforcement of patient progress. Patients likely will need to be provided long-term support and taught principles of relapse prevention (48). The reader interested in guidelines for setting up a chronic pain rehabilitation program is referred to the *Standards Manual* published by CARF (18), which includes general requirements for all rehabilitation programs as well as ones specific for chronic pain management programs. Roles of major disciplines at MPCs are as follows:

Physician's Role

The role of the physician initially includes evaluation of the patient's medical condition and of the appropriateness of MPC treatment for that condition. During treatment, the physician becomes largely an educator and reinforcer of patients' rehabilitation efforts and a guide to other professionals. Medical education groups also can be very helpful and often address such topics as medical causes and contributants to pain, how behavior and emotion affect medical factors, proper use of medications, and the role of medical treatments for pain. The physician also typically plays a major role in evaluating impairments and defining physical limitations, which can be critical for successful return to work and/or fair settlement of disability issues. Medical interventions can help relieve pain so as to enhance function, and medications can assist with problems such as sleep loss, depression, and anxiety.

Psychologist's Role

The basic role of the psychologist is to work with patients to develop skills that will enhance their behavioral, cognitive, and emotional functions as they relate to pain and related problems. Though long-term maintenance of behavior is so critical for successful management of pain, Lutz, Silbret, and Olshan (49) found that only 18% of patients seen at an MPC reported daily compliance with each of five suggested treatment modalities at 23-month followup. Thus, psychologists need to help patients develop skills leading to such maintenance, such as self-monitoring of behavior, realistic goal setting, and self-reward, as well as principles of relapse prevention. Education and involvement of the patient's support system are often critical for the long-term compliance with needed behaviors.

Often led by psychologists, groups often can be very powerful for education, therapy, and support. They can help patients understand and cope with the many common problems associated with chronic pain, such as sleep loss, depression, problems with relationships, and sexual dysfunction. Patients' isolation is often reduced, and they can benefit from giving and receiving suggestions with other group members. Many initially need the support and encouragement of the group to make difficult changes, and seeing that others with similar problems are benefiting from treatment can be a powerful motivator. Groups also can play a major educational role in helping patients understand the role of attitudes, cognitions, and behaviors in chronic pain management. Patients often need to learn to accept and grieve through losses, yet still maintain appropriate optimism and determination to improve their function. Doing so may involve working through the stages of grief initially proposed by Elisabeth Kubler-Ross (50), encompassing denial, anger, bargaining (or anxiety), depression, and acceptance without resignation.

Because pain can be worsened by stress and is such a stressor itself, stress management therapy is important in pain rehabilitation. The group context is often ideal for such treatment. Patients with pain may need to alter stressful events in their lives, such as responsibilities that now are beyond limitations; however, the most important aspect often involves identifying and modifying their own behaviors, thoughts, and emotions. Many patients have to learn to reduce anger and to focus away from pain, dysfunction, and negative and pessimistic thinking, attending instead to the recognition, development, and use of positive skills and abilities. These changes may encompass improving assertiveness and communication and regaining one's use of humor. Maintaining appropriate pacing, regular exercise, adequate sleep, good nutrition, and balance among work, enjoyable activities, and rest are other behaviors that often help to reduce stress.

Taught in groups or individually, relaxation techniques are staples in pain management programs. Methods of relaxation are diverse and may involve progressive muscle relaxation (sequentially tensing and letting go of muscles throughout the body), deep (diaphragmatic) breathing, imagery, focusing intensively on positive images or memories, and meditation. Patients generally are given a tape and are instructed to practice such methods daily, with the goal of eventually learning to relax deeply through application of brief relaxation methods throughout the day. Maintaining a relaxed state often reduces pain, anxiety, muscle tension, and sleep problems and thus also reduces the need for many medications.

Biofeedback increases the credibility of relaxation by allowing patients to see its physiological effects. It may be most effective in its enhancement of patient perceptions of control and self-efficacy, which can serve as a powerful antidote to pain-related depression and helplessness. The astute clinician will employ the form(s) of biofeedback that enhances the individual patient's goals for increased pain control and function. Biofeedback often is most effective as an adjunct to other therapies; by no means does evidence support the idea that every patient or no patient should undergo biofeedback, nor that a large number of repetitive sessions is needed for most patients to have optimal outcome (46,47). Patients most likely to benefit may be those who have a specific problem for which the biofeedback parameter is employed or those who need the external feedback to enhance their relaxation skills or their perceived control of pain and related problems.

Many patients with chronic pain also need individual and/or marital psychotherapy to deal intensively and most effectively with their problems. The individual setting allows more intensive feedback and working through of individual issues that affect coping with and controlling pain. These problems can involve many aspects of function, such as dealing with previous abuse issues or family or marital disharmony. The individual setting also allows close supervision of patient responses to treatment and reevaluating of goals and treatments.

Physical Therapist's Role

The physical therapist often faces a dilemma in that many chronic pain patients report that physical activity directly aggravates their pain; however, there is excellent evidence that many patients with chronic pain can increase activity substantially and report reduced pain in the long term (51,52). Clearly, different forms of exercise are appropriate for different patients, depending on the nature of their medical impairments. Parameters to consider in designing an exercise plan are many, including general medical condition and fitness, the current level of exercise, and factors important in patient compliance, including patient goals, enjoyment of activity, and the effect of activity on pain. These factors affect the nature, duration, frequency, and recommended setting of physical activity. Many patients with arthritic and musculoskeletal problems can be much more active in a well-heated pool, where the buoyancy of the water reduces stress on joints and muscles and the warmth helps to relieve pain (53). Principles for activity programs often include staying within assigned limitations, working on increasing levels gradually from the current level, pacing activities with breaks throughout the day, and staying consistent rather than changing activity levels each day depending on pain.

Because patients often report increased pain in the short term with reactivation, the physical therapist and treatment team must provide support and make sure that patients understand the role of activity in pain management and set realistic goals. Daily guidance and reinforcement often are critical ingredients of success, particularly as patients first increase activities, and activity programs may need to be modified frequently based on patient response. Teaching proper posture and body mechanics is critical to allow patients to perform activities with the minimum of pain. Exercises to increase strength and range of motion help to restore function needed for optimal performance of activities of daily living.

An additional role of the physical therapist is evaluation of how the patient's environment can be modified to best enhance function, including such factors as optimum sleeping surfaces, ergonomic furniture, and assistive devices. The therapist also may employ techniques for relief of pain, such as massage, application of heat and cold, and electrical stimulation methods, such as transcutaneous electrical nerve stimulation (TENS). These techniques can be powerful for relieving pain and thus helping patients to function; however, like medical procedures, they can reinforce a passive patient role or encourage the patient to focus on pain and disability. Furthermore, repetition of such treatments in the office can be endless and expensive. Teaching family members to perform massage, if needed, and teaching the patient to apply TENS or heat and/or cold may be far more cost effective than simply applying these therapies in the professional setting.

Role of Nursing and Other Disciplines

Nursing personnel often play the role of "program managers," keeping in close touch with the patient and his/her progress and helping to coordinate treatment among the disciplines. They also play critical roles in patient education, quality review, and program evaluation. Quality programs include systems for evaluating the success of their programs versus objectives and include followup as well as posttreatment data and measures of patient satisfaction. Many other disciplines, too many to list exhaustively, provide important treatment for patients. A few examples include the occupational therapist, for arranging adaptive devices and helping patients with work simplification, energy conservation methods, use of leisure time, and proper activity management; the nutritionist, for proper diet and weight loss; multiple medical specialists for consultations; and such disciplines as recreational specialist, social worker, kinesiologist, massage therapist, pharmacologist, and chaplain.

Return to Employment

Many disciplines need to be involved in helping patients return to work: the physician to define medical limitations, the psychologist to assess and treat work-related attitudes, and the physical therapist and the vocational specialist to evaluate work potential and guide the patient toward feasible employment. Rehabilitation programs need to establish at the onset that a goal is to return to maximum productivity within whatever limitations are present and then to guide the patient to work step by step to achieve maximum function related to work tasks. Documentation of work abilities through functional capacity evaluation and close observation of patient performance are critical takeoff points for work planning. This planning needs to encompass not only physical skills, but also cognitive abilities, work attitudes and interests, and the availability of appropriate jobs in the community. The patient's job-finding skills may need to be improved, and the work site and job schedule may need to be evaluated and modified to be suitable for his/her needs. Finally, the patient's family, rehabilitation provider (if applicable), attorney, and prospective employer all need to be included, and recruited, if possible, to support the return to productivity.

TREATMENT OUTCOME IN REHABILITATION

Comprehensive pain programs provided at MPCs have been well studied. Indeed, Flor, Fydrich, and Turk (51) reviewed findings from 65 outcome studies from such programs, all of which provided empirical clinical outcome data on groups of patients using multiple measures, generally including subjective pain intensity, mood, medication use, activity level, return to work, and use of the healthcare system. Their review compared mean outcome from these programs with that found for patients who received either single-discipline approaches, such as conventional medical treatment or physical therapy, or no treatment at all. Outcomes were assessed with a recognition that patients undergoing MPC treatment often had failed to report or show benefit with many other treatments and had experienced pain and dysfunction of very significant magnitude for long periods of time. Findings revealed significant improvements with MPC treatment in all the measures evaluated, with the vast majority of studies showing superior outcome at MPCs compared to conventional or no treatment. Furthermore, maintenance of positive changes was demonstrated in studies ranging from 7 months to 7 years after treatment.

In a more comprehensive and recent review, Turk and Okifuji (54) summarized findings with patients at MPC programs as follows: mean 20% to 40% reduction in subjective pain intensity, reduction in opioid use so that 65% of patients are opioid free a year after treatment, significant activity increase in 65% of treated patients, return to some form of employment in approximately two thirds of patients for whom return to work was a goal, no additional treatment sought by 62% to 90% of patients for periods ranging from 3 to 12 months posttreatment, and 31% fewer surgeries following MPC treatment than following conventional medical approaches. MPC treatment also was less costly than many alternative approaches; for example, Turk and Okifuji quoted the average cost of MPC pain programs as $8100 (using research from an organization called Marketdata Enterprises) versus a typical expense of $40 000 for surgical treatment of back pain. Though one can criticize some of the studies included in the review for imperfect data-gathering techniques, reliance on self-reports, and varying means of assessing outcome measures across studies, many were well controlled with careful data analyses.

Reviewers who have formulated clinical practice guidelines for chronic pain management also have concluded that many patients with chronic pain require multidisciplinary and coordinated treatment rather than single-disciplinary approaches (55–57). Sanders et al. (56) defined "chronic pain syndrome patients" as having at least two of the following four features: deterioration in function, progressive increase in health-care use, mood disturbance, and clinically significant anger and hostility. Analyzing outcome only from studies using a prospective controlled research design with quantifiable objective outcome measures, they found that such patients "are best treated in an integrated interdisciplinary program." They reported a lack of convincing evidence for the efficacy of opioid-based analgesics, sedative-hypnotic medications, or procedures such as implantable spinal stimulators, continuous infusion devices, and brain stimulation. Using similar criteria for inclusion and analysis of effective treatments for chronic low back pain, Compas et al. (55) also concluded that operant therapy and cognitive-behavioral therapy, the backbones of interdisciplinary rehabilitation, clearly were efficacious.

PATIENT HELPFULNESS RATINGS

These conclusions fit with patients' ratings of the perceived helpfulness of treatments received at an MPC. Chapman et al. (58,59) devised the Treatment Helpfulness Questionnaire (THQ) to assess the level of perceived helpfulness of the many types of treatment administered to patients at comprehensive MPCs. The THQ consists of visual analog scales for different treatment modalities, with end points labeled "extremely harmful" and "extremely helpful," with "neutral" at the midpoint. Patient responses for any given treatment can range from a score of –5 (representing "extremely harmful") to +5 (representing "extremely helpful"). Mean posttreatment and followup ratings of treatments for subjects at four comprehensive MPCs are presented in Table 52-1.

The mean fee represents the average gross billing of the listed treatment for those patients who rated it on the THQ. As seen in the table, patients rated group psychological and educational approaches as among the most helpful both at posttreatment and followup, whereas they rated as least helpful injections for pain relief and transcutaneous electrical nerve stimulation. Aquatics, provided at one of the four centers, also was rated highly at posttreatment. Significantly, those treatments that were the most costly were not rated the most helpful: The group and educational approaches bore lower costs than procedures, despite their higher ratings. Given that the authors did find significant relationships between helpfulness ratings on the THQ and outcome measures (58), it may be that pain treatment centers could improve their outcomes by modifying those components of their programs with low comparative ratings so that they more closely resemble the corresponding components in programs with higher ratings.

Some caveats are needed in the interpretation of these findings from the THQ. The data came from a very selected subject population, namely those who generally had failed to report benefit from previous medical interventions for pain control. Furthermore, the emphasis of the programs studied was on using methods to gain greater control of pain and related problems through education and therapy.

CONCLUSION

Comprehensive pain rehabilitation provided at MPCs has been one of the most carefully and thoroughly researched forms of treatment for patients with chronic pain. Despite failure to benefit from many alternative approaches, many patients undergoing such treatment significantly increase their emotional and physical functioning, return to work, and save costs by ending disability and reducing reliance on the health-care system. One can hope that the politics of health-care reimbursement does not override science and put an end to such needed programs.

TABLE 52-1. *Mean THQ* ratings and mean total fees at four MPCs***

	Posttreatment			3–6-month followup	
	N	THQ rating	Fee	N	THQ rating
Aquatics	27	3.33	$210	—	—
Individual psychological therapy	241	3.17	$653	159	2.63
Group counseling	250	3.15	$529	143	2.46
Education groups	248	2.93	$374	143	2.23
Relaxation therapy	262	2.82	$204	169	2.15
Physical therapy	203	2.59	$1230	149	1.66
Drug prescriptions	242	2.42	—	137	2.07
M.D. office visits	150	2.31	$648	114	2.20
Drug withdrawal	68	2.14	—	31	0.80
Biofeedback	91	1.93	—	61	1.76
Trigger point injections	133	1.61	$503	108	1.40
TENS	65	1.22	—	54	1.09
Sympathetic nerve blocks	62	0.65	$997	56	0.73
Epidural steroid injections	42	0.00	$1249	42	0.36

*THQ, Treatment Helpfulness Questionnaire.
**MPCs, multidisciplinary pain centers.

REFERENCES

1. International Association for the Study of Pain (Subcommittee on Taxonomy): Pain terms: a list with definitions and notes on usage. *Pain* 1979;6:249–252.

2. Loeser J, Bigos SJ, Fordyce WE, et al. Low back pain. In: Bonica JJ, ed. *Management of pain*. Philadelphia: Lea and Filbiger, 1990;2: 1448–1483.

3. Flor H, Turk DC. Etiological theories and treatments for chronic back pain. I. Somatic models and interventions. *Pain* 1984;19: 105–121.

4. Frymoyer JW, Durett CL. The economics of spinal disorders. In: Frymoyer JW, Ducker TB, Hadler NM, et al., eds. *The adult spine*, 2nd ed. Philadelphia: Lippincott-Raven, 1997:143–150.

5. Spitzer WO, LeBlanc FE, Dupius M. A scientific approach to the assessment and management of activity-related spinal disorders: a monograph for clinicians. Report of The Quebec Task Force on Spinal Disorders. *Spine* 1987;12:S1–S59.

6. Spengler DM, Bigos SJ, Martin NA, et al: Back injuries in industry: a retrospective study. I. Overview and cost analysis. *Spine* 1986;11: 241–251.

7. Bonica JJ. *The management of pain*. Philadelphia: Lea and Filbiger, 1953.

8. Melzack R, Wall PD. Pain mechanism: a new theory. *Science* 1965; 150:971–979.

9. Fordyce WE: *Behavioral methods for chronic pain and illness*. St. Louis: Mosby, 1976.

10. Chapman SL, Brena SF, Bradford LA. Treatment outcome in a chronic pain rehabilitation program. *Pain* 1981;11:255–268.

11. Peters JL, Large RG. A randomized control trial evaluating in and outpatient pain management programs. *Pain* 1990;41:283–293.

12. Keefe FJ, Crisson J, Urban BJ, et al. Analyzing chronic low back pain: the relative contribution of pain coping strategies. *Pain* 1990; 40:293–301.

13. Turk DC, Meichenbaum D, Genest M. *Pain and behavioral medicine: a cognitive-behavioral perspective*. New York: Guilford, 1983.

14. Melzack R. The tragedy of needless pain. *Scientif Amer* 1990;262: 27–33.

15. Portenoy RK. Chronic opioid therapy for nonmalignant pain: from models to practice. *Amer Pain Soc J* 1992;1:285–288.

16. Abram SE. Systemic opioid therapy for chronic pain. In: Abram SE, Haddox JD, eds. *The pain clinic manual,* 2nd ed. Philadelphia: Lippincott, Williams, and Wilkins, 135–141.

17. Fishbain DA, Rosomoff HL, Rosomoff RS. Drug abuse, dependence and addiction in chronic pain patients. *Clin J Pain* 1992;8:77–85.

18. Commission on Accreditation of Rehabilitation Facilities: *Standards manual for organizations serving people with disabilities*. Tucson, 1991.

19. Morse RH. Pain and emotions. In Brena SF, Chapman SL, eds. *Management of patients with chronic pain*. New York: SP Medical and Scientific Books, 1983:47–54.

20. Kerns RD, Turk DC, Rudy TE. The West-Haven-Yale Multidimensional Pain Inventory (WHYMPI). *Pain* 1985;23:345–356.

21. Turk DC, Rudy TE. Toward an empirically derived taxonomy of chronic pain patients: integration of psychological assessment data. *J Consult Clin Psychol* 1988;56:233–238.

22. Block AR. *Presurgical psychological screening in chronic pain syndromes: a guide for the behavioral health practitioner*. Mahwah, NJ, Lawrence Erlbaum Associates, 1996.

23. Beck AT, Beck RW. Screening depressed patients in family practice. *Postgrad Med* 1972;32:81–85.

24. Rosensteil AK, Keefe FJ. The use of cognitive coping strategies in chronic low back pain patients: relationship to patient characteristics and current adjustment. *Pain* 1983;17:33–44.

25. Jensen MP, Karoly P, Huger R. The development and preliminary validation of an instrument to assess patients' attitudes toward pain. *J Psychosom Res* 1987;31:393–400.

26. Heaton RK, Getto CJ, Lehman RA, et al. A standardized evaluation of psychosocial factors in chronic pain. *Pain* 1982;12:165–174.

27. Melzack R. The McGill Pain Questionnaire: major properties and scoring methods. *Pain* 1976;1:277–299.

28. Scott J, Huskisson EC. Graphic representation of pain. *Pain* 1976;2: 175–184.

29. Bergner M, Bobbitt RA, Carter WB, et al: The sickness impact profile: development and final revision of a health status measure. *Med Care* 1981;19:787–805.

30. Ware JE, Sherbourne CD. The MOS 36-item short-form health survey (SF-36). Conceptual framework and item selection. *Med Care* 1992;30:473–483.

31. DeRogatis LR, Rickels K, Rock AF. The SCL-90 and the MMPI: A step in the validation of a new self-report scale. *Brit J Psychiat* 1976;128:280–289.

32. Keefe FJ, Block AR. Development of an observational method for assessing pain behavior in chronic low back pain patients. *Behav Ther* 1982;13:363–375.

33. Keefe FJ, Wilkins RH, Cook WA. Direct observation of pain behavior in low back pain patients during physical examination. *Pain* 1984; 20:59–68.

34. Bortz JM The disuse syndrome. *West J Med* 1984;141:691–694.

35. Mayer TG, Gatchel RJ, Mayer H, et al: A prospective two-year study of functional restoration in industrial low back injury. *JAMA* 1987; 258:1763–1767.

36. Basbaum AI, Fields HL. Endogenous pain control mechanisms. *Annals Neurol* 1978;4:699–716.

37. Bigos SJ, Spengler DM, Martin NA, et al. Back injury in industry: a retrospective study. III. Employee-related factors. *Spine* 1986;11: 252–256.

38. Dworkin RW, Handlin DS, Richlin DM, et al. Unraveling the effects of compensation, litigation, and employment on treatment response in chronic pain. *Pain* 1985;23:49–59.

39. Gallagher RM, Williams RA, Shelly J. Workers' compensation and return-to-work in low back pain. *Pain* 1995;61:299–307.

40. Fillingim RB, Wilkinson CS, Powell T. Self-reported abuse history and pain complaints in young adults. *Clin J Pain* 1999;15:85–91.

41. Wurtele SK, Kaplan GM, Keavines M. Childhood sexual abuse among chronic pain patients. *Clin J Pain* 1990;6:110–113.

42. Jensen MP, Turner JA, Romano JM. Self-efficacy and outcome expectancies: relationship to chronic pain coping strategies and adjustment. *Pain* 1991;44:263–269.

43. Jensen MP, Turner JA, Romano JM. Correlates of improvement in multidisciplinary treatment of chronic pain. *J Consult Clin Psychol* 1994;62:172–179.

44. Brown, BB. *Stress and the art of biofeedback*. New York: Harper & Row, 1977.

45. Belar CD, Kibrick SA. Biofeedback in the treatment of chronic back pain. In: Holzman AD, Turk DC, eds. *Pain management: a handbook of psychological treatment approaches*. New York: Pergamon Press, 1986:131–150.

46. Chapman SL. A review and clinical perspective on the use of EMG and thermal biofeedback for chronic headaches. *Pain* 1986;27:1–44.

47. Grzesiak R, Ciccone DS. Relaxation, biofeedback, and hypnosis in the management of pain. In: Lynch NT, Vasudevan SV, eds. *Persistent pain: psychosocial assessment and intervention*. Boston: Kluwer Academic Publishers, 1988:163–168.

48. Wilson PH. *Principles and practice of relapse prevention*. New York: Guilford, 1992.

49. Lutz RW, Silbret M, Olshan N. Treatment outcome and compliance with therapeutic regimens: long-term follow-up of a multidisciplinary program. *Pain* 1983;17:301–308.

50. Kubler-Ross E. *On death and dying*. New York: Macmillan, 1969.

51. Flor H, Fydrich T, Turk DC. Efficacy of multidisciplinary pain centers: a meta-analytic review. *Pain* 1992;49:221–230.

52. Waddell G. A new clinical model for the treatment of low-back pain. *Spine* 1987;12:632–644.

53. Cole AJ, Eagleston RE, Moschetti M, et al. Spine pain: aquatic rehabilitation strategies. *J Back Musculoskel Rehabil* 1994;4:273–286.

54. Turk DC, Okifuji A. Efficacy of multidisciplinary pain centres: an antidote to anecdotes. *Bailliere's Clin Anesthesiol* 1998;12:103–119.

55. Compas BE, Haaga DAF, Keefe FJ, et al. Sampling of empirically supported psychological treatments from health psychology: smoking, chronic pain, cancer, and bulimia nervosa. *J Consult Clin Psychol* 1998;66:89–112.

56. Sanders SH, Rucker KS, Anderson KO, et al. Clinical practice guidelines for chronic non-malignant pain syndrome patients. *J Back Musculoskel Rehabil* 1995;5:115–120.

57. Sanders SH, Harden RN, Benson SE, et al. Clinical practice guidelines for chronic non-malignant pain syndrome patients. II. An evidenced-based approach. *J Back Musculoskel Rehabil* in press.

58. Chapman SL, Jamison RN, Sanders SH. Treatment helpfulness questionnaire: a measure of patient satisfaction with treatment modalities provided in chronic pain management programs. *Pain* 1996; 68:349–361.

59. Chapman SL, Jamison RN, Sanders SH, et al. Perceived treatment helpfulness and costs in chronic pain rehabilitation. *Clin J Pain* 2000;16:169–177.

CHAPTER 53

Hospital-based Inpatient Treatment Programs

Renee Steele Rosomoff and Hubert L. Rosomoff

It is conceded that pain programs very often will take on the characteristics of the medical director. This may bias programs toward a given discipline but obviously does not preclude a multidisciplinary approach, despite the emphasis. In the same manner, programs may be influenced by the patient population that presents to the given center or clinic. The more complex, the more complicated, the more drug dependent, to name a few characteristics, the more likely it is that a hospital-based program will be necessary. Aside from the medical necessity there are major issues concerning reimbursement for hospital-based programs. As such, validation of medical necessity becomes important, but rejection can occur and does quite frequently. Despite the most cogent arguments, reimbursement will still be denied. In most recent years, the criteria, labeled medical necessity, have become more demanding. Aside from the criteria that follow, there has been a major shift to the consideration of function, regardless of the intensity or characteristic of the pain. The emphasis is on impairment in the activities of daily living that affects the patient's ability to function independently and that requires assistance for self-care and mobility and on the potential for risks of injury like falling due to poor coordination and strength.

We have found the following criteria to be the most powerful to support the request for hospitalization in a chronic pain patient. At least one of the following criteria must be present: (a) The pain must be sharp, severe, and incapacitating, having a rapid onset with severe symptoms over a short course, even though this might be an acute exacerbation within a chronic condition. (b) The pain must be happening repeatedly at short intervals at least once every 8 hours or more. (c) It will be necessary to observe, evaluate, and specifically record observations about the patient's condition. These observations are nec-

essary to the diagnosis or treatment of the patient's medical problem.

A second set of criteria may also be necessary: (a) observation or treatment in a special care unit and (b) a specific need for daily physician monitoring and full-time availability. This primarily refers to instances in which patients have associated significant medical problems or comorbidities that would have required an acute care setting for diagnosis or treatment. In this setting, patients may require acute treatment that refers to specific drug therapy, such as anticoagulants, psychopharmacologic agents, chemotherapy, anticonvulsants, antihypertensives, and cardiac medications that, during the initial phases of observation and treatment, require regulation of dosage. Furthermore, failure of nonsurgical interventions and conservative treatment at home must be fully documented, usually meaning previous treatment as an outpatient in physical medicine. In more recent times, this may now include failure of interventional techniques like nerve blocks, epidural steroids, lysis of adhesions, and percutaneous rhizotomies. To support the need for rehabilitation physical medicine in an acute setting, it may follow that the authorization will be restricted to the initial phases only, anywhere from 1 to 2 weeks. During this time, the patient must have documented rehabilitation potential and must demonstrate progress during therapy. Again, the emphasis on loss of function, aside from the pain, has become the foremost consideration for medical necessity.

Another set of criteria refers to the severity of illness. Functional impairment of a body part may need to be demonstrated, as well as the need for medications that are changing in dosage and that need to be regulated no less than every 2 days. Radiologic studies may show pathology such as a herniated disc or spinal stenosis, for which "conservative treatment" had not been attempted and which does not yet meet the criteria for surgical intervention, so a decision may be made to attempt nonsurgical treatment, particularly in the acute setting. Treatments must require skilled physical therapy on a daily basis, and rehabilitation, evaluation, goal setting, and management must be initiated within 24 hours of admission. Psychiatric criteria are those of a suicide attempt, suicidal ideation, or assaultive behavior. Disturbances such as seizures from withdrawal or toxic circumstances or impending loss of impulse control are other standards. Manic behavior, incapacitating anxiety or depression, severe incapacitation with obsessive thinking and/or compulsive behavior, and disabling paranoia are other conditions that may dictate hospitalization. The evaluations for drug tolerance and/or abuse, drug detoxification, and overdose were almost always acceptable for inpatient treatment, but now with the increasing availability of substance abuse clinics, the payers are more resistant to authorizing inpatient management. It is their contention that substance abuse can most often be managed in an outpatient setting and that, therefore, hospitalization may not be required and is often denied unless the other criteria for comorbidities pertain.

Lastly, intensity of service must be documented with the administration of medications at least daily, intravenously or intramuscularly, or the regulation and monitoring of high-risk medication. The management of a noncompliant patient or a patient with potential medical complications also speaks to intensity, wherein comprehensive therapy planning requires close supervision because of concomitant medical conditions and the requirement of skilled around-the-clock observation, supervision, and/or treatment. When these criteria can be cited, hospitalization can be considered reasonable and necessary: When a diagnosis of a physical cause has been established, the usual methods of treatment have not been successful, and there is a *significant loss* of ability to function independently, predominantly for activities of daily living (ADLs). These criteria have become increasingly applicable to all payer classes from Medicare through industrial injuries to commercial and managed care contracts.

Most insurers accept that a hospital-level pain rehabilitation program is one that employs a coordinated multidisciplinary team to deliver, in a controlled environment, a concentrated program designed to modify pain behavior through the treatment of the psychological, physical, and social aspects of pain. Such programs generally include diagnostic testing, skilled nursing, psychotherapy, structured progressive withdrawal from pain medications, and physical and occupational therapy to restore physical fitness including mobility, strength, and endurance to a maximal level within the constraints of a patient's physical condition. The use of mechanical devices and/or activities to relieve pain or modify a patient's reaction, such as massage, ice, hydrotherapy, nerve stimulation, and neuromuscular reeducation, are usually part of the treatment plan. The nurse is a member of this team and has a respon-

sibility to observe and assess, on a continuing basis, a patient's condition and response to medication and the treatment during therapy or on the nursing unit. The nurse must report these responses to the applicable disciplines to assure that the atmosphere within the unit is not supportive of pain behavior. Further, the nurse should reinforce the teachings of other disciplines and observe the patients carrying out their therapeutic assignments. This means that nurses on a pain treatment unit must be cross-trained to at least appreciate the therapeutic assignments, specifically those that patients are instructed to carry out after treatment hours and that, so to speak, represents "homework." The day-to-day activities involve carrying out the program under the general supervision and, as needed, direct supervision of a physician. It is universally accepted that an inpatient program generally takes at least 4 weeks with a range of 2 to 4 weeks to modify or control pain. In fact, the first 7 to 10 days of such an inpatient program constitute, in effect, an evaluation period. If the patient is unable to carry out the program due to physical infirmity within this period, it may be concluded that it is unlikely that the program will be effective and that the patient should be discharged from the program. Another criterion is the inability to carry out the program due to the effect of the medical comorbidities that may preclude the intensity of participation that will be necessary to assure success. Occasionally a program longer than 4 weeks may be required, and generally this is considered to be possible by transfer to an outpatient status. In such a case, there should be documentation to substantiate that care beyond the 4-week period is reasonable and necessary, although it still may be difficult to obtain payer approval beyond 4 weeks.

PROGRAM DESCRIPTION

An inpatient treatment program should be multidisciplinary and designed to provide individualized, intensive, aggressive physical, behavioral, and avocational/vocational rehabilitation for persons with acute or chronic intractable pain whose level of function and productivity and lifestyle are moderately to severely impaired. Patients should have been judged to require observation and treatment in a hospital setting on completion of a comprehensive multidisciplinary evaluation. The program should provide a safe, therapeutic environment with constant supervision for physically impaired, not totally independent, depressed, anxious, or otherwise disturbed or drug/alcohol-dependent patients who may or may not have underlying or associated medical problems that require observation and/or treatment.

PROGRAM GOALS AND OBJECTIVES

An inpatient program should be designed to physically recondition and restore the patient to a level of function that includes full range of motion, acceptable strength requirements, decreased pain level, and increased tolerances in preparation for transfer to an outpatient program or discharge home. The program should physically recondition and restore patients who require close nursing and medical inpatient supervision to full levels of function with minimal to no pain, with minimal to no limitations, and minimal to no disability on discharge to home. It should detoxify dependent patients from alcohol, narcotics, barbiturates, and analgesics and educate patients to use alternative methods to alleviate pain, although some patients will need psychopharmacology due to previously undetected behavioral or psychiatric problems and, at times, will be seen to be taking more total medication at discharge even though they have been tapered from dependence-inducing or addictive drugs. Patients should be able to self-administer any medication needed at the time of transfer or discharge to maintain health. Patients should be educated to manage pain episodes that may arise so they may be totally able to self-administer any modalities or exercises required in order to be discharged to a motel or home and be totally independent. Patients with spinal pain are expected to maintain their optimal weight to avoid exacerbation of pain due to excessive loading of the spine and hips. The need for assistive devices such as braces, corsets, canes, crutches, walkers, wheelchairs, and stimulators, which serve to perpetuate deconditioning and are counterproductive in the alleviation of pain, should be eliminated when possible. Realignment of the spine and extremities to eliminate poor posture and maladaptive gait, which contribute to intractable pain and perpetuate the cycle, must be achieved. Stress management, relaxation, psychological support, and family counseling should be provided so that patients are able to function appropriately in the outpatient setting or after return to their own environment. A positive behavioral change must be effected so that patients will be independent of the health-care system and be in control of their situation. Patients must learn to substitute for inappropriate behavior and responses behavior that is appropriate to reduce pain-producing stress. Patients must come to understand self and be totally responsible for their actions and rehabilitation. Patients must regain confidence to return to employment without fear or anxiety and to perceive themselves as well persons. Constructive coping strategies must be developed to reduce stress, and biofeedback and relaxation techniques must be mastered so that patients understand the relationship between muscle tension, anxiety, and pain in order to reduce stress and prevent reinjury. The program must alleviate and teach control of anxiety, depression, fear, anger, and interpersonal problems so that patients may function in an emotionally healthy manner, thereby maintaining the physical and mental gains made. Disability-oriented attitudes in patients and families must be eliminated, and patients' families must be educated to support wellness behavior and attitude. Patients must learn to relate to their families and others appropriately; patients' families must understand the patients' problem and abilities, as well as their role in their rehabilitative process, so that they may offer positive reinforcement and foster open communication within the family structure. Patients must learn to function at a high level and enjoy optimal wellness through training to instinctively use good body mechanics, pacing, and energy-saving techniques. Patients must be taught how to maintain rehabilitation gains and prevent reinjury without reliance on health-care professionals, medication, and appliances. The program should enable patients to participate in leisure activities, including active sports, in a safe and planned manner so that patients may prevent injury or reinjury and enjoy a complete, well-rounded, and satisfying life. The program should restore patients' capacity to return to previous employment with minimal to no limitations or modifications to the workplace immediately upon discharge, having the ability to physically, psychologically, and vocationally return to full-time employment, heavy labor not precluded, with confidence and with the ability to do the job in a safe manner. Patients must learn to overcome any obstacle that may interfere with return to employment through instructions in job-seeking skills, resume writing, and application and interview techniques. Rehabilitation should allow patients to return to previous employment or to a new work setting through the use of job simulation and functional restoration to full capacity based on an ergonomic and vocational analysis. Patients must learn to avoid situations that would contribute to a reoccurrence of the chronic pain cycle through knowledge of ergonomics and know how to make simple adjustments to the home and workplace setting.

In summary, the overall goal is to interrupt the chronic pain cycle; to optimally rehabilitate the patient physically, behaviorally, avocationally, vocationally, and socially; and to teach responsibility, control, awareness of reinjury mechanisms, and total independence from drug use, appliances, and the health-care system, thus enabling the patient to return to home, employment, and community as a fully rehabilitated, productive member of society.

PATIENT PROFILE

The type of patient who presents to a pain center has usually suffered from chronic pain for many months or years. The patient has had multiple physicians, undergone numerous diagnostic procedures and interventions, and has failed those treatments. Unfortunately, many patients have not had the opportunity to be knowledgeable of all of their treatment options and may not have tried those that could have been pain relieving and function improving due to failure of the treating physicians to recognize pain as a medical specialty and to refer patients to pain specialists when the treatment options of the provider have been exhausted. These patients have been on large amounts of medication and may still be in significant pain despite the heavy use of narcotics, which do not relieve but only "take the edge off" the pain. They have had multiple surgeries. They trust no one, and they see themselves as being crippled and suffering for the rest of their life. In addition, they may have a self-defeating background. They may focus on body cues and pain. They usually have a poor work history, poor interpersonal relationships, a low sense of self-esteem, poor skills, and little job satisfaction. They may have never liked their job, may blame their employer for their plight, and may be angry with the insurance company. Their families may have a history of low back pain, so their empathy makes them attentive to the patients' needs, and they assume the patients' responsibilities at home. These frightened families are protective, angry, and supportive of disability.

The other contributors to these "losers" are the medical community, the attorneys, the rehabilitation specialists, the insurance companies, and the employers. The doctor of such a patient has put the patient in bed with traction, passive therapy, pain medication, and muscle relaxants. The patient has been radiographed, imaged, myelogrammed, frightened by the results, and told that if he doesn't have an operation, he will be paralyzed and in a wheelchair. The insurance company joins with an uncaring attitude, supporting usually the least costly and, sometimes, the poorest kind of therapy without questioning recommendations; thus, operations mount one after another. The patient is blamed if he or she either refuses the risky surgery or does have the operation and doesn't get better. The surgeon claims the surgery to be successful, so it is the patient who has failed. The adjuster becomes hostile, delaying benefits, which compounds the anger and the now-developing behavioral problems of the patient.

The employer remains basically uncaring. He or she doesn't bother to call the patient to inquire how he is. Actually, the employer may have wanted to be rid of that employee before all this started and thus is happy. If an attorney is involved, he or she may tell the client to not trust, not cooperate, not communicate, not rehabilitate, and, by all means, not go back to work.

The result is a patient who has chronic pain, who is physically impaired, weak, drug dependent, alcohol dependent, hostile, untrusting, frightened, helpless, hopeless, and socially dependent, with sexual problems, anxiety, fear, anger, depression, no job, no future, totally disabled, and potentially suicidal and homicidal. He or she has marital problems, has no motivation, and is disability oriented. Everyone is angry. The patient is angry at himself or herself, the family, the boss, the employer, the physician, the lawyer, the insurance company, the disability system, and the law.

Moreover, the patient believes that he or she is entitled to a monetary award for the disability, and, of course, this is not forthcoming. He or she is fearful and doesn't know if he/she will ever get better or can ever be productive again. The patient is afraid of reinjury and further loss of function, especially if frightened by the warnings of physicians.

Most of all, patients fear the loss of benefits because they are still in pain and physically impaired and are fearful that they cannot perform the job. Therefore, they may maintain this disabled pose. They are dependent on alcohol, narcotics, barbiturates, psychotropics, muscle relaxants, and, often, street drugs. This type of patient may appear not to be cooperative or well motivated and to be interested only in what appears to be secondary gain. The real issues are fear and anger, which must be addressed if a successful outcome is to be achieved.

THE PROGRAM

The University of Miami Comprehensive Pain and Rehabilitation Center is a hospital-based program. It has more than 60 full-time personnel in six divisions. Neurologic surgery is noninvasive but minds the nervous system. Physical medicine and rehabilitation direct the physical and occupational therapists in the application of all physical medicine modalities and treatments. Nurses, trained in rehabilitation and behavior, monitor patient progress and serve as case managers. The behavioral division has both a psychiatrist and psychologists who are assigned as counselors to each patient and who administer biofeedback, behavioral modification, or other applicable techniques. A vocational rehabilitation division evaluates, counsels, and directs job placement; and an ergonomics division simulates the job and adapts the patient and/or work site while computing daily achievement goals. Incidentally, orthopedics falls within the division of physical medicine and rehabilitation. Interventional anesthesiology may have a role, particularly, in the acute phase where interventional techniques like epidural steroids and nerve blocks may be either diagnostic or therapeutic, the latter usually for a limited period of time. In the chronic pain patient such interventions have very limited application except for maintenance techniques when everything else fails. This may be the cancer patient who may need a morphine pump or a patient with a vascular problem, including intractable angina, where a spinal cord stimulator implant may have applicability. The use of the stimulator for failed back pain remains an open issue.

To enter the system, the patient must undergo multidisciplinary evaluation over a 1 to 3-day period. A problem-solving group attempts to identify the medical, behavioral, vocational, financial, social, and other significant problems of the patient. The approach is comprehensive and holistic. Patient selection criteria are broad. The patient must have the ability to understand and carry out instructions, must be compliant and cooperative, and must not have aggressive or disruptive behavior that would disturb the milieu. Patients with schizophrenia, manic-depression, or other major psychiatric disorders are not precluded as long as they are compensated. Lastly, the patient, the family, and significant others such as the lawyer, the employer, and the insurer must agree to the program.

Worker's compensation, liability cases, multiple surgeries, long histories of invalidism, or drug abuse are not exclusionary conditions.

The average program will last 4 weeks on an inpatient or outpatient basis or a combination thereof. Inpatient status is preferred for the difficult, complicated case, but it is not always feasible, as dictated by reimbursement status. It should be understood clearly that, in a tertiary referral center, few "simple" early primary cases are seen. We receive the most complex "court of last resort" salvage cases.

PHYSICAL MEDICINE AND REHABILITATION

Physical medicine has the goal of restoring body function to normal or to its closest equivalent. Because myofascial contracture is the common denominator in the low back disorders that we see, the first phase of management is muscle stretching and restoration of full range of motion in the joints of the hips, back, and lower extremities. This therapy includes gait retraining because of acquired maladaptive patterns, postural adjustment, proper use of effective modalities, elimination of adjunct equipment when possible, strength and endurance conditioning with instruction of body mechanics, prevention of reinjury, vocational or avocational requirements, sexual counseling, and, lastly, a home maintenance program.

Modalities, when evaluated individually, may not show clear-cut evidence of effectiveness (1). They appear to be useful in combination, however, which unfortunately makes statistical evaluation more difficult. Nonetheless, scientific rationale exists for some. Ice application with lowering of temperature is known to decrease nerve conduction to the point of anesthesia, and inflammatory reaction is contained with a reduction of chronic changes (2,3). To be effective, the body part must be packed in ice for periods in excess of 30 minutes. Heat does seem to soften muscle preparatory to stretching. An adjunct vapocoolant may help to block the stretch reflex and makes lengthening easier (4).

Traction is useful for certain specific indications. Conceptually, we apply traction to stretch muscle groups, not to distract the spine or to release nerve entrapment. We do not believe that distraction of the spine can be effected with the weights that are commonly used, and the principle of entrapment is not tenable. Therefore, traditional pelvic or leg traction is not employed. Gravity traction is applied for iliopsoas contractures in the patient with a spinal flexion deformity and/or failure to extend the back.

Autotraction is an important technique that allows three-dimensional placement of the spine by rotating, flexing, or extending the unit as the patient imposes his or her own body force by pushing and pulling (5). The self-applied force of autotraction will not exceed that which could be potentially injurious, but it will release tight paraspinal muscles. Autotraction does not decompress the nerve root, as was the concept of its originators (6,7).

Trigger-point desensitization is indicated. Liberal use of ice is the preferred method of treatment, but—like the modalities of ultrasonography, electrical stimulation, and neuroprobe—it is only an adjunct to stretching. Heat and neuromuscular massage also are used as adjunct treatment to enhance muscle lengthening and supple movement. Neuromuscular massage is utilized to eliminate trigger points from taut bands, reduce muscle irritability, and readjust postural abnormalities.

Transcutaneous electrical neural stimulation (TENS) is used infrequently and only with patients who are TENS responders and who can be assisted with a difficult detoxification for which TENS will give short-term relief as the drugs are withdrawn. TENS will not be given to the patient beyond this period; it has no role in long-term therapy. Conceptually, it is to be emphasized that we are aiming for resolution of the painful disorder by physical restitution, not by an attempt at distraction or at coping by "learning to live with pain."

Intramuscular stimulation has been a new and helpful technique to release tight muscles that the therapists find difficult to stretch. The technique includes the insertion, with electrical resistive mapping, of fine number 30 stainless steel needles into the identified muscle. The muscle is then stimulated at a low-frequency, 20 Hz, alternating the polarity every 5 minutes. It is most fascinating to see a taut ballooned muscle suddenly release midway into the stimulation period and, with this, a marked relief of pain. However, it still should be noted that this is not a pain-relieving technique, per se, but rather one to make muscle stretching easier and, thereby, to deliver a route for pain relief. Patients may choose to compare this method with acupuncture, but it is not considered an acupuncture technique despite the use of the fine-type acupuncture needles (8).

Passive, then active, ranging of motion is essential, especially about the hips and, in particular, the hip rotators. Hamstring lengthening is another mandate because hamstring tightness will affect back movement. Full ranges of back motion are the ultimate goal, so flexion and extension exercises are instituted without prejudice for the proponents of either type. Both flexion and extension exercises are needed.

A full compendium of exercises is employed, as described in any standard physical therapy textbook, to establish full ranges of motion throughout the lower body with supple muscles and fluid movement. As this is being achieved, muscle strengthening and cardiovascular conditioning are added to the regimen with monitoring of those patients who have associated medical problems.

Movement therapy using musical input is an interesting adjunct because patients with pain will often perform to music when seemingly they cannot move their bodies on command. When a specific muscle group is weak, functional electrical neuromuscular stimulation (FES) and muscle reeducation are implemented (9). This technique can produce rapid and dramatic increases in muscle recruitment patterns and muscle strength; foot-drop braces can be discarded.

Occupational therapy concentrates on proper body mechanics and function. Tolerances of activities of daily living, including sitting, standing, walking, lifting, and driving, are established and brought to normal levels of function. Pacing of activity is taught. Assistive equipment is used infrequently and only with specific indications. Energy-saving techniques are taught. Posture and gait are corrected; importantly, most patients are found to have poor posture and maladaptive gaits. Diversionary activities are reviewed, and eye/hand/leg coordination and tolerances are established. Educational and vocational goals are set, and job simulation is begun.

Job simulation and work conditioning are another concept that we introduced to pain center management more than 2 decade ago. This is the ultimate goal for the working-age group, but it does not exclude students or elderly persons, who receive instruction for their needs. With respect to these problems, the occupational and physical therapists team with vocational counselors and ergonomists to develop the treatment plan.

NURSING CARE

Nurses are cross-trained and play a vital and varied role in this hospital-based inpatient treatment program. They are involved in every aspect of the program from program direction, admission screening, case management, patient assessment and monitoring, counseling education, coordination, medication, and nutritional management to preadmission and discharge planning and followup. They are reinforcers of multidisciplinary team concepts and instructions.

VOCATIONAL REHABILITATION

Vocational rehabilitation counselors analyze factors of employment, such as age, educational level, work history, supervisory and peer relationships, job requirements, job skills, transferable skills, date and circumstances of injury, return to work since injury, and, most important, motivation and compliance. This type of program cannot be successful without the patient's full attention or effort. If the patient will not give both, he or she is not accepted. The vocational goal is full functional activity and return to previous employment when applicable. Retraining is recommended rarely. Even the heaviest physical capacities can be achieved in most patients.

BEHAVIORAL MANAGEMENT

Behavioral management is a key issue. Nearly 20% of Americans suffer from one or more emotional disorders, so the low back injury patient may be harboring such a problem. The psychiatric profile is inherited by the treatment team, insurer, and all others concerned. Our study of

pain population patients found 62.5% to have anxiety disorders and 56.2% to have current depression (10). These conditions were commingled with other, less prevalent disorders. Only 5.3% of 283 patients were found to have no psychiatric diagnosis. Further, this study questions the criteria for the diagnosis of psychogenic pain. Pure psychogenic pain is probably rare when presented as mental events giving rise to pain. Even so, all pain, as perceived by the patient, is real, regardless of cause. Most bodily pain is the result of a combination of factors, e.g., physical stimuli and mental events. Mental and emotional states may be due to circumstances of the moment, a background of past personal experiences with pain, such as physical or mental abuse, or personality characteristics.

Behavioral analysis considers compliance, achievement level before injury, activity level after injury, functional capacities, anxiety, depression, personality disorders, marital status, role reversal, and family history. Psychological services offer biofeedback and relaxation training and group and family therapy that deals with social interactions, return to environment, employment, and disability versus wellness with an emphasis on function, not pain.

Individual counseling is given when needed, including sexual counseling. Every patient has an assigned counselor who monitors daily progress and reinforces the goal of physical restoration. Relaxation training includes coping approaches, muscle reeducation, meditation and distraction, guided imagery, autosuggestion (especially to be used with physical activity), and tape supplements that enhance "live" therapy. This approach has proven very successful in the reduction of pain. Stress management is incorporated into the behavioral sessions.

Weekly family groups explore the goals of the patient with the spouse and/or other family members. How to respond to pain without fear is discussed. Communication is an important subject. The roles of the various family members are defined, both as to distribution and as to responsibility. Experiences and frustrations are shared. These sessions facilitate the return home to an environment that, it is hoped, will now foster wellness, not disability.

Biofeedback is an effective pain control method when used as a muscle tension/relaxation technique. Electromyographic feedback is used to regulate muscle tension, especially when an activity may, by past experience, have been pain provoking. Reduction of muscle tension correlates well with reduction of pain (11).

Our psychological assessment instrument choice has varied through the years. We have never used the Minnesota Multiphasic Personality Inventory (MMPI) because this was designed to detect behavioral abnormalities in a predominantly Scandinavian population in Minnesota. The test uses archaic language and is long. It is not very suitable for pain patients. It certainly cannot be used as a predictor of outcome, nor should any other instrument of this nature. For many years, we had used the Millon Behavioral Health Inventory Assessment. This instrument tests psychogenic attitudes, such as chronic tension, recent stress, premorbid pessimism, future despair, social alienation, and somatic anxiety. It was normed on pain patients and, therefore, has more applicability than the MMPI.

Through the years, we have come to replace this test with four instrument assessments. The first is the Beck Depression Inventory. The score results of this test indicate that the patient is either functioning within the normal range or experiencing varying degrees of depression. The second test is the Catastrophizing Scale of the Coping Strategies Questionnaire. This scale measures negative self-statements and catastrophizing thoughts and ideations so common to pain patients. The third test is the Pain and Impairment Relationship Scale. This measures the extent to which a patient believes that pain is linked to physical activity. If these beliefs are prominent, they can severely disrupt one's ability to participate in treatment or to function normally. For our rehabilitation model program, this test is most important. The fourth test is the Pain Beliefs and Perceptions Inventory (PBPI). This is a measure of a set of beliefs that patients have about pain. Maladaptive beliefs about pain have been shown to predict treatment compliance and psychological distress. Because our psychologists are working with behavioral modification, it is easy to understand why these four measures could provide important information. The psychologist also does a personal interview as well as an attempt to contact significant others who may add to the behavioral background of the patient

Lastly, the psychiatrist regulates tapering or detoxification from drugs. As stated earlier, this process is carried out rapidly while pursuing intense activation. Endorphin release will help ameliorate withdrawal, and symptoms are generally minimal. The psychologists address the fear of detoxification and promote wellness. Most important of all, we do not teach people how to live or cope with their pain. We look for relief of pain. We attempt to reverse the somatic changes and, with behavioral modification, bring these patients back to equilibrium with their previous lifestyles.

ISSUE OF "OBJECTIVE FINDINGS"

A particular body of literature alleges that many patients suffering from chronic low back pain cannot be assigned a diagnosis conforming to a specific defined disease. The lack of "objective" physical findings in such patients has led to the designation of chronic intractable benign pain (12). This type of pain was thought to be a "central" phenomenon, which was made worse by sensory input. Poor adaptation made pain the focus of the patient's life. Patients so classified were often evaluated for behavioral abnormalities and often became candidates for the diagnosis of psychogenic pain. Presumably, no physical findings indicative of an organic dysfunction or pathologic process

were present. Such a presumption is not supported by facts.

In a study that addressed this issue, 90 patients with back pain were isolated from a group of 283 mixed chronic pain patients who conformed to the diagnosis of chronic intractable benign pain (13). None had neurologic deficit; all radiologic studies were unremarkable. Almost all (97.6%) had tender/trigger points and multiple other nonneurologic abnormalities. Seven categories of abnormalities were identified: tender/trigger points, decreased range of motion, nondermatomal sensory abnormalities, contracted muscles, abnormal gait, miscellaneous physical signs, and decreased range of motion at the hips. Patients had an average of three of the seven categoric findings, led by myofascial syndromes and other soft tissue changes. Almost half (45.6%) had nondermatomal sensory changes; this condition is a physiologic dysfunction, as cited earlier, not malingering or hysteria (14).

The investigators made the following conclusions:

1. Chronic intractable benign pain patients without "objective findings" can be shown regularly to have musculoskeletal disorders.
2. Myofascial syndromes are the source of nociception in these patients.
3. Criteria for the specific diagnosis of myofascial pain syndrome are demonstrable in 97.6% of the patients.
4. Multiple physical findings (average, 3.1) are usual.
5. The demonstrations of such physical findings invalidate the chronic intractable benign pain concept.
6. The *DSM-III* diagnosis of psychogenic pain is overstated, and the criteria now need to be revised.

The investigators added an important comment: With respect to the nondermatomal sensory change, the decreased sensation is commonly "stocking" in distribution; but, often, the perception may appear to involve the lateral or medial foot. Careful examination, however, will demonstrate loss in only half of the dorsum of the foot, with escape of the plantar surface or vice versa. This condition looks more like a peripheral nerve alteration, consistent with possible sciatic entrapment, as might be seen with the gluteal or piriform myofascial syndromes.

ERGONOMICS

In 1982, industrial engineering and ergonomics were invited to join the pain team. We are learning much together because ergonomics has much to teach us (15). Ergonomics studies the human factors and how persons fit into their environments, trying to match the physical capabilities to the required tasks. This process may require designing or limited redesigning of the workplace or home and tools that are used. The goal is to condition the person with regard to strength, posture, and flexibility while eliminating fatigability.

The engineers see the human body as a machine, working with levers and acting as a mechanical crane. They validate the need for proper body mechanics. Proper lifting dictates carrying the weight close to the body; the more bulky the weight, the more difficult it is to carry, and the less efficient the handling of materials. The objectives are human comfort, optimal efficiency of the human-machine system, safety and prevention, health, and work satisfaction. Work satisfaction is a very important issue.

Measuring outcome is a complex problem. To account for psychophysical variants, a measure of back strength in back pain patients was developed called AME—acceptable maximum effort (16). This measure is highly reliable and useful in determining treatment outcome. Reliability coefficients for all strength measurements are greater than 0.90.

The level of voluntary muscular effort beyond which the patient's level of pain becomes unacceptable is the principle. Patients are tested before, during, and after treatment. Back and leg strength may more than double in a 4-week treatment period, which is also true for composite strength. Human performance evaluations track overall strength, pacing, reactions, hand steadiness, flexibility, level of cooperation, level of effort, ranges of motion, gait, posture, and pain level. The bottom line is to make the achievement level match or exceed the task demand.

The ergonomists also analyze the patient's anthropometric measurements, from which ideal layouts for chairs, desks, home furniture, work site equipment, and condition can be developed and printed out by computer.

The inpatient pain program is a 7-day/week program for approximately 2 to 4 weeks. The patient is in treatment from 8 a.m. until 4 p.m. Evening assignments are carried out on the inpatient unit. Therapeutic time schedules allow the individual to have alternating but consecutive periods of exertional and nonexertional activity. By the time of discharge, patients may have achieved the best physical condition of their life. Usually, by 1 week, patients are ambulatory and becoming independent in activities of daily living (ADL) with decreasing levels of pain. They are approaching full ranges of motion with increasing strength in 2 to 3 weeks. Assistive devices can usually be eliminated. Function, not relief of pain, is the end point. At the end of 4 weeks, sometimes, in extreme cases, 6 weeks, the patients have achieved full functional levels of activity, now with decrease or relief of pain. If a neurologic deficit has been present, motor strength may recover in 2 to 3 weeks, sensation in 2 to 3 months, and reflexes in 3 months. Complete pain relief is attained in one third of patients at discharge; in the remainder, the pain usually dissipates over time or becomes easily controlled for functional comfort. The majority are fully functional at discharge and able to resume prepain lifestyles despite some residual pain (20).

COST EFFECTIVENESS/CONTAINMENT

Are pain programs cost effective? We think they are (17). An average cost benefit of $238 000 per patient was demon-strated in a study of 53 patients with industrial injuries (18). If only a 1% change in awards for Social Security disability were to be reversed over a 5-year period, this nation would save $900 000 000. That's truly cost effective. Several meta-analyses have demonstrated the cost effectiveness of the multidisciplinary pain center approach. The potential savings are enormous. In one study, based on the treatment of 3080 patients, the savings in medical expenditures were $9 548 000, and the savings and indemnity expenditures were $175 225 000. This made for a total savings of $184 772 050. Clearly, containment and effectiveness can be demonstrated, but there still remains the psychological barrier for insurers who look at the multidisciplinary center approach as being expensive and potentially more money thrown away for failure. They do not appreciate that if the multidisciplinary approach had been initiated early on, potentially as early as 6 weeks, the large number of dollars expended for nonproductive treatments would have been avoided, and, thereby, the multidisciplinary center costs seem relatively small. The goal, therefore, is to educate the insurer and the provider to seek early referral to pain specialists and pain treatment facilities, thereby avoiding cost and, more importantly, the suffering of the patient and failure of productivity, both socially and economically.

SUMMARY AND CONCLUSIONS

The primary objective of the program described is restoration to full function. Other objectives include relief or decrease in pain with the abolition of pain medication, elimination of assistive devices, low or zero disability rating, job satisfaction with return to work and leisure activities without limitations, independence from the healthcare system, prevention of reinjury, and optimal wellness. The intense, multidisciplinary program described involves a full-time multidisciplinary staff, complete patient involvement, weight control, physical restoration and conditioning, home program maintenance, pacing, body mechanics, energy-saving techniques, reinjury prevention education, drug detoxification, behavioral elimination or control of pain, modification, biofeedback, relaxation, imagery, individual and group therapy, family therapy, assertiveness training, stress management, coping skills, vocational counseling, job planning/development/simulation, achievement of maximal function, immediate return to work at discharge, and followup care.

It is possible to return 86% of these patients to full function and work; they may have some residual pain, which should eventually remit. The 14% who "fail" are hard-core patients with major behavioral problems; although, to be fair, there are still unanswered questions to resolve. These people have problems that cannot be eliminated within the time we have to work with them. Lastly, these patients can be disturbed and dangerous, as evidenced by the headline of "A Former Patient Shoots, Kills, New York Neurosurgeon, Self, Wife" (19).

In the new millennium, all hospitals are struggling for survival. Pain centers must be mindful of reimbursement issues and deliver treatment programs by managing resources when delivering care. Attention must be paid to the amount of reimbursement to be realized against what it will cost to deliver the care. If this is not done on a case-by-case basis, the pain center will no longer be economically viable. We can no longer give everyone all of the services described in this chapter, as cost constraint and reimbursement will play a major role in pain health-care delivery. Unfortunately, this may prove to be adverse to the best interests of many patients who will be disadvantaged by their health-care contracts and policies. Few hospitals can afford to support cost centers that are not viable despite their exemplary work. Unprofitable centers will be replaced by those that are profitable. Many pain centers have learned this valuable lesson too late, and they no longer exist.

REFERENCES

1. Deyo RA. Conservative therapy for low back pain: distinguishing useful from useless therapy. *JAMA* 1983; 250:1057–1062.
2. Rosomoff HL. The effects of hypothermia on the physiology of the nervous system. *Surgery* 1956;49:328–336.
3. Rosomoff HL, Clasen RA, Hartstock R, et al. Brain reaction to experimental injury after hypothemria. *Arch Neurol* 1960;13:337–345.
4. Travell JG, Simons D. *Myofascial pain and dysfunction: the trigger point manual*. Baltimore: Williams & Wilkins, 1983.
5. Larsson U, Choler U, Lidstrom A, et al. Autotraction for treatment of lumbago-sciatica: a multi centre controlled investigation. *Acta Orthop Scand* 1980;51:791–798.
6. Lind GAM. *Auto-traction: treatment of low back pain and sciatica*. Sweden: Sturetryckeriet, 1974:62.
7. Natchev E. *A manual on auto-traction treatment for low back pain*. Folksam Scientific Council Publ. B 171,1984:319.
8. Gunn CC. *The Gunn approach to the treatment of chronic pain, intramuscular stimulation for myofascial pain of radiculopathic origin*. New York, Edinburgh, London, Madrid, Melbourne, San Francisco and Tokyo: Churchill Livingston, 1996:165.
9. Abdel-Moty E, Khalil TM, Rosomoff RS, et al. Computerized electromyography in quantifying the effectiveness of functional electrical neuromuscular stimulation In: Asfour Ss, ed. *Ergonomics/human factors IV*. New York: Elsevier, 1987;1057–1065.
10. Fishbain, DA, Goldberg M, Meagher P, et al. Male and female chronic pain patients categorized by DSM-III psychiatric diagnostic criteria. *Pain* 1986;26:181–197.
11. Khalil I, Asfour SS, Waly SM, et al. Isometric exercise and biofeedback in strength training. In: Asfour SS, ed. *Trends in ergonomics/human factors IV*. New York: Elsevier, 1987:1095–1101.
12. Crue BL, Pinsky IJ. An approach to chronic pain of nonmalignant origin. *Postgrad Med J* 1984;60:858–864.
13. Rosomoff HL, Fishbain D, Goldberg M, et al. Physical findings in patients with chronic intractable benign pain of the back and/or neck. *Pain* 1989;37:279–287.
14. Wall P. The role of the substantia gelatinosa as a gate control. In: Bonica JJ, ed. *Pain*. New York: Raven Press, 1980:205–231.
15. Khalil TM, Asfour SS, Motv EA, et al. New horizons for ergonomics research in low back pain. In: Eberts PE, Eberts CC, eds. *Trends in ergonomic/human factors II*. New York: Elsevier, 1985;591–598.
16. Khalil TM, Goldberg ML, Asfour SS, et al. Acceptable maximum effort (AME). A psychosocial measure of strength m back pain patients. *Spine* 1987;12:372–376.
17. Steele P. Is the pain program cost effective? *Pain* 1984;(Suppl 2):438.
18. Stieg RL, Williams RC, Timmermans-Williams G, et al. Cost benefits of multidisciplinary chronic pain treatment. *Clin J Pain* 1985;1:189–193.
19. Pinckney D. A former patient shoots, kills, New York neurosurgeon, self, wife. *Am Med News* Mar 20, 1987:1.
20. Cutler R, Fishbain D, Rosomoff HL, et al. Does nonsurgical pain center treatment of chronic pain return patients to work? a review and meta-analysis of the literature. *Spine* 1994;19:643–652.

CHAPTER 54

Providing Pain Management Services under the Managed Care Paradigm

Steven D. Waldman and Katherine A. Waldman

As the specialty of pain management continues to grow, it faces many new challenges. Beginning as a primarily anesthesiology-based, self-taught discipline, the specialty of pain management has evolved into a complex multispecialty endeavor with organized certification examinations and recognition by the American Board of Medical Specialties as a legitimate specialty. In a manner analogous to plastic surgery, one may enter the pain management board examination process via a number of medical specialties, including anesthesiology and physical medicine and rehabilitation, suggesting the diverse nature of the knowledge base of the specialty. Unfortunately, whereas the educational aspects of the specialty of pain management have matured, many of the organizational, logistical, and administrative aspects have not. The reasons for this are twofold: First, most of the development of the specialty of pain management has occurred at academic institutions, which have been slow to adapt to the paradigm shift from the traditional professional-based paradigm to practice under the managed care paradigm. Second, until recently, the specialty of pain management has been primarily anesthesiology based. This has resulted in the insulation of the majority of pain practitioners to many of the administrative issues unique to the managed care paradigm, e.g., precertification and medical necessity determinations, as the specialty of anesthesiology, at least so far as operating room anesthesia is concerned, remains largely unaffected by them. This chapter will examine the effect that managed care has had on the specialty of pain management and will provide practical suggestions as how to best practice under the managed care paradigm.

DEFINING THE MANAGED CARE PARADIGM

In order to understand the impact of the managed care paradigm on the specialty of pain management, it is first necessary to explore the forces that led to the paradigm shift in the first place. Health care in the United States can be characterized as historically having operated under a professional paradigm (4). The hallmark of the professional paradigm is physician control and dominance. This physician empowerment occurred in large part as the result of efforts in the late nineteenth and early twentieth centuries to standardize medical education and to make it more scientific. As the practice of medicine changed from an art to a science, the physician's assertion that patients had a limited ability to make informed decisions about their health was further legitimized, as was the assertion that the physician's judgment should be substituted for that of patients.

In economic terms, this knowledge asymmetry and its resultant disempowerment of the consumer is called *market substitution* (5). Economists generally hold that such market substitution leads to the impairment of traditional market forces for two reasons:

1. The consumer lacks adequate information to make informed choices about health care.
2. The tradeoffs of increments of quality to lower cost inherent in the traditional economic marketplace are attenuated because the professionally imposed standards govern.

State efforts at professional regulation and licensure requirements, as well as hospital accreditation standards, have served to further strengthen the physician's control and dominance of health care in the United States. This duty of professional self-regulation, which emphasizes quality and deemphasizes the economic aspects of health care, further reinforced the professional paradigm.

In large part, the professional paradigm, with its paternalistic physician-oriented decision making, can be seen as being responsible for health care as we know it today. The professional decision-making hegemony that had been fostered by the professional paradigm forced those who wanted to improve health care for the elderly and indigent to allow the physician decision makers to design programs to meet these lofty goals. The result was Medicare and Medicaid. These vast social welfare programs have served to further shift control from the consumer to the physician fiduciaries. These programs have also served to insulate physician services from the economic realities of a true market-based system because a third-party payer (in this case, the government), rather than the patient, was responsible for the bill. As a result the resource constraints of the normal economic marketplace were greatly attenuated.

Under the professional paradigm, patients implored their physicians to spare no cost to find a cure. Although this approach has undoubtedly led to improved health care for the majority of Americans, it has allowed a belief to develop that any restraint on health-care resources will automatically lead to lower-quality health care. This quality threat has been termed the physician's "silver bullet" in any debate about health-care reform.

Linked to the perception that resource constraints will decrease quality is the strong belief that the patient should have the freedom to choose his or her own physician. This belief has been in part fostered by the professional paradigm, but in part may be due to the very nature of the physician-patient relationship.

It was Bill Clinton's first-term push toward health-care reform that brought the health-care debate into the hearts and minds of the American people (6). Although the U.S. health-care system is arguably the best, albeit most expensive, in the world, polls suggested that most Americans were concerned about the perceived high cost of this care and the fact that 35 million were uninsured (7). In spite of the fact that Clinton's "Health Security Act" lost momentum and drifted into legislative obscurity, its imprint remains (8).

Many health-care reform experts credit Clinton's efforts as the driving force that led to the shift from the professional paradigm (which had dominated health-care policy for almost 100 years) to the new managed care-based paradigm. Central to this managed care paradigm is the belief that managed care alternatives will provide the mechanism to cure most of the perceived wrongs of the current health-care marketplace (9). Touted as a cure-all, managed care achieves its purported cost savings by striking at the very foundations of the professional paradigm; this concept addressed the cost/quality relationship as well as the freedom of patients to choose their own physicians.

As the managed care paradigm has matured, the very limitations on access and choice that led to its initial success have now conspired to destroy it. Perceived limitations on access to needed care and arbitrary refusals to allow patients to see specialists, combined with the public revelations of huge salaries and bonuses paid to managed care executives, have led both the public and politicians to turn on the managed care industry. In order to improve their public image, some managed care plans have eliminated costly precertification procedures and loosened restrictions on access to out-of-network care. Whether these changes represent a real effort by the managed care industry to correct these perceived abuses or whether these changes are just a public relations ploy remains to be seen. Regardless of the motivation behind these changes, one must surmise that the marketplace may in fact work better than its detractors ever believed it would at least in terms of protecting the consumer. Furthermore, these changes may represent the beginning of a paradigm shift away from the managed care paradigm to a new construct of health care in this country.

STRATEGIES TO SUCCEED UNDER THE MANAGED CARE PARADIGM

Because managed care is the predominant type of health-care coverage currently purchased in the United States, it behooves the pain management specialist to fully understand the steps he or she must take to successfully practice under the managed care paradigm. The following discussion will provide the pain management specialist with a practical guide through the administrative barriers put in place by the managed care paradigm and steps to overcome them. It should be noted as we embark on the following discussion that patient care considerations should always take precedence over the administrative limitations placed on the pain management specialist by managed care plans, but it is the very unreasonableness of many of the limitations that has led to dissatisfaction with the managed care paradigm by both patients and practitioners alike.

Insurance Verification

From an administrative viewpoint, the starting point for any patient interaction is the insurance verification process. Without this crucial first step, the pain management specialist is completely in the dark as to what he or she may not do in terms of the treatment plan for any given patient. Barring pain management emergencies, the insurance verification process should take place prior to the patient being seen by the pain management specialist. Figure 54-1 is an example of an insurance verification sheet that will serve well for this purpose. Key points in the patient verification process are listed in Table 54-1 and include the gathering of: (a) accurate demographic data; (b) Social Security number; (c) employer information; (d)

TABLE 54-1. *Key points in the insurance verification process*

Accurate demographic data
Social Security number
Employer information
Primary insurance information
Secondary insurance information
Emergency contact numbers
Accident or worker's compensation information

primary insurance information; (e) secondary insurance information; (f) emergency contact numbers; (g) accident or worker's compensation information. Each will be discussed individually.

Demographic Data

It is often said that you can't tell the players without a scorecard, and this certainly applies to patients and their third-party payers under the managed care paradigm. Without accurate demographic data, it is impossible to identify patients and successfully get paid for the care provided. Accurate spelling of patient names with special attention to middle names, *Jr.*, *Sr.*, etc. is the first step in the patient identification process. Problem areas in this regard include nicknames, aliases, maiden names, hyphenated last names, and situations where the patient name is different from that of the policy holder. Foreign names, where it may be impossible to determine which is the first

INSURANCE VERIFICATIONS

Appt Date________ Place of Service________

Patient Name________ ID #________

DATE OF BIRTH________ Group#________

Insured's Name________

Mailing Address for claims ________

Primary____ Secondary____ Secondary ID #________

EFFECTIVE DATE________ TIMELY FILING________

INN Benefits________

OON Benefits________

INN Deductible________ OON Deductible________

Referral Required________ PCP________

Precert for: EPI____ EMG____ MRI____ BONE DENSITY____

Precert phone#________ VERIFIED BY________

SDW________ REHAB________ HAC________ MRI________

MEDICAID: Missouri/Kansas Eligible____ Date Spec____

Lockin________ Precert________

Notes:________

FIG. 54-1. Insurance verification sheet

and which is the last name, can also present difficulties when trying to verify insurance benefits. Careful attention to the date of birth of both the policy holder and the patient is important because both can serve as another way to help identify who actually received the care. Accurate phone numbers, including those of cell phones and beepers, are also useful not only in contacting the patient during care, but also in making collection efforts after the care is rendered. When possible, obtain a copy of the patient's driver's license. The license will provide a picture of the patient and will also be useful in proving that the patient seen was actually the insured.

Social Security Number

Although not originally intended as a unique identification number by the federal government, the Social Security number is often used exactly as that. The Social Security number offers another point from which to search for and help identify the patient. When possible, obtain the Social Security number of the insured if different from that of the patient.

Employer Information

Employer information should include not only the name and address of the employer, but also the patient's and insured's work phone numbers as well. Often the pain management physician will receive denials of payment asserting that the patient's insurance has been canceled or the premium has not been paid. Proof of insurance coverage or payment of premium is often most easily obtained by contacting the employer directly. In order to do this, the pain management specialist must obtain a valid release of information to talk directly with third parties regarding the patient's care. Such a release may be included in the assignment of insurance benefits (see following). Accurate employer information is especially useful if a worker's compensation claim is asserted.

Primary Insurance Information

Under the professional-based paradigm, most insurance companies offered a limited number of product lines that were easily identifiable and presented limited problems for the handful of pain management specialists practicing at the time. However, just as our specialty has changed, so has the way in which managed care plans market their products. Not only do most managed care plans offer a myriad of product lines, but also they often name them similarly, making easy identification all but impossible. For example, Blue Cross and Blue Shield offer over 30 product lines, all with similar-sounding names such as Preferred Care, Preferred Care Blue, and BlueCare. Each of the plans has specific limitations and precertification requirements, deductibles, etc. A failure to accurately identify the specific plan that the patient has can lead only to lost revenues for the pain management specialist.

Secondary Insurance Information

Many patients are covered by more than one insurance policy or managed care plan. Each state has rules as to which plan is primary and which is secondary. Additionally, Medicare has specific rules as to its obligation when Medicare is determined to be the secondary payer. Failure to identify which insurer or managed care plan is primary will lead to denied claims and may lead to timely filing denials if the wrong plan is filed as primary due to the delay in receiving a denial. The pain management specialist should also be aware that special rules apply if the primary insurer is paying for injuries due to a worker's compensation claim or motor vehicle accident. These rules are even more complex if Medicare or Medicaid is involved because any payment from these payers may be subrogated to any ultimate damages a patient may receive in court, and the money may have to be returned to Medicare, Medicaid, and other third-party payers.

Emergency Contact Numbers

It is important to obtain alternative ways to contact a patient should his or her claim be denied by a third-party payer. Often, there can be significant delays before the pain management specialist is advised that a claim has been denied, and by that time the patient may have moved, changed phone numbers, etc. The emergency contact number can then serve as a ready way to contact family members or significant others to help learn the patient's whereabouts. As mentioned, the pain management specialist should obtain a signed release of information from the patient to avoid breach of patient confidentiality (see "Assignment of Insurance Benefits" following).

Worker's Compensation and Accident Information

Every patient verification process should include an inquiry as to whether the patient's presenting complaint is the result of an accident or on-the-job injury. As mentioned, if the patient's problem is related to a motor vehicle accident, the patient's insurance or managed care plan benefits may be subrogated to the patient's auto insurance personal injury protection (PIP) or any ultimate court judgment he or she may receive. Furthermore, in most states, worker's compensation claims require prior authorization, and in some instances precertification, for treatment. Failure to obtain authorization and/or precertification will result in claims denials.

ASSIGNMENT OF INSURANCE BENEFITS AND STATEMENT OF SERVICE

I hereby assign and authorize payment made directly to
the covered insurance benefits, including major medical benefits, whether payable to me by Blue
Cross/Blue Shield, Medicare, Medigap, and/or commercial insurance companies. I understand
that my health insurance provider may not cover part or all of the medical services rendered,
**I fully understand that I am financially responsible for and agree to pay all charges not paid
by my health care coverage, including deductibles, co-insurance, and payments from insurance companies sent directly to me. In consideration of the medical services furnished
to me, I hereby agree to pay**   **any balance due within nine-
ty days from presentation of my bill. If my account should become delinquent and collection efforts become necessary, I agree to pay any reasonable collection or attorney's fees
incurred.**

This assignment shall apply to all services now rendered and to be rendered in the future until
it is revoked.

I have disclosed the names of all of my health insurance providers including tie-in-coverage
and I represent that such health care coverage is in full force and effect at this time.

If prior authorization or certification for medical services is required under my health care
coverage, I agree to obtain and furnish such authorization or certification.

I authorize the release of medical information as may be required to process the claims for
payment of the medical services rendered and it is expressly understood that the right of such
information to be privileged is hereby waived.

I have had an opportunity to discuss with the physician or his staff to my satisfaction the nature
of the services provided. **I acknowledge that no guarantees have been made to me as to the
results.** I am satisfied that I fully understand this assignment and its significance.

I agree to promptly notify your office of any change of address.

A copy of this assignment shall be considered as valid as the original.

X _____   X _____
Signature of Patient   Signature of Insured (if applicable)

Date _____

Social Security # _____   Social Security # _____

Employer-Firm _____   Employer-Firm _____

Insurance   Insurance
Company _____   Company _____
(Primary)   (Secondary)

SIGN BELOW IF YOU HAVE A MEDIGAP INSURANCE POLICY.
MEDICARE LIFETIME MEDIGAP ASSIGNMENT

I assign and authorize payment of Medigap benefits to
any services furnished to me by him. I authorize any holder of medical information about me
to release to the Health Care Financing Administration and its agents any information needed
to determine these benefits or the benefits payable for related services.

X _____   Date _____
Signature of Patient

FIG. 54-2. Assessment of insurance benefits

Assignment of Insurance Benefits

In order for the pain management specialist to be paid directly by Medicare, Medicaid, insurance companies, and managed care plans, the patient must assign his or her insurance benefits to the pain management specialist. The effect of an assignment of insurance benefits is to allow the pain management specialist to "step into the shoes" of the insured. Not only does this allow the pain management specialist (the assignee) to be paid directly by the third-party payer, but it also allows the assignee to partake of the other benefits of the patient's coverage, e.g., deductible information, denial appeals processes, and the like. Figure 54-2 is an example of a well-crafted assignment of insurance benefits. The reader should note that

this document not only serves to assign the patient's benefits, but also serves as an additional proof of informed consent and a release of patient information.

The Authorization and Precertification Process

Authorization and precertification are cornerstones of the managed care paradigm and serve to help managed care plans limit access and choice as well as to allow managed care plans to avoid paying claims. Authorization and precertification are often confused as being one and the same, but this is not the case. Authorization for treatment is formal approval by the third-party payer that allows the pain management physician to see a specific patient. It is used

Patient Account No.	Provider:	☐ O
		☐ OS
		☐ IH
		☐ OH

1. PATIENT'S NAME: _____
2. DATE OF SERVICE: _____
3. LOCATION:

☐ A. VENCOR	☐ F. NORTH KC	☐ N. CSC	☐ S. LAWRENCE MEMORIAL	☐ Y. CASS MED. CTR.
☐ B. BAPTIST	☐ J. MED. CTR. INDEP.	☐ O. KAISER BR	☐ T. RANSOM MEMORIAL	☐ Z. MENORAH MED. CTR.
☐ C. LEE'S SUMMIT	☐ K. INDEP. REGIONAL	☐ P. PROV. MED.	☐ U. MIAMI	☐ 1. OLMC
☐ D. TRINITY LUTHERAN	☐ L. OVERLAND PARK	☐ Q. CUSHING MEM.	☐ V. MID-AMERICA REHAB.	☐ 5. RAY COUNTY
☐ E. SURGICENTER OF KC	☐ M. HEADACHE & PAIN CTR	☐ R. ST. JOHN	☐ X. EXCELSIOR SPRINGS	☐ 7. KAISER BAP
				☐ 8. KAISER PKWY
				☐ OTHER _____

4. ICD-9

	DIAGNOSIS CODE	DESCRIPTION
☐	053.9	Acute Herpes Zoster
☐	354.4	* Causalgia – Upper Limb
☐	355.71	* Causalgia – Lower Limb
☐	723.1	Cervicalgia
☐	723.4	* Cervical Radiculopathy
☐	786.52	Chest Wall Pain
☐	346.2	Cluster Headache
☐	724.5	Facet Syndrome
☐	729.1	Fibromyositis
☐	722.0	* Herniated Disc – Cervical
☐	722.11	* Herniated Disc – Thoracic
☐	722.10	* Herniated Disc – Lumbar
☐	355.8	Ilioinguinal Neuralgia
☐	719.46	Knee Pain
☐	724.4	* Lumbar Radiculopathy
☐	_____	Malig Neoplasm _____
☐	355.1	Meralgia Paresthetica
☐	354.8	* Mononeuritis Arm Incl. Shingles
☐	355.8	* Mononeuritis Leg Incl. Shingles
☐	729.2	* Neuralgia, Neuritis, & Radiculitis
☐	729.2	Occipital Neuralgia
☐	443.9	Periph Vascular Insufficiency
☐	353.6	Phantom Limb Pain
☐	349.0	Post Dural Puncture Headache
☐	053.19	Postherpetic Neuralgia
☐	337.20	RSD – Unspecified
☐	337.21	RSD Upper Limb
☐	337.22	RSD Lower Limb
☐	337.29	RSD Of _____
☐	719.41	Shoulder Pain
☐	739.4	SI Joint Dysfunction
☐	350.1	Trigeminal Neuralgia
☐	724.4	* Thoracic Radiculopathy
☐	784.0	Vascular Headache
☐	805.6	* Vertebral Fracture
☐	_____	Other _____

5. CPT-2000

	PROCEDURE CODE	DESCRIPTION
OUTPATIENT SERVICES		
☐	99243	Initial Consult
☐	99244	Initial Consult Complex
☐	99203	Initial Consult-Self Ref
☐	99204	Initial Consult-Self Ref-Complex
☐	99243	Reconsult
☐	99214	Reconsult-Self Referred
☐	99212	Follow-Up Est Patient
INPATIENT SERVICES		
☐	99253	Initial Consult
☐	99254	Initial Consult Complex
☐	99253	Reconsult
☐	99231	Follow-Up Visit
PROCEDURES		
☐	62310	* Cervical Steroid Epidural
☐	62310	* Thoracic Steroid Epidural
☐	62311	* Lumbar Steroid Epidural
☐	62311	* Caudal Steroid Epidural
☐	62273	Epidural Blood Patch
☐	64400	Trigeminal Nerve Block
☐	64405-50	Occipital Nerve Block – Bilateral
☐	64415	Brachial Plexus Block
☐	64421	Mult. Intercostal Block
☐	64425	Ilioinguinal Nerve Block
☐	64470	Facet Cerv. or Thor. Single
☐	64472	_____ Facet Cerv. Or Thor. Add'l
☐	64475	Facet Lumbar Single
☐	64476	_____ Facet Lumbar Add'l
☐	20610	Intra-Artic Shoulder ___ R ___ L
☐	20610	Intra-Artic Knee ___ R ___ L
☐	27096	Intra-Artic SI Joint
☐	20550	Trigger Point Injection X _____
☐	64505-50	Sphenopal Gang. Block-Bilat.
☐	64510	Stellate Ganglion Block
☐	64520	Lumbar Sympathetic Block
☐	64530	Celiac Plexus-Diagnostic
☐	62310	Cervical Epidural w/o steroid
☐	62310	Thoracic Epidural w/o steroid
☐	62311	Lumbar Epidural w/o steroid
☐	62311	Caudal Epidural w/o steroid
☐	64680	Celiac Plexus-Neurolytic
☐	76005	Fluoro Needle Guidance-Spine
☐	_____	Other _____
☐	BILL INS.	_____
6.	REFERRING DR.	_____

I certify that I personally saw the above patient and performed the indicated procedures and in my opinion they are medically necessary.

FIG. 54-2. *Continued*

commonly as a gate-keeping function to limit a patient's access to specialists, even if they are part of a managed care network. The pain management specialist should determine if authorization is required on every patient as part of the insurance verification process *prior* to the patient being seen. If authorization is required, and it is not obtained prior to seeing the patient, claims denial will almost always result.

Even if authorization to see the patient is obtained, it does not necessarily mean that the pain management specialist may do any more than provide cognitive services, i.e., a consultation. In order to perform a nerve block or order testing such as an electromyogram or magnetic resonance scan, precertification may be required. The pain management specialist should determine if precertification is required on every patient as part of the insurance verification process *prior* to the patient being treated. If precertification is required, and it is not obtained prior to treating the patient, claims denial will almost always result. The pain management specialist should be aware that both authorization and precertification may be date, provider, and location specific and that such restrictions must be followed or else payment denial will result.

Timely Filing

One of the new ways that third-party payers use to deny claims is by shortening the time in which the pain management specialist has to file a claim for services rendered. Thirty- to ninety-day timely filing limitations are becoming the rule rather than the exception. Because third-party payers will often claim that they did not receive a claim during the timely filing period, it is incumbent on the pain management specialist to keep proof of the date of filing to refute such denials. It may often be necessary to seek the help of the state insurance commissioner to resolve such erroneous claims denials.

Out-of-Network and Point-of-Service Benefits

Determination of out-of-network and/or point-of-service benefits should be part of the insurance verification process on every patient. Rather than arbitrarily deciding that patients with certain managed care plans cannot be seen because the pain management physician does not participate in a given managed care plan, it should be ascertained whether the patient has out-of-network or point-of-service benefits that would allow the pain management specialist to be paid should he or she decide to see the patient. As a general rule, these out-of-network benefits and point-of-service benefits pay to a pain management specialist at a lower rate than to an in-network physician.

Copayments

Most managed care plans require patients to pay a portion of the cost of their care at the time of service. Such a payment is called a copayment. Amounts range from $10 to $20 per cognitive service and may be as much as $75 for surgical procedures such as nerve blocks. Determination of the patient's obligation to submit a copayment at the time of service should be part of the insurance verification process on every patient. An organized plan to collect copayments prior to the patient being seen should be part of every pain management physician's practice. Such a plan should include how cash and checks are handled to avoid the potential for embezzlement.

CONCLUSION

Practicing under the managed care paradigm has presented a myriad of challenges to the pain management physician. Careful attention to the preceding practice management techniques is mandatory to ensure a financially healthy practice to allow our patients to continue to be served. The health-care field is a dynamic rather than a static environment, and no doubt additional changes will occur. It is hoped that these changes will benefit society, the patient, and the pain management specialists.

SUGGESTED READING

1. Waldman SD, Waldman KA. Interventional pain management programming for success. In: Waldman SD, Winnie AP, eds. *Interventional pain management*. Philadelphia: WB Saunders, 1996:69–72.
2. Waldman SD. Setting up a pain treatment facility. In: Warfield C, ed. *Principles & practice of pain management*. New York: McGraw Hill, 2001:In Press.
3. Waldman SD. On Inappropriate utilization review. *Pain Practice Management* 1989; 1:2–3.
4. Waldman SD. Joining a managed care pare: a guide to the pain management specialist. *Amer J Pain Mgmt* 1992;2:215–218.
5. Waldman SD. Reimbursement for chronic pain management service—the cloud's silver lining. *Regional Anesthesia* 1993;18:227–28.
6. Waldman SD. Providing pain management services—Part I: basic considerations. *Amer J Pain Mgmt* 1994;4:86–88.
7. Waldman SD. Providing pain management services—Part II: specific considerations. *Amer J Pain Mgmt* 1994;4:132-135.
8. Waldman SD. Lessons from academia don't translate into medicine. *American Medical News* March 27, 1995. (Letter).
9. Waldman SD. Any willing provider laws-paradox or panacea—Part I. *Amer J Pain Mgmt* 1996;6:54–61.
10. Waldman SD. Any willing provider laws-paradox or panacea—Part II. *Amer J Pain Mgmt* 1996;6:93–96.
11. Waldman SD. Medical staff credentialing—physician constitutional rights & remedies—Part I: the law and public policy of medical staff credentialing. *Amer J Pain Mgmt* 1997;7:100–104.
12. Waldman SD. Medical staff credentialing—physician constitutional rights & remedies —Part II: the law and public policy of medical staff credentialing. *Amer J Pain Mgmt* 1997;7:146–150.
13. Waldman SD. The antitrust implications of medical staff credentialling—Part I. *Amer J Pain Mgmt* 1997;7:22–27.
14. Waldman SD. The antitrust implications of medical staff credentialling—Part II. *Amer J Pain Mgmt* 1997;7:66–69.

Index

806 / Index

Computed tomography (CT)
  low back pain, differential diagnosis of
    structural lesion methods, 405–406, 406f
  radiographic assessment, cancer pain, 638
Connective tissue
  diseases, 558
    mixed connective tissue disease, 558
    progressive systemic sclerosis, 558
    systemic lupus erythematosus (SLE), 558
    systemic vasculitides, 558
  pain, 546–560
    diagnosis approach, 547
    history, 547–548
    laboratory analyses of, 548–549
    physical examination, 547–548
Conscious laparoscopic pain mapping (CLPM), 475
Constipation
  drug-related side effects, neuroaxial opioid therapy, 149
  prevention/treatment of
    terminally ill patient, 338
Consultations, hospital, 760–768
  Current Procedural Terminology (CPT) handbook, 767t
  postsurgical pain management, 763
Consultations, office, 760–768, 761–763, 761t
  Current Procedural Terminology (CPT) handbook, 767t
  disability issues, 763
  medication issues, 761–762
  nerve blocks, 761–762
  psychological issues, 762–763
Continuous paravertebral sympathetic block
  complex regional pain syndrome (CRPS), nerve blocks, 514
Continuous somatic blockade
  complex regional pain syndrome (CRPS), nerve blocks, 514–515
Contributory negligence, 679–680
Conversion disorder, somatizing disorders, 586–587, 723, 723t
Coping, psychological factors of pain, 35
Corticosteroids (CS)
  complex regional pain syndrome (CRPS), treatment for, 509
  inflammatory joint disease, drug therapy, 551–552, 551t
  nociceptive transmission, interventions to modulate, 20
  peripheral sites of injury, 16
COX-2 inhibitors (COXIBS)
  analgesic medications, 248–250, 249t
    anticonvulsants, 250
    capsaicin, 249–250
    celecoxib, 248–250
    efficacy in acute pain, 249
    efficacy in chronic pain, 249
    rofecoxib, 248–250
    serotonin, 250
    toxicity of, 249
  antiinflammatory agents
    chronic pain, medications for, 259
COX-I, cyclooxygenase enzymes, peripheral site of injury, 15, 15f
COX-II, cyclooxygenase enzymes, peripheral site of injury, 15, 15f
Cracked tooth syndrome
  odontogenic origin, orofacial pain of, 370
Cranial nerves, neuralgias of, 364–369
  craniofacial pain of musculoskeletal origin, 365–369

geniculate neuralgia (VIIth cranial nerve), 364
glossopharyngeal neuralgia (IXth cranial nerve), 364
occipital neuralgia, 365
raeder's paratrigeminal neuralgia, 365
sphenopalatine neuralgia, 365
Cranial neuralgias, cancer pain management, 609
Craniofacial pain of musculoskeletal origin
  cranial nerves, neuralgias of, 365–369
    bone infections, 368–369
    osteoarthritis of temporomandibular joint, 367–368, 368t
    specific myofascial disorders, 367, 367t
    temporomandibular pain and dysfunction syndromes (TMPDS), 365–367, 367t
    tumors, 368–369
Criminal False Claims Act, the, 691
CRPS Type I
  complex regional pain syndrome (CRPS), types of, 500
    criteria for, 507t
CRPS Type II
  complex regional pain syndrome (CRPS), types of, 500
    criteria for, 507t
Cryoglobulinemia
  immunoglobulinemias, neuropathic pain, 438
Cryptogenic neuropathies, 440–441
  complex regional pain syndromes (CRPS), 440–441
  glossopharyngeal neuralgias, 441
  idiopathic polyneuropathy, 440
  sympathetically maintained pain, 441
  trigeminal neuralgias, 441
Crystal-induced arthritis, 555–556
  gout, 555
  hydroxyapatite deposition disease, 555–556
  pseudogout, 555
  treatment of, 556
    colchicine, 556
    indomethacin, 556
    phenylbutazone, 556
    probenecid, 556
    sulfinpyrazone, 556
Current Procedural Terminology (CPT), 766–768
  hospital consultations, 767t
  office consultations, 767t
  pain diagnosis by location, 766t
  pain diagnosis by presumed etiology, 766t
  pain management, 767t
Cyclobenzaprine
  muscle relaxants, chronic pain, 283–284
Cyclooxygenase enzymes, peripheral site of injury, 15
  COX-I, 15, 15f
  COX-II, 15, 15f
Cyclophosphamide
  rheumatoid arthritis, drug treatment, 554
Cystic fibrosis pain
  pediatric chronic pain, 297
Cytarabine, management of herpes zoster, 535

Danazol
  endometriosis, gynecologic diseases, 479
Dantrolene
  antispastic medication, chronic pain, 272–273
De Quervain's tendinitis, extra-articular pain syndromes, 559